Klaas (N) M.A. Bax
Keith E. Georgeson
Steven S. Rothenberg
Jean-Stéphane Valla
CK Yeung

Editors

Endoscopic Surgery in Infants and Children

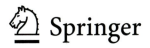 Springer

Klaas (N) M.A. Bax, MD, PhD, FRCS (Ed)
Department of Pediatric Surgery
Sophia Children´s Hospital
Erasmus Medical Center Rotterdam
3000 CB Rotterdam, The Netherlands

Keith E. Georgeson, MD
Division of Pediatric Surgery
Children's Hospital of Alabama
1600 7th Avenue South
Birmingham, AL 35233, USA

Steven S. Rothenberg, MD
The Rocky Mountain Hospital for Children
1601 E 19th Ave, Suite 5500
Denver, Colorado 80218, USA

Jean-Stéphane Valla, MD, PhD
Hôpital Lenval
Department of Pediatric Surgery
Fondation Lenval
57, Avenue de la Californie
06200 Nice, France

CK Yeung, MD, PhD
Department of Surgery
Chinese University of Hong Kong
Prince of Wales Hospital
Shatin, Hong Kong

ISBN   978-3-540-00115-7 Springer Berlin Heidelberg New York

Library of Congress Control Number: 2005938804

Springer is a part of Springer Science+Business Media
springer.com

© Springer-Verlag Berlin Heidelberg 2008

Editor: Gabriele M. Schröder, Heidelberg, Germany
Desk Editor: Stephanie Benko, Heidelberg, Germany
Production: LE-TEX Jelonek, Schmidt &. Vöckler GbR, Leipzig, Germany
Illustrations: Dr. Michael von Solodkoff, Christiane von Solodkoff, Neckargemünd, Germany
Cover Design: Frido Steinen-Broo, eStudio Calamar, Spain
Typesetting and Reproduction: am-productions GmbH, Wiesloch, Germany
Printing and Binding: Stürtz GmbH, Würzburg, Germany

Printed on acid-free paper   19/3180YL – 5 4 3 2 1 0

Dedication

"Love for children through technology"

Dedication

Preface

Since the breakthrough of endoscopic surgical procedures in medicine at the end of the 1980s and the beginning of the 1990s, there has been an enormous evolution in endoscopic surgery, not only in general surgery but also in pediatric surgery. By now most of the operations that were classically performed in an open way have been described in an endoscopic surgical variant. Concomitantly the equipment, telescopes and instruments have evolved very much as well. More recently robot endoscopic surgery has entered the field.

The present book is the successor of the book "Endoscopic Surgery in Children", which appeared in 1999 and which was also published by Springer. The present book has expanded, not only in format but also in the number of procedures described and in its layout. The main intention of the book is to give surgeons a reference for when they want to embark on endoscopic surgical procedures that they have not carried out before. The book concentrates on the technique, which is explained and illustrated in detail. Experts from all over the world have contributed to the book. The Editorial Board would like to thank them for the excellent job they have done. Some differences in techniques between the authors may emerge as the various authors present their personal techniques. They may also have different views regarding indications. These differences reflect reality in medicine.

The cooperation between the Editorial Board and Springer has been outstanding. In particular, the editors thank Ms. Gabriele M. Schröder, Editorial Director of Clinical Medicine at Springer for her efforts in publishing books in the field of pediatric surgery.

Klaas (N) M.A. Bax, Rotterdam
Keith E. Georgeson, Birmingham
Steven S. Rothenberg, Denver
Jean-Stéphane Valla, Nice
CK Yeung, Hong Kong

Contents

Abdomen
Liver and Biliary Tree

Abdomen
Spleen

Abdomen
Pancreas

Abdomen
Shunts and Catheters

Adrenal Gland

Urogenital Tract

Contributors

Craig T. Albanese
Stanford University Surgery - Pediatric Surgery
780 Welch Road, Suite 206
Stanford, CA 94305-5733, USA

Hossein Allal
Lapeyronie Hospital
Department of Visceral Pediatric Surgery
371, Avenue du Doyen Gaston Giraud
34295 Montpellier Cedex 5
Montpellier, France

Steven R. Allen
Cincinnati Children's Hospital Medical Center
Department of Pediatric Surgery
3333 Burnet Avenue
Cincinnati, OH 45229-3039, USA

Antonio Aquino
Clinica Chirurgica Pediatrica
U.O. di Chirurgia Pediatrica
Padiglione 13
Via Massarenti 11
40124 Bologna, Italy

Anthony Atala
The W. Boyce Professor and Chair
Department of Urology
Wake Forest University School of Medicine
Medical Center Boulevard
Winston Salem, NC 27156, USA

Cindy S.T. Aun
Department of Anesthesia and Intensive Care
The Chinese University of Hong Kong
Shatin NT, Hong Kong SAR, Republic of China

Maria Marcela Bailez
Hospital Aleman – Deutsches Hospital
Av. Pueyrredn 1640
1118 Buenos Aires, Argentina

Douglas C. Barnhart
University of Alabama-Birmingham
The Children's Hospital
1600 7th Avenue South, ACC 300,
Birmingham, AL 35233, USA

Klaas (N) M.A. Bax
Department of Pediatric Surgery
Sophia Children's Hospital, Room SK 1264
Erasmus Medical Center
P.O. Box 2060
3000 CB Rotterdam, The Netherlands

John F. Bealer
Presbyterian/St. Luke's Medical Center
Department of Pediatric Surgery
1719 East 19th Avenue
Denver, CO 80218, USA

Francois Becmeur
Hôpitaux Universitaires de Strasbourg
Service de Chirurgie Infantile
67098 Strasbourg Cedex, France

Francisco J. Berchi
c/Margarita 69
28109 Soto de la Moraleja
Madrid-Alcobendas, Spain

Thane A. Blinman
The Children's Hospital of Philadelphia
Philadelphia, PA 19104, USA

Peter Borzi
St. Andrews War Memorial Hospital
Department of Pediatric Surgery
457 Wickham Terrace,
Brisbane, Queensland, Australia

Rajen Butani
The Childrens Hospital of Pittsburgh
3705 5th Avenue
Pittsburgh, PA 15213, USA

Marco Castagnetti
Chirurgia e Urologia Pediatrica
IRCCS G. Gaslini
Universit di Genova
Largo G. Gaslini, 5
16100 Genova, Italy

S.K. Chowdhary
Prince of Wales University Hospital,
Shatin, Hongkong SAR

Randall M. Clark
The Rocky Mountain Hospital for Children
Department of Anesthesiology, Box B090
1601 East 19th Avenue
Denver, CO 80218, USA

Zahavi Cohen
Department of Pediatric Surgery
P.O. Box 151
Beer-Sheva 84101, Israel

Alfred Cuschieri
Ninewells Hospital & Medical School
University of Dundee
Surgical Skills Unit
Dundee Tayside DD1 9SY, Scotland, UK

Steven G. Docimo
The Children's Hospital of Pittsburgh
The University of Pittsburgh Medical Center
Pittsburgh, PA 15213, USA

Marcello Dòmini
Clinica Chirurgica Pediatrica
U.O. de Chirurgia Pediatrica
Padiglione 13
Via Massarenti 11
40138 Bologna, Italy

Haluk Emir
Division of Pediatric Urology
Department of Pediatric Surgery
Cerrahpasa Medical Faculty
Istanbul University
34303 Istanbul, Turkey

Ciro Esposito
Department of Clinical and Experimental Medicine
Pediatric Surgery
"Magna Graecia" University of Catanzaro
School of Medicine
88100 Catanzaro, Italy

Fabio Ferro
U.O. Chirurgia Andrologia e Ginecologia
Ospedale Pediatrico Bambino Gesu
00165 Rome, Italy

Philip K. Frykman
Cedars-Sinai Children's Hospital
8700 Beverley Boulevard
Los Angeles, CA 90048, USA

Keith E. Georgeson
The Children's Hospital of Alabama
1600 7th Avenue South, ACC 300,
Birmingham, AL 35233, USA

Alaa El Ghoneimi
Hôpital Robert Debré
48 Boulevard Serurrier
Paris, France

Stéphane Grandadam
Hôpitaux Universitaires de Strasbourg
Service de Chirurgie Infantile
1 Place de l'Hôpital, BP 426
67091 Strasbourg Cedex, France

Christine Grapin
Service de chirurgie visceral pediatrique
Hopital Armand Trousseau
26 Rue du docteur Arnold Netter
75012 Paris, France

Frederic Hameury
Service d'Urologie Pediatrique
Centre Hospitalier Debrousse
29 rue Soeur Bouvier
69322 Lyon Cedex 05, France

George B. Hanna
Department of Biosurgery and Surgical Technology
Divison of Surgery, Oncology, Reproductive Biology
and Anesthetics Imperial College London
St. Mary's Hospital, Imperial College of Science
10 th Floor, QEQM Wing, Praed Street
London W2 1NY, UK

Carroll M. Harmon
Children's Hospital of Alabama
300 Ambulatory Care Center
1600 7th. Avenue South
Birmingham, AL35233, USA

Yves Heloury
Service de chirurgie infantile
HME - CHU Hotel Dieu
7, quai Moncousu
44 093 Nantes Cedex 1, France

George W. Holcomb
Children's Mercy Hospital
2401 Gillham Road
Kansas City, MO 64108, USA

Thomas H. Inge
Comprehensive Weight Management Center
Division of Pediatric General and Thoracic Surgery
Cincinnati Children's Hospital Medical Center
3333 Burnet Avenue, MLC 2023
Cincinatti, OH 45229-3039, USA

Tadashi Iwanaka
Department of Pediatric Surgery
The University of Tokyo
Graduate School of Medicine
7-3-1 Hono, Bunkyo-ku, Tokyo 113-8655, Japan

Vincenzo Jasonni
Chirurgia e Urologia Pediatrica
IRCCS G. Gaslini
Universit di Genova
Largo G. Gaslini, 5
16100 Genova, Italy

D. Denison Jenkins
Stanford University School of Medicine
Department of Surgery, Division of Pediatric Surgery
780 Welch Road, Suite 206
Stanford, CA 94305-5733, USA

Natalie K. Jesch
Hannover Medical School
Department of Pediatric Surgery
Carl-Neuberg-Strasse 1
30625 Hannover, Germany

Timothy D. Kane,
University of Pittsburgh and
School of Medicine
Children's Hospital of Pittsburgh
Division of Pediatric Surgery
3705 Fifth Avenue
Pittsburgh, PA 15213-2583, USA

Manoj K. Karmakar
The Chinese University of Hong Kong
Department of Anesthesia and Intensive Care
Hong Kong, China SAR

Saundra M. Kay
The Mother and Child Hospital at Presbetyrian
St Lukes
1601 East 19th Avenue, Suite 5500,
Denver, CO 80218, USA

Tamir Keshen
Cottage Children's Hospital
2403 Castillo St.
#202 Santa Barbara, CA 93105, USA

Michael D. Klein
Children's Hospital of Michigan
3901 Beaubien Boulevard,
Detroit, MI 48201, USA

Colin G. Knight
205 Montclair Avenue,
Pittsburgh, PA 15237, USA

Curt S. Koontz
Emory University School of Medicine
Emory Children' Center
Division of Pediatric Surgery
2015 Uppergate Drive NE
Atlanta, GA 30322, USA

Scott E. Langenburg
Children's Hospital of Michigan
Wayne State University, Department of Surgery
3901 Beaubien Boulevard
Detroit, MI 48201, USA

Marc David Leclair
Service de Chirurgie Infantile
HME CHU Hotel Dieu
7, Quai Moncousu
44 093 Nantes Cedex 1, France

K.H. Lee
Chinese University of Hong Kong
Shatin, New Territories, Hong Kong SAR, China

Mario Lima
Università di Bologna "Alma Mater Studiortum"
Clinica Chirurgica Pediatrica
40126 Bologna, Italy

Thom E. Lobe
Blank Children's Hospital
1200 Pleasant Street
Des Moines, IA 50309, USA

Gordon A. MacKinlay
The University of Edinburgh
The Royal Hospital for Sick Children
Sciennes Road
Edinburgh, EH9 1LF, Scotland UK

N. Magsanoc
Chinese University of Hong Kong
Shatin, New Territories, Hong Kong SAR, China

Jacques Marescaux
European Institute of Telesurgery
1 Place de l'Hôpital,
67091 Strasbourg, France

Marcelo Martinez-Ferro
Private Children's Hospital
Buenos Aires Argentina
Cramer 4601 (14290
3er Piso. Oficina de Cirurgia
Ciudad Autonoma de Buenos Aires, Argentina

Girolamo Mattioli
Chirurgia e Urologia Pediatrica
IRCCS G. Gaslini
Universit di Genova
Largo G. Gaslini, 5
16100 Genova, Italy

Philippe Montupet
Bicêtre Hospital
Pediatric Surgical Unit, Paris XI University
CHU Bicêtre
78 Rue du Gal Leclerc
94275 Le Kremlin-Bicêtre, France

Oliver J. Muensterer
Department of Pediatric Surgery
Children's University Hospital of Leipzig
Liebigstrasse 20
04103 Leipzig, Germany

Calvin S.H. Ng
Chinese University of Hong Kong
Prince of Wales Hospital
Department of Surgery
Shatin, N.T., Hong Kong SAR, China

Rainer Nustede
Hannover Medical School
Department of Pediatric Surgery
Carl-Neuberg-Strasse 1
30625 Hannover, Germany

Jacques Paineau
Service de Chirurgie
Centre Ren Gauducheau
Bd J Monod
44805 St Herblain Cedex, France

Craig A. Peters
Children's Hospital
Department of Urology
300 Longwood Avenue
Boston, MA 02115, USA

Shawn D. Peter St.
Department of Surgery
Children's Mercy Hospital
2401 Gillham Road
Kansas City, MO 64108, US

Alessio Pini Prato
Chirurgia e Urologia Pediatrica
IRCCS G. Gaslini
Universit di Genova
Largo G. Gaslini, 5
16100 Genova, Italy

Guillaume Podevin
Service de Chirurgie Infantile
HME, CHU Hôtel Dieu
7, quai Moncousu
44093 Nantes, France

Thomas Pranikoff
Wake Forest University School of Medicine
Section of Pediatric Surgery
Medical Center Boulevard
Winston Salem, NC 27157, USA

Olivier Reinberg
Department of Pediatric Surgery
University Hospital of Lausanne (CHUV)
1011 Lausanne-CHUV, Switzerland

Frederick J. Rescorla
JW Riley Hospital for Children
702 Barnhill Drive, Rm. 2500,
Indianapolis, IN 46202, USA

Steven S. Rothenberg
The Rocky Mountain Hospital for Children
1601 East 18 Avenue
Suite 5500
Denver, Colorado 80218, USA

Francesco Rubino
European Institute of Telesurgery
1 Place de l'Hopital
67091 Strasbourg, France

Daniel F. Saad
Emory University School of Medicine
Division of Pediatric Surgery
Emory Children's Center
2015 Uppergate Drive NE
Atlanta, GA 30322, USA

Jacqueline M. Saito
Division of Pediatric Surgery
University of Alabama, Birmingham
1600 7th Avenue South, ACC-300
Birmingham, AL 35233-1711, USA

Klaus Schaarschmidt
HELIOS Klinikum Berlin Buch
Schwanebecker Chaussee 50
13125 Berlin, Germany

Felix Schier
Universitätsklinikum Mainz
Department of Pediatric Surgery
Langenbeckstrasse 1
55101 Mainz, Germany

Jürgen Schleef
Children's Hospital
IRCCS Burlo Garofolo
Via dell'Istria 65/1
34137 Trieste, Italy

Manoj U. Shenoy
Department of Pediatric Urology
Nottingham University Hospitals
City Hospital Campus
Hucknall Road
Nottingham NG5 1PB, UK

J.D. Sihoe
Chinese University of Hong Kong
Prince of Wales Hospital
Department of Surgery
Shatin, N.T., Hong Kong SAR, China

Perry W. Stafford
Children's Hospital of Pennsylvania
34th. & Civic Center Blvd
Philadelphia, 34th & Civic PA 19104, USA

Henri Steyaert
Fondation Lenval
Department of Paediatric Surgery
57 Av. de la Californie
06200, Nice, France

Karl G. Sylvester
Stanford University School of Medicine
Department of Surgery
780 Welch Road, Suite 206,
Stanford, CA 94305-5733, USA

Y.H. Tam
Chinese University of Hong Kong
Shatin, New Territories, Hong Kong SAR, China

Holger Till
Children's University Hospital
Oststrasse 21-25
04317 Leipzig, Germany

Benno M. Ure
Department of Pediatric Surgery
Hannover Medical School
Carl-Neuberg-Strasse 1
30625 Hannover, Germany

K. Uschinsky
HELIOS Klinikum Berlin Buch
Schwanebecker Chaussee 50
13125 Berlin, Germany

Jean-Stéphane Valla
Hôpital Lenval
Department of Pediatric Surgery
Fondation Lenval
57, Avenue de la Californie
06200 Nice, France

David C. van der Zee
Department of Pediatric Surgery
Wilhelmina Children's Hospital
University Medical Center Utrecht
P.O.Box 85090
3508 AB Utrecht, The Netherlands

Bryan C. Weidner
PMG Pediatric Surgical Group
201 Cedar Street SE, Suite 503,
Albuquerque, NM 87106, USA

Duncan T. Wilcox
Department Pediatric Urology
Children's Medical Center
2350 Stemmons Frwy Syute D-4300
Dallas, TX 75207, USA

Mark L. Wulkan
Emory University School of Medicine
Emory Children's Center
Division of Pediatric Surgery
2015 Uppergate Drive NE,
Atlanta, GA 30322, USA

Aydin Yagmurlu
University of Ankara School of Medicine
Dogol Caddesi
06100 Tandogan, Ankara, Turkey

C.K. Yeung
Chinese University of Hong Kong, Prince of Wales
Hospital
Department of Surgery
Shatin, N.T., Hong Kong

Anthony P.C. Yim
Chinese University of Hong Kong
Prince of Wales Hospital
Department of Surgery
Shatin, N.T., Hong Kong

Basics

Chapter 1

Why Endoscopic Surgery?

Klaas (N) M.A. Bax

Until the introduction of general anesthesia into medicine in 1846, surgery was limited to external conditions. When general anesthesia became available, it became possible for the surgeon to enter body cavities. The problem had, however, to be exteriorized and a large exposure was usually required to accomplish this. No wonder that the adage "large incision big surgeon, small incision little surgeon" governed surgery for over 100 years. When muscle relaxants became available, smaller incisions in combination with retraction of the wound edges could provide good exposure. However, the relationship between the length of the incision and the magnitude of the exposure remained. Moreover, the smaller the incision the more retraction onto the wound edges.

Even in the absence of complications, opening of a body wall results in morbidity such as stress and pain. The larger a wound, the more skin, fascia, muscles and nerves are transected, and the more morbidity can be expected. Pain related to the access wound may not only be related to the early postoperative period but may become chronic. Some paresthesia is virtually always present around a scar and long-term pain after a classic posterolateral thoracotomy is a well-known phenomenon. The consequences of abnormal wound healing are usually much more serious in large access wounds, for example wound infection, dehiscence, and incisional hernia.

Wide opening of the body wall results in loss of water and heat, which especially threatens small children. Drying out of the tissues and handling causes trauma to them and impaired healing. Organs covered with gauze often show petechiae and fibrin as a result of the rubbing caused by the gauze. No wonder that adhesions develop, with their intrinsic predisposition for complications such as strangulation of bowel.

The wish to look into the body cavities has existed for over a century. One of the major problems in the past has been the lack of a lens system through which enough light could be transmitted. It was the British scientist Hopkins, who invented the now classic Hopkins rod lens system (Hopkins 1953). This system has revolutionized image transmission and is still very much in use today. Karl Storz was the first to combine the Hopkins lens system with cold light illumination through glass fibers (Berci and Cushieri 1996). Two

pediatric surgeons have been very much in the frontline of the development of endoscopy in children: while Stephen Gans was active in the field of bronchoscopy and laparoscopy, Bradley Rodgers was and still is active in the field of thoracoscopy (Gans 1983; Gans and Berci 1973; Rodgers et al. 1979).

Until the mid 1980s, most endoscopic surgical procedures were diagnostic. This is not surprising as the surgeon had to hold the telescope with one hand and look with one eye through the telescope close to the patient, which was not ideal from the ergonomic point of view and also not from the point of view of sterility. Moreover the surgeon had only one hand left for instrumentation.

The real breakthrough in endoscopic surgery came when chip cameras became available allowing for real-time video transmission of the endoscopic picture onto a TV screen (Berci et al. 1986). From then onward, the surgeon had a binocular picture as well as his assistant. The view obtained with such a system was and is far better than the view obtained through a large incision. Laparoscopic cholecystectomy was first described in 1989 by Dubois et al. (1989), and laparoscopic Nissen fundoplication in 1991 by Dallemagne et al. (1991).

While endoscopic surgery was embraced in general surgery from the outset, the breakthrough in endoscopic surgery in children lagged behind. A number of pioneers, however, have been involved in the field since its introduction into medicine (Alain et al. 1990; Bax and van der Zee 1995, 1998, 2002; Bax et al. 2000; Borzi 2001; Georgeson et al. 1995, 2000; Holcomb et al. 1991; Lobe et al. 1993, 1999; Montupet 2002; Montupet and Esposito 1999; Rothenberg 1999, 2000a,b, 2002; Schier 1998; Smith et al. 1994; Tan and Roberts 1996; Tulman et al. 1993; Valla et al. 1991, 1996; van der Zee and Bax 1995, 1996; van der Zee et al. 1995; Waldschmidt and Schier 1991; Yeung et al. 1999). The general backlog in endoscopic surgery in children is decreasing and, by now, most of the operations in children that are classically done in an open way have been described using endoscopic surgical techniques. Even hepatoportojejunostomy for choledochal cyst (Shimura et al. 1998) and biliary atresia (Esteves et al. 2002) have been carried out, as well as transvesical reimplantation of ureters (Gill et al. 2001). Not only have classic operations been translated into an endoscopic surgical variant, but also complete new operations have been introduced such as the creation of a hole in the floor of the fourth ventricle of the brain to drain hydrocephalus.

There is consensus that endoscopic surgery is more difficult than open surgery: the view obtained is two-dimensional, the entrance ports are fixed, and instruments have to be inserted through narrow cannulae into the body, causing resistance and decreased tactile feeling. Moreover the tips of the instruments have only a very limited number of degrees of freedom of movement making the tasks to be exerted much more difficult than during open surgery. No wonder that most endoscopic surgical operations take longer and are more fatiguing for the surgeon. There is also the matter of the CO_2 insufflation and of extreme Trendelenburg and reversed Trendelenburg position. These factors have an influence on the general and locoregional hemodynamics and on lung physiology.

The question "Is it worth the trouble?" is certainly a valid one and has to be answered. The traditional Hippocratic ethos provides for the background of the idea that the less invasive a procedure, the better it is (van Wilgenburg 1995). Also modern parents dislike scars being inflicted on their children and each scar on a child is a scar on the soul of the parents. A question often asked by parents before the operation is how long the incision is going to be. Not only the parents but also the children themselves do not like scars. Even the slight touch of acne can cause severe psychological problems. Scars do grow with the child. Moreover scars in infants often adhere to the fascia because of lack of subcutaneous fat. This results in retraction of the scar, giving it an ugly aspect. Not surprisingly more and more children nowadays have their childhood scars corrected when they are grown up. Bergmeijer looking at the long-term results after a Nissen fundoplication in childhood found that 37.5% of patients were not happy with the upper laparotomy scar (Bergmeijer 2002).

There is more to it than Hippocrates and the feelings of the parents and the children. There is also a scientific basis for endoscopic surgery. The relationship between the degree of operative trauma and the magnitude of the stress response as well as the degree of immunosuppression has been shown over and over again (Gutt et al. 1998). It leaves no doubt that the stress response, as well as the changes in the inflammatory and antiinflammatory parameters, are less pronounced after laparoscopic surgery (Neudecker et al. 2002; Neugebauer et al. 1991), when compared with the same procedure performed through a laparotomy. The clinical relevance of these results is not clear at present.

Any new method should be superior or at least equal to the conventional technique (Neugebauer et al. 1991). Comprehensive technology assessment includes four steps that have been described by Jennett (1986):

1. Feasibility and safety
2. Efficacy (benefit for the patient)
3. Efficiency (benefit for the general population)
4. Economic appraisal (does it save money)

But how do we measure this? There is no doubt that randomized controlled trials (RCT) are the gold standard to study these various steps, but such studies are difficult to perform, especially in surgery. In a study of all 760 abstracts that have been accepted for presentation by the British Association of Paediatric Surgeons in the period 1996–2000, only 9 abstracts concerned clinical randomized studies (Curry et al. 2003). None mentioned the method of randomization. Only 4 studies had relevant endpoints, and sample size in all was inadequate. Only one study has been published so far in the English literature. As is the case in pediatric surgery in general, evidence-based studies on endoscopic surgery in children are rare. Most RCTs regarding laparoscopic surgery in children relate to appendectomy (Lejus et al. 1996; Lintula et al. 2001; Pedersen et al. 2001). Recently two randomized trials on endoscopic surgery in children were published one comparing open with laparoscopic inguinal hernia repair (Chan et al. 2005) and one comparing laparoscopic with open pyloromyotomy (St. Peter et al. 2006). RCT concerning thoracoscopic procedures are even more scarce. Even for a relatively frequent condition such as pleural empyema, insufficient good studies are available to draw definite conclusions (Colice et al. 2000; Coote 2002).

There are other levels of evidence than the evidence provided by good RCT (Sackett et al. 2000). In order to obtain the best available evidence, the European Association for Endoscopic Surgery holds regular Consensus Development Conferences (Neugebauer et al. 2000). The era of feasibility studies in endoscopic surgery has reached its end, even in pediatric surgery. In order to do prospective randomized studies, a large volume of pathology is usually required and this is hard to achieve in pediatric surgery. Multicenter studies are an option but the participating centers need to have an equal level of expertise and, moreover, such studies are difficult to conduct logistically.

The major impact of endoscopic surgery onto modern surgery has been that surgeons are now thinking in terms of invasiveness. As a result open surgery has evolved as well and there is a tendency to avoid large incisions. The smaller the exposure, the less stress response and the more difficult to prove that the endoscopic surgical variant is superior (Geiger et al. 1998; Kennedy et al. 1998; Majeed et al. 1996; Miller et al. 2000a,b). It leaves no doubt that minimal access surgery in its broad sense is going to develop further. Pediatric surgeons should be able to provide their patients with the best available treatment options, including the endoscopic surgical approach.

Endoscopic surgical techniques will become easier with further technical development. Good three-dimensional vision in endoscopic surgery already exists, for example in the da Vinci robot system, making the surgery easier. Unfortunately the size of the actual scope prohibits its use in small children. The more we understand matters of ergonomics and the more we introduce these ergonomic principles into our surgery, the easier the surgery will be. But we should be aware that technology waits for no one and that new technology has the potential to replace established organizations such as corporations, businesses, and professions (Satava 2002).

References

Alain JL, Grousseau D, Terrier G (1990) Extra-mucosa pylorotomy by laparoscopy. Chir Pediatr 31:223–224

Bax NMA, van der Zee DC (1995) Laparoscopic removal of aganglionic bowel using the Duhamel-Martin method in five consecutive infants. Pediatr Surg Int 10:226–222

Bax NMA, van der Zee DC (1998) Laparoscopic treatment of intestinal malrotation in children. Surg Endosc 12:1314–1316

Bax KMA, van Der Zee DC (2002) Feasibility of thoracoscopic repair of esophageal atresia with distal fistula. J Pediatr Surg 37:192–196

Bax NMA, Ure BM, van der Zee DC, et al (2000) Laparoscopic duodenoduodenostomy for duodenal atresia. Surg Endosc 15:217

Berci G, Cuschieri A (1996) Karl Storz, 1911–1996. A remembrance. Surg Endosc 10:1123

Berci G, Brooks PG, Paz-Partlow M (1986) TV laparoscopy. A new dimension in visualization and documentation of pelvic pathology. J Reprod Med 31:585–588

Bergmeijer JHLJ (2002) Diagnosis and treatment of gastro-esophageal reflux in patients with esophageal atresia. Optima Grafische Communicatie, Rotterdam, pp 21–30

Borzi PA (2001) A comparison of the lateral and posterior retroperitoneoscopic approach for complete and partial nephroureterectomy in children. BJU Int 87:517–520

Chan KL, Hui WC, Tam PK (2005) Prospective randomized single-center, single-blind comparison of laparoscopic vs open repair of pediatric inguinal hernia. Surg Endosc 19:927–32

Colice GL, Curtis A, Deslauriers J, et al (2000) Medical and surgical treatment of parapneumonic effusions: an evidence-based guideline. Chest 118:1158–1171

Coote N (2002) Surgical versus non-surgical management of pleural empyema. Cochrane Database Syst Rev CD001956

Curry JI, Reeves B, Stringer MD (2003) Randomized controlled trials in pediatric surgery: Could we do better? J Pediatr Surg 38:556–559

Dallemagne B, Weerts JM, Jehaes C, et al (1991) Nissen fundoplication: preliminary report. Surg Laparosc Endosc 1:138–143

Dubois F, Berthelot G, Levard H (1989) Cholecystectomie par coelioscopie. Presse Med 18:980–982

Esteves E, Clemente Neto E, Ottaiano Neto M, et al (2002) Laparoscopic Kasai portoenterostomy for biliary atresia. Pediatr Surg Int 18:737–740

Gans SL (1983) Pediatric Endoscopy. Grune and Stratton, New York

Gans SL, Berci G (1973) Peritoneoscopy in infants and children. J Pediatr Surg 8:399–405

Geiger JD, Dinh VV, Teitelbaum DH, et al (1998) The lateral approach for open splenectomy. J Pediatr Surg 33:1153–1156

Georgeson KE, Fuenfer MM, Hardin WD (1995) Primary laparoscopic pull-through for Hirschsprung's disease in infants and children. J Pediatr Surg 30:1017–1021

Georgeson KE, Inge TH, Albanese CT (2000) Laparoscopically assisted anorectal pull-through for high imperforate anus: a new technique. J Pediatr Surg 35:927–930

Gill IS, Ponsky LE, Desai M, et al (2001) Laparoscopic cross-trigonal Cohen ureteroneocystostomy: novel technique. J Urol 166:1811–1814

Gutt CN, Kuntz C, Schmandra T, et al (1998) Metabolism and immunology in laparoscopy. Surg Endosc 12:1096–1098

Holcomb GW 3rd, Olsen DO, Sharp KW (1991) Laparoscopic cholecystectomy in the pediatric patient. J Pediatr Surg 26:1186–1190

Hopkins HH (1966) US Patent 3,257,902. Optical system having cylindrical rod-like lenses

Jennett B (1986) High technology medicine. Benefits and burdens. Oxford University Press, Oxford

Kennedy AP Jr, Snyder CL, Ashcraft KW, et al (1998) Comparison of muscle-sparing thoracotomy and thoracoscopic ligation for the treatment of patent ductus arteriosus. J Pediatr Surg 33:259–261

Lejus C, Delile L, Plattner V, et al (1996) Randomised, single-blinded trial of laparoscopic versus open appendectomy in children: effects on postoperative analgesia. Anesthesiology 84:801–806

Lintula H, Kokki H, Vanamo K (2001) Single-blind randomized clinical trial of laparoscopic versus open appendicectomy in children. Br J Surg 88:510–514

Lobe TE, Schropp KP, Lunsford K (1993) Laparoscopic Nissen fundoplication in childhood. J Pediatr Surg 28:358–360

Lobe TE, Rothenberg SS, Waldschmidt J, Stroeder L (1999) Thoracoscopic repair of esophageal atresia in an infant: a surgical first. Pediatr Endosurg Innov Tech 3:141–148

Majeed AW, Troy G, Nicholl JP, et al (1996) Randomised, prospective, single-blind comparison of laparoscopic versus small-incision cholecystectomy. Lancet 347:989–994

Miller JD, Urschel JD, Cox G, et al (2000a) A randomized, controlled trial comparing thoracoscopy and limited thoracotomy for lung biopsy in interstitial lung disease. Ann Thorac Surg 70:1647–1650

Miller JD, Simone C, Kahnamoui K, et al (2000b) Comparison of videothoracoscopy and axillary thoracotomy for the treatment of spontaneous pneumothorax. Am Surg 66:1014–1015

Montupet P (2002) Laparoscopic Toupet's fundoplication in children. Semin Laparosc Surg 9:163–167

Montupet P, Esposito C (1999) Laparoscopic treatment of congenital inguinal hernia in children. J Pediatr Surg 34:420–423

Neudecker J, Sauerland S, Neugebauer E, et al (2002) The European Association for Endoscopic Surgery clinical practice guideline on the pneumoperitoneum for laparoscopic surgery. Surg Endosc 16:1121–1143

Neugebauer E, Troidl H, Spangenberger W, et al (1991) Conventional versus laparoscopic cholecystectomy and the randomized controlled trial. Br J Surg 78:150–154

Neugebauer E, Sauerland S, Troidl H (2000) Recommendations for evidence-based endoscopic surgery: the updated EAES consensus development conferences. Springer, Paris

Pedersen AG, Petersen OB, Wara P, et al (2001) Randomised clinical trial of laparoscopic versus open appendicectomy. Br J Surg 88:200–205

Rodgers BM, Moazam F, Talbert JL (1979) Thoracoscopy in children. Ann Surg 189:176–180

Rothenberg SS (1999) Experience with 220 consecutive laparoscopic Nissen fundoplications in infants and children. J Pediatr Surg 33:274–278

Rothenberg SS (2000a) Thoracoscopic lung resection in children. J Pediatr Surg 35:271–274

Rothenberg SS (2000b) Thoracoscopic repair of a tracheoesophageal fistula in a newborn infant. Pediatr Endosurg Innov Tech 4:289–294

Rothenberg SS (2002) Thoracoscopic repair of tracheoesophageal fistula in newborns. J Pediatr Surg 37:869–872

Sackett DL, Strauss SE, Richardson WS, et al (2000) Evidence based medicine: how to practice and teach EBM, 2nd edn. Churchill Livingston, London

Satava RM (2002) Disruptive visions. Surgeon responsibility during era of change. Surg Endosc 16:733–734

Schier F (1998) Laparoscopic herniorrhaphy in girls. J Pediatr Surg 33:1495–1497

Shimura H, Tanaka M, Shimizu S, et al (1998) Laparoscopic treatment of congenital choledochal cyst. Surg Endosc 12:1268–1271

Smith BM, Steiner RB, Lobe TE (1994) Laparoscopic Duhamel pull-through procedure for Hirschsprung's disease in childhood. J Laparoendosc Surg 4:273–276

St. Peter SD, Holcomb GW, Calkins CM, et al (2006) Open versus laparoscopic pyloromyotomy for pyloric stenosis. A prospective, randomized trial. Ann Surg 244:363-370

Tan HL, Roberts JP (1996) Laparoscopic dismembered pyeloplasty in children: preliminary results. Br J Urol 77:909–913

Tulman S, Holcomb GW 3rd, Karamanoukian HL, et al (1993) Pediatric laparoscopic splenectomy. J Pediatr Surg 28:689–692

Valla JS, Limonne B, Valla V, et al (1991) Laparoscopic appendectomy in children: report of 465 cases. Surg Laparosc Endosc 1:166–172

Valla JS, Guilloneau B, Montupet P, Geiss S, et al (1996) Retroperitoneal laparoscopic nephrectomy in children. Preliminary report of 18 cases. Eur Urol 30:490–493

van der Zee DC, Bax NM (1995) Laparoscopic repair of congenital diaphragmatic hernia in a 6-month-old child. Surg Endosc 9:1001–1003

van der Zee DC, Bax NM (1996) Laparoscopic Thal fundoplication in mentally retarded children. Surg Endosc 10:659–661

van der Zee DC, van Seumeren IG, Bax KM, et al (1995) Laparoscopic approach to surgical management of ovarian cysts in the newborn. J Pediatr Surg 30:42–43

van Wilgenburg T (1995) Laparoscopic surgery: systematic appraisal of moral pros and cons. Book of abstracts. International Symposium on the Occasion of 121/2 years Paediatric Surgery. Laparoscopic Procedures in Children: Sense and Nonsense, Utrecht, 7–8 April 1995, p 14

Waldschmidt J, Schier F (1991) Laparoscopic surgery in neonates and infants. Eur J Pediatr Surg 1:145–1450

Yeung CK, Liu KW, Ng WT, et al (1999) Laparoscopy as the investigation and treatment of choice for urinary incontinence caused by small "invisible" dysplastic kidneys with infrasphincteric ureteric ectopia. Br J Urol Int 84:324–328

Chapter 2

Equipment and Instruments

Carroll M. Harmon

Introduction

The evolution and development of minimally invasive (minimal access) pediatric endosurgery has depended on the evolution and development of equipment and instrumentation technology. Our past, current, and future successes in the field of endoscopic pediatric surgery – for even our smallest, most delicate patients – has been, and will be, dictated not so much by the willingness and talents of pediatric surgeons, but by the equipment available to them.

History of Pediatric Minimally Invasive Surgical Equipment

The desire to look inside the human body is as old as medicine. Minimally invasive pediatric surgical technology used today started with that same desire. However, the history of endoscopy is relatively young, just the past 200 years. For thousands of years, easily accessible bodily cavities such as the mouth, vagina, and anus have been inspected using a speculum. However, endoscopy and endoscopic surgery in general, and pediatric endoscopy surgery in particular, needed to overcome severe technical problems with lighting, image transmission, and space.

Credit goes to Philipp Bozzini (1773–1809) of Germany as the father of modern endoscopy. In 1804, he first reported the creation of his endoscopic instrument, the *Lichtleiter*, which utilized a wax candle for lighting and a system of mirrors and tubes. This apparatus allowed limited visualization of the upper and lower gastrointestinal tract (Bozzinni 1806). In 1853, Antonin Desormeaux (1830–1894) demonstrated a new instrument he dubbed *l'endoscope* for the examination of the urethra, bladder, vagina, bowels, and wounds (Reuter et al. 1999). The Desormeaux endoscope was accompanied by accessory devices such as a lamp, attachable scopes, sound, a knife, and a grasper. For lighting, the instrument utilized a flame from a mixture of alcohol and turpentine, which occasionally resulted in burns to the face of the physician and the legs of the patient. In 1876, Maximilian Nitze (1848–1906), following Thomas Edison's invention of the light bulb, created the first optical magnifying view endoscope with built-in electrical light bulb as the source of illumination (Modlin et al. 2004; Reuter et al. 1999).

In 1901, Dimitri Oskarovich Ott (1859–1929) performed the first documented human laparoscopy in St Petersburg, Russia, using a gynecologic head mirror, an external light source, and speculum (Ott 1901). In 1902, George Kelling (1866–1945) of Dresden, Germany, used the Nitze cystoscope to examine the abdominal cavity of dogs (Modlin et al. 2004). Kelling also described the insufflation of air into the abdominal cavity in order to create a *lufttamponade* or tamponade pneumoperitoneum, with the goal of stopping intra-abdominal bleeding from conditions such as ectopic pregnancy, bleeding ulcers, and hemorrhagic pancreatitis (Modlin et al. 2004). By 1910, he had undertaken many successful diagnostic laparoscopies on humans and he coined the term *coelioskopie* to describe his technique.

H.C. Jacobaeus, from Stockholm, used the term *laparothorakoskopie* in 1910 to describe procedures on the human thorax and abdomen, and was particularly enthusiastic about thoracoscopic cauterization of pleural adhesions in respiratory tuberculosis (Jacobaeus 1910). In 1920, Benjamin Orndoff developed a sharp pyramidal-shaped point on the laparoscopic trocar to facilitate puncture (Orndoff 1920). The following year, Korbsch (Korbsch 1921) introduced the first needle for peritoneal insufflation and Goetze (Goetze 1921) published details of his novel device, the insufflator. In 1924, Richard Zollikofer was the first to recognize the value of using carbon dioxide to obtain a pneumoperitoneum (Modlin et al. 2004). In 1929, Heinz Kalk, considered the founder of the German School of Laparoscopy, developed a 135° lens system allowing laparoscopic diagnostic and biopsy evaluation for liver disease (Kalk 1929).

In 1934, John Ruddock of Los Angeles, California, collaborated with American Cystoscope Makers, Inc. (ACMI) to modify a cystoscope and develop a fore-oblique visual system that greatly facilitated peritoneoscopy (Ruddock 1934). In his 1957 manuscript reviewing his results with 5,000 cases of peritoneoscopy, Ruddock included almost 100 cases of using this technology in infants and children (Ruddock 1957). The Hungarian J. Veress developed the spring-loaded needle for performance of therapeutic pneumothorax to

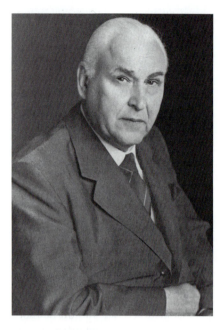

Fig. 2.1. Karl Storz

treat pulmonary tuberculosis in 1938; he then applied this technique to cases of pneumoperitoneum (Veress 1938).

In 1952, N. Fourestier introduced the use of a quartz light rod to replace the distal lamp in the rigid bronchoscope and its application in laparoscopy became immediately apparent (Fourestier et al. 1952; Modlin et al. 2004). This method of light delivery drastically improved illumination and obviated the heat and electrical problems associated with the typical distal lamp (Modlin et al. 2004). The technology also facilitated the development of color cinematography and television imaging in the peritoneal cavity (Modlin et al. 2004). However, quartz rod technology was expensive and fragile (Modlin et al. 2004). Therefore, the advancement of fiberoptic technology revolutionized both rigid and flexible endoscopic surgery. In 1954, Harold Hopkins and Narinder Kapany of Imperial College in London, UK, first reported a useful fiberoptic system (Hopkins and Kapany 1954). From 1957 to 1961, Basil Hirschowitz of the University of Alabama at Birmingham, working with ACMI, developed glass-coated fibers that could function in a flexible "fiberscope" to be used in gastroscopy, as he demonstrated upon himself at the American Gastroscopic Society meeting in 1957 (Hirschowitz 1961; Modlin et al. 2004).

In 1959, Harold H. Hopkins also described the rod lens telescope system for image transmission and by 1967, Karl Storz, working with Hopkins, developed a rigid endoscope that utilized rod lens and fiberoptic light transmission (Reuter et al. 1999). Also, in 1960 Karl Storz (■ Fig. 2.1) patented the first extracorporeal cold light source, which allowed the light source to

be separated from the endoscope and allowed intense light to be transmitted from the light source through the endoscope via fiberoptic fibers (Reuter et al. 1999).

In the 1960s, the German gynecologist, Kurt Semm contributed significantly to laparoscopic surgery by inventing an electronic automatic carbon dioxide insufflator. On 13 September 1980, Professor Semm also performed the world's first laparoscopic appendectomy (Hasson 1978; Semm 1983). Hasson described his blunt-tipped peritoneal access cannula attached to an olive-shaped sleeve in 1978, introducing an alternative method of trocar placement (Hasson 1978).

In 1982, the first solid-state camera was introduced, opening the era of "video-laparoscopy." This advance allowed for a real-time binocular video image transmission to a video monitor. By 1989, the first three-chip video camera was produced allowing enhanced resolution and image brilliance.

It has been the development and manufacture of novel endoscopic surgical instruments that catapulted laparoscopy from a role in diagnostics to therapeutics. Endoscopic instrument production allowing for pediatric-specific application is relatively recent. Since 1995, several companies including Karl Storz Endoscopy and Jarit Instruments, in particular, have developed many high-quality pediatric-specific instruments.

Technology Challenges of Pediatric Endosurgery

There are a number of technical and technological challenges that are specific for pediatric endosurgery. Below is a list of some of the technology hurdles in advanced pediatric endosurgery:
- Small instruments (short and narrow)
- Carbon dioxide insufflator sensitivity (volume and rate)
- Trocar slippage
- Abdominal wall flexibility
- Small cavity working space
- Light intensity (small scope produces white spot)
- Advanced suturing techniques

Visualization/Video Technology

Introduction

It is a fundamental ability of the surgeon to be able to visualize organs and tissues that has allowed success with pediatric endosurgery. Loss of tactile feedback and decreased degrees of movement inherent, to date, in endoscopic surgery make quality of video image

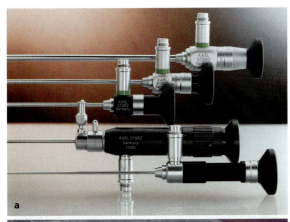

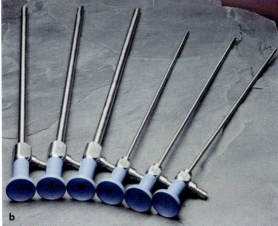

Fig. 2.2. a Telescopes (Karl Storz Endoscopy). **b** Telescopes (Stryker Endoscopy)

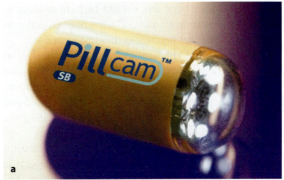

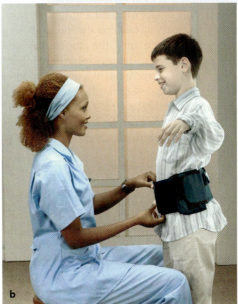

Fig. 2.3. PillCam. **a** Wireless camera. **b** Belt with recording device

most critical. A bright, clear image is mandatory. Therefore, the development of small, reliable, high-resolution imaging systems has been essential for the pediatric surgeon's acquisition of detailed information about the tissues being manipulated. The quality of the image depends on each component of the laparoscopic imaging unit and is only as good as the weakest component of the system.

Telescopes

The development of a rod lens optical system by Harold H. Hopkins in 1959 and the coupling of this system with fiberoptic light transmission technology by Karl Storz in 1960 marked a breakthrough in modern endoscopic surgery. The Hopkins rod lens endoscope system consists of a series of glass rod lenses separated by air and fiberoptic bundles surrounding the lens for transmission of light. The first laparoscopes were too large for widespread application in infants and young children. However, by the mid 1990s, several companies were producing small-diameter rigid telescopes

that could provide enough light and clarity of image for use in infants.

Currently, most pediatric endosurgeons utilize telescopes ranging from 1 to 5 mm in diameter and from 18 to 25 cm in length (■ Fig. 2.2a,b). However, as technologies advance (high-definition digital cameras and improved light transmission) 1- to 2 mm-diameter telescopes should be more functional in the future. Telescopes in the 2.5- to 5 mm-diameter range are available with angled lenses (30°, 45°, and 70°) allowing better visualization for most intra-abdominal and intrathoracic procedures. The use of an angled lens (30–45°) allows the tip of the operating lens to be above the operating field within the chest or abdomen. This position is very helpful in most standard pediatric endosurgical procedures; it helps prevent "sword fighting" of the scope with other instruments and allows a better working view than that achieved with a straight viewing telescope. One problem with angled telescopes is that there is some loss of light transmission. Most pediatric endosurgery sets should include at least 3- and 5 mm-diameter, 0° and 30° telescopes in order to perform procedures on infants to adolescents.

The eyepiece of the telescope typically attaches to the camera head by means of a C-mount coupler that allows for easy telescope changes if needed. An important accessory item is a stainless steel thermos filled with hot sterile water that can be used for cleaning the tip of the telescope and prevents it from fogging.

A recent innovation that has promising application in pediatric diagnostics and possibly endosurgery, is capsule endoscopy (PillCam Capsule Endoscopy, Yoqneam, Israel). This device includes a miniature camera mounted in a clear capsule that can be swallowed or endoscopically placed into the duodenum and allowed to pass through the gastrointestinal tract (■ Fig. 2.3a). Images are recorded in a small computer data recording device housed in a belt worn around the abdomen during the 8- to 12-h examination (■ Fig. 2.3b). This device provides endoscopic images of the small bowel, in particular, and can be used in children 10 years of age or older.

Light Source and Light Cables

A high-intensity light source is required for satisfactorily bright images. Most commercially available units utilize a halogen, xenon, or metal halide bulb (150–300 W). Halogen light sources produce a slightly yellow light that requires compensation during "white balancing." Xenon light is whiter and the most natural in color. These sources of light provide a color temperature (hue or color appearance of a specific type of light) that is in the range of average daylight (5,500 K). Bulbs typically have a life span of 250–500 h. In most surgical endoscopic video systems, the illumination intensity is automatically adjusted via interaction of the camera and light source so that the level of light detected at the camera CCD surface allows for reduced glare. The automatic modulation of light intensity is a particular problem in pediatric endosurgery where the small telescope through which the light passes focuses the light over a smaller area than the larger telescopes. Thus, as the telescope approaches the tissue surface a central glare, or whiteout, is common. Light sources that are optimal for pediatric endosurgery may require different specifications than those for adult laparoscopic surgery.

Light from the light source lamp is transmitted to the telescope through a fiberoptic light cable. Optical fibers are long, thin strands of glass that are bundled together to form "cables." Light is passed from the light source through the optical fibers and flexible cable, utilizing the principle of total internal reflection without much degradation of the light signal. The light cable is

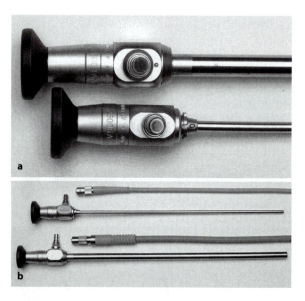

Fig. 2.4. Smaller telescopes (**a**) together with smaller light cords (**b**)

attached to the telescope and thus transmission of the light continues through fiberoptic fibers of the rigid telescope. Larger telescopes have more fibers for light transmission than smaller scopes and the diameter of the light cable should be adapted to the size of the scope. Using a larger cable according to the size of the telescope will just produce more heat at the connection site with no improvement in the amount of light reaching the target (■ Fig. 2.4a,b). If a fiberoptic light cable has greater than 15% of the fibers broken then it should be replaced.

Video Camera

The rapid expansion of videoendoscopic surgery in general and pediatric in particular has resulted from the technical development of the small charge-coupled device (CCD) video camera (■ Fig. 2.5a,b). Prior to the development of the video camera, operating surgeons had to look down the lens of the telescope to directly view thoracic or peritoneal organs. The ability to attach a relatively small video camera to the telescope allowed the surgeon to stand upright and operate while looking at a video image on a monitor. The CCD contains an imaging chip that is composed of a thin, flat silicone wafer that measures only about half an inch in diameter. The CCD matrix is composed of a series of horizontal and vertical rows of light sensors called "pixels" (picture elements). Camera-specific resolution is dictated by the density of the pixels. Initial surgical cameras contained a single "chip" on which a color mosaic produced reds (R), greens (G), and blues (B) for an image. Most current surgical CCD cameras

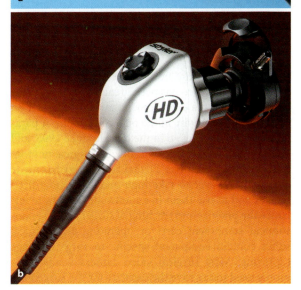

Fig. 2.5. a CCD camera Karl Storz (Karl Storz Endoscopy.
b CCD camera Stryker (Stryker Endoscopy)

now contain three chips and use prisms that split the image into three paths which pass through R, G, and B filters onto the three separate chips that then provide a red, green, and blue output signal. Many excellent three-chip cameras are available today. The next generation of cameras will integrate high-definition signals allowing for image resolution of greater than 1,000 lines. Camera light sensitivity is measured in lux and indicates the amount of light that is required to produce an image.

The camera head coupler that attaches the telescope also typically has a focusing knob. In addition, most camera heads contain control buttons that can be programmed to enable the surgeon to control and adjust the white balance, gain, digital zoom, and image capture. The camera head attaches via a cable to the camera box or power unit. This unit also typically contains controls for white balance, gain, shutter, digital enhancements, and preset specialty settings (orthopedic, general surgery, etc.).

An alternative to the telescope attached to a three-chip camera head configuration has been developed (Olympus) and is advocated by some non-pediatric surgeons. The "chip on a stick" technology places a small single-chip camera in the tip of a semirigid tele-

scope, eliminating the rod lens system for relay of image from the tip of the telescope back to the camera. The flexible tip compensates for the lack of an angled lens and allows for oblique views. Advocates argue that digitizing the image at the tip of the telescope allows for superior image quality. However, this technology has not been of practical use in most pediatric endosurgery because until recently the size of the telescope required was 10 mm in diameter. Recently, a 5 mm-diameter rigid version of this device has become available and should have broader application in children and adolescents.

The development of an acceptable three-dimensional camera and the necessary accessories continues. These devices are often showcased by companies at endosurgical meetings; however, to date this technology has not been widely adopted in adult or pediatric endosurgery. It should be expected that with refinement of three-dimensional technology there will be systems that are useful in the future.

Monitors

The most common monitor found in operating rooms today is still the cathode ray tube (CRT)-type surgical video monitor which operates similarly to consumer television sets (Fig. 2.6a). Images are reproduced using a horizontal electron scanning beam (horizontal linear scanning) aimed at the surface of a picture tube. The minimum required number of lines has been standardized in the USA at 525 lines for one complete picture or frame by the National Television System Committee (NTSC). The NTSC standard is used by many countries on the American continent as well as many Asian countries including Japan. The time required to complete one frame with 525 scanning lines is 1/30 s. To overcome flicker, each frame is divided into two parts such that 60 views, with odd or even lines, is presented each second. Each view of odd or even lines is called a field. The process of alternate-line field scanning is called interlacing. Another standard is the Phase Alternating Line (PAL) standard, which is used is most European countries except France. This standard has 625 lines per picture and has an interlacing frequency of 60 Hz. France uses the SECAM (Sequential Couleur Avec Memoire or Sequential Colour with Memory) standard, which has the same bandwidth as PAL but does transmit the color information sequentially.

In most cases, it is the resolution of the surgical monitor that is the limiting factor in providing the highest quality image for the surgeon. Lines of resolution refer to the number of alternate black and white lines that a system is able to discriminate. Horizontal resolution is the number of vertical lines and vertical

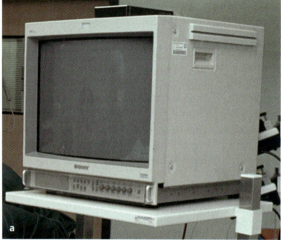

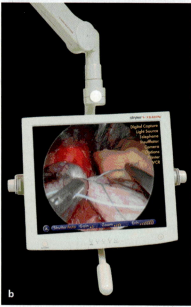

Fig. 2.6. a Classic monitor. **b** Flat panel monitor

picture is a pixel and the number of pixels governs the detail of the picture. A row of pixels is the digital equivalent of a scanning line. This image is non-interlaced because the scan rate can be very high and is sometimes referred to as progressive scanning. High-quality medical LCD monitors are now available from several companies with resolution of 1,280 × 1,024 pixels per inch and greater.

Image Capture

The ability to capture both single surgical images as well as surgical video has been greatly enhanced in recent years with the development and implementation of digital photography in the operating room. A paradigm shift has occurred in the decade since 1995, and digital technology has revolutionized surgical photography and presentations. Digital technology has made it easier than ever to take high-quality, standardized images and to use them in a multitude of ways to enhance the practice and teaching of surgery. Most endosurgical equipment carts or operating endosurgical suites contain equipment specific to surgical image capturing. Most surgical video camera heads commonly used today have the capacity for the surgeon to push a button on the camera head that will take a picture and send the image to a printer (■ Fig. 2.7a). Other methods for taking a picture include pendant control by the surgeon or nurse or voice activation control by the surgeon (■ Fig. 2.7b). Many endosurgical companies produce digital image capture devices that allow for intraoperative images to be stored on a computer in the operating room; these images can then be transferred to other portable media such as USB thumb drives, compact discs (CD), or digital video discs (DVD). Ideally, however, images and video taken in the operating suite can be transmitted to and stored in the hospitals archiving data base. Typically, these still images are compressed and stored in a standard digital picture format such as Joint Photographic Experts Group (JPEG), Tag(ged) Image File Format (TIFF), or Bitmap (BMP) which can be easily edited using personal computers and readily available software (Adobe Photoshop) and directly imported into presentation software such as PowerPoint.

Many endosurgical systems also have the capacity to record video directly to an analog tape (VHS), digital tape, or routed through a computer and transferred ("burned") to a digital video device such as a CD/DVD. Digital video is easily and usually automatically compressed (Moving Picture Experts Group: MPEG 1 or 2, Audio Video Interleave: AVI) and stored on digital tape, CD, or DVD. Many surgeons use their personal computers and video editing software to produce operative video for training, teaching, and presentations.

resolution is the number of horizontal lines. As mentioned the vertical resolution is limited by the number of scanning lines which is fixed according to the standard used (in standard NTSC monitors at 525 lines) and, therefore, cannot be improved by better camera resolution quality. However, horizontal resolution can be improved by increasing camera and monitor quality.

In recent years, as with computer monitors, liquid crystal display (LCD) monitors have appeared in the operating room (■ Fig. 2.6b). In the operating room LCD monitors are versatile. They can be light weight and flat allowing for use of ceiling-mounted booms and swing arms to position the monitor in multiple positions, thus improving visual and physical ergonomics for the surgeon. LCD monitors are not evaluated for resolution based on scanned lines, but instead on pixels per area. Each point of information of a given

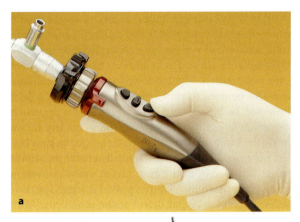

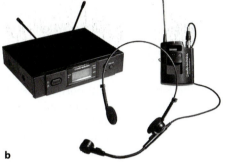

Fig. 2.7. a Camera head with image capturing button (Karl Storz Endoscopy). **b** Voice activation control for image capturing (Stryker Endoscopy)

Insufflators

In laparoscopic surgery, exposure is primarily achieved by insufflation of the peritoneal cavity with carbon dioxide to achieve a pneumoperitoneum. Although other gases have been studied, carbon dioxide continues to the preferred gas for laparoscopic surgery in adults and children because it is inexpensive, readily available, and highly soluble, allowing for large volumes to be absorbed and excreted by the lungs. The device that delivers and regulates the gas is the insufflator. The insufflator regulates the flow of carbon dioxide from a pressurized reservoir, through plastic insufflation tubing, and into the patient. Importantly, the insufflator also monitors the patient's intra-abdominal pressure. The flow of gas stops automatically when a preset intra-abdominal pressure is achieved. The panels on most available insufflators display the current and preset level of intra-abdominal pressure, the preset and current gas flow rate, the volume of gas infused (and leaked), and the residual volume of carbon dioxide in the tank.

Importantly, alarms signal and gas flow is stopped when intra-abdominal pressure exceeds the preset pressure. This is particularly important in infants and younger children where high intra-abdominal pressure can result in decreased venous return to the heart,

decreased peripheral perfusion, hypotension, and rapid rise in $PaCO_2$. Several manufacturers of insufflators have produced devices that are particularly helpful in infants and young children where the flow rates can be controlled at a low level, and where the measurement of intra-abdominal pressure is in real time (while gas is flowing) by utilizing a separate tube connected from the insufflator box to another trocar valve. The second tube does, however, add to the operating field clutter. For most insufflators that are on the market, the gas flow must stop briefly to measure the intra-abdominal pressure. In the later case, flow and "puff" volume can "overshoot" the preset pressure limit and the intra-abdominal pressure can exceed safe levels before the device can read the pressure and shut off the flow of gas. Even when overpressure is sensed and gas flow is halted, the system does not immediately or automatically reduce the critically high pressure, requiring the surgeon to recognize the problem and vent the intraperitoneal cavity, typically by opening a trocar valve. Neonatal-specific insufflators are now being developed to allow for very small, rapid puff volumes, with very rapid accurate pressure measurements between puffs.

In most infant laparoscopic operations, we start with a low flow rate of carbon dioxide (2 L/min) and advance to 5 L/min once the child and abdomen have acclimated. Preset pressures of 8–10 mmHg for infants and young children are usually safe. For older children and adolescents, settings of 20–40 L/min for flow rate and 15 mmHg for pressure are common. The higher flow rates are particularly helpful in operations where gas leak due to intra-abdominal suctioning, instrument exchanges, or port site leak is high.

Most insufflation tubing contains an in-line, hydrophobic filter which filters debris from the gas cylinder tank such as rust, metal filings, and other inorganic particles, and, in addition, the filter prevents backflow of body fluids and microorganisms into the insufflator, thus reducing the risk of cross-contamination and equipment damage. Some companies are now also manufacturing insufflators or component systems that provide for warmed and humidified insufflation gas in order to theoretically stabilize the patient's core temperature, improve postoperative pain, and decrease telescope lens fogging. However, clear benefits have not been established and, in infants, these potential benefits are weighed against the increased weight and bulk of the insufflator tubing and increased filter size which clutter the small operative field (Farley et al. 2004; Nguyen et al. 2002).

Insufflation is also helpful in thoracoscopic pediatric endosurgery in order to compress the ipsilateral lung slightly. However, the preset pressure and flow rates should be low (2–4 mmHg and 2–5 L/min).

The use of gasless laparoscopy using wires, corkscrews, or metal struts as body wall lifting devices has not been widely adopted in pediatric endosurgery. Although this technology has theoretical advantages of simplification of trocars (no valves), no collapse of operative field with suctioning or gas leak, and decreased cost, less ideal visualization and few choices for the variety of pediatric patient sizes have made these devices uncommon in pediatric operating suites.

Instruments

The acceleration of the adoption of pediatric endosurgical procedures has paralleled the development and production of appropriate small-diameter surgical instruments. Pediatric surgeons who pioneered minimal access videoendoscopic operations in children in the late 1980s and early 1990s were limited by the choice of large adult surgical laparoscopic instruments. The use of 10- to 15 mm-diameter trocars and 10 mm × 32 cm instruments for common pediatric surgical procedures, such as appendectomy or fundoplication, resulted in skeptical pediatric surgeons adding up the length of the traditional open incision and comparing this to the additive lengths of the combined trocar incisions and concluding that laparoscopic opera-tions where just as, or more invasive than, the open procedure in terms of the cumulative size of the incision.

Adult endoscopic instruments were too wide and too long for widespread pediatric application. The ideal position of an endosurgical instrument during a procedure is to have two thirds of the instrument inside the body cavity, and one third outside the body. When using adult-size instruments in infants, it was common to have 75% of the instrument outside and 25% inside, resulting in awkward manipulation, less precise movements, and poor ergonomics. However, since 1995, several companies (Karl Storz Endoscopy, Richard Wolf, Jarit Instruments) have been willing to work with pediatric surgeons to develop instruments that were appropriate in size and function to allow significant success in developing and applying minimal access surgery to infants and small children. Because of the diversity in size of patients most pediatric surgeons require several sets of instruments including sets appropriate for infant, young child (toddler), older child, and teenager. In addition, reusable instruments are preferred to most disposable instruments since reusable ones are made of higher quality materials and are less expensive in the long term.

Access Instruments and Trocars

The first step in most laparoscopic operations requires intraperitoneal access and insufflation. In most pediatric laparoscopic operations the umbilicus is chosen as the first site of intraperitoneal access. A Veress needle can be used safely in infants and children; however, the intra-abdominal viscera are a short distance from the abdominal fascia and skin and can be injured if great care is not taken. The cutdown, or Hasson technique can also be used to gain safe initial peritoneal access; however, in infants and thin children this approach can result in significant gas leak around the trocar. We have, therefore, used a modified technique to gain initial peritoneal access, where a small vertical incision is made in the skin at the base of the umbilicus and a small blunt mosquito clamp is passed through the consistently present fascial defect at the umbilicus. After blunt instrument access, a 14-gauge Veress-type needle covered by a radially expandable sheath is easily introduced into the peritoneal cavity and the abdomen insufflated followed by removal of the needle and insertion of a 5 mm cannula through the expandable sheath (STEP Access System; Autosuture/Tyco Healthcare) (■ Fig. 2.8a,b). The 5 mm umbilical port is typically the largest access device used in infants and smaller children unless stapling or other devices are required. Additional trocars can be placed under direct endoscopic visualization. The expandable sheath cannula system is relatively safe and allows for trocar stability (less slippage in and out), at least in patients with a thicker abdominal wall; however, this system is, at least partially, disposable, and therefore results in increased hospital costs. If reusable or small-diameter trocars are desired, several metal devices are available (2.5–5 mm) (Richard Wolf, Karl Storz Endoscopy). After a small skin incision, these are placed using a sharp-bladed trocar insert to penetrate the abdominal fascia under direct endoscopic visualization or by scalpel incision through the fascia and then sliding the trocar through this fascial defect, again, under direct endoscopic visualization.

Both reusable and disposable trocars can be used in pediatric endosurgery. The reusable trocars are less expensive but typically lack safety shields and require more forceful insertion. Many adult-style reusable trocars are frequently "top heavy" making their use as working ports awkward. Light plastic ports or metal ports with small light heads are much easier to use. Trocar valves should also be carefully considered. Trocars with manual trumpet valves or very stiff valves decrease the working dexterity of pediatric endoscopic surgeons and can diminish task performance. Other than the expandable sheath system mentioned above, most trocars utilize an insertion spike. The spike can have a conical or cutting tip. The cutting tip allows for easier insertion but leaves a larger fascial defect than the conical tip, which requires more force to place but leaves a small fascial defect and fits more tightly in the tissue.

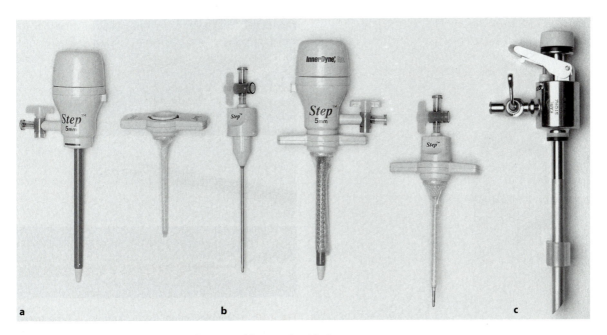

Fig. 2.8. a,b Expandable sheath cannula. **c** Reusable cannula with sleeve

Trocar stability (sliding in or out) can be a particular problem in thin children and infants because of the thickness of the abdominal wall. This problem can be lessened by suturing the cannula to the skin. This can be accomplished by utilizing a 1 cm rubber or silicone catheter segment slid tightly over the metallic reusable trocar to allow placement of a silk suture through the skin and the rubber/silicone ring around the catheter to keep the trocar from sliding (■ Fig. 2.8c). This method also allows for adjustment of the trocar's position during the operative procedure, if needed, by sliding the trocar within the sleeve. Another important consideration when choosing trocar design for endoscopic surgery in infants is the fact that the abdominal surface area for trocar placement and the working space above the abdomen is quite small. Most adult-size trocars, even those that are 5 mm in diameter, have very large "heads" which fill much of the working area above the abdomen and collide during instrument manipulation, limiting hand motion and position. Therefore, care should be taken in choosing trocars and cannulae with small heads, including heads without insufflation ports if necessary, in order to maximize the working space for instruments.

Recent experience with trocarless peritoneal access in pediatric surgery is gaining enthusiasm. In this setting, a trocar is typically passed through the umbilicus for initial access, and then under direct vision a small scalpel or a size 11 blade is used to "stab" through the skin and abdominal wall, allowing the subsequent passage of a working instrument without a trocar. This approach has been commonly utilized for laparoscopic pyloromyotomy where the need for frequent instrument change is rare and the operation is relatively short. However, the trocarless approach is being more widely applied to other common laparoscopic procedures (Ostlie and Holcomb 2003). The suggested advantages of trocarless access include a superior cosmetic result and a significant cost saving related to the elimination of accessory cannulae.

Laparoscopic Retractors

In order to expose the upper abdomen (esophageal hiatus for fundoplication) or deep pelvis (for endorectal pull-through procedures) retracting devices are often helpful and necessary. Retracting techniques may be simple, such as a thick suture on a large needle passed under endoscopic vision through the abdominal wall, around the falciform ligament, and out through the abdominal wall in order to lift the liver up for better exposure of the pylorus during laparoscopic pyloromyotomy. Transabdominal suture retraction is also helpful in lifting and positioning viscera, such as bladder for exposure in the pelvis or the stomach for gastrostomy-tube placement or retrogastric exposure (pancreas).

Retraction and manipulation of solid viscera, such as the liver for esophageal hiatal exposure, can often be accomplished using a locking grasper which can slip under the left lobe of the liver and grasp the anterior rim of the hiatus. This maneuver drapes the left lobe of the liver over the grasper. If the liver is large or fragile, a flexible retractor (3–5 mm in diameter) which can be configured into a triangle or a circle (Diamond-Flex;

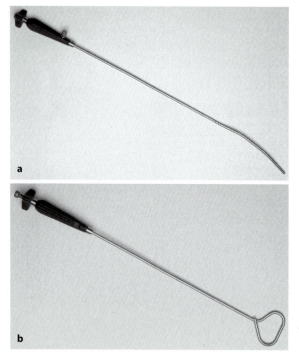

Fig. 2.9 a,b. Flexible retractor

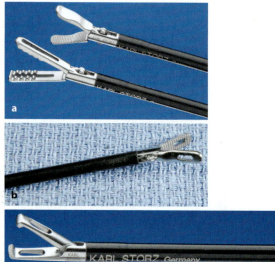

Fig. 2.10. a Double action tissue grasper. **b** Fenestrated duckbill grasper. **c** Single action Allis grasper (Karl Storz Endoscopy)

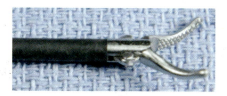

Fig. 2.11. Kelly dissector (Karl Storz Endoscopy)

Snowden Pencer) (■ Fig. 2.9a,b) can be used to elevate the liver and is typically held stationary by means of an external holding device attached to the operating table.

Tissue Graspers and Dissectors

High-quality tissue graspers are necessary for any functional set of pediatric endosurgical instruments. Many complex pediatric endosurgical operations are carried out with the surgeons assisting hand (left hand for a right-handed surgeon) utilizing tissue graspers for most of the operation while the right hand holds dissecting, cutting, and suturing instruments. The most functional atraumatic tissue grasper provides good grasping strength for tissue, such as stomach or bowel, without tearing. Considering currently available pediatric instruments, most tissue graspers that can provide this function are 2–5 mm in diameter and 19–32 cm in length. There are a wide variety of tissue grasper jaw and teeth configurations including double- and single-action hinges, and a number of "teeth" designs that allow for a secure, yet gentle grip of tissue, such as duckbill, "DeBakey-style," or "crocodile" tips. In general, double-action jaws open wider and are easier to manipulate during tissue dissection, but have a groove that can trap suture during knot tying. An appropriately designed grasper should be chosen for a particular task. For instance, the grasper that may work

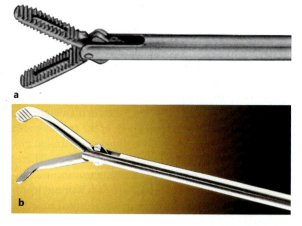

Fig. 2.12. a Straight pyloric spreader. **b** Angled pyloric spreader (Karl Storz Endoscopy)

best to manipulate a thick omentum, may be too vigorous for small bowel manipulation. In addition to standard atraumatic tissue graspers, there are also a variety of specialty tip graspers available in a range of sizes, such as Babcock, Hunter, and Allis-style clamps (■ Fig. 2.10a–c).

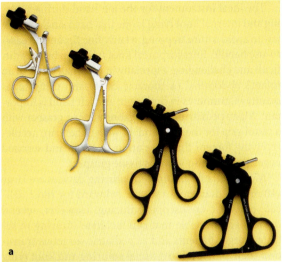

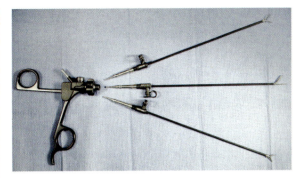

Fig. 2.14. Modular instruments (Karl Storz Endoscopy)

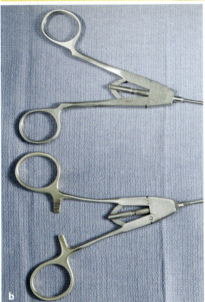

Fig. 2.13. a Pistol grip handles (Karl Storz Endoscopy). b In-line handles

The type of handle design that is deemed most effective depends on the surgeon. The gun or pistol grip type handle has been popular and widely used as this style was prominent in most of the earliest handle designs for laparoscopic instruments (■ Fig. 2.13a). "In-line" style handles are also popular and include a variety of configurations, such as rings that are similar to a traditional "open" needle driver to cylindrical handles with thumb- or finger-controlled release mechanisms (■ Fig. 2.13b).

Regardless of the chosen tip (jaws and teeth) or handle, the most functional graspers have finger-controlled shaft rotation capability, allowing for fine control of the tip orientation and preferable handle location in the external operating space. Graspers (and other instruments in general) with locking mechanisms that require two hands to unlock should be avoided for safely reasons.

Recently, several manufacturers have produced reusable instrument sets that are modular and allow for exchangeable tips and handles (CLICK line from Karl Storz Endoscopy, Micro Line, Stryker Endoscopy). A set of instruments can have many more tips than handles (■ Fig. 2.14). In addition to flexibility, this approach theoretically should also cut costs since it allows for more choices of type of grasping or dissecting tip applied to a specific handle design.

Needle Drivers

The development of small, but strong needle drivers has been critical for the advancement of pediatric endosurgery from extirpative (appendectomy, for example) to reconstructive (fundoplication and intestinal atresia repair, as examples). Although there are several alternative automated suturing devices on the market, suturing and knot-tying skills are critical for successful advanced pediatric endosurgery. Ideally, most pediatric endosurgical instrument sets would contain several needle drivers, including short (19–20 cm) and narrow

In addition to tissue graspers designed for holding tissue, pediatric instrument sets also require delicate tissue dissectors. The curved Maryland or Kelly-style dissector is the most common and versatile dissecting forceps allowing for gentle dissection of small structures such as blood vessels, cystic or common bile duct, pulmonary hilar structures, etc. (■ Fig. 2.11). Other dissecting forceps that can be helpful include blunt or dolphin-nosed tips and Mixter-style right-angled tips. Several companies now produce very acceptable laparoscopic pyloric spreaders for performing laparoscopic pyloromyotomy for hypertrophic pyloric stenosis (■ Fig. 2.12a,b). These grasper/dissectors are 3 mm in diameter and have serrations on both the outer and inner surface of the double-action spreader.

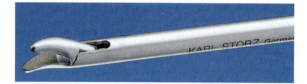

Fig. 2.15. Curved jaw needle driver (Karl Storz Endoscopy)

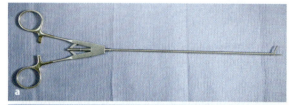

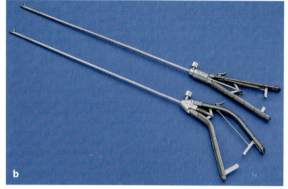

Fig. 2.16. a In-line coaxial needle driver. **b** Angled and straight Castro-Viejo needle driver handles (Karl Storz Endoscopy)

(2.5–3.0 mm) and long (28–32 cm) and wide (5 mm). The preferred shape of the jaws (curved or straight) and handle (pistol or in-line, Castro-Viejo or ring grip) of the needle driver is very surgeon dependent. However, angled jaws are typically superior for internal knot tying (■ Fig. 2.15). The Castro-Viejo-type locking mechanism that is preferred by many instrument companies is typically awkward for internal knot tying. Self-righting needle drivers are preferred by some surgeons; however, these devices eliminate the ability to angle the needle as is needed in complex suture applications. It is important that the driver utilize a single jaw action that securely holds the chosen needle and that the handle mechanism allows for easy ratcheting and unratcheting (■ Fig. 2.15). The in-line ring handle coaxial needle driver (3.5 mm × 24 cm) with an easy locking and unlocking mechanism typical of open needle drivers is an excellent choice for both suturing and intracorporeal knot tying (Jarit Instruments) (■ Fig. 2.16a). There are also 2 mm × 20 cm and 3 mm × 30 cm needle drivers with a Castro-Viejo-type ratcheting mechanism that are popular (Karl Storz Endoscopy) (■ Fig. 2.16b).

The ideal instrument for the left hand during suturing and internal knot tying is one that has a single-action jaw to avoid suture trapping, a fairly fine tip, and an easy-to-use handle. Intracorporeal knot tying can be very difficult and challenging, especially in the small space of an infant's abdominal or thoracic cavity and using high-quality instruments in both right and left hand is important. Many pediatric endosurgeons prefer a grasper with a pistol grip for the left hand; however, there are needle-receiving forceps that have an in-line grip and serrated edges that can also serve as tissue graspers.

Most available automated suturing devices are large (10 mm in diameter) and are awkward for most delicate pediatric endoscopic suturing. However, several devices are available that can facilitate suturing in selected larger patients and as pediatric surgeons transition their skill level to manual suturing and knot tying (Endo Stitch device; Autosuture/Tyco Healthcare).

Knot Pushers and Needles

Knot pushers for external knot tying come in a variety of configurations. Rapid application and reliability are important factors when selecting knot pushers. Ideally the external knot is tied without having to disengage the suture from the knot pusher, and the tip design minimizes suture twisting (■ Fig. 2.17).

Needles for pediatric endosurgical suturing come in three basic configurations: curved, straight, and "ski"-shaped. Straight needles are the easiest to manipulate and pass through small-diameter trocars; however, they do not utilize standard surgical wrist rotation/supination and are typically inadequate for complex suturing. Curved needles are difficult to pass through small trocars though they can be passed directly through the abdominal wall and be grasped internally in most children. Ski (or canoe)-shaped needles are frequently used by endoscopic pediatric surgeons because they can pass through small trocars, be easily grasped and aligned using the straight part of the needle behind the curved tip, and allow for rotational suturing (■ Fig. 2.18a,b). Most ski-shaped needles (19 mm long) on the market can pass through a 4 mm-diameter trocar. However, because of their length these needles are sometimes difficult to maneuver in the small space of a neonatal abdomen. Therefore, a shorter (13- to 15 mm-long) regular curved tapered needle can be "unbent" (using two open needle drivers) into a ski- or canoe-shaped needle. To pass the needle through the trocar, the left-hand grasper (for a right-handed surgeon) should hold the sweged on suture several millimeters behind the needle. Once the needle is through the trocar the right-handed needle driver can often grasp the needle in the desired location and begin suturing without "fumbling" and chasing the needle around in the abdomen.

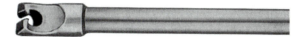

Fig. 2.17. Knot pusher (Karl Storz Endoscopy)

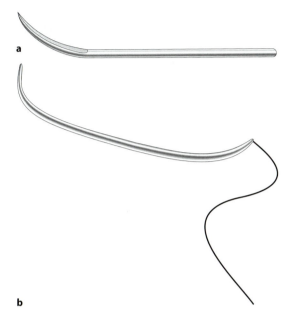

Fig. 2.18. **a** Ski needle. **b** Canoe needle

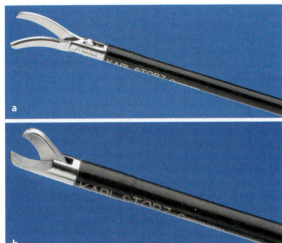

Fig. 2.19. **a** Metzenbaum scissors. **b** Hook scissors (Karl Storz Endoscopy)

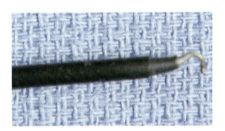

Fig. 2.20. J-hook (Karl Storz Endoscopy)

Cutting, Coagulation, and Sealing Devices

As in open pediatric surgery, delicate, sharp endoscopic scissors are important in pediatric endosurgery. Curved Metzenbaum tips are commonly used for tissue cutting, dissecting, and electrocautery in many common pediatric laparoscopic procedures. Several brands of endoscopic scissors have both monopolar and bipolar electrocautery capability. When using the scissors with monopolar current it is usually best to close the scissors and use the tip as a "cautery wand." Activating cautery while cutting tissue dulls the cutting surfaces of the scissors. Several companies now manufacture component instruments such that the scissor insert can be exchanged as the scissor dulls, while preserving the insulation sheath and instrument handle (Fig. 2.19a). In addition to Metzenbaum scissors, pediatric endosurgical sets should contain less delicate type scissors, such as Mayo or hook-type tips that allow for cutting suture and dense tissue as well as fine-tipped microscissors for very fine tissue division (Fig. 2.19b).

Insulated J hook or L-shaped electrocautery probes are very versatile instruments (Fig. 2.20). They come in a variety of sizes ranging from 2 to 5 mm and can be effectively used in tissue dissection, vessel coagulation, and tissue division. Even moderately large vessels can be controlled and divided by turning the hook in line with the vessel and applying cauterizing current (typically via a foot pedal) along a segment of vessel and then turning the hook at right angle to the vessel and pulling through the tissue. Clear visualization is very important during electrocautery in order to avoid inadvertent collateral injury. Electrocautery applied through insulated fine-tipped graspers or dissectors, such a Maryland-type instrument, is also a helpful sealing technique for blood vessels, or actively bleeding tissue or vessels. In addition, electrocautery bipolar forceps for fine coagulation are occasionally helpful.

Ultrasonic scalpels and scissors are now readily available to pediatric surgeons. Several companies now produce a 5- to 5.5 mm instrument that can control and divide fairly large blood vessels (SonoSurg Ultrasonic Cutting and Coagulation System, Olympus and the Harmonic Scalpel, Ethicon Endo-Surgery) (Fig. 2.21). This technology converts ultrasonic vibrations into energy that enables rapid coagulation and cutting at a low temperature and without an elec-

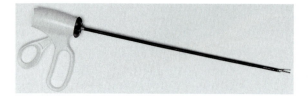

Fig. 2.21. Ultrasonic device

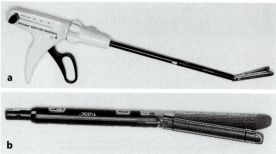

Fig. 2.22. a Endolinear stapling device. **b** Stapling cartridge

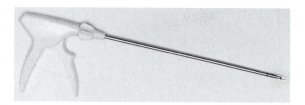

Fig. 2.23. Clipping device

trical current passing through the body. The 5 mm instrument tip is relatively large, however, when performing endosurgical procedures on infants and small children. The LigaSure Vessel Sealing System (Valleylab, Tyco Healthcare) is another helpful innovative technology that permanently seals tissue bundles and vessels up to 7 mm in diameter by fusing collagen and elastin. The most recent version of this device is 5 mm in diameter, uses a fine Maryland-type tip that is helpful for tissue dissection, and provides a cutting mechanism as well as sealing. Another recent technology for tissue sealing uses focused heat and pressure, or "thermal welding" (Thermal Ligating Shears, Starion Instruments).

In addition to endoscopic instruments for controlling bleeding from tissue or vessels, several sealant products are also now available for endoscopic application. Fibrin-based sealant kits such as Tisseel VH (Baxter) can provide physiologic hemostasis by combining fibrinogen and thrombin at the tissue surface.

The next generation of anastomosis technology, including new energy sources that will allow for tissue welding for vascular and intestinal anastomoses and other tissue cooptation techniques, are currently being developed (Coalescent Surgical's U-CLIP Anastomotic Device, Medtronic). These specialized instruments could revolutionize many pediatric endosurgical procedures allowing for more practical, safe, and expedient tissue reconstruction.

Staples and Clips

Stapling devices that allow for tissue resection and intestinal anastomoses are very useful in many pediatric endosurgical procedures (■ Fig. 2.22a,b). Endoscopic stapling devices are available for tissue approximation alone and approximation and division from several manufacturers (Endo GIA, Autosuture, United States Surgical and Endopath Endoscopic Staplers and Cutters, Ethicon Endo-Surgery). Most devices use titanium staples placed in two triple rows of staggered staples and contain an internal knife that divides the tissue between the rows. Staplers are available in several configurations for specific types of tissue or thickness. The staples come in different sizes/depth (2, 2.5, and 3.5 mm) and variable staple cartridge lengths (30, 45, and 50 mm). The most flexible devices allow rotation along the shaft, articulation (20–45°) of the stapling cartridge on the shaft, and reloading of cartridges on the single shaft and handle. Unfortunately, the stapling devices available are still quite large (12–15 mm diameter) and are difficult to utilize in small children and infants. The temptation to use electrocautery along a staple line that is bleeding should be resisted. Cauterization can cause retraction of tissue through the staples and worsening of bleeding or intestinal or pulmonary leak.

Several multiload clip application devices, reusable and disposable, are also available (Endoclip, Autosuture, United States Surgical and LigaClip, Ethicon Endo-Surgery) (■ Fig. 2.23). These devices have been downsized to 5 mm and are, therefore, now helpful in some pediatric endosurgical procedures although the energy source devices mentioned in this chapter that control fairly large vessels have largely replaced the use of titanium clips. More recently absorbable endoscopic clips have been introduced and are reported to be safe for applications such as cystic duct ligation in cholecystectomy (Bencini et al. 2003; Yano et al. 2003). The device (Biomedicon) is a reusable 8 mm clip applier that deploys bioabsorbable polyglyconate and polyglycolic acid polymer clips that absorb within 6 months.

Other Instruments

The following is a list of other endosurgical instruments that are commonly helpful in pediatric endosurgical procedures and are available through several vendors:

- *Endoretrieval bags* allow for the protected removal of tissue such as the appendix, gall bladder, spleen, bowel resection specimens, and tumors. These instruments are typically 10–15 mm in diameter and, therefore, quite large for smaller children and infants (■ Fig. 2.24).

- *Endoscopic loop ties* for tissue ligation are cost effective and multifunctional devices used for tissue ligation and retraction. They are small-diameter rod-type devices that hold a loop of suture on the distal tip which can be place over/around tissue to be ligated or manipulated (■ Fig. 2.25). The loop is tightened by snapping or breaking the plastic rod externally and pulling to tighten the loop around the tissue. Several manufacturers make loop ligating devices utilizing varied suture materials including chromic, gut, and polyglycolic acid as well as some non-absorbable suture materials.

- *Endoscopic biopsy forceps, scalpels, probes, and needles* are occasionally very helpful during the course of pediatric endosurgical procedures. Biopsy forceps are available in a variety of sizes and designs and are useful for solid tumor biopsy. A particularly important instrument for laparoscopic pyloromyotomy is a retractable arthroscopic scalpel. Simple probe devices are often helpful to "palpate" tissue as well as to measure the true size of objects and tissue (such as the length of a fundoplication) that are otherwise magnified. A variety of endoscopic needle devices are available for aspirating cysts or injecting saline or dye.

- *Endoscopic suction–irrigation devices* (3–5 mm in diameter) allow for washing and aspirating the peritoneal and thoracic cavity and are very useful instruments for several common pediatric endosurgical conditions, including ruptured appendicitis and empyema. These devices are available in a variety of configurations including a finger-controlled "trumpet valve" mechanism that regulates suction and irrigation flow.

- *Endoscopic balloon dissection devices* are used commonly in adult endoscopic hernia repair, to create an extra peritoneal space in which to operate; however, they can have a role in pediatric retroperitoneal procedures to establish exposure of structures such as the kidney.

- *Endoscopic tacking or anchor fixation devices.*

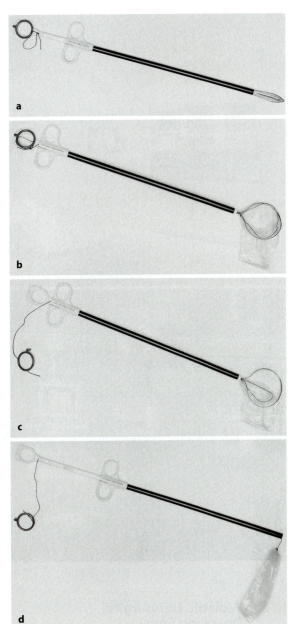

Fig. 2.24 a–d. Removal bag

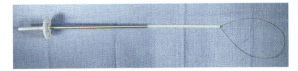

Fig. 2.25. Preformed loops

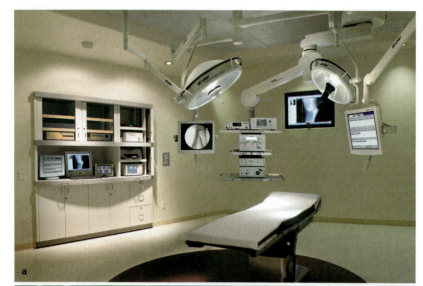

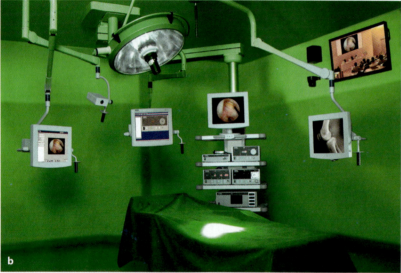

Fig. 2.26. a EndoSuite (Stryker Endoscopy). b OR1 (Karl Storz Endoscopy)

Pediatric Endosurgical Operating Suites

As more technology has been brought into the operating room, the need for changes in operating room design has emerged. Many hospitals are now constructing operating rooms specifically designed to facilitate video-assisted endosurgery as well as other advanced technology surgical applications (■ Fig. 2.26a,b). These "endosuites" are designed to accommodate the latest surgical technology and improve overall operating room efficiency and safety. This new operating environment requires integration of old and new surgical technology with digital, information technology. The old cart-based equipment paradigm restricts the ergonomic configuration of the operating room for surgeon, nurse, anesthesia team, and patient. This model creates potential mechanical, electrical, and biological hazards to the patient and operating room staff. The endosurgery suite is designed to decrease clutter, ease personnel movement, improve ergonomics, maintain the sterile field, and facilitate the use of advanced imaging, communication, and display devices. Using touch panels or voice control technology, surgeons can now control much of their operating environment including the operating table, room and surgical lighting, camera, insufflator, light source, and image capturing.

For pediatric endosurgeons, the newest endosurgical suites can be designed to meet the specific diverse needs of neonatal to adolescent bariatric surgery. The benefit of having high-resolution, thin, LCD monitors that can be mounted on a boom that allows exact positioning for optimal visualization and ergonomics is keenly appreciated during an operation such as a colectomy and endorectal pull-though for Hirschsprung's disease or ulcerative colitis during which the surgeon must move to different positions around the operating table. The ability to route images from the hospital data base up onto one of three or four monitors positioned around the patient allows for easy visual comparison between preoperative radiographic images and operative findings, such as with pulmonary biopsy for metastatic malignant disease. With surgeon voice control of equipment, it is easy to make fine-tuned adjustments of light brightness, insufflator pressure and flow, and camera settings and to record still and video images without having to ask, wait for, and instruct a circulating nurse in making the adjustments or hitting the "capture image" button.

However, problems do exist with current endosurgical suite technology. They are expensive and there are frequent technology glitches that must be endured and solved. Just as with computing technology in general, surgical technology is evolving rapidly, and the "OR of the Future" that a hospital decides to build today can be obsolete by the time it is built. In the future, it is probable that specialized endosurgical suites will integrate imaging and visualization modalities that are now considered components of flexible endoscopy, interventional radiology, or interventional cardiovascular suites.

Robotics

The application of robotics in adult endosurgery has received an enormous amount of attention since 1995 (mitral valve repair, radical prostatectomy, gastric bypass). The potential role of robotics in pediatric endosurgery in now under significant investigation; however, to date a clear added benefit of robotics for common pediatric endosurgical procedures has not been established. As robotic technology evolves, it should be expected that there will be robotic applications that facilitate some of the most delicate and challenging pediatric endosurgical procedures.

The first robot that found some acceptance in both adult and pediatric endosurgery was the voice controlled AESOP, developed by Computer Motion in Santa Barbara, California. This robotic arm attaches to the side of the operating table and replaces the camera/telescope holder. The surgeon is able to control the movements of the telescope in the operative field using voice control technology and thus perform many operations without the need of an assistant. In addition, the robotic control of the surgical video image provides improved stability of the image and avoids "motion sickness" in the operative team.

Computer Motion went on to develop the more comprehensive multiple arm Zeus robotic system, while Intuitive Surgical developed the da Vinci surgical system. Both systems provide extraordinary sensitivity, technical accuracy, and visualization. The surgeon is seated at a console, which can be in or outside the operating theater, providing three-dimensional electronic interface and controls the robotic arms which can, depending on the instrumentation, transfer wrist movements from the surgeon to the tips of the robotic instruments. When initially assessed by pediatric surgeons, both systems had promising features. The Zeus system was more flexible in terms of instrumentation, size, footprint, and voice control, while the da Vinci system provided a very instinctive surgeon–robot interface and a better three-dimensional visualization system. However, both systems have had significant deficiencies for widespread application in pediatric endosurgery, including the size and bulk of the footprint, cost, lack of haptic feedback, instrument and telescope size, and the need for additional degrees of instrument wrist freedom. When Intuitive Surgical and Computer Motion merged as Intuitive Surgical in 2003, the development of the Zeus platform was largely abandoned. The da Vinci robotic platform has continued to evolve and the number of da Vinci-assisted operations on adults are growing. Several robotically assisted successful pediatric endosurgical procedures have been performed in infants and children, including fundoplication (Heller et al. 2002; Knight et al. 2004), hepatobiliary procedures (Mariano et al. 2004), and pediatric urologic procedures (Peters 2004). At the present date (2005), the wider pediatric endosurgery community awaits continued evolution of robotic technology including downsizing of the platform, instruments, and telescope and further development of instrument tips and enhancement of the instrument wrist mechanism.

References

Bencini L, Boffi B, Farsi M, et al (2003) Laparoscopic cholecystectomy: retrospective comparative evaluation of titanium versus absorbable clips. J Laparoendosc Adv Surg Tech A 13:93–98

Bozzinni P (1806) Lichtleiter, eine Erfindung Zur Anschauung innerer Teile und Krankheiten. J Prak Heilk 24:107

Farley DR, Greenlee SM, Larson DR, et al (2004) Double-blind, prospective, randomized study of warmed, humidified carbon dioxide insufflation vs standard carbon dioxide for patients undergoing laparoscopic cholecystectomy. Arch Surg 139:739–743; discussion 743–744

Fourestier N, Gladu A, Vulmiere J (1952) Perfectionnements a l'endoscopie medical: realization bronchoscopique. Presse Med 60:1292

Goetze O (1921) Die neues Verfabren der Gasfullung fur das Pneumoperitoneum. Munchen Med Wochenschr 51:233

Hasson HM (1978) Open laparoscopy vs. closed laparoscopy: a comparison of complication rates. Adv Plan Parent 13:41–50

Heller K, Gutt C, Schaeff B, et al (2002) Use of the robot system da Vinci for laparoscopic repair of gastro-oesophageal reflux in children. Eur J Pediatr Surg 12:239–342

Hirschowitz BI (1961) Endoscopic examination of the stomach and duodenal cap with the fiberscope. Lancet 1:1074–1078

Hopkins H, Kapany NS (1954) A flexible fiberscope using static scanning. Nature 173:39–41

Jacobaeus HC (1910) Ueber die Moglichkeit die Zystoskopie bei Untersuchung Seroser Hohlungen Anzuwenden. Munchen Med Wochenschr 57:2090–2092

Kalk H (1929) Erfafungen mit der Laparoskopie. Z Klin Med 111:303–348

Knight CG, Lorincz A, Gidell KM et al (2004) Computer-assisted robot-enhanced laparoscopic fundoplication in children. J Pediatr Surg 39:864–856; discussion 864–866

Korbsch R (1921) Die Laparoskopie nach Jakobaeus. Berl Klin Wochenschr 38:696

Mariano ER, Furukawa L, Woo RK, et al (2004) Anesthetic concerns for robot-assisted laparoscopy in an infant. Anesth Analg 99:1665–1667

Modlin IM, Kidd M, Lye KD (2004) From the lumen to the laparoscope. Arch Surg 139:1110–1126

Nguyen NT, Furdui G, Fleming NW, et al (2002) Effect of heated and humidified carbon dioxide gas on core temperature and postoperative pain: a randomized trial. Surg Endosc 16:1050–1054

Orndoff BH (1920) The peritoneoscope in diagnosis of diseases of the abdomen. J Radiol 1:307

Ostlie DJ, Holcomb GW III (2003) The use of stab incisions for instrument access in laparoscopic operations. J Pediatr Surg 38:1837–1840

Ott D (1901) Illumination of the abdomen (ventroscopy). J Akush Zhensk Boliez 15:1045–1049

Peters CA (2004) Robotically assisted surgery in pediatric urology. Urol Clin North Am 31:743–752

Reuter MA, Reuter HJ, Engel RM (1999) History of Endoscopy. Karl Storz, Tuttlingen

Ruddock JC (1934) Peritoneoscopy. West J Surg 42:392

Ruddock JC (1957) Peritoneoscopy: a critical clinical review. Surg Clin North Am 37:1249–1260

Semm K (1983) Endoscopic appendectomy. Endoscopy 15:59–64

Veress J (1938) Neues Instrument zur Ausfuhrung von Brust-oder Bauchpunktionen und Pneumothoraxbehandlung. Dtsch Med Wochenshr 41:1480–1481

Yano H, Okada K, Kinuta M, et al (2003) Efficacy of absorbable clips compared with metal clips for cystic duct ligation in laparoscopic cholecystectomy. Surg Today 33:18–23

Chapter 3

Robotics

Colin G. Knight, Michael D. Klein, and Scott E. Langenburg

Introduction

With the advent of laparoscopic surgery, surgeons have lost what had been within their reach for centuries: direct visualization of the area upon which they work and direct tactile feedback from the tissues. Additionally, laparoscopic surgeons have surrendered a fair amount of dexterity in order to accomplish operations laparoscopically. With their hands distant from the operative site, they must use long, inflexible instruments to operate. Surgical robotics attempts to regain these lost senses and skills in order to enhance laparoscopic surgery. Although the term "robot" implies a degree of autonomy, the systems commercially available actually function as tools for telepresence surgery and do not move autonomously. Telepresence surgery is surgery done with a collection of instruments that function to place the surgeon where he or she is not present. Surgeons may be across the room or across the world, but they will feel like, and operate as if, they were standing at the operating room table. Today's surgical robots are a collection of tools that allow telepresence surgery and offer some degree of dexterity enhancement to overcome some of the hurdles of laparoscopic surgery. The technology is still in its infancy, but surgeons will expand the role of surgical robots in the operating room and laboratory, and engineers will continue to enhance them.

History

The term robot, first used in 1924 by Karl Capek in his play, *Rossum's Universal Robots*, comes from the Czech word *robota*, meaning forced labor. Although robots and robotics began in the realm of fiction, they have become commonplace in modern factories and industrial operations. It was not, however, until the late 1980s that researchers began to work on applying robotic technology to surgery.

In the early 1990s, the NASA-Ames Research Center, SRI International, and the US Army began collaborating on a telepresence system that would go on to be developed into Intuitive Surgical's (www.intuitivesurgical.com) da Vinci system. At the same time, a group from the IBM T.J. Watson Research Center started to develop the RoboDoc system, which is used for boring out the femoral shaft for hip replacement surgery. Also during that period, Computer Motion (www.computermotion.com) was founded and began to develop a robotic endoscope holder, the AESOP (Automatic Endoscopic System for Optimal Positioning) device (Fig. 3.1). They received US Food and Drug Administration (FDA) approval for the device in 1994, the first FDA-approved surgical robotic device (Satava 2002).

On 3 March 1997 in Dendermonde, Belgium, surgeons used Mona, a predecessor of the da Vinci system, to perform a cholecystectomy, the world's first robotic surgery on a human (Himpens et al. 1998). In 2001, a group made headlines by using the Zeus system to perform a laparoscopic cholecystectomy on a patient in France, while the operating surgeon sat at the master console in New York (Marescaux et al. 2001). From these milestones, robotic surgery has grown into a field that has spread around the globe to all surgical specialties. Surgical robotic systems are no longer experimental; they are available commercially and have been employed clinically. Their safety and efficacy have been established and their role in the operating room will expand as their use increases.

Available Systems

The two commercially available robotic surgery systems share a similar design. The surgeon sits across the room from the patient at a master console, while slave instruments at the patient's bedside carry out the operation by mirroring the surgeon's movements. Both systems have instruments with a wrist-like articulation at the distal end, allowing additional freedom of movement over standard laparoscopic instruments (Fig. 3.2). Both offer motion scaling, where gross movements of the surgeon are translated into smaller movements at the effector instrument. This scaling can be adjusted to the surgeon's preference based on the nature of the operation. Both systems also offer tremor filtration. The long-handled instruments used for minimally invasive surgery act as levers magnifying the natural tremor found in all surgeons. Because these systems digitize the surgeon's movements, this tremor

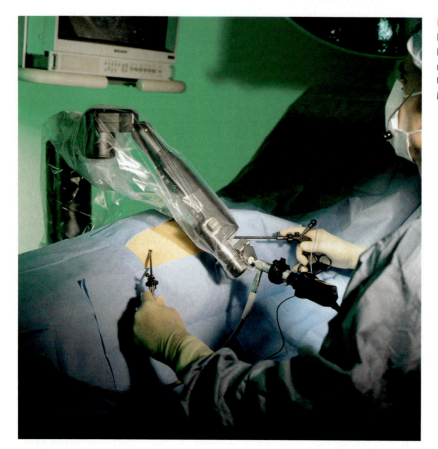

Fig. 3.1. AESOP (Automatic Endoscopic System for Optimal Positioning) was the first surgical robot approved for use in the USA. Courtesy of Computer Motion

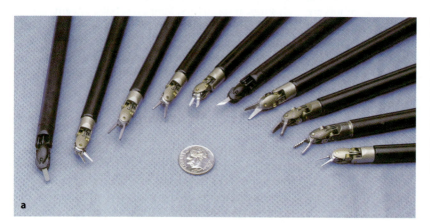

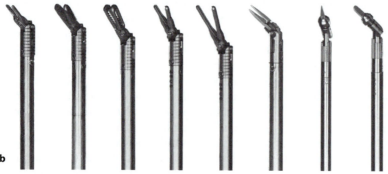

Fig. 3.2. Intuitive Surgical's da Vinci system instruments (a) are 8 mm in diameter and Computer Motion's Zeus system instruments (b) are 5 mm in diameter. Note the wrist found on the distal portion of the instruments from both systems and that the two photographs are not to the same scale. Courtesy of Computer Motion and Intuitive Surgical

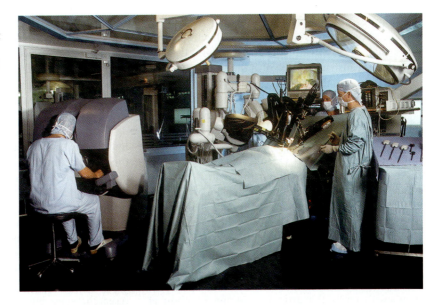

Fig. 3.3. The da Vinci system at work. The surgeon sits on the left at the master console while the slave instruments are suspended from the cart at the operative table. Courtesy of Intuitive Surgical

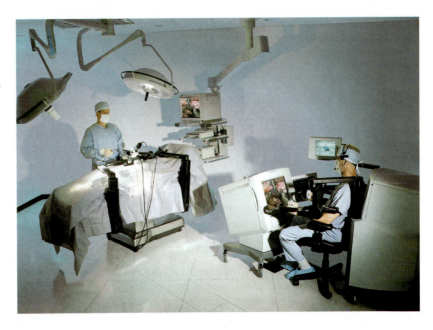

Fig. 3.4. The Zeus system with the surgeon at the master console on the right and the slave instruments mounted directly on the rails of the operative table. Courtesy of Computer Motion

can be eliminated and allows the tips of the surgical instruments to move precisely and without visible tremor, even at high magnification. At times during laparoscopic procedures, surgeons can find their hands and arms in uncomfortable and unnatural positions. Both systems allow surgeons to freeze the instruments by releasing a clutch. At that point, the surgeon can adopt a more comfortable position and then reengage the instruments. This process is called indexed movement. Both systems were designed to place the video screen in a position where it is in line with the surgeon's arms thus enhancing the feeling that the instruments' movements in the patient's body are the surgeon's own

movements. Finally, both feature a video interface that provides a three-dimensional (3D) view for the surgeon.

The da Vinci system (■ Fig. 3.3) is made by Intuitive Surgical. An immersive system, the surgeon sits face down in the master console where a separate video display for each eye provides a 3D view of the operation. The effector arms are mounted on a cart that rolls to the patient's bedside for the operation. Because the instruments are cart-mounted, the instruments must be disengaged before adjusting the operating room table. There are two instrument-holding arms that require 10 mm ports and an endoscope-holding arm that requires a 12 mm port. The operative instruments provide seven degrees of freedom by having a wrist that articulates in two directions. The system's design is such that the instruments pivot at the trocar site, eliminating the use of the patient's abdominal or chest wall as a fulcrum.

The Zeus system (■ Fig. 3.4), made by Computer Motion, is more open than the da Vinci system. Although the master console is also across the room from the patient, the surgeon's video display is open to the room. The Zeus system is compatible with a variety of visualization options, both two-dimensional (2D) and 3D. The effector arms of the Zeus system are independently mounted on the side rails of the table yielding flexibility in arm position. Since the arms are mounted directly on the operative table, there is no need to disengage the instruments when adjusting the operating room table. The Zeus system can use 5 mm instruments with a wrist that articulates in one direction, allowing six degrees of freedom, or it can use 3.5 mm instruments that do not have a wrist. Unlike the da Vinci system, the distal joints on the robotic arm are passive. Thus the Zeus system requires a fulcrum (usually the trocar site) for proper operation.

Robotic Endoscope Holders

The purpose of a robotic endoscope holder is to free the surgeon, or surgical assistant, from holding the endoscope. Since these holders do not fatigue or tremor, they can provide a much steadier field of view than with a human holding the endoscope. Also, they give the operating surgeon direct control over the endoscope, eliminating the potential for miscommunication between the surgeon and the assistant who is holding the endoscope.

Two of the robotic endoscope holders on the market are AESOP and EndoAssist. AESOP, made by Computer Motion, uses a voice-control interface to command movement of the surgical endoscope, enabling the surgeon to control the view of the operation while working with both hands on surgical instruments. The device clamps to the side rail of the operating room table and uses a magnetic coupler to attach to a collar that holds the endoscope. The EndoAssist, made by Armstrong Healthcare (www.armstrong-healthcare.com), is a floor-standing cart with an autoclavable camera-holding arm. An infrared sensor in a headband worn by the surgeon allows the robot to follow the surgeon's head movements. One group has compared the two systems by measuring response time and movement accuracy in a variety of *ex vivo* movement tasks, and found that the AESOP responds more quickly and accurately (Yavuz et al. 2000).

Application of Robots in Pediatric Surgery

The additional dexterity built into robotic surgery systems, the extra precision allowed through motion scaling and tremor filtration, and the superior ergonomics provided by the master consoles of the Zeus and da Vinci platforms make surgical robotics attractive to many pediatric surgeons. As the reader can see from the other chapters in this book, there are few, if any, procedures out of the reach of an experienced pediatric laparoscopist. Many of these advanced procedures, however, are beyond the skill of today's mainstream pediatric surgeon. The enhancements of robotic surgery may make it possible for a greater number of these surgeons to attempt advanced laparoscopic procedures in children and infants. Several pioneers have begun to use surgical robots for surgery in these patients and researchers are pursuing new applications in animal laboratories.

The initial use of surgical robots has been to duplicate procedures that are widely performed laparoscopically. Both the Zeus and the da Vinci systems have been used to perform laparoscopic cholecystectomies and laparoscopic fundoplications in children. Procedures like this have served to demonstrate the safety and efficacy of the robotic systems. Although no one has demonstrated a clinical benefit of using the robotic systems for these cases, many times the surgeons feel more comfortable using the robot for the case, and feel that they have better control of the surgical instruments. The first report of robotic surgery in infants was recently presented as a series of six patients who underwent a robot-assisted pyloromyotomy. When these patients were compared with historic controls, the robotic cases took significantly longer (94 versus 137 min of anesthesia time), but the clinical outcomes were the same (Hollands et al. 2003).

One team, using an early, un-wristed version of Zeus, has performed enteroenterostomy, hepaticojejunostomy, esophagoesophagostomy, and portoenterostomy in a non-survival animal model using 6- to 8-kg piglets. Importantly, they also performed all of these procedures using standard laparoscopic techniques, as a way of comparison. There was no difference between the two techniques in the enteroenterostomy group, when looking at surgical time, anastomotic size, and leak rate. In the hepaticojejunostomy group, there also was no difference in operative times; however, there were fewer complications in the robotic cases. In the portoenterostomies, the robotic cases took significantly longer than the laparoscopic cases, but the complication rates were similar for both techniques. For the esophagoesophagostomies, the times for the two techniques were statistically similar and there were no complications in the robotic group and one in the laparoscopic group (Hollands and Dixey 2002). These experiments illustrate that the extra precision provided by surgical robots can lead to fewer complications in complex cases. All of these procedures have great potential for application in pediatric surgery.

At our institution, we have performed a series of portoenterostomies using Zeus in infant-sized piglets (2.5–8 kg) as a survival model. Of the eight cases we performed, five survived for 1 month while gaining weight appropriately without becoming jaundiced. The other three animals had to be killed before a month was out. The first became septic and was found to have a biloma. The second developed peritonitis and was found to have an anastomotic leak. The third developed an incomplete bowel obstruction from a stricture at the enteroenterostomy. We have also performed a series of esophagoesophagostomies in infant-sized piglets (2.0–3.3 kg) using Zeus, again allowing the animals to survive for 1 month. Five of seven survived for the duration. One died during an esophageal dilatation and another had to be euthanized for enteritis of unknown origin. We found that the tremor-free motion and small, articulated instruments allowed us to effectively perform these complex procedures in a small working volume. For example, the operative space for the esophagoesophagostomies was as small as $2 \times 2 \times 2$ cm. Cases like these demonstrate one of the advantages of the smaller Zeus instruments.

One group has looked at patent ductus arteriosus ligation with da Vinci (Le Bret et al. 2002) and another has performed lung resections in pigs with Zeus (Weigel et al. 2003). These excursions into robotic cardiothoracic surgery raise the possibility of performing robotic surgery for conditions such as pulmonary sequestration in infants and children. There has been a case report of repair of a traumatic diaphragmatic injury in an adult patient using da Vinci (Kaul et al. 2003). Our group has performed two Morgagni hernia repairs in children using Zeus. We found that the extra dexterity provided by the robotic instruments made it relatively simple to perform the numerous suture placements required to close the hernia defect without a patch. These children ate dinner the evening after surgery, and went home the next day. Without the robotic system at our institution, these defects would have required a laparotomy to close.

The problem of ureteropelvic junction obstruction in infants and children is often corrected with an operation performed retroperitoneally through a flank incision or transabdominally through a laparotomy incision. One group has performed nine pyeloplasties in adults using da Vinci (Gettman et al. 2002). Our group has begun using Zeus for proximal ureteroureterostomiesnnn in piglets as a model for pyeloplasty in children. In non-survival piglets, we have performed several of these procedures though both a transabdominal

and retroperitoneal approach. Despite the small size of the piglets' ureters, often less than 3 mm in diameter, we have found our anastomoses to be patent on postmortem examination. We anticipate that after demonstrating the procedure in a survival model, we will begin applying it in humans at our institution in 2006nnn.

Several institutions are performing fetoscopic surgery (FETENDO), but these procedures are limited in complexity by the limited dexterity of laparoscopic instruments. For example, in utero myelomeningocele repair is now routinely performed through a uterine incision. Early attempts at FETENDO myelomeningocele repair were limited to placing a patch over the defect rather than performing a surgical repair (Bruner et al. 1999). One group has used da Vinci in an ovine model to explore the application of surgical robotics to a more complex in utero myelomeningocele repair (Aaronson et al. 2002). At our institution, we have performed 25 operations on fetal sheep using Zeus. Six cases were in a survival model and five of the six fetuses survived until necropsy at 2 weeks. Although these studies are only the beginning of applying robotics to FETENDO, the potential to increase the number of cases possible by FETENDO is large. For example, non-lethal conditions such as gastroschisis and cleft lip might be repaired in utero using robot-assisted FETENDO.

Many pediatric surgeons operate with magnifying loupes for open cases, and many pediatric subspecialists, such as neurosurgeons, use operative microscopes for their open cases. Surgeons using such magnification find their natural tremor is magnified. The tremor filtration and motion scaling of robotic surgery may have a role in these open cases performed under magnification. Researchers have used three different systems for open microsurgery in animal models.

One group used a specially designed robotic system, a precursor to the da Vinci system (Li et al. 2000). This system had force feedback, a 3D display, microsurgical forceps, but only four degrees of freedom. Overall, microsurgery with this system took about three times as long to complete when compared with standard microsurgery techniques. Other groups have worked with another experimental system: the Robot Assisted MicroSurgery (RAMS) workstation. RAMS has a single arm, controlled with a joystick, with six degrees of freedom. One of these groups (Le Roux et al. 2001) that tested this system for microvascular surgery in rats found that although technically similar to standard techniques, the system doubled the length of time of the procedures. Our group has adapted Zeus for open microsurgery (Knight et al. 2003). We compared anastomoses of 1 mm-diameter rat femoral arteries, performing 30 by hand and 30 with Zeus. There was no difference in patency or leak rates between the two techniques but anastomotic time was 1.4 times longer with Zeus. The surgeon found the tremor filtration remarkable and felt that he had more precision with placing sutures when using Zeus. We attribute the difference in anastomotic time to the size difference between the tips of the Zeus microneedle driver (1 mm) and the tips of the jeweler's forceps (0.3 mm) routinely used.

The Future

Our operative carts and Mayo stands are covered with instruments that bear the name of the surgeon who invented them. With the increase in complexity of surgical instruments, which is at its most extreme in surgical robotics, gone are the days where the surgeon alone can invent these instruments. Now, biomedical engineers and surgeons must collaborate to enhance these devices. For example, at our institution we have established a formal collaboration with an engineering team at our sister university and we have an engineer employed directly by our research team for the purpose of enhancing this liaison. As we indicated earlier, robotic surgery technology, although being used clinically, is still in development.

One of the key areas for development is the addition of haptics, or force feedback to the systems. Currently, surgeons must rely on visual cues to know how much tension and pressure they are applying to tissues, needles, and suture when operating with the surgical robot. For example, advanced video games and flight simulators provide resistance in the steering wheel, yolk, or joystick that is appropriate for the amount of resistance a driver or pilot would experience while driving a car or flying an airplane. This feedback enhances the realism of these games or training modalities, and would certainly enhance the feeling of "being there" in robotic surgery. Whether the addition of haptics to robotic surgery systems would result in any clinical advantage remains to be seen.

Since entire operations are now being performed though a computer interface, surgeons' movements can be digitized. This digitization has two possible applications. One is that master surgeons can perform operations and have their movements recorded. This recording could then be used as a comparison for evaluating surgical residents or recent graduates or as a basis for training. Also, this digitization could serve as the beginning for automating some tasks of surgery that are repetitive and require minimal judgment, such as knot-tying.

Engineers will continue to work on shrinking the robotic instruments. For example, as our team has applied Zeus to open microvascular surgery, we have found that the 1 mm tips of the most delicate needle holder available for Zeus to be cumbersome. So, we are working directly with Computer Motion to shrink the size of the instrument. There is also room for further miniaturization of the endoscopes. For example, the endoscope that ships with the da Vinci system provides a remarkably clear 3D view, but requires a 12 mm port which is clearly too large for surgery in many pediatric cases. In our laboratory, we have had an opportunity to try a prototype endoscope that used two 2 mm lenses encased in a 5 mm endoscope that provided an equally impressive 3D view in a package less than one half the diameter of the endoscope from the da Vinci system. The end result of increased miniaturization may be that microscopic robots will swarm through the body of a patient, much like the operation imagined by Isaac Asimov in *Fantastic Voyage*.

Conclusion

Surgical robotics is an exciting new field. The enhancements in robotic surgery systems of additional degrees of freedom, tremor-free surgery, improved ergonomics, better visualization, indexed motion, and motion scaling hold great promise for increasing the breadth of operations offered to patients laparoscopically. We anticipate that, as the number of complex laparoscopic cases performed with robotic enhancement grows, there will be a measurable improvement in patient outcomes. Additionally, as the biomedical engineers and surgeons continue to collaborate to enhance the current robotic surgery technology, and to invent new ones, we expect this field to grow.

References

Aaronson OS, Tulipan NB, Cywes C et al. (2002) Robot-assisted endoscopic intrauterine myelomeningocele repair: a feasibility study. Pediatr Neurosurg 36:85–89

Bruner JP, Richards WO, Tulipan NB et al. (1999) Endoscopic coverage of fetal myelomeningocele *in utero*. Am J Obstet Gynecol 180:153–158

Gettman MT, Neururer R, Bartsch G et al. (2002) Anderson-Hynes dismembered pyeloplasty performed using the da Vinci robotic system. Urology 60:509–513

Himpens J, Leman G, Cadiere GB (1998) Telesurgical laparoscopic cholecystectomy. Surg Endosc 12:1091

Hollands CM, Dixey LN (2002) Applications of robotic surgery in pediatric patients. Surg Laparosc Endosc Percutan Tech 12:71–76

Hollands C, Johnson A, Jefferson E et al. (2003) Robotic-assisted pyloromyotomy. [abstract] Pediatr Endosurg & Innov Tech 7:98

Kaul A, Bilaniuk J, Sullivan T, et al (2003) Use of da Vinci robot in repair of a diaphragmatic injury [abstract]. Surg Endosc 17: S290

Knight CG, Cao A, Lorincz A et al. (2003) Application of a surgical robot to open microsurgery: the equipment. Pediatr Endosurg Innov Tech 7:227–232

Le Bret E, Papadatos S, Folliguet T et al. (2002) Interruption of patent ductus arteriosus in children: robotically assisted versus videothoracoscopic surgery. J Thorac Cardiovasc Surg 123:973–976

LeRoux PD, Das H, Esquenazi S et al. (2001) Robot-assisted microsurgery: a feasibility study in the rat. Neurosurgery 48:584–589

Li RA, Jensen J, Bowersox JC (2000) Microvascular anastomoses performed in rats using a microsurgical telemanipulator. Comput Aided Surg 5:326–332

Marescaux J, Leroy J, Gagner M et al. (2001) Transatlantic robot-assisted telesurgery. Nature 413:379–380

Satava RM (2002) Surgical robotics: the early chronicles. Surg Laparosc Endosc Percutan Tech 12:6–16

Weigel T, Quick D, Agarwal S et al. (2003) Robotic lung resection with Zeus in a pig model [abstract]. Surg Endosc 17:S294

Yavuz Y, Ystgaard B, Skogvoll E et al. (2000) A comparative experimental study evaluating the performance of surgical robots Aesop [sic] and Endosista. Surg Laparosc Endosc Percutan Tech 10:163–167

Chapter 4

Future Technology

Jacques Marescaux and Francesco Rubino

Introduction

While during the decade since 1995 the computer has represented an essential tool for the surgeon mostly because of its use as a support for storage of patient data or for scientific presentations at meetings, more recently the ability to obtain rapid data processing and exchange through computer-generated programs is having a tremendous impact on all aspects of surgery, creating the basis for a true revolution of diagnosis, therapy, and the teaching of surgery.

Although there is the inevitable tendency to consider computer-generated virtual reconstructions as fascinating laboratory work with small actual impact on the routine of the general surgeon, some applications are emerging from the scrutiny of scientific investigations and will very reasonably become commonplace in the foreseeable future. Computer-generated three-dimensional (3-D) images that reconstruct anatomical and pathological structures and the possibility to translate medical information contained in images into a set of 3-D models, allow to visualize structures from multiple points of view as well as to develop an actual interaction of virtual instruments with the virtual organs. Applications of these virtual reality systems provide new potentialities for education and training, preoperative diagnostics, preoperative planning, and intraoperative and postoperative applications. The computer also allows digitization of the surgical movements and images. Once digitized, this information can be modified to filter and exclude non-finalized movements, for example physiological tremor of the surgeon (Garcia-Ruiz et al. 1998), resulting in greater dexterity and higher precision for performance of difficult tasks (Damiano et al. 2000; Falcone et al. 2000; Reichenspurner et al. 1999), which is one of the advantages of robotic surgery. Furthermore, computer programs can be used to convert video images and surgical movements into electronic signals, which, after being appropriately compressed with algorithms, can be transmitted to distant sites enabling the performance of remote surgery.

In this chapter we discuss the role of new technologies in surgery by reporting the main applications currently under evaluation at the European Institute of Telesurgery of Strasbourg (EITS) as well as trying to pinpoint current limitations and possible future developments.

Education and Training

The major technological advantage of virtual reality is the real-time interactivity in full 3-D space and real-time changes of tissues in response to specific actions, which is the fundamental concept of surgical simulation.

Virtual reality provides a safe training environment where errors can be made without consequences to a patient and the learning process is based upon learning the cause of failure. Just as military and commercial pilots who perform a considerable amount of their training in simulated environments and must be certified in their technical skills, the surgeons of the future may train with the aid of realistic surgical simulators and their skills assessed repeatedly and objectively.

This new way for surgical training has several possible advantages; in fact, in addition to improving educational opportunities, it may shorten residency training programs and lower educational expenses. The possibility to avoid the detrimental consequences of the early phases of the learning curve is perhaps the most important among the potential advantages.

Another new aspect of the changes that surgical education is undergoing over recent years is the possibility to obtain expert assistance from a distance in the form of teleproctoring, telementoring, and teleconsultation.

Surgical education can also be boosted by the great potentialities offered by the Internet. At the EITS surgeons, engineers, information technology specialists, and computer medical artists have worked together to develop the Virtual University concept, realized in the Websurg. The purpose of using the Internet for education is twofold: one aim is to enhance the teaching efficacy through the use of multimedia tools and interactivity, and the second aim is to increase access to surgical education by eliminating geographical and time constraints.

The Internet is ideal for the creation of a truly comprehensive encyclopedia of surgery, where operative techniques, discussion of interesting clinical cases, literature reviews, and experts' opinions on special topics or technical issues can be easily accessed. The Internet, more than other traditional tools, allows rapid updating of chapters, and this feature is particularly suitable

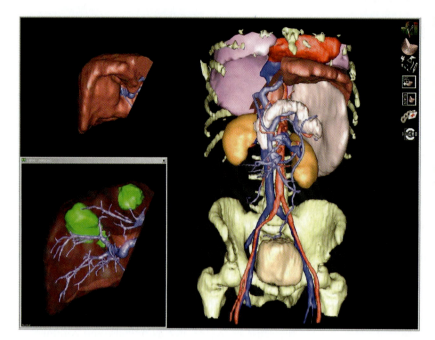

Fig. 4.1. Three-dimensional anatomical reconstruction of different abdominal organs based on data obtained by a CT scan. For instance, the virtual reconstruction of the liver allows enhanced visualization of lesions and inner structures by using transparencies. The virtual reality system also allows navigation inside the lumen of vascular and biliary vessels

for the teaching of minimally invasive techniques, due to the rapid and important changes associated with them.

Continuing medical education can greatly benefit from using interactivity as a teaching approach. Coupling the interactivity to multimedia and ease of access we believe that surgical education will have a greater impact than in the past in terms of modification of professional practice.

Preoperative Diagnostics

Current applications of virtual reality in preoperative diagnostics include gastroscopy, bronchoscopy, and colonoscopy. Some authors suggested that virtual colonoscopy may be better than barium enema for detection of colon polyps (Halligan and Fenlon 1999). In addition, virtual colonoscopy has the unique advantage to allow "navigation" in the lumen of the bowel and viewing of the mucosa from any angle, as well as the possibility to pass through a stenosis and even across the colonic wall into adjacent structures (Halligan and Fenlon 1999). These advantages might render virtual colonoscopy especially suitable for use in screening programs for colorectal cancer.

At the EITS, we have developed systems based on the automatic reconstruction of anatomical and pathological structures from medical imaging such as computed tomography (CT) and magnetic resonance imaging (MRI). These systems automatically delineate anatomical structures with high contrast by combining the use of thresholding, mathematical morphology,

and distance maps for liver, upper airways, colon, and biliary tracts (■ Fig. 4.1). We are currently evaluating the clinical applicability and possible advantages of using such systems. Preliminary results of our 3-D virtual cholangiography system in 26 consecutive patients with suspected lithiasis of the common bile duct seem to indicate that this procedure is feasible and sufficiently accurate for non-invasive preoperative diagnosis of lithiasis of the biliary tract.

The development of systems for 3-D reconstruction of liver anatomy and hepatic lesions has been shown to improve tumor localization ability and to increase precision of operation planning. Lamade et al. (2000) have reported a clinical study showing that the ability to adequately assign a tumoral lesion to a liver segment was significantly increased by 3-D reconstruction when compared with two-dimensional (2-D) CT scans. The target area of the resection proposal was also improved by up to 31% when using the 3-D model.

At the EITS we have developed fully automated software that provides, in less than 5 min from CT scan and MRI images, an accurate 3-D reconstruction of anatomical and pathological structures of the liver as well as invisible functional information such as portal vein labeling and anatomical segment delineation according to the Couinaud definition. Using a computer mouse, the surgeon can select various segmental resections to determine the optimum procedure. After clinical application in more than 30 patients this methods shows that automated delineation of anatomical structures is more sensitive and more specific than manual delineation performed by a radiologist.

Fig. 4.2. Simulation of a laparo-scopic abdominal operation based on the reconstruction of a single patient's anatomy. Using a "virtual laparoscope" it is possible to obtain an internal view of the patient's abdomen and predict difficulties, anatomical abnormalities, as well as plan the ideal positioning of trocar and instruments

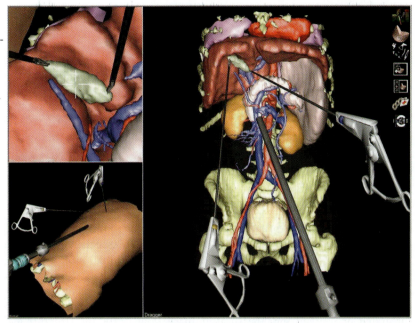

An important impact that virtual reality imaging can have on liver tumor resection is the calculation of risk. The calculation of the remaining liver volume subsequent to partial hepatectomy is considered to be essential in predicting the future development of postoperative liver failure. On the basis of the 3-D imaging and a patient-oriented risk analysis using objective parameters, virtual planning of hepatic resections could be helpful in improving patient selection, and reduce the postoperative liver failure rate (Rau et al. 2000).

Preoperative Planning

Traditionally, preoperative planning of interventions has always taken place in the surgeons' mind, and it was not too long ago when surgeons derived most of their information from the physical examination of their patients. Besides the appropriate diagnosis, precise preoperative planning of the surgical procedure is essential for the success of complex surgical procedures. Preoperative planning requires precise location of the lesions and their anatomical relation to the adjacent tissues and vessels.

The development of digitized medical images from CT scan and MRI represents a major advancement in medicine; however, the detection of lesions or localization of vessels is sometime difficult to process due to a variable image contrast between parenchymas and vessels as well as due to an important image anisotropy, the slice thickness being three times larger than the

pixel width. Moreover, with conventional 2-D medical images it is not easy to address important issues such as the spatial relationship of tumors with crucial structures, the evaluation of anatomical variants regarding vascular supply, and a volumetric and functional analysis to predict the risk of organ failure after resections.

Although it has been nearly a decade since surgical simulation was first attempted, computer-assisted planning and simulation of operations have mostly been used in some subspecialties such as craniofacial surgery, neurosurgery, and orthopedic surgery. While in neurosurgery and orthopedic surgery a firm bony reference frame is available, for most procedures in general surgery the virtual operation planning on the basis of 3-D reconstruction of soft tissues has to overcome the obstacles of the inherent mobility and flexibility of the target organs.

However, more recent virtual reality systems that reconstruct in 3-D the patient-specific anatomical structures and lesions as well as surgical anomalies help surgeons to better comprehend and practice the proposed procedure for each single patient, and be able to repeat individual steps to improve surgical technique (■ Fig. 4.2). Whether or not this will result in the best surgical outcomes is not possible to say at the present time; however, the potential is huge. In craniofacial surgery, the use of 3-D solid models for preoperative planning for craniosynostosis has been reported to reduce operating time and blood transfusion (Imai et al. 1999).

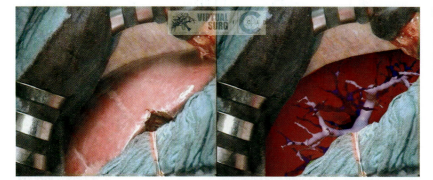

Fig. 4.3. Concept of augmented reality (AR). With AR computer-generated images are superimposed onto the real view of the liver in real time. The vessels appear on the visible surface of the liver through a virtual transparency

Intraoperative Application: the Concept of Augmented Reality

Usually surgeons use CT, ultrasound (US), or MR images to provide additional information reviewed during surgery. These images, however, cannot be readily integrated or overlaid into the surgical space. Augmented reality (AR) superimposes computed-generated images onto the real view of the world in real time. In surgery, the 3-D reconstruction can be superimposed onto the real patient, providing additional help and facilitating the operative procedure. For instance, with augmented reality 3-D reconstruction of the vessels can appear on the visible surface of the liver through a virtual transparency.

Augmented reality can be used to provide additional visual input, by labeling certain structures or allowing visualization of otherwise hidden structures. At our institute we have developed a real-time augmented reality system for hepatic surgery. Two cameras provide a 3-D video view of the physical model; by superimposing the virtual model we obtain a virtual transparency of the physical model (■ Fig. 4.3).

Robotic Surgery

Surgical robots are an application of the concept of computer-assisted surgery, where the processing of data and the digitization of surgical movements are important. We fully agree with the view of Rick Satava, that "surgical robots are not a mechanical system, but an information system." Robotic systems have computer programs that filter out hand tremors, while the chair's arm at the surgeon's console adds stability and comfort during the procedure, improving endurance. These features and the possibility to modulate the amplitude of surgical motions by downscaling and stabilization translate into smooth and precise surgical maneuvers, which have great potential for improvement of dexterity and enhanced precision (Buckingham and Buckingham 1995; Haluck and Krummel 2000; Satava 1999.

Enhanced dexterity is suitable in many instances, especially when operating on anatomical structures of small size, a task for which even the physiological tremor can render the performance troublesome. For example, robotic systems have been successfully used for retinal vein cannulation, involving cannulation of a 100-μm structure with a needle for administration of local therapy for retinal vein thrombosis (Riviere and Jensen 2000). Others have reported efficient performance of sutured coronary artery bypass anastomoses in a plastic model using robotic enhancement technology (Garcia-Ruiz et al. 1997).

Clinical trials verifying the potential advantages of robotic over conventional surgery are not yet available; despite this, feasibility and safety of robotic surgery has been reported by several independent groups. Our group performed laparoscopic robotic cholecystectomy in 25 patients, with no robot-related morbidity and with operative time and patient recovery similar to those of conventional laparoscopy (Marescaux et al. 2001b). Cadiere et al. (2001) have recently reported a series of 146 patients undergoing robot-assisted laparoscopic surgeries, including antireflux procedures, gastroplasties, cholecystectomies, inguinal hernias, hysterectomies, and prostatectomies. Falcone et al. (2000) reported successful robotic assistance for reversal of tubal ligation using 8-0 sutures. Robotic assistance has also been used for laparoscopic nephrectomy (Cadiere et al. 2001) and laparoscopic radical prostatectomy (Guillonneau et al. 2001; Pasticier et al. 2001).

Endoscopic cardiac surgery, including coronary artery bypass and mitral valve repair (Carpentier et al. 1999; LaPietra et al. 2000), is a further important field of application of robotic surgery, and will probably benefit, in the future, from the possibility to operate on a beating heart through motion compensation; this would allow the surgeon to manage any moving structure with the same precision as if it was perfectly still (Mack 2001).

Remote Surgery

In addition to enhancing human performance, robotic systems provides the unique ability to perform surgery in remote locations. Challenges to this concept are several, but the most important limitations have been the reliability (or quality of service) of the telecommunication lines and the issue of latency (the delay time from when the hand motion is initiated by the surgeon until the remote manipulator actually moves and the image is shown on the surgeon's monitor). Due to the latency factor it was believed that the feasible distance for remote surgery was no more than a few hundreds miles over terrestrial telecommunications (Mack 2001) while geosynchronous satellite systems, which have a latency of nearly 1.5 s, are considered unsuitable for performing long-distance surgery (Satava 1999).

Since 1994 at the EITS surgeons and computer scientists as well as telecommunication and robotic engineers from Computer Motion (Santa Barbara, CA) have joined in a common effort aimed to verify the feasibility of surgery through long distances. This project was articulated in several steps including: (1) testing the effect of artificially introduced time delays between the surgeon's manipulations and the robotic effectors; (2) the experimental performance of laparoscopic cholecystectomy from a remote distance on a pig model (Marescaux et al. 2001a); and (3) the performance of a remote robot-assisted surgical operation on a human. The project led to the performance, on 7 September 2001, of the first robot-assisted laparoscopic cholecystectomy in a human, between New York (surgeons) and Strasbourg (patient) (Marescaux et al. 2002).

The first series of our experiments estimated at about 300 ms the maximum time delay compatible with safe performance of surgical manipulations. Subsequently, we measured a mean time delay of 155 ms over transoceanic distances when using dedicated asynchronous transfer mode (ATM) fibers (Marescaux et al. 2001a). This extremely short delay has allowed the safe performance of remote laparoscopic cholecystectomy in six pigs and has provided the basis for the clinical application that was carried out successfully without specific difficulties or complications due to the use of the teletransmission of the surgical procedure (Marescaux et al. 2002).

These results support the use of existing high-bandwidth, dedicated telecommunication lines for performing intercontinental surgery on humans with adequate efficacy and safety. Technical feasibility and clinical safety, however, are not the only issues to solve to permit implementation of remote surgery into routine clinical practice. The use of remote surgery will indeed depend upon a balance between real benefits and limitations.

Limitations are several. First, high-speed terrestrial ATM fibers are not yet available in most hospitals. Second, the cost of remote operations may represent a reasonable concern. In addition to the cost of the robotic system, which approximates US$1 million, other costs are derived from the use of the teletransmission. There is no doubt that, if evaluated solely as the expansion of existing surgical practice, remote surgery it is not cost effective. However, considering that the cost of technologies is expected to reduce with time, and there is a potential to improve training and efficiency with enhanced outcomes, it is possible that remote surgery may prove less costly to healthcare systems in the future. Third, since remote surgery may involve more than one state or country, conflicts of jurisdictions and legal issues may arise, such as whether the surgeon should or should not be liable for errors related to delays in transmission or equipment failure or whether a special consent should be obtained.

Despite these serious concerns, potential benefits are multiple and encourage the efforts to develop remote surgery. For instance patients will be able to receive the type of treatment best suited to their condition ideally in any part of the world. Lack of expertise will not prevent, for example, exposure of the patient to new minimally invasive techniques. Furthermore, healthcare volunteers in developing countries may benefit from the assistance of experts from elsewhere. Likewise, challenging emergency operations in small rural hospitals could be performed by a young surgeon on call under the guidance of a distant expert from a major center. Availability of expert surgeons might also very well help in remote areas where military or scientific missions are being performed or on remote islands.

In theory, remote surgery could also be useful to improve teaching and mentoring in order to reduce the learning curve of surgeons for new procedures.

Future Developments

Virtual and augmented reality systems can be used not only to teach surgical skills and judgment or facilitate intraoperative maneuvers, but also to rehearse procedures before performing them. With more perfected surgical simulators, in the near future, surgeons may work out the best operative procedure for each single patient and being able to repeat individual steps to improve surgical technique. The procedures can also be recorded and replayed from a robot automatically and at a distance.

Combining augmented reality with advanced robotics could guide the surgeons through technically challenging procedures and avoid injury to vital structures. The integration of physiology and anatomy in virtual 3-D systems and simulators may also have a significant impact on research since new procedures could be performed in a virtual patient and functional consequences or possible complications anticipated.

References

Buckingham RA, Buckingham RO (1995) Robots in operating theatres. BMJ 311:1479–1482

Cadiere GB, Himpens J, Germay O et al. J (2001) Feasibility of robotic laparoscopic surgery: 146 cases. World J Surg 25:1467–1477

Carpentier A, Loulmet D, Aupecle B et al. (1999) Computer-assisted cardiac surgery. Lancet 353:379–380

Damiano RJ Jr, Ehrman WJ, Ducko CT, et al (2000) Initial United States clinical trial of robotically assisted endoscopic coronary artery bypass grafting. J Thorac Cardiovasc Surg 119:77–82

Falcone T, Goldberg JM, Margossian H et al. (2000) Robotic-assisted laparoscopic microsurgical tubal anastomosis: a human pilot study. Fertil Steril 73:1040–1042

Garcia-Ruiz A, Smedira NG, Loop FD et al. (1997) Robotic surgical instruments for dexterity enhancement in thoracoscopic coronary artery bypass graft. J Laparoendosc Adv Surg Tech A 7:277–283

Garcia-Ruiz A, Gagner M, Miller JH et al. (1998) Manual vs robotically assisted laparoscopic surgery in the performance of basic manipulation and suturing tasks. Arch Surg 133:957–961

Guillonneau B, Jayet C, Tewari A, Vallancien G (2001) Robot assisted laparoscopic nephrectomy. J Urol 166:200–201

Halligan S, Fenlon HM (1999) Virtual colonoscopy. BMJ 319:1249–1252

Haluck RS, Krummel TM (2000) Computers and virtual reality for surgical education in the 21st century. Arch Surg 135:786–792

Imai K, Tsujiguchi K, Toda C, et al (1999) Reduction of operating time and blood transfusion for craniosynostosis by simulated surgery using three-dimensional solid models. Neurol Med Chir (Tokyo) 39:423–426

Lamade W, Glombitza G, Fischer L et al. (2000) The impact of 3-dimensional reconstructions on operation planning in liver surgery. Arch Surg 135:1256–1261

LaPietra A, Grossi EA, Derivaux CC et al. (2000) Robotic-assisted instruments enhance minimally invasive mitral valve surgery. Ann Thorac Surg 70:835–838

Mack MJ (2001) Minimally invasive and robotic surgery. JAMA 285:568–572

Marescaux J, Leroy J, Gagner M et al. (2001a) Transatlantic robot-assisted telesurgery. Nature 413:379–380

Marescaux J, Smith MK, Folscher D et al. (2001b) Telerobotic laparoscopic cholecystectomy: initial clinical experience with 25 patients. Ann Surg 234:1–7

Marescaux J, Leroy J, Rubino F et al. (2002) Transcontinental robot-assisted remote telesurgery: feasibility and potential applications. Ann Surg 235:487–492

Pasticier G, Rietbergen JB, Guillonneau B et al. (2001) Robotically assisted laparoscopic radical prostatectomy: feasibility study in men. Eur Urol 40:70–74

Rau HG, Schauer R, Helmberger T et al. (2000) Impact of virtual reality imaging on hepatic liver tumor resection: calculation of risk. Langenbecks Arch Surg 385:162–170

Reichenspurner H, Boehm D, Reichart B (1999) Minimally invasive mitral valve surgery using three-dimensional video and robotic assistance. Semin Thorac Cardiovasc Surg 11:235–240

Riviere CN, Jensen PS (2000) A study of instrument motion in retinal microsurgery. Abstract presented at 21st Annual Conference of IEEE Eng Med Biol Soc, Chicago, 26 June 2000

Satava RM (1999) Emerging technologies for surgery in the 21st century. Arch Surg 134:1197–1202

Chapter 5

Ergonomics of Task Performance in Endoscopic Surgery

George B. Hanna and Alfred Cuschieri

Introduction

Ergonomics is the scientific study of people at work in terms of workplace layout, equipment design, the work environment, safety, productivity and training. Ergonomics is based on multiple disciplines such as anatomy, physiology, psychology and engineering combined in a systems approach. The ergonomic approach has been used in industry and the military to improve the safety and productivity of the work environment. By contrast in surgical practice, morbidity and mortality are used as an index of safety but this approach does not address adequately the causation of surgical complications or the measures that increase efficient delivery of surgical care.

Since 1995 there has been widespread use of endoscopic surgical techniques in almost all surgical specialities, and the laparoscopic approach has become the gold standard management of many surgical disorders. Both industry and surgeons have responded positively to the new endoscopic era. The medical technology industry has developed and marketed a whole range of new endoscopic instrumentation and video equipment, while surgeons have developed or modified existing techniques and, more recently, instituted measures to audit the benefit, safety and impact of the new endoscopic surgical management. This rapid advancement of endoscopic surgery has encountered and still faces some problems. Most of the endoscopic equipment and instruments in current usage are adaptations from other areas of technology and from open surgery without adequate considerations to the demands of endoscopic techniques. The ergonomic layout of the current operating theatres, designed for conventional open practice, is also not ideal for the needs of endoscopic surgery where a variety of high technology ancillary devices are necessary for the conduct of endoscopic interventions. Despite the increasing complexity of these technologies used in the operating theatre, ergonomic progress and design has laggednnn behind these developments. Only a few surgeons maintain interest in recent advances in medical technology and in ergonomic studies.

Constraints in Endoscopic Surgery in General

In endoscopic surgery, the surgeon utilises a limited access to approach the operative field. Instruments and endoscopes are passed into the body cavity via cannulae, which are inserted through the body wall to provide narrow channels of fixed positions but of variable directions. This minimal access approach creates a set of mechanical and visual restrictions on the execution of surgical tasks. Some of these are considered below.

Mechanical Restrictions

These are the restrictions encountered on the handling of tissues by endoscopic instruments (summarised in ■ Table 5.1). Standard endoscopic instruments have four degrees of freedom of movement (DOFs). A DOF is the potential for movement in a single independent direction, or a rotation around one axis. The surgeon can move the endoscopic instrument in and out along the z-axis, rotate the instrument in the line of the z-axis, move it from side to side pivoted at a point on the y-axis and move it up and down about the x-axis (■ Fig. 5.1a–e). By contrast, the body-limb-fingertips movements in open surgery have more than 36 DOFs. There are six DOFs for the position of the trunk, three rotations at the shoulder, one at the elbow, one in the forearm and two at the wrist. There is also a complex mobility from several types of protraction and retraction by the precision grip of the hand, as well as rotation of instruments within the fingertips. These constitute two DOFs at each of the five metacarpophalangeal joints and one DOF for each of the nine interphalangeal joints giving a total of 19 DOFs for the hand and a total of 32 DOFs at the finger tips (Patkin and Isabel 1995). The limited number of DOFs of endoscopic in-

Table 5.1 Mechanical restrictions

1. Limited number of DOFs
2. Diminished tactile feedback
3. Small and long endoscopic instruments
4. Problems of tissue retrieval

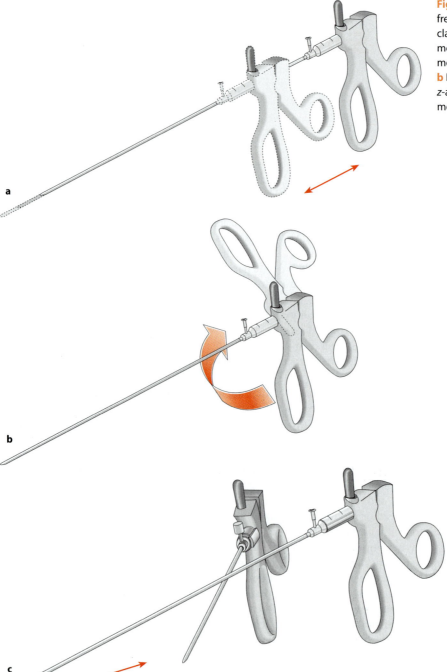

Fig. 5.1 a – c. Degrees of freedom of movement with classic endoscopic instruments. **a** In and out movement along the *z*-axis. **b** Rotation in the line of the *z*-axis. **c** Side to side movement along the *y*-axis.

struments makes handling of tissues in endoscopic procedures more difficult than during conventional open surgery.

In endoscopic surgery, direct tactile feedback (hand to tissue) is lost and the indirect tactile feedback (through the instrument) is markedly diminished due to the length of endoscopic instruments and the friction between the instruments and the ports. This de-

grades the ability of the surgeon to identify the nature of component tissues and tissue planes. It can also lead to tissue damage from excessive instrument grip, poorly appreciated, by the surgeon.

The small size of endoscopic ports dictates the size of endoscopic instruments. This causes several difficulties in the design of endoscopic instruments to perform the same function as their open counterparts.

Fig. 5.1 d, e. Degrees of freedom of movement with classic endoscopic instruments. **d** Up and down movement along the *x*-axis. **e** Combined movements

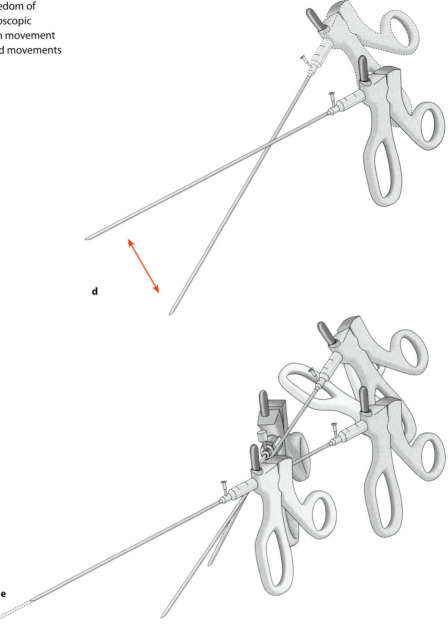

Long thin instruments have a poor mechanical advantage. The narrow end of instruments may cause tissue damage either accidentally if the instruments are not moved under direct endoscopic vision or during gripping the tissues with the small jaws. The length of endoscopic instruments exaggerates hand tremors especially in a magnified endoscopic field.

Another intrinsic problem in endoscopic surgery is tissue retrieval after detachment from adjacent tissues. This problem has two aspects: (1) the tissue must be reduced to the size of the access wounds with preservation of tissue architecture and (2) the risk of contamination including spillage of cancer cells must be eliminated.

Visual Limitations

The use of an image display system as the visual interface between the surgeon and the operative field has several visual limitations compared to conventional open surgery (summarised in ■ Table 5.2). These limitations of current image display systems are responsible for the degraded task performance in endoscopic surgery compared to direct normal vision (Crosthwaite et al. 1995; Tendick et al. 1993).

Standard monitors in current use in surgical practice are two-dimensional (2-D) imaging systems. They present only 2-D depth (pictorial) cues of the operative field to the surgeon (■ Table 5.3). For controlled endoscopic manipulations, the surgeon has to reconstruct a three-dimensional (3-D) picture from a 2-D image. This entails intense perceptual and mental processing which has to be sustained by the surgeon throughout the operation.

The current ergonomic layout of operating theatres with crowding of free-standing equipment often precludes optimal placement of the viewing monitor in front of the surgeon who usually operates from one or other side of the patient. In consequence, the visual axis between the surgeon's eyes and the monitor is no longer aligned with the hands and instruments. Furthermore, the monitor is often far removed from the surgeon and thus the spatial location of the display system (sensory information) is remote from the manipulation area at the hand level of the operator (motor space). These factors degrade task performance in endoscopic surgery.

The current generation of rigid endoscopes have a coaxial alignment of the lens system and the illuminating optical light fibres. This arrangement produces no shadow in the endoscopic field and hence the current

2-D video endoscopic imaging systems are totally devoid of shadow, which constitutes an important depth cue for 3-D perception.

Reduced field of endoscopic vision compared to ordinary unrestricted sight results in a decrease of the sensory input from the periphery of the operative field. The viewing angle of the endoscope refers to the angle formed by the two outer visual limits and determines the diameter of the field of view and the size of the objects seen. The field of view describes the area inspected by the objective of the endoscope (Berci 1976). At a given distance from the objective lens, the larger the field of view, the greater the area that can be observed. The restricted field of endoscopic vision accounts for the incidental tissue injury when instruments move outside the field of view.

The position of the instrument ports in relation to each other and to the optical port is an important determinant of the ease of performance of an endoscopic procedure and its execution time. For bimanual tasks, manipulation, azimuth and elevation angles govern optimal port sites (■ Fig. 5.2). The manipulation angle is the angle between the active and assisting instruments, while the azimuth angle describes the angle between either instrument and the optical axis of the endoscope. The elevation angle of the instrument is defined as the angle between the instrument and the horizontal plane. These angles determine optimal port location.

The display of the same manipulation angle on a 2-D monitor depends on the angle between the optical axis of the endoscope and the instruments' plane. The frame of the monitor provides the reference for the entry of the instruments to the operative field. The instruments appear to enter the image field from the side of the surgeon (real side) when the endoscope views the instruments from above whereas instruments enter the field from the opposite side (unintuitive) when the endoscope views the instruments from below (Patil et al. 2004).

Table 5.2 Visual limitations

1. Loss of normal binocular vision
2.. Decoupling of motor and sensory spaces (monitor location)
3. Coaxial alignment of lens system and light fibres
4. Reduced size of endoscopic field of view
5. Disturbed endoscope-instrument-tissue relationship (port location)
6. Angle between the optical axis of endoscope and instruments' plane
7. Reverse alignment of the endoscope and instruments
8. Limitations of the quality of endoscopic image

Table 5.3 Depth cues

Pictorial cues	Kinetic cues	Physiological cues	nnn
– Linear perception	– Motion parallax	– Convergence	– Retinal disparity
– Interposition	– Kinetic depth effect	– Accommodation	
– Height in the plane			
– Light and shadow			
– Relative size			
– Familial size			
– Arial perspective			
– Proximity-luminance covariance			
– Texture gradients			

Fig. 5.2. Angles govern port placement:
1 manipulation angle, *2* azimuth angle,
3 elevation angle

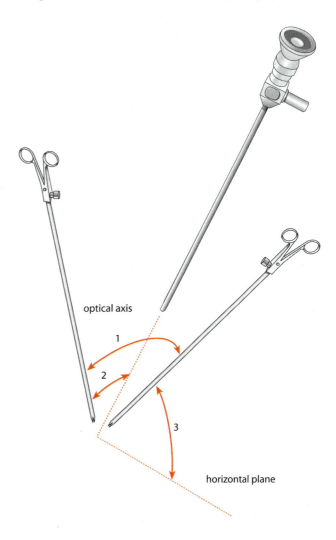

At times during the performance of endoscopic procedures, the surgeon may operate with the optical axis of the endoscope subtended 180° to the axis of the instruments, i.e. the surgeon manipulates the instruments opposite to the endoscope-camera assembly. This reverse alignment produces an inverted mirror image of the instruments' movements. This situation creates intersensory and sensorimotor discordance (Howard 1971) because the visual and proprioceptive inputs do not equate. The processing and manipulation of a mirror image is difficult (Corballis and McMaster 1996) and although some individuals can adapt to reverse alignment, this adaptation requires increased mental processing, thereby accelerating mental fatigue.

There are three major components that determine the quality of the image: resolution, luminance and chroma (Satava et al. 1988). Resolution determines the clarity of the image, luminance measures the amount of light available in the image signal and the chroma represents the intensity or saturation of the colour. In addition to the quality of the monitor, the final image

produced by the endoscopic system depends on the optical characteristics of the endoscope and quality of the camera.

Constraints in Endoscopic Paediatric Surgery

Endoscopic paediatric surgery has inherited all the mechanical and imaging constraints of adult endoscopic surgery. Moreover, there are some special considerations that relate to paediatric surgery since the patient's size and physiology markedly varies from standard adult surgery. The operative field is significantly reduced in children due to the small working spaces and the minimal distension created by low pressure pneumoperitoneum. In addition, particularly in neonates, the liver is relatively larger and the abdomen is greater transversely than it is lengthwise. Moreover the bladder in children is a much more intra-abdominal organ than in adults. Further difficulties may occur in kyphoscoliotic patients because of distortion of the working space.

In addition to the restricted peritoneal space, the small size of neonates and children limits the workspace outside the patients. There is a restricted surface area for trocar insertion and instrument manipulation outside the patient. The surgical team also has to operate within this restricted workspace. Surgeons have to adopt awkward positions especially in advanced paediatric endoscopic procedures that need more than one assistant in a limited workspace.

The diminished tactile feedback in using laparoscopic instruments through access ports, together with the delicacy of neonatal tissues, increases the risk of tissue damage. These problems are heightened by the use of standard laparoscopic instruments developed for adult surgery. The shaft length and the active tip (jaw) of adult-sized instrument are often not appropriate for the neonatal laparoscopic approach. This results in a higher operative risk and a reduced efficiency of operative performance, which in conjunction with the lack of training modules, limits the expansion of endoscopic paediatric surgery.

Smaller and shorter instruments have become available. The beak of these instruments has remained relatively long, predisposing for collateral damage when monopolar high-frequency energy is applied. The smaller diameter makes them more pointed increasing the likelihood of accidental perforation. Moreover, as higher pressures are generated in the beak of smaller instruments, the likelihood of trauma during grasping is increased. It leaves little doubt that the length of the instrument used should be adjusted to the size of the working space. In neonates and small infants 20 cm-long instruments should be used.

Lastly the body walls in children are thin, offering much less grip onto the cannulae than in adults. Especially in children, in whom the available working space is small, the internal part of the trocar should be kept as short as possible. These factors predispose for cannula displacement in both directions: in and out. Cannulae in endoscopic surgery in children should therefore be well fixed by sutures anchored either to a sleeve or to the hub in combination with tape (Bax and van der Zee 1998; Georgeson 1999). When the trocar is only sutured to the skin, pulling out can still occur as the skin is loosely attached to the underlying fascia.

For this reason the suture should take the fascia instead of the skin. Radially expanding trocars are an alternative; they are inserted via a Veress needle and the polymer can be stretched up to 12 mm with dilators.

Ergonomics of the Set-up in Endoscopic Surgery

For a particular operation, the surgeon has to select the appropriate endoscope and place the ports and the monitor in optimum locations. The principles of the set-up of endoscopic equipment are summarised in ■ Table 5.4.

Endoscope Selection

Direction of view of the endoscope describes the angle between the centre of the visual field (optical axis) and the physical axis of the endoscope. Endoscopes can be of forward-viewing (0°) or forward-oblique direction of view (30°, 45°). The angle between the optical axis of the endoscope and the plane of the target is referred to as the optical axis-to-target view angle (OATV) (■ Fig. 5.3). The best task performance during endoscopic work is obtained with an OATV angle of 90° and relatively small decreases in this viewing angle are attended by a significant degradation of task performance. In addition a significant increase in the execution time and the force applied on the target with the decrease in the OATV angle were observed in this study (Hanna and Cuschieri 1999).

Endoscopes of different directions of view have no significant effect on the execution time or the quality of task performance when the optical axis of the endoscope subtends the same OATV angle (Hanna et al. 1997a). In practice, however, only oblique-viewing endoscopes or ones with flexible tips (chip on stick technology) can achieve an adequate OATV angle approximating to 90°. For this reason, forward-oblique endoscopes are preferable despite the easier deployment of forward-viewing types. In addition, the visual field changes when the forward-oblique endoscope is rotated, whereas the operative field of the forward-view-

Table 5.4 Principles of videoendoscopic set-up

Endoscope selection	Port placement	Monitor location
– OATV angle of 90°	– Manipulation angle 60°	– In front of the surgeon
– Visual field changes on rotating forward-oblique endoscopes	– Equal azimuth angles	– At the level of manipulation work space
– Endoscopes of different directions of view have no significant effect on task performance with the same OATV angle	– Narrow manipulation angle necessitates narrow elevation angle	

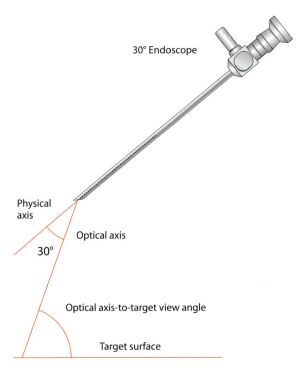

30° Endoscope

Physical
axis

Optical axis

30°

Optical axis-to-target view angle

Target surface

Fig. 5.3. Direction of view of the endoscope and target-to-endoscope distance

ing endoscope is unaltered. Different perspectives can be obtained by rotation of the forward-oblique endoscopes, which provide more visual information for the execution of advanced laparoscopic procedures.

There are two factors that determine optimum OATV angle: the location of the optical port in relation to the centre of the operative field and the direction of view of the endoscope. Variations in the build of patients necessitate a careful selection of the location of the optical port in the individual patient to obtain both an optimum OATV angle and the correct target-to-endoscope distance for a specific endoscopic operation. The endoscope should be selected to obtain an OATV angle approximating to 90°.

To achieve the optimal balance between light availability and endoscope diameter, 3.3- or 5 mm endoscopes are recommended for general paediatric use. Several miniscopes, even of 1.9 mm or less diameter, are currently being marketed. In general it can be said that the smaller the scope, the less light is transmitted and the less good the optical image. More research is required to investigate the field of vision, resolution and illumination provided by miniscopes and their influence on task performance in advanced endoscopic surgery.

Port Placement

The maximal efficiency and quality performance of intracorporeal knotting are obtained with a manipulation angle ranging between 45° and 75° with the ideal angle being 60°. Manipulation angles below 45° or above 75° are accompanied by increased difficulty and degraded performance. Therefore, on placing the operating ports for the active and assisting instruments, for example needle drivers, these should subtend a manipulation angle within the 45–75° range and as close to 60° as possible. A better task efficiency is also achieved with equal rather than wide unequal azimuth angles on either side of the optical port (■ Fig. 5.4). In practice, equal azimuth angles may be difficult to achieve but wide azimuth inequality should be avoided since this degrades task efficiency irrespective of the side, right or left, of the azimuth angle predominance. When a 30° manipulation angle is imposed by the anatomy or build of the patient, the elevation angle should be also 30° as this combination carries the shortest execution and an acceptable knot quality score. Likewise with a 60° manipulation angle, the corresponding optimal elevation angle that yields the shortest execution time and optimal quality performance is 60°. Thus, within the range of angles that ensure adequate task efficiency, a good rule of thumb is that the elevation angle should be equal to the manipulation angle (Hanna et al. 1997b).

The angle between the optical axis of the endoscope and instruments' plane determines how the instruments appear to enter the operative field. The monitor display angle between the instruments is different from the real angle unless the angle of the optical axis-to-instruments' plane is near 90°. The apparent entry of instruments into the operative field becomes intuitive for the surgeon only if the endoscope is viewing from above or the same plane as the instruments. Hence, the best performance is obtained with this configuration.

The planning of port location should avoid operating in the reverse alignment condition, i.e. the surgeon operating against the endoscope-camera assembly as the reverse alignment markedly reduces task performance (Cresswell et al. 1999). Some surgeons would not be able to operate looking at an inverted mirror image while others have intense mental processing to perform a simple task. Moving the endoscope to another port or the surgeon changing his or her position to the other side of the operating table are other useful tactics that can be used during the course of the operation to avoid operating in the reverse alignment condition.

The trocar length should generally be less than 6 cm. For operations that do not involve significant tissue extraction, a trocar diameter of less than 5 mm is adequate. For most operations in children, instruments with a 3 mm diameter in conjunction with a 3.5 mm cannulae suffice.

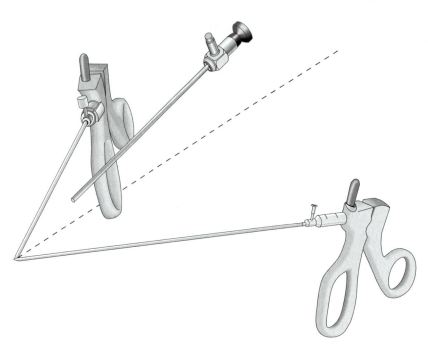

Fig. 5.4. Unequal azimuth angle decreases task efficiency

Monitor Location

The best task performance is obtained with the monitor located in front of the operator at the level of the manipulation work space (hands), permitting 'gaze-down viewing' and alignment of the visual and motor axis (■ Fig. 5.5) (Hanna et al. 1998b). Gaze-down viewing by the endoscopic operator allows both sensory signals and motor control to have a close spatial location and thus bring the visual signals in correspondence with instrument manipulations, similar to the situation encountered during conventional open surgery. In practice, the location of the monitor is determined by the site of the operation. For advanced upper abdominal procedures, such as fundoplication, the child is placed in a frog leg position with the surgeon standing between the patient's knees looking at the monitor above the patient's head. During appendectomy, the monitor is located over the right iliac fossa and the surgeon stands on the left side near the patient's hypochondrium.

To obtain the optimum monitor location, alterations in the design of the operating room and operating table are necessary to improve the ergonomic layout. In addition, technology that projects the image onto the manipulation work space is needed. This could be achieved by head-up display systems that project the image on collimating glass although these systems are known to cause eye accommodation problems (Edgar et al. 1994). The best technical solution would project the image back on top of the patient above but close to the 'real operative field'. The use of a flat thin transistor screen may allow better placement

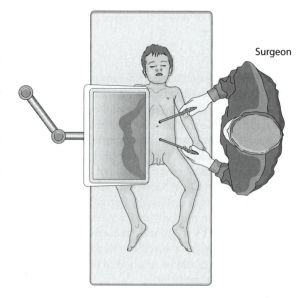

Surgeon

Fig. 5.5. Flat monitor gaze-down viewing increases task efficiency

of the display closer to the workspace and thereby more physical and psychological comfort for the operator even though it gives inferior technical performance compared with a standard monitor (Veelen et al. 2002). The Dundee Projection System is another alternative to permit gaze-down stance. It projects the endoscopic image on a sterile screen placed on the patient without any distortion in a close proximity to the operative area. This development was based on the ViewSite system (■ Fig. 5.6) (Karl Storz, Tuttlingen,

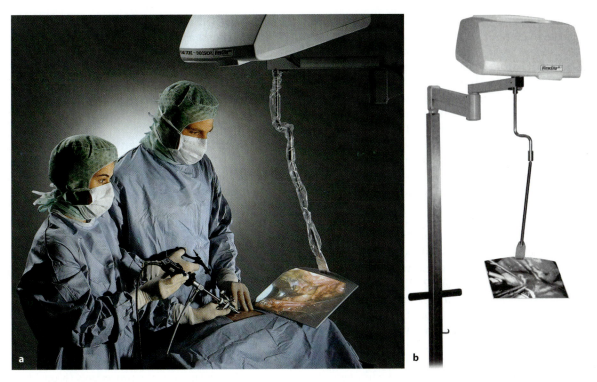

Fig. 5.6. Projection system for gaze-down viewing. The endoscopic image is projected on a sterile screen placed on the patient, (Karl Storz Endoscopy)

Germany), which has the same principle but suffers from lower resolution compared to a standard monitor (Brown et al. 2003). Laboratory experiments with the Dundee Projection System confirmed that the gaze-down stance reduces task execution time and error rate compared to a gaze-up stance. This improvement in task performance becomes more pronounce as the task complexity increases (Omar 2004).

Modality of the Imaging System

Since 1995, 3-D imaging systems have been introduced in an attempt to improve depth perception during endoscopic surgery. The vast majority are based on rapid sequential imaging, alternating between the two eyes by means of optical shutters (active or passive) thus presenting two slightly different images in an alternating sequence to each of the two eyes separated by a few milliseconds. Image fusion for 'stereopsis' is made from the after image in one retina (shutter closed) with current image in the other retina (shutter open). This is, of course, quite different from normal stereoscopic vision which requires co-instantaneous images on each retina with the image falling on different sectors of the two retinas (retinal disparity), eyeball convergence, accommodation and input from the vestibular system.

These 'quasi 3-D' systems have a major disadvantage: there is significant reduction of light transmitted through the optical shutters to the retina, so that the image is distinctly darker and the colour is degraded (von Pichler et al. 1996a). Nevertheless, several reports have suggested that these 3-D systems improve task efficiency in endoscopic manipulations (Becker et al. 1993; Pietrabissa et al. 1994; Satava 1993; von Pichler et al. 1996a,b) while others did not find any superiority of the 3-D systems over 2-D systems (Chan et al. 1997). There was also no significant difference in intracorporeal knot tying (Crosthwaite et al. 1995), endoscopic bowel suturing (Hanna and Cuschieri 2000) or the performance of laparoscopic cholecystectomy in a randomised controlled trial (Hanna et al. 1998a) between 3-D and 2-D imaging systems.

There are several limitations of the current 3-D videoendoscopic systems, which are not, strictly speaking, real stereoscopic displays. The 3-D display does not reconstruct the scene's pattern of light rays in 3-D space, and hence does not present vertical, longitudinal and horizontal parallax as the observer's viewpoint changes. If the surgeon's head moves, the two retinal images do not transform as they normally would in direct viewing of the operative field (Merritt 1987). Furthermore, the current 3-D videoendoscopic systems have a single disparity which yields different magnitudes of depth depending on the viewing distance, in contrast to the human visual system which perceptually rescales disparity information for different distances to produce valid depth, a process called stereoscopic depth constancy (Coren and Ward 1989). The depth perceived by the current 3-D systems is valid if it corresponds to the predicted depth by geometry (Cormack and Fox 1985). As a result, there is a limited operational distance such that a 3-D effect is obtained, but outside this range the surgeon operates from non-valid depth information. In addition, flatness (or anti-cues) emanating from the monitor frame and surface reflections degrade depth perception (Yeh and Silverstein 1991).

The use of optical shuttering glasses results in a substantial loss of photons transmitted to each retina causing significant degradation of the sensory input especially with respect to brightness and colour (von Pichler et al. 1996a). Therefore, 2-D imaging has better sharpness and contrast than a 3-D system. Visual strain on using 3-D systems may result from the decoupled relationship between accommodation and vergence and from interocular crosstalk between the two eye-views (Yeh and Silverstein 1991). Accommodation tends to remain at the screen distance while vergence follows the induced retinal disparity and thus visual strain results from the sustained force vergence effort during prolonged viewing (Tyrrell and Leibowitz 1990). The visual strain and headache may account for the surgical fatigue syndrome during endoscopic operations.

An alternative approach to 3-D videoendoscopic systems is to enhance monocular depth cues in current 2-D display systems. The use of a shadow-inducing endoscopic system would improve task performance (Hanna et al. 2002). This can be achieved by using a single or multipoint illumination/image capture system. The single-point approach is to employ the optical port to provide illumination and to capture the image. A shadow-inducing endoscope has been developed by Buess' technology group (Kunert et al. 1997; Schurr et al. 1996) (MGB Endoscope, Seoul, Korea). This employs additional illumination fibres at a distance behind the front lens resulting in an angle between illumination and view direction with shadow production. However, the angle between the incident light and the optical axis is fixed and thus so is the shadow. A better solution producing variable natural shadows requires a system that provides multipoint balanced illumination of the operative field that is separate from the imaging system contained in the endoscope.

Laboratory experiments showed that the best performance is obtained with overhead shadow-casting illumination as opposed to side illumination (Mishra et al. 2004). This observation is not unexpected because several studies in visual psychology have confirmed that the human visual system prefers overhead illumination (Berbaum et al. 1983, 1984; Howard et al. 1990; Ramachandran 1988) as it is accustomed to overhead lightening by the sun and other sources of artificial light. A balanced degree of shadow and illumination is required for maximum gain in endoscopic task performance (Mishra et al. 2004).

Surgeon–Instrument Interface

The use of laparoscopic instruments results in greater forearm discomfort, possibly due to the need for increased forearm flexor muscle contractions compared to conventional surgical instruments (Berguer et al. 1997a). The handling of the current generation of laparoscopic instruments during grasping motions entails flexion and ulnar deviation of the wrist, which decrease maximum grip force. The handle configuration of laparoscopic instruments also requires the operator to use the opposing muscles of the thenar and hypothenar compartments for gripping rather than the more powerful grasping grip that uses the deep forearm flexors. Some reports have documented thumb paraesthesia in surgeons during laparoscopic procedures (Kano et al. 1995; Majeed et al. 1993; van der Zee and Bax 1995). New handle designs, such as the rocker and ball handles, improve endoscopic task performance (Emam et al. 1999, 2001). Ergonomic assessment using motion analysis of joint movement and electromyography showed that the use of rocker and ball handles is associated with reduced muscle workload and angular velocity at the shoulder and elbow joints compared with the finger-loop handle.

Furthermore, surgeons exhibit decreased mobility of the head and neck and less anteroposterior weight shifting during laparoscopic manipulations despite a more upright posture. This more restricted posture during laparoscopic surgery may induce fatigue by limiting the natural changes in body posture that occur during open surgery (Berguer et al. 1997b). Also, operating from the side of the patient results in muscle fatigue in the shoulder region.

In addition to physical fatigue, laparoscopic surgery requires more mental concentration than open surgery. The surgeon has to reconstruct a 3-D picture from a 2-D image and to perform the task under several mechanical and visual restrictions. The physical, mental and visual demands of endoscopic manipulations may be responsible for the surgical fatigue syndrome encountered in endoscopic surgery (Cuschieri 1995). After a variable but finite time, the surgical fatigue syndrome sets in, manifested by mental exhaustion, increased irritability, impaired surgical judgement and reduced the level of psychomotor performance.

Table 5.5 Recommendations of the Advisory Council on Science and Technology

- All new medical devices or novel applications/treatments used within the National Health Service (NHS) should be developed under controlled conditions
- Only procedures and equipment that have been subjected to assessment and approval should be used within NHS
- Novel surgical procedures and surgical teams practising them should be registered with a committee on the safety and efficacy of procedures
- The NHS should adopt codes of agreed practice in deciding the most cost-effective way of introducing novel devices, applications and treatment
- Specific centres specialising in appropriate diseases and techniques should be resourced to develop, evaluate and educate the rest of the profession

Safety Considerations

Safety aspects in endoscopic surgery should include: (1) control measures to regulate the introduction of new equipment into clinical practice and (2) sound principles of handling of tissues during laparoscopic procedures. It is crucial to control the rate of diffusion of new technologies into surgical practice according to the evidence related to their safety and benefits. In this respect, the Advisory Council on Science and Technology in the UK has several recommendations (■ Table 5.5). New equipment should be the subject of ergonomic studies to evaluate the influence of such technology on task performance. There will always be room for personal preference but basic safety requirements are essential. Instrument design has to be as 'fail-safe' as possible, i.e. when the surgeon fails to use the instrument correctly it should remain in a safe, non-injurious state.

Basic endoscopic training should aim at teaching the principles required for safe surgical practice rather than the techniques of different procedures. Acquisition of skills required for generic tasks should be an essential part of training in endoscopic surgery. Accurate movements of instruments under direct endoscopic vision prevent incidental tissue injury. Controlled endoscopic manipulations require hand-to-eye coordination, two-hand coordination, visuospatial ability, aiming ability and steadiness of the hand in a magnified field. In addition to the development of psychomotor skills, surgeons should be aware of the hazards of surgical equipment. For instance, the temperature at the end of fibre optic light cables may reach 240°C which is enough to ignite surgical drapes or cause skin burns (Hensman et al. 1998). Finally, surgeons should be acquainted with the physics governing the function of ancillary equipment/devices used in endoscopic surgery, and this aspect should form an integral part of the surgical training programme.

References

Bax NMA, van der Zee DC (1998) Trocar fixation during endoscopic surgery in children. Surg Endosc 12:181–182
Becker H, Melzer A, Schurr MO et al. (1993) 3-D video techniques in endoscopic surgery. Endosc Surg Allied Technol 1:40–46
Berbaum K, Bever T, Chung CS (1983) Light source position in the perception of object shape. Perception 12:411–416
Berbaum K, Bever T, Chung CS (1984) Extending the perception of shape from known to unknown shading. Perception 13:479–488
Berci G (1976) Instrument I: rigid endoscope. In: Berci G (ed) Endoscopy. Appleton-Century-Crofts, New York pp 74–112
Berguer R, Remler M, Beckley D (1997a) Laparoscopic instruments cause increased forearm fatigue: a subjective and objective comparison of open and laparoscopic techniques. Minim Invasive Ther Allied Technol 6:36–40
Berguer R, Rab GT, Abu-Ghaida H et al. (1997b) A comparison of surgeons' posture during laparoscopic and open surgical procedures. Surg Endosc 11:139–142
Brown SI, Frank TG, Shallaly G, Cuschieri A (2003) Comparison of conventional and gaze down imaging in laparoscopic task performance. Surg Endosc 17:586–590
Chan ACW, Chung SCS, Yim APC et al. (1997) Comparison of two-dimensional vs. three-dimensional camera systems in laparoscopic surgery. Surg Endosc 11:438–440
Corballis MC, McMaster H (1996) The roles of stimulus response compatibility and mental rotation in mirror image and left to right decisions. Can J Exp Psychol 50:397–401
Coren S, Ward LM (1989) Space. In: Sensation and Perception, 3rd edn. Harcourt Brace Jovanovich College Publishers, Florida, pp 274–303
Cormack R, Fox R (1985) The computation of disparity and depth in stereograms. Percept Psychophys 38:375–380
Cresswell AB, Macmillan AIM, Hanna GB et al. (1999) Methods for improving performance under reverse alignment conditions during endoscopic surgery. Surg Endosc 13:591–594
Crosthwaite G, Chung T, Dunkley P et al. (1995) Comparison of direct vision and electronic two- and three-dimensional display systems on surgical task efficiency in endoscopic surgery. Br J Surg 82:849–851
Cuschieri A (1995) Whither minimal access surgery: tribulations and expectations. Am J Surg 169:9–19
Edgar GK, Pope JCD, Craig IR (1994) Visual accommodation problems with head-up and helmet-mounted displays? Displays 15:68–75
Emam TA, Frank TG, Hanna GB et al. (1999) Rocker handle for endoscopic needle drivers: technical and ergonomic evaluation. Surg Endosc 13:658–661

Emam TA, Frank TG, Hanna GB et al. (2001) Influence of handle design on the surgeon's upper limb movements, muscle recruitment and fatigue during endoscopic suturing. Surg Endosc 15:667–672

Georgeson KE (1999) Instrumentation. In: Bax NMA, et al (eds) Endoscopic surgery in children. Springer, Berlin Heidelberg New York, pp 7–13

Hanna GB, Cuschieri A (1999) Influence of optical axis-to-target view angle on endoscopic task performance. Surg Endosc 13:371–375

Hanna GB, Cuschieri A (2000) Influence of two- and three-dimensional imaging on endoscopic bowel suturing. World J Surg 24:444–449

Hanna GB, Shimi S, Cuschieri A (1997a) Influence of direction of view, target-to-endoscope distance and manipulation angle on endoscopic knot tying. Br J Surg 84:1460–1464

Hanna GB, Shimi S, Cuschieri A (1997b) Optimal port locations for endoscopic intracorporeal knotting. Surg Endosc 11:397–401

Hanna GB, Shimi S, Cuschieri A (1998a) Randomised study of influence of two-dimensional versus three-dimensional imaging on performance of laparoscopic cholecystectomy. Lancet 351:248–251

Hanna GB, Shimi S, Cuschieri A (1998b) Task performance in endoscopic work is influenced by location of the image display. Ann Surg 227:481–484

Hanna GB, Cresswell AB, Cuschieri A (2002) Shadow depth cues and endoscopic task performance. Arch Surg 137:1166–1169

Hensman C, Hanna GB, Drew T et al. (1998) Total radiated power, infra-red output and heat generation by cold light sources at the distal end of endoscopes and fibre optic bundle of light cables. Surg Endosc 12:335–337

Howard IP (1971) Perceptual learning and adaptation. Br Med Bull 27:248–252

Howard IP, Bergstrom SS, Ohmi M (1990) Shape from shading in different frames of reference. Perception 19:523–530

Kano N, Yamakawa T, Ishikawa Y, et al. (1995) Prevention of laparoscopic surgeon's thumb. Surg Endosc 9:738–739

Kunert W, Flemming E, Schurr MO et al. (1997) Optik natürlich wirkender Zusatzbeleuchtung. Langerbecks Arch Suppl II Seiten 114:1232–1234

Majeed AW, Jacoub G, Reed MW et al. (1993) Laparoscopist's thumb: an occupational hazard. Arch Surg 128:357

Merritt JO (1987) Visual-motor realism in 3D teleoperator display systems. SPIE True Three-dimensional Imaging Techniques and Display Technologies 761:88–93

Mishra RK, Hanna GB, Brown SI, et al. (2004) Optimum shadow-casting illumination for endoscopic task performance. Arch Surg 139:889–892

Omar AM (2004) Interaction between display location, display alignment and task complexity. Master in Minimal Access Surgery, University of Dundee

Patil PV, Hanna GB, Cuschieri A (2004) Effect of angle between the optical axis of endoscope and instruments' plane on monitor image and surgical performance. Surg Endosc 18:111–114

Patkin M, Isabel L (1995) Ergonomics, engineering and surgery of endosurgical dissection. J R Coll Surg Edinb 40:120–132

Pietrabissa A, Scarcello E, Carobbi A et al. (1994) Three dimensional versus two dimensional video system for the trained endoscopic surgeon and the beginner. Surg Endosc 2:315–317

Ramachandran VS (1988) Perception of shape from shading. Nature 331:163–165

Satava RM (1993) 3-D vision technology applied to advanced minimally invasive surgery systems. Surg Endosc 7:429–431

Satava R, Roe W, Joyce G (1988) Current generation video endoscopes: a critical evaluation. Am Surg 54:73–77

Schurr MO, Buess G, Kunert W et al. (1996) Human sense of vision: a guide to further endoscopic imaging systems. Minim Invasive Ther Allied Technol 5:410–418

Tendick F, Jennings RW, Tharp G et al. (1993) Sensing and manipulation problems in endoscopic surgery: experiment, analysis and observation. Presence 2:66–81

Tyrrell RA, Leibowitz HW (1990) The relation of vergence effort to reports of visual fatigue following prolonged near work. Hum Factors 32:341–357

van der Zee DC, Bax NM (1995) Digital nerve compression due to laparoscopic surgery. Surg Endosc 9:740

Veelen MA, Jakimowicz JJ, Goossens RH et al. (2002) Evaluation of the usability of two types of image display systems during laparoscopy. Surg Endosc 16:674–678

von Pichler C, Radermacher K, Boeckman W (1996a) The influence of LCD shatter glasses on spatial perception in stereoscopic visualisation. In: Weghorst SJ, Sieburg HS, Morgan KS (eds) Medicine meets virtual reality: health care in the information age. IOS Press, Amsterdam, pp 523–531

von Pichler C, Radermacher K, Rau G (1996b) The state of 3-D technology and evaluation. Minim Invasive Ther 5:419–426

Yeh Y-Y, Silverstein LD (1991) Human factors for stereoscopic colour displays. SID 91 Digest 826–829

Chapter 6

Training in Pediatric Endoscopic Surgery

David C. van der Zee and Klaas (N) M.A. Bax

Introduction

In the past surgical training has always been one of master and apprentice. Although this approach has produced many skilled surgeons, in recent years more attention has been paid to standardization and credentialing of surgical training. Skills laboratories have been established where surgical procedures can be practiced and postgraduate courses have been instituted to keep the surgeon updated with recent developments and new techniques. Training in pediatric surgery has followed a similar course.

As pediatric endoscopic surgery is being more generally accepted, an increasing number of centers are willing to start up minimally invasive procedures in children. This implies that an increasing number of complications will occur when no proper training is offered. This could ultimately result in peer groups turning away from endosurgery, as has occurred in adult surgery (van der Zee and Bax 2003).

Prerequisites for pediatric endoscopic surgery are a structured organization with a well-trained staff, adequate acquaintance with the devices and instruments used, proper training for all personnel involved, and a thorough consultation with the anesthesiology department.

Training of Personnel in the Operating Room

As many pediatric surgical procedures will be performed outside regular hours it is imperative to familiarize all operating room (OR) personnel with endoscopic devices and instruments, including where they are stored and how they should be assembled and/or connected. A checklist of an endoscopy tower with all its connections, and a tray with instruments and cables, was published in *Pediatric Endosurgery & Innovative Techniques* (van der Zee 2003) and may be useful as an overview for OR personnel. Regular (fresh-up) courses should keep OR personnel updated with the available equipment and/or new developments. Investment by the endoscopic surgeon in this field will be repaid during night hours.

The initial reluctance sometimes met by OR personnel can be overcome by actively involving them in the surgical procedures. Additional monitors can be helpful to facilitate them to keep up with the procedure and stay motivated. Co-responsibility in the maintenance of instruments and devices increases motivation to stay involved in endoscopic surgery.

When endoscopic surgery is started it is important to continue the regimen both during the day and overnight to avoid discussions whether endoscopic procedures should only be performed during daytime.

Operating room personnel should be encouraged to create protocols for the different procedures concerning instrumentation, positioning of the patient and the OR team, the endoscopy tower, and other devices.

Training of Pediatric Surgical Staff

Apprenticeship

Training in pediatric endoscopic surgery by means of apprenticeship is under debate (Bergamaschi 2001), because of:
1. Loss of tactile feeling
2. Disruption of the constrained coupling between the surgeon's hand and eyes
3. Therapy complexity
4. Lack of endoscopic experience by senior pediatric surgeons

These factors also put a greater intellectual strain not only on the residents, but also on the senior staff member.

Training Courses

Over the years numerous training courses have been available for pediatric minimal access surgery (MAS). Due to the limited time factor training courses usually are only a first acquaintance with endoscopic surgery. Furthermore there is no follow-up or after sales.

Nussbaum stated in 2002 that at that time general surgery training programs as a whole failed to provide residents with significant surgical experience in advanced laparoscopic procedures. The American Board of Surgery in 1999 inventoried that the mean number of advanced laparoscopic procedures performed by graduating trainees was less than 10. In response to this perceived shortcoming at least 50 laparoscopic fellowships have been established in the USA. However, these fellowships are totally devoid of programmatic oversight or mechanisms to guide the trainers' educational agendas (van der Zee and Bax 2003). There is so far no insight in pediatric endoscopic surgery training programs.

Fellowships

When properly described and protocolized it is obvious that fellowship or residency in an expert center provides the best option to acquire skills in endoscopic pediatric surgery. Expert centers can offer coaching during skills training on pelvic trainers (PT) and/or virtual reality trainers (VRT), practicing on animal models, and coaching during endoscopic surgical procedures. In order to fulfill the criteria set for technical competence, fellows and residents should have a prolonged exposure to endoscopic procedures. Mastering of skills should not only be obtained by holding the camera (Nussbaum 2002), but above all by progressive active participation, depending on acquired skills on PT and/or VRT. Pitfalls can be explained and taught to be avoided, and difficulties can be demonstrated and shown how to get around, thus reducing the learning curve.

Pediatric surgery is a specialty of rarities. It may therefore be difficult to condition the required skills for specific procedures by number. Exposure to a broad range of pediatric procedures that is feasible is the crux not only in endoscopy but also in open surgery (van der Zee and Bax 2003). In the future validation of VRT tests (Dawson 2002; Gallagher et al. 2003) may provide additional tools to define accreditation for pediatric endoscopic surgery.

Laboratory Training
Pelvic Trainer
The PT forms a good means to practice endoscopic techniques, from basic procedures, such as spatial definition, camera handling, and simple maneuvers like picking up small particles and putting them into a matchbox, to more specific procedures, such as suturing and using specific devices like the Endo-GIA, as a preparation for surgical endoscopic procedures. The advantage of the PT is its availability throughout the day and the low-cost budget. Sessions on the PT can also be programmed into the OR program for residents. The PT has proven its benefit (Powers et al. 2002).

Virtual Reality Trainer
In recent years virtual reality training is becoming a practical, affordable technology for the teaching and practice of clinical medicine (Bergeron 2003). It is believed that objective methods of skills evaluation, such as the VRT, may be useful as part of a residency skills curriculum and as a means of procedural skills testing (Bloom et al. 2003). Several studies show the benefit of virtual reality training. It has been demonstrated that there may be a difference in learning curves and impact of previous operative experience on performance on a VRT, i.e., more experienced surgeons have a shorter learning curve (Grantcharov et al. 2003a; Seymour et al. 2002). The VRT and the PT are equally efficient (Kothari et al. 2002) in improving endoscopic maneuvering. The advantage of the VRT is its capability of objectively measuring the outcomes.

Although already used for more than a decade, endoscopy is the technique of the new generation. Grantcharov et al. (2003b) were able to demonstrate that residents that had experience with computer games performed better with the VRT. Apparently right-handed persons seem to do better in the tests. Sessions on the VRT can also be programmed into the OR program for residents.

Virtual reality training is becoming a more and more important tool in the training for endoscopic surgery. There are several different VRT on the market. They are far from ideal at present, for example, most of them lack force feedback. There is no doubt, however, that major progress in this field will be made in the foreseeable future. Preoperative imaging of the specific patient with 3-D reconstruction will make many specific operations trainable before the actual operation is carried out (see also Chapter 4).

Practical Training
All the training on the PT and the VRT has the ultimate goal of applying the experience clinically. Practical training consists of stepwise progressive tasking. Maneuvers learned in the skills laboratory can be brought into practice during the surgical procedure (■ Table 6.1). On the one hand, adequate training on the PT and the VRT is rewarded with progressive participation in endoscopic procedures. On the other hand, if gaps occur in endoscopic tissue handling the fellow can return to the skills laboratory to practice further on the issue concerned before returning to the OR.

Training programs can differentiate between basic and advanced courses, depending on the level of expertise and/or endpoints set out. Basic procedures may vary from appendectomy to antireflux procedures, while advanced procedures include esophageal atresia and anorectal malformation. Fellows can actively participate in more complex procedures from the begin-

Table 6.1 Endoscopic procedures

Camera holding
(Open) introduction of first trocar
Introduction of trocar under direct vision
Diagnostic laparoscopy of four quadrants
Introduction of instruments such as liver retractor
Ergonomics
Simple tissue preparation
More extensive dissection
Suturing
Vascular ligation and section
Use of appliers such as clipping device, stapler
Endoscopic procedures

ning as long as the tasks they are asked to perform are adapted to the level of expertise they have acquired. For example, they can start relatively early with the dissection in antireflux surgery or esophageal atresia, while the suturing should be done at a later stage.

Usually fellows are being integrated into the department of the expertise center and may thus profit from the opportunities to participate in scientific studies from the expert center (van der Zee and Bax 2003).

Training for the Senior (Pediatric) Surgeon

Training for the senior pediatric surgeon is difficult for several reasons. First of all it will be almost impossible to go to a training center for a prolonged period of time. Second it will be harder for the senior pediatric surgeon to become adapted to the endoscopic technique than younger surgeons. However, with perseverance and having other colleagues in either pediatric or adult surgery around who are familiar with endoscopic techniques the senior pediatric surgeon can carefully expand his or her expertise in endoscopic surgery. Starting off with diagnostic procedures, slowly more advanced endoscopic procedures can be performed. For example, a Meckel's diverticulum can be mobilized laparoscopically and then be exteriorized through the umbilicus for resection. Conversion is not a complication, as it is only a transformation from one laparoscopic procedure to another laparoscopically assisted, i.e., partly "open," procedure. However, when a complication does occur, the threshold for conversion should be low.

The advantages of endosurgery in pain control and shortened hospitalization make the technique deserving of commitment by the senior pediatric surgeon (Chang et al. 2001).

Non-pediatric surgeons with experience in endoscopic procedures who also operate on children can, in good conjunction with the anesthetist, expand on the endoscopic procedures in children as long as they are familiar with the pediatric surgical pathology they are dealing with and with the principles for pediatric instrumentation. Endoscopic appendectomy, splenectomy, or antireflux surgery in children are principally similar to adult procedures.

References

Bergamaschi R (2001) Editorial. Farewell to see one, do one, teach one? Surg Endosc 15:637
Bergeron BP (2003) Virtual reality applications in clinical medicine. J Med Pract Manage 18:211–215
Bloom MB, Rawn CL, Salzberg AD et al. (2003) Virtual reality applied to procedural testing: the next era. Ann Surg 237:442–448
Change JH, Rothenberg SS, Bealer JF et al. (2001) Endosurgery and the senior pediatric surgeon. J Pediatr Surg 36:690–692
Dawson S.L (2002) A critical approach to medical simulation. Bull Am Coll Surg 87:12–18
Gallagher AG, Ritter EM, Satava RM (2003) Fundamental principals of validation and reliability: rigorous science for the assessment of surgical education and training. Surg Endosc 17:1525–1529
Grantcharov TP, Bardram L, Funch-Jensen P et al. (2003a) Learning curves and impact of previous operative experience on performance on a virtual reality simulator to test laparoscopic surgical skills. Am J Surg 185:146–149
Grantcharov TP, Bardram L, Funch-Jensen P et al. (2003b) Impact of hand dominance, gender, and experience with computer games on performance in virtual reality laparoscopy. Surg Endosc 17:1082–1085
Kothari SN, Kaplan BJ, Demaria EJ et al. (2002) Training in laparoscopic suturing skills using a new computer-based virtual reality simulator (MIST-VR) provides results comparable to those with an established pelvic trainer system. J Laparoendosc Adv Surg Tech A 12:167–173
Nussbaum MS (2002) Surgical endoscopy training is integral to general surgery residency and should be integrated into residency and fellowship abandoned. Semin Laparosc Surg 9:212–215
Powers TW, Murayama KM, Toyama M et al. (2002) Housestaff performance is improved by participation in a laparoscopic skills curriculum. Am J Surg 184:626–629
Seymour NE, Gallagher AG, Roman SA et al. (2002) Virtual reality training improves operating room performance: results of a randomized, double-blinded study. Ann Surg 236:458–463
Soper NJ (2001) Editorial. SAGES and surgical education. Surg Endosc 15:775–780
van der Zee DC (2003) Prevention of complications in pediatric minimal invasive surgery. Pediatr Endosurg Innov Tech 7:1–4
van der Zee DC, Bax NMA (2003) The necessity for training in pediatric endoscopic surgery. Pediatr Endosurg Innov Tech 7:27–31

Chapter 7

Physiologic Responses to Endoscopic Surgery

Benno M. Ure, Natalie K. Jesch and Rainer Nustede

Introduction

The impact of surgery is reflected by the function of specific organs, and hormonal, immunologic, and metabolic changes. The limited number of reports on the effects of minimally invasive techniques in children is focused in particular on organ functions or cell products, but the complex responses have not been investigated as a whole yet. Today, up to 60% of abdominal procedures in children can be performed laparoscopically (Ure et al. 2000) and there is an increasing use of minimally invasive techniques in children with specific conditions, such as in premature babies and newborns (Fujimoto et al. 1999b), and children with cancer (Holcomb 1999; Warmann et al. 2003). However, very little is known about the impact on specific organs and on endocrinologic and immunologic parameters in this age group. The present chapter summarizes the available data.

Specific Organs and System Function

Cardiovascular

Cardiovascular changes are mainly the result of hypercarbia from an increase in intra-abdominal pressure, peritoneal absorption of carbon dioxide (CO_2), and a stimulation of the neurohumoral vasoactive system. These conditions result in a decrease in venous return, preload, cardiac output and an increase in heart rate, mean arterial pressure, and systemic and pulmonary vascular resistance. These effects have been documented in numerous series of adults (Neudecker et al. 2002).

Also in infants, the heart rate, mean arterial pressure, left ventricular end-systolic and end-diastolic volumes, and meridional wall stress increase (de Waal and Kalkman 2003; Gentili et al. 2000; Laffon et al. 1998). However, Bozkurt et al. (1999) reported on transient arrhythmias in 10 out of 27 children aged 1–12 months, but they did not find significant alterations of cardiovascular parameters and the base excess during and after laparoscopy. In a prospective study on 33 children undergoing laparoscopic fundoplication, no significant changes in the heart rate, blood pressure, partial oxygen saturation, or base excess were detected when the insufflation pressure did not exceed 10 mmHg (Mattioli et al. 2003). Fujimoto et al. (1999b) reported no cardiac decompression or fluid and electrolyte balances in 65 laparoscopically operated neonates. De Waal and Kalkman (2003) reported that low pressure CO_2 pneumoperitoneum did not alter the cardiac index in a series of 13 children aged 6–36 months. Therefore, in otherwise healthy infants and children cardiovascular changes during pneumoperitoneum may be expected to be without clinical consequences and to vanish after desufflation (Gueugniaud et al. 1998).

Since hemodynamic effects of pneumoperitoneum are volume dependent, adequate pre- and intraoperative loading is essential, in particular in patients with cardiac diseases (Neudecker et al. 2002). Tobias and Holcomb (1997) concluded from two cases with decreased myocardial function that avoiding agents with negative inotropic effects and including those that dilate the peripheral vasculature allows laparoscopic procedures to be performed. However, the authors observed a substantial increase in arterial and end-tidal CO_2. Van der Zee et al. (2003) retrospectively analyzed 20 neonates with various cardiac anomalies, such as tetralogy of Fallot, defects of the ventricular or atrial septum, or open ductus Botalli. No adverse effects were encountered during and after laparoscopy.

Lung Physiology and Gas Exchange

Carbon dioxide pneumoperitoneum causes considerable hypercarbia and respiratory acidosis, reduces pulmonary compliance, and increases airway resistance (Neudecker et al. 2002). Manner et al. (1998) found that head-down tilt in children induced a mean decrease of 17% in lung compliance, which was further decreased by 27% during pneumoperitoneum. The peak airway pressure increased by 32%. Hsing et al. (1995) investigated 126 children during brief pneumoperitoneum of 15 min. Although the airway pressure and end-tidal CO_2 tension were increased, this did not differ between age groups. Tobias et al. (1995) investigated 55 children with brief pneumoperitoneum. An increase in ventilatory parameters was not required.

Information on the impact of long pneumoperitoneum on lung physiology and gas exchange in small children and newborns is lacking. Relaxation of the diaphragm in combination with increased abdominal pressure may lead to compression of the lower lung lobes. In particular in small children, this may result in a decreased tidal volume, ventilation-perfusion mismatch, increased dead space, and decreased pulmonary compliance (Rayman et al. 1995). The clinical impact in children with impaired lung function remains to be determined.

Renal Function

Numerous experimental studies and some clinical trials in adult patients showed a significant and reversible decrease in renal blood flow, urinary output, and the glomerular filtration rate during pneumoperitoneum (Dunn and McDougall 2000; Schäfer and Krähenbühl 2001). These effects were pressure dependent (Kirsch et al. 1994). Several underlying mechanisms, such as decreased cardiac output, compression of the renal vein and parenchyma, ureteral obstruction, and hormonal effects have been proposed.

However, normalizing cardiac output with plasma expanders failed to improve diminished renal blood flow and glomerular filtration (Harman et al. 1982). In experimental studies, ureteral stents (McDougall et al. 1996) and intraoperative urograms (Kirsch et al. 1994) during pneumoperitoneum confirmed the absence of ureteral obstruction. Kirsch et al. (1994) found a decrease of 92% in vena cava blood flow in rats and concluded that the renal effects were caused by renal vascular insufficiency from central venous compression. Additional compelling evidence for the cause of renal effects is that of direct renal parenchymal compression (Razvi et al. 1996). Hamilton et al. (1998) confirmed that catecholamines may play an additional role. Endothelin, a potent vasoconstrictor, was increased in response to renal vein compression during pneumoperitoneum.

These effects have not been investigated in infants and children. They may not be clinically relevant in otherwise healthy children, but research on the renal effects of pneumoperitoneum in children with impaired renal function remains mandatory.

Hepatoportal and Splanchnic Function

Intestinal circulation of hollow viscus and solid organs reveals a decrease, similar to that of hepatic blood flow. Schilling et al. (1997) found a decrease in blood flow of up to 54% in the stomach, 32% in the jejunum, and 44% in the colon during laparoscopy in patients. In rats (Schäfer et al. 2000), microcirculation in solid organs compared to bowel was even more suppressed. This was a pressure-related phenomenon. When using mechanical retractors to lift the abdominal wall, no impairment of intestinal blood flow was detected (Koivusalo et al. 1997).

It remains unclear whether the impairment of microcirculation may cause clinically relevant damage to the mucosal barrier with subsequent translocation, in particular in small children. Alterations in organ perfusion could have detrimental effects in children with comorbidities or preexisting organ disorders. Bozkurt et al. (2002) reported a considerable increase in arterial and end-tidal CO_2 in children with portal hypertension as compared to systemically healthy children.

Cerebral Function/Intracranial Pressure

Experimental studies using a small animal model showed that laparoscopy is associated with an elevation of basilar artery velocity and a decrease in resistance index values (Erkan et al. 2001). Malone dialdehyde values as an indicator for ischemia-reperfusion injury of brain tissue were not altered. In adults, CO_2 pneumoperitoneum induced hypercapnia with a subsequent increase in cerebral blood volume (Kitajima et al. 1996) and cerebral blood flow velocity (Fujii et al. 1994).

It has been advocated that infants have a greater cerebrovascular sensitivity to changes in P_{CO_2} (Wyatt et al. 1991). De Waal et al. (2002) tried to quantify the impact of CO_2 pneumoperitoneum on cerebral oxygenation and blood flow by near-infrared spectroscopy, a method for determination of relative changes in regional cerebral oxygen saturation. There was a significant increase in cerebral blood volume and oxygen saturation, the latter not returning to normal 10 min after desufflation. However, all children had normal intracranial compliance and there was no indication of a clinically relevant increase in intracranial pressure. To counteract these CO_2-induced effects, the authors advocate more aggressive hyperventilation during CO_2 insufflation. However, Huetteman et al. (2002) found an increase of cerebral blood flow velocity by Doppler sonography in young children independent from hypercapnia, whereas CO_2 reactivity remained normal.

There are reports on an increase of intracranial pressure from 9 mmHg to over 60 mmHg within 10 min in patients with head injury undergoing diagnostic laparoscopy (Mobbs and Yang 2002). Similar data were reported from children with ventriculoperitoneal shunts undergoing laparoscopy (Uzzo et al. 1997). Clinically, laparoscopic surgery was well tolerated in several series of children with ventriculoperitoneal shunts (Jackman et al. 2000; Walker and Langer

2000). Therefore, it has been postulated that these shunts do not represent a contraindication to laparoscopy. However, it is advocated not to perform laparoscopy in patients with head injury or other intracranial mass lesions with reduced compensatory mechanisms to decrease intracranial pressure (Holthausen et al. 1999; Mobbs and Yang 2002).

Hormonal Stress Response

Conflicting data on the perioperative humoral stress response exist. An experimental study using a canine model indicated lower postoperative levels of cortisol after laparoscopic versus open surgery (Marcovich et al. 2001). Lower serum levels of adrenaline, noradrenaline, and cortisol after laparoscopic compared to conventional surgery have been reported from randomized controlled trials in adults (Karayiannakis et al. 1997; Le Blanc-Louvry et al. 2000), but another study did not confirm these data (Hendolin et al. 2000). Bozkurt et al. (2000) compared the hormonal response in 15 laparoscopically and 14 conventionally operated children with acute abdominal pain. The serum levels of insulin, cortisol, prolactin, epinephrine, lactate, and glucose were not significantly different between the groups.

Immunologic Response

Surgery alters the function of the immune system by triggering the production of cytokines, reactive oxygen species, and nitric oxide. There is an impact on the function of various cell populations, such as monocytes, macrophages, polymorphonuclear leucocytes (PMN), and lymphocytes. Because laparoscopic surgery reduces the magnitude of the surgical insult, it may be associated with less local and systemic immune impairment. Better preservation of immune function might contribute to a faster recovery.

Most research on the immunologic impact of pneumoperitoneum and laparoscopic surgery focused on cytokines and other cell products. These parameters are highly variable in children. No significant changes between pre- and postoperative plasma cytokines, such as tumor necrosis factor (TNF-alpha), interleukin (IL)-1, IL-6, IL-10, and interferon-gamma were determined in infants and young children after major surgery (Hansen et al. 1998). Parameters of the cell function itself may be more conclusive, but they have not been systematically determined in patients.

Ure et al. (2002) investigated the cytokine release and cell functions in a pediatric pig model. Laparoscopy compared to laparotomy led to a lower abdominal IL-6 release and a lower migration of polymorphonuclear cells to the abdominal cavity. Carbon dioxide compared to air contamination led to similar effects. After contamination of the abdominal cavity with air, but not with CO_2, the production of reactive oxygen species of pulmonary macrophages was increased. The authors concluded that both the laparoscopic approach and the use of CO_2 versus air led to a lower immune response. The results of a randomized clinical trial of Neuhaus et al. (2001) suggested that CO_2 laparoscopy preserves the production of cytokines by lowering the abdominal pH, but that the insufflation gas does not affect macrophage phagocytosis. However, these effects have not been investigated in pediatric models.

Reduced cytokine levels (IL-1, IL-6, C-reactive protein) and a better preserved cell-mediated immunity were shown after laparoscopy in numerous controlled trials (Neudecker et al. 2002). Differences in the activation of other cytokines such as IL-8 and TNF-alpha and changes in the levels of acute phase proteins were less clear (Gupta and Watson 2001). Fujimoto et al. (1999a) investigated 65 neonates, who underwent laparoscopic procedures and compared the immunologic response to conventionally operated children. Serum IL-6 was significantly lower after laparoscopic nephrectomy and salpingo-oophorectomy. The highest differences were detected 4 h postoperatively. The IL-6 levels returned to normal after 48 h in both groups. The same workgroup found a significantly lower systemic IL-6 response after laparoscopic versus conventional pyloromyotomy. However, patients were not randomized, but matched for clinical data. The impact of pneumoperitoneum on PMN, which play a key role in the host defense against microorganisms, is unknown in pediatric patients. The lack of increase in the number of leucocytes, the reduction in their phagocytic activity, and other parameters of cellular activation, such as surface expression of CD11b and concentration of elastase (Gupta and Watson 2001), have not yet been investigated in children.

There have been numerous studies on pneumoperitoneum and the growth of various types of cancer cells. The data are not conclusive (Jacobi et al. 2002b). Data on pediatric tumors are scarce and clinical reports do not indicate an increase in tumor growth or metastases (Holcomb 1999; Warmann et al. 2003). Iwanaka et al. (1998) investigated port-site metastases of a neuroblastoma cell line in a mouse model. There was no difference in the incidence of metastases between biopsies taken by CO_2 laparoscopy, gasless laparoscopy, or open surgery. Fondrinier et al. (2001) found no significant differences in carcinomatosis between CO_2 laparoscopy, laparotomy, and controls 2 weeks after peritoneal implantation of an aneuploid tumor cell line in rats. Nothing is known about effects on lymphoma, hepatoblastoma, or rhabdomyosarcoma cells.

Experimental work indicates that pneumoperitoneum alters the peritoneal host response in septic patients. Hajri et al. (2000) found an enhancement of TNF-alpha, IL-6, and inducible synthase gene transcription in white blood cells, and a depression in peritoneal immune cells after laparoscopy. During CO_2 insufflation, the intra- and extracellular pH values dramatically decreased, and the regulation of oxidative phosphorylation, cell proliferation, and the onset of apoptosis was altered (Wildbrett et al. 2003). Basic research on the impact of pneumoperitoneum in pediatric patients with abdominal sepsis is lacking.

Conclusions

Clinical and experimental studies support the view that laparoscopic surgery is well tolerated by otherwise healthy infants and children. The technique seems to be associated with better preservation of postoperative systemic immune function than conventional surgery, but evidence has not been derived from well-designed studies. The essential clinical outcomes after surgery concerning immunologic functions are infections and cancer growth. Until now, there has been no compelling clinical evidence that the advantages of pneumoperitoneum or laparoscopic surgery are due to differences in the immunologic response (Neudecker et al. 2002). There is no study demonstrating an association between changes of immune function and a lower incidence of complications after laparoscopic surgery (Jacobi et al. 2002a). Intraperitoneal immunity is complex and systemic benefits may not extend to the peritoneal interface. Little is known about the impact of pneumoperitoneum in children with septic conditions or cancer. It remains a major task for endoscopic pediatric surgeons to investigate the pathophysiologic consequences of minimally invasive procedures and to determine whether potentially adverse effects are clinically relevant.

References

Bozkurt P, Kaya G, Yeker Y, Tunali Y et al. (1999) The cardiorespiratory effects of laparoscopic procedures in infants. Anaesthesia 54:832–834

Bozkurt P, Kaya G, Altintas F et al. (2000) Systemic stress response during operations for acute abdominal pain performed via laparoscopy or laparotomy in children. Anaesthesia 55:5–9

Bozkurt P, Kaya G, Yeker Y et al. (2002) Arterial carbon dioxide markedly increases during diagnostic laparoscopy in portal hypertensive children. Anesth Analg 95:1236–1240

de Waal EEC, Kalkman CJ (2003) Haemodynamic changes during low-pressure carbon dioxide pneumoperitoneum in young children. Paediatr Anaesth 13:18–25

de Waal EEC, de Vries JW, Kruitwagen CLJJ et al. (2002) The effects of low-pressure carbon dioxide pneumoperitoneum on cerebral oxygenation and cerebral blood volume in children. Anesth Analg 94:500–505

Dunn MD, McDougall EM (2000) Laparoscopic considerations. Renal Physiol 27:609–614

Erkan N, Gokmen N, Goktay AY et al. (2001) Effects of CO_2 pneumoperitoneum on the basilar artery. Surg Endosc 15:806–811

Fondrinier E, Boisdron-Celle M, Chassevent A et al. (2001) Experimental assessment of tumor growth and dissemination of a microscopic peritoneal carcinomatosis after CO_2 peritoneal insufflation or laparotomy. Surg Endosc 15:843–848

Fujii Y, Tanaka H, Tsuruoka S, et al (1994) Middle cerebral arterial blood flow velocity increases during laparoscopic cholecystectomy. Anesth Analg 78:80–83

Fujimoto T, Lane GJ, Segawa O et al. (1999a) Laparoscopic extramucosal pyloromyotomy versus open pyloromyotomy for infantile hypertrophic pyloric stenosis: which is better? J Pediatr Surg 34:370–372

Fujimoto T, Segawa O, Lane GJ et al. (1999b) Laparoscopic surgery in newborn infants. Surg Endosc 13:773–777

Gentili A, Iannettone CM, Pigna A et al. (2000) Cardiocirculatory changes during videolaparoscopy in children: an echocardiographic study. Paediatr Anaesth 10:399–406

Gueugniaud PY, Abisseror M et al. (1998) The hemodynamic effects of pneumoperitoneum during laparoscopic surgery in healthy infants: assessment by continuous esophageal aortic blood flow echo-Doppler. Anesth Analg 86:290–293

Gupta A, Watson DI (2001) Effect of laparoscopy on immune function. Br J Surg 88:1296–1306

Hajri A, Mutter D, Wack S et al. (2000) Dual effect of laparoscopy on cell-mediated immunity. Eur Surg Res 32:261–266

Hamilton BD, Chow GK, Inman SR et al. (1998) Increased intra-abdominal pressure during pneumoperitoneum stimulates endothelin release in a canine model. J Endourol 12:193–197

Hansen TG, Tonnesen, Andersen JB et al. (1998) The peri-operative cytokine response in infants and young children following major surgery. Eur J Anaesth 15:56–60

Harman PK, Kron IL, McLachlan HD, et al (1982) Elevated intra-abdominal pressure and renal function. Ann Surg 196:594–597

Hendolin HI, Paakonen ME, Alhava EM et al. (2000) Laparoscopic or open cholecystectomy: a prospective randomised trail to compare postoperative pain, pulmonary function, and stress response. Eur J Surg 166:394–399

Holcomb GW 3rd (1999) Minimally invasive surgery for solid tumors. Semin Surg Oncol 16:184–192

Holthausen UH, Nagelschmidt M, Troidl H (1999) CO(2) pneumoperitoneum: what we know and what we need to know. World J Surg 23:794–800

Hsing CH, Hseu SS, Tsai SK et al. (1995) The physiological effect of CO_2 pneumoperitoneum in pediatric laparoscopy. Acta Anaesthesiol Sin 33:1–6

Huettemann E, Terborg C, Sakka SG et al. (2002) Preserved CO_2 reactivity and increase in middle cerebral arterial blood flow velocity during laparoscopic surgery in children. Anesth Analg 94:255–258

Iwanaka T, ;Arya G, Ziegler MM (1998) Mechanism and prevention of port-site tumor recurrence after laparoscopy in a murine model. J Pediatr Surg 33:457–461

Jackman SV, Weingart JD, Kinsman SL et al. (2000) Laparoscopic surgery in patients with ventriculoperitoneal shunts: safety and monitoring. J Urol 164:1352–1354

Jacobi CA, Bonjer HJ, Puttick MI et al. (2002a) Oncologic implications of laparoscopic and open surgery. Surg Endosc 16:441–445

Jacobi CA, Wenger F, Opitz I et al. (2002b) Immunologic changes during minimally invasive surgery. Dig Surg 19:459–463

Karayiannakis AJ, Makri GG, Mantzioka A et al. (1997) Systemic stress response after laparoscopic or open cholecystectomy: a randomized trial. Br J Surg 84:467–471

Kirsch AJ, Hensle TW, Chang DT (1994) Renal effects of CO_2 insufflation: oliguria and acute renal dysfunction in a rat model. Urology 43:453–459

Kitajima T, Shinohara M, Ogata H (1996) Cerebral oxygen metabolism measured by near-infrared laser spectroscopy during laparoscopic cholecystectomy with CO_2 insufflation. Surg Laparosc Endosc 6:210–212

Koivusalo AM, Kellokumpu I, Ristkari S et al. (1997) Splanchnic and renal deterioration during and after laparoscopic cholecystectomy: a comparison of the carbon dioxide pneumoperitoneum and the abdominal wall lift method. Anesth Analg 85:886–891

Laffon M, Gouchet A, Sitbon P et al. (1998) Difference between arterial and end-tidal carbon dioxide pressures during laparoscopy in paediatric patients. Can J Anaesth 45:561–563

Le Blanc-Louvry I, Coquerel A, Koning E et al. (2000) Operative stress response is reduced after laparoscopic compared to open cholecystectomy: the relationship with postoperative pain and ileus. Dig Dis Sci 45:1703–1713

Manner T, Aantaa R, Alanen M (1998) Lung compliance during laparoscopic surgery in paediatric patients. Paediatr Anaesth 8:25–29

Marcovich R, Williams AL, Seifman BD et al. (2001) A canine model to assess the biochemical stress response to laparoscopic and open surgery. J Endourol 15:1005–1008

Mattioli G, Montobbio G, Pini Prato A et al. (2003) Anesthesiologic aspects of laparoscopic fundoplication for gastroesophageal reflux in children with chronic respiratory and gastroenterological symptoms. Surg Endosc 17:559–566

McDougall EM, Monk TG, Wolf JS, et al (1996) The effect of prolonged pneumoperitoneum on renal function in an animal model. J Am Coll Surg 182:317–328

Mobbs RJ, Yang MO (2002) The dangers of diagnostic laparoscopy in the head injured patient. J Clin Neurosci 9:592–593

Neudecker J, Sauerland S, Neugebauer E et al. (2002) The European Association for Endoscopic Surgery clinical practice guideline on the pneumoperitoneum for laparoscopic surgery. Surg Endos 16:1121–1143

Neuhaus SJ, Watson DI, Ellis T et al. (2001) Metabolic and immunologic consequences of laparoscopy with helium or carbon dioxide insufflation: a randomized clinical study. Aust N Z J Surg 71:447–452

Rayman R, Girotti M, Armstrong K et al. (1995) Assessing the safety of pediatric laparoscopic surgery. Surg Laparosc Endosc 5:437–443

Razvi HA, Fields KLD, Vargas JC, et al (1996) Oliguria during laparoscopic surgery: evidence for direct renal parenchymal compression as an etiologic factor. J Endourol 10:1–4

Schäfer M, Krähenbühl L (2001) Effect of laparoscopy on intra-abdominal blood flow. Surgery 129:385–389

Schäfer M, Sägesser H, Krähenbühl L (2000) Liver and splanchnic hemodynamic changes in rats during laparoscopy. Surg Endosc 14:S216

Schilling MK, Redaelli C, Krähenbühl L et al. (1997) Splanchnic microcirculatory changes during CO_2 laparoscopy. J Am Coll Surg 184:378–382

Tobias JD, Holcomb GW (1997) Anesthetic management for laparoscopic cholecystectomy in children with decreased myocardial function: two case reports. J Pediatr Surg 32:743–746

Tobias JD, Holcomb GW 3rd, Brock JW 3rd et al. (1995) Cardiorespiratory changes in children during laparoscopy. J Pediatr Surg 30:33–36

Ure BM, Bax NMA, van der Zee DC (2000) Laparoscopy in infants and children: a prospective study on feasibility and the impact on routine surgery. J Pediatr Surg 35:1170–1173

Ure BM, Niewold TA, Bax NMA et al. (2002) Peritoneal, systemic, and distant organ immune responses are reduced by a laparoscopic approach and carbon dioxide vs air. Surg Endosc 16:836–842

Uzzo RG, Bilsky M, Mininberg DT et al. (1997) Laparoscopic surgery in children with ventriculoperitoneal shunts: effect of pneumoperitoneum on intracranial pressure-preliminary experience. Urology 49:753–757

van der Zee DC, Bax KMA, Sreeram N et al. (2003) Minimal access surgery in neonates with cardiac anomalies. IPEG oral abstracts

Walker DH, Langer JC (2000) Laparoscopic surgery in children with ventriculoperitoneal shunts. J Pediatr Surg 35:1104–1105

Warmann S, Fuchs J, Jesch NK et al. (2003) A prospective study on minimally invasive techniques in pediatric surgical oncology: preliminary report. Med Pediatr Oncol 40:155–157

Wildbrett P, Oh A, Naundorf D, Volk T et al. (2003) Impact of laparoscopic gases on peritoneal microenvironment and essential parameters of cell function. Surg Endosc 17:78–82

Wyatt JS, Edwards AD, Cope M, et al (1991) Response of cerebral blood volume to changes in arterial carbon dioxide tension in pre-term and term infants. Pediatr Res 29:553–557

Chapter 8

Complications of Endoscopic Surgery in Infants and Children

Jürgen Schleef

Introduction

A surgeon should be aware of the potential hazards, complications, and other morbidity of the operation that he or she is going to perform. Many potential complications are easy to avoid and are preventable.

Complications of surgery can be the result of mistakes or pitfalls which can occur during the procedure or are related to the indication itself. Unfortunately many complications related to the technique and the intervention are not recognized during the procedure. A critical discussion of the indication and a careful preoperative preparation of the surgeon, the team, and of course of the patient prevent many complications. Nevertheless even with careful preparation, complications can arise.

Problems arising during an endoscopic operation can be divided into four groups:

1. Problems related to instrumentation and equipment
2. Problems related to the intervention
3. Problems related to the creation of a working space, for example the insufflation of CO_2 and anesthesia
4. Problems related to the surgeon and the team

As was mentioned above, surgery can be influenced by different problems and aspects. In the beginning endosurgery was affected by many technical and strategic problems. We have been able to solve many of them, and endosurgery has become a real and valuable alternative to many open procedures. Nevertheless, there are still some problems and complications related to the endoscopic approach and intervention. Furthermore some differences exist between the typical risks of endoscopic surgery in the newborn and the adolescent (Fujimoto et al. 1999; Holland and Ford 1998; Waldschmidt and Schier 1991). ▄ Table 8.1 shows some special aspects of endoscopic surgery in the newborn and very small children. These relate to the limited working space, anatomical considerations, and anesthesia in the small child.

Table 8.1. Side effects and causes of possible complications in the very young infant

Anesthesia
– Potentially patent ductus arteriosus Botalli
– Ductus arteriosus may reopen during a laparoscopic/thoracoscopic procedure
– High intra-abdominal pressure decreases contractility and compliance of the left cardiac ventricle, which decreases the cardiac output
– High gas flow decreases body temperature and might cause hypothermia

Surgery
– Small working spaces
– Risk of tissue damage introducing cannulas
– Tiny abdominal structures (sliding of trocars)
– Fragile tissue
– Risk of omental prolapse (if trocar incisions are not closed properly)

Complications Related to Instrumentation and Equipment

Compared to traditional surgery endosurgery is highly technical and needs sophisticated equipment and instrumentation. This kind of "high tech surgery" is more sensitive to drop outs and malfunction. Technical failures can be potentially hazardous or might just lead to a longer operative time. Defects in the control of CO_2 flow and pressure can impair the ventilation and O_2 exchange and can be life threatening. Uncontrolled coagulation can lead to organ damage, perforation, or bleeding. Minor defects, for example a defective trocar valve, can lead to a constant loss of pressure which might reduce the overview and the ability to proceed in an appropriate and safe way with the procedure and often unnecessarily prolongs the operation time. A defective light cable might reduce the luminosity of the image and can impair the view of the operative field.

Cutting and Sealing by Energy Application

Severe complications due to defective instruments are rare. Typical problems related to the application of monopolar cautery may arise. The exact frequency of accidents with monopolar cautery is not known but the literature review gives some reports and episodically reported accidents (Swank et al. 2002). The general rule "do not handle instruments if you do not see them" is probably the most important one. Coagulation should be performed only under view and with instruments without insulation break (Berci 1994; Capelouto and Kavoussi 1993; Esposito et al. 2002). The contact to the tissue should be controlled and limited to the point where coagulation should take place. It should be remembered that the consequence of damage to tissue, for example the bowel, will depend not only on the degree of damage but also on whether the damage has been recognized or not. If recognized a repair can be carried out either endoscopically or open and most likely the patient will do well. In contrast unrecognized damage to the bowel may lead to severe complications (e.g. sepsis, peritonitis) (Jansen et al. 1997; Swank et al. 2002).

Different techniques for coagulation, cutting, and sealing of tissue are available: monopolar and bipolar electrocoagulation, ultrasonic energy, Ligasure®, and laser. The appropriate use of all these techniques seems to be safe. But we should be aware that the temperature of the tip of any of these instruments can be elevated and can cause unintended, uncontrolled burns (Awwad and Isaacson 1996). We experienced in one of our patients a temporary dysfunction (thermal damage?) of a phrenic nerve due to the use of ultrasonic energy to adjacent tissue (damage using the harmonic scalpel) without touching the nerve directly.

The author's own preference in routine surgery is bipolar coagulation. Other surgeons are using monopolar electrocoagulation, ultrasonic energy, Ligasure, and laser and feel comfortable and safe. Whichever method is used, we should remember that we are applying high energy and are using instruments that might become hot and destroy tissue, even if there is no application of energy at the time. Compared to bipolar cautery, monopolar cautery might be faster and easier to apply. Laser can be used in very small diameters (less than 1 mm) in non-contact or contact use.

Instruments

In recent years many different companies have offered a vast number of instruments of different length, size, and diameter. The smallest ones have a diameter of 2 mm and are suggested for use in newborns. But small instruments do not necessarily mean they are less trau-

matic. Touching bowel and other fragile tissue with 2 mm instruments might lead to greater damage to tissue than using, for example, soft 4- or 5 mm forceps. The pressure applied grasping the tissue is similar with both instruments, but as it is spread over a smaller area with the 2 mm forceps, it leads to more local tissue trauma than with the larger instruments (Becmeur and Besson 1998; Borer et al. 1999). In particular, in the situation of inflamed dilated bowel the trauma caused by grasping the bowel can lead to local ischemia followed by perforation.

Clip Applier and Stapler

Due to technical difficulties with knotting and suturing in endosurgery, clipping and stapling is very popular and used frequently. Many companies supply different kinds of instruments, non-disposable as well as disposable. Each stapler or clipping device is different in handling, therefore the surgeon should be aware how to use the instrument before it is applied.

Furthermore care should be taken in clipping vessels and similar tissue structures. The vessels should be carefully isolated and identified and blind clipping should always be avoided. Retracted vessels can cause occult bleeding. In one patient, the author experienced a severe bleeding from a cystic artery during a cholecystectomy due to dislocation of clips.

Staplers are supplied for different purposes, such as vessel occlusion and bowel anastomoses. Bowel staplers may be circular or linear. They are usually indicated for special situations and can be ordered with staples of different length. These staplers are however too big and too large to be used in small children. Linear staplers require a port of 12 mm! Moreover as these staplers are made for use in adults, the size of the staples in the cartridge is made for thick adult tissue. When applied in children the device may not staple or cut properly. Anastomotic leakage and again bleeding from retracted vessels may be the consequence (Niebuhl et al. 1993; Nord 1992; Peters 1995).

Clips or staples may drop during clipping or stapling. A few reports have been published in which bowel and choledochal perforations have been attributed to a lost clip (Tsumara et al. 2002; Yao et al. 2001). The exact incidence of this complication is not known, but one should be aware that lost clips may cause trouble and that they should be removed. For this reason dropped clips should be removed whenever possible. Some companies offer magnetic metal retrievers, which can be used for this purpose but only for magnetic metal clips.

Trocars

A wide variety of trocars both in size and as well as in technique of insertion do exist (Oshinsky and Smith 1992). Many of them are disposable and have a sliding security shield, which means that the knife is protected once the trocar is passed trough the parietal wall of the thorax or abdomen. Unfortunately in some instances this protection does not work properly, especially with the elastic peritoneum of small children. The consequence can be inadvertent damage to vessels, bowel, or lung tissue as it is documented by different authors (Almeida and Val-Gallas 1998; Champault et al. 1996; Geers and Holden 1996). If a blind puncture is performed as the first step in gaining access to a body cavity, the operative field should be checked immediately and meticulously for occult damage.

Devices for Specimen Removal

During many procedures, such as splenectomy, cholecystectomy, colon resection, tumor resection, and biopsies for different purposes, specimens have to be removed. For all these interventions there is a common problem: how to get a specimen through the parietal wall without a large incision. Many harvesting devices and specimen bags are available. Nevertheless, in small children these devices are to big to be used in the reduced abdominal or thoracic space. It is tempting to pull smaller specimens out through a trocar or even through a bare incision without protection. Typical complications are spillage of contaminated debris, loss of stones or tissue fragments, and in malignant disease probably implanted cells in the port incisions. The exact incidence is not known, but reports do exist (Anderson and Steven 1995), therefore careful handling of tissue during the extraction phase is mandatory. Specimen bags should be checked carefully for small holes or lacerations to avoid one of these very unpleasant complications (Esposito et al. 2001; Schleef and Morcate 2001).

Complications Related to the Intervention

General Complications

The approach via small incisions and trocars to the abdomen, the thorax, or extrapleural or extraperitoneal space is basically different in endosurgery from traditional incisions. The instillation of a pneumoperitoneum or even pneumothorax with mostly CO_2 is a special aspect of endoscopic procedures. Furthermore the surgeon misses three-dimensional (3-D) vision and lacks direct tactile sensation with direct palpation and feeling of tissue consistency, pulsation of vessels, and limits of organ structures.

Insertion of Trocars

Access to body cavities can be gained by blind puncture or open access. The blind puncture is usually performed with a Veress needle. Large studies in adult patients exist in the literature comparing complications (damage to vessels and parietal organs) between closed and open access (Begin 1993; Kazemier et al. 1999). According to these experiences "open laparoscopy" is safer than any closed method (Hasson 1971).

In order to avoid possible damage to persistent embryological structures such as an open omphaloenteric duct or open urachus, we perform a periumbilical incision on the left side of the umbilicus. Some surgeons gain access directly through the umbilicus, while others prefer an infraumbilical incision. When using direct access through the umbilicus, the author experienced a case of a small umbilical hernia with fixed bowel in it.

Once the peritoneum is open, a purse-string suture is established and a blunt trocar is introduced (Fig. 8.1). During the procedure the suture fixes the trocar and is helpful in closing the incision at the end after removing the trocar, thus avoiding a peritoneal problem with omental prolapse. Omental prolapse, mostly umbilical, presents in many series, as in our own with small children, as the most frequent abdominal wall complication (Bloom and Ehrlich 1993; Schleef 2002; Ure et al. 2000). This complication usually requires careful wound inspection and closure under general anesthesia.

After the introduction of the first trocar and installation of a CO_2 pneumoperitoneum, secondary trocars can be inserted. The introduction of these secondary trocars is performed generally under direct puncture of the abdomen and should be performed under direct endoscopic vision and control. Especially in small children a secondary trocar can be placed by introducing it in the direction of the first cannula to avoid damage to bowel and vessels (Fig. 8.2).

Port Site Complications

These complications can be either primary or secondary.

Primary Complications

Primary complications are problems occurring during puncture of the abdomen, changing of trocars, or reintroducing of trocars during the procedure (Apelgren and Scheeres 1994; Esposito et al. 1997; Oza et al. 1992). A rare problem is bleeding from the port site. This can be detected immediately or later during the procedure and can cause bothersome bleeding after

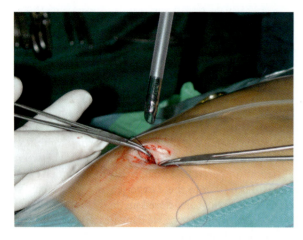

Fig. 8.1. Open laparoscopy using a paraumbilical incision. Introduction of the first trocar. For better viewing during this procedure in small children we use a transparent disposable trocar, which is fixed by a purse-string suture

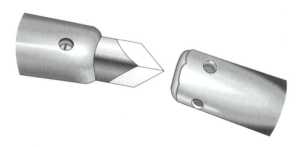

Fig. 8.2. A trocar is introduced while another trocar is used as a guide and protection shield to avoid tissue damage

the operation. Our own experienced of this was the port site bleeding (from a trocar incision) after a laparoscopic cholecystectomy in a very obese boy with a secondary infected hematoma.

Ports should be placed where no abdominal wall vessels can be expected or seen in thin abdominal walls in small children. A knife should be used only for the skin incision. Cutting with the knife down through the peritoneum is not recommended since a vessel might be cut and occluded during the procedure by the pressure on the surrounding tissue by the trocar. Repositioning a slipped trocar is better performed over a blunt instrument introduced through the trocar incision first to avoid the creation of a second wall incision near to the original one. Such repositioning, like any endoscopic procedure, should of course be performed under endoscopic control. Also the removal of trocars should be controlled under direct vision. A bleeding might be discovered retracting the trocar. Many of these bleedings from port sites will disappear during the procedure due to the compression of the vessels by the trocar. If the bleeding persists a suture should be

placed in order to close the bleeding structure. In severe cases a suture through the abdominal wall might be placed and tied over the skin, for example with an Endoclose (Tyco). After 3 days the suture can be removed.

Secondary Complications

A typical secondary port site complication is herniation (Holzinger and Klaiber 2002). It can be a palpable hernia only without herniated tissue or even an incarcerated hernia. Many reports exist in the literature. Mostly 10 mm trocars have been in place but, especially in smaller children, hernias might occur also with smaller ports (Nakajima et al. 1999). The author's own experiences include a 5 mm port site hernia after laparoscopic splenectomy, being asymptomatic at the beginning and showing signs of incarceration after 2 years (requiring a surgical intervention), and a 3 mm port site hernia without symptoms in a baby after fundoplication. Adaptation of the fascia should be attempted whenever possible in order to reduce the risk of this bothersome problem. In adult patients special needles are used by some authors to close the fascia as well as the peritoneum. Unfortunately these devices are usually too large for the use in children.

Care has to be taken if children complain of pain in the region of port sites. This can be due to irritation of an adjacent nerve and is a very difficult problem to handle. Another cause can be an adhesion of the bowel, mesentery, or omentum to the former peritoneal incision of a port site. In these cases an ultrasound might be helpful to clarify the situation, as we experienced in two children after appendectomy. There was no palpable hernia but there was a peritoneal adhesion which needed to be removed.

A very difficult subject is the problem of port site metastasis. There are case reports in the adult literature (Champault et al. 1996), but none in the pediatric surgical literature. The reason for this could be that the number of laparoscopic procedures for malignant disease in children is small. Moreover the indication in adults is usually carcinoma. In children the indication is usually tissue diagnosis for suspected lymphoma or resection of small neuroblastomas, which usually require vigorous consecutive chemotherapy. In any case there is no evidence to substantiate that endosurgery is contraindicated in children with solid tumors (Holcomb et al. 1995; Saenz et al. 1997; Schleef et al. 1998; Waldhausen et al. 2000). In the practical guidelines of the European Association for Endoscopic Surgery (EAES) regarding pneumoperitoneum, it is put forward that there are no contraindications to pneumoperitoneum in patients with intra-abdominal malignancy provided that a number of precautions are taken, such as protecting the port site holes from direct contact with the specimen (Neudecker et al. 2002).

Retraction of Tissue and Organs

In endosurgery the retraction and handling of tissue and organs is an unsolved problem in many instances. Many different devices for organ retraction are available, but many of them are traumatic or insufficient. Forceps are used to retract bowel, stomach, or the liver. In small children this might cause organ damage, bleeding, and, in the worst case, perforation of intestinal structures. These incidents are not reported frequently, but have to be regarded as a rare but very serious problem. We experienced a gastric perforation during a Heller myotomy after grasping and retracting the stomach. The hole was detected during the procedure and could be closed.

A liver retractor might be displaced during the procedure and perforate the liver capsule. This can cause bleeding which might need conversion, especially in small children. We usually use a forceps to retract the liver, grasping the diaphragm. This might reduce the risk of perforation by dislocation during the operation. All tissue and organs that have been retracted or grasped should be checkednnn at the end of the procedure to avoid unrecognized damage (Esposito et al. 2001a,b).

Specific Complications

Minimal access (invasive) surgery is usually performed under similar circumstances as open, conventional surgery regarding the indication and the surgical strategy. Nevertheless there are differences between the open and the minimal access approach. These differences also account for specific complications, which occur rarely or occur in different forms during open surgery. The endoscopic operation does not always mimic the conventional open approach, and this can sometimes be advantageous and sometimes disadvantageous. In the following sections the most frequently performed procedures will be discussed concerning specific and typical complications.

Appendectomy

Laparoscopic appendectomy in children is performed in different ways. Many surgeons favorite the "in" technique, while others perform the "out" technique (El-Ghoneimi et al. 1994). A few reports exist of damage to vessels and bleeding during and after a laparoscopic appendectomy (Juricic 1994). In particular, when the appendix is embedded in an inflammatory mass, care should be taken and even experienced surgeons report a number of conversions to open surgery (Ure et al. 2000). According to the literature there is a higher risk of intra-abdominal abscess formation in the laparoscopic group, while the overall infection rate is reduced in the laparoscopic group (Eypasch et al. 2002). The

matter of an increased incidence of intra-abdominal abscesses after laparoscopic appendectomy has not been settled yet. In a recent Cochrane review it was concluded that there may be an increased incidence of intra-abdominal abscesses after laparoscopic removal of gangrenous or perforated appendix. Is was said, however, that the quality of the available research data was mediocre (Sauerland et al. 2002). As in open surgery the spillage of contaminated material should always be avoided at every step of the procedure. In some conditions early stump abscesses can be observed. This situation should be kept in mind in complicated postoperative courses after a laparoscopic appendectomy (Chikamori et al. 2002). Recurrent appendicitis (appendicitis after appendicectomy) has also been described, which underscores that the appendix should be prepared to its basis and removed completely.

Fundoplication

Fundoplication has several complications, both intraoperative and postoperative, with short- and long-term sequelae (Pessaux et al. 2002). They are well known and described in the literature (Esposito et al. 2000). The laparoscopic approach is not affected by "typical" access-related complications. During the learning curve many surgeons described a higher incidence of esophageal perforation, postoperative dysphagia, and problems with gastrostomies performed in the same session (Allal et al. 2001). But in the meantime results are comparable to the open technique and there is no specific laparoscopic complication (Hüttl et al. 2002; Mattioli et al. 2003).

Pyloromyotomy

The endoscopic treatment of pyloric hypertrophy is still not comparable concerning the rate of complication to the conventional surgery. A higher rate of perforation and incomplete myotomy is described by many authors. This incidence of complications is falling in all series as experience is gained and as better knives and spreaders for performing the procedure become available. But it is still slightly higher even in experienced groups (Campbell et al. 2002; Sitsen et al. 1998).

Splenectomy

With gaining experience the incidence of conversion due to injury of vessels, the stomach, and the spleen itself is constantly decreasing. The handling of the tissue and vessels – in the past a severe problem especially with larger organs – is no longer a problem due to new cutting and sealing devices and more sophisticated grasping instruments (Schleef et al. 1997). The laparoscopic approach does not have a typical complication concerning the operative technique, which is very similar to open surgery. Splenosis due to a hole in the harvesting bag or a laceration of the capsule with spillage of splenic tissue are described. Nevertheless the author's own series and series of other groups do not reflect a higher rate of complications in laparoscopic versus open splenectomy (Rescorla et al. 1998). The detection of accessory spleens has to be performed very carefully to avoid recurrent disease (Esposito et al. 2001b). In the adult literature splenic vein thrombosis is described after laparoscopic splenectomy. This has not been observed in the pediatric literature so far.

Cholecystectomy

The numbers of cholecystectomies in children are much lower than in adults. The technique of surgery is comparable (Esposito et al. 2001a). Large studies exists in adult patients comparing the incidents of complications between the laparoscopic and the open approach. A difference exists concerning the rate of damage to the choledochal duct, which is higher in all major studies in the laparoscopic group (Svanvik 2000). This damage could be related to the use of cautery during preparation near to the choledochal structures or to incorrect application of the clip, but patient-related factors such as severe cystitis with scar formation also play a role. Arterial bleeding and blind clamping predisposes for common bile duct injury (Buell et al. 2002). The number of cholecystectomies in children is too small to verify this finding in the pediatric age group. The conclusion should be to avoid preparation of the vascular and biliary structures during a cholecystectomy if the anatomy is not clear.

Other Procedures

Many other procedures are performed using an endosurgical approach in small infants and children. Thoracoscopy as well as retroperitoneal surgery for renal and adrenal pathology are becoming more and more popular (Diamond et al. 1995; Peters 1995; Rassweiler et al. 1998; Rogers et al. 1992). Nevertheless there are insufficient published cases to give a clear answer concerning "typical" procedure-related complications (El-Ghoneimi et al. 1994).

Interaction Between the Pneumoperitoneum and Anesthesia

To provide an adequate view in different cavities of the human body (abdomen, retroperitoneum) insufflation of gas is required. Even in the chest CO_2 may be insufflated in order to create working space.

A pneumoperitoneum is a non-physiological condition with many possible side effects, related both to pressure and to the use of CO_2. The general effects of the pneumoperitoneum on respiratory function and hemodynamic parameters are discussed elsewhere.

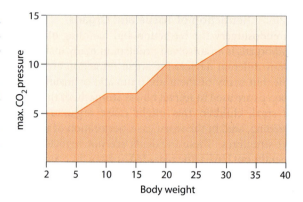

Fig. 8.3. Diagram showing the maximum CO_2 pressure (expressed in mmHg) in relation to the bodyweight of the patient, as has been used by the author for many years

Other consequences are an increased intracranial pressure and decreased perfusion of splanchnic organs. Moreover backflow to the heart can be reduced and stasis in the venous system of the lower limbs might be possible (Pennant 2001; Wazz et al. 2000). All these mentioned side effects can not be regarded as complications but have to be observed as a source of possible complications in high-risk patients [newborns, cardiac insufficiency, elevated cranial pressure, patients with coagulopathy (Dabrowiecki et al. 1997)]. All these side effects are pressure related and increase with increased abdominal pressure and with the duration of the operation. Therefore the pressure should be limited and adjusted according to the operative space and the size, age, and status of the patient (Mattioli et al. 2003). De Waal et al. published recently that a pressure of 5 mmHg does not affect the respiratory and cardiac function in small infants. We found that in a 3-month-old child even a pressure of 5 mmHg was not tolerated and the procedure, a fundoplication, had to be converted. This child had respiratory problems due to recurrent aspirations and prolonged ventilator therapy after birth. Generally, pneumoperitoneum, adjusted to the size and age of the patient, is well tolerated. For many years we have used the diagram shown in ■ Fig. 8.3 as a guideline for the maximal applied abdominal pressure. This guideline is based on our own experience, but correlates well with data published by others (de Waal and Kalkman 2003; de Waal et al. 2002).

We have very limited experience with mechanical abdominal wall lifting, which appears to be very traumatic especially in small children. According to the EAES guideline regarding pneumoperitoneum, abdominal wall lifting has no clinically relevant advantages above low pressure (5–7 mmHg) pneumoperitoneum (Neudecker et al. 2002).

A further problem might be the heat loss of the patient during longer procedures. Especially in small children and newborns adjusting the room temperature, using tools such as warming pads, and warming the gas might avoid severe complications (Fujimoto et al. 1999; Sugi et al. 1998). The most important factor in the prevention of hypothermia during endoscopic surgery is to avoid the use of high volumes of CO_2. In the extraperitoneal approach and situations where a subcutaneous emphysema is present, a higher absorption of CO_2 might be possible and is described in adults (Wolf et al. 1995). This is certainly not the experience of pediatric surgeons who use this approach regularly.

The Surgeon and the Team

There is little doubt that the experience and skills of a particular surgeon are of the utmost importance in the outcome. Some risk factors are always related to the skills and experience of the surgeon and the team in the operation room. But even a skilled surgeon with considerable experience in classic pediatric surgery starts as a beginner in endosurgery, and due to the different situations (e.g., operating without direct view; having a two-dimensional image; working at a distance with different instruments; no finger–tissue contact and lack of tactile feedback; different suturing and knotting technique) an easy procedure might become difficult surgery. Every surgeon who performs endosurgery has to realize that these special aspects, as mentioned above, are mandatory for performing secure endosurgical procedures and obtaining results comparable with conventional surgery. The learning curve for demanding endoscopic surgery is fairly long and some authors (Chang et al. 2001) believe that about 100 endoscopic operations are necessary to gain the experience for performing routine endosurgery in newborns. Nevertheless, every surgeon starts with simple diagnostic and therapeutic interventions and, as experience is gained, more demanding procedures can be performed.

Typical complications related to the inexperienced surgeon are tissue damage while introducing instruments without view, uncontrolled coagulation due to confused reaction using the wrong pedal, and hazardous preparation due to the lack of experience in the interpretation of the two-dimensional image (Soot et al. 1999). Not only can the surgeon be a risk factor but also the assisting team. A camera operator who is impatient and not familiar with the procedure might cause even a trained endosurgeon trouble.

Therefore the following recommendations should be followed:

1. The steps of the operation to be performed should be familiar to all members of the surgical team.
2. Instruments and equipment and their handling have to be checked before the procedure.
3. The surgeon should be familiar with the instruments that are available, especially coagulation equipment, clip applier, and complex instruments such as laser or ultrasound scalpel.
4. A first case would be better operated in the presence of or with the help of an experienced endosurgeon, even if the surgeon is very familiar with the open technique.
5. The parents should be informed about the experience of the surgeon carrying out the scheduled procedure and the possibility of conversion. The consent form should include typical and specific aspects and sequelae of the endoscopic approach.
6. A conversion to open surgery should be considered before an intraoperative complication occurs.

Conclusion

The field of endosurgery in children is constantly expanding and growing. Many reports in the literature can be found about new procedures, new techniques, and modified approaches. Prospective studies are rare and numbers of patients are small. Accordingly, an analysis of complications is difficult, since it is based usually on retrospective, multicenter observations. Many studies represent an overview over a long period of time including the individual learning curve. But this dynamic process shows that problems, which occurred more often during the early period of endosurgery, are reduced by changing techniques, better equipment, and naturally gained experience.

Nevertheless complications related to instruments and surgical technique (open access, trocar placement) will always exist in relation to the standard of accuracy and experience with which a procedure is performed. As was mentioned before, many of the complications observed might be avoidable. If we follow the recommendations and if we analyze our complications by reviewing videos, there will be a process of constant learning which will result in prevention.

References

Allal H, Captier G, Lopez M et al. (2001) Evaluation of 142 consecutive laparoscopic fundoplications in children: effects of the learning curve and technical choice. J Pediatr Surg 36:921–926

Almeida OD Jr, Val-Gallas JM (1998) Small trocar perforation of the small bowel: a case report. J Soc Laparoendosc Surg 2:289–290

Anderson JR, Steven K (1995) Implantation of metastasis after laparoscopic biopsy of bladder cancer. J Urol 153:1044–1048

Apelgren KN, Scheeres DE (1994) Aorta injury, a catastrophic complication of laparoscopic cholecystectomy. Surg Endosc 8:689–691

Awwad JT, Isaacson K (1996) The harmonic scalpel: an intraoperative complication. Obstet Gynecol 8:718–720

Becmeur F, Besson R (1998) Treatment of small-bowel obstruction by laparoscopy in children a multicentric study. GECI. Groupe d'Etude en Coeliochirurgie Infantile. Eur J Pediatr Surg 8:343–346

Begin FG (1993) Création du pneumopéritoine sous contrôle visuel. J Coeliochir 5:18–20

Berci G (1994) Complications of laparoscopic surgery. Surg Endosc 8:165–168

Bloom DA, Erhlich RM (1993) Omental evisceration through small laparoscopy port sites. J Endourol 7:31–32

Borer JG, Cisek LJ, Atala A et al. (1999) Pediatric retroperitoneoscopic nephrectomy using 2 mm instrumentation. J Urol 162:1725–1730

Buell JF, Cronin DC, Funaki B et al. (2002) Devastating and fatal complications associated with combined vascular and bile duct injuries during cholecystectomy. Arch Surg 137:703–708

Campbell BT, McLean K, Barnhart DC et al. (2002) A comparison of laparoscopic and open pyloromyotomy at a teaching hospital. J Pediatr Surg 37:1068–1071

Capelouto CC, Kavoussi LR (1993) Complications of laparoscopic surgery. Urology 42:2–12

Champault G, Cazacu F, Taffinder N (1996) Serious trocar accidents in laparoscopic surgery: a French survey of 103,852 operations. Surg Laparosc Endosc 6:367–370

Chang JH, Rothenberg SS, Bealer JF et al. (2001) Endosurgery and the senior pediatric surgeon. J Pediatr Surg 36:690–692

Chikamori F, Kuniyoshi N, Shibuya S et al. (2002) Appendiceal stump abscess as an early complication of laparoscopic appendectomy: report of a case. Surg Today 32:919–921

Dabrowiecki S, Rosc D, Jurkowski P (1997) The influence of laparoscopic cholecystectomy on perioperative blood clotting and fibrinolysis. Blood Coagul Fibrinolysis 8:1–5

De Waal EE, Kalkman CJ (2003) Hemodynamic changes during low-pressure carbon dioxide pneumoperitoneum in young children. Paediatr Anaesth 13:18–25

De Waal EE, de Vries JW, Kruitwagen CL et al. CJ (2002) The effect of low-pressure carbon dioxide pneumoperitoneum on cerebral oxygenisation and cerebral blood volume in children. Anesth Analg 94:500–505

Diamond DA, Price HM, McDougall EM et al. (1995) Retroperitoneal laparoscopic nephrectomy in children. J Urol 153:1966–1968

El-Ghoneimi A, Valla JS, Limonne B et al. (1994) Laparoscopic appendectomy in children: report of 1379 cases. J Pediatr Surg 29:786–789

El-Ghoneimi A, Valla JS, Steyaert H et al. (1998) Laparoscopic renal surgery via a retroperitoneal approach in children. J Urol 160:1138–1141

Esposito C, Ascione G, Garipoli V et al. (1997) Complications of pediatric laparoscopic surgery. Surg Endosc 11:655–657

Esposito C, Montupet P, Amici G et al. (2000) Complications of laparoscopic antireflux surgery in childhood. Surg Endosc 4:622–624

Esposito C, Gonzalez Sabin MA et al. (2001a) Results and complications of laparoscopic cholecystectomy in childhood. Surg Endosc 15:890–892

Esposito C, Schaarschmidt K, Settimi A, et al. (2001b) Pitfalls and secrets of laparoscopic splenectomy. J Pediatr Surg 5:970–973

Esposito C, Mattioli G, Monguzzi GL et al. (2002) Complications and conversions of pediatric videosurgery: the Italian multicentric experience on 1689 procedures. Surg Endosc 16:795–798

Eypasch E, Sauerland S, Lefering R et al. (2002) Laparoscopic versus open appendectomy: between evidence and common sense. Dig Surg 19:518–522

Fujimoto T, Segawa O, Lane GJ et al. (1999) Laparoscopic surgery in newborn infants. Surg Endosc 13:773–777

Geers J, Holden C (1996) Major vascular injury as a complication of laparoscopic surgery: a report of three cases and review of the literature. Am Surg 62:377–379

Hasson H (1971) Modified instrument and method for laparoscopy. Am J Obstet Gynecol 110:886–887

Holcomb GW 3rd, Tomita SS, Haase GM et al. (1995) Minimally invasive surgery in children with cancer. Cancer 76:121–128

Holland AJA, Ford WDA (1998) The influence of laparoscopic surgery on perioperative heat loss in children. Pediatr Surg Int 13:350–351

Holzinger F, Klaiber C (2002) Trokarhernien, eine seltene, potenziell gefährliche Komplikation nach laparoskopischen Eingriffen. Chirurg 73:899–904

Hüttl TP, Hohle M, Meyer G et al. (2002) Antirefluxchirurgie in Deutschland. Ergebnisse einer repräsentativen Umfrage mit Analyse von 2540 Antirefluxoperationen. Chirurg 73:451–461

Jansen FW, Kapiteyn K, Trimbos-Kemper T et al. (1997) Complications of laparoscopy: a prospective multicentre observational study. Br J Obstet Gynaecol 104:595–600

Juricic M, Bossavy JP, Izard I et al. (1994) Laparoscopy appendectomy: case report of vascular injury in two children. Eur J Pediatr Surg 4:327–328

Kazemier G, Hazebroek EJ, Lange JF et al. (1999) Needle and trocar injury during laparoscopic surgery in Japan. Surg Endosc 13:194

Mattioli G, Montobbio G, Pini Prato A et al. (2003) Anesthesiologic aspects of laparoscopic fundoplication for gastroesophageal reflux in children with chronic respiratory and gastroenterological symptoms. Surg Endosc 17:559–566

Nakajima K, Wasa M, Kawahara H et al. (1999) Revision laparoscopy for incarcerated hernia at a 5 mm trocar site following pediatric laparoscopic surgery. Surg Laparosc Endosc Percutan Tech 9:294–295

Neudecker J, Sauerland S, Neugebauer E et al. (2002) The European Association for Endoscopic Surgery clinical practical guideline on the pneumoperitoneum for laparoscopic surgery. Surg Endosc 16:1121–1143

Niebuhl H, Nahrestedt U, Ruckert K et al. (1993) Laparoscopic surgery: mistakes and risks when the method is introduced. Surg Endosc 7:412–415

Nord HJ (1992) Complications of laparoscopy. Endoscopy 24:693–700

Oshinsky G, Smith AD (1992) Laparoscopic needle and trocar: an overview of design and complications. J Laparoendosc Surg 2:117–125

Oza KN, O'Donnell N, Fisher JB (1992) Aortic laceration: a rare complication of laparoscopy. J Laparoendosc Surg 2:235–237

Pennant JH (2001) Anesthesia for laparoscopy in the pediatric patient. Anesthesiol Clin North Am 19:69–88

Pessaux P, Arnaud JP, Ghavami B et al. (2002) Morbidity of laparoscopic fundoplication for gastroesophageal reflux: a retrospective study about 1470 patients. Hepatogastroenterology 49:447–450

Peters CA (1995) Complications in pediatric urological laparoscopy: results of a survey. J Urol 155:1070–1073

Rassweiler JJ, Seemann O, Frede T et al. (1998) Retroperitonoscopy: experience with 200 cases. J Urol 160:1265–1269

Rescorla FJ, Breitfeld PP, West KW et al. (1998) A case controlled comparison of open and laparoscopic splenectomy in children. Surgery 124:670–675

Rogers DA, Philippe PG, Lobe TE et al. (1992) Thoracoscopy in children: an initial experience with an evolving technique. J Laparoendosc Surg 2:7–14

Saenz NC, Conlon KC, Aronson DC et al. (1997) The application of minimal access procedures in infants, children, and young adults with pediatric malignancies. J Laparoendosc Adv Surg Tech A 7:289–294

Sauerland S, Lefering R, Neugebauer EA (2002) Laparoscopic versus open surgery for suspected appendicitis. Cochrane Database Syst Rev CD001546

Schleef J, Morcate JJ (2001) Laparoscopic splenectomy in children. Present state and future aspects. J Coelio Chir 37:59–65

Schleef J, Morcate JJ, Steinau G et al. (1997) Technical aspects of laparoscopic splenectomy in children. J Pediatr Surg 32:615–617

Schleef J, Morcate JJ, Wagner A et al. (1998) Laparoscopia diagnóstica en tumores abdominales infantiles: una alternativa a la laparotomiá. Cir Pediatr 11:109–111

Sitsen E, Bax NM, van der Zee DC (1998) Is laparoscopic pyloromyotomy superior to open surgery? Surg Endosc 12:813–815

Soot SJ, Eshraghi N, Farahmand M (1999) Transition from open to laparoscopic fundoplication: the learning curve. Arch Surg 134:278–281

Sugi K, Katoh T, Gohra H et al. (1998) Progressive hyperthermia during thoracoscopic procedures in infants and children. Paediatr Anaesth 8:211–214

Svanvik J (2000) Results of laparoscopic compared with open cholecystectomy. Eur J Surg 585:12–15

Swank DJ, van Erp WFM, Repelaer van Driel OJ et al. (2002) Complications and feasibility of laparoscopic adhesiolysis in patients with chronic abdominal pain. A retrospective study. Surg Endosc 16:1468–1473

Tsumara H, Ichikawa T, Kagawa T, et al. (2002) Failure of endoscopic removal of common bile duct stones due to endo-clip migration following laparoscopic cholecystectomy. J Hepatobiliary Pancreat Surg 9:274–277

Ure BM, Bax NM, van der Zee DC (2000) Laparoscopy in infants and children: a prospective study on feasibility and the impact on routine surgery. J Pediatr Surg 35:1170–1173

Waldhausen JH, Tapper D, Sawin RS (2000) Minimally invasive surgery and clinical decision-making for pediatric malignancy. Surg Endosc 14:250–253

Waldschmidt J, Schier F (1991) Laparoscopical surgery in neonates and infants. Eur J Pediatr Surg 1:145–150

Wazz G, Branicki F, Taji H et al. (2000) Influence of pneumoperitoneum on the deep venous system during laparoscopy. J Soc Laparoendosc Surg 4:291–295

Wolf JS, Monk TG, McDougall EM (1995) The extraperitoneal approach and subcutaneous emphysema are associated with greater absorption of carbon dioxide during laparoscopic renal surgery. J Urol 154:959–963

Yao CC, Wong HH, Chen CC et al. (2001) Migration of endoclip into the duodenum. A rare complication after laparoscopic cholecystectomy. Surg Endosc 15:217

Neck

Cervicoscopy, a Minimally Invasive Approach for the Thyroid, Parathyroid, and Thymus in Children

Olivier Reinberg

Introduction

Since the beginning of the 1990s minimally invasive endoscopic techniques have been applied for surgery in natural body cavities such as the thorax and abdomen of children. The pediatric surgeon had to be trained to work in limited spaces. With the improvement in technical skills in endoscopic surgery and the development of thinner and shorter instruments, new spaces have become accessible to endoscopic surgery. With the aid of CO_2 pneumodissection virtual spaces, for example the retroperitoneum, can be turned into to real spaces allowing for endoscopic surgery in these areas.

In 1996, Gagner published the first case of subtotal resection of the parathyroids via a cervical endoscopic approach in a 37-year-old man. The operation lasted five hours, and the only problems encountered were hypercarbia and tachycardia. Other such experiences have been reported, both in animal experiments as well as in human adults (Naitoh et al. 1998; Norman and Albrink 1997). In 1997, at the first course of endocrine endosurgery at the European Institute of Telesurgery (EITS) in Strasbourg, France, Gagner, Marescaux, and colleagues demonstrated their technique of endoscopic neck operations both in animals as well as in adult human patients, and discussed the potential hazards as well as the measures to avoid them.

In 1997, Hüscher et al. reported their first endoscopic right thyroid lobectomy for a 4 mm adenoma. A year later Yeung (1998) reported his experience on three endoscopic parathyroidectomies for adenomas and five endoscopic hemithyroidectomies, which were carried out without any complication. These preliminary experiences demonstrated that endoscopic dissection and surgical intervention of the neck were technically feasible and safe.

After having performed two video-assisted thymectomies in children in 1996 (Reinberg 1998) we changed to a totally closed approach in five additional cases by so-called cervicomediastinoscopy (Reinberg and Montupet 1999, 2000). Meanwhile this minimally invasive method has been successfully used for thyroid and parathyroid surgery as well. The surgical technique for both the thyroid and parathyroids as well as for the thymus will be described in detail.

Cervicoscopic Thyroidectomy and Parathyroidectomy

Preoperative Preparation

General anesthesia with endotracheal intubation is used. The end-tidal CO_2 is monitored with special care, and the ventilator settings are adjusted accordingly.

Positioning

Patient
The patient is placed in a supine position (■ Fig. 9.1). The neck is slightly hyperextended, but less than in conventional surgery, as has been advocated by Gagner (■ Fig. 9.2).

Crew and Equipment
The surgeon stands to the right of the patient with the scrub nurse to his right and the assistant opposite (■ Fig. 9.1). Two monitors are used, one at each side of the head of the patient.

Special Equipment
Short 3 mm-diameter instruments are used. Bipolar electrocoagulation is essential.

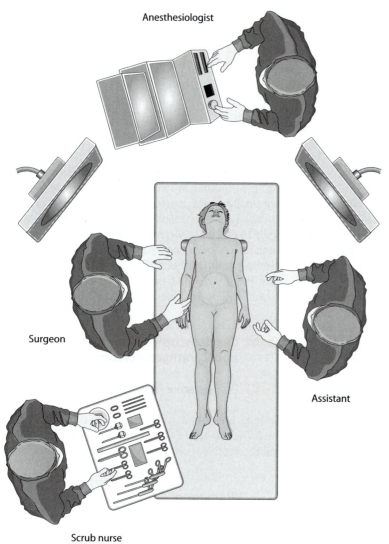

Anesthesiologist

Surgeon

Assistant

Scrub nurse

Fig. 9.1. Position of patient, crew, and equipment for thyroidectomy and parathyroidectomy

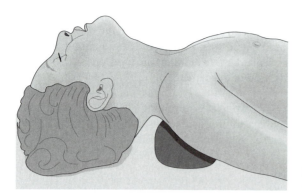

Fig. 9.2. Hyperextension of the neck, but less than in conventional surgery

Technique

Cannulae

Cannula	Method of insertion	Diameter (mm)	Device	Position
1	Open	5	Optic 25°	Suprasternal notch
2	Closed	3	Babcock, bipolar, scissors	Right lower sternomastoid muscle
3	Closed	3	Babcock, bipolar, scissors	Left lower sternomastoid muscle

Procedure

A 10 mm transversal incision is made just above the suprasternal notch (■ Fig. 9.3). An open dissection is performed first through the superficial fascia and then through the deeper fascia of the neck, between the anterior borders of the sternohyoid muscles and down to the pretracheal space (■ Fig. 9.4a,b). The midline venous structures have to be avoided, or ligated and divided if necessary, to prevent any bleeding.

A 5 mm cannula with a 45° beveled end is inserted into the wound under direct vision (■ Fig. 9.5). A purse-string suture, taking the platysma as well as the skin, is tied around the cannula in order to achieve an airtight seal and to prevent the cannula from slipping out (■ Fig. 9.6). A 4 mm 25° 170 mm-long telescope is inserted and CO_2 is insufflated at an initial pressure of 12 mmHg in order to initiate surgical emphysema (■ Fig. 9.7). Once a good space has been created, the

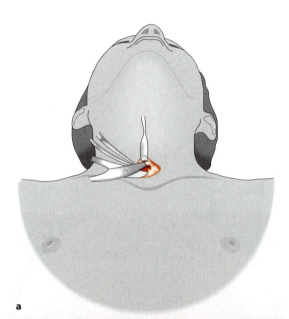

a

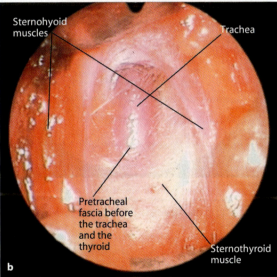

Sternohyoid muscles

Trachea

Pretracheal fascia before the trachea and the thyroid

Sternothyroid muscle

b

Fig. 9.4. a Dissection of the platysma on the median line. **b** Severing the cervical muscles on the median line. The trachea becomes visible

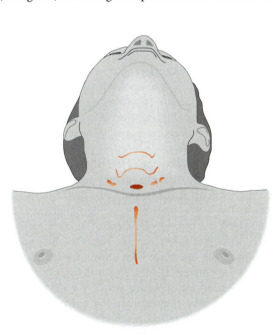

Fig. 9.3. Position of incision

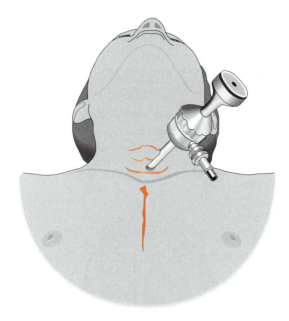

Fig. 9.5. Insertion of first port in close contact with the trachea

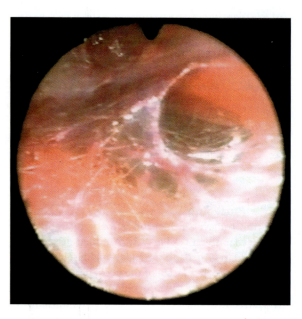

Fig. 9.7. The soft prethyroidal fascia as it appears before insufflation

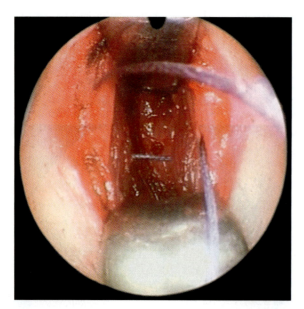

Fig. 9.6. Securing the telescope's trocar by a purse-string suture taking in the superficial fascia (platysma layer) and the skin

pressure can be decreased to 6–8 mmHg. Pneumodissection separates the soft prethyroidal fascia and lifts the anterior cervical muscles away from the thyroid, thus developing a working space. Pneumodissection is further facilitated by the gentle motion of the telescope. During the creation of the working space, the surgeon has to be patient as this step of the procedure takes a few minutes.

Once enough space has been created, two 3 mm-diameter short reusable Teflon ports for the working instruments are inserted 3 cm from the midline on each side through the sternomastoid muscle, but under endoscopic control thus avoiding injury to the internal jugular vein (■ Fig. 9.8a,b). Such Teflon ports are advantageous as they are light weight (■ Fig. 9.9). Eighteen-centimeter-long pediatric atraumatic instruments are passed through them. Gentle backward and forward movements with these instruments facilitate further pneumodissection and widen the working space. With a 3 mm monopolar hook, or scissors, remaining firm fibers are cut. Crossing veins are coagulated with a 3 mm bipolar electrocautery. The dissection needs to be bloodless as any blood will obscure the image.

Attention is paid to one of the thyroid lobes, for example the left one. First, the inferior pole is approached. A 3 mm Babcock forceps is inserted through the right port and serves as a retractor while the gland is dissected with a 3 mm bipolar electrocautery forceps inserted through the left port (■ Fig. 9.10). The magnification of the operative field allows for an excellent view of the different tissues. Pneumodissection eliminates the need for an active search for the recurrent laryngeal nerves as they can easily be seen (■ Fig. 9.11). By turning the 25° telescope, the thyroid gland can be clearly seen from the lateral and posterior side as well. The lateral edge of the thyroid gland can be elevated without dividing the vascular pedicle, which greatly facilitates the identification of the parathyroid glands. They look like buff-colored glands against the pink

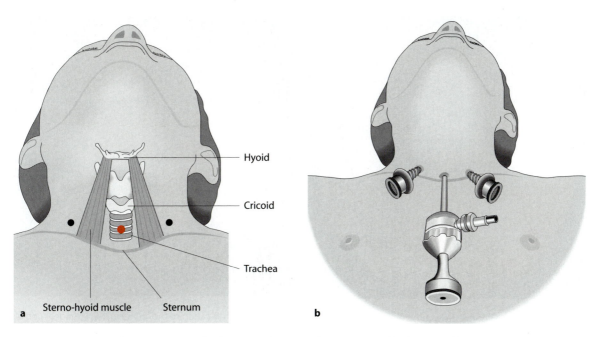

Fig. 9.8 a,b. Position of the ports. *O* Port for the 4 mm-diameter telescope. *I* Ports for the 3 mm-diameter instruments

Fig. 9.9. Ports. *Top* Light reusable 3 mm-diameter Teflon port for instruments. *Bottom* A 45° port for telescope

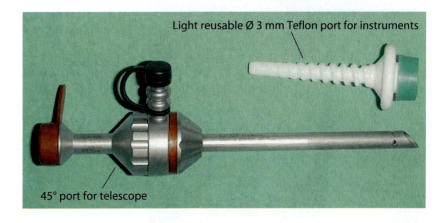

thyroid background, at least in a bloodless field (■ Fig. 9.12). Once a parathyroid is identified, it is gently lifted from its bed and its blood supply divided with bipolar electrocoagulation. To remove the parathyroid we insert the finger of a glove through a port, place the gland inside it, grab the finger and pull it into the port, and remove the port and the bag together applying traction and circular movements at the same time.

Then the opposite side is dissected. The port is repositioned so that the other parathyroids can be removed

in the same way. Each parathyroid is histologically examined after removal to confirm that it has been taken out in its entirety.

At the end of the procedure, the instrument ports are removed under visual control, to make sure that there is no bleeding when the working space is being deflated. No drainage is required. The median muscles are adapted in the midline with a running absorbable suture through the suprasternal incision, and the remaining wound is closed with a 5-0 monofilament non-absorbable suture.

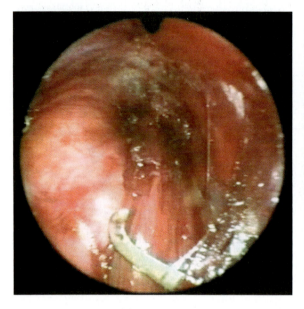

Fig. 9.10. Dissection of the thyroid

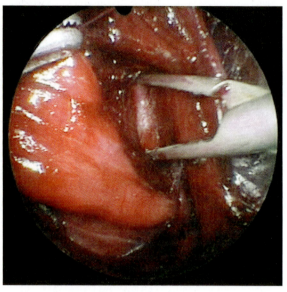

Fig. 9.11. Identification of the left recurrent laryngeal nerve

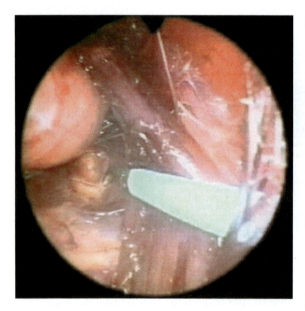

Fig. 9.12. Exposure of lower left parathyroid gland

Surgical Technique for the Thymus and the Mediastinum

Preoperative Preparation

General anesthesia with endotracheal intubation is used. The end-tidal CO_2 is monitored with special care, and the ventilator settings are adjusted accordingly.

Positioning
Patient
The patient is put in a supine position on the operating table, which is tilted in the Trendelenburg position (■ Fig. 9.13). The head of the patient should not be fixed as gentle rotation may help in avoiding collision between the telescope and the chin.

Crew and Equipment
The surgeon is at the head of the patient with the camera operator to his left and the scrub nurse to his right (■ Fig. 9.13). Two monitors are used.

Special Equipment
The same equipment as for thyroid and parathyroid surgery is used.

Technique

Cannulae
The same landmarks for insertion of the ports as for endoscopic thyroid and parathyroid surgery are chosen (■ Fig. 9.14). If the ports were to be introduced closer to the suprasternal notch, the large veins in this area may be injured

Procedure
The telescope port is inserted, in close contact with the trachea, but in a reverse position, i.e., looking downward to the mediastinum (■ Fig. 9.14).

Carbon dioxide insufflation is started at a pressure of 12 mmHg in order to create the initial surgical em-

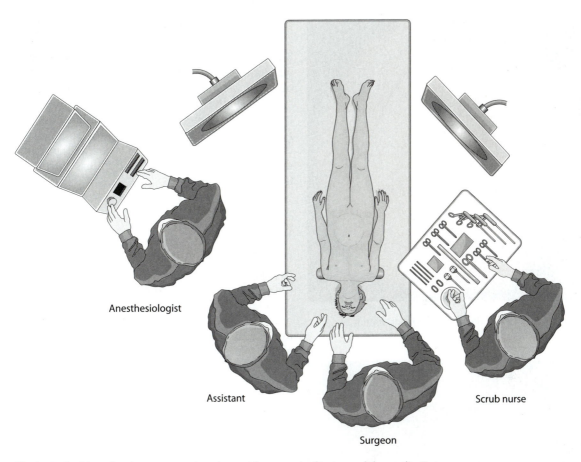

Fig. 9.13. Position of patient, crew, and equipment for access to thymus and the mediastinum

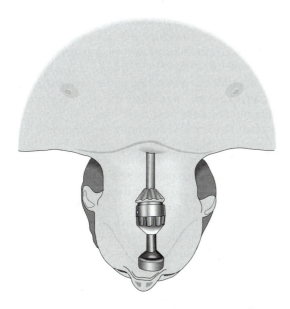

Fig. 9.14. Positioning the patient for thymectomy by cervicoscopy. The first port is placed in close contact with the trachea, facing downward

physema. It does not interfere with ventilation as the patient has been intubated. Once a good space has been developed, pressure can be decreased to 6–8 mmHg. Pneumodissection in the anterior mediastinum is easier than in the neck as the perithymic fascia is softer and the working space is wider. Pneumodissection is helped by gentle movement with the optical system. Then the working ports are inserted under endoscopic control.

The two upper lobes of the thymus are easily identified. Gentle traction with the contralateral instrument helps to expose a lobe and the homolateral instrument is used for dissection and coagulation, i.e., the patient's left lobe is held by the surgeon's right hand. The two lobes are asymmetrical, the right being usually larger than the left. They are easily separated from each other and so they are dissected separately. Bipolar coagulation is mostly used, but clips can be useful for large pedicles, which are located at the medial side of both lobes and at the lower poles. Unfortunately, 3 mm clips are not as commonly available as for 5 mm ones.

The wide working space gives good vision of the internal jugular vein and of the carotid artery. Moreover the vagal and the recurrent laryngeal nerves are easily

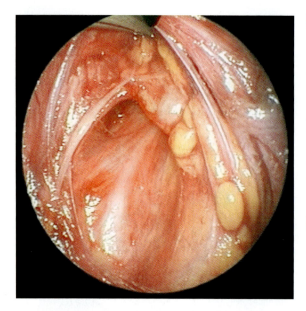

Fig. 9.15. Downward view of the left mediastinum

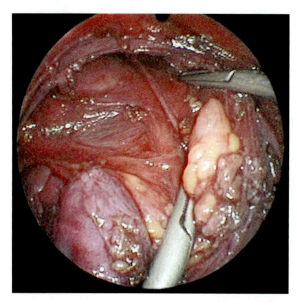

Fig. 9.16. End of dissection in the mediastinum

identified (■ Fig. 9.15). The innominate vein (left brachiocephalic vein) spreads in front of the telescope and can be dissected out if the thymus overlaps it to reach the pericardium. Even then, the thymus can be approached well (■ Fig. 9.16). A subcarinal dissection can be carried out if lymph nodes have to be removed.

Postoperative Course

There should not be peroperative or postoperative hypercapnia. Some postoperative emphysema may be observed, but this disappears completely within 24 h.

Postoperative pain can easily be controlled with paracetamol and mefenamic acid. After thymic or thyroid surgery, the patient is discharged on postoperative day one or two. After parathyroidectomy, the patient is discharged once the level of calcium has been stabilized.

Results

So far we have performed eight parathyroidectomies, two resections of ectopic adenomas, two partial thyroidectomies, and five so-called cervicomediastinoscopic thymectomies. We have not encountered peroperative or postoperative complications, for example hypercapnia or laryngeal nerve injury. Cervical emphysema may be present but is usually mild and disappears within 24 h.

Discussion

Parathyroidectomy is one of the most commonly performed endocrine procedures in adults and, as its technique is well known, it is considered to be a relatively safe procedure. However iatrogenic injuries of the laryngeal nerve are not uncommon: there is a 0.5–3% chance of nerve paralysis, even for experienced surgical teams. Early dissection and visualization of this nerve is considered mandatory for its preservation. Anatomical variations are well known and may be the cause of accidental transection of the laryngeal nerve.

Several attempts to facilitate the surgical approach and to minimize the hazards of dissection have been described: localization of the lesion by technetium 99m methoxyisobutyl isonitrile imaging (Tc 99m MIBI = sestamibi scan) or by magnetic resonance imaging (MRI); percutaneous preoperative needle localization of the parathyroid; and minimal bilateral access. However, reoperation for recurrent hyperparathyroidism is not uncommon, being necessary in 3–10% of cases. Theoretically the incidence of reoperation after (non-endoscopic) minimal access procedures may be higher as these techniques do not allow extensive exploration of the operating field.

The most important benefit of the endoscopic surgical approach is the detailed anatomic view. This extended microsurgical view prevents damage being inflicted on the surrounding vascular and nervous structures, and the recurrent laryngeal nerves in particular.

Most of the thymectomies performed by pediatric surgeons are for myasthenia gravis. The prognosis is better if the removal is total. As in open surgery, and even after complete removal of all adipose tissue, a completeness of the thymectomy cannot be guaranteed as there may be ectopic thymic tissue. For this reason, we recommend a preoperative MRI: it allows identification of ectopic tissues in contiguity with the thymus and may sometimes be helpful in identifying isolated ectopic tissue.

In spite of a rather limited operative field, the endoscopic technique allows for easy access of hidden areas as well as for extensive exploration of the neck without full-scale open surgical dissection: the total length of the wounds is even smaller than those caused by minimal open surgical approaches.

As mentioned by Gagner, placing the patient in a supine position with the neck slightly extended prevents the cervical muscles along the trachea being stretched. This facilitates pneumodissection and creates the widest space possible.

No hypercarbic episode was recorded, contrary to what was previously reported by Gagner, possibly because our insufflation pressure is much lower (12 mmHg initially, 6–8 mmHg after the working space has been created). As was experimentally demonstrated for the retroperitoneum, pneumodissection in the neck would not appear to induce an increased P_{CO2} at low pressure and using modulation of insufflation. Nevertheless, we believe that continuous endtidal CO_2 monitoring is mandatory for such a procedure.

Capillary bleeding is avoided with pneumodissection. Hemostatic vascular control was efficiently achieved by bipolar electrocoagulation.

We have not been using 2 mm instruments as they are not rigid enough to lift up the thyroid. Moreover 2 mm bipolar electrocoagulation forceps or scissors are too sharp to be used as dissectors. For this reason we used a 3 mm bipolar forceps (Micro-France) which has smooth spatulated ends and can be used either to coagulate or to dissect.

As the procedure is bloodless, no suction probe or gauze pads are needed. Suction in such a small working space would certainly cause collapse of the working space and hinder further surgery.

As with other minimally invasive techniques, less pain, fewer wound-related complications, and better cosmetic results may be expected from this procedure. Transection of neck muscles, and the subsequent functional loss that may result, is also avoided. The small size of incisions is good enough for the extraction of small specimens such as parathyroids, thyroid, or thymic lobes.

Conclusion

The technique for thyroidectomy and parathyroidectomy described is a minimally invasive technique giving a view of the parathyroids that is even better than the view with an open approach. These benefits must be weighed against the relative drawbacks such as the duration of the operation, the use of expensive specialized instruments, and the need for expertise in performing such endoscopic operations. Careful evaluation on a case by case basis is therefore mandatory.

Cervicoscopic thymectomy avoids a sternotomy, gives a wide and nearly microsurgical view of the thymic area and of the surrounding structures, and provides as good or even better proof of total removal of the thymus than by open surgery. The technique differs from the lateral thoracoscopic surgical approach as described in adults, which has the disadvantage that the thymus is approached from one side.

References

Gagner M (1996) Endoscopic subtotal parathyroidectomy in patients with primary hyperthyroidism (letter). Br J Surg 83:875

Hüscher CS, Chiodini S, Napolitano C, et al (1997) Endoscopic right thyroid lobectomy. Surg Endosc 11:877

Naitoh T, Gagner M, Garcia-Ruiz A, et al (1998) Endoscopic endocrine surgery in the neck. An initial report of endoscopic subtotal parathyroidectomy. Surg Endosc 12:202–205

Norman J, Albrink MH (1997) Minimally invasive videoscopic parathyroidectomy: a feasibility study in dogs and humans. J Laparoendosc Adv Surg Tech A 7:301–306

Reinberg O (1998) Thymectomie vidéo-assistée par voie cervicale. Expérience préliminaire de 2 cas pédiatriques. Eur J Coelio Surg 28:7–11

Reinberg O, Montupet P (1999) Parathyroidectomie totale par cervicoscopie chez l'enfant (Video Version Française, 7 minutes). Endoscopic total parathyroidectomy in a child (English Video Version, 7 minutes) Realisation: CEMCAV

Reinberg O, Montupet P (2000) Endoscopic total parathyroidectomy in a child. Pediatr Endosurg Innov Tech 4:301–306

Seminar Book of the First International Post-Graduate Course of Endocrine Tele-Surgery (1997) European Institute of Tele-Surgery (EITS) Hôpitaux Universitaires BP 426, F 67091 Strasbourg, France. 13–15 February 1997

Yeung GH (1998) Endoscopic surgery of the neck: a new frontier. Surg Laparosc Endosc 8:227–232

Chapter 10

Anesthesia for Pediatric Thoracoscopic Surgery

Randall M. Clark

Introduction

Thoracoscopic surgery in infants and children is a rapidly progressing discipline. Advances in endoscopic equipment and technique have led to the use of minimally invasive thoracic surgery in an ever-increasing number of pediatric surgical procedures. As the field has expanded, there has been a concomitant need for pediatric anesthesiologists to meet the challenge of caring for the infants and children undergoing these demanding procedures.

The goal of this chapter is to help surgeons and others understand the issues involved in delivering a safe anesthetic for thoracoscopic procedures in infants and children. It is also intended to help surgeons understand how the anesthesiologist can facilitate the successful completion of the surgical procedure and how the surgeon can help recognize and assist in anesthetic issues that may arise during the operation.

Preoperative Evaluation

The overriding goal in the preoperative evaluation is to ascertain whether or not the patient is in the best condition possible given the relative urgency of the planned procedure. Questions to be asked include, "Can the medical condition of this patient be optimized before we go to the operating room?" For elective procedures in patients with complicated medical histories, this may require the assistance of pediatric medical specialists prior to the scheduling of the operation. For urgent or emergency procedures, the surgeon and anesthesiologist must work together to ensure that the patient is in the best condition possible for the anticipated surgery.

For elective procedures in healthy pediatric patients, no preoperative laboratory testing is indicated. Routine "screening" examinations have almost no value in this population. For patients with complicated medical problems, laboratory examination should be focused on known or suspected physiologic derangements.

Some thoracoscopic procedures involve or are near the great vessels of the chest. These patients should have blood available in the operating room. Since preoperative blood draws can be a traumatic experience for pediatric patients, some have suggested that blood for type and crossmatch can be drawn after the induction of anesthesia (Tobias 2001). Obviously this type of recommendation depends on the ability of the local blood bank to have blood available quickly.

The anesthesiologist must endeavor to understand the nature and location of the thoracic pathology. With the exception of neurosurgery, no other surgical interventions interact with the organ systems and patient physiology most critical to the conduct of a safe anesthetic as does thoracic surgery. For example, mediastinal and pulmonary masses have significant impact on the choice of anesthetic technique as well as the planning for the immediate postoperative period. Preoperative consultation with the surgeon is imperative.

Preoperative Preparation/ Premedication

Anesthesia for pediatric thoracoscopic surgery is equipment intensive. Items not usually found inside an individual operating room include:

- Special endotracheal tubes: Univent, double lumen tubes, etc.
- Bronchial blockers
- Long suction catheters
- Flexible fiberoptic scope and light source
- Medical grade silicon lubricant
- Pediatric-sized beanbag
- Extra padding for positioning
- Equipment for regional anesthetic techniques

The anesthetic and surgical plan must be discussed with nursing and technical personnel in the operating room. Quality patient care demands that all involved know and understand their role and what is expected of them. The need for discussion and proper preparation with other operating room personnel is equally as true for the anesthesiologist as it is for the surgeon.

Judicious use of preoperative sedation, usually accomplished with oral midazolam 0.5–0.7 mg/kg from 10 to 30 min before the start of the procedure, can greatly facilitate separation from parents and ease the transition of the pediatric patient into the operating room (Kain et al. 2000). Not every pediatric patient requires preoperative sedation, however. Pediatric anesthesiologists successfully use many non-pharmacologic techniques such as distraction accomplished by simple magic tricks or by simply talking to the child at his or her intellectual and emotional level.

Induction and Maintenance of Anesthesia/Positioning

The induction of anesthesia can be accomplished by the methods customary to the practice of the individuals involved. In most elective procedures this will be by inhaled induction of a volatile agent. For the older patient or one with an intravenous line already in place, intravenous induction may be more appropriate.

Depending on the institution involved, the individuals helping the anesthesiologist at the time of induction may not be familiar with the special demands of pediatric patients with thoracic pathology. In these circumstances the surgeon may be the one best able to assist the anesthesiologist while lung isolation is obtained. Techniques for achieving one-lung ventilation will be explored in detail below.

Proper positioning and padding is critical for the prevention of serious postoperative morbidity in these patients. Most pediatric thoracoscopic procedures will require the patient to be placed in the lateral decubitus position. A chest roll must be placed under the thoracic cage to elevate the down shoulder and relieve traction on the brachial plexus. Care must be taken so that the chest roll is not placed so high in the axilla as to cause direct compression of the brachial plexus and its branches. The lateral side of the down knee should be padded to relieve pressure on the common peroneal nerve. Care must be observed if tape is used across the hip or shoulder in an attempt to keep the child from rocking on the table. Tape used in this way, even over padding, can cause shearing stress in the skin sufficient to cause blistering or skin loss. There should be no pressure on the eyes.

Nitrous oxide (N_2O) is commonly used during inhaled induction in pediatric patients. It is used because it is an anesthetic in its own right and because it increases the concentration and onset of other volatile agents through mechanisms known as the concentration and second gas effects (Taheri and Eger 2002). Continued nitrous oxide administration after induction is not advisable because of its ability to rapidly diffuse into closed gas spaces. The nitrous oxide attempts to achieve equilibrium across these spaces. However the nitrogen cannot escape as rapidly as the nitrous oxide moving in. The result is that these closed spaces expand in volume. This principle applies just the same to gas pockets inside the bowel and chest as to the small pocket inside the endotracheal tube cuff.

Attention must be directed toward maintaining patient temperature. Much body heat can be lost during the first 30 min of anesthesia while the patient is exposed and the patient's thermoregulation is blunted by general anesthetics. Patient temperature can be maintained by the appropriate use of radiant warming lights, warm water mattresses, and forced-air warming devices. Care must be taken that forced-air tubing remains connected to the appropriate perforated blanket. Leaving the air hose open and blowing on the patient under the drapes (termed "hosing") can lead to a devastating burn (Augustine 2002). The use of warmed insufflation gasses also helps maintain patient temperature.

Preemptive analgesia is the concept of blocking pain pathways before the creation of a painful stimulus. As the neurohumoral mechanisms of pain became better understood, it was postulated that preemptive analgesia might block some of the physiologic feedback mechanisms that contribute to and intensify acute and chronic pain. Initial animal studies of this concept were encouraging but conclusive data in humans were elusive. More recently, however, pain research in humans has generally supported the concept of preemptive analgesia.

Techniques for Achieving One-lung Ventilation

Surgical thoracoscopy can be aided greatly by deflation of the lung on the operative side. Numerous techniques are used to obtain selective one-lung ventilation including endobronchial intubation with standard endotracheal tubes (either uncuffed or cuffed), placement of double lumen tubes, and placement of bronchial blockers.

Despite what may appear as adequate positioning by direct fiberoptic guidance, variations in individual patient anatomy may lead to an inability to isolate one lung from the other (Lammers et al. 1997). Alternate methods must be planned and available when initial efforts fail to achieve the desired result.

Bronchial blocker use in children has been described since at least 1969 (Vale 1969). These techniques consist of the placement of a balloon-tipped catheter into the bronchus on the operative side. Fogarty, atrial septostomy, and Swan-Ganz catheters have all been used as blockers. In the blocker technique the catheter may be placed within the lumen of the endotracheal tube. This is accomplished by passing the catheter through a self-sealing port such as the type used during fiberoptic bronchoscopy in the intubated patient. Alternatively, the blocker may reside outside the endotracheal tube by being placed into the trachea prior to intubation. Blocker positioning may be facilitated by the use of wire-guided placement and direct observation with the fiberoptic endoscope.

A special type of purpose-built blocker, the Univent tube, was introduced in 1985 (Kamaya and Krishna 1985). In a Univent tube the blocker is incorporated into a separate channel within the lumen of the endotracheal tube. Advantages include easy manipulation of the blocker, easy deployment and retraction of the blocker when two-lung ventilation is needed, the ability to allow gas in the blocked lung to escape through the lumen of the blocker, and the ability to use the same tube used in the operation for postoperative ventilation if needed (with the blocker retracted). The Univent is especially useful in patients over the age of 6 years needing collapse of the right lung. Traditional double lumen tubes may be too large for placement in these patients and endobronchial intubation into the left main stem bronchus with a standard tube may be difficult (Hammer et al. 1999). In these situations the Univent is placed into its normal tracheal position and the blocker balloon is inflated in the right main stem bronchus under fiberoptic guidance. Care must be taken to prevent the blocker balloon from obstructing the orifice of the right upper lobe bronchus.

Larger size is the primary disadvantage of the Univent tube. The smallest Univent has an inside diameter (ID) of 3.5 mm and an outside diameter (OD) of 7.5–8 mm (Univent tubes are oval in cross-section). This size tube corresponds to the approximate OD of a standard 5.5 mm endotracheal tube and would typically be used in children 5 or 6 years old. The small luminal size in relation to overall diameter also makes the use of standard (3.5 mm) fiberoptic endoscopes difficult if not impossible.

Arndt has described an ingenious method for placement of a specialized bronchial blocker (Arndt 1999). In this technique, a loop protruding from the end of the blocker is placed around the flexible fiberoptic endoscope. When the endoscope is positioned in the proper bronchus, the blocker follows the loop as it slides down over the endoscope and into position. Commercial kits for this device are now available.

When techniques for achieving one-lung ventilation fail or the patient is simply too small or too ill to tolerate lung isolation, surgical approach with two-lung ventilation and modest (4–8 m of H_2O) insufflation of CO_2 on the operative side can be attempted. Most patients tolerate this level of "tension pneumothorax" without difficulty.

Monitoring

Thoracoscopic surgery and anesthesia can induce significant physiologic changes. In addition to the usual monitors used in pediatric anesthesia, special consideration should be given to the areas of acid-base status, auscultation, and capnography. Monitoring should be focused on intended and anticipated changes in the patient's physiologic status.

Derangements of normal respiratory physiology induced by the surgical approach and the installation of carbon dioxide into the thoracic cavity can lead to alterations of normal acid-base status. Tobias (2001) and others have measured these changes in children undergoing endoscopic surgery and have found that most of the changes related to carbon dioxide absorption are small.

Continuous capnography is invaluable for evaluating changes related to tube position or airway collapse during thoracoscopic surgery. Early changes in the exhaled carbon dioxide waveform can help the anesthesiologist anticipate problems related to gas exchange. One must also keep in mind that end-tidal carbon dioxide levels in these procedures can have a much greater difference from arterial carbon dioxide tension owing to the significantly different physiology of one-lung ventilation and carbon dioxide insufflation. Despite this, routine placement of intra-arterial catheters with repeated measurement of arterial blood gasses does not appear necessary for most of these cases.

Complications and Issues Arising During Thoracoscopic Surgery

Hypoxemia

Transient hypoxemia is common during one-lung ventilation and surgical procedures in the chest. Initial investigation should include examination of the position of the endotracheal or endobronchial tube. It is fairly common for bronchial blocker balloons or the tube itself to occlude the upper lobe bronchus, especially on the right. Repositioning frequently corrects the desaturation.

Attention should then be turned to other causes of hypoxemia. Surgical traction or insufflation pressures can impair venous return or cardiac function. Volume expansion or inotropic support may assist in correcting these situations.

Persistent hypoxemia unresponsive to more conservative measures may be treated by the application of small amounts of oxygen supplied under low pressure to the collapsed lung. Care must be taken so that the lung on the operative side is not reexpanded into the surgical field. Intermittent two-lung ventilation can be used if no other option works to relieve the hypoxia.

Bronchial Injury

All bronchial blocker techniques are susceptible to causing bronchial injury. Once inflated past their resting volume, the balloons on these catheters become high-pressure devices. Mucosal ischemia and bronchial rupture (usually posteriorly) can occur. Several methods to prevent excessive cuff pressure have been described (Hannallah and Benumof 1992).

Hypercarbia

Carbon dioxide absorption, one-lung ventilation, and surgical manipulation can lead to hypercarbia. This can usually be treated by increasing alveolar minute ventilation in the ventilated lung. In a small group of patients, end-tidal carbon dioxide levels may remain elevated despite increases in minute ventilation. Fortunately, moderate levels of hypercarbia are well tolerated.

Persistent and significantly elevated carbon dioxide levels can be treated by interruption of the surgical procedure and reinstitution of two-lung ventilation. Several cycles of two-lung ventilation may be necessary to bring carbon dioxide levels back to acceptable levels.

Special Challenges

Patent Ductus Arteriosus

Thoracoscopic patent ductus arteriosus ligation carries some additional risks compared to other procedures. These are primarily related to the fragile nature of the ductal tissue, especially at earlier ages. Plasma expanders and blood should be available in the operating room while performing this surgery. Adequate intravenous access is a must.

Tracheoesophageal Fistula

Tracheoesophageal fistula repair in the newborn is an especially challenging and rewarding endeavor. Visualization of the fistula and close-up observation of the esophageal anastomosis show the tremendous advantage of these video-assisted techniques.

The fistula location can vary widely. The anesthesiologist must consider where he or she will place the tip of the endotracheal tube and discuss with the surgeon how the patient will be managed until the fistula is ligated. In addition, the anesthesiologist may be asked to assist the surgeon with the placement of a nasopharyngeal tube to serve as a stent over which the esophageal anastomosis is performed.

Nuss Repair

Thoracoscopic-assisted Nuss repair for pectus excavatum also has special considerations. The anesthesiologist must be vigilant for physiologic derangements or injury during the placement of the Nuss bar across the anterior mediastinum. In addition, the desired changes to the cartilaginous and bony anatomy that the Nuss bar creates seem to induce a level of postoperative pain unlike any other. Planning for postoperative pain control must be given just as much consideration as the conduct of the anesthetic itself.

Emergence and Extubation

The nature of endobronchial intubation is such that the tip of the endotracheal tube may traumatize the mucosa of the bronchial tree. Movement of the mediastinum and lungs may aggravate this during the course of the surgery. In these patients it is prudent to gently suction the endotracheal tube prior to extubation. A significant number of pediatric patients will have inspissated mucus or even a frank blood clot at the tip of the endotracheal tube. In some instances, such as a continued ball-valve-type obstruction despite apparently adequate suctioning, an endotracheal tube change may be necessary if intubation is planned to continue postoperatively.

Postoperative Pain Management

There are numerous techniques for obtaining adequate postoperative pain control in pediatric patients undergoing thoracic surgery. By its nature, thoracoscopic surgery is much less traumatizing than traditional open procedures, especially lateral thoracotomies. However, despite the "minimally invasive" label, these patients may still have significant postoperative pain.

Epidural analgesia with local anesthetics and narcotics is frequently used to provide postoperative pain relief in children undergoing thoracoscopic surgery. Local anesthetics can reach the thoracic dermatomes from single injections at the caudal canal, but large volumes of potentially toxic local anesthetics would be required to obtain adequate blockade via this route. Catheter techniques have been used with entry at both the caudal canal and in the thoracic spine. The threading of the catheter from the caudal canal can be facilitated by fluoroscopy and flexion/extension of the spine in infants and small children.

Some pediatric anesthesiologists advocate the placement of thoracic epidural catheters under general anesthesia (Krane et al. 1998). However, case reports of devastating neurologic injury from such techniques are beginning to appear (Bromage and Benumof 1998; Kasai and Yaegashi 2003). This debate centers on the wisdom of pointing a large-bore needle toward the thoracic spinal cord in a unresponsive patient for what is essentially a purely elective procedure. (For epidurals above the level of the conus medullaris, adult patients almost always have these catheters placed in the awake state so that if paresthesias are elicited, the needle and catheter can be redirected.) Other pediatric anesthesiologists note that the quality of pain relief obtained by caudal or lumbar epidural catheters infused with narcotics is almost as good as that obtained from thoracic epidurals but without the risk of cord injury.

Other techniques should also be considered. These include intrapleural infusion of local anesthetics, intercostal blocks, and stellate ganglion blocks. Obviously, continuous infusions with local anesthetics, narcotics, or alpha agonists give much longer pain relief than single injections. In appropriately selected patients, patient-controlled analgesia and non-steroidal anti-inflammatory agents may also be employed. Careful coordination with the pediatric nurses caring for the child postoperatively is mandatory.

Conclusion

No class of surgical procedures demonstrates the advantages of team effort more than does thoracoscopic surgery in infants and children. By understanding the issues that each discipline faces and working together to meet the challenges as they arise, surgeons, anesthesiologists, and nurses can accomplish what heretofore had been considered impossible.

References

Arndt GA, DeLessio ST, Kranner PW, et al (1999) One-lung ventilation when intubation is difficult: presentation of a new endobronchial blocker. Acta Anaesthesiol Scan 43:356–358

Augustine S (2002) Misuse of forced air warming devices causes burns. APSF Newsletter. Spring:17

Bromage PR, Benumof JL (1998) Paraplegia following intracord injection during attempted epidural anesthesia under general anesthesia. Reg Anesth Pain Med 23:104–107

Hammer GB, Fitzmaurice BG, Brodsky JB (1999) Methods for single-lung ventilation in pediatric patients. Anesth Analg 89:1426–1429

Hannallah MS, Benumof JL (1992) Comparison of two techniques to inflate the bronchial cuff of the Univent tube. Anesth Analg 75:784–787

Kain ZN, Hofstadter MB, Mayes LC, et al (2000) Midazolam: effects on amnesia and anxiety on children. Anesthesiology 93:676–684

Kamaya H, Krishna PR (1985) New endotracheal tube (Univent tube) for selective blockade of one lung. Anesthesiology 63:342–343

Kasai T, Yaegashi K (2003) Spinal cord injury in a child caused by an accidental dural puncture with a single-shot thoracic epidural needle. Analg Anesth 96:65–67

Krane EJ, Dalens BJ, Murat I, et al (1998) The safety of epidurals placed under general anesthesia. Reg Anesth Pain Med 23:433–438

Lammers CR, Hammer GB, Brodsky JB, et al (1997) Failure to isolate the lungs with an endotracheal tube positioned in the bronchus. Anesth Analg 85:946–947

Taheri S, Eger EI (2002) A demonstration of the concentration and second gas effects in humans anesthetized with nitrous oxide and desflurane. Anesth Analg 94:765–766

Tobias JD (2001) Thoracoscopy in the pediatric patient. Anesthesiol Clin North Am 19:173–186

Vale R (1969) Selective bronchial blocking in a small child. Br J Anaesth 41:453–454

Chapter 11

Thoracoscopy in Infants and Children: Basic Techniques

Steven S. Rothenberg

Introduction

Thoracoscopy is a technique that has been in use since the early 1900s but has undergone an exponential increase in popularity and growth since the early 1990s. The first experience in humans was reported by Jacobeus in 1910 and consisted of placing a cystoscope inserted through a rigid trocar into the pleural space to lyse adhesions and cause complete collapse of a lung as treatment for a patient with tuberculosis. He later reported the first significant experience with a series of over 100 patients (Jacobeus 1921). During the next 70 years thoracoscopy gained some favor, primarily in Europe, for the biopsy of pleural-based tumors and limited thoracic explorations in adults, however widespread acceptance was minimal (Bloomberg 1978; Page et al. 1989).

In the 1970s and 1980s the first significant experience in children was reported (Rodgers et al. 1979; Ryckman and Rodgers 1982). Equipment modified for pediatric patients was used to perform biopsies, evaluate various intrathoracic lesions, and perform limited pleural debridement in cases of empyema (Kern and Rodgers 1993). However even though there was an increasing recognition of the morbidity associated with a standard thoracotomy, especially in small infants and children, there was little acceptance or adoption of these techniques (Rothenberg and Pokorny 1992). It was not until the early 1990s with the dramatic revolution in technology associated with laparoscopic surgery in adults that more advanced diagnostic and therapeutic procedures have been performed in children (Rodgers 1993). The development of high-resolution microchip and now digital cameras, smaller instrumentation, and better optics has enabled pediatric surgeons to perform even the most complicated intrathoracic procedure thoracoscopically (Rothenberg 1994).

Indications

Today there are a wide variety of indications for thoracoscopic procedures in children (■ Table 11.1) and the number continues to expand with advances and refinements in technology and technique. Currently, thoracoscopy is being used extensively for lung biopsy

Table 11.1. Indications for thoracoscopy in infants and children

– Lung biopsy	– Patent ductus arteriosus (PDA) ligation
– Lobectomy	– Thoracic duct ligation
– Sequestration resection	– Esophageal atresia repair
– Cyst excision	– TEF repair
– Decortication	– Aortopexy
– Foregut duplication resection	– Mediastinal mass excision
– Esophageal myotomy	– Thymectomy
– Anterior spine fusion	– Sympathectomy
– Diaphragmatic hernia/ plication	– Pericardial window

and wedge resection in cases of interstitial lung disease (ILD) and metastatic lesions (Rothenberg et al. 1996; Smith et al. 2002). More extensive pulmonary resections including segmentectomy and lobectomy have also been performed for infectious diseases, cavitary lesions, bullous disease, sequestrations, lobar emphysema, congenital adenomatoid malformations, and neoplasm (Hazelrigg 1993; McKenna 1994; Rothenberg 2003; Walker 1996). Thoracoscopy is also extremely useful in the evaluation and treatment of mediastinal masses (Mack 1993). It provides excellent access and visualization for biopsy and resection of mediastinal structures such as lymph nodes, thymic and thyroid lesions, cystic hygromas, foregut duplications, ganglioneuromas, and neuroblastomas (Holcomb 2001; Kogut et al. 2000; Patrick and Rothenberg 2001). Other advanced intrathoracic procedures, such as decortication for empyema, patent ductus arteriosus closure, repair of hiatal hernia and congenital diaphragmatic defects, esophageal myotomy for achalasia, thoracic sympathectomy for hyperhidrosis, anterior spinal fusion for severe scoliosis, and most recently primary repair of esophageal atresia, have also been described in children (Laborde et al. 1993; Mack et al. 1995; Pellegrini et al. 1992; Rothenberg 2001, 2002; Rothenberg et al. 1995, 1998, 2001; Sartorelli et al. 1996).

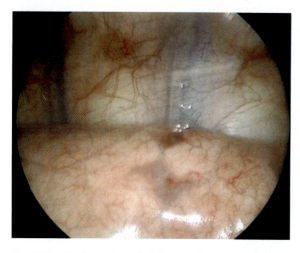

Fig. 11.1. Small blood patch visible on pleural surface marking the underlying nodule

Preoperative Workup

The preoperative workup varies significantly depending on the procedure to be performed. Most intrathoracic lesions require routine radiographs as well as a computed tomography (CT) or magnetic resonance imaging (MRI) scan. A thin-cut high-resolution CT scan is especially helpful in evaluating patients with ILD as it can identify the most affected areas and help determine the site of biopsy, as the external appearance of the lung is usually not helpful. CT-guided needle localization can also be used to direct biopsies for focal lesions which may be deep in the parenchyma and therefore not visible on the surface of the lung during thoracoscopy. This is usually performed just prior to the thoracoscopy with the radiologist marking the pleura overlying the lesion with a small blood patch or dye (Fig. 11.1). On occasion a wire may be placed, as in breast biopsies, but these may become dislodged during collapse of the lung at the time of surgery. As intraoperative ultrasound imaging improves this may provide a more sensitive way for the surgeon to detect lesions deep to the surface of the lung and make up for the lack of tactile sensation. Unfortunately in its current state this technology is still unreliable (Waldenhausen et al. 2000). An MRI scan may be more useful in evaluating vascular lesions or masses, which may arise from or encroach on the spinal canal, or in the case of vascular rings. These studies can be extremely important in determining positioning of the patient and initial port placement.

Another major consideration for the successful completion of most thoracoscopic procedures is whether or not the patient will tolerate single-lung ventilation thus allowing for collapse of the ipsilateral lung to ensure adequate visualization and room for

manipulation. Unfortunately there is no specific preoperative test that will yield this answer. However, most patients, even those who are ventilator dependent, can tolerate short periods of single-lung ventilation. This should allow adequate time to perform most diagnostic procedures such as lung biopsy. In cases where single-lung ventilation cannot be tolerated other techniques may be used and these will be discussed later.

Anesthetic Considerations

While single-lung ventilation is achieved relatively easily in adult patients using a double-lumen endotracheal tube, the process is more difficult in the infant or small child. The smallest available double-lumen tube is a 28 French, which can generally not be used in a patient under 30 kg. Another option is a bronchial blocker. This device contains an occluding balloon attached to a stylet on the side of the endotracheal tube. After intubation this stylet is advanced in the bronchus to be occluded and the balloon is inflated. Unfortunately size is again a limiting factor as the smallest blocker currently available is a 6.0 tube. For the majority of cases in infants and small children a selective mainstem intubation of the contralateral bronchus with a standard uncuffed endotracheal tube is effective. This can usually be done blindly without the aide of a bronchoscope simply by manipulating the head and neck. It is also important to use an endotracheal tube one half to one size smaller than the anesthesiologist would pick for a standard intubation or the tube may not pass into the mainstem bronchus, especially on the left side.

At times this technique will not lead to total collapse of the lung as there may be some overflow ventilation because the endotracheal tube is not totally occlusive. This problem is overcome by the routine use of a low flow (1 L/min), low pressure (4 mmHg) CO_2 infusion during the procedure to help keep the lung compressed. If adequate visualization is still not achieved then the pressure and flow can be gradually turned up until adequate lung collapse is achieved. Pressures of 10–12 mmHg can be tolerated without significant respiratory or hemodynamic consequences in most cases. This requires the use of a valved trocar rather than a non-valved port (Thoracoport). This technique can also be used on patients who cannot tolerate single-lung ventilation. By using small tidal volumes, lower peak pressures, and a higher respiratory rate, enough lung collapse can be achieved to allow for adequate exploration and biopsy. In neonates with tracheoesophageal fistula (TEF) or other congenital malformations, CO_2 alone can be used to deflate the lung. Once the lung is collapsed it will stay that way until the anesthesiologist makes a conscious effort to reexpand it. The surface tension of the collapsed alveoli in the newborn keeps the lung collapsed without excessive pressures being used.

This technique is also useful if bilateral procedures are being performed such as in the case of sympathectomy (Cohen et al. 1995). A slight tension pneumothorax gives adequate exposure to visualize the sympathetic chain without the need to change the lung that is isolated. Whatever method is chosen it is imperative that the anesthesiologist and surgeon have a clear plan and good communication to prevent problems with hypoxia and excessive hypercapnia, and to ensure the best chance of a successful procedure (Tobias 2002).

Technique

Positioning

Positioning depends on the site of the lesion and the type of procedure. Most open thoracotomies are performed with the patient in a lateral decubitus position. Thoracoscopic procedures should be performed with the patient in a position that allows for the greatest access to the areas of interest and uses gravity to aid in keeping the uninvolved lung or other tissue out of the field of view.

For routine lung biopsies or lung resections, the patient is placed in a standard lateral decubitus position (■ Fig. 11.2a). This position provides for excellent visualization and access to all surfaces of the lung. This position is also the most beneficial setup for decortications, pleurodesis, and other procedures where the surgeon may need access to the entire pleural or lung surface. For anterior mediastinal masses the patient should be placed supine with the affected side elevated 20–30° (■ Fig. 11.2b). This allows for excellent visualization of the entire anterior mediastinum while allowing gravity to retract the lung posteriorly without the need for extra retractors. The surgical ports may then be placed between the anterior and midaxillary lines giving clear access to the anterior mediastinum. This position should be used for thymectomy, aortopexy, or biopsy or resection of anterior tumors or lymph nodes. For posterior mediastinal masses, foregut duplications, esophageal atresia, and work on the esophageal hiatus, the patient should be placed in a modified prone position with the affected side elevated slightly (■ Fig. 11.2c). This maneuver again allows for excellent exposure without the need for extra retractors. The patient can then be placed in Trendelenburg or reverse Trendelenburg as needed to help keep the lung out of the field of view.

Once the patient is appropriately positioned and draped, the monitors can be placed in position. For

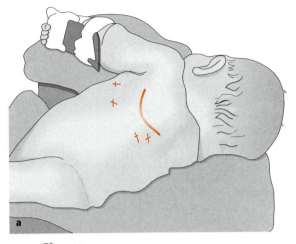

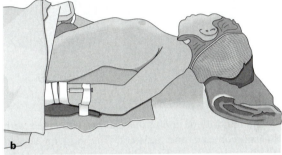

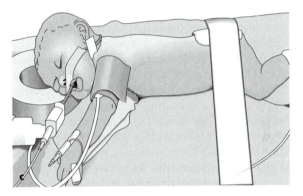

Fig. 11.2. a Patient placed in right lateral decubitus position for lung biopsy. **b** Standard setup for anterior mediastinal structure. **c** Standard setup for posterior mediastinal structure

most thoracoscopic procedures it is advantageous to have two monitors, one on either side of the table. The monitors should be placed between the patient's shoulders and hips depending on the site of the lesion. The goal as always with endoscopic procedures is to keep the surgeon in line with the camera, in line with the pathology, and finally in line with the monitor. This allows the surgeon to work in the most efficient and ergonomic way. In some cases, such as decortication, the field of interest may constantly change. In this case the monitors should be placed at shoulder level and moved as necessary.

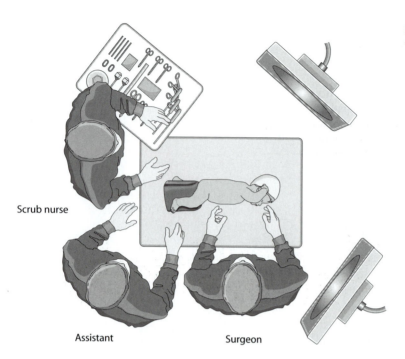

Fig. 11.3. Standard room setup for thoracoscopic procedure

Scrub nurse

Assistant   Surgeon

The majority of operations can be performed with the surgeon and one assistant. The surgeon should stand on the side of the table opposite the area to be addressed so that he or she can work in line with the camera as he or she performs the procedure. In most lung cases such as biopsies, it is preferential to have the assistant on the same side of the table as the surgeon so that he or she is not working in a paradox (against the camera), as he or she is responsible for operating the camera and providing retraction as necessary (■ Fig. 11.3). This concept is even more important when the field of dissection is primarily on one side. Cases such as a mediastinal masses, esophageal atresia, or more complicated lung resections require greater surgical skill. It is imperative that both the surgeon and the assistant are working in line with the field of view to prevent clumsy or awkward movements. In cases such as decortication where the field of view and dissection are constantly changing and the majority of movements are relatively gross, having the surgeon and assistant on opposite sides of the table is appropriate and may actually expedite the procedure.

Trocar Placement

Positioning of the trocars varies widely with the procedure being performed and the site of the lesion. Thoughtful positioning of the trocars is more important than with laparoscopic surgery because the chest wall is rigid and therefore the mobility of the instruments will be somewhat restricted as compared to in the abdomen. The most commonly performed procedures, such as

lung biopsy for ILD or decortication for empyema, may require wide access to many areas in the thoracic cavity and therefore the ports are placed in such a fashion as to facilitate this. However this may result in some degree of paradox during portions of the procedure. Other operations are directed toward a very restricted area and therefore the trocars are placed to allow for the best visualization and access to this specific spot. In general the camera port should be placed slightly above and between the working ports to allow the surgeon to look down on the field of view, much as in open surgery. This will also minimize instrument dueling, which can be a significant problem in smaller infants.

For example with lung biopsies the trocars should usually be placed between the 4th and 8th intercostal spaces. The camera port is usually in the midaxillary line at the 5th or 6th interspace. If an endoscopic stapler is being used it requires a 12 mm port which therefore should be placed in the lowest interspace possible, especially in smaller children, as these are the widest and better able to accommodate the larger port. If the lesion is anterior the port should be positioned closer to the posterior axillary line and vice versa. This is to allow the greatest amount of space between the chest wall insertion and the lesion as the working head of the stapler requires at least 45–50 mm of space. The third or grasping port is placed closer to the lesion and provides traction on the lesion during biopsy. This arrangement allows the surgeon, camera, and primary working port to be in line with the area to be biopsied. The midaxillary port should be placed first to allow for modification of the other two ports once an initial survey of the chest cavity has been completed. A triangular arrangement of the trocars has also been recommended because it allows for rotation of the telescope and instruments between the three ports giving excellent access to all areas. However the surgeon can find himself working against the camera, a situation which can make the simplest procedure very difficult. Also, especially in children, the number of large ports should be limited. Therefore careful planning should go into port placement, to limit the number and size of ports needed. Generally trocar placement can be tentatively planned based on preoperative imaging studies and then modified once the initial trocar is placed.

Instrumentation

The equipment used for thoracoscopy is basically the same as that for laparoscopy. In general 5- and 3 mm instrumentation is of adequate size and therefore 5 mm and smaller trocars can be used. In most cases valved trocars are used for the reasons previously discussed. Basic equipment should include 5 mm 0° and 30° lenses (most procedures are best performed with a 30° lens). If procedures are being performed in smaller children and infants it is also helpful to have smaller lenses such as a short (16- to18 cm-long), 3- or 4 mm-diameter, 30° scopes and specifically designed shorter instruments. These tools enable the surgeon to perform much finer movements and dissection allowing advanced procedures to be performed in infants as small as 1 kg. A high resolution microchip or digital camera and light source are also extremely important to allow for adequate visualization especially when using smaller scopes which transmit less light. Basic instrumentation should include curved dissecting scissors, curved dissectors, atraumatic clamps (i.e., 3- and 5 mm atraumatic bowel clamps), fan retractors, a suction/irrigator, and needle holders. Disposable instrumentation which should be available includes hemostatic clips, endoloops (pretied ligatures), and an endoscopic linear stapler. The linear stapler is an endoscopic version of the GIA used in open bowel surgery. It lays down six to eight rows of staples and divides the tissue between them, providing an air and watertight seal. This is an excellent tool for performing wedge resections of the lung but unfortunately its current size requires placement of a 12 mm trocar precluding its use in patients much under 10 kg because of the limited size of their thoracic cavity. There are also a number of energy sources available, which provide hemostasis and divide tissue. These include monopolar and bipolar cautery, the ultrasonic coagulating shears, and the Ligasure (Valleylab), all of which can be helpful in difficult dissections. It is also helpful to have one of the various tissue glues available for sealing lung and pleural surfaces.

Postoperative Care

Postoperative care in the majority of patients is straightforward. Most patients following biopsy or limited resection can be admitted directly to the surgical ward with limited monitoring (i.e., a pulse oximeter for 6–12 h). These patients are generally 23 h observation candidates and a number are actually ready for discharge the same evening. If a chest tube is left in it can usually be removed on the first postoperative day. Pain management has not been a significant problem. Local anesthetic is injected at each trocar site prior to insertion of the trocar and then one or two doses of IV narcotic is given in the immediate postoperative period. By that evening or the following morning most patients are comfortable on oral codeine or acetaminophen. It is very important, especially in the patients with compromised lung function, to start early and aggressive pulmonary toilet. The significant decrease in postoperative pain associated with a thoracoscopic approach results in much less splinting and allows for more effective deep breathing. This has resulted in a decrease in postoperative pneumonias and other pulmonary complications.

Conclusions

The recent advances in technology and technique in endoscopic surgery have dramatically altered the approach to intrathoracic lesions in the pediatric patient. Most operations can now be performed using a thoracoscopic approach with a marked decrease in the associated morbidity for the patient. This has allowed for an aggressive approach in obtaining tissue for diagnostic purposes in cases of ILD or questionable focal lesions in immunocompromised patients without the fear of significant pulmonary complications previously associated with a standard thoracotomy. In general, a lung biopsy can now be done with little more morbidity than a transbronchial biopsy, yet the tissue obtained is far superior. The same is true for mediastinal masses or foregut abnormalities. Patients undergoing limited biopsy can even be done as same day surgery and lesions such as esophageal duplications can be excised thoracoscopically with the patient ready for discharged the following day. Even patent ductus arteriosus closures are now performed safely thoracoscopically with a hospitalization of less than 24 h. While a thoracoscopic approach may not always result in a significant decrease in hospital days it may result in a significant decrease in the overall morbidity for the patient, such as in the case of severe scoliosis patients in whom a thoracoscopic anterior spinal fusion results in earlier extubation, a decreased intensive care unit stay, and in general earlier mobilization. Thoracoscopic surgery has clearly shown significant benefits over standard open thoracotomy in many cases and with continued improvement and miniaturization of the equipment the procedures we can perform and the advantages to the patient should continue to grow.

References

Bloomberg HE (1978) Thoracoscopy in perspective. Surg Gynecol Obstet 147:433–443

Cohen Z, Shinar D, Levi I, Mares AJ (1995) Thoracoscopic upper sympathectomy for primary hyperhidrosis in children and adolescents. J Pediatr Surg 30:471–473

Hazelrigg SR (1993) Thoracoscopic management of pulmonary blebs and bullae. Semin Thorac Cardiovasc Surg 5:327–331

Holcomb GW III (2001) Indications for minimally invasive surgery in pediatric oncology. J Laparoendosc Adv Surg Tech B 6:299–304

Jacobeus HC (1921) The practical importance of thoracoscopy in surgery of the chest. Surg Gynecol Obstet 4:289–296

Kern JA, Rodgers BM (1993) Thoracoscopy in the management of empyema in children. J Pediatr Surg 28:1128–1132

Kogut KA, Bufo AJ, Rothenberg SS (2000) Thoracoscopic thymectomy for myasthenia gravis in children. J Pediatr Surg 35:1576–1577

Laborde F, Noirhomme P, Karam J, et al. (1993) A new video assisted technique for the interruption of patent ductus arteriosus in infants and children. J Thorac Cardiovasc Surg 105:278–280

Mack MJ (1993) Thoracoscopy and its role in mediastinal disease and sympathectomy. Semin Thorac Cardiovasc Surg 5:332–336

Mack MJ, Regan JJ, McAfee PC, et al (1995) Video assisted thoracic surgery for the anterior approach to the thoracic spine. Ann Thorac Surg 54:142–144

McKenna RJ (1994) Lobectomy by video-assisted thoracic surgery with mediastinal node sampling. J Thorac Cardiovasc Surg 107:879–882

Page RD, Jeffrey RR, Donnelly RJ (1989) Thoracoscopy: a review of 121 consecutive surgical procedures. Ann Thorac Surg 48:66–68

Partrick DA, Rothenberg SS (2001) Thoracoscopic resection of mediastinal masses in infants and children: an evolution of technique and results. J Pediatr Surg 36:1165–1167

Pellegrini C, Wetter A, Patti M, et al (1992) Thoracoscopic esophagomyotomy: initial experience with a new approach for the treatment of achalasia. Ann Surg 216:291–299

Rodgers BM (1993) Pediatric thoracoscopy. Where have we come, what have we learned? Ann Thorac Surg 56:704–707

Rodgers BM, Moazam F, Talbert JL (1979) Thoracoscopy in children. Ann Surg 189:176–180

Rothenberg SS (1994) Thoracoscopy in infants and children. Semin Pediatr Surg 3:277–288

Rothenberg SS (2001) Thoracoscopic closure of patent ductus arteriosus in infants and children. Pediatr Endosurg Innov Tech 5:109–112

Rothenberg SS (2002) Thoracoscopic repair of tracheo-esophageal fistula and esophageal atresia in newborns. J Pediatr Surg 37:869–872

Rothenberg SS (2003) Experience with thoracoscopic lobectomy in infants and children. J Pediatr Surg 38:102–104

Rothenberg SS, Pokorny WJ (1992) Experience with a total muscle sparing approach for thoracotomies in neonates, infants and children. J Pediatr Surg 27:1157–1160

Rothenberg SS, Chang JHT, Toews WH, et al (1995) Thoracoscopic closure of patent ductus arteriosus: a less traumatic and more cost effective technique. J Pediatr Surg 30:1057–1060

Rothenberg SS, Wagener JS, Chang JHT, et al (1996) The safety and efficacy of thoracoscopic lung biopsy for diagnosis and treatment in infants and children. J Pediatr Surg 31:100–104

Rothenberg SS, Erickson M, Eilert R, et al (1998) Thoracoscopic anterior spinal procedures in children. J Pediatr Surg 33:1168–1171

Rothenberg SS, Partrick DA, Bealer JF et al. (2001) Evaluation of minimally invasive approaches to achalasia in children. J Pediatr Surg 36:808–810

Ryckman FC, Rodgers BM (1982) Thoracoscopy for intrathoracic neoplasia in children. J Pediatr Surg 17:521–524

Sartorelli KH, Rothenberg SS, Karrer FM, et al (1996) Thoracoscopic repair of hiatal hernia following fundoplication: a new approach to an old problem. J Laparoendosc Surg 6:S91–S93

Smith JJ, Rothenberg SS, Brooks, M, et al (2002) Thoracoscopic surgery in childhood cancer. J Pediatr Hematol Oncol 24:429–435

Tobias JD (2002) Anesthesia for minimally invasive surgery in children. Best Pract Res Clin Anaesthesiol 16:115–118

Waldenhausen JH, Tapper D, Sawin RS (2000) Minimally invasive surgery and clinical decision making for pediatric malignancy. Surg Endosc 14:250–253

Walker WS (1996) Video assisted thoracic surgery: pulmonary lobectomy. Semin Laprosc Surg 3: 233–244

Chapter 12

Implantation of a Nuss Bar Under Thoracoscopic Guidance

Klaas (N) M.A. Bax and David C. van der Zee

Introduction

In 1998 Nuss et al. described a new procedure for the correction of pectus excavatum. The procedure basically consists of implantation of an anteriorly prebent metal bar in such a way that the median one third of the bar lies underneath the sternum and pushes it up, while the lateral thirds lie subcutaneously on the lateral chest wall. For inserting this bar a minimal access technique is used. Originally the passage of the bar between the sternum and the pericardium was made in a blind way but accidental puncture of the heart has occurred (Hebra et al. 2000). It is now common practice to make the passage between the sternum and the pericardium under thoracoscopic control. This chapter concentrates on the thoracoscopic part of the procedure.

Preoperative Preparation

Before Induction of General Anesthesia

We only operate on children at an age when they can decide for themselves whether they want to have a correction of their deformity, which is usually around puberty. Many patients, however, present later, as the deformity has often not received adequate medical attention. Preoperatively the deformity is documented with photographs and an anteroposterior (AP) as well as a lateral chest X-ray. Additional investigations are carried out on indication only.

After Induction of General Anesthesia

There is no need for unilateral lung ventilation. After induction of general anesthesia and intubation, a high thoracic epidural catheter is inserted and bupivacaine in combination with clonidine given. Epidural analgesia (bupivacaine in combination with sufentanil) is given postoperatively for at least 72 h. To avoid over-distention of the urinary bladder, in relationship with the epidural anesthesia, a urinary catheter is inserted and left in place for the same period of time as the epidural catheter. Antibiotics are given intravenously and continued postoperatively for 72 h.

Positioning

Patient

The patient is placed in a flat supine crucifix position on the operating table (■ Fig. 12.1). Asymmetry is avoided. It is advantageous to elevate the chest with a folded up towel (■ Fig. 12.2) as this gives a better approach to the midaxillary line. The midaxillary lines on both sides are marked. Immediately anterior to these lines but at the level of the maximal sternal depression 3 cm-long transverse lines are also drawn. Moreover we mark the intercostal sites were the bar will enter and leave the chest, which is where the depression begins and ends. Care is taken that the bar will be underneath the distal sternum and not underneath the xiphoid process.

The anterior bi-midaxillary distance at the level of the maximal depression is measured (■ Fig. 12.3). This length minus one inch will be the appropriate length of the bar to be inserted. In obese patients an even shorter bar may be required as the bar is inserted under the subcutaneous fat.

Crew, Monitors, and Equipment

The surgeon stands on the right of the operating table with the camera operator to his right and the scrub nurse further down (■ Fig. 12.1). This is at variance with the usual position of the (right-handed) camera operator, which is to the left of the surgeon, because there is not enough room to accommodate two persons between the incision to be made and the abducted arm of the patient. As we always have two monitors available, the tower is positioned behind the surgeon with the second monitor opposite to the surgeon on the patient's left. By having the tower behind the surgeon, all cables come from behind him or her and along his or her left side and run along the patient's right side. By doing so the cables do not have to cross to the other side. The thoracoscopy can also be carried out from the left, but we prefer to do it from the right as the heart may be in the way.

Special Equipment

No special energy applying systems are needed, but the Nuss instrumentarium should be available (■ Fig. 12.4).

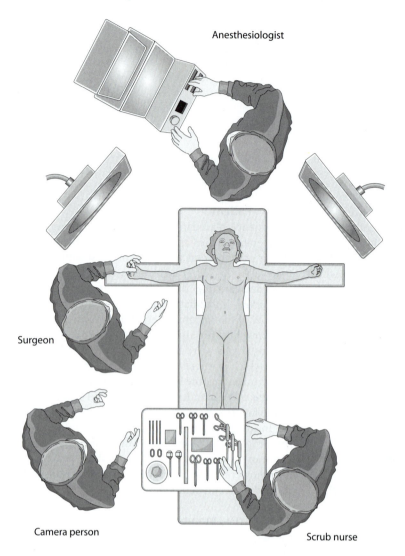

Anesthesiologist

Surgeon

Camera person

Scrub nurse

Fig. 12.1. Position of the patient, crew, and equipment. The patient is placed in a flat supine crucifix position on the operating table. Asymmetry is avoided. The surgeon stands on the right of the operating table with the camera operator to his right and the scrub nurse further down. The tower is positioned behind the surgeon with the second monitor opposite to the surgeon on the patient's left

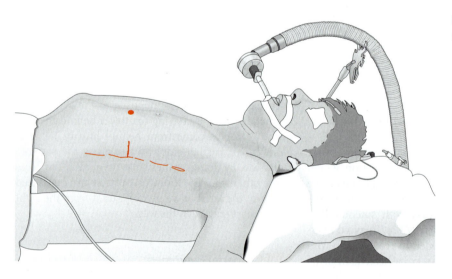

Fig. 12.2. Elevation of the chest with a folded up towel

Fig. 12.3. The anterior bi-midaxillary distance at the level of the maximal depression is measured. This length minus one inch will be the appropriate length of the bar to be inserted

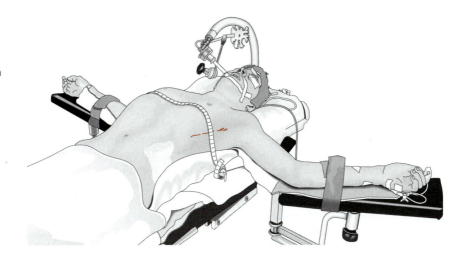

Fig. 12.4. The Nuss instrumentarium should be available. This includes different bar lengths and templates, elongated stabilizers, a bar bender, an S-shaped instrument to create the substernal tunnel, and two bar flippers

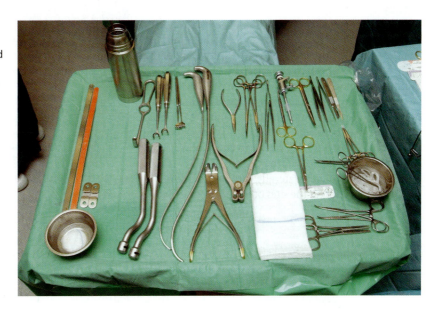

Technique

Cannulae

Cannula	Method of insertion	Diameter (mm)	Device	Position
1	Open	6	Telescope 30°, 30 cm long	Seventh intercostal space, anterior axillary line

The cannula (■ Fig. 12.8) has a siliconized sleeve for suture fixation to the skin and underlying fascia. As we scope the entire substernal passage, we may need the full length of the scope, depending on the size of the patient. In the adolescent it may become necessary to glide the cannula further inside the chest in order to reach the other side.

Carbon Dioxide Pneumothorax

Carbon dioxide is insufflated at a pressure of 5–8 mmHg, and at an initial flow of 0.5 L/min. This does not causes major cardiorespiratory problems. If the lung stays in the way, one can ask the anesthesiologist to decrease ventilatory pressure or to increase the frequency when volume ventilation is used.

Once the chest is entered using the S-shaped instrument to make the substernal passage, an important CO_2 leak occurs and insufflation flow needs to be is increased. We usually set flow then at 5 L/min, but the leak may be so significant that we occlude the leaking tunnel with a finger.

Procedure

The chest is disinfected widely from the suprasternal notch to the umbilicus and laterally until well behind the midaxillary line. Attention should be paid to draping. When disposable sheets are used one should use sheets with adhesive bands of good quality. Several times we have experienced these disposable sheets becoming loose during the operation which jeopardizes sterility.

A template bar of appropriate size (one inch shorter than the measured length) is chosen and bent into the desired shape (■ Fig. 12.5). Next a definitive bar of the same length is bent with the special instruments into the shape of the template (■ Fig. 12.6). As the bar has a tendency to wing out laterally because of downward pressure of the pushed up sternum, we bend the lateral ends more than needed at first glance. We then put the bar externally onto the chest wall to check how its fits. The bar ends should "grab" the chest.

Incisions are made bilaterally through the skin and subcutaneous fascia at the sites of the transverse marks.

Next subcutaneous epifascial tunnels are made until the previously marked intercostal sites are included in the tunnel (■ Fig. 12.7). As we always use one or two stabilizers to glide laterally over the bar, we undermine the skin with subcutaneous fascia widely at the site where the stabilizers will be inserted. It is especially important to extend this well anteriorly so that the stabilizer can be pushed up against the chest wall. To make the tunnels and to undermine the skin we use heavy Mayo scissors, as such blunt dissection avoids bleeding.

Somewhat distal to the incision on the right (7th intercostal space) and somewhat more anteriorly (an-

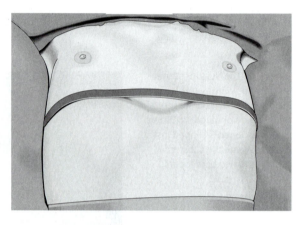

Fig. 12.5. A template of appropriate length is bent into the desired shape

Fig. 12.6. The bar is bent according to the shape of the template

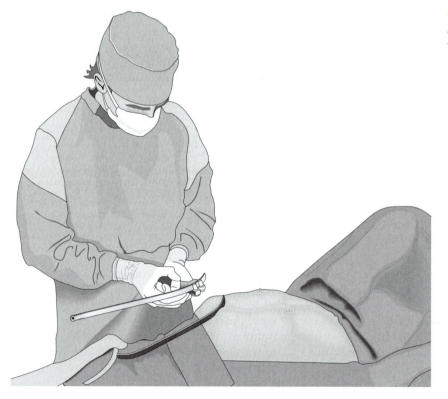

Fig. 12.7. Bilateral subcutaneous tunnels are made through small transverse incisions just anterior to the midaxillary line at the level of the maximal depression of the sternum

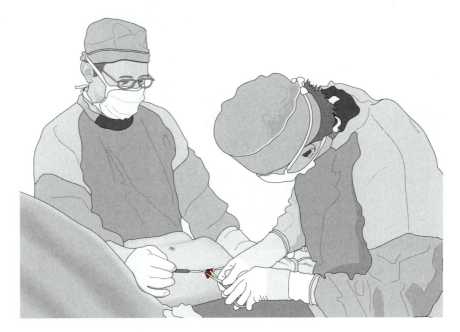

Fig. 12.8. A 6 mm cannula has been inserted slightly below and anterior to the incision. CO_2 is insufflated at a maximal pressure of 8 mmHg and an initial flow of 0.5 L/min. The S-shaped instrument is introduced into the tunnel and pierces the anterior chest wall at the beginning of the funnel

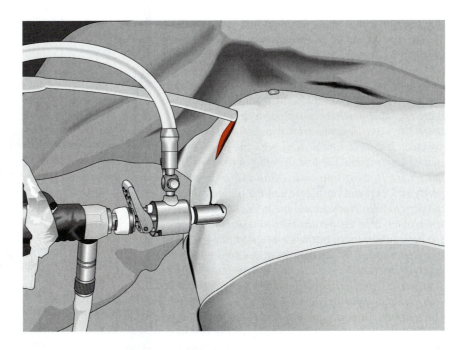

terior axillary line), a 6 mm cannula for a 5 mm 30° telescope is inserted (■ Fig. 12.8). To do this we make a 6 mm incision in the direction of the skin folds and make a small hole just cranial to the rib with a Mosquito forceps in the same way as we do when we insert a chest drain. Next a 6 mm cannula with blunt trocar is inserted and fixed to the skin. The intrathoracic position is checked before commencing insufflation. The first structure one sees is the diaphragm which moves with respiration. After creation of the CO_2 pneumothorax the chest cavity is scoped to verify that the lung is nicely pushed posteriorly and that there are no adhesions that may be in the way. The 30° scope is turned anteriorly and the place where the chest will be entered is identified. Next the S-shaped instrument is inserted in the right tunnel and turned over 180° with the point at the site where it should enter the chest (■ Fig. 12.8). The tip of the instrument now pierces the intercostal space in the middle and is pushed further until the lung is almost reached (■ Fig. 12.9). The instrument is then turned back over 180° and advanced to reach the groove between the sternum and pericardium. The

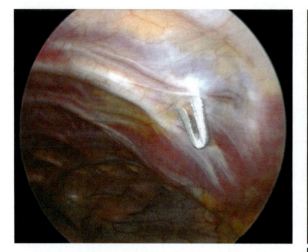

Fig. 12.9. The piercing of the anterior chest wall with the S-shaped instrument is watched endoscopically with a 5 mm 30° telescope

place of entry is always lateral to the internal mammary vessels which should be identified and saved.

Now the dissection of the substernal groove starts (■ Fig. 12.10a–c). The tip of the instrument should aim in the direction of the intercostal site at the other side where the instrument should come out. There is a tendency to direct the instrument more cranially as there are fat appendices lower down that tend to obscure the view. A more cranial direction should be avoided. The dissection is done with the tip of the S-shaped instrument. The first opening of the mediastinal pleura is most important. One can differentiate pretty well between the pleura and the pericardium as the pericardium is whiter and much thicker. Moreover when one is onto the pericardium, one does not pierce the pericardium once but twice as a fold of pericardium is entrapped. When the tip of the instrument is gently pushed downward in the groove between the sternum and pericardium, the mediastinal pleura will thin out and separate; this will not happen with the pericardium. Once a small opening is made the tip is inserted and now moved tangentially to the sternum thus enlarging the opening. CO_2 pressure will develop the substernal space further, much in the same way as during retroperitonoscopy. Soon the other side will be reached and the left lung can be seen through the mediastinal pleura of the other side. When the thin opposite mediastinal pleura is pierced, CO_2 will enter the opposite chest and will push the lung posteriorly. Finger pressure is exerted at the site where the S-shaped instrument should leave the chest and this place can be identified well endoscopically. The opposite skin incision is then pulled medially over the tip of the piercing S-shaped instrument (■ Fig. 12.11).

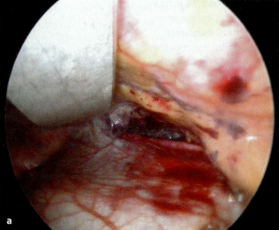

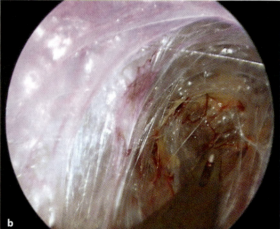

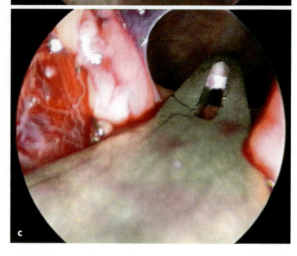

Fig. 12.10. **a** The groove between the sternum and pericardium is opened with the S-shaped instrument. **b** Next a substernal tunnel is created using CO_2 insufflation and blunt dissection. **c** The contralateral mediastinal pleura is pierced. As a result of CO_2 insufflation into the opposite chest cavity, the contralateral lung falls backward

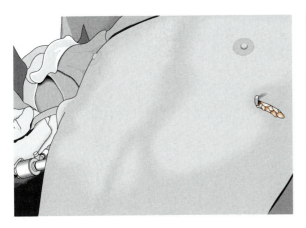

Fig. 12.11. The S-shaped instrument pierces the opposite chest wall at the side where the funnel ends

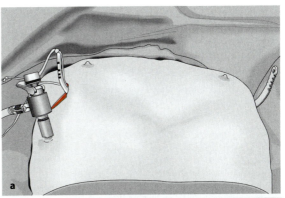

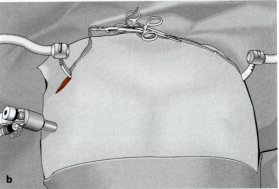

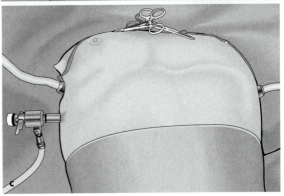

Fig. 12.12. **a** The bar has been pulled through from the left to the right with the concavity directed anteriorly. **b** The bar is being rotated through 180° posteriorly. **c** The rotation is completed

Next an umbilical tape is moistened and put through the eye of the tip of the S-shaped instrument after which the tape is pulled through as a loop. The loop is then divided leaving two separate tapes in the substernal tunnel. One tape will be used for pulling the bar through and the second one is used as a spare. They are marked with separate clamps at the ends. The prebent bar is tied to one of the tapes on the left side, after which the bar is pulled through with the concavity directed anteriorly (▬ Fig. 12.12a). It is important to pull rather than to push the bar in order to avoid the creation of a false passage. For initial entrance of the bar on the left it is advantageous to turn the bar so that the concavity is directly caudally. By doing so the bar enters the intercostal space on its side and not with its full transverse diameter. To pull the bar out on the right side the pulling force should not be laterally but anteriorly. Otherwise the intercostal space may be opened further laterally which does not contribute to good fixation and is more traumatizing.

Next the bar is turned over 180° posteriorly in such a way that the concavity passes caudally and not cranially (▬ Fig. 12.12b,c).

To avoid turning of the bar we glide a stabilizer over one of the ends, usually on the right. It is important that the stabilizer glides far enough over the bar so that the stabilizer rests on the chest wall over its entire length. We fix the stabilizer onto the bar with one diagonally placed metal suture (▬ Fig. 12.13a–c). If we are not sure that one stabilizer is enough we will use a second one on the other side as well. Some bars tend to turn because they are forced to do so by posterior angulation of the distal sternum. When this is the case, it seems wise to insert a second bar. If a second bar is inserted we use one stabilizer on each bar but on opposite sides.

At the end of the procedure, the spare tape is removed and remaining CO_2 is aspirated by connecting the hub of the cannula to the suction tube. We do not routinely insert chest drains (▬ Fig. 12.14).

If there are intrathoracic problems such as adhesions as a result of previous surgery, more ports can be inserted to deal with these using a two-handed dissection. Under such circumstances a second cannula can be inserted at the side of the lateral incision. The telescope is then changed to this position. A third port can be inserted two intercostal spaces higher up for the surgeon's left-hand instrument.

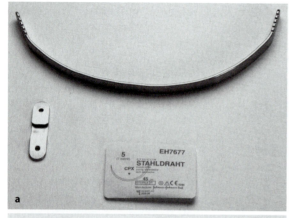

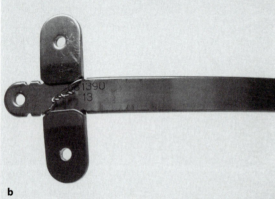

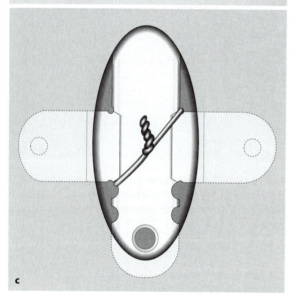

Fig. 12.13. **a** Bent bar with stabilizer and metal suture. **b** The stabilizer will be fixed to the bar with a diagonally placed metal suture. **c** Stabilizer with metal suture in place

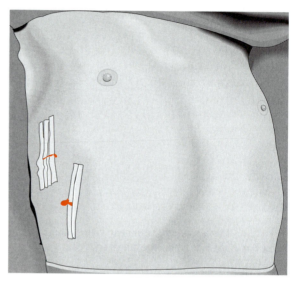

Fig. 12.14. End of the operation

Postoperative Care

A postoperative chest X-ray is made to evaluate lung expansion and residual pneumothorax as well as the position of the bar(s). A small residual pneumothorax, sometimes bilateral may be present but is clinically irrelevant.

Nuss bar correction of pectus excavatum is certainly not a minimally invasive procedure. The procedure is very painful, especially in older children and even more so in adults. Epidural analgesia for at least 72 h should therefore be given to all patients unless specific contraindications, for example coagulation disturbances, are present. At the same time as epidural analgesia we give the patients acetaminophen and diclofenac. In patients having epidural analgesia for this indication we often see a unilateral Horner syndrome and paresthesia or even paresis of an arm. Depending on the severity and complaints the dosage is adjusted. It is important to warn the patients of these side effects. After discontinuation of the epidural anesthesia, we add tramadol for the night for at least a week or even also for the day, when necessary. The patient is seen as an outpatient about 10 days after discharge. Pain medication is then adjusted as required. We stop first the tramadol during the day, then the tramadol during the night, then diclofenac, and finally acetaminophen.

A number of individuals continue to complain of pain for months, even for longer, and may need medication. We always tell them that we are prepared to take the bar out whenever they feel that they can not live with the pain. Of course we will tell them that we cannot guarantee the result when the bar is taken out too soon. We try to leave the bar in for 3 years and remove the bar then in daycare surgery.

Results

So far we have treated 57 children with the Nuss procedure for pectus excavatum. In one patient, difficulties in thoracoscoping the right chest were encountered. It appeared impossible to introduce a cannula. Finally we made a 2 cm-long minithoracotomy at the side of the transverse skin incision on the right and found a completely occluded pleural space. The history revealed severe pneumonia when the patient was very young. With digital dissection the lung was freed from the chest wall. Two more cannulae were inserted and further lysis of the lung was carried out thoracoscopically until the groove between the mediastinal pleura and pericardium was reached. The rest of the procedure was uneventful.

In a 15-year-old boy with severe pectus excavatum, but who had received an arterial switch procedure for transposition of the great vessels shortly after birth, dense adhesions were present between the sternum and underlying heart. The substernal space was freed without problems by bilateral thoracoscopic dissection, using a triangular configuration of the telescope cannula and two working cannulae. A pediatric cardiac surgeon was on standby.

Helping a thoracic surgeon performing a Nuss procedure in an adult patient, the pericardium was pierced twice, in and out, but this was diagnosed immediately, as some clear fluid leaked into the right chest, and was corrected.

Three patients have developed bar infection. The infection settled in all patients with antibiotics and none of them required bar removal (Van Renterghem et al. 2005).

The most important drawback of the operation is the pain it causes. The pain may persist for weeks or even months and deserves attention. In the early postoperative period side effects of the high epidural analgesia, such as Horner syndrome and paresthesia or even paresis of the arm, are frequently observed. These side effects do not seem harmful but the patients should be informed about them.

Discussion

There is no doubt that Nuss has revolutionized the treatment of pectus excavatum. The best results are achieved in patients with a symmetrical deep deformity. The results, as can be expected, are less good in patients with asymmetrical deformities and in patients with a flat chest. In the latter patients the Nuss procedure can be seen either as an initial repair to be followed by further more classic corrective surgery, or as an adjuvant during initial full correction. We have used the Nuss bar with success in patients in which we corrected a pectus carinatum but in which the sternum sank too deep after extensive subperichondrial resection of the involved ribs.

A 9.5% incidence of displacement of the bar has been reported (Hebra et al. 2000). Several methods to prevent this complication have been tried out. By using lateral stabilizers, Croitoru et al. (2002) were able to reduce the incidence of bar displacement from 15% to 6%. Thoracoscopic pericostal fixation of the bar either parasternally or more laterally has also been described (Hebra et al. 2001; Schaarschmidt et al. 2002). We are not in favor of pericostal sutures as they may cause damage to the intercostal nerve.

Thoracoscopy is an essential part of the procedure and complications related to a more or less blind creation of the substernal tunnel are unacceptable. Bilateral thoracoscopy has been advocated by some (Schaarschmidt et al. 2002), but we feel that this is unnecessary in most patients as a complete substernal tunnel can be easily created from the right. If there is any problem in creating the tunnel, a second cannula can be inserted at the site of the lateral skin incision allowing for formal dissection of the tunnel. Thoracoscopic clearance of the sternum has been advocated for patients requiring reiterative sternotomy in order to avoid complications during the opening of the sternum (Gazzaniga and Palafox 2001). We also were impressed by the easiness of the substernal dissection in the patient who had an arterial switch procedure in the neonatal period.

We have not had any complication related to the thoracoscopy, and the creation of a bilateral CO_2 pneumothorax seems to be well tolerated. There is no need for leaving a drain behind unless there is a suspicion that the lung has been damaged. Postoperative AP and lateral chest X-rays are taken to document the position of the bar and stabilizer(s) and to check lung expansion.

A major drawback of the procedure is the pain it causes and protocolized pain management is imperative. The term minimal invasive is not appropriate here and should be replaced by minimal access.

References

Croitoru DP, Kelly RE Jr, Goretsky MJ, et al (2002) Experience and modification update for the minimally invasive Nuss technique for pectus excavatum repair in 303 patients. J Pediatr Surg 37:437–445

Gazzaniga AB, Palafox BA (2001) Substernal thoracoscopic guidance during sternal reentry. Ann Thorac Surg 72:289–290

Hebra A, Swoveland B, Egbert M, et al (2000) Outcome analysis of minimally invasive repair of pectus excavatum: review of 251 cases. J Pediatr Surg 35:252–257

Hebra A, Gauderer MW, Tagge EP, et al (2001) A simple technique for preventing bar displacement with the Nuss repair of pectus excavatum. J Pediatr Surg 36:1266–1268

Nuss D, Kelly RE, Croitoru DP, et al (1998) A 10-year review of a minimally invasive technique for the correction of pectus excavatum. J Pediatr Surg 33:545–552

Schaarschmidt K, Kolberg-Schwerdt A, et al (2002) Submuscular bar, multiple pericostal bar fixation, bilateral thoracoscopy: a modified Nuss repair in adolescents. J Pediatr Surg 37:1276–1280

Van Renterghem KM, von Bismarck S, Bax NMA et al. ME (2005) Should an infected Nuss bar be removed? J Pediatr Surg 40:670–673

Chapter 13

Thoracoscopic Drainage and Debridement of Empyema

Saundra M. Kay and Steven S. Rothenberg

Introduction

In the past, empyema was treated with antibiotics, prolonged chest tube drainage, and, if this failed, open thoracotomy for debridement. This was associated with long hospitalizations and significant morbidity due to the delayed referral to a surgeon and to the surgical procedure itself. With the expanded use of endoscopic techniques, thoracoscopy has been increasingly used in the treatment of empyema and much earlier in the course of disease (Gandhi and Stringer 1997; Kercher et al. 2000; Kern and Rodgers 1993; Klena et al. 1998; McGahren 2001; Merry et al. 1999; Rodgers 2003; Rothenberg and Chang 1997). The minimal morbidity associated with this procedure makes it ideal for the treatment of empyema in children.

Preoperative Preparation

Before Induction of General Anesthesia

Confirmation that the pleural fluid collection is indeed loculated, and therefore much less likely to respond to chest tube drainage alone, can be accomplished with a lateral decubitus chest radiograph, thoracic ultrasound, or chest computed tomography (CT). Deteriorating pulmonary function should be considered an indication rather than a contraindication for quicker intervention.

After Induction of General Anesthesia

The patient has generally been started on antibiotics and these are continued. The anesthetist can perform a selective contralateral bronchial intubation, but this is not necessary. If done, prior to finishing the procedure the endotracheal tube will need to be pulled back to ensure full expansion of the released lung. If the patient already has a chest tube in place, this can be removed prior to patient positioning and preparation and the site may be used for placement of one of the ports. A suction trap should be prepared to obtain a sample of the pleural fluid for cell count, gram stain, and culture [± lactate dehydrogenase (LDH), glucose, and protein], if this has not been done previously. Injection of port sites with a local anesthetic agent such as 0.25% Marcaine ± epinephrine may help decrease postoperative discomfort (maximum dose: 2 mg/kg = 0.8 cc/kg).

Positioning

Patient

The patient is placed in a lateral decubitus position with the affected side up. An axillary roll and appropriate protective padding are used and the patient secured with tape or straps. In an older child, support can be provided by a beanbag. The upper arm is extended upward and outward and secured in position (Fig. 13.1) If the patient does not tolerate this position (persistent desaturation), s/he may be placed more supine, at a 30–45° angle.

Crew, Monitors, and Equipment

As the surgeon will need to access the entire chest cavity, s/he may stand on either side of the patient. The surgical assistant is usually positioned on the other side of the table to hold the camera. Alternatively, the assistant may stand on the same side of the operating table as the surgeon, either cranially or caudally. The scrub nurse is toward the patient's feet, on either side.

Two monitors are used with one placed on each side of the patient at the level of the patient's chest near the shoulders to allow unobstructed views by the surgeon and assistant (Fig. 13.2).

Special Equipment

No special energy applying system is required. A suction-irrigation system should be present as well as a Pleurovac and an appropriate-sized chest tube.

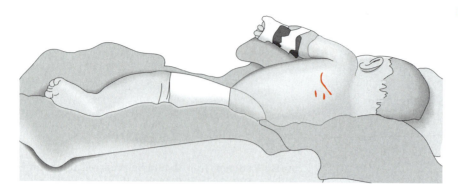

Fig. 13.1. Patient position

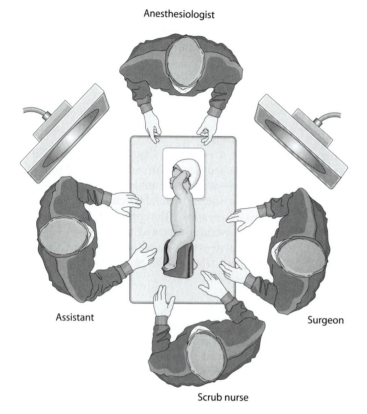

Anesthesiologist

Assistant

Scrub nurse

Surgeon

Fig. 13.2. Positioning of the crew and equipment.

Technique

Cannulae

Cannula	Method of insertion	Diameter (mm)	Device	Position
1	Closed (or open)	5	4- or 5 mm 30° endoscope	Just anterior to midaxillary line at approximately the 5th interspace
2	Closed	5	Suction-irrigator and grasping forceps	Just posterior to midaxillary line at approximately the 6th interspace

The two port sites (■ Fig. 13.3) can be used interchangeably to reach all pleural surfaces. A 10 mm port can be used instead of a 5 mm port at one site to facilitate removal of the fibrinous debris. Also, a third 5 mm port can be added if the two existing ports do not allow access to all the pleural surfaces. This is rarely needed.

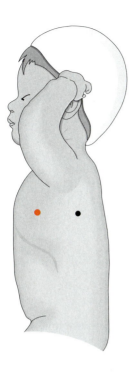

Fig. 13.3. Positioning of the ports

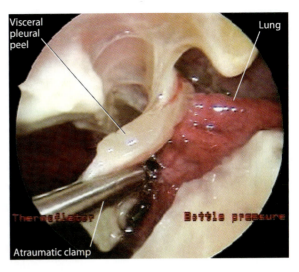

Fig. 13.4. Intraoperative view of pleural peel

Procedure

A Veress needle is placed just anterior to the midaxillary line at approximately the 4th or 5th interspace after infiltrating the site with local anesthetic and making a small transverse incision. Alternatively, an open approach may be used for placement of the first trocar. If there is an identified site on ultrasound or CT with a big fluid pocket close to one of the proposed port sites, this should be chosen as the point of entry. Insufflation with low flow CO_2 to a pressure of 4–5 mmHg may help collapse the lung and improve visualization as the fibrinous adhesions are taken down. A 5 mm trocar is then placed and the 30° scope is introduced.

The endoscope can be used to bluntly take down adhesions and break up loculations, especially inferoposteriorly to allow for placement of the second trocar under thoracoscopic vision. This 5 mm port is placed more posteriorly and inferiorly at approximately the 6th interspace along the posterior axillary line.

A suction-irrigator is introduced to aspirate the free pleural fluid and further break down loculations with blunt dissection. A sample of the fluid can be collected at this time with a trap. A grasping forceps can then be used to peel off and remove the fibrinous debris through the trocar (■ Fig. 13.4). A bowel clamp works well for this purpose.

The scope and operating instrument can be interchanged from one port site to another to ensure that all of the pleural surfaces are reached. A systematic approach within the chest also helps ensure that no surface is left untouched.

Once the lung has been completely freed, all of the pleural fluid drained, and most of the fibrinous peel removed, the thoracic cavity is irrigated with warm normal saline that is subsequently aspirated out. The suction-irrigator is removed and the pneumothorax dissipated. The lung is allowed to expand fully with the help of positive pressure breaths from the anesthetist. Once full expansion is confirmed, the lower trocar is removed and a chest tube, appropriate to the child's size, is placed and positioned posteroinferiorly under thoracoscopic vision and secured in place. The scope and remaining trocar are removed. This site is closed in two layers. The chest tube is attached to a Pleurovac and appropriate dressings are placed.

Postoperative Care

The chest tube is initially left to suction at −10 to −20 cm H_2O pressure. Once drainage becomes minimal, there is no evidence of an air leak, and the child is improving, the chest tube can be removed, usually after a trial of underwater seal. This is usually by the 3rd or 4th postoperative day. Antibiotics are continued and, if cultures are positive, adjusted accordingly. Chest X-rays are obtained at intervals to follow progress. Analgesia is necessary and most often given as intravenous morphine boluses in the first 24–48 h postoperatively. Oral analgesia may be adequate thereafter. The patient is usually discharged to home on antibiotics after s/he has been afebrile for 48 h. Follow-up chest X-rays are obtained as an outpatient to insure complete resolution.

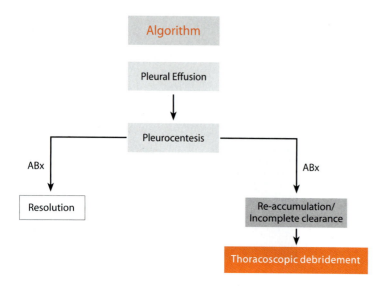

Fig. 13.5. Algorithm for management of empyema

Results

Over a 10-year period we have performed 117 thoracoscopic drainage and debridements. Ages have ranged from 5 months to 20 years and weights from 6 to 110 kg. Operative times have been from 15 to 135 min with the average being 48 min. There were no conversions to open. Chest tubes were left in for 2–10 days with an average of 3.2 days. One patient required reexploration for drainage of loculated abscesses. Two patients had small intraparenchymal abscesses which developed after their initial debridement; these were drained with small pigtail catheters under CT guidance. Three patients underwent reexploration with formal lobectomy for severe necrotizing pneumonia and continued deterioration after their thoracoscopic debridement.

Discussion

Thoracoscopic debridement has significantly changed the algorithm for the treatment of empyema in children (■ Fig. 13.5). The ability to quickly clean out infected fluid and debris through minimal incisions and with minimal morbidity has lowered our threshold for intervention. In general any child thought to need a chest tube for adequate drainage of an empyema is taken to the operating room for a thoracoscopic debridement. Earlier intervention has resulted in quicker recovery with minimal complications. The procedure is relatively straightforward and does not require advanced endoscopic skills. Also excessive time should not be taken in debriding the chest as the goal should be to break down all loculations and remove the majority of the inflammatory peel. Excessive operative times will add to the morbidity of the procedure.

A little bleeding is to be expected as the inflamed fibrinous adhesions are taken down and the peel is removed. This is usually minor and self-limited. If there is a localized bleeding point, monopolar cautery may be used with care.

Small air leaks may also result from the blunt dissection. These are also usually self-limited and will seal early in the postoperative period with full lung expansion and a chest tube. Occasionally, a persistent bronchopleural fistula may necessitate reoperation but this is rare.

An added advantage of the procedure is that the lung parenchyma may itself be easily evaluated. In the three cases of severe necrotizing pneumonia requiring later lobectomy, direct visualization of necrotic lung at the time of thoracoscopy helped in the decision to resect the lung.

If surgical consultation is delayed and the patient has been symptomatic for a prolonged period of time, thoracoscopic drainage and debridement may not be possible and an open decortication may be the patient's only option. This can, however, be assessed by the thoracoscope. With increased awareness of the success of thoracoscopic debridement, surgeons are now generally consulted early on in the course of disease and the need for open decortication is rarely seen.

References

Gandhi RR, Stringel G (1997) Video-assisted thoracoscopic surgery in the management of pediatric empyema. JSLS 1:251–253

Kercher KW, Attorri RJ, Hoover JD, et al (2000) Thoracoscopic decortication as first-line therapy for pediatric parapneumonic empyema: a case series. Chest 118:24–27

Kern JA, Rodgers BM (1993) Thoracoscopy in the management of empyema in children. J Pediatr Surg 28:1128–1132

Klena JW, Cameron BH, Langer JC, et al (1998) Timing of video-assisted thoracoscopic debridement for pediatric empyema. J Am Coll Surg 187:404–408

McGahren ED (2001) Use of thoracoscopy for treatment of empyema in children. Pediatr Endosurg Innov Tech 5:117–125

Merry CM, Bufo AJ, Shah RS et al. (1999) Early definitive intervention by thoracoscopy in pediatric empyema. J Pediatr Surg 34:178–181

Rodgers BM (2003) The role of thoracoscopy in pediatric surgical practice. Semin Pediatr Surg 12:62–70

Rothenberg SS, Chang JHT (1997) Thoracoscopic decortication in infants and children. Surg Endosc 11:993–994

Chapter 14

The Thoracoscopic Approach to Pneumothorax in Children

Klaus Schaarschmidt and K. Uschinsky

Introduction

Spontaneous pneumothorax has an occurrence of 3.4 in 10,000 hospitalized infants and of 1 in 10,000 hospitalized children (Alter 1997), whereas the incidence in cystic fibrosis above the age of ten rises to 5.1% (Kuster et al. 1988).

The first symptom of spontaneous pneumothorax is a sudden, sharp, "burning" pleuritic pain out of perfect well being, sometimes treated as "back pain" or ipsilateral shoulder pain. Underlying pathologies are cystic fibrosis, asthma, cystic malformations, postinfectious bullae, infectious pneumonias, Ehlers-Danlos syndrome, Marfan syndrome, or endometriosis, i.e., catamenial pneumothorax (Hässler et al. 1999), while in developing countries tuberculosis, acquired immunodeficiency syndrome (AIDS), or parasites such as hydatid disease and *Ascaris lumbricoides* are reported causes.

Indications

The primary therapy in every case is thoracic drainage preferably placed in the 2nd intercostal space (ICS) and a medioclavicular line with its tip in the apical thorax. Drainage in the 4th ICS (mamillar level) carries the risk of placing the drain into the interlobar fissure, which renders the drainage insufficient.

Persistent air bubbles in the drainage system indicate a parenchymatous fistula. Thoracoscopy is indicated if a fistula persists beyond 72 h (maximum 1 week) of sufficient suction, in recurrent or bilateral spontaneous pneumothorax, in large cystic malformations with any proven bullae (e.g., postinfectious), or with any significant apical adhesions of the lung because they predispose to bulla formation in the fixed parts of the lung (Fackeldey et al. 2002).

Preoperative Preparation

High-resolution multislice computed tomography (CT) of the thorax is superior to X-rays because 50% of the bullae go unrecognized on conventional thorax X-rays in two planes. Epidural anesthesia is helpful and usually double lumen endotracheal intubation or single lung main stem intubation is required, but a bronchoscopically placed Fogarty catheter for intermittent blockage is satisfactory for very young children although pleurectomy is a typical operation of adolescence.

The child is fitted with a nasogastric tube and is given a single injection of cephalosporin. The port site holes are injected with 1 ml of 0.5% mepivacaine (Schaarschmidt et al. 1996).

Positioning

The patient is placed in a lateral position as for an anterolateral thoracotomy with the surgeon standing at the patient's ventral side and the assistant and scrub nurse opposite. In reversed Trendelenburg position the lung is kept out of the operative field by gravity, when the operating table is turned. The child is securely fixed with supports for the scapular and pelvic regions (■ Fig. 14.1a).

Energy Sources and Equipment

Energy source	Equipment
High-frequency electro-coagulation (HFE)	Monopolar hook and bipolar scissors
Ultrasonic energy	Ultrasonic shears
Argon	Argon beamer
Laser	Nd-YAG 1,064 nm or KTP laser
Other	Infrared coagulator 10 mm
Hydrojet 5 mm	Rarely for water jet dissection of adhesions
Ligasure, Biclamp	For the treatment of blebs
Clips	10 mm for last tissue bridges in stapler resection
Staplers	Endolinear staplers (-GIA)
Other	Roeder loops, mineral sponge (Sponge Ethicon)

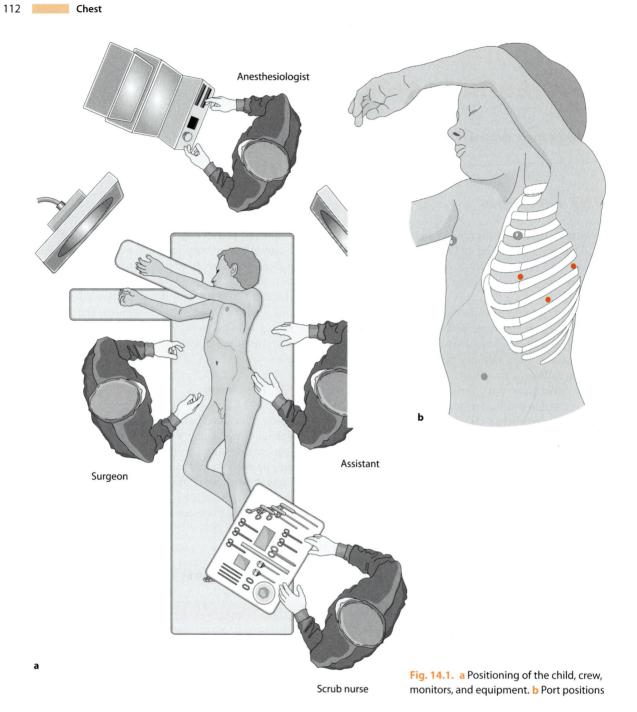

Anesthesiologist

Surgeon

Assistant

Scrub nurse

b

Fig. 14.1. a Positioning of the child, crew, monitors, and equipment. **b** Port positions

Technique

Cannulae

Cannula	Method of insertion	Diameter (mm)	Device	Position
1	Open	5–10	30° lens, 5–10 mm	Seventh intercostal space, axillary line
2	Open	5, flexible	Satinsky clamp	Sixth intercostal space, posterior axillary line
3	Open	10–12	Clamp/sponge/GIA	Fifth intercostal space, anterior axillary line

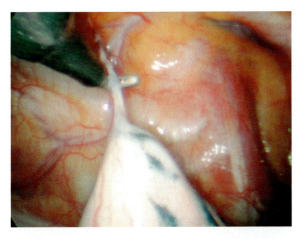

Fig. 14.2. Apical adhesion in spontaneous pneumothorax resected by hook cautery

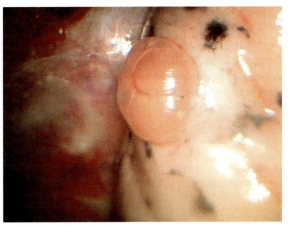

Fig. 14.3. Single apical bulla in an 18-year-old girl with spontaneous pneumothorax

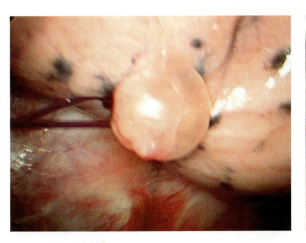

Fig. 14.4. Ligation of an isolated bulla

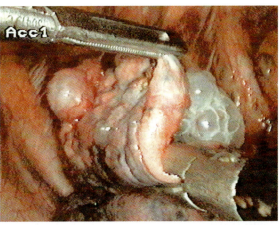

Fig. 14.5. Stapler resection of multiple bullae in the pulmonary apex

Three trocars are required: one in the 5th or 6th intercostal space at the anterior axillary line, one lower in the midaxillary line, and one in the 6th intercostal space at the posterior axillary line (■ Fig. 14.1b). The basal port is commonly used for the 30° telescope, the ventral port for dissecting forceps or the forceps holding the mineral sponge, and the dorsal for dissecting forceps or preferably Satinsky clamp.

Pleurodesis

Pleurodesis consists of three essential steps: thorough inspection of the lung, resection of adhesive bands and bullae, and finally apical pleurodesis.

The first step of pleurodesis is a thorough inspection of the whole hemithorax including the diaphragm, ventral and dorsal parts of the lung, and particularly the lower lobe. Inspection of the lung must detect all adhesions and bullous changes.

Adhesions are vascularized and cut by monopolar or ultrasonic hook or bipolar scissors (■ Fig. 14.2), while, for example, tearing apical adhesions may induce severe hemorrhage. Bullae are most frequent in the dorsal parts of segment one, the apex of segment six along the edges of the lobes, and occasionally in the middle lobe (■ Fig. 14.3). Some patients have bullae in all these regions, but in children and adolescents they are often limited to segment one. We ligate single bullae (■ Fig. 14.4) by Roeder loops (Yim and Liu 1996; Liu et al. 1999), although not all authors recommend this (Cardillo et al. 2000). Although we prefer ultrasonic scissors, the Ligasure has been increasingly used for bullae and in many centers has become a preferential instrument for lung reduction surgery. Areas with multiple bullae are resected by Endo-GIA (■ Fig. 14.5) taking care that the border line of the resection is free of bullae predisposing to leaks and persisting fistulae along the staples (this danger can be reduced by reinforcing the stapling line with strips of bovine pericardium (e.g., Peristrips). Marked scars in the pulmonary apex are resected, even if they do not display unequivocal bullous changes, because similar to pleural adhesions they induce bulla formation in their periphery (Fackeldey et al. 2002).

Pleurectomy

The concept of apical pleurodesis is based on two facts. First, bullous changes are usually restricted to the supramamillar thorax. Second, complete pleurodesis to the diaphragm results in severe restrictive ventilation disorders, which are the problems in talcum poudrage or chemical pleurodesis and which are difficult to control (e.g., supramycin, acting by excessively lowering the pH).

Basically the complete pleura cranially of the mamilla is removed circumferentially (■ Fig. 14.6). Pleurectomy is started on the dorsal aspect of the thorax from the 6th rib upward to the thoracic apex. Ventrally the pleura is dissected off the thoracic wall from the 3rd or 4th rib (corresponds to the mamilla) up to the apex again. The most problematic part is the mediastinal pleura, which must be removed completely above the mamillar plane, i.e., close to the hilum of the lung. Here nervous (phrenic nerve, sympathetic chain) and vascular injuries are possible, and this is why the procedure is often done incompletely in this area, which results in the particularly frequent mediastinal recurrences of the pneumothorax. Even performing pleurectomy very meticulously, we experienced two hemorrhages.

Pleural Abrasion

Consequently we have favored pleural abrasion in recent years, which we perform by means of a mineral sponge (diathermy cleaner) (■ Fig. 14.7). The sponge is held by a clamp and rubbed over the pleura until visible superficial bleeding indicates pleural injury sufficient to induce effective pleurodesis (■ Fig. 14.8). Pleural abrasion is started dorsolaterally on the 6th rib and followed upward to the pleural apex. Small bleeding points should be visible all over the abraded pleura, however excessive pressure may injure the intercostal veins (■ Fig. 14.9). Rubbing the pleura with a dry sponge, however, will not lead to sufficient pleurodesis.

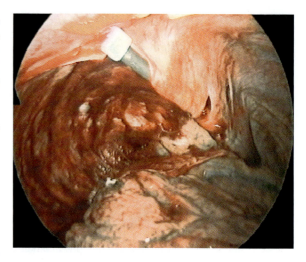

Fig. 14.6. Pleurectomy of the complete apical thorax by the "roll off" technique

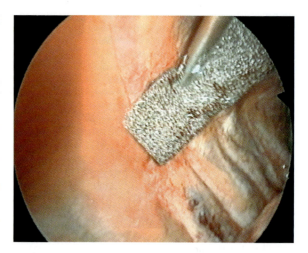

Fig. 14.7. Pleural abrasion by mineral sponge rubbed firmly over the pleura

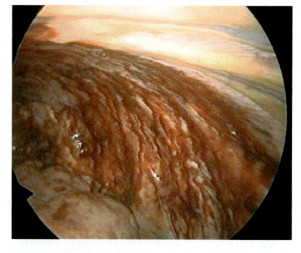

Fig. 14.8. Pleural abrasion from dorsal 6th rib; note border between abraded and native pleura

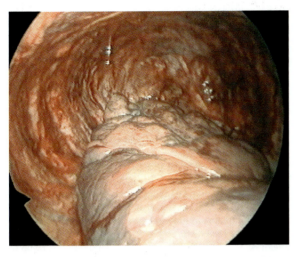

Fig. 14.9. Apical pleural abrasion completed with effective superficial lesions of the apical pleura

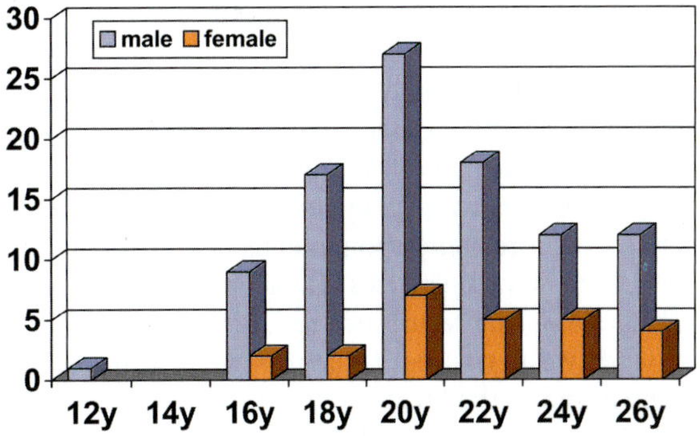

Fig. 14.10. Age and sex distribution of 121 pediatric and adolescent patients with pneumothorax undergoing thoracoscopic pleurodesis: a 10-year experience, Berlin-Buch 1993–2002

Postoperative Care

Consequent and sufficient thoracic suction is indispensable for complete expansion of the lung and full success of pleurodesis. We use two drains with multiple holes and at least a 24-French lumen, one up the dorsal thoracic wall and the second from the ventral access, which must reach the apex to avoid residual pneumothorax or a residual cavity. Sufficient suction means that under spontaneous breathing no pressure changes can be observed in the drainage system. As a rule 40 cm of H_2O and more for at least 72 h (time until first phases of wound healing occur) will be required to achieve effective pleurodesis. The patient can eat a regular diet once awake from anesthesia, and the urine catheter is removed the next day. In young patients dystelectasis or atelectasis of the lower lobe is not rare, therefore, even with suction, they should be mobilized early and vigorously by portable accu-pump. Pleurectomy and suction in young patients can be very painful and requires peridural anesthesia or liberal analgesics.

The next day an X-ray should show complete lung expansion, correct drain position, and no residual atelectasis. In uncomplicated cases the thoracic drains are removed, but not before 72 h of suction because in redo procedures within 72 h the visceral pleura can be easily peeled of the abraded areas. A further X-ray control after drain removal sometimes displays residual basal pleural effusion. The patients can be discharged from hospital after 5–6 days and have a final X-ray 4–7 days after discharge.

Results

None of our 121 patients treated thoracoscopically, 56 for left-sided, 66 for right-sided, and 1 for bilateral pneumothorax, died. Six patients had underlying disease such as cystic fibrosis, Stevens-Johnson syndrome, Marfan syndrome, histiocytosis X, Hodgkin's disease, or a posttraumatic pneumothorax. Ten patients had previously been treated for a contralateral pneumothorax by drainage elsewhere (■ Fig. 14.10).

Four patients needed a thoracotomy for complications: one for recurrent pneumothorax, one for a persisting fistula, one for postoperative hemorrhage, and one for a parenchymal tear at the stapler line. Two patients required a rethoracoscopy: one for recurrent pneumothorax and one for postoperative hemorrhage. Moreover eight patients required a subsequent tube thoracostomy drainage: three for recurrent pneumothorax, one for a persisting fistula, and four for pleural infection following long-standing tube thoracostomy drainage. In the these latter cases we recommend 2% povidone-iodine rinsing of the pleural cavity prior to thoracoscopy in order to prevent dissemination of bacteria.

Discussion

Chest tube drainage alone is indicated for spontaneous pneumothorax exceeding 20% of the pleural space (Effeldt et al. 1994; Weissberg and Refaely 2000) and is successful in about 70% of the cases (Cook et al. 1999; Schmelz et al. 1996; Wilcox et al. 1995). As a pathogenetic factor often small bullae or adhesions in the apical regions are seen. Large bullae usually develop in older patients. Some spontaneous pneumothoraces occur without detectable local pathological changes. In children, however, an obvious reason for spontaneous pneumothorax is found more frequently (42%) than in adults (<20%; Wilcox et al. 1995). The recurrence rate after tube drainage is 50% (Poenaru et al. 1994), second recurrences occur in up to 75% of cases, and there is risk of contralateral spontaneous pneumothorax in 50% of the first recurrences (Cook et al. 1999). Thus at 7/121 (5.8%) our recurrence rate (five pneumothoraces and two persisting fistulae) is well within in the range found in the literature (9% Cook et al. 1999; 0–7.9% Casadio et al. 2001, 2002)

Apical pleurodesis may be performed in four ways:
1. Pleurectomy
2. Abrasion of the parietal pleura in the apical thoracic cavity
3. Electropleurodesis by cautery (spray mode) or argon beamer along the ribs
4. Talcum poudrage of the apical thoracic cavity

Sufficient injury to the pleura, the fundamental mechanism, can be achieved by all four methods. However, pleurectomy is the most radical method, with a substantial incidence of hemorrhage (up to 10%). Abrasion is often not performed in a meticulous manner, but is reliable if done properly. Electropleurodesis is only performed along the ribs and therefore prone to recurrences of bullae and pneumothorax in between the coagulated areas (we had two recurrences).

Our complications of thoracoscopic pleurectomy were two hemorrhages (after pleurectomy), two persisting fistulae, for example from missed bullae (both following electropleurodesis), and a leaking stapler line erroneously placed through emphysematous pulmonary tissue. In continuously leaking fistulae or hemorrhage from the pleural edge, rethoracoscopy or thoracotomy may be inevitable. Thoracic hemorrhages covered by a coagulum do not stop until the hematoma has been removed. Infection of the access sites is rare.

After long persisting collapse of the lung and rapid expansion, very rarely a reexpansion edema (Yim and Liu 1996; Wong et al. 2000) may occur which can be life-threatening (clinical presentation as a unilateral pulmonary edema).

The most secure method of apical pleurodesis with the least complications is talcum poudrage (Rodgers et al. 1979), but it induces such firm scars that a subsequent thoracotomy may be virtually impossible (Cardillo et al. 2000; McGahren et al. 1990). Therefore talcum poudrage should be avoided for pleurodesis in young patients and is contraindicated if later lung transplantation is considered, for example in patients with cystic fibrosis.

Presently we use pleural abrasion as the standard technique and pleurectomy in rare problem cases.

References

Alter SJ (1997) Spontaneous pneumothorax in infants a 10-year review. Pediatr Emerg Care 13:401–403

Cardillo G, Facciolo F, Giunti R, et al (2000) Videothoracic treatment of primary spontaneous pneumothorax: a 6-year experience. Ann Thorac Surg 69:357–362

Casadio C, Rena O, Giobbe R, et al (2001) Primary spontaneous pneumothorax. Is video-assisted thoracoscopy stapler resection with pleural abrasion the gold-standard. Eur J Cardiothoracic Surg 20:897–898

Casadio C, Rena O, Giobbe R, et al (2002) Stapler blebectomy and pleural abrasion by video-assisted thoracoscopy for spontaneous pneumothorax. J Cardiovasc Surg 43:259–262

Cook CH, Melvin WS, Groner JI, et al (1999) A cost-effective thoracoscopic treatment strategy for pediatric pneumothorax. Surg Endosc 13:1208–1210

Effeldt RJ, Schröder DW, Thies DJ (1994) Long-term follow-up of different therapy procedures in spontaneous pneumothorax. J Cardiovasc Surg 35:229–233

Fackeldey V, Schöneich R, Otto A, et al (2002) Recurrence of apical blebs after surgical treatment of primary spontaneous pneumothorax.. Chirurg 73:348–352

Hässler K, Uschinsky K, Engelmann C (1999) Catamenial pneumothorax: report of three cases and review of the literature. Z Herz Thorax Gefässchir 13:78–82

Kuster P, Bender SW, Posselt HG, et al (1988) Spontaneous pneumothorax in cystic fibrosis. Monatsschr Kinderheilkd 136:251–255

Liu HP, Yim APC, Izzat MB, et al (1999) Thoracoscopic surgery for spontaneous pneumothorax. World J Surg 23:1133–1136

McGahren ED, Teague WG, Flanagan T, et al (1990) The effect of talc poudrage on growing swine. J Pediatr Surg 25:1147–1151

Poenaru D, Yazbeck S, Murphy S (1994) Primary spontaneous pneumothorax in children. J Pediatr Surg 29:1383–1385

Rodgers BM, Moazam F, Talbert J (1979) Thoracoscopy in children. Ann Surg 189:176–180

Schaarschmidt K, Schleef J, Kerremanns I, et al (1996) Laparoscopic and thoracoscopic surgery in infancy and childhood: the Münster/Gent experience. Technol Health Care 4:263–271

Schmelz HU, Becker HP, Gerngross H (1996) Spontaneous pneumothorax: what is the treatment of choice? Evaluation of 7820 published cases. Z Herz Thorax Gefässchir 10:177–184

Weisberg D, Refealy Y (2000) Pneumothorax: experience with 1199 patients. Chest 117:1279–1285

Wilcox DT, Glick PL, Karamanoukian HL et al. (1995) Spontaneous pneumothorax: a single-institution, 12-year experience in patients under 16 years of age. J Pediatr Surg 30:1452–1454

Wong KS, Liu HP, Yeow KM (2000) Spontaneous pneumothorax in children. Acta Paediatr TW 41:263–265

Yim APC, Liu HP (1996) Complications and failures of video-assisted thoracic surgery: experience from two centers in Asia. Ann Thorac Surg 61:538–541

Chapter 15

Thoracoscopic Lung Biopsy

Steven S. Rothenberg

Introduction

One of the most common thoracic procedures performed in children today is a lung biopsy. This can be for diagnostic reasons, in the case of interstitial lung disease (ILD), or for therapeutic and diagnostic reasons in the case of pulmonary nodules (Fan et al. (1997). Lung biopsy was one of the first procedures to be performed using thoracoscopic techniques (Rodgers 1993). New equipment and techniques now allow this to be performed in even the sickest and smallest patients with excellent results and with minimal morbidity. This technique has largely replaced open lung biopsy as the standard of care in infants and children.

Preoperative Preparation

Before Induction of General Anesthesia

Little preoperative intervention is usually necessary, even in the sickest patients. For ILD and cases of possible metastatic disease, a preoperative computed tomography (CT) scan is indicated to help identify the areas of interest. Biopsies in patients with ILD are usually directed to the most involved area on CT scan, as visual inspection often fails to identify discrete abnormalities. Pulmonary nodules that are peripherally placed and larger than 5 mm can usually be seen on the pleural surface once the lung is collapsed. In the case of smaller nodules or those that appear deeper in the lung parenchyma, preoperative localization may be necessary as visual inspection may fail to pinpoint the nodule. In these cases the patient should undergo preoperative CT localization. The patient is brought to the CT suite just prior to the thoracoscopy. Under CT guidance a small needle is inserted through the chest wall into the lung parenchyma directly overlying the nodule. One cubic centimeter of the patients own blood is then inserted into the pleura to create a blood patch which can be visualized at the time of thoracoscopy. This acts as a marker under which the surgeon can perform the wedge resection.

Respiratory failure requiring ventilator support is not a contraindication to a thoracoscopic approach. Even the sickest patients will tolerate a limited period of partial lung collapse required to perform the biopsy.

After Induction of General Anesthesia

Once the patient is under general anesthesia an attempt to obtain one-lung ventilation is usually made. In general, a mainstem intubation of the contralateral side is a quick and efficient way to obtain lung collapse of the side to be biopsied. Other techniques can be used if necessary and have already been discussed. In some cases the patient cannot tolerate collapse of one lung, and in these cases a tracheal intubation is used together with CO_2 insufflation to help partially collapse the lung. Pulse oximetry and an end-tidal CO_2 monitor are used during the case. Invasive monitoring is generally not needed.

A dose of cefazolin is generally administered, but may be held until after the biopsy in cases where the biopsy is being performed to look for a possible infectious cause.

Positioning:

Patient

In general the patient is placed in a lateral decubitus position with the side to be biopsied placed up. If a specific lesion is the target the patient may be placed in a more supine or prone position to give greater exposure to that area (■ Fig. 15.1). The patient can be placed on a beanbag for support, or in infants small

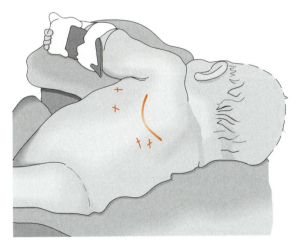

Fig. 15.1. Position of patient

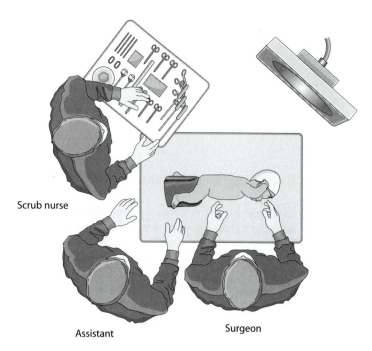

Fig. 15.2. Room setup for lung biopsy

Scrub nurse

Assistant

Surgeon

roles and pads can be used. An axillary role should be placed in all cases.

Crew, Monitors, and Equipment

The room should be set up to maximize exposure and ergonomics for the surgeon. If the site of biopsy is in the anterior portion of the lung then the monitor is placed across from the front of the patient and the surgeon and assistant stand at the patient's back (■ Fig. 15.2). The reverse is done if the site to be biopsied is posterior. If multiple sites are to be biopsied,

monitors may be necessary on both sides to facilitate the procedure.

Special Equipment

Usually no special energy applying systems are required. Endoloops may be used in children less than 10 kg bodyweight and staplers in patients over 10 kg. In selected cases a bag is inserted to retrieve the specimen.

Technique

Cannulae

Cannula	Method of insertion	Diameter (mm)	Device	Position
1	Closed	3 or 5	30° scope	Fifth or 6th intercostal space, midaxillary line
2	Closed	5 or 12	Endoloops, scissors, stapler	Varies depending on site to be biopsied
3	Closed	3 or 5	Maryland dissector, Babcock	Varies depending on site to be biopsied
4	Closed/ optional	3	Blunt grasper, retractor	

Figure 15.3 shows port placement.

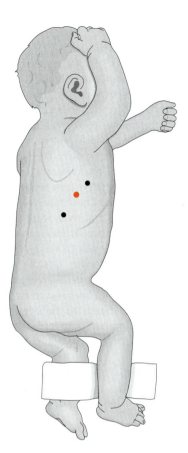

Fig. 15.3. Port placement for lung biopsy

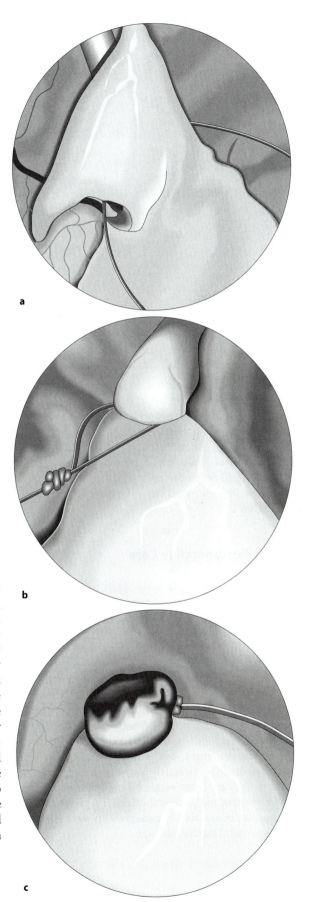

Procedure

After the patient is prepared and draped a Veress needle is inserted in the midaxillary line in the 5th or 6th interspace and the pleural cavity is insufflated with a low flow low pressure of CO_2 to help collapse the lung. A 3- or 5 mm trocar is then inserted and a 30° lens is used to survey the chest. If a specific lesion is being biopsied it is located, or in the case of preoperative localization the blood patch is identified. The second and third ports are placed to optimize the approach for the biopsy. If an anterior site is being biopsied the larger port (5 or 12 mm) is placed more posteriorly to allow for adequate room for the endoloops or stapler. It is placed in the lowest interspace that gives an acceptable approach to the biopsy site. The larger trocars are more easily placed through the lower interspaces especially in smaller infants. The third trocar is placed more anteriorly, closer to the biopsy site. A grasper is used through this site to grasp the biopsy site and facilitate the wedge resection. In smaller patients a series of two endoloops (0 Ethibond or a similar braided suture) are passed around the tongue of tissue to be biopsied and snared at the base (■ Fig. 15.4). The specimen is then

Fig. 15.4 a–c. Lung biopsy using endoloops

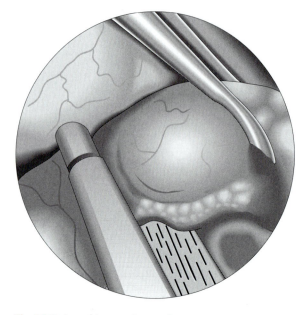

Fig. 15.5. Lung biopsy using staples

resected distally to the loops. In larger patients the endoscopic stapler is used to cut out the wedge of tissue (■ Fig. 15.5). If other sites are to be biopsied the same procedure is duplicated. The specimens can be removed through either the trocar itself or the trocar incision. If there is a concern for malignancy and the specimen will not fit through the trocar then it should be placed in a specimen bag to prevent trocar site recurrences.

Postoperative Care

A chest tube is left in place, usually through the lowest trocar site. This is set to suction at 15–20 cm of water pressure. The other sites are closed with absorbable suture. The endotracheal tube is then pulled back into the trachea and the lung is reinflated. If there is no evidence of an air leak the chest tube can be pulled out and an occlusive dressing applied prior to extubation in the operating room. If a small air leak is present the chest tube can be left in until it has resolved. Pain is usually adequately controlled with intermittent intravenous narcotic during the first 12–24 h and patients are rapidly switched to oral pain medication. A regular diet is resumed immediately. Patients are discharged as soon as they are comfortable on oral pain medication and tolerating adequate oral intake. This is usually the first postoperative day in patients who were admitted to the hospital for their biopsy.

Results

From January 1992 to July 2003, 194 thoracoscopic lung biopsies were performed in infants and children. Ages ranged from 3 weeks to 18 years and weight from 3.2 to 100 kg. Biopsy were performed for ILD, metastatic lung disease, and infectious etiology. Patients with ILD underwent biopsy of two different sites, in different lobes if possible. Most patients were done under single-lung ventilation achieved by mainstem intubation of the contralateral side. Operative time for lung biopsy (two sites) averaged 26 min. Chest tubes were left in place in only 5% of patients and most were removed in the first 24 h. Average hospital stay in patients admitted for their lung biopsy was 1.1 days. Adequate tissue for diagnosis was obtained in 98% of patients with ILD and 95% with malignancy. There were no intraoperative complications and there were two conversions to open because of extensive metastatic disease. There was one postoperative complication, a delayed pneumothorax on the third postoperative day.

Discussion

Lung biopsy is a commonly performed procedure in children. It is used for diagnosis and treatment of undiagnosed solitary nodules, in cases of metastatic lesions to the lung, and in cases of ILD or infectious infiltrates of unknown etiology. The ability to perform this procedure thoracoscopically has broadened the indications and applications of this technique and lowered the threshold for obtaining lung tissue to better direct therapy (Fan et al. 1997).

Thoracoscopic biopsy has several advantages over a standard or minithoracotomy. First, the entire surface of the lung and pleura can be evaluated through very limited access ports, and biopsies from multiple areas can easily be obtained. Second, the postoperative pain and recovery associated with a thoracoscopic biopsy is significantly less than that associated with a thoracotomy, to the extent where some patients may be done on an outpatient basis. The techniques of using an endoscopic stapler or endoloops have proven to be relatively simple and reliable allowing us to refrain from leaving chest tubes in, which are responsible for the majority of the pain following a thoracoscopic biopsy. The quality and size of the biopsies has been excellent allowing us to achieve over 95% diagnostic yield. Because of the rapidity of the procedure and ease with which it can be performed, we recommend obtaining two biopsies from divergent areas in all cases of ILD (Rothenberg 2000; Rothenberg et al. 1996).

The greatest controversy surrounds the use of this technique in the case of metastatic lung disease, especially with soft tissue sarcomas. The concern is that CT scan is not sensitive enough to detect all the nodules in the lung (especially in cases of soft tissue sarcomas) and therefore some may be missed at the time of surgery because the lung cannot be palpated. Also lesions which are significantly deep to the pleura cannot be visualized even with the lung collapsed. Preoperative CT localization has proved to be a good adjunct in these cases and we have only missed one lesion using this technique (the blood patch could not be seen on exploration). The issue of lesions not seen by CT is somewhat of a philosophical debate. The question arises that if there are lesions not seen by CT and removing these affects the patient's survival then should not all patients undergo bilateral open thoracotomy. And what of the lesions that are too small to be palpated: is leaving them behind clinically significant. We have elected to approach these cases thoracoscopically if there are three or fewer lesions on CT, and then we follow them with serial scans and repeat the thoracoscopy if new lesions arise (Smith et al. 2002). We feel the low morbidity associated with this procedure warrants this approach. If there are more than three nodules or are multiple nodules on both sides then we favor an open approach. Using this algorithm our survival rate in sarcoma patients with metastatic disease is similar to that of previous reports using open techniques.

References

Fan LL, Kozmetz CA, Rothenberg SS (1997) The diagnostic value of transbronchial thoracoscopic and open lung biopsy in immunocompetent children with chronic interstitial lung disease. J Pediatr 131:565–569

Rodgers BM (1993) Pediatric thoracoscopy. Where have we come, what have we learned? Ann Thorac Surg 56:704–707

Rothenberg SS (2000) Thoracoscopic lung resection in children. J Pediatr Surg 35:271–275

Rothenberg SS, Wagener JS, Chang JHT, et al (1996) The safety and efficacy of thoracoscopic lung biopsy for diagnosis and treatment in infants and children. J Pediatr Surg 31:100–104

Smith JJ, Rothenberg SS, Brooks M, et al (2002) Thoracoscopic surgery in childhood cancer. J Pediatr Hematol Oncol 24:429–435

Chapter 16

Thoracoscopic Lobectomy in Infants and Children

Steven S. Rothenberg

Introduction

While many thoracoscopic procedures have become commonplace, anatomic or formal thoracoscopic lobectomy in children has been a relatively rarely described procedure. Initial reports suggested that these procedures were best performed using a video-assisted thoracoscopic or VATS approach combining a mini-thoracotomy with two or three thoracoscopic ports (Mattioli et al. 1998; Rothenberg 1998). The procedure was performed using a combination of standard and laparoscopic instrumentation. Others have described non-anatomic dissections, primarily for lower lobectomies, performing essentially a mass ligature of structures crossing the major fissure using an endoscopic stapler. However anatomic variation makes this a riskier and less attractive alternative. The primary limitation has been the relatively small working space available in the thorax of an infant or small child (especially in the case of large cystic lesions), and the difficulty of isolating and safely ligating the main pulmonary vessels. Recent technologic advances in instrumentation, energy sources, and technique have now made formal anatomic lobectomy using thoracoscopic techniques a much more feasible and safe procedure. Indications for thoracoscopic lobectomy include intralobar sequestration, congenital adenomatoid malformation (CAM), congenital lobar emphysema (CLE), severe bronchiectasis, and, on rare occasions, malignancy (Albanese et al. 2003; Rothenberg 2000, 2003).

Preoperative Preparation

Before Induction of General Anesthesia

Extensive preoperative workup is generally not necessary. The lesions should be evaluated with a computed tomography (CT) scan to determine the location and probable etiology of the lesion. Many of the patients are now diagnosed *in utero* on prenatal ultrasound. In these cases a confirmatory CT scan should be performed after birth. The timing of the operation is dependent on the surgeons' experience, the physiologic condition of the infant or child, the etiology of the disease, and to a lesser extent the size of the child. Because of the potential for significant bleeding, blood should be typed and crossmatched and available in the operating room at the time of surgery. Routine magnetic resonance imaging (MRI), angiography, ventilation perfusion scan, and pulmonary function studies are generally not necessary but can be obtained on an individual basis depending on the type of lesion suspected.

After Induction of General Anesthesia

The procedures are best performed with single-lung ventilation of the opposite side. In larger patients a double lumen endotracheal tube or a bronchial blocker can be placed. In infants and smaller children single-lung ventilation is obtained by mainstem intubation of the contralateral side. Routine pulse oximetry is used but formal arterial lines, central venous monitoring, or other invasive monitoring is rarely needed. If single-lung ventilation cannot be obtained, the procedure can be performed with just CO_2-induced pneumothorax. However this can make the dissection somewhat more difficult. A nasogastric tube is routinely placed to help identify and avoid injury to the esophagus, and a single preoperative dose of cefazolin is generally sufficient except in cases of ongoing infection. Spinal or epidural anesthesia is rarely indicated and the port sites are all infiltrated with 0.25% Marcaine prior to an incision being made.

Positioning

Patient

For most cases the procedure is best performed with the patient in a lateral decubitus position (■ Fig. 16.1). The patient should be supported on a bean bag with an axillary role and sufficient padding of pressure points (i.e., knee or ankle). In neonates the patient may be supported with just small roles. The table can then be tilted toward or away from the surgeon as necessary to facilitate the operation.

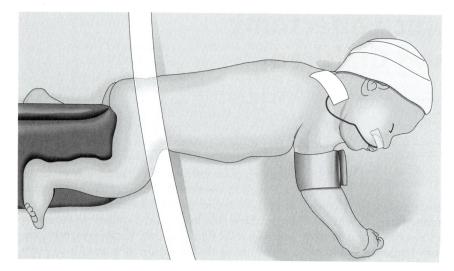

Fig. 16.1. Patient is placed in a lateral decubitus position for a thoracoscopic lobectomy

Scrub nurse

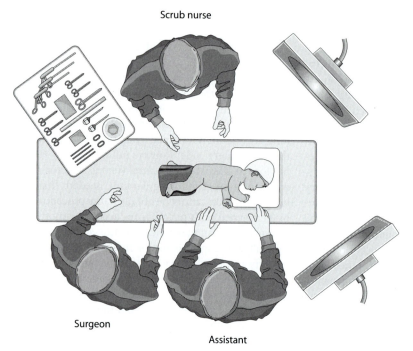

Fig. 16.2. Standard setup for thoracoscopic lobectomy

Surgeon

Assistant

Crews, Monitors, and Equipment

In general a single video monitor is used although a second monitor can be helpful occasionally. The surgeon and assistant are positioned at the front of the child with the monitor directly across from them, generally at midchest level. The assistant is usually above the surgeon who stands toward the head of the patient. The scrub nurse is across the table below the video monitor. It is imperative that the setup is as ergonomically efficient and comfortable for the surgeon as possible as the procedure involves fine dissection of major vascular structures (■ Fig. 16.2).

Special Equipment

Bipolar high frequency electrocautery and ultrasonic energy are optional but Ligasure is a very important tool. A 5 mm clipping device should be at hand and staplers can be useful in larger children. A retrieval bag will be needed in selected cases.

Technique

Cannulae

Cannula	Method of insertion	Diameter (mm)	Device	Position
1	Closed	5	30° scope	Fifth or 6th intercostal space, midaxillary line
2	Closed	5 or 12	Ligasure, scissors, stapler, clips	Seventh intercostal space, anterior axillary line
3	Closed	3	Maryland dissector	Fourth intercostal space, anterior axillary line
4	Closed/optional	3	Blunt grasper, retractor	Third or 4th intercostal space, midaxillary line

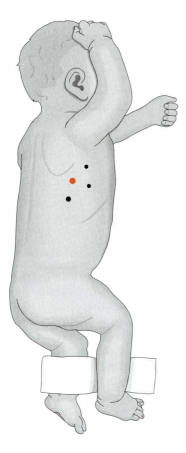

Fig. 16.3. Port placement for right upper lobectomy in an infant with a CAM. Camera port is in the midaxillary position and operating ports are in the anterior axillary line

Port Placement

The procedure is started by inserting a Veress needle in the midaxillary line in the 5th or 6th intercostal space. A low flow (1 L/min) low pressure (4 mmHg) of CO_2 is started to help collapse the lung. A 5 mm trocar is then inserted and a 4 mm 30° telescope is used to perform an initial survey. This initial positioning should avoid injury to the diaphragm and other intrathoracic structures. From this position the exact location of the major fissure is determined and this aids in placement of

the other ports. For lower lobectomies a 5 mm port is placed in the anterior axillary line in approximately the 7th or 8th interspace. This port should be placed to give the best access to structures in the major fissure as this is where the most complicated dissection will occur. In larger children where an endoscopic stapler may be used to divide the pulmonary vessels or bronchus, a 12 mm port may be placed at this site. The left hand port is then placed in the 4th or 5th intercostal space to compliment the lower port for dissection. In upper lobectomies the two ports may be shifted superiorly one or two interspaces to give better access to the superior pulmonary vessels (■ Fig. 16.3). If necessary a fourth port may be added above the telescope port to allow for retraction of the lung.

Lower Lobectomy

A lower lobectomy is the easiest to perform because structures distal to the major fissure are the end vessels and bronchus and may be divided without risk of compromising the upper or middle lobe. The surgery begins with a quick survey of the chest to evaluate the adequacy of lung collapse, anatomic variations, and completeness of the major fissure. In cases of CAM or CLE the collapse of the lung is often incomplete because of trapped air in the cyst or lung alveoli, making visualization very difficult. In these cases the Ligasure device can be used to decompress the cysts or lung tissue, causing the lung to deflate like a collapsed balloon (■ Fig. 16.4). This is accomplished simply by grasping the cysts with the device and activating the energy source. The cyst/lung tissue collapses and involutes creating space within the thoracic cavity in which to work.

Once adequate space is obtained the inferior pulmonary ligament is mobilized. This can be done sharply or with hook cautery or the Ligasure. There is usually a small vein in the ligament which should be sealed

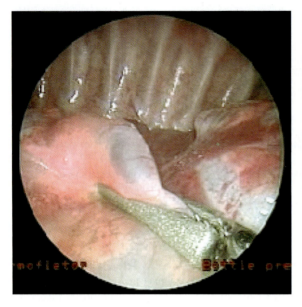

Fig. 16.4. Using the Ligasure device to collapse large cysts in a type 1 CAM to create intrathoracic space. *LUL* Left upper lobe

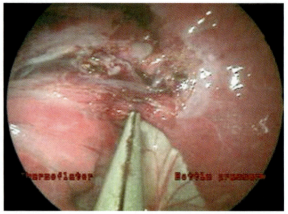

Fig. 16.5. Use of Ligasure for incomplete fissures

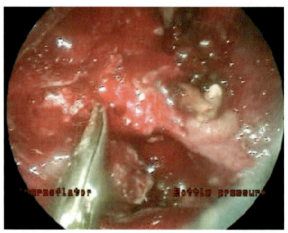

Fig. 16.6. Identification of bifurcation of right lower and middle lobe bronchi. This ensures the middle lobe is not compromised by division of the lower lobe bronchus

preemptively to avoid troublesome bleeding. The inferior pulmonary vein is dissected out for later ligation. It is preferable to ligate the vein after the artery especially in small infants as the lung may otherwise become congested making it more difficult to manipulate the lobe with endoscopic instruments.

Attention is then turned to the major fissure. Dissection proceeds from anterior to posterior in an orderly fashion, so it is imperative that the surgeon has a good understanding of the three-dimensional relationships of the major structures as they pass through the fissure. Attempts to constantly evaluate the lung from both the anterior and posterior aspects should be avoided as this will cause a repeated loss of exposure and needlessly prolong the procedure.

If the fissure is incomplete the Ligasure can be used to compress, seal, and divide the lung in the presumed anatomic division between the upper and lower lobe (■ Fig. 16.5). If the lung tissue is quite thick this can be done in layers, taking sequential bites of the lung. In larger patients an endoscopic stapler maybe used to achieve completion of the fissure; however, this requires a 12 mm port and it is usually not necessary.

As dissection proceeds posteriorly the pulmonary artery is encountered as it passes through the fissure. The vessel is isolated as it passes through the fissure and ligated. This is easily accomplished with the Ligasure but can also be performed with clips, suture, and in larger patients a stapler with a vascular load. When using the Ligasure, it maybe preferable in larger patients to trace the vessel distally to where it divides into the segmental branches, to allow sealing of slightly smaller vessels. The Ligasure is ideal for this type of work, as

opposed to other energy sources, because it seals the vessels without dividing them. Therefore the vessel can be sealed in two places and then cut between the seals under direct vision. If the seal appears to be incomplete there is time to reapply the Ligasure or other device prior to completely dividing the vessel and losing vascular control. Whatever device is used care should be taken not to divide the artery to the lingula or middle lobe as these vessels may originate near the major fissure but then pass superiorly.

With the artery divided, the bronchus to the lower lobe is now readily apparent. It should be mobilized making sure the dissection is carried distally enough to similarly avoid compromise to the middle or upper lobe bronchus. Since the bifurcation of the bronchus cannot be palpated easily, it must be clear to visual inspection (■ Fig. 16.6). Prior to dividing the bronchus the posterior aspect of the fissure is completed in a similar fashion to the anterior portion. The inferior pulmonary vein is then sealed with the Ligasure or other device either at its base or at the first bifurcation, depending on the size of the vessel. With the vein divided the only remaining structure is the bronchus. This is divided sharply and the resultant bronchial stump is closed with 3-0 PDS suture on an R-B 1 needle. In larger patients an endoscopic stapler may be used but again care must be taken not to compromise the upper or middle lobe bronchus.

The specimen is removed through the lowermost trocar site as this is the largest interspace. If the lesion is not infected the lobe can be removed bluntly though a slightly widened site (1 cm). If the patient is large enough or the lobe is infected an endoscopic specimen bag should be inserted. The specimen can then be removed in a piecemeal or morselized fashion as with a spleen.

Upper Lobectomy

An upper lobectomy is a more complicated procedure because the lung must be dissected off the main pulmonary artery as it passes to the lower lobe. The patient is positioned in a lateral decubitus position and again the chest cavity is insufflated with CO_2. The initial port is placed in the anterior axillary line in the 4th or 5th intercostal space. The upper lobe is examined and cysts decompressed if necessary as described above. The dissection starts anteriorly. The pleura overlying the superior pulmonary vein is incised and the vein is mobilized. Usually it is easier to seal and divide the vein after the first bifurcation. The same techniques as discussed for the lower lobe are used. With the vein divided the lung is gently stripped off the superior portion of the main pulmonary artery (■ Fig. 16.7). This is done by gently retracting the lung posteriorly exposing the plane between the main pulmonary trunk and the upper lobe. The segmental branches to the upper lobe can be sequentially identified, isolated, and divided. By retracting the lung posteriorly the vessels are slightly stretched making them easier to identify and dissect out.

After division of the arterial branches attention is turned to the major fissure. The fissure is completed using the techniques described above. Occasionally identification and division of the lower arterial branches is aided by completing the fissure first. With this completed the upper lobe bronchus can be isolated and divided. Again care must be taken to avoid compromise to the lower or middle lobe bronchus.

Middle Lobectomy

The techniques are the same as described above. The dissection is started anteriorly with division of the branches of the vein to the middle lobe. The minor and

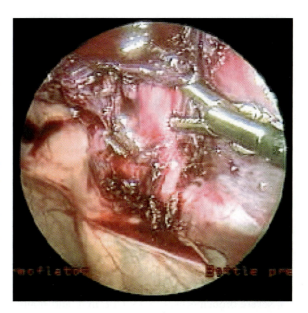

Fig. 16.7. Upper lobe is stripped off the main trunk of the pulmonary artery after division of the superior pulmonary vein

major fissures are then completed. The arterial branches to the middle lobe are located in the posterior portion of the minor fissure near the confluence with the major fissure. Once these branches are divided the bronchus becomes readily apparent. It can easily be divided and sealed as described above.

Postoperative Care

A chest tube is left in place, usually through the lowest trocar site. This is left to suction at 15–20 cm of water pressure. Pain is usually adequately controlled with intermittent intravenous narcotic. Occasionally a patient-controlled analgesia (PCA) pump is necessary but rarely is a thoracic epidural needed. A regular diet is resumed immediately. If no air leak is present the chest tube is removed on the first postoperative day. Patients are discharged as soon as they are comfortable on oral pain medication and tolerating adequate oral intake. This is usually the second postoperative day.

Results

From January 1995 to September 2003 all patients with lung pathology requiring resection were considered for a video-assisted thoracoscopic (VATS) approach. The only patients excluded were those with solid mass lesions occupying over 50% of the chest or those with extreme respiratory compromise suggesting they would not tolerate any length of single-lung ventilation. Ages ranged from 2 days to 18 years of age (mean 4.2 years) and weight from 2.8 to 78 kg (mean 18.7 kg). Preoperative evaluation suggested upper lobe pathology in 6, middle lobe in 3, and lower lobe in 39. Presumed diagnosis included sequestration or CAM in 30, severe bronchiectasis in 15, CLE in 1, and malignancy in 2. Seventeen of the CAMs and sequestrations were prenatal diagnoses. Six of the patients with bronchiectasis had cystic fibrosis; the others had chronic aspiration and pneumonia. The two malignancies were in patients with metastatic osteogenic sarcoma.

Forty-six of 48 lobectomies were completed endoscopically. Operative times ranged from 35 to 210 min (mean 125 min). There were 6 upper, 3 middle, and 39 lower lobectomies. Six of the lobectomies, 5 lower and 1 upper, were extralobar sequestrations. Pathology of the other specimens included sequestration/CAM in 23, severe bronchiectasis in 13, CLE in 4, and malignancy in 2. There were no bleeding complications and only one intraoperative complication (2.2%). This was in a case of severe bronchiectasis the left lower lobe. The bronchus was divided with an Endo-GIA and the firing resulted in compromise of the left upper lobe bronchus. The procedure was converted to open to perform a bronchoplasty on the left upper lobe bronchus. The other conversion was in a patient with metastatic osteosarcoma with a large centrally located tumor. She required a left lower lobectomy to remove the mass. The procedure was converted because of the size and location of the mass, and so as not to violate the tumor. Chest tubes were left in place in 39 of 48 cases and remained in for 1–5 days postoperatively (average 1.6 days). There were two postoperative complications. The first was a pneumothorax on postoperative day 7 in a patient with cystic fibrosis. A chest tube was placed with immediate expansion of the lung and no evidence of air leak. The tube was removed after 72 h without incident. The second was a postoperative pneumonia which resolved with antibiotics and aggressive respiratory care.

Hospital stay ranged from 1 to 5 days (average 2.4 days) in the 46 patients whose surgery was completed successfully thoracoscopically. There was one prolonged hospitalization of 12 days in the patient who required a bronchoplasty; this was primarily to treat a postoperative pneumonia.

Discussion

Over the decade since 1995 thoracoscopy has become an increasingly important tool in the armamentarium of the pediatric surgeon. The limited explorations, biopsies, and debridements described by Rodgers in the mid to late 1970s have become replaced by extensive, technically demanding resections and reconstructive procedures. These procedures have also shown extremely promising results. The application of thoracoscopic techniques in performing a formal lobectomy presents several unique and difficult problems and can be broken down into three different areas. The first is anesthetic considerations. For the majority of cases it is necessary to obtain single-lung ventilation primarily to create space for adequate visualization and dissection. We have found that the majority of infants and children, even with significant parenchymal disease, can tolerate this for the length of the procedure without significant compromise. This ties into the second hurdle, creating adequate space to work. For solid tumors there is little that can be done other than to have the normal lung collapsed as much as possible. However in cases of CAM or CLE, where a cyst or cysts are occupying a large portion of the intrathoracic cavity, space can be created by rupturing the cyst.

The third major hurdle is control of the vascular structures. The methods for doing this have been described extensively above and vary with the size of the child. Needless to say new sealing devices such as the Ligasure have improved the safety and efficiency with which this can be accomplished. Control of the bronchus has not been a major problem and can be accomplished with either an Endo-GIA or sharp division and suture closure. There have been no cases of stump leak or bronchopleural fistula. The one case requiring bronchoplasty may have been the result of a stenotic left upper lobe bronchus not recognized preoperatively. This complication probably could have been avoided if the lower lobe bronchus had been divided sharply and sutured closed.

Our results show that thoracoscopic lobectomy is feasible, safe, and effective. Recent technologic advances have made the procedures technically easier with operative times similar to, or in some cases faster than, those associated with an open thoracotomy. The surgeon must have a clear understanding of the regional anatomy and three-dimensional relationships in order to safely perform these procedure as the thoracoscopic approach provides only a two-dimensional picture. While a thoracoscopic approach results in decreased postoperative pain, a shorter hospital stay, and a superior cosmetic result, the greatest advantage is the avoidance of a formal thoracotomy with its inherent long-term morbidity of scoliosis, shoulder muscle girdle weakness, and chest wall deformity (Vaiquez et al. 1985). However, basic surgical principles should not be compromised and a formal anatomic lobectomy should be performed in all cases.

References

Albanese CT, Sydorak RM, Tsao K et al. (2003) Thoracoscopic lobectomy for prenatally diagnosed lung lesions. J Pediatr Surg 38:553–555

Mattioli G, Buffa P, Granata C et al. (1998) Lung resection in pediatric patients. Pediatr Surg Int 13:10–13

Rothenberg SS (1998) Thoracoscopy in infants and children. Semin Pediatr Surg 7:194–201

Rothenberg SS (2000) Thoracoscopic lung resection in children. J Pediatr Surg 35:271–275

Rothenberg SS (2003) Experience with thoracoscopic lobectomy in infants and children. J Pediatr Surg 38:102–104

Vaiquez JJ, Murcia J, Diez Pardo JA (1985) Morbid musculoskeletal sequelae of thoracotomy for tracheoesophageal fistula. J Pediatr Surg 20:511–514

Thoracoscopic Management of Esophageal Duplications, Bronchogenic Cysts, and Extralobar Sequestration

Steven S. Rothenberg

Introduction

The traditional approach to the evaluation and treatment of posterior mediastinal masses has been a standard lateral or posterolateral thoracotomy. These procedures can be associated with significant surgical morbidity and recovery. Since the early 1990s thoracoscopy, or video-assisted thoracic surgery (VATS), has been utilized to perform increasingly complex diagnostic and therapeutic procedures in the chest (Colt 1998; Rothenberg 1998). These techniques are perfectly suited for dealing with foregut duplications as these lesions tend to be well circumscribed, have a limited vasculature, and in general are easily dissected off the esophagus, bronchus, and lung. Extralobar sequestration will also be discussed here as these lesions are generally separate structures attached to the mediastinum by only its feeding systemic vessels. This chapter describes using a thoracoscopic approach as the primary modality for the diagnosis and therapy of these lesions (Bousamra et al. 1996; Demmy et al. 1998; Martinod et al. 2000; Michel et al. 1998; Patrick and Rothenberg 2001; Sandoval and Stringer 1997).

Preoperative Preparation

Before Induction of General Anesthesia

Patients with these lesions may present with evidence of esophageal or airway compression. Symptoms may include dysphagia, obstructed foreign body, stridor, or recurrent respiratory infections. The initial workup is usually a plain chest X-ray (CXR) that shows a mass effect in the posterior mediastinum. In cases of esophageal duplication a barium swallow can show compression of the esophageal lumen, and this is usually in the lower third of the esophagus. In general a computed tomography (CT) scan of the chest is the most helpful test and usually the only test needed to define the anatomy prior to exploration. This helps determine which side of the chest to approach the lesion from as well as what structures it may be intimately attached to. In general other testing and laboratory work is not necessary but should be obtained on an individual basis dependent on the case.

After Induction of General Anesthesia

Whenever possible, single-lung ventilation is obtained as previously discussed, to allow better exposure of the posterior mediastinum. When this is not possible CO_2 insufflation will generally give enough lung compression to provide adequate exposure. A single intravenous line is appropriate in most cases along with pulse oximetry and blood pressure monitoring. Central lines and arterial lines are not necessary. A single preoperative dose of a cephalosporin is given unless there is evidence of an active infectious process. A nasogastric tube or an esophageal bougie should be placed to help define the esophagus during the dissection. In some cases of suspected bronchogenic cysts, bronchoscopy just prior to thoracoscopy may be helpful in further defining the lesion.

Positioning

Patient

In most cases the lesion is a posterior mediastinal structure, therefore the patient is positioned in a modified prone position with the affected side elevated 30–45° (■ Fig. 17.1). An axillary role should always be placed and larger patients may be supported on a bean bag. The table can be rotated left or right to help increase exposure.

Crew, Monitors, and Equipment

The surgeon and assistant stand on the same side directly across from the lesion (■ Fig. 17.2). For example, with an esophageal duplication in the right chest the patient is placed prone with the right side elevated 30°. The surgeon and assistant are on the left side of the table with the monitor on the right, at the level of the lesion. This allows the surgeon and assistant to work in line with the lesion and the monitor avoiding any paradox. The scrub nurse is positioned toward the patient's back on the right side of the table. A second monitor may be placed on the left side of the table for the nurse to be able to observe the procedure.

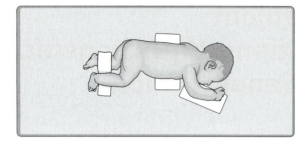

Fig. 17.1. Positioning of the patient for foregut duplication or other posterior mediastinal mass. A modified prone position allows gravity to retract the lung

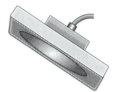

Fig. 17.2. Standard setup for posterior mediastinal structure

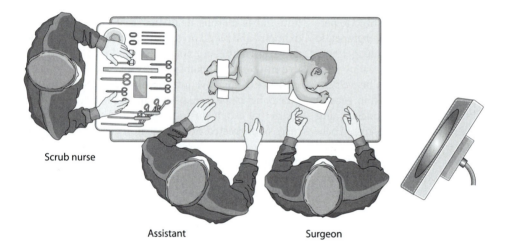

Scrub nurse

Assistant

Surgeon

Special Equipment

No special energy applying systems are required. En-doloops, 5 mm clips, and staplers in larger children, may sometimes be useful. In selected cases a bag is required for specimen removal.

Technique

Cannulae

Cannula	Method of insertion	Diameter (mm)	Device	Position
1	Closed	3 or 5	30° scope	Fifth to 7th intercostal space, midaxillary to posterior axillary line
2	Closed	3 or 5	Ligasure, scissors, stapler, clips	Fourth to 6th intercostal space, midaxillary line
3	Closed	3 or 5	Maryland dissector	Sixth to 8th intercostal space, midaxillary line
4	Closed/optional	3 or 5	Blunt grasper, retractor	Variable

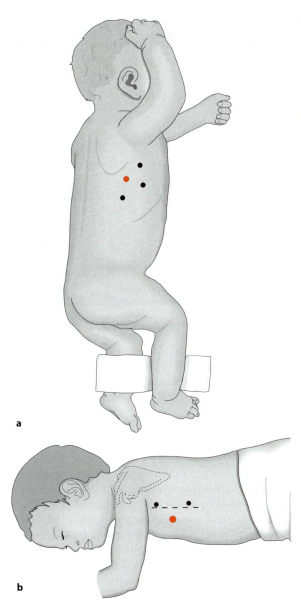

Fig. 17.3. a Port placement for esophageal duplication. **b** Port placement for sequestration

Cases are started with the insertion of a Veress needle in the midaxillary line and the insertion of a low pressure, low flow of CO_2 to help collapse the ipsilateral lung. Three or four ports are placed between the anterior and posterior axillary lines; valved ports are used in all cases to help maintain a slight tension pneumothorax (Fig. 17.3a,b). A nasogastric tube, esophageal bougie, or flexible gastroscope is placed to help identify the esophagus.

Procedure

A survey of the posterior mediastinum is performed and the mass identified (Fig. 17.4). The pleura overlying the mass is incised and the duplication is gradually mobilized. This is done with a combination of blunt and sharp dissection as this is a relatively avascular plane. It is done in a circumferential fashion until the base or stalk of the cyst is reached. In general this is easily accomplished as the attachments are loose and it is an avascular plane. Usually there is a central but relatively small stalk attaching the duplication to either the esophagus or the bronchus (Fig. 17.5).

In the case of an esophageal duplication the attachment often extends to the submucosa of the esophagus. Therefore it is necessary to dissect the cyst off the esophagus creating a defect in the muscular wall. This defect should be sutured closed in order to prevent later diverticulum formation. This can be accomplished with a few interrupted absorbable sutures. In the rare case where there is a common lumen this can be divided with an endoscopic stapler in larger patients or divided sharply and sutured closed in two layers. However it is important to not compromise the native esophageal lumen.

In cases of bronchogenic cysts there is usually a common wall with the back wall of the bronchus or trachea. An attempt to completely excise this common wall will often result in a tear in the wall of the primary airway. Therefore the mucosa in the wall of the cyst, at this common area, should be excised sharply leaving the common wall intact. If necessary the exposed mucosal lining can be ablated with cautery or other energy ablation if the mucosa cannot be removed.

Once the cyst is removed the area is carefully examined to ensure there is no injury to the native esophageal or tracheal wall. The lung is then reexpanded by pulling back the end of the endotracheal tube if single-lung ventilation was used. If there is no evidence of an air leak the tube is removed prior to extubation in the operating room.

Extralobar sequestrations are approached in exactly the same fashion. The only difference is that their primary attachment tends to be the feeding vessel coming directly off the aorta. These lesions tend to be inferior near the diaphragm. Some may even be associated with a diaphragmatic defect or may be completely intra-abdominal. The first step is to identify and then carefully dissect out the systemic artery. It is usually easily seen (Fig. 17.6). The vessel can be ligated either using sutures, clips, or sealed with the Ligasure device. It is important that the vessel be completely ligated/sealed before division otherwise the stump can retract below the diaphragm resulting in uncontrolled bleeding. For this reason a device which seals and divides simultaneously is not recommended. Once the

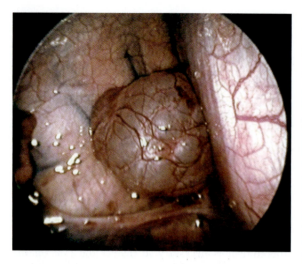

Fig. 17.4. Visualization of foregut duplication. Lung is retracted away from the cyst by gravity

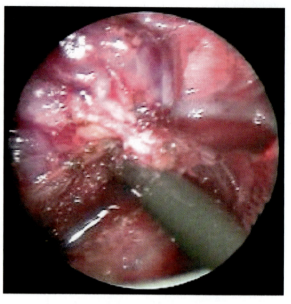

Fig. 17.5. Stalk attaching a duplication to the esophagus

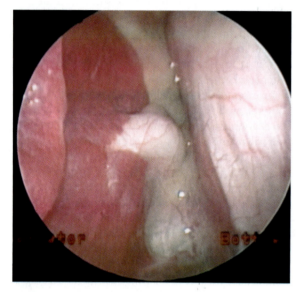

Fig. 17.6. Feeding vessel to sequestered lobe seen coming off aorta

vessel is divided the rest of the attachments tend to be limited and flimsy and can be divided with scissors or a hook cautery.

Specimen Removal

Once the specimen is free it can be removed through a slightly enlarged trocar site. Generally the lowest trocar site is used as these interspaces are the largest. Most cysts and duplications can be decompressed to limit the size of the opening needed to remove it. Sequestrations can usually be removed piecemeal. If there is any question of infection in the cyst or sequestration the specimen should be placed in a bag to prevent contamination of the pleural space.

Postoperative Care

A CXR is obtained in the recovery room and only repeated if there was an abnormality. Liquids were started immediately unless the esophageal lumen was breached. Intravenous narcotics are given in the initial postoperative period but most patients are on oral pain medication and a regular diet on the first postoperative day. Most patients are discharged on the first postoperative day once they are comfortable on oral pain medication and tolerating adequate oral intake. A contrast study should be obtained if there is any concern about the integrity of the esophagus.

Results

Between 1993 and 2003 nineteen foregut duplications were approached thoracoscopically. All were completed successfully using VATS. Operative times ranged from 20 to 90 min (mean 52 min). All patients were extubated in the operating room. Chest tubes were left in 3/19 cases and 2/3 were removed in the first 24 h. There was a single intraoperative complication, a tear of the posterior tracheal wall. This was repaired primarily thoracoscopically with no postoperative sequelae. Hospital stay ranged from 12 h to 2 days (mean 1.6 days). There were no postoperative complications or recurrences.

Discussion

The role of thoracoscopy in the evaluation and treatment of pediatric patients with foregut duplications has taken on an increasingly important role. These lesions, which are usually cystic in nature, are perfectly suited for a minimally invasive approach. The most important technical point in these cases is identification of the esophagus and trachea to prevent inadvertent injury. There is often a common inner wall and care must be taken to maintain the integrity of the native tracheal or esophageal wall. Positioning is also critical as placing the patient prone allows gravity to retract the collapsed lung giving clear access to the lesion. The tendency is for the surgeon to place the patient in a lateral decubitus position. However the advantages and exposure obtained by having the patient nearly prone far out way any possible disadvantages. Chest drains are not routinely left in place in these cases and all patients are started on oral feeds the same day, with all patients in this study being discharged in less than 2 days. Because of the low morbidity and quicker recovery period thoracoscopic resection should probably be considered the treatment of choice for benign conditions such as foregut duplication.

References

Bousamra M, Haasler GB, Patterson GA, et al (1996) A comparative study of thoracoscopic vs. open removal of benign mediastinal tumors. Chest 109:1461–1465

Colt HG (1998) Therapeutic thoracoscopy. Clin Chest Med 19:383–394

Demmy TL, Krasna MJ, Detterbeck FC, et al (1998) Multicenter VATS experience with mediastinal tumors. Ann Thorac Surg 66:187–192

Martinod E, Pons F, Azorin J, et al (2000) Thoracoscopic excision of mediastinal bronchogenic cyst: results in 20 cases. Ann Thorac Surg 69:1525–1528

Michel JL, Revillon Y, Montupet P, et al (1998) Thoracoscopic treatment of mediastinal cysts in children. J Pediatr Surg 33:1745–1748

Partrick DA, Rothenberg SS (2001) Thoracoscopic resection of mediastinal masses in infants and children: an evolution of technique and results. J Pediatr Surg 36:1165–1167

Rothenberg SS (1998) Thoracoscopy in infants and children. Semin Pediatr Surg 7:194–201

Sandoval C, Stringer G (1997) Video-assisted thoracoscopy for the diagnosis of mediastinal masses in children. J Soc Laparoendosc Surg 1:131–133

Chapter 18

The Role of Thoracoscopy for the Resection of Pulmonary Metastasis

Thom E. Lobe

Introduction

Since thoracoscopy first appealed to pediatric surgeons as a potentially useful technique for oncological cases, the concept of resection of pulmonary metastatic lesions was foremost in the minds of the many surgeons who pioneered the field. While the advantages to the patients were obvious, there were many obstacles to overcome and there was broad resistance from the conservative base of medical oncologists and surgeons whose principal concern was the reliability of this new technique compared to known outcomes from tried and true, if not somewhat more extensive or at least more invasive, surgery. The basic techniques are similar to others well described in this book, so we will not dwell on them here other than to add some helpful hints that are specific to metastatectomy.

Preoperative Preparation

Before Induction of General Anesthesia

We believe that to be most effective, one must plan ahead. While this may seem obvious, there are a couple of simple steps that can make your life more straightforward as a surgeon and result in a more satisfying outcome for all concerned. The highest quality image possible should be obtained as close in time to the planned resection as possible; this preoperative image is critical.nnn

There is some evidence to suggest that two relatively new modalities may provide some improved results here. One is the use of one of the newer 16-channel multidetector computerized tomography machines that can see amazing detail (Gilkeson et al. 2003). This device has the promise of being able to focus on smaller lesions than before and potentially can enable us to see lesions that were previously missed. The other device that can help us intraoperatively is ultrasound. This now takes two forms: one is the use of an endoscopic ultrasound probe to use thoracoscopically (Gruppioni et al. 2000; Smith et al. 1996; Yamamoto et al. 2003), and the other is a transbronchial ultrasound. Between the two techniques, more detail and better localization, particularly of central lesions, is possible, particularly when color Doppler ultrasound is used (Falcone et al. 2003).

After Induction of General Anesthesia

We like to use double lumen endotracheal tubes in children older than about 12 years and bronchial blockers in younger children and infants in order to allow the lung to collapse on the side on which we are operating. While many believe the placement of bronchial blockers to be difficult or intimidating, nothing could be further from the truth. A brief description of our technique is as follows.

We and others use a standard Fogarty catheter (Mitsui et al. 2002), usually a 4 or 5 French in size depending on the child's age or size, and introduce this through the vocal cords, into the trachea immediately before introducing the endotracheal tube. We then use a pediatric flexible bronchoscope (or fluoroscopy if a bronchoscope is not available), and position the balloon just inside the mainstem bronchial orifice to be blocked. We test the system by inflating the balloon and listen to the lungs. If the desired lung is blocked and we can still ventilate the opposite lung, we tape the endotracheal tube in place and proceed to tape the Fogarty catheter to the secure endotracheal tube. We then position the patient as desired and retest the bronchial blocker in case the tube or catheter have shifted. If indeed the lung is not adequately blocked, we reposition the balloon and repeat the process until we are satisfied. The entire process usually takes a few minutes to complete.

The advantage of blocking the bronchus is significant. This maneuver enables you to see a wider variety of smaller lesions, both superficial and deep within the lung parenchyma. With the air out of the lung, the lung parenchyma appears more solid and is more amenable to inspection with ultrasound devices, either applied pleurally or via the endobronchial route. And with the lung collapsed, you simply have more room to see and to carry out any complex dissection necessary for mediastinal dissection, node sampling, and segmental resection necessary for pulmonary metastatectomy.

Positioning

Patient

An important part of the planning is the position of the patient on the operating table. We find it beneficial to use gravity to our advantage whenever possible and plan to position the patient accordingly so that the collapsed lung will fall dependently, out of the field of vision. It is often helpful to use a "beanbag" or other positioning device to make it easier to secure the patient in position, especially if you plan, as we usually do, to tilt the table from side to side and from head to foot so that the lung will further gravitate away from the field of view.

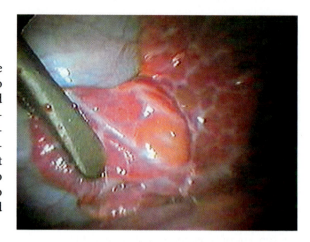

Fig. 18.1. Lingula of a 6-year-old girl 2 years after amputation and treatment for a sarcoma of her leg. Note the fleshy lesion on the pleural surface. This was easily resected for diagnosis of recurrent sarcoma. Immediately superior to this is a smaller lesion that was not visible on the diagnostic imaging. There were many such smaller lesions seen at thoracoscopy

Crew, Monitors, and Equipment

The team or crew necessary for thoracoscopic resection of pulmonary metastases is essentially the same as for any thoracoscopy. The surgeon should have a clear understanding of the location of the lesion, know whether there exists more than one lesion, and know whether the disease in the chest is bilateral. With this in mind, the surgeon will plan to stand facing the lesion with the lesion between him or herself and the main monitor. This principle is basic to all endoscopic surgery and should not be new to the reader.

It may be helpful to have a monitor on either side of the patient, positioned either at the patient's head or at the level of the patient's pelvis, depending on whether the lesion is apical or basilar. For midlobar lesions, the monitors can be placed at the level of the midthorax on either side. The two monitors are necessary so that the assistant who usually stands opposite the surgeon, can see.

Today, one should use the highest resolution camera/monitor system available. High-definition, or so-called high-definition systems, with pure digital signals seem to offer the best resolution if one expects to detect the small metastatic lesions studding the visceral pleura in patients with osteosarcoma. Many surgeons now have integrated operating theaters instead of towers. Whatever you use, if you plan to search for small metastatic lesions, you need the best optics you or your hospital can afford.

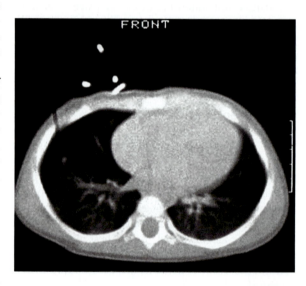

Fig. 18.2. A CT scan documenting a "solitary" pulmonary metastasis in a 2-year-old boy after treatment for hepatoblastoma

Special Equipment

The lung is best examined for metastasis when it is completely collapsed and evacuated of air (Fig. 18.1). Initially, we gently rub a blunt grasper back and forth over the surface of the lung to "feel" any lesions deep to the surface that cannot be seen visually.

Another technique used by some is endoscopic ultrasound (Figs. 18.2–18.4). This technique can be used on collapsed lung for detecting deep parenchymal lesions, lymph nodes in the hilum, and differentiating solid structures from vascular channels. Laparoscopic ultrasound probes of 1 cm in diameter are readily available in many centers that deal with cancer. They are used in conjunction with cryotherapy of metastatic lesions to the liver and other solid organs. They do not work at all well if there is air in the lung, thus the lung must be completely collapsed and devoid of air for this technique to be useful. When preoperative imaging

Fig. 18.3. Intraoperative ultrasound of the patient in ■ Fig. 18.2 at which a new perihilar lesion was discovered. The ultrasound image can be seen in the *upper left* of the figure

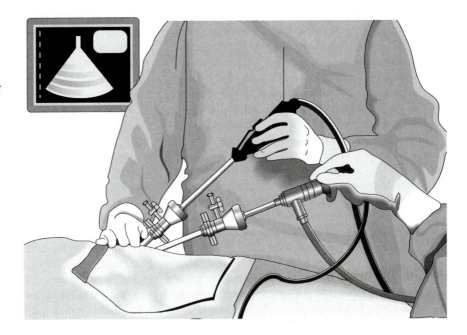

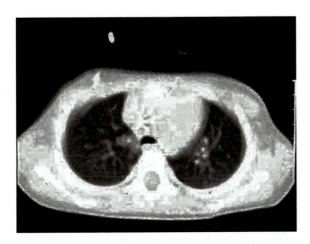

Fig. 18.4. A CT scan of the same patient looking at a second perihilar pulmonary lesion. This was initially read as a normal part of the left hilum. Had it not been for the ultrasound, this second metastatic lesion in the lung would have been missed

has detected a central lesion, a wire can be left in situ to help localize the lesion that otherwise would be difficult to find.

However the lesions are localized, one must remove them safely and leave the lung without an air leak. We believe that there are two effective ways to do this today. I will mention the use of endoloops only to say that, in our hands at least, they often fail to hold the lung securely after it is reexpanded. Many in the past would put two endoloops securely on a collapsed segment of infant lung to be removed and cut beyond the

endoloops. This works sometimes. At other times, when the lung reexpands, the loops cut through the lung parenchyma and a significant air leak ensues. Because of this, we have abandoned this technique.

The two approaches that work nearly without fail are the use of the endoscopic stapler and the use of the Ligasure device. The former places six rows of staples and cuts between the middle two. The later seals or melts the cut surface of the lung and prevents air leaks.

Lasers can be used to do the same as the Ligasure and have been used successfully in many centers around the world for years. The Nd:YAG laser is particularly useful for this because of its coagulating characteristics. The CO_2 laser is primarily a vaporizing laser and will not seal the lung. The problem with the laser is the risk of a fire in the chest with the patient who has an high O_2 requirement.

Many surgeons have access to a harmonic scalpel or similar devices using ultrasonic energy. While this device is excellent for cutting and dividing the lung tissue and for providing hemostasis, it does not seem to do a very good job of sealing the lung and preventing air leaks. The same can be said for conventional electrocautery.

Technique

Our preference is to begin with 5 mm telescopes, usually 0° or 30°, placed through 5 mm cannulae. The initial insertion of the first cannula depends on the location of the lesion. Generally, I prefer to think of the operative, thoracoscopic field as a diamond-shaped configuration with the telescope at one point, the lesion at the opposite point, and the two working instruments entering at approximately 45° from the lateral two points of the diamond.

Because there may be some adhesions to the lateral pleura, we prefer to enter the chest bluntly in the following manner. We first make a 5 mm incision at the desired spot in an intercostal space. We then use a hemostat to bluntly enter the pleural space so that the cannula can be inserted gently. Once this is done, we insert the telescope and inspect the pleural cavity to make certain that we are in a free space as opposed to the chest wall or somewhere buried in the lung parenchyma. When we know that we are free in the pleural cavity, we begin to insufflate with CO_2. The pressure limit of insufflation depends on the age of the child, the patient's pulmonary status, and whether we have a bronchial blocker in place. In general, lower pressures, between 4 and 10 torr are adequate for infants, while 10–15 torr may be acceptable in older teens.

After the initial cannula is inserted and the telescope is in place the chest is inspected. The metastatic lesions may be obvious, or none may be seen. If you expect only a single lesion and multiple lesions are seen, your plan may change depending on the patient's primary disease. Some diseases, such as osteosarcoma, may benefit from excising all the lesions, while multiple lesions in a patient with Wilms' tumor have a different prognosis and if seen on your initial inspection may change your operative plans.

When only one lesion is seen or you do not see the expected lesion, at least two additional ports are introduced at the lateral points of the diamond configuration described above. The location of these depends on the expected location of the metastatic lesion and your initial trocar placement. Your goal is to have the two hand-driving instruments, one in each hand, entering at about a 45° angle toward the lesion as you look at the lesion and monitor directly, head-on. The monitors should, ideally, be at eye level, and your arms should hang comfortably at your sides with your elbows flexed at a 90° angle. The camera holder generally should stand at the side of your non-dominant hand.

We initially manipulate the lung with 5 mm blunt, atraumatic graspers. We avoid graspers that tend to cut and tear the lung, particularly when there has been some inflammation. When lesions are centrally located, the surgeon has several options. First, a simple, segmental resection can be performed if the segment is easily resected and the lesion is not too large. This can be done with the Ligasure in an infant or a stapler in an older patient. Often we will begin the dissection using the Ligasure until the stapler can be used to its best advantage. To use the endoscopic stapler, one of the trocar sites must be enlarged to a 12 mm size to accept the larger cannula required. Which cannula depends on the location of the lesion and the direction from which the stapler seems best applied. This may not be obvious at first but will become clear when the time for stapler application is at hand. An additional feature of the staplers today is that they can be angled once inside the chest so that they can be applied at the optimal angle, even in a relatively young child of 4 years old as well as in older children.

When a lesion is deep in the center of the lung and segmental resection is not practical, we use a similar technique. We begin dissecting through the parenchyma, immediately over the lesion, then continue to "core" the lesion out with a rim of normal parenchyma, all using the Ligasure. This is a technique that we used to do using a laser fiber, but the Ligasure today is safer and gives us greater control.

Once the lesion is free in the chest cavity, we remove it by placing it in a sac or bag for removal through a trocar site that we have enlarged for that purpose.

Postoperative Care

Postoperative care is rather straightforward. Whenever lung is resected it is safest to place a thoracostomy tube through one of the trocar sites. Usually we do this through the posteriormost site. Our reason for this is not so much for drainage as for air leak. Accordingly, a tube that will just fit the hole should suffice. Thus a 16 or 18 French chest tube usually works fine. We leave this in place until there is no further air leak, which is often just overnight.

Postoperative pain is handled in the standard fashion. Its management varies from region to region. We routinely administer a posterior rib block with 0.25% bupivacaine with epinephrine, above and below the field of trocar sites, and offer the patient oral analgesics as they desire. This is usually sufficient for their discomfort.

The patients ambulate and eat the day of the procedure unless their tumor therapy requires otherwise.

Results

Our initial experience is as follows. Of 131 patients under the age of 18 years, 101 were white and 75 were male. The preoperative diagnoses were: undiagnosed mass (33), leukemia (16), Hodgkin's and non-Hodgkin's lymphoma (13 each), Ewing's sarcoma (12), Wilms' tumor (7), brain tumor (6), osteosarcoma (6), rhabdomyosarcoma (5), and a variety of other miscellaneous tumors (20).

Several patients were converted to thoracotomy (13.7%). This occurred due to: failure to gain safe access (6), unresectability of the lesion (6), failure to locate the suspected lesion (3), non-diagnostic tissue (1), inadequate sample (1), and one patient was too unstable to continue with thoracoscopy. One should note that the goal for these procedures is to make certain that you have adequate material for the pathologist to examine. If we are convinced on the preoperative imaging that a lesion exists and cannot find it at thoracoscopy, we will open the chest to find the lesion. In all three cases where this happened, no lesion could be found at thoracotomy either. Additionally, we will not leave the operating theater until we are told by the pathologist that we have sufficient material for diagnosis. We routinely obtain a frozen section to confirm that we have diagnostic tissue. If there is doubt and we believe that we can do no better with continued thoracoscopy, we will convert to an open procedure. Those patients in whom access was unable to be obtained had received preoperative radiation and/or had had multiple thoracotomies and safe thoracoscopy was not possible.

In our experience there were some operative complications noted (4%). One patient desaturated severely and had to be converted to thoracotomy. One patient who had undergone previous radiation and whose access was difficult had an inadvertent esophagotomy that was repaired thoracoscopically and had an uneventful postoperative course. Another patient had a difficult selective intubation. One patient's lesion was unresectable and a final patient suffered hemorrhage requiring transfusion.

Postoperative complications were as you might expect (7%). There were three lymphatic leaks, two pneumothoraces in patients who did not have postoperative chest tubes placed initially, one delayed pneumothorax after the initial chest tube was removed in a patient on positive pressure ventilation, two patients with bronchopleural fistulae (one of these patients – an infant with severe respiratory insufficiency – ultimately died of her respiratory insufficiency), and one implant in a trocar site in a patient with a sarcoma.

Discussion

Several early authors recognized the potential value of thoracoscopy for the resection of metastatic disease (Congregado Loscertales et al. 2002; Mutsaerts et al. 2001a; Partrick and Rothenberg 2001; Rao 1997; Saenz et al. 1997; Sailhamer et al. 2003; Warmann et al. 2003). The usual advantages are cited and include smaller incisions, less pain, shorter hospitalization, and fewer complications. Resection of pulmonary metastasis has shown promise in several adult tumors including: breast (Shiraishi et al. 2003), colon (Watanabe et al.

1998), melanoma (Leo et al. 2000), and renal cell carcinoma (Shiraishi et al. 2003; Tajiri et al. 2000). One of the early problems that established a mood of caution was the high incidence of port site implants noted by some authors with some common tumors (Ang et al. 2003; Fondrinier et al. 1998; Mutsaerts et al. 2001b; Wille et al. 1997). This principally occurred with sarcomas and led us and others to the conclusion that thoracoscopy was not an appropriate option for the management of children with osteosarcoma (Sartorelli et al. 1996; Wille et al. 1997). Another reason for this conclusion is that the existing data supported the concept that the best results with osteosarcoma are achieved with excision of all existing lesions. One of the problems with thoracoscopy is the inability to palpate tiny lesions between the surgeon's fingers as can be done with open surgery. Since you cannot do this at thoracoscopy, the likelihood of missing tiny lesions the size of grains of sand is high. Thus, since you are likely to miss these lesions, thoracoscopy is relatively contraindicated in these sarcomas in this author's opinion.

Regarding surgical attempts to minimize tumor implantation and spread, it is appealing to place the specimen in a bag or sac of some kind so as not to drag the specimen through the trocar wound in the chest wall. There are many commercially available devices designed to facilitate this. Despite this, there are no data to suggest that this is of any value, no matter how careful you are as a surgeon. I suspect that tumor cells scatter in the process of resection if you cross a tumor margin. They may also disseminate through lymphatics and vascular channels. This is not to recommend sloppy technique. One can never be too careful. Nor can one be too complacent or rely solely on some device to protect your patient. Careful attention to every aspect of operative detail and tumor biology should be foremost in the mind of any surgeon operating on a child with cancer.

One of the major technical difficulties with pulmonary metastasis, and a problem that dissuaded many from attempting thoracoscopy for metastatectomy, is the issue of finding central lesions, deep within the parenchyma. Recently, there have been some serious attempts at better localizing deep-seated lesions by using more sophisticated imaging modalities. One such technique uses computed tomography (CT)-guided imaging with injection of some methylene blue dye-stained blood from the patient to be imaged. Partrick et al. (2002) used this technique for 13 thoracoscopic procedures on 12 children who presented with pulmonary nodules that were less than 1 cm in diameter or were deep to the pleural surface. Preoperative needle localization was performed under CT guidance and methylene blue dye was injected into the lung parenchyma. All 13 biopsies were performed successfully, 12 yielded diagnoses, and 7 were curative.

While another technique, similar in approach, is to localize breast lesions using a "J-wire" placed at the time of CT-guided imaging, McConnell et al. (2002) compared a variety of dyes and wires and ultimately concluded that their best results were obtained when 3 ml of autologous blood was mixed with 0.3 ml of methylene blue dye and injected into the lesion under CT guidance. Nineteen procedures were performed in 17 children averaging 11 years in age. All material was diagnostic.

Despite the best efforts, you will still have the occasional case in which it seems impossible to localize the lesion in question. In those cases, you have two options. One is to perform a blind biopsy, based on an educated guess as to where the lesion is. You can then perform a frozen section or wait for permanent sections. The second is to convert the case to an open thoracotomy for a more thorough exploration. When we have done this, however, the results have been disappointing in that we routinely failed to identify a lesion if we could not identify something at thoracoscopy.

Overall, the experience with thoracoscopic metastasectomy is favorable (Delgrado Munoz et al. 2000). Mutsaerts et al. (2002) evaluated the long-term survival in these patients and concluded that patients undergoing metastasectomy by the thoracoscopic route experienced significantly fewer complications than those undergoing thoracotomy for the same procedure with similar disease-free and overall survival rates.

The data suggest that, to some extent at least, the pathology determines the aggressiveness with which a surgeon should pursue thoracoscopic resection of pulmonary metastases. Solitary metastatic lesions for most of the pediatric tumors are nearly always worth resecting. For some of the tumors, such as Wilms' tumors and hepatoblastoma, the evidence suggests that if there exist only a few metastatic lesions or a solitary lesion in each lung, it is probably worth the effort.

Osteosarcoma presents a special case. The data suggest that resection of all palpable lesions makes a difference in length of survival. Usually you can feel many more lesions than you can see when you hold the lung tissue in your hands as the sarcoma is studded on the parietal pleural surface. While you can certainly resect many of these lesions thoracoscopically, you cannot "feel" the lung tissue between your fingers and it is doubtful that you can detect many of the small lesions that exist that are not visible on the diagnostic imaging. For this reason, we do not advocate thoracoscopic resection of pulmonary metastatic disease for osteosarcoma. Another reason for this is the risk of port site metastasis that exists for this disease. The only patient in our series with port site metastasis was a patient with sarcoma.

References

Ang KL, Tan C, Hsin M, Goldstraw P (2003) Intrapleural tumor dissemination after video-assisted thoracoscopic surgery metastasectomy. Ann Thorac Surg 75:1643–1645

Congregado Loscertales M, Giron Arjona JC et al. (2002) Usefulness of video-assisted thoracoscopy for the diagnosis of solitary pulmonary nodules. Arch Bronconeumol 38:415–420

Delgado Munoz MD, Anton-Pacheco JL et al. (2000) Surgery of lung metastasis. Cir Pediatr 13:7–10

Falcone F, Fois F, Grosso D (2003). Endobronchial ultrasound. Respiration 70:179–194

Fondrinier E, Lorimier G, Cellier P et al. (1998) Parietal tumor seeding after thoracoscopic surgery: apropos of a case. Chirurgie 123:612–615

Gilkeson RC, Ciancibello L, Zahka K (2003) Pictorial essay. Multidetector CT evaluation of congenital heart disease in pediatric and adult patients. AJR Am J Roentgenol 180:973–980

Gruppioni F, Piolanti M, Coppola F et al. (2000) Intraoperative echography in the localization of pulmonary nodules during video-assisted thoracic surgery. Radiol Med (Torino) 100:223–228

Leo F, Cagini L, Rocmans P et al. (2000) Lung metastases from melanoma: when is surgical treatment warranted? Br J Cancer 83:569–572

McConnell PI, Feola GP, Meyers RL (2002) Methylene blue-stained autologous blood for needle localization and thoracoscopic resection of deep pulmonary nodules. J Pediatr Surg 37:1729–1731

Mitsui T, Kakinuma T, Niiyama K et al. (2002) Anesthetic management of pediatric video-assisted thoracoscopic surgery with Fogarty catheter. Masui 51:1120–1122

Mutsaerts EL, Zoetmulder FA, Meijer S et al. (2001a) Outcome of thoracoscopic pulmonary metastasectomy evaluated by confirmatory thoracotomy. Ann Thorac Surg 72:230–233

Mutsaerts EL, Zoetmulder FA, Rutgers EJ (2001b) Port site metastasis as a complication of thoracoscopic metastatectomy. Eur J Surg Oncol 127:327–328

Mutsaerts EL, Zoetmulder FA, Meijer S et al. (2002) Long term survival of thoracoscopic metastasectomy vs metastasectomy by thoracotomy in patients with a solitary pulmonary lesion. Eur J Surg Oncol 28:864–868

Partrick DA, Rothenberg SS (2001) Thoracoscopic resection of mediastinal masses in infants and children: an evaluation of technique and results. J Pediatr Surg 36:1165–1167

Partrick DA, Bensard DD, Teitelbaum DH et al. (2002) Successful thoracoscopic lung biopsy in children utilizing preoperative CT-guided localization. J Pediatr Surg 37:970–973

Rao BN (1997) Present day concepts of thoracoscopy as a modality in pediatric cancer management. Int Surg 82:123–126

Saenz NC, Conlon KC, Aronson DC et al. (1997) The application of minimal access procedures in infants, children, and young adults with pediatric malignancies. J Laparoendosc Adv Surg Tech A 7:289–294

Sailhamer E, Jackson CC, Vogel AM et al. (2003) Minimally invasive surgery for pediatric solid neoplasms. Am Surg 69:566–568

Sartorelli KH, Partrick D, Meagher DP Jr (1996) Port-site recurrence after thoracoscopic resection of pulmonary metastasis owing to osteogenic sarcoma. J Pediatr Surg 31:1443–1444

Shiraishi Y, Nakajima Y, Katsuragi N et al. (2003) Metastatic lung tumor: report of two cases. Kyobu Geka 56:47–50

Smith MB, Lobe TE, Schropp KP et al. (1996) A prospective evalua-
    tion of an endoscopic ultrasonic probe to detect intraparen-
    chymal malignancy at pediatric thoracoscopy. J Laparoendosc
    Surg 6:233–237

Tajiri M, Sakoh A, Ishii H et al. (2000) A thoracoscopic resection of
    pulmonary metastasis from breast cancer: a case report with a
    27-year disease-free interval. Kyobu Geka 53:242–245

Warmann S, Fuchs J, Jesch NK et al. (2003) A prospective study of
    minimally invasive techniques in pediatric surgical oncology:
    preliminary report. Med Pediatr Oncol 40:155–157

Watanabe M, Deguchi H, Sato M et al. (1998) Midterm results of
    thoracoscopic surgery for pulmonary metastases especially
    from colorectal cancers. J Laparoendosc Adv Surg Tech A
    8:195–200

Wille GA, Gregory R, Guernsey JM (1997) Tumor implantation at
    port site of video-assisted thoracoscopic resection of pulmo-
    nary metastasis. West J Med 166:65–66

Yamamoto M, Takeo M, Meguro F et al. (2003) Sonographic evalu-
    ation for peripheral pulmonary nodules during video-assisted
    thoracoscopic surgery. Surg Endosc 17:825–827

Chapter 19

Thoracoscopy and Hydatid Cyst of the Lung

François Becmeur and Stéphane Grandadam

Introduction

Hydatid disease of the lung (HDL) can occur without any other, particularly abdominal, localization. HDL in childhood most frequently occurs by inhalation.

In the case of a large isolated young cyst surgical treatment is usually simple (■ Fig. 19.1). There are, however, also complicated cases, for example, rupture of a cyst in the bronchus with partial disappearance of the membrane (■ Fig. 19.2). Contamination of a large part of the bronchial tree is then highly probable. After such a rupture, the cyst becomes infected with involvement of the pericystic area and even of the surrounding compressed and rather stiff pulmonary parenchyma. Surgical treatment consists of clearance of the cavity, removal of the proligerous membrane, closure of bronchial fistulas, and drainage of the cavity, which helps the cavity to collapse.

Thoracoscopic treatment of HDL was first proposed in 1993 (Becmeur et al. 1994). It follows the same principles as in open surgery, to be remembered with the acronym "PAIRE," which stands for: Puncture of the cyst, Aspiration, Instillation of hypertonic saline (10%), Reaspiration 15 min later, and finally Extraction of the membrane of the cyst. Hypertonic saline destroys the scoleces by osmotic dehydration (Cangir et al. 2000; Munzer 1991; Smego et al. 2003).

Preoperative Preparation

Before Induction of General Anesthesia

Other hydatid localizations should be excluded by computed tomography (CT) scan and abdominal ultrasonography. Medical treatment with albendazole is indicated for 6 weeks before surgery if there are concomitant small cysts.

After Induction of General Anesthesia

Epidural analgesia in combination with general anesthesia is given unless the cyst is infected. In all cases prophylactic broad-spectrum antibiotics are started.

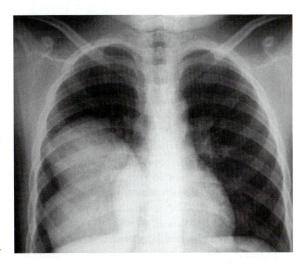

Fig. 19.1. An anteroposterior (AP) chest X-ray shows a young cyst in the inferior right lobe

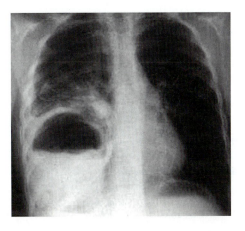

Fig. 19.2. An AP chest X-ray of a cyst that has ruptured into the bronchus. An air/fluid level is seen. Note the proligerous membrane, or Belot membrane

One-lung ventilation is mandatory in order to prevent spillage of material and drowning of the other healthy lung either by cystic material from the diseased lung or by aspiration of the hypertonic saline used to kill the scoleces. The selective lung ventilation is pursued until all major bronchial fistulae have been closed

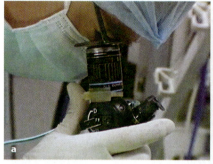 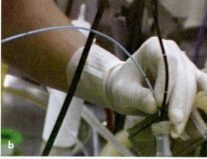 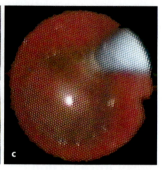

Fig. 19.3 a–c. Introduction of a Fogarthy catheter into the bronchus of the diseased lung under bronchoscopic control. The balloon has been inflated

after removal of the pericyst. Fistulae may go unnoticed until the diseased lung is reinsufflated.

Single lung ventilation in teenage children can be achieved by inserting a double lumen Carlens' tube. In children above 8 years of age and weighing about 25 kg, a left-sided Robert Shaw 26 French probe can be used. In children below 8 years of age, we use either a standard endotracheal tube in combination with a 5 or 6 French Fogarthy catheter, which is put into the main bronchus of the diseased lung under endoscopic control (▬ Fig. 19.3a–c), or we selectively intubate the healthy lung under guidance with a flexible endoscope.

A nasogastric tube is also inserted.

Positioning

Patient

The patient is put in a lateral decubitus position as for a standard thoracotomy.

Technique

Cannulae

Crew, Monitors, and Equipment

The surgeon and the assistant both stand in front of or behind the patient, depending on the localization of the cyst. The surgeon stays close to the head of the patient, while the assistant stays lower down. The scrub nurse also stands on the same side but even lower down.

The monitor is placed in front of the surgeon at the level of the patient's leg. Surgeon, operative field, and monitor should be in line.

Special Equipment

Standard equipment is used. We use monopolar scissors but a bipolar forceps should be at hand as well. An endobag for removal of the pericyst and three large chest drains should be available. A large-diameter chest drain is advantageous but the actual choice will depend on the width of the intercostal space.

Cannula	Method of insertion	Diameter (mm)	Device	Position
1	Open	5	Optic	A short distance in front of the cyst. The actual position will depend on the preoperative CT localization of the cyst
2	Closed	3 or 5	Forceps, electrocoagulation, needle holder	In triangular configuration with the optic and port 3
3	Closed	3 or 5	Forceps, suction and irrigation	In triangular configuration with the optic and port 2
4	Closed		Veress needle	In front of the cyst

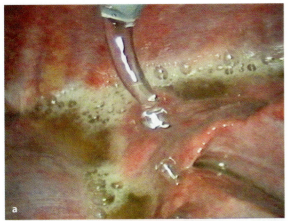

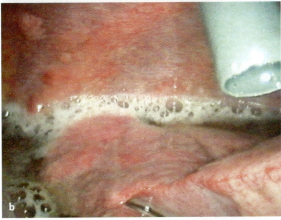

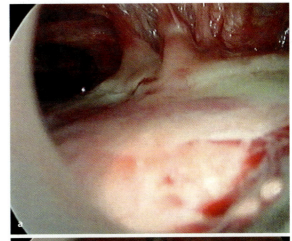

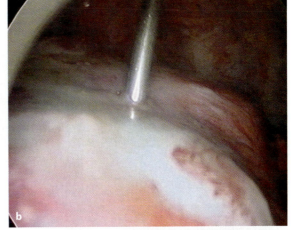

Fig. 19.4 a,b. The pleural cavity is filled with hypertonic saline

Port Placement

The preoperative CT scan allows for an optimal positioning of the optic. As the vault of the cyst frequently sticks to the parietal pleura, the optic should be placed at a little distance from the vault. The other trocars are placed in triangular configuration under concomitant thoracoscopic surveillance.

Procedure

The cyst is easily located as the it usually adhers to the parietal pleura. This adhesion is kept in place during the whole procedure until the pericyst has been removed and all bronchial fistulae have been closed. After insertion of the trocars and inspection, the pleural cavity is filled with hypertonic saline (10%) to protect the pleura from infestation (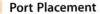 Fig. 19.4a,b).

A Veress needle, or another big needle, is used for the first steps of the PAIRE procedure. The needle must be inserted right into the vault of the cyst, even inside the adhesions in order to prevent leakage of the con-

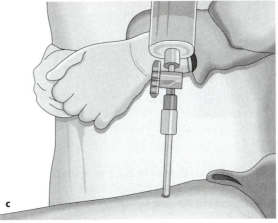

Fig. 19.5 a–c. The superficial part of the cyst has been located and is punctured

tents of the cyst into the pleural space. Some material is aspirated for parasitological and bacteriological study (■ Fig. 19.5a–c).

If the cyst were to be emptied completely the cyst would collapse, which could cause dislodgement of the tip of the needle to the outside of the cyst. If hyper-

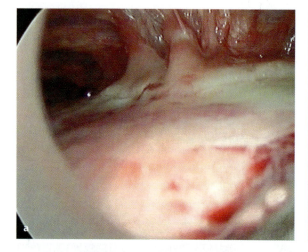
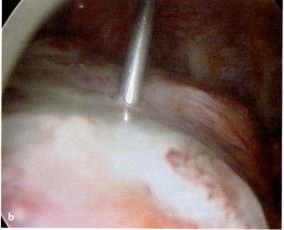

Fig. 19.6 a,b. After sterilization, the cyst is opened and the membrane is detached and put into a bag

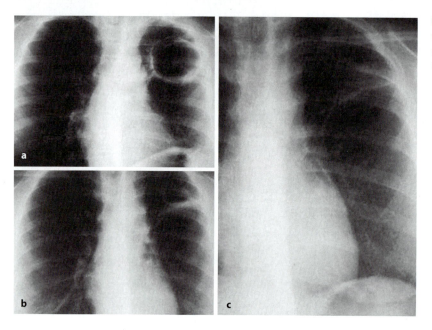

Fig. 19.7 a–c. Serial postoperative X-rays: spontaneous regression of a pneumatocele in the left upper lobe

tonic saline were then to be injected it would flow into the pericystic space, not killing the scoleces and potentially damaging the lung by leakage through bronchial fistulae. To prevent this, the cyst is only partially aspirated and partially refilled with saline. This procedure is repeated until one is sure that what remains in the cyst is only hypertonic saline. It takes about 15 min for an optimal scolecidal action of the hypertonic saline. After that period of time the cyst can be emptied completely after which the pericyst can be removed.

To do this, the vault of the cyst is opened with monopolar scissors and the pericyst is removed. To remove the pericyst without contamination of the surrounding tissues and without fragmentation, we put the pericyst into an endobag and remove it; it is then sent to the pathologist (■ Figs. 19.6a,b).

After ventilating the deflated lung, possible air leaks through bronchial fistulae can be seen and are closed with sutures or clips. The time spent doing this is valuable because persistent air leaks require prolonged tube drainage and sometimes even repeat surgery.

Drainage of the residual cyst cavity is important as it permits the lung to collapse within 5 or 7 days. If not done, a pneumatocele may form. Anterior and posterior lung drains are also placed to ensure good expansion of the lung.

Postoperative Care

Physiotherapy is started within a few hours after the surgery, but pain relief is essential. Albendazole is given for 6 weeks.

 Results

Bronchial inhalation of hypertonic saline induced drowning after the surgery in one patient, requiring intensive care. Hypertonic saline is very aggressive for the pleura, sometimes inducing exudation of the pleura for several days and requiring drainage for that period. A pneumatocele can be seen several months later. The postoperative course is almost always good. Occasionally a fistula induces the occurrence of a pneumatocele, or causes abscess formation. In these cases physiotherapy is very important. Chest X-rays are sufficient to monitor the disappearance of a pneumatocele (■ Fig. 19.7a–c). None of our cases required repeat surgery for a pneumatocele.

Discussion

The thoracoscopic approach is of interest (Becmeur et al. 1994; Cangir et al. 2000; Keramidas et al. 2004) not only for a young cyst, but also for a secondary infected cyst or for a ruptured cyst. The main advantage of this procedure is the minimal invasiveness not only regarding the thoracic wall but also regarding the pulmonary parenchyma. Bronchial exclusion is mandatory for this form of surgery thereby decreasing the risk of inhalation of cystic material and anaphylactic shock and the risk of inhaling hypertonic saline. All fistulas must be closed. The remaining cyst cavity has to be drained, especially when the wall is rigid, as is often the case in old cysts.

References

Becmeur F, Chaouachi B, Dhaoui R et al. (1994) Video-assisted thoracic surgery of hydatid cysts of the lung in children. J Chir (Paris) 131:541–543

Cangir AK, Sahin E, Enon S et al. (2000) Surgical treatment of pulmonary hydatid cysts in children. J Pediatr Surg 36:917–920

Keramidas D, Mavridis G, Soutis M et al. (2004) Medical treatment of pulmonary hydatidosis: complications and surgical management. Pediatr Surg Int 19:774–776

Munzer D (1991) New perspectives in the diagnosis of Echinococcus disease. J Clin Gastroenterol 13:415–423

Smego RA Jr, Bhatti S, Khaliq AA et al. (2003) Percutaneous aspiration-injection-reaspiration drainage plus albendazole or mebendazole for hepatic cystic echinococcosis: a meta-analysis. Clin Infect Dis 37:1073–1083

Chapter 20

Thoracoscopic Closure of Patent Ductus Arteriosus in Infants and Children

Steven S. Rothenberg

Introduction

The incidence of a patent ductus arteriosus (PDA) in the general population has been described as being as high as 0.7%, and in low birth weight infants (<1,500 g) may reach up to 50%. Treatment in neonates has consisted of time, allowing the PDA to close spontaneously, or the use of Indocin in those PDAs that are hemodynamically significant. The consequences of a persistent PDA include heart failure, pulmonary hypertension, and an increased risk of spontaneous bacterial endocarditis (SBE). When medical management and time have failed to result in closure of the PDA or when there has been significant hemodynamic instability, surgical ligation (TSL) through a posterolateral thoracotomy incision had been considered the option of choice for dealing with these lesions.

Since the early 1995s this algorithm has changed dramatically. Two relatively new options are available for the treatment of these lesions (Radtke 1998). One option is the placement of a transcatheter occlusive (TCO) device placed in the angio-suite by the cardiologist. The first report of this technique was in 1971 by Portsman, but there have been significant modifications and improvements in this technique during the 1990s. The second option involves the thoracoscopic closure of the PDA (TCP). This method adheres to the same basic tenets as open surgical closure but uses minimally invasive techniques. Laborde reported the first experience of a video-assisted thoracoscopic (VATS) closure in 1993 (Laborde et al. 1993). Modifications in technique and instrumentation since 1995 have refined this technique making it quicker, safer, and more cost efficient. At centers performing one or both of these new techniques, thoracotomy and surgical closure has become an infrequently used technique (Burke et al. 1999; Hines et al. 1998; Laborde et al. 1997; Rothenberg et al. 1995).

Preoperative Preparation

Before Induction of General Anesthesia

In most patients the only preoperative study necessary is an echocardiogram to verify and document the presence of a PDA. This, in conjunction with consultation with a pediatric cardiologist, is generally the only workup necessary. Occasionally, if there is a question of other congenital defects, a more invasive study such as a cardiac catheterization maybe indicated. All patients are typed and crossmatched for blood prior to the procedure and the blood should be available in the operating room at the start of the procedure. It is unlikely that blood will be needed but if the ductus tears it needs to be available immediately while the surgeon converts to open.

After Induction of General Anesthesia

Once the patient is anesthetized single-lung ventilation is obtained with a right mainstem intubation as described in Chapter 11. Usually a single peripheral intravenous (IV) line is adequate for the procedure and the patient should have a pulse oximetry probe placed on a lower limb distal to the ductus. If the patient has more complex congenital heart disease, a central venous line or arterial line may be indicated. The patient is given preoperative IV antibiotics in accordance with SBE prophylaxis protocols.

Positioning

Patient

The patient is placed in a modified prone position with the left side elevated just 20–30° (■ Fig. 20.1). This allows gravity to retract the lung out of the way and eliminates the need for one trocar. Larger patients (>10 kg) are placed on a beanbag for support. Smaller patients are stabilized and padded with small roles and sheepskin. An axillary role is placed in all patients.

Crew, Monitors, and Equipment

The surgeon and the assistant stand on the right side of the table, toward the patient's front (■ Fig. 20.2). This keeps both the surgeon and the assistant in line with the camera eliminating paradoxical motion. A single monitor is used and is placed behind the patient's back so that the surgeon, area of dissection, and monitor are all in line. A second monitor can be placed above the surgeon's left shoulder for the scrub nurse to monitor, when the nurse is positioned on the left of the table.

Special Equipment

No special energy applying systems are required. A 5 mm clipping device is at hand. The availability of transesophageal or standard echocardiography is optional.

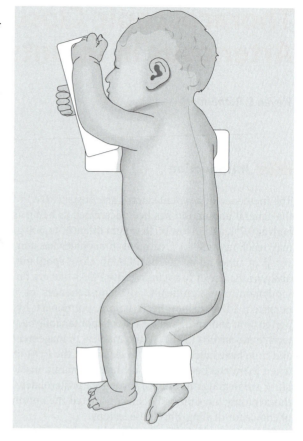

Fig. 20.1. Patient is placed in a modified prone position for thoracoscopic PDA ligation

Technique

Cannulae

Cannula	Method of insertion	Diameter (mm)	Device	Position
1	Closed	3 or 5	30° scope, 3 or 4 mm	Fourth intercostal space, posterior axillary line
2	Closed	5	Clip applier, scissors	Sixth intercostal space, slightly posterior to scope port
3	Closed	3 or 5	Maryland dissector	Third intercostal space in midaxillary line (anterior to scapula)

■ Figure 20.3 shows port positions.

Procedure

After the patient is prepared and draped, the chest is insufflated with a Veress needle at the camera trocar site. A low flow, low pressure of CO_2 is used to help collapse the lung and diminish the risk of lung injury with trocar insertion. In infants less than 5 kg a 3 mm port and 3 mm telescope are used. In children over 5 kg a 5 mm port and 4 mm telescope are selected. The CO_2 insufflation is continued throughout the proce-

dure. After an initial survey of the chest the other two ports are placed. The upper port is basically in the axilla and used for a grasper. The lower port is placed primarily to give the best access to the ductus for the clip applier.

The first step is to identify and cauterize the small vein which usually transverses the aorta at the level of the ductus. The pleura is then incised over the aorta and a pleural flap is developed which is mobilized medially, exposing the ductus. This allows the surgeon to pull the vagus and recurrent laryngeal nerves out of the field of dissection without grasping them. With the pleura mobilized medially the lower border of where

Fig. 20.2. Room setup for thoracoscopic PDA ligation

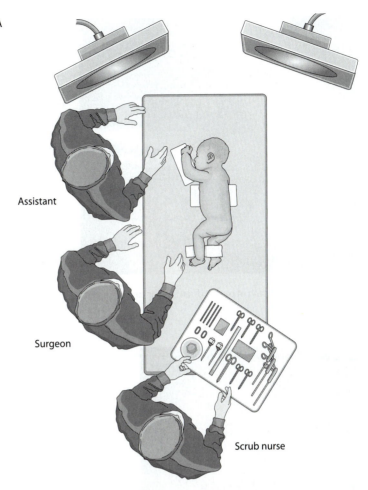

Assistant

Surgeon

Scrub nurse

Fig. 20.3. Port placement for thoracoscopic PDA ligation

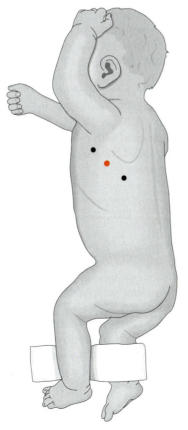

the ductus meets the aorta can easily be seen and a Maryland dissector is used to bluntly develop this plane. Dissection is continued posteriorly, gently mobilizing the back wall of the ductus. A similar technique is used on the upper crotch in order to create a safe plane between the ductus and aorta. This portion of the dissection is more difficult because the ductus often lies adjacent and parallel to the aorta making it hard to develop this plane. Once adequate mobilization is achieved a Maryland dissector is used to test clamp the ductus to ensure the right structure is being ligated (■ Fig. 20.4). The distal pulse oximeter should remain stable and in larger PDAs an increase in systolic blood pressure may be noted. After the test clamping, the clip applier is passed through the lower port. A test firing of the device should always be performed first to ensure proper firing of the mechanism and clips. If the jaws do not meet appropriately then the clip may scissor causing a tear of the duct. The applier is inserted and the angler should allow easy insertion of the clip around the PDA, going from inferior to superior (■ Fig. 20.5). In general the tips of the clip applier cannot be seen. The pleural flap should be retracted medially to help keep the recurrent laryngeal nerve out of the jaws of the clip. Once the clip is applied the

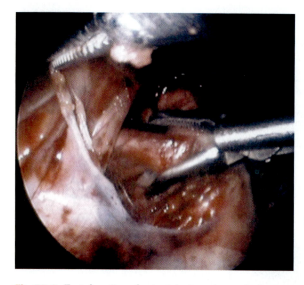

Fig. 20.4. Test clamping of patent ductus prior to placing surgical clip

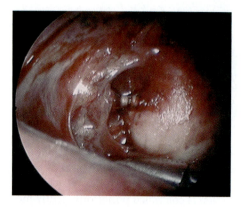

Fig. 20.5. Insertion of titanium clip on ductus. Care must be taken to avoid recurrent laryngeal nerve

applier is gently withdrawn and the clip is inspected. If there is concern that the ductus is not completely occluded then a second clip can be applied. Generally the anesthesiologist can detect a change in the murmur. Esophageal or standard echocardiography can also be performed in the operating room if there is significant concern that the ductus may not be completely occluded.

Once the clip applier is removed all other instruments and the upper two trocars are removed. The endotracheal tube is then brought back into the trachea and the left lung inflated. The upper trocar incisions are closed with absorbable suture. Once the lung is re-inflated, and with the patient still intubated, the lower port is removed under positive pressure and an occlusive dressing is applied, a procedure similar to removing a chest tube. The patient is then awoken from general anesthetic and extubated.

Postoperative Care

The patient is taken to the recovery room and a chest X-ray is obtained. A small residual pneumothorax is not unusual and can be generally watched. The patient is given IV narcotics for the first 12 h but is rapidly switched to oral pain medication. Feedings are resumed immediately and the patient is discharged to home when tolerating adequate oral intake. Routine follow-up is at 10 days and repeat echocardiography is performed at 1 month to ensure complete closure.

Results

Between November 1994 and December 2003 we have performed 86 TCPs. Ages ranged from 5 days to 48 years of age (all but four patients were less than 4 years of age) and weights ranged from 1.5 to 62 kg. Eighty-three procedures were completed successfully thoracoscopically. The first procedure took 2 h. The average operative time for the last 30 has been 22 min. Chest tubes were left in only 4 cases. Three patients were converted to open because of bleeding, one from an intercostal vessel injured with the initial trocar insertion, one from a partial tear of the ductus during an attempt to suture ligate the vessel, and one tear from a clip. There was one incomplete closure (the clip partially slipped off) that required a second procedure and there was one temporary injury to the recurrent laryngeal nerve, which resolved after 9 months. The average hospital stay for those patients admitted the day of surgery has been 1.2 days.

Of great help has been the development of a reliable 5 mm endoscopic clip (USSC, Norwalk, CT). This obviates the need for removing the trocar and makes insertion and application of the clip much smoother and quicker. We have also switched to 2.7 mm instruments and a 2.7 mm 30° lens so that the procedure is now performed with two 3 mm trocars and one 5 mm trocar placed between the midaxillary and posterior axillary lines.

Discussion

The need for the closure of a persistent PDA, even in an asymptomatic child, has been well documented but the treatment options have changed dramatically. Since Gross first described surgical ligation in 1939 the procedure has been associated with a very low mortality and a nearly 100% success rate. Therefore any procedure which hopes to compete with TSL must have similar success but should avoid the short- and long-term morbidity of a posterolateral thoracotomy incision.

Since 1971 the interventional cardiologists have been perfecting a technique of placing an intraluminal occlusive device. The initial reports had a significant failure and device migration rate. A multicenter report by Gray in 1993 found that TCO was more costly and less efficacious than TSL, with up to 10% of the devices migrating. However since 1999, with improvement in technique and a greater use of coils rather than the Rashkind occluder, migration problems have diminished and successful occlusion has approached 95%. The procedure still requires a special angio-suite and is not suitable to all sizes of patients and PDAs. TCO still has a higher failure rate than TSL and coil migration and incomplete closure is still a significant concern.

Laborde et al. first reported thoracoscopic closure of a PDA in 1993 and Burke reported a second series in 1994. Both used techniques similar to that described earlier and had little morbidity and no mortality with a high success rate. The major concern of uncontrolled bleeding has never materialized and in the few cases of bleeding, conversion to an open thoracotomy was quickly and safely achieved. Incomplete occlusion has been a rare complication and only a handful of patients have required a secondary procedure. Burke (1994), Laborde et al. (1993), and others have now reported on over 800 cases with no mortality and minimal morbidity. Burke has also reported on a series of low birth weight infants 575–2,500 g (Burke et al. 1999). Although the surgical times and conversion rate are slightly higher the technique is still safe and effective even in this select group.

In our series the operative times and technique have improved greatly over the course of time. Perhaps the biggest advance was the development of a reliable 5 mm endoscopic clip applier, which has greatly simplified the procedure. Our experience with other thoracoscopic procedures in small neonates has also enhanced and modified our technique. To date we have not performed the procedure in infants under 1,500 g primarily because we perform these procedures in the neonatal intensive care unit (NICU) and because of the still relatively large size of the instruments and clips.

At our institution all three methods of closure are available. In those cases that the cardiologists feel are amenable to any of the techniques, the parents are given a detailed description of the procedures along with the risks and benefits. The parents are then allowed to make an informed decision as to which technique is used. Approximately two thirds choose TCO and the rest TCP. Few parents opt for TSL. However in our previous report (Rothenberg et al. 1995) we did document that TCP resulted in the lowest hospital charges as compared to the other two.

References

Burke RP (1994) Video-assisted thoracoscopic surgery for patent ductus arteriosus. Pediatrics 93:823–825

Burke RP, Jacobs JP, Cheng W, et al (1999) Video assisted thoracoscopic surgery for patent ductus arteriosus in low birth weight neonates and infants. Pediatrics 04:227–230

Hines MH, Bensky AS, Hammon JW, et al (1998) Video-assisted thoracoscopic ligation of patent ductus arteriosus: safe and outpatient. Ann Thorac Surg 66:853–858

Laborde F, Noirhomme P, Karam J et al (1993) A new video assisted thoracoscopic surgical technique for interruption of patent ductus arteriosus in infants and children. J Thorac Cardiovasc Surg 87:870–875

Laborde F, Folliguet TA, Etienne PY, et al (1997) Video-thoracoscopic surgical interruption of patent ductus arteriosus. Routine experience in 332 pediatric cases. Eur J Cardiothorac Surg 11:1052–1055

Radtke WA (1998) Current therapy of the patent ductus arteriosus. Curr Opin Cardiol 13:59–65

Rothenberg SS, Chang JH, Toews WH, et al (1995) Thoracoscopic closure of patent ductus arteriosus: a less traumatic and more cost-effective technique. J Pediatr Surg 30:1057–1060

Chapter 21

Aortosternopexy for Tracheomalacia

Klaas (N) M.A. Bax and David C. van der Zee

Introduction

Tracheomalacia is a condition in which the trachea is not rigid enough to prevent airway collapse during expiration (Baxter and Dunbar 1963). Tracheomalacia may be localized or diffuse, congenital or acquired. It may be idiopathic or occur in association with vascular rings or slings, an aberrant innominate artery, esophageal atresia with distal fistula, mediastinal masses, prolonged intubation, and bronchopulmonary dysplasia. Gross and Neuhauser (1948) proposed aortosternopexy as a treatment option in the belief that a compressing innominate artery was the cause. Although it is now recognized that tracheomalacia, at least in esophageal atresia, is mainly caused by an intrinsic anomaly of the trachea at the site of the distal fistula (Griscom and Martin 1990; Qi et al. 1997; Wailoo and Emery 1979), aortosternopexy has remained the cornerstone of the treatment of symptomatic tracheomalacia. This has been classically performed through a left thoracotomy, a median sternotomy, or a cervical approach (Blair et al. 1986; Schwarz and Filler 1980; Vaishnav and MacKinnon 1986). An aortosternopexy can, however, be performed well using a thoracoscopic technique (de Cou et al. 2001; Schaarschmidt et al. 2002).

Preoperative Preparation

The definitive diagnosis is usually made by bronchoscopy under general anesthesia but under spontaneous breathing (Azizkham et al. 1997). Helical computed tomography (CT) has been advocated in order to define the exact location and extent of the tracheomalacia (Inoue et al. 1998). Aortic arch anomalies as a cause for the tracheomalacia have to be excluded.

Anesthesia

General anesthesia is used. It is the custom in our hospital to add locoregional techniques as well. The child is endotracheally intubated and no attempt for single-lung ventilation is made. Instead a CO_2 pneumothorax is created.

Positioning

Patient

The patient is placed in a supine position on the operating table. The left chest is elevated 15°, and the table is put in 15° reversed Trendelenburg (■ Fig. 21.1). The child's head is positioned in such a way that a concomitant bronchoscopy can be carried out during the tying of the transsternal aortopexy sutures at the end of the operation in order to have visual control of the effect of the pulling sutures on the anteroposterior diameter of the trachea at the level of the tracheomalacia. The midsternal line is marked for the future insertion of sutures (■ Fig. 21.2).

Crew, Monitors, and Equipment

The surgeon stands at the patient's left side with the camera operator to his or her left and the scrub nurse at the bottom end of a shortened operating table. One monitor stands to the left of the patient's head, and this monitor can be used by the bronchoscopist at the end of the operation. The second monitor stands to the right of the patient's head and is the monitor that the surgeon watches (■ Fig. 21.3).

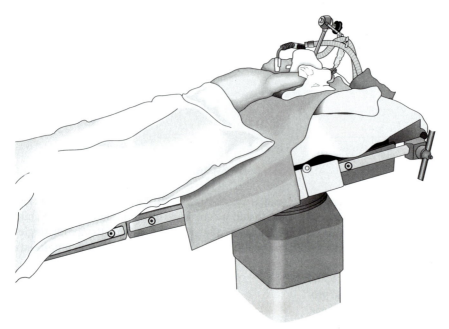

Fig. 21.1. Position of the patient on the table: supine, 15° tilt to the left, 15° reversed Trendelenburg

Fig. 21.2. Marking of the midsternal line

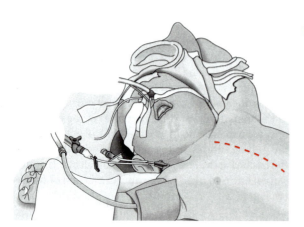

Technique

Cannulae

Cannula	Method of insertion	Diameter (mm)	Device	Position
1	Open	6	Telescope 30°, 24 or 30 cm long	Midaxilla, 4th intercostal space 1 cm below the inferior tip of the scapula
2	Closed	3.5	Surgeon's right-hand instrument	Midaxilla, more cranially than the telescope cannula
3	Closed	3.5	Surgeon's left-hand instrument	More caudally and more anteriorly than the telescope cannula

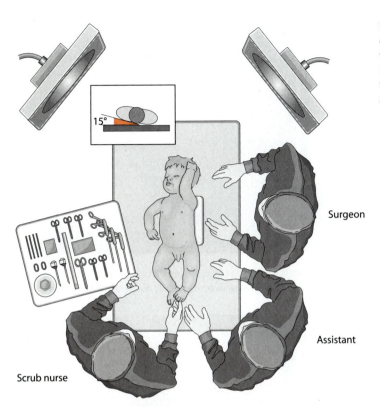

Carbon Dioxide Pneumothorax

Carbon dioxide is insufflated at a pressure of 5 mm Hg and a flow of 0.5 L/min. This is usually well tolerated in the older child but may be more troublesome in the newborn. Close collaboration between the anesthesiologist and surgeon is always needed but the more so when the CO_2 pneumothorax is not well tolerated. Increasing the ventilation rate while keeping the minute volume unchanged may be helpful, as is the temporary decrease in the pneumothorax pressure. A saturation drop is counteracted by an increase in fractional intake of oxygen (FIO_2). It is most important that the surgeon is not impatient. After a few minutes, the ipsilateral lung collapses and will stay so even when almost no further pneumothorax pressure is given. During thoracoscopic correction, lung retraction is not usually needed.

Procedure

Three cannulae are inserted, a 6 mm cannula for a 5 mm 30° telescope, and two 3.5 mm cannulae for the working instruments. The cannulae are inserted in a triangular configuration in the midaxillary region on the left (■ Fig. 21.4).

The procedure is only started when the baby has reached a stable condition. A magnificent view of the

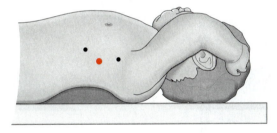

Fig. 21.4. Position of the cannulae. Triangular with the telescope in the midaxillary line and the working cannulae more anteriorly

anterior mediastinum is obtained (■ Fig. 21.5a). Care is taken not to injure the phrenic nerve which lies in front of the left pulmonary pedicle on the left pericardium. The mediastinal pleura is opened longitudinally, midway over the edge of the thymic gland pleura (■ Fig. 21.5b). The thymus is freed first posteriorly to expose the ascending aorta inclusive of the pericardial reflection, the aortic arch, and the innominate artery (■ Fig. 21.6). The gland is then detached from the sternum anteriorly and is pushed to the right (■ Fig. 21.7). Alternatively the left lobe of the thymic gland may be resected (Schwarz and Filler 1980). The aortic arch as well as the innominate artery are clearly visible. The adventitia of these structures should not be stripped off as the adventitia is needed for the insertion

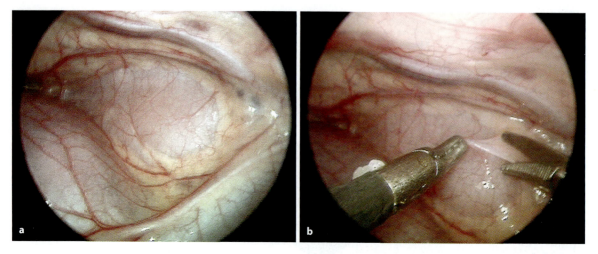

Fig. 21.5. View of the anterior mediastinum. **a** The thymic gland is clearly seen as is the pericardium which bulges on the left. The phrenic nerve runs over a persistent left superior caval veinn. **b** The pleura over the thymic gland is opened longitudinally

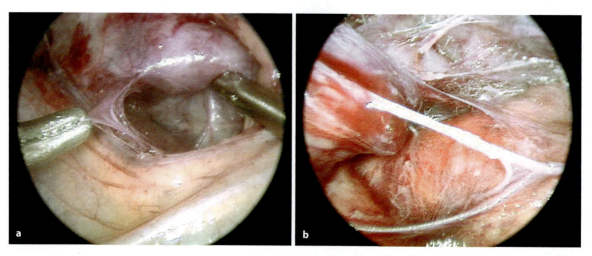

Fig. 21.6 a,b. The thymic gland is dissected free posteriorly until the ascending aorta with pericardial reflection and innominate artery are seen

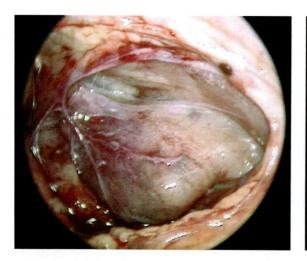

Fig. 21.7. The thymic gland has been detached from the sternum as well and is pushed to the right

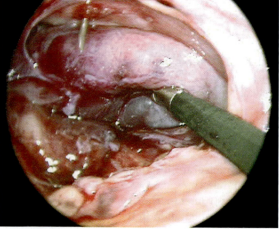

Fig. 21.8. A needle has been pushed through the sternum in the midsternal line for identification of the correct position of the sutures

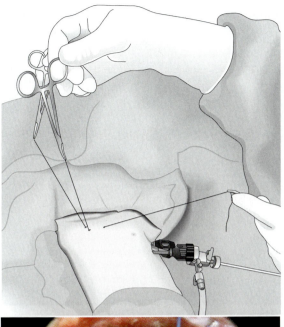

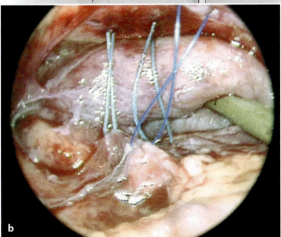

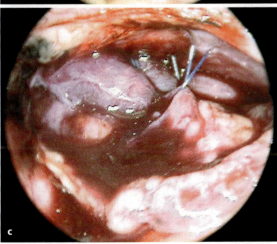

Fig. 21.9 a,b,c Three sutures have been passed through stab incisions through the midsternum. The adventitia has been taken and the needles have been passed out through the same stab incisions. Traction is exerted on the sutures under concomitant tracheoscopy control. Note that the distance between the aorta and sternum decreased during traction

of the pulling sutures. To obtain stronger tissue for the pulling sutures an anterior pericardial flap can be made at the pericardial reflection on the anterior ascending aorta with its base attached to the ascending aorta (Applebaum and Wooley 1990; Schaarschmidt et al. 2002). Alternatively the pericardial reflection itself can be taken in the sutures. It is said that the area to be suspended is rather the ascending aorta than the innominate artery or the aortic arch.

For identification of the right position of the future traction sutures, a straight needle is passed through the sternum in the midline (■ Fig. 21.8). The sternum in children is rather soft and it is not very difficult to push a needle through it. The position of the entering tip of the needle in relation to the part of the aorta to be pulled up is verified. If the position is all right, then a 2- or 3 mm transverse incision is made in the skin at the entrance of the needle, and a 3 × 0 Ethibound suture on a round-bodied needle with sharp point is introduced. The needle is somewhat straightened in order to allow easy entrance. After taking the pericardial flap or pericardial reflection or adventitia of the ascending aorta or innominate artery, the needle is passed through the sternum in the opposite direction and out through the same incision. In general three sutures are placed over the length of the ascending aorta and innominate artery (■ Fig. 21.9 a-c). Under concomitant bronchoscopic control, the sutures are tied (■ Figs. 21.9, 21.10). If necessary, additional sutures can be placed. There is no need to pull the ascending aorta and innominate artery completely against the sternum. The lung is reexpanded and remaining CO_2 is aspirated. Portholes are closed, adhesive strips are applied to the skin, and no drain is left behind.

Postoperative Care

A postoperative chest X-ray is made for appreciation of lung expansion and for evaluation of remaining CO_2. Small amounts of remaining CO_2 are irrelevant.

The procedure is very well tolerated and the patient can be rapidly extubated. The effect of the procedure on the tracheomalacia is immediately obvious.

Results

Three children with tracheomalacia and acute life-threatening events have received a thoracoscopic aortosternopexy. They were, respectively, 3, 6, and 12 months old. The procedure in all children proved easy, and it was effective in the two older children. Symptoms in the youngest child did not subside and at repeat tracheoscopy it seemed that the most distal part of the trachea was nicely open but that the more prox-

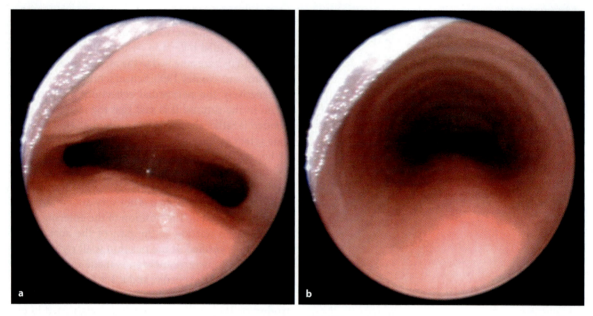

Fig. 21.10 a,b. Tracheoscopic images before (a) and after traction (b). A greatly enlarged diameter is visible

imal part was still narrow. This patient had the first procedure at the age of 3 months and the redo procedure 1 month later. During the first operation the pericardial reflection onto the ascending aorta was sutured to the sternum. During the redo procedure the innominate artery was sutured to the sternum as well. The redo procedure was not very difficult.

Discussion

There is little doubt that thoracoscopic aortosternopexy is far superior when compared with a comparable procedure using either a thoracotomy or an anterior mediastinal approach. As the thoracoscopic approach allows relatively simple exposure of the major intrathoracic vessels, the thoracoscopic approach may also be beneficial in patients with tracheobronchomalacia in whom suspension of the pulmonary artery is required (Kamata et al. 1998).

References

Applebaum H, Wooley MM (1990) Pericardial flap aortopexy for tracheomalacia. J Pediatr Surg 25:30–32

Azizkham RG, Caty MG (1997) Subglottic airway. In: Oldjam KT, Colombai PM, Foglia RP (eds) Surgery of Infants and Children. Lippincott-Raven, Philadelphia, pp 897–913

Baxter JD, Dunbar JS (1963) Tracheomalacia. Ann Otol Rhinol Laryngol 77:1013–1023

Blair GK, Cohen R, Filler RM (1986) Treatment of tracheomalacia: eight years' experience. J Pediatr Surg 21:781–785

DeCou JM, Parsons DS, Gauderer MWL (2001) Thoracoscopic aortopexy for severe tracheomalacia. Pediatr Endosurg Innov Tech 5:205–208

Griscom NT, Martin TR (1990) The trachea and esophagus after repair of esophageal atresia and distal fistula: computed tomographic observations. Pediatr Radiol 20:447–450

Gross RE, Neuhauser EBD (1948) Compression of the trachea by an anomalous innominate artery: an operation for its relief. Am J Dis Child 75:570–574

Inoue K, Yanagihara J, Ono S et al. (1998) Utility of helical CT for diagnosis and operative planning in tracheomalacia after repair of esophageal atresia. Eur J Pediatr Surg 8:355–357

Kamata S, Usui N, Sawai T et al. (2000) Pexis of the great vessels for patients with tracheobronchomalacia in infancy. J Pediatr Surg 35:454–457

Qi BQ, Merei J, Farmer P, Hasthorpe S et al. (1997) Tracheomalacia with esophageal atresia and tracheoesophageal fistula in fetal rats. J Pediatr Surg 32:1575–1579

Schaarschmidt K, Kolberg-Schwerdt A, Bunke K et al. (2002) A technique for thoracoscopic aortopericardiosternopexy. Surg Endosc 16:1639

Schwarz MZ, Filler RM (1980) Tracheal compression as a cause of apnea following repair of tracheoesophageal fistula: treatment by aortopexy. J Pediatr Surg 15:842–848

Vaishnav A, MacKinnon AE (1986) New cervical approach for tracheopexy. Br J Surg 73:441–442

Wailoo MP, Emery JL (1979) The trachea in children with tracheomalacia. Histopathology 3:329–338

Chapter 22

Thoracoscopic Venous Vascular Access

Klaas (N) M.A. Bax and David C. van der Zee

Introduction

Vascular access is very important in modern medicine in general and in the care of sick children in particular (Coran 1992; Gauderer 1992). Some children are very dependent on long-term vascular access, for example in cases of hemodialysis for end-stage renal disease, total parenteral nutrition for short bowel syndrome, chemotherapy for malignancy, or ventriculoatrial shunting for hydrocephalus. When the classic access sites have become exhausted, vascular access becomes a major problem. Procedures such as lumbar venous access to the inferior vena cava through a lumbotomy (Boddie 1989), access of the azygos vein through a thoracotomy (Malt and Kempster 1983; Redo et al. 1992), and direct right atrial cannulation after sternotomy (Hayden et al. 1981) have been described, but such procedures are quite invasive and there is a continuous search for making these procedures less invasive. Percutaneous ultrasound-guided catheterization of the inferior vena cava either through the lumbar region or through the liver is an example of this (Azizkhan et al. 1992; Robertson et al. 1990). Another possibility is to cannulate the azygos vein by percutaneous puncture under thoracoscopic vision (Bax and van der Zee 1996) or to cannulate the remaining open superior caval vein just above the right atrium also by percutaneous puncture under thoracoscopic control.

Preoperative Preparation

Before embarking on more complicated procedures for vascular access, imaging studies should be performed to make sure that the classic venous access sites, for example the subclavian or internal jugular veins, are no longer available and that the intended site is available.

Positioning of Patient, Crew, Monitors, and Equipment

Cannulation of the Azygos Vein

The child is placed in a semiprone left lateral decubitus position on the operating table (■ Fig. 22.1), which is tilted in reversed Trendelenburg. The table is bent underneath the chest in order to increase the intercostal spaces of the right chest (■ Fig. 22.2). Alternatively a sandbag is placed underneath the left chest. The position of the chest on the table is such that it allows for fluoroscopy to check the position of the guide wire and, later on, the tip of the catheter. The right arm is abducted over the head. The principal video monitor (the second one) stands to the left of the patient's head. The surgeon stands to the right of the patient, the scrub nurse to the right of the surgeon and the assistant to the left of the patient (■ Fig. 22.1). The stack with the first video monitor is positioned behind the surgeon.

Cannulation of the Remaining Superior Caval Vein

For an intended cannulation of the remnant of the superior caval vein, the patient is placed in a three quarter posterior left lateral position. The principal monitor is then placed more distally in front of the abdomen of the patient, while the surgeon stands at the upper end of the table (■ Fig. 22.3).

Special Equipment

No special equipment is needed. An appropriately sized central venous catheter with or without a chamber is chosen together with an appropriate Seldinger-type introduction system. Fluoroscopy is at hand.

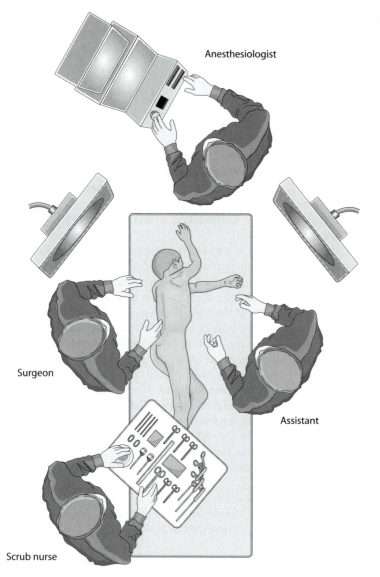

Anesthesiologist

Surgeon

Assistant

Scrub nurse

Fig. 22.1. Positioning for cannulation of the azygos vein. The patient lies in a semiprone left lateral decubitus position on the table, which is tilted in reversed Trendelenburg. The surgeon stands behind the patient, with the scrub nurse to his or her right. The camera operator stands on the opposite side. The two monitors are placed at either side of the head of the patient

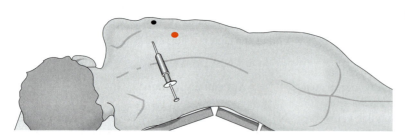

Fig. 22.2. The telescope cannula is inserted 1 cm below the inferior tip of the scapula in an open way. A second cannula is inserted more proximally in the midaxillary line for lung retraction

Fig. 22.3. Positioning for cannulation of the superior caval vein. The patient is placed supine on the operating table with the neck in hyperextension. The table is in the Trendelenburg position. The surgeon stand at the top of the operating table, with the camera operator on the right side of the patient. The stack is located behind the surgeon with the principal monitor at the patient's left but facing the surgeon

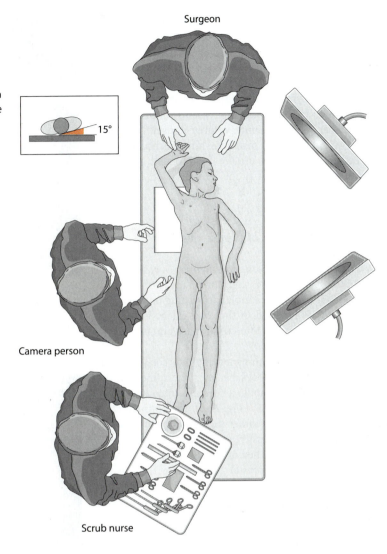

Surgeon

15°

Camera person

Scrub nurse

Procedure

Cannulae

Azygos Vein Cannulation

Cannula	Method of insertion	Diameter (mm)	Device	Position
1	Open	6	Telescope	1 cm below the tip of the scapula
2	Closed	3.5–6	Lung retractor	Midaxillary line, 3rd or 4th intercostal space

Superior Caval Vein Cannulation

Cannula	Method of insertion	Diameter (mm)	Device	Position
1	Open	6	Telescope	Midaxillary line, high in the axilla
2	Closed	3.5–6	Lung retractor	Midaxillary line, 3rd or 4th intercostal space

Carbon Dioxide Pneumothorax

Carbon dioxide is insufflated at a pressure of 5–8 mmHg and at a flow of 0.5 L/min. This is usually well tolerated, but it may require some time to obtain a steady hemodynamic and respiratory state. If the lung is too much in the way, an increase in ventilation rate while keeping the minute volume constant is often very helpful. Once the ipsilateral lung has become collapsed, pressure can usually be reduced to about 3 mmHg. A palpation probe may be used as a lung retractor.

Cannulation of the Azygos Vein

A 6 mm cannula is inserted in an open way below the tip of the scapula and is used for a 5 mm 30° scope. A second 3.5- or 6 mm cannula, depending on the age of the patient, is inserted in the midaxillary line at the level of the 3rd or 4th intercostal space and is used for a lung retractor.

The azygos vein with its feeding intercostal veins is visualized. From the back between the spine and the medial edge of the scapula a needle is introduced into the extrapleural space (■ Fig. 22.4). The optimal intercostal space is chosen under thoracoscopic control by exerting external pressure onto adjacent intercostal spaces. The needle is then advanced extrapleurally either into a large intercostal vein or directly into the azygos vein. The tip of the needle can be seen in the particular vein and blood is easily aspirated. Next a guide wire is inserted into the vessel and the needle is withdrawn (■ Fig. 22.5). The position of the tip of the guide wire is positioned fluoroscopically and the length of the intracorporeal part of the guide wire is measured. An appropriate plastic dilator with a peel a way sheet is introduced over the guide wire. After tunneling of the appropriate catheter along the lower anterior chest wall to the place of insertion of the peel a way system, the catheter length is adjusted according to the measured length of the guide wire, and the catheter introduced into the peel a way sheet and further pushed into place. The place of the tip of the catheter is checked fluoroscopically in two directions. The catheter is then fixed to the chest wall or assembled to a subcutaneously placed chamber. The CO_2 is aspirated under thoracoscopic control and the cannulae are removed. There is no need to close the holes except for application of adhesive tape to the skin. No drain is left behind.

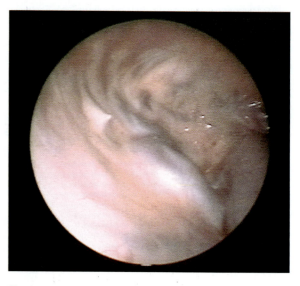

Fig. 22.4. Cannulation of the azygos vein. A needle has been pushed through the thoracic wall but is withdrawn into the extrapleural space. There are dilated intercostal veins

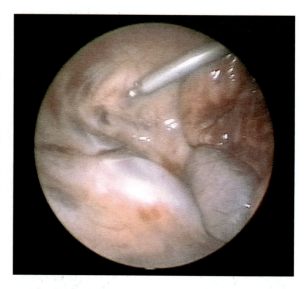

Fig. 22.5. The needle has been advanced in an intercostal vein after which a guide wire has been brought in. The guide wire is seen through the wall of the vein. Next a tunneled catheter is brought in using a Seldinger technique. Fluoroscopy is used to verify the correct position of the catheter

Cannulation of the Remaining Superior Caval Vein

The caval vein between the entrance of the azygos vein and the right atrium usually remains patent just above the right atrium. This part of the caval vein can be punctured from the right side of the neck in much the same way as the internal jugular vein is punctured at that side. The needle can then be advanced underneath the mediastinal pleura until the remaining open caval vein is reached. The caval vein is punctured and a catheter is brought in via a Seldinger-type technique.

The telescope cannula is inserted high in the axilla. A second cannula may be inserted for an instrument to retract the lung. The catheter is tunneled in a classic way and may be hooked up to a chamber. No drain is left behind.

Postoperative Care

As the procedure is carried out under thoracoscopic guidance there is no need for a postoperative chest X-ray. We keep the patients in the hospital overnight.

Results

This technique of azygos vein cannulation was used in an 8-year-old boy with severe combined immunodeficiency and chronic diarrhea from birth. He had had multiple central venous lines over the years, but both the upper and lower caval vein became occluded. Cannulation of the azygos vein as described proved easy and no complications in direct relationship with the insertion occurred. As a result of repetitive septicemia with *Xanthomonas maltophilia*, however, the catheter had to be removed 3 months later. Happily enough, the patient has not required a new central line since then.

The technique of superior caval vein cannulation was attempted in a 7-year-old girl with congenital diarrhea and dependent on parenteral supplementation of nutrition. The azygos vein was rather small. As the superior caval vein just above the heart appeared open, it was punctured from the right side of the neck. Unfortunately there was a stenosis of the entrance of the superior caval vein into the right atrium and the procedure had to be abandoned.

Discussion

The technique presented is simple and safe. The advantage is obvious: one sees what one is doing.

References

Azizkhan RG, Taylor LA, Jaques PF, et al (1992) Percutaneous translumbar and transhepatic inferior vena cava catheters for prolonged vascular access in children. J Pediatr Surg 27:165–169
Bax NMA, van der Zee DC (1996) Percutaneous cannulation of the azygos vein. Surg Endosc 10:863–864
Boddie AW Jr (1989) Translumbar catheterization of the inferior vena cava for long-term angioaccess. Surg Gynecol Obstet 168:55–56
Coran AG (1992) Vascular access and infusion therapy. Semin Pediatr Surg 1:173–241
Gauderer MWL (1992) Vascular access techniques and devices in the pediatric patient. Surg Clin North Am 71:1267–1284
Hayden L, Stewart GR, Johnson DC, et al (1981) Transthoracic right atrial cannulation for parenteral nutrition. Anaesth Intensive Care 9:53–57
Malt RA, Kempster M (1983) Direct azygos vein and superior vena cava cannulation for parenteral nutrition. J Parenter Enter Nutr 7:580–581
Redo SF, Ciccarelli A, Ghajar J, et al (1992) Ventriculoatrial shunt utilizing the azygos vein. J Pediatr Surg 27:642–644
Robertson LJ, Jaques PF, Mauro MA, et al (1990) Percutaneous inferior vena cava placement of tunneled Silastic catheters for prolonged vascular access in children. J Pediatr Surg 25:596–598

Chapter 23

Thoracoscopic Treatment of Palmar Hyperhidrosis

Zahavi Cohen

Introduction

Upper thoracic sympathectomy is indicated in the treatment of a variety of sympathetic disorders, including palmar hyperhidrosis, facial blushing, Raynaud's disease, splanchnic pain, and reflex sympathetic dystrophy. In my experience, hyperhidrosis was the only indication for surgical intervention in children. Primary hyperhidrosis is considered a very distressing and embarrassing condition affecting the hands and sometimes axillae and feet. Conservative treatment may be effective only in the mild forms (Cullen 1975; Scholes et al. 1978; White 1986). Operative treatment is the method of choice in severe cases (Adar et al. 1977; Bogokowski et al. 1983; Mares et al. 1994), its goal being to achieve a constant anhidrotic state of the palms. Various surgical approaches have been described for conventional "open" thoracic sympathectomy (Adson et al. 1935; Atkins 1954; Ellis and Morgan 1971; Gask 1933; Telford 1935). The thoracoscopic technique has simplified surgery on the upper thoracic chain and, indeed, proved to be superior in almost every respect (Cohen et al. 1995, 1996; Kao et al. 1994; Kux 1977; Malone 1986). The therapeutic aim in the treatment of hyperhidrosis is to interrupt the sympathetic impulse transmission from the lower sympathetic ganglia through the stellate ganglion to the hands. Thoracoscopic electrocautery transection of the sympathetic chain at the level of T2 and T3 has been the preferred treatment in my experience with more than 600 thoracoscopic sympathectomies.

Preoperative Workup

Since upper thoracic sympathectomy is primarily indicated in idiopathic primary palmar hyperhidrosis it is important to exclude other disease entities that include ("secondary") local or generalized hyperhidrosis among other manifestations, for example a variety of neurological diseases, thyrotoxicosis, pheochromocytoma, etc. A preoperative chest X-ray is taken to exclude any lung pathology, particularly one that causes adhesions. Simple adhesions can be easily divided thoracoscopically, but severe adhesions may require conversion. However, we have seldom encountered adhesions in the pediatric age group.

Routine complete blood count is performed in all patients. Blood should be typed and crossmatched. The operation is performed bilaterally, sequentially, under general anesthesia using an ordinary endotracheal intubation.

Positioning

Patient

The patient is placed in a supine position slightly elevated at the shoulders with both arms abducted to 90° and a 45° reversed Trendelenburg position (■ Fig. 23.1). The chest and axillae are prepared and draped widely in case conversion to open thoracotomy becomes necessary.

Crew, Monitors, and Equipment

The surgeon stands at the side of the sympathetic chain to be coagulated. The scrub nurse stands on the right side of the surgeon, when operating on the right side, and on the left side of the surgeon, when operating on the left side (■ Fig. 23.1). There are two monitors, one on each side of the head of the patient (■ Fig. 23.1).

Special Equipment

An endoscope with a built-in operating channel is used (■ Fig. 23.2). The diameter of the device is 10 mm and that of the operating channel 6 mm.

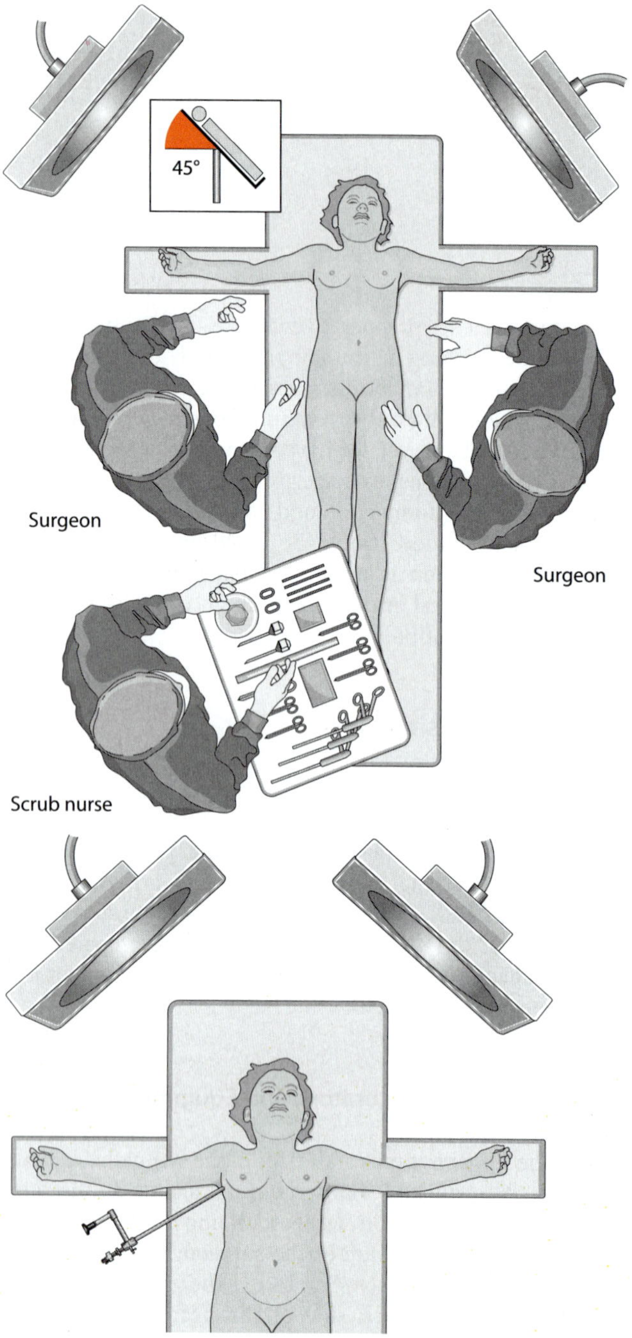

Fig. 23.1. Position of the patient, crew and monitors

45°

Surgeon

Surgeon

Scrub nurse

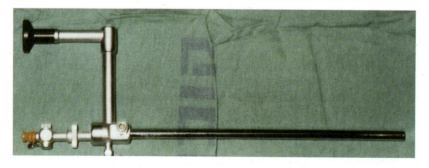

Fig. 23.2. Endoscope with a built-in operating channel

Fig. 23.3. Placement of operating thoracoscope

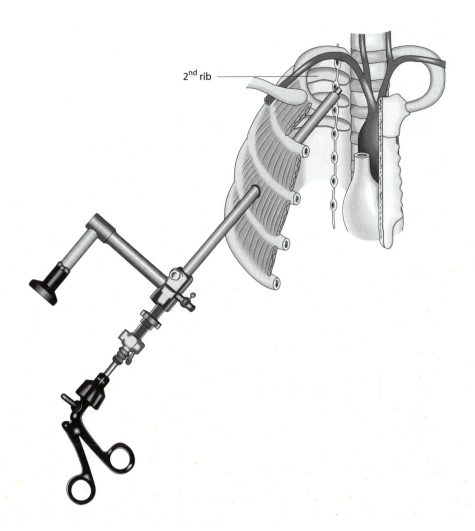

2nd rib

Technique

Cannulae

A 10 mm anterior axillary incision in the 4th or 5th intercostal space is performed. The anesthesiologist is requested to stop ventilation for a few seconds while the Veress needle is inserted into the pleural cavity and CO_2 is insufflated up to a pressure of 10–12 mmHg. The Veress needle is then removed and an 11 mm trocar is inserted through which a 10 mm 0° operating thoracoscope (Fig. 23.3) with a built-in working channel is introduced.

Procedure

The sympathetic chain is easily identified under the parietal pleura, running vertically over the neck of the ribs in the upper costovertebral region (Fig. 23.4). Occasionally the sympathetic chain is difficult to visualize, but it can be identified by rolling it under the grasping forceps. Sometimes the apex of the lung does not allow adequate visualization at the level of the 3rd or 4th sympathetic ganglia. The operating thoracoscope can be used to push the lung apex in a downward direction. Alternatively, the CO_2 pressure can be increased by 2 or 3 mmHg. A 45 cm grasping forceps connected to electrocoagulation is introduced through the working channel. The sympathetic chain is coagulated and resected at the level of T2 and T3 (Fig. 23.5). If severe axillary hyperhidrosis is present, the T4 ganglion should be ablated as well. Special care is taken to make sure that complete ablation of ganglia and discontinuity of the sympathetic chain is achieved. The grasping forceps is removed and the lung reexpanded under direct vision. The operating thoracoscope is removed and the skin is promptly closed by using two skin hooks and applying a few drops of Histoacryl (cyanoacrylate glue), or metal clips. It is important to have the anesthesiologist exert continuous positive pressure for the few seconds when the skin is closed to avoid a residual pneumothorax. Hence, no thoracic drain is necessary. The same procedure is repeated on

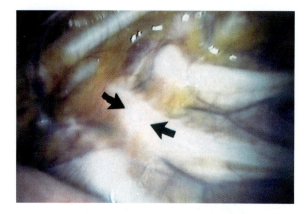

Fig. 23.4. Sympathetic chain (*arrows*) seen running vertically over the neck of the ribs under the parietal pleura

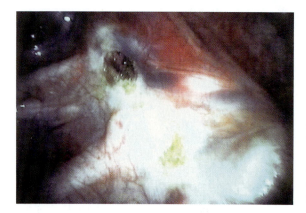

Fig. 23.5. Coagulation and resection of the sympathetic chain at the level of T2 and T3

the contralateral side. A chest radiograph is immediately requested postoperatively to prove complete lung expansion.

Results

We have been using this thoracoscope procedure for approximately ten years, and over 600 sympathectomies have been performed. No conversion to the open technique was ever necessary. The operative time for bilateral procedures is 30 min on average. No intraoperative complications were detected.

Ninety-eight percent of patients had an uneventful postoperative course and were discharged the following day. Seven patients had a subsequent residual pneumothorax that required intercostal drainage and were discharged on the third postoperative day. Ninety-eight percent of patients were completely satisfied with the operative results (palmar anhidrosis). Seven patients were dissatisfied claiming only minimal im-

provement. One patient was moderately satisfied complaining of excessive dryness of the palms. Some degree of "compensatory" sweating (chest and back) was the only side effect in approximately one third of all patients, but this did not decrease their overall satisfaction.

Discussion

The obvious advantage of the thoracoscopic approach to sympathectomy is the feasibility of performing bilateral procedures at the same time, as well as the minimal operative trauma, easy postoperative course, short hospitalization, excellent cosmetic results, and a quick return to school and normal activities.

Ordinary endotracheal intubation has replaced double lumen one-lung intubation, which is occasionally difficult and time-consuming and is not available in the small sizes for children under 10 years of age. A CO_2 pressure of approximately 10 mmHg enhances visualization and is safely tolerated.

Traditionally, upper thoracic sympathectomy included resection of the lower portion of the T1 ganglion down to the 4th and even the 5th ganglion. Our experience gained over 20 years (Cohen et al. 1995, 1996; Mares et al. 1994) as well as others (Hehir and Brady 1993; Kao et al. 1994) led us to perform a limited sympathectomy resecting only the 2nd and 3rd thoracic ganglia, thus diminishing considerably the compensatory sweating and avoiding the occasional occurrence of Horner's syndrome. This limited resection is all that is necessary to achieve the palmar anhidrotic effect. Once the sympathetic chain is visualized, there is no need to incise the pleura. The sympathetic chain is strongly grasped, elevated over the ribs, coagulated, and ablated to the point of complete disconnection of the chain at the level of T2 and T3.

The main complication of upper thoracic sympathectomy, Horner's syndrome, is almost non-existent with the endoscopic technique. The stellate ganglion is not seen endoscopically as it is covered by a characteristic yellow fat pad. Caution must be taken during electrocoagulation of the 2nd thoracic ganglion to avoid retrograde propagation of the coagulation to the stellate ganglion.

In order to avoid bleeding, the sympathetic chain should be elevated from its bed and then coagulated until complete discontinuity of the chain is achieved. Blood loss during the procedure is negligible and we have never encountered a major bleeding episode that required transfusion. However, to be on the safe side, it is advisable to have blood typed and crossmatched for every eventuality.

References

Adar R, Kurchin A, Zweig A, et al (1977) Palmar hyperhidrosis and its surgical treatment. A report of 100 cases. Ann Surg 186:34–41

Adson AW, Craig W, Brown GE (1935) Essential hyperhidrosis cured by sympathetic ganglionectomy and trunk resection. Arch Surg 31:794

Atkins HJB (1954) Sympathectomy by the axillary approach. Lancet 1:538–539

Bogokowski H, Slutzki S, Bacalu L, et al (1983) Surgical treatment of primary hyperhidrosis. Arch Surg 118:1065–1067

Cohen Z, Shinar D, Levi I, et al (1995) Thoracoscopic upper thoracic sympathectomy for primary palmar hyperhidrosis in children and adolescents. J Pediatr Surg 30:471–473

Cohen Z, Shinar D, Mordehai J, et al (1996) Thoracoscopic upper thoracic sympathectomy for primary palmar hyperhidrosis. Harefuah 131:303–305

Cullen SI (1975) Topical methenamine therapy for hyperhidrosis. Arch Dermatol 111:1158–1160

Ellis H, Morgan MN (1971) Surgical treatment of severe hyperhidrosis. Proc R Soc Med 64:16–18

Gask GE (1933) The surgery of the sympathetic nervous system. Br J Surg 21:113–130

Hehir DJ, Brady C (1993) Long term results of limited thoracic sympathectomy for palmar hyperhidrosis. J Pediatr Surg 28:909–911

Kao MC, Lee WY, Hip KM, et al (1994) Palmar hyperhidrosis in children: treatment with video endoscopic laser sympathectomy. J Pediatr Surg 29:387–391

Kux M (1977) Thoracic endoscopic sympathectomy for treatment of upper limb hyperhidrosis. Lancet 1:1320

Malone PS, Cameron AEP, Rennie JA (1986) Endoscopic thoracic sympathectomy in the treatment of upper limb hyperhidrosis. Ann R Coll Surg Engl 68:93–94

Mares AJ, Steiner Z, Cohen Z, et al (1994) Transaxillary upper thoracic sympathectomy for primary palmar hyperhidrosis in children and adolescents. J Pediatr Surg 29:382–386

Scholes KT, Crow KD, Ellis JP, et al (1978) Axillary hyperhidrosis treated with alcoholic solution of aluminium chloride hexahydrate. Br Med J 2:84–85

Telford ED (1935) The technique of sympathectomy. Br J Surg 23:448–450

White JW (1986) Treatment of primary hyperhidrosis. Mayo Clin Proc 61:951–956

Chapter 24

Thoracoscopic Treatment of Chylothorax

Steven S. Rothenberg

Introduction

Chylothorax in infants and children can arise from congenital causes, trauma, or iatrogenic injury. The treatment usually consists of chest tube drainage and giving the patient nothing by mouth (NPO) or maintaining them on a fat-free diet to limit the production of chyle. This treatment may often take weeks to resolve a chylothorax. If these conservative measures fail or if chyle losses are so large that the patient's protein and fat losses cannot be kept up with, then surgical intervention is indicated. This used to involve a major posterolateral thoracotomy and attempted ligation of the thoracic duct where it arises through the diaphragm. Advances in thoracoscopy now allow this procedure to be performed using a minimally invasive approach (Graham et al. 1994; Hillerdal 1997; Peillon et al. 1999; Wurnig et al. 2000). There are certain advantages to this technique including a magnified view of the area of the posterior thorax at the level of the diaphragm where the thoracic duct passes into the chest. This area is hard to visualize through an open thoracotomy, especially in an infant. The magnified view may aid in identification of the chyle leak and direct sealing at this point.

Preoperative Preparation

Before Induction of General Anesthesia

Few specific requirements are necessary prior to thoracoscopic exploration. If the patient has had significant chyle drainage for a prolonged period of time, care should be taken to ensure their nutritional and volume status are corrected. Occasionally ingestion of a fatty substance just prior to the procedure (e.g. olive oil) may aid in identifying the site of the leak.

After Induction of General Anesthesia

Once the patient is intubated, appropriate lines can be placed. Usually these patients already have central venous access for their hyperalimentation. An arterial line is rarely necessary as these patients have no intrinsic lung disease. The approach is through the right chest so

it is helpful if the anesthesiologist can obtain single-lung ventilation by performing a left mainstem intubation.

Positioning

Patient

The patient is placed in a modified prone position with the right side elevated 30–45°. Depending on the size of the child this can be accomplished with padded roles or a beanbag. An axillary role should be placed in all cases. The right arm should be placed up toward the head. Care should be taken to ensure access to the areas between the anterior and posterior axillary lines down to the iliac crest (■ Fig. 24.1).

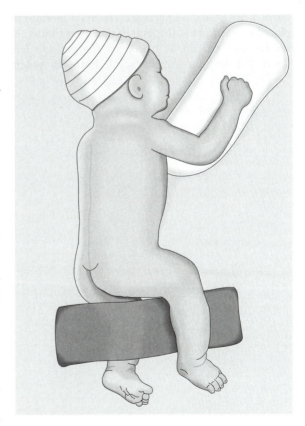

Fig. 24.1. Patient positioning. A modified prone position allows gravity to retract the lung out of the operative field

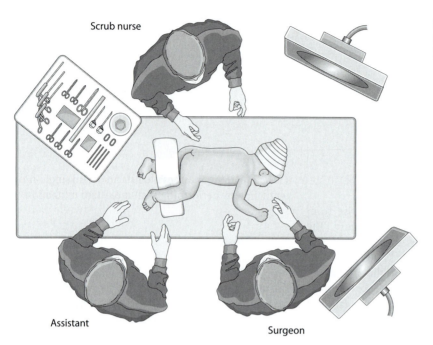

Scrub nurse

Assistant

Surgeon

Fig. 24.2. Room setup for thoracoscopic thoracic duct ligation

Crew, Monitors, and Equipment

The surgeon and assistant are positioned on the left side of the table toward the patient's front. The scrub nurse is positioned on the right. The main monitor is placed on the right at the level of the lower thorax. A second monitor can be placed on the patient's left above the surgeon for the scrub nurse to watch (■ Fig. 24.2).

Special Equipment

Energy applying systems:

Equipment	Required
Monopolar high-frequency electrocoagulation (HFE)	Yes
Bipolar HFE	Optional
Ultrasonic energy	No
Ligasure	Optional (recommended)
Argon	No
Laser	No
Other	No
Other equipment:	

Equipment	Required
Clips	Optional
Staplers	No
Bag	
Endoscopic peanuts	Yes
X-ray	
Fibrin glue or other sealant	Yes

Technique

Cannulae

Cannula	Method of insertion	Diameter (mm)	Device	Position
1	Closed	3 or 5	30° optic	Posterior axillary line, 6th or 7th intercostal space
2	Closed	5	Dissector, Ligasure, clips, curved scissors	Midaxillary line, 6th interspace
3	Closed	3 or 5	Dissector/grasper	Midaxillary line, 8th or 9th interspace

▪ Figure 24.3 shows port positions.

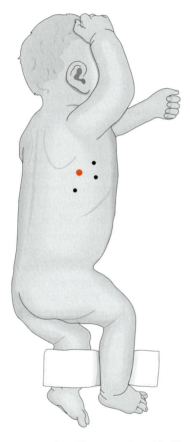

Fig. 24.3. Ports are placed between the midaxillary and posterior axillary line

Procedure

The procedure is started by inducing a slight tension pneumothorax to help collapse the lung. A Veress needle is inserted in the midaxillary line in approximately the 6th interspace and the pleural cavity is insufflated with a low flow low pressure of CO_2. A 5 mm port is placed, the telescope is inserted, and a quick survey of the chest performed. In most cases a chest tube will have already been in place. If so the chest tube is removed prior to the preparation and the first cannula can be placed through this site. There may be some mild adhesions secondary to the chest tube but these are of little consequence. However they should be divided to allow the lung to completely expand at the end of the procedure.

Under direct vision the other cannulae are placed. The optic is moved to the posterior trocar so it can look down on the working ports and give the best view of the posterior thorax. A thorough examination of the lower thoracic vertebrae and diaphragm is then performed. The inferior pulmonary ligament can be divided to give better exposure of this area. With the added magnification and direct view afforded by the thoracoscope the site of the chyle leak can often be visualized. If this is the case the site of the pleural rent is sealed. This can be accomplished in several ways. The site can be cauterized with monopolar or bipolar cautery. In some cases a clip can be applied or a suture ligature can be placed. In most cases we prefer to use the Ligasure to seal the pleural tear (▪ Fig. 24.4).

If there is no discreet tear or obvious leak site seen, a blind ligation of the thoracic duct is performed. This is done at the level of the esophageal hiatus where the thoracic duct should pass posterior and lateral to the esophagus. One or two suture ligatures can be placed in this area or the Ligasure can be used to mass seal the tissues at the posterolateral attachments of the diaphragm. Whichever method is used care must be taken to not injure the wall of the esophagus.

If there is an active leak the chyle will continue to accumulate during the procedure. If the ligation is successful the surgeon should note a marked decrease in the amount of fluid accumulating in the pleural space.

Once the ligation is complete an extensive pleurodesis is performed of the lower half of the thorax, especially the posterolateral area around the esophageal hiatus, aorta, and diaphragm. This can be done with a 5 mm endoscopic peanut, or a small sponge can be placed through one of the trocar sites and used to

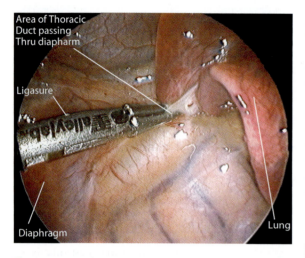

Fig. 24.4. Use of the Ligasure device to seal the area where the thoracic duct passes through the diaphragm into the right thoracic cavity

abrade the pleura. As a last step one of the tissue glues (Tisseel, etc.) is applied at the area of ligation and along the base of the diaphragm to act as an added sealant. With this accomplished the lower port is removed and a chest tube is placed under direct vision along the diaphragm and into the posterior gutter. A single chest tube is generally sufficient. The other ports are then removed and closed in layers with absorbable sutures. All port sites are injected with 0.25% Marcaine.

The endotracheal is pulled back into the trachea and the left lung reexpanded. In most cases the child should be extubated at the end of the procedure.

Postoperative Care

The patient is kept NPO postoperatively and intravenous (IV) hyperalimentation is continued. Pain control is achieved with small doses of IV morphine or other suitable narcotic for the first 24–48 h and then oral pain medication should be adequate. The chest tube is kept to 15–20 mm of continuous suction until the drainage has decreased to less than 5–10 ml/day. This may take up to a week although in most cases the drainage decreases almost immediately. The drain is then placed to water seal for 24 h and if there is no reaccumulation of fluid on chest X-ray oral feeds are resumed. If the drainage remains minimal the tube is removed.

Results

As this is a relatively rare problem and most cases are treated by chest tube drainage alone, experience with this procedure is relatively limited. Over an 8-year pe-

riod we have treated eight cases thoracoscopically. Seven cases were in infants and one in a 5-year-old who had fallen off the back of a truck. All procedures were completed thoracoscopically and one patient also underwent a lung biopsy. This patient ended up having congenital lymphangiomatosis (on lung biopsy) and later died. Of the other seven the site of the leak was visualized in four and a blind ligation was performed in the other three. Tisseel was used only in the last three cases. Operative time averaged 50 min. The chyle leak was sealed in all seven cases. Chest tubes were left in for 2–10 days (average 4.6 days). There were no recurrences and no postoperative complications.

Discussion

Congenital or acquired chylothorax is a complex problem to deal with and treatment can be a difficult. There is a significant hidden morbidity because of the large fluid and nutritional losses associated high volume leaks. While conservative therapy with chest tube drainage is often successful it may be prolonged resulting in long-term hospitalization and associated morbidity. Thoracoscopic ligation of the thoracic duct offers a more invasive but perhaps less morbid way of treating this disease. A combination of direct sealing, local pleurodesis, and now tissue glue has resulted in successful sealing of the leak in all cases. In a few cases drainage did persist for up to a week, but then it diminished and sealed. There is little morbidity from this minimally invasive approach and the treatment. It may be that the success of this approach may warrant earlier surgical intervention. The key, as with all thoracoscopic procedures, is to be quick and efficient to avoid a prolonged anesthetic. If the site of the leak is not readily apparent a blind ligation and pleurodesis should be performed quickly and efficiently. The new tissue glues add the extra insurance to provide a complete seal. Even if unsuccessful there is little to be lost by an initial thoracoscopic approach.

References

Graham DD, McGahren ED, Tribble CG, et al (1994) Use of video-assisted thoracic surgery in the treatment of chylothorax. Ann Thorac Surg 57:1507–1511

Hillerdal G (1997) Chylothorax and pseudochylothorax. Eur Respir J 10:1157–1162

Peillon C, D'Hont C, Melki J, et al (1999) Usefulness of video thoracoscopy in the management of spontaneous and postoperation chylothorax. Surg Endosc 13:1106–1109

Wurnig PN, Hollaus PH, Ohtsuka T, et al (2000) Thoracoscopic direct clipping of the thoracic duct for chylopericardium and chylothorax. Ann Thorac Surg 70:1662–1665

Chapter 25

Video-assisted Thoracic Surgery for Thymectomy

Calvin S.H. Ng and Anthony P.C. Yim

Historical Perspective

Myasthenia gravis (MG) has a history that dates back over three centuries (Pascuzzi 1994 and references therein). It was first described in 1672 by an Oxford clinician, Thomas Willis. The first thymectomy was performed by Ferdinard Sauerbruch in Zurich in 1911 and reported by Shumacher and Roth the following year. The patient was a 21-year-old woman with hyperthyroidism and MG. Thymectomy was performed in an attempt to treat her hyperthyroidism. The thymus was hyperplastic and, following surgery, both conditions were reported to improve temporarily. Mary Walker (1934) noted the similarity in clinical features between MG and curare poisoning and introduced treatment with the anticholinesterase, physostigmine. Alfred Blalock (1944) reported improvement in MG patients following resection of *normal* thymus and introduced this as a surgical therapy for this condition. Clinical use of endrophonium was introduced around 1950 and followed a few years later by pyridostigmine. John Simpson (1960) first proposed that MG might be an autoimmune disease. This was later confirmed experimentally by Patrick and Lindstrom (1973) who immunized rabbits with purified acetylcholine receptors.

Introduction

It is now common knowledge that MG is an autoimmune disorder of the postsynaptic nicotinic acetylcholine receptor, and is characterized by weakness and fatigability of voluntary muscles. The ocular muscles are frequently involved, rendering ptosis and diplopia the most common mode of presentation. Despite the fact that the condition has been recognized for more than three centuries, considerable controversies still remain over its diagnosis, natural history, and therapy. This chapter is primarily focused on the surgical therapy.

Thymectomy is now an established therapy in the management of generalized MG in conjunction with medical treatment. However, a randomized, prospective study investigating the role of thymectomy has never been undertaken, and is unlikely to ever happen.

A recent meta-analysis of 28 controlled studies showed that MG patients undergoing thymectomy were twice as likely to attain medication-free remission, 1.6 times as likely to become asymptomatic, and 1.7 times as likely to improve. Different demographics and baseline characteristics however existed between groups (Gronseth and Barohn 2000). Uncertainties remain over the role of thymectomy for patients with purely ocular symptoms and those with late onset of disease.

Several surgical approaches to thymectomy exist. The most commonly adopted surgical approach to thymectomy is via a median sternotomy. Other thymectomy techniques include the transcervical, the combine median sternotomy with a transcervical incision (T-incision), video-assisted thoracic surgery (VATS) (unilateral) (Yim 2002; Yim et al. 1995b), partial sternotomy involving either the upper (Milanez de Campos et al. 2000) or lower sternum (Granone et al. 1999), and the bilateral thoracoscopic approach combined with a cervical incision (video-assisted thoracoscopic extended thymectomy; VATET) (Novellino et al. 1994). This chapter reviews our technique regarding VATS for thymectomy, discusses the perioperative management in our institution and our criteria for patient selection, and reports on our intermediate results.

Patient Selection

For young patients with generalized MG, it is now fairly well accepted that thymectomy should be offered. However, uncertainties remain over the role of thymectomy for patients with purely ocular symptoms and those with late onset of disease. On the one hand, arguments have been put forward not to operate on ocular symptoms alone because ocular MG is not only less likely to respond to thymectomy but also carries a better prognosis, compared with generalized MG. On the other hand, it has been shown that between 30% and 70% of patients with initial ocular symptoms will eventually develop generalized MG. It is on that basis that we advised some of our young patients to undergo surgery even though their presentation was purely ocular (■ Fig. 25.1a,b). Although some patients with purely ocular symptoms improve following thymectomy, the patients have to clearly understand that the

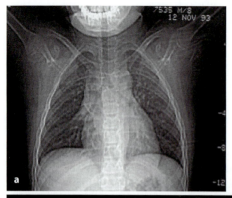

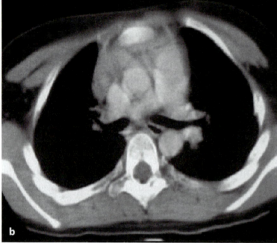

Fig. 25.1. Large mediastinal mass on chest radiograph (**a**) and computed tomography (**b**) of a 9-year-old boy with thymic hypertrophy and stage I MG

rationale for surgery here is not based on symptomatic improvement, but rather on the expectation of halting disease progression. It is vital that the thoracic surgeons work closely with the neurologists and anesthesiologists to achieve optimal results.

Preoperative Preparation

Myasthenia gravis causes weakness of voluntary muscles, including those involved in respiration, so that patients are at risk of developing postoperative respiratory failure. If bulbar palsy is present, they may also develop aspiration pneumonia. Medical treatment is associated with its own complications. Anticholinesterase treatment increases vagal tone, enhances oral secretion, and potentiates laryngeal spasm. Prolonged steroid use could result in electrolyte imbalance and increase the susceptibility to infections.

Before elective surgery, it is important that the distribution and severity of muscle weakness are carefully assessed. Respiratory function and nutritional status

should also be documented and medical treatment optimized. Patients with severe weakness may require preoperative plasmapheresis, together with steroid and anticholinesterase therapy. Admission to the intensive care unit for ventilatory support is indicated for patients who are already in respiratory failure, but it is not necessary to wait until the patient is extubated before surgery can proceed. Intravenous immunoglobulin is an alternative to plasmapheresis, but there is no clear evidence that one is better than the other. The patient should be warned of the possibility of postoperative ventilation. The operation is usually arranged as the first case on the elective list. Premedication is prescribed as appropriate, but respiratory depressant drugs are avoided. "Stress" doses of steroids may be required (Yim et al. 1999).

Induction of General Anesthesia

Selective one-lung ventilation to the left lung is required to facilitate the operation (Yim et al. 1999). General anesthesia with left-sided double-lumen endobronchial tube is used. Patients are induced with 2 mg/kg of propofol and 2 µg/kg of fentanyl. Intubation can usually be achieved without muscle relaxants. Pretreatment of the tracheobronchial tree with local anesthetics will facilitate intubation (Chan et al. 1995). Proper positioning of the endobronchial tube is confirmed with the use of the fiberoptic bronchoscope after intubation and reconfirmed after positioning. However, it is generally held that a body weight of at least 30–35 kg is necessary for the patient's airway to accommodate the smallest double-lumen device (28 French). This size limitation essentially precludes the use of these devices for patients younger than approximately 8 years of age. Other techniques to achieve one-lung ventilation, such as placement of a bronchial blocker or intentional intubation of a main stem bronchus with an endotracheal tube, should be used (Krucylak 2000).

Hypoxemia during one-lung ventilation is usually caused by shunting of blood. In case of hypoxemia, the position of the double-lumen endobronchial tube and hemodynamic stability should be confirmed. A low level of continuous positive airway pressure (CPAP) applied to the collapsed right lung may improve saturation. Applying positive end expiratory pressure (PEEP) to the ventilated lung can also raise oxygen saturation during one-lung ventilation.

Anesthesia is maintained with isoflurane 1–2%, 60% nitrous oxide in oxygen, and a single bolus of 0.1 mg/kg of morphine. Ventilation is controlled to achieve normocarbia. Patients with MG are usually more susceptible to the neuromuscular blocking effect of volatile anesthetics so that non-depolarizing muscle

Fig. 25.2. Operating room setup for VATS thymectomy

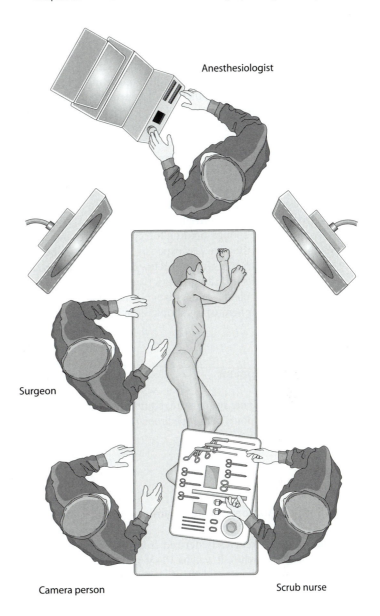

Anesthesiologist

Surgeon

Camera person

Scrub nurse

relaxants are usually not required (El-Dawlatly and Ashour 1994).

Patients with MG are usually also very sensitive to non-depolarizing muscle relaxants. If muscle relaxation is necessary during the course of anesthesia, a reduced dose of an intermediate-acting non-depolarizing muscle relaxant should be used followed by a carefully titrated intravenous infusion. Monitoring neuromuscular transmission is mandatory to adjust the dose of muscle relaxant used and to ensure complete reversal of neuromuscular blockade after the surgery.

The electrocardiogram, non-invasive blood pressure, pulse oximetry, end-tidal carbon dioxide, airway pressure, ventilatory volume, inspired oxygen, and neuromuscular transmission are routinely monitored and continuously displayed. An arterial line and a cen-

tral venous catheter for invasive pressure monitoring may be required for coexisting medical conditions.

Positioning

Patient

Under general anesthesia with selective one-lung ventilation, the patient is positioned in the full left lateral decubitus position for the approach to the anterior mediastinum. Some surgeons prefer to place the patient in a 45° lateral decubitus position to allow for greater posterior displacement of the lung. The operating table is flexed to 30° with the fulcrum just inferior to the level of the nipples, to open up the upper intercostal spaces for thoracoscope insertion and instrumentation (Yim 1995).

Crew, Monitors, and Equipment

The team of the principal surgeon, an assistant, scrub nurse, and the anesthesiologist will remain in the same positions during the whole procedure. The operating room setup consists of the anesthetic unit, video-thoracoscopy unit (TV monitor, video image printer, video recorder, light source), TV monitor, electrocautery, and instrument trolley (■ Fig. 25.2).

Mostly conventional instruments are utilized such as sponge-holding forceps (for retraction), dental pledget mounted on a curved clamp (for dissection), and right-angled clamp (for dissection of vascular branches). We advocate the use of conventional thoracic instruments, such as the sponge-holding forceps, whenever possible because they are less expensive and are more familiar to the surgeon. However, a few dedicated endoscopic instruments including endoscissors for incising the mediastinal pleura, endograsper, and endoclip applier for vascular hemostasis should be available to aid surgery.

Special Equipment

No special energy applying systems are required. A clip applier and bag for removal of the specimen should be available.

Technique

Surgical Anatomy of the Thymus

The thymus is embryologically derived from the 3rd and 4th branchial pouches. It weighs 10–35 g at birth, grows to 20–50 g at puberty, and after that slowly involutes to 5–15 g in the adult. With the process of involution, the thymic parenchyma is gradually replaced by fibroadipose tissue. The fully developed gland is bilobed, but its exact shape is largely molded by the adjacent structures and is highly variable. It occupies the anterior mediastinum, with the superior horns often extending into the neck, lying deep to the sternothyroid muscle. The body of the gland is related anteriorly to the sternum and the upper four costal cartilages; posteriorly to the pericardium, the ascending aorta, the brachiocephalic veins, and superior vena cava; and laterally to the mediastinal pleura. Its relationship with the veins is of great surgical importance. Its fibrous capsule blends in with the pretracheal fascia. The arterial supply is derived laterally from branches of the internal mammary artery, and venous drainage is through two or three tributaries posteriorly to the left brachiocephalic vein.

There are two technical considerations regarding thymectomy in the prepubertal population. First, the thymus is relatively large compared to the body weight and, second, the chest is relatively small. Attention has to be given to achieve selective one-lung ventilation and to use finer instruments (5 mm external diameter or less).

Operative Principles

The chest is the most suitable body cavity for the minimal access approach because once the lung is collapsed (with selective one-lung ventilation) there is plenty of room for instrument maneuvering. The use of carbon dioxide insufflation, and hence valved ports, is therefore unnecessary. In fact, there is evidence that thoracic carbon dioxide insufflation during VATS has an adverse effect on the patient's hemodynamics compared with selective one-lung ventilation.

There are additional strategies in VATS that can assist in minimizing chest wall trauma, avoid intercostal nerve compression, and hence minimize postoperative pain:
- Avoiding the use of trocar ports by introducing instruments directly through the wound
- Avoiding torquing of the thoracoscope by visualizing with an angled lens (30° scope)
- Using smaller telescopes (5 mm) when clinically allowed
- Delivering specimens through the anterior port because the anterior intercostal spaces are wider (Yim 1995)

Cannulae and Position

Cannula	Method of insertion	Diameter (mm)	Device	Position
1	Open	10	0° (or 30°) telescope	In front of tip of scapula, posterior axillary line
2	Open	5	Atraumatic endograsper	Third intercostal space, mid-axillary line
3	Open	5	Endoscissors, grasper, clip	Sixth intercostal space, anterior axillary line

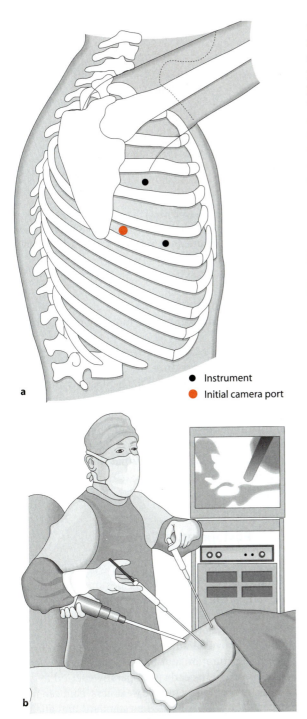

● Instrument
● Initial camera port

Fig. 25.3. Positions of the thoracic ports (**a**) and their utilization during VATS for thymectomy (**b**)

vocate a right-sided approach and a three-port technique for the procedure. The thoracoscope port incision should be in front of the tip of the scapula along the posterior axillary line for the insertion of the 10 mm port and 0° telescope (Yim et al. 1995a). The second and third 5 mm instrument ports should be inserted by open technique under direct thoracoscopic vision at the 3rd intercostal space on the midaxillary line, and at the 6th intercostal space on the anterior axillary line (■ Fig. 25.3a,b). Additional ports are made for lung retraction as necessary. In young female patients, the instrument ports should be strategically placed over the submammary fold for cosmetic consideration.

Procedure

Exploration

The entire hemithorax is carefully examined with particular attention to the mediastinum. Blunt instruments may be used to help collapse the lung, and for manipulation to complete the exploration. The major structural landmarks should be identified, including the superior vena cava, brachiocephalic vein, and right phrenic nerve. It is of paramount importance that the right phrenic nerve should be carefully preserved throughout the dissection because phrenic nerve palsy represents a major complication for patients with MG. Pleural adhesions may be present and require adhesiolysis to facilitate complete lung collapse and achieve a good operating field.

Dissection and Vascular Control

The right inferior horn of the thymus can be identified draping over the pericardium. The mediastinal pleura over the free edge of the right inferior thymic horn is sharply incised. The thymus can then be lifted up and bluntly dissected off the underlying pericardium extending onto the aorta in a cephalad manner until the left brachiocephalic vein is exposed. We have found it useful to apply deliberate and gentle traction on the thymus to allow blunt dissection using a pledget. The thymic venous tributaries (usually two or three) draining into the left brachiocephalic vein can be identified, clipped, and divided. It is important to obtain vascular control before further manipulation of the thymus. Dissection is then carried behind the sternum. With gentle traction on the thymus using a sponge-holding forceps, the left inferior horn can be identified and likewise dissected up to the thymus isthmus.

Dissection of Superior Horns

The most difficult part of the operation is to dissect the superior horns. The right internal mammary vein is divided in most cases to facilitate exposure. With gentle and deliberate inferior traction on the thymus,

Under general anesthesia, selective one-lung ventilation should be confirmed with the anesthesiologist prior to port incision. In small children, it is not feasible to use a double-lumen tube. We prefer an endotracheal tube placed in the left main bronchial position to achieve one-lung ventilation (Krucylak 2000). We ad-

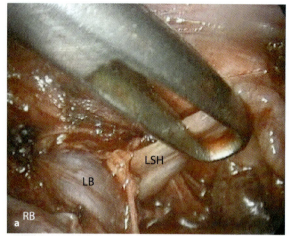

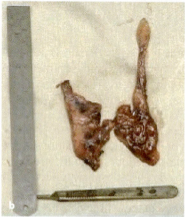

Fig. 25.4. Dissection of left superior horn behind the left bra-chiocephalic vein (a) and the resected complete specimen (b). *LSH* Left superior horn of thymus, *LB* left brachiocephalic vein, *RB* right brachiocephalic vein

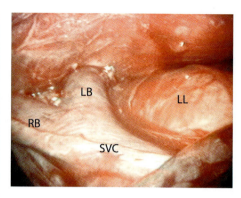

Fig. 25.5. Thymic bed following thymectomy clearly demonstrating the venous anatomy. *LL* Left lung, *SVC* superior vena cava, *LB* left brachiocephalic vein, *RB* right brachiocephalic vein [Yim et al. 1999]

the superior horns can be carefully dissected free from their fascial attachments. The positions of the thoraco-scope and inferior instrument port may be exchanged to allow better reach toward the superior parts of the thymus, particularly when conventional instruments are used. The left superior horn may occasionally pass behind, instead of in front of, the brachiocephalic vein, and this anatomic variation has to be looked for (we have encountered this in one case and thoracoscopic dissection was successfully accomplished) (■ Fig. 25.4a,b).

Extraction

The thymus, as a free specimen, can be removed in a plastic bag through the most anterior port, because the intercostal space is wider anteriorly. After thymectomy, the anterior mediastinal soft tissue including the pericardial fat is separately removed. The specimen is inspected for completeness of resection. In small children with hyperplastic thymus, we have found it useful

to retract part of the gland out of an anteriorly placed wound. The maneuver creates more room for further dissection.

End of Procedure

The thymic bed is inspected for hemostasis and completeness of resection. The brachiocephalic veins should have been skeletonized and the junction to form the superior vena cava should be clearly visualized (■ Fig. 25.5). The insertion of tube thoracostomy is optional. The lung is then reinflated under direct vision, and layered closure of the stab wounds completes the operation.

Postoperative Care

The patient should resume full diet when fully awake from the general anesthesia. A postoperative sitting chest radiograph is taken to detect pneumothorax, hemothorax, and any significant atelectasis. Postoperative chest physiotherapy and incentive spirometry should be provided and encouraged. Regular checks on oxygen saturation and bedside spirometry should be performed in the early postoperative period to give warning of respiratory muscle weakness. Pain can usually be adequately controlled by standard oral analgesics. Tube thoracostomy can be removed on day 1 after confirming no air leak or bleeding.

Limitations of Video-assisted Thoracic Surgery for Thymectomy

There are relatively few contraindications to VATS. In addition to the general contraindications such as severe coagulopathy, specific ones include pleural symphysis and patients with severe underlying lung disease or poor lung function who are unable to tolerate the selective one-lung ventilation during general anesthesia.

Prior operation in the ipsilateral chest should not be regarded as a contraindication. Adhesions can usually be taken down using a combination of sharp and blunt dissection under videoendoscopic vision. However, patients with difficult adhesions to take down may be more suitable for open procedure.

Results

In our institution, we have so far attempted 41 VATS thymectomies. Three were not related to MG. Two patients required conversion to a small lateral thoracotomy for control of bleeding. Therefore, 36 VATS thymectomies were successful performed for MG (23 females, and ages ranged from 9 to 75 years with a mean age of 35.2 years). The final pathology results were 4 thymomas, 16 hyperplastic thymus, 8 atrophic thymus, and 8 normal thymus. There was no surgical mortality. The median hospital stay was 5 days. Preoperatively, 3 patients were in stage I, 12 in stage IIA, 12 in stage IIB, 6 in stage III, and 3 in stage IV MG, according to the modified Osserman and Genkins classification (1971) (■ Table 25.1). After a mean period of 40 months (range 12–84 months), 5 patients (13.9%) were in complete remission (class I), 23 patients (63.9%) were asymptomatic on decreased medication (class III), 7 patients (19.4%) had little or no change in symptoms (class IV), and 1 patient (2.8%) had worsening of symptoms (class V) according to the classification by DeFilippi et al. (1994).

The last patient was an elderly man who presented with pure ocular symptoms when he was 73 years old. However, within one year, his symptoms progressed to involve the bulbar muscles. At this point, he was referred for surgery. Thoracoscopic thymectomy was performed, and an atrophic thymus was removed without complication. Postoperatively, his symptoms never improved and, after 8 months, he developed acute respiratory failure leading to death within 2 days of admission. This was clearly a case of "thymectomy failure," which was not related to any particular surgical approach, but to the unpredictable natural history in patients with "late-onset" MG. He represented the only death in our series.

All patients except two were extubated within 24 h. The first patient was a 29-year-old woman with Down's syndrome and a history of asthma who experienced postoperative pneumonia and required prolonged ventilation and a tracheostomy. The second patient was a 22-year-old woman who was already on mechanical ventilation before surgery for MG. Other potential postoperative complications not encountered in

Table 25.1. Modified Osserman and Genkins classification of MG

Stage	Symptoms
I	Ocular MG: involvement restricted to extraocular muscles
IIA	Mild generalized MG: generalized weakness without respiratory muscle involvement
IIB	Moderately generalized MG: more severe generalized involvement, bulbar symptoms common and relative sparing of respiratory muscles
III	Acute fulminating MG: rapid onset (within 6 months) of respiratory muscle involvement
IV	Late severe MG: severe symptoms that have progressed for more than 2 years after onset of ocular or mild generalized MG

our series include wound infection, hypocalcemia, pneumothorax, surgical emphysema, intercostal neuralgia, and phrenic nerve palsy.

Discussion

Considerable uncertainties remain over the optimal treatment of MG. The best surgical approach to thymectomy remains controversial. Regardless of technique, it is generally agreed that thymectomy for MG should be complete. The Columbia-Presbyterian group advocated "maximal" thymectomy (Jaretzki et al. 1988) involving a combination of median sternotomy with cervical incision to achieve en bloc thymectomy and anterior mediastinal exenteration, which includes mediastinal pleura from the level of the thoracic inlet to the diaphragm, pericardial fat pad, and all the mediastinal fat. However, despite this radical approach, when compared with sternotomy alone (Olanow et al. 1987) or the transcervical approaches (Cooper et al. 1988), results in terms of clinical improvement did not seem to be significantly different. In addition, a detailed autopsy study identified ectopic thymic tissue in areas (like the retrocaval fat) which are not accessible via a median sternotomy (Fukai et al. 1991). Although it may seem intuitive to remove as much mediastinal soft tissue as possible to avoid leaving behind ectopic thymus, these remnants have never been conclusively shown to be clinically relevant, and even the most radical surgical approach does not result in a remission rate greater than 40%.

The VATS approach is similar to the transcervical approach in that both are associated with minimal chest wall trauma, low postoperative morbidity, short hospital stay, and, perhaps more importantly, improved patient acceptance for surgery earlier in the disease compared with the transsternal approach. However,

VATS has additional advantages over the conventional transcervical approach because the visualization is much better and there is no crowding of instruments through a single access site. The thymus, being largely an anterior mediastinal structure, can be more directly approached through the chest than the neck. Video assistance provides a wide, magnified operative field. In addition, VATS may be a helpful approach for completion thymectomy in patients with refractory MG who have already undergone resection, with the potential advantage of avoiding previously dissected tissue planes and facilitating the search for residual thymic tissue. We believe that we are performing the same operation thoracoscopically compared with the transsternal approach by examination of the thymic beds and the resected specimens (Yim et al. 1995a). The cosmetic appearance of the surgical scars is seldom used to argue for a particular surgical approach. However, thymectomy may be a notable exception considering that the majority of patients are young girls, and the superior cosmetic appearance of VATS should be considered. In addition, it has recently been shown in a small randomized prospective study that the pulmonary function is significantly better preserved in the immediate postoperative period following VATS compared to the median sternotomy approach to thymectomy for MG (Rückert et al. 2000).

However, even among the surgeons performing VATS for thymectomy, there is controversy over the exact technique and, in particular, whether the thymus should be approached from the left or the right. On the one hand, Mineo et al. (2000) from Rome advocated a left-sided approach and the use of pneumomediastinum to facilitate dissection. On the other hand, we advocate the right-sided approach for the following reasons (Yim 1997). First, the superior vena cava, easily identified from the right, provides a clear landmark for further dissection of the innominate veins. Second, the confluence of the two innominate veins to form the superior vena cava is an area most difficult to dissect well. This could be more easily accomplished from the right. Third, from the ergonomic standpoint, it is easier for right-handed surgeons performing VATS to start at the inferior poles and work cephalad from the right side. The ultimate surgical goal of thymectomy is to completely remove the gland and the anterior mediastinal tissue. Which side to approach remains largely the surgeon's preference, which is ultimately influenced by his/her experience and training.

We have shown that, in our institution, patients who underwent thoracoscopic thymectomy had significantly less analgesic requirement and shorter hospital stays compared with a historical group who underwent transsternal thymectomy (Yim et al. 1995a). Collective experience on 33 patients from four centers (Columbia Hospital in Dallas, University of Pittsburgh, Southern Illinois University, and our own) has been previously reported. Clinical improvement was observed in 88% of patients who underwent thoracoscopic thymectomy after a mean follow-up of 23 months. Meta-analysis compared with nine published series performed by other approaches showed no difference in clinical improvement after thymectomy between series (Cooper et al. 1988; DeFilippi et al. 1994; Jaretzki et al. 1988; Mack et al. 1996; Mulder et al. 1989; Nussbaum et al. 1992).

Concerns have been raised regarding using the VATS approach for thymoma with or without associated MG. We are careful in restricting this technique to small, completely encapsulated, stage I thymoma (Masaoska et al. 1981). Clinical judgment is of paramount importance in thymic surgery, and any sign of tissue plane invasion mandates conversion to an open dissection (Yim et al. 1999).

Conclusion

Video-assisted thoracic surgery for thymectomy is a safe operation in experienced hands and represents a new, viable alternative approach for patients with MG. The right-sided approach is preferred because visualization of the venous anatomy for dissection is essential. Our own as well as collective experience so far shows that this approach produces results comparable to other conventional surgical techniques. By minimizing chest wall trauma, the thoracoscopic approach causes less postoperative pain, shortens hospital stay, better preserves lung function in the early postoperative period (which may be particularly important for patients with MG), and gives superior cosmesis. It is hoped that this patient-friendlier approach would lead to wider acceptance by MG patients and their neurologists for earlier thymectomies.

References

Chan MTV, Ng SK, Low JM (1995) A non muscle-relaxant technique for video-assisted thoracoscopic thymectomy in myasthenia gravis (letter). Anaesth Intensive Care 23:256–257

Cooper JD, Al-Jilaihawa AN, Pearson FG et al. (1988) An improved technique to facilitate transcervical thymectomy for myasthenia gravis. Ann Thorac Surg 45:242–247

DeFilippi VJ, Richman DP, Ferguson MK (1994) Transcervical thymectomy for myasthenia gravis. Ann Thorac Surg 57:194–197

El-Dawlatly AA, Ashour MH (1994) Anesthesia for thymectomy in myasthenia gravis: a non-muscle-relaxant technique. Anaesth Intensive Care 22:458–460

Fukai I, Funato Y, Mizuno T et al. (1991) Distribution of thymic tissue in the mediastinal adipose tissue. J Thorac Cardiovasc Surg 101:1099–1102

Granone P, Margaritora S, Cesario A et al. (1999) Thymectomy in myasthenia gravis via video assisted infra-mammary cosmetic incision. Eur J Cardiothorac Surg 15:861–863

Gronseth GS, Barohn RJ (2000) Practice parameter: thymectomy for autoimmune myasthenia gravis (an evidence-base review). Report of the Quality Standards Subcommittee of the American Academy of Neurology. Neurology 55:7–15

Jaretzki A III, Penn AS Younger DS et al. (1988) "Maximal" thymectomy for myasthenia gravis. Results. J Thorac Cardiovasc Surg 95:747–757

Krucylak CP (2000) Anesthetic considerations for pediatric thoracoscopic procedures. In: Yim APC, Hazelrigg SR, Izzat MB, et al (eds) Minimal Access Cardiothoracic Surgery. Saunders, Philadelphia, pp 281–289

Mack MJ, Landreneau RJ, Yim AP et al. (1996) Results of video-assisted thymectomy in patients with myasthenia gravis. J Thorac Cardiovasc Surg 112:1352–1360

Masaoka A, Monden Y, Nakahara K, Tanioka T (1981) Follow up study of thymoma with references to their clinical stages. Cancer 48:2485–2492

Milanez de Campos JR, Filomeno LTB, Marchiori PE et al. (2000) Partial sternotomy approach to the thymus. In: Yim APC, Hazelrigg SR, Izzat MB, et al (eds) Minimal Access Cardiothoracic Surgery. Saunders, Philadelphia, pp 205–208

Mineo TC, Pompeo E, Lerut TE et al. (2000) Thoracoscopic thymectomy in autoimmune myasthenia gravis: results of left sided approach. Ann Thorac Surg 69:1537–1541

Mulder DG, Graves M, Hermann C (1989) Thymectomy for myasthenia gravis: recent observations and comparisons with past experience. Ann Thorac Surg 48:551–555

Novellino L, Longoni M, Spinelli L et al. (1994) "Extended" thymectomy without sternotomy, performed by cervicotomy and thoracoscopic techniques in the treatment of myasthenia gravis. Int Surg 79:378–381

Nussbaum MS, Rosenthal GJ, Samaha FJ et al. (1992) Management of myasthenia gravis by extended thymectomy with anterior mediastinal tumor. Surgery 112:681–688

Olanow CW, Wechsler, AS, Sirontkin-Roses M et al. (1987) Thymectomy as primary therapy in myasthenia gravis. Ann N Y Acad Sci 505:595–606

Osserman KE, Genkins G (1971) Studies in myasthenia gravis: review of a 20-year experience in over 1200 patients. J Mt Sinai Hosp N Y 38:497–537

Pascuzzi R (1994) The history of myasthenia gravis. Neurol Clin 12:231–242

Rückert JC, Wlater M, Müller JM (2000) Pulmonary function after thoracoscopic thymectomy versus median sternotomy for myasthenia gravis. Ann Thorac Surg 70:1656–1661

Yim AP (1995) Minimizing chest wall trauma in video assisted thoracic surgery. J Thorac Cardiovasc Surg 109:1255–1256

Yim APC (1997) Thoracoscopic thymectomy: which side to approach? (letter) Ann Thorac Surg 64:584

Yim APC (2002) Paradigm shift in surgical approaches to thymectomy. Aust N Z J Surg 72:40–45

Yim APC, Ho JKS, Chung SS, et al (1994) One hundred and sixty-three consecutive video thoracoscopic procedures: the Hong Kong experience. Aust N Z J Surg 64:671–675

Yim APC, Kay RLC, Ho JKS (1995a) Video-assisted thoracoscopic thymectomy for myasthenia gravis. Chest 108:1440–1443

Yim APC, Low JM, Ng SK et al. (1995b) Video-assisted thoracoscopic surgery in the paediatric population. J Paediatr Child Health 31:192–196

Yim APC, Kay RLC, Izzat MB et al. (1999) Video-assisted thoracoscopic thymectomy for myasthenia gravis. Semin Thorac Cardiovasc Surg 11:65–73

Chapter 26

Thoracoscopic Removal of Neurogenic Mediastinal Tumors

Jean-Stéphane Valla, Marc D. Leclair, and Yves Heloury

Introduction

Neurogenic tumors are the most frequent solid mediastinal tumors in children. They are located in the posterior mediastinum and arise from the sympathetic chain in the posterior paravertebral gutter (Lemoine and Montupet 1990). They can be benign or malignant and are usually resected by classic thoracotomy.

A minimally invasive endoscopic technique for resection of these tumors can be used in selected cases (Akashi et al. 1997; Hazelrigg et al. 1999). The aim of such an approach is to ensure the same complete resection as with open thoracotomy but to reduce thoracotomy-related morbidity by avoiding muscle transection and rib retraction.

There are two minimally invasive ways to proceed. First, there is video-assisted thoracic surgery (VATS) in which video imaging is used for visualization and dissection of the pathology but in which the procedure itself is performed through a minithoracotomy using not only thoracoscopic but also standard surgical instruments; it has the advantage that the specimen is easily removed through the minithoracotomy at the end of the procedure. Second, there is closed videothoracoscopic surgery (CVTS) in which the entire operation is performed through ports, but in which one of the portholes is enlarged at the end of the procedure in order to allow for tumor extraction.

Preoperative Preparation

Before the operation, complete clinical (symptoms related to compression), radiological (X-ray, computed tomography [CT] scan, methyliodobenzoguanidine [MIBG] scintigraphy), and biological (vanylmandelic acid [VMA], homovanillic acid [HVA], dihydroxyphenylalanine [DOPA]) tumor assessment is essential for selection of the surgical approach. Bulky malignant tumors extending over the midline are contraindications for a minimally invasive approach. The preoperative assessment will exclude other rare tumefactions such as teratoma, aneurysm, osteosarcoma, and others. Moreover the preoperative imaging will allow for adjustment of the procedure according to the size and position of the tumor.

The operation is performed under general anesthesia. For a good exposure of mediastinal structures, the ipsilateral lung should be collapsed. This can be achieved by single-lung ventilation using a double lumen endotracheal tube in older children or by endotracheal ventilation in combination with bronchial blocking. Alternatively the lung can be pushed aside by CO_2 insufflation (5–8 mmHg). A single injection of antibiotics is given before port placement. Future port sites are infiltrated with bupivacaine.

In the case of a small tumor (4 cm or less) neither a nasogastric tube nor a bladder catheter are inserted. In the case of larger tumors (4–7 cm) or when it is suspected that the dissection could be difficult, and therefore long lasting or bloody, a nasogastric tube should be inserted for easy identification of the esophagus, while a bladder catheter will allow for monitoring of the diuresis.

Positioning

Patient

The child is placed in an anterolateral decubitus position with the diseased side upward and slightly forward. A roll is placed under the thorax in order to enlarge the intercostal spaces. The upper arm is elevated and abducted in order to ensure a maximum superior displacement of the scapula (■ Fig. 26.1).

Crew, Monitors, and Equipment

The surgeon, the assistant, and the scrub nurse usually stand on the ventral side of the child with the monitor in front of the surgical team (■ Fig. 26.1). The respective position of the surgeon and the assistant depends on whether the tumor is located in the upper or lower part of the thorax. The table is tilted in such a way that gravity drags the collapsed lung out of the operative field, for example reversed Trendelenburg when the tumor is located in the upper part of the thorax or Trendelenburg when the tumor is in the lower part of the chest. This will avoid the need for active lung retraction, which would require an extra port. Moreover active lung retraction is traumatic for the lung.

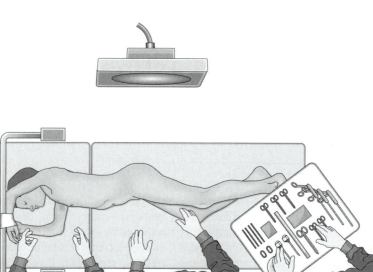

Assistant   Surgeon   Scrub nurse

Fig. 26.1. Position of the patient and surgical team for a left-sided lesion. The patient is placed in a left lateral decubitus position with the arm elevated and abducted. The surgical team stays at the ventral side of the patient with the most important monitor opposite

Equipment

Unless CO_2 insufflation is used, in which event the ports have to be valved, special thoracoscopic ports, which are short, have no valves, and are flexible, are used. Flexible ports allow for more movement and for the introduction of curved instruments which is especially advantageous when the tumor is located at the apex of the thoracic cavity. Once a stable working space has been created, ports can be removed and instruments can be passed directly through the chest wall openings.

The size of instruments depends on the size of the patient. As far as energy applying systems are concerned a 5 mm port is required for the introduction of ultrasonic energy or for the Ligasure. These two energy applying systems are very useful for precise dissection of the tumor avoiding adjacent nervous and vascular structures. They have limited the used of clips.

All specimens should be removed in a bag to avoid tumor contamination during extraction. Morcellation of the tumor in the bag is possible but extreme care should be exerted not to rupture the bag. The pathologist may demand a non-morcellated specimen in order to define completeness of the resection.

The type of telescope is chosen according to the lesion and the size of the child. For a lesion located in the middle of the chest a 0° telescope is well suited but for lesions located in the upper or lower part a 30° telescope is a better choice. When possible a 10 mm telescope is used, but in infants this will not fit between the ribs and may damage the intercostal neurovascular bundle. Moreover in infants a 5 mm telescope suffices.

In the case of a "dumbbell" tumor, the intrathoracic part is removed at the level of the foramina using a curette. During the curettage, the dura can be injured and sealing wax should be at hand.

Technique

Port Insertion and Placement

There are no standard trocar insertion sites but usually the ports are inserted in the axillary triangle bordered anteriorly by the lower edge of the pectoralis major muscle, posteriorly by the anterior edge of the latissimus dorsi, and inferiorly by the diaphragmatic insertions (■ Fig. 26.2). The first trocar is placed in the midaxillary line in the 5th or 6th intercostal space; it is introduced under direct vision, after blunt dissection and opening of the pleural space creating a pneumothorax. After an initial inspection of the chest cavity, the other two ports are placed respecting the triangulation principle and under videoendoscopic control thereby avoiding the risk of lung tear.

Fig. 26.2. Port positions for an upper mediastinal lesion. Triangle configuration of the ports. The first port is inserted in the midaxillary line

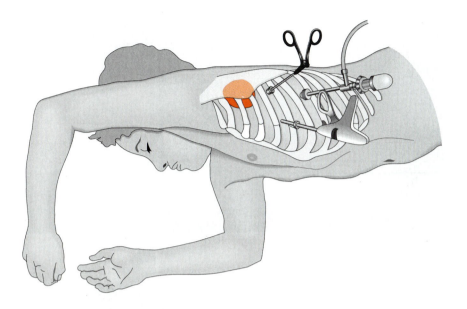

Dissection of the Tumor

The entire thoracic cavity is inspected first and then the parietal and mediastinal pleura is grasped and incised around the tumor with the hook electrocautery or with the ultrasonic scalpel; tumor dissection is performed in the extrapleural plane (■ Fig. 26.3a,b).

In the case of a tumor in the middle of the chest, the sympathetic trunk is dissected above and below the tumor and divided, after which the tumor is dissected from the posterior thoracic wall (■ Fig. 26.3c,d). Hemostasis must be carefully done at the level of each intercostal space (■ Fig. 26.3e,f). It is better not to grasp the tumor directly but to pull on it or retract it with an atraumatic device such as an endoscopic peanut. In the case of a completely mature neurogenic tumor, the neoplasm is well encapsulated and close dissection is easy. Sometimes, however, the tumor is strongly fixed to adjacent structures, especially ribs and spine at the level of foramina. It is sometimes im-

possible to resect the whole tumor en bloc. Under such circumstances the main part is removed, providing a much better view, after which the small residual parts that stick to bone are removed at each level. Tumor division must not be regarded as a technical mistake and may facilitate a safer resection.

The tumor is placed in an endobag and extracted through a limited "utility thoracotomy" (■ Fig. 26.4a–c). For cosmetic reasons, the highest port hole incision in the axilla is used for that purpose, at least when feasible.

The operative field is irrigated, hemostasis is checked under endoscopic control, and the intercostal spaces concerned are infiltrated with bupivacaine. Depending on the situation a chest tube is left in place or not. The lung is reinflated under direct vision. The intercostal spaces and muscles are closed at the extraction site and the 5 mm incisions are closed subcutaneously.

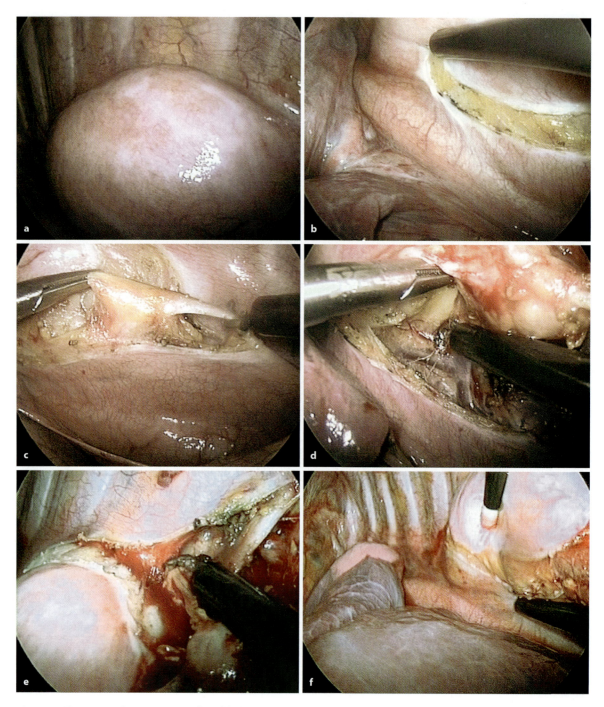

Fig. 26.3. Dissection of a tumor; an incidental finding in a 14-year-old girl. **a** Middle mediastinum, left-side lesion. **b** Opening of the pleura around the tumor with electrocautery or ultracision. **c** Transection of the sympathetic chain above the tumor. **d** Transection of the sympathetic chain below the tumor. **e,f** Opening the pleura around the tumor with electrocautery or ultracision on the external side (**e**) and on the internal side (**f**)

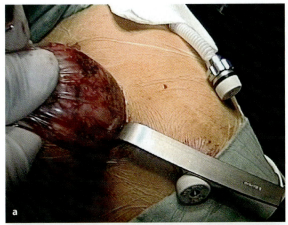

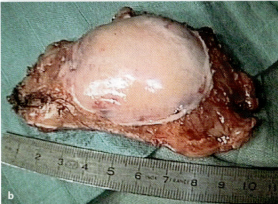

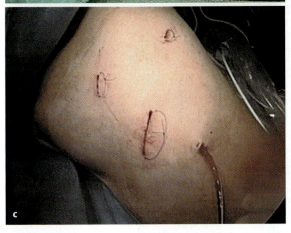

Fig. 26.4. a Extraction of the tumor in an endobag through a slightly extended porthole. **b** Exteriorized specimen. **c** Closed wounds and chest drain after completion of the operation.

Special Tumor Locations

Tumors Arising in the Upper Mediastinum

These tumors usually enter the thoracic inlet and involve the subclavian artery, the C8 to T1 nerve roots, the right recurrent laryngeal nerve, and the lower cervical sympathetic ganglia. Under such circumstances, the tumor is usually removed through a thoracic approach (■ Figs. 26.5, 26.6). Thoracoscopy offers a much better view than that obtained by an open approach (Pons et al. 2003). A combined supraclavicular approach is seldom required to spare all these structures (Lemoine and Montupet 1990) except for the sympathetic chain, which is transected in all cases. The resulting Horner's syndrome usually does not improve with time. This possibility should always be discussed with the patient's family prior to surgery.

Tumors Arising in the Lower Mediastinum

Although low tumors may extend through the diaphragmatic foramen into the abdomen, complete resection is usually possible through the thoracoscopic approach (■ Fig. 26.7). Care should be taken not to injure the aorta, esophagus, or thoracic duct. Small tumor extensions into the intervertebral foramina are easy to remove employing VATS (■ Fig. 26.7f); however, deeper invasion into the spinal canal requires neurosurgical involvement, which could also be carried out using minimally invasive techniques (Negri et al. 2001).

Tumors Arising in the Middle Part of the Mediastinum

When the tumor is located in the middle part of the left side, care should taken not to interfere with the anterior spinal artery, thus avoiding paraplegia. The best way to avoid this complication is to localize this artery preoperatively by selective arteriography (■ Fig. 26.8), and to perform a precise dissection close to the aorta branches by using Ligasure or ultrasonic scalpel (Patrick and Rothenberg 2001; Pons et al. 2003).

Results

Our experience is limited to nine cases. Seven patients were asymptomatic and two suffered intercostal pain. Ages varied between 6 months and 15 years. Tumor localization was as follows: upper part five cases, middle part three cases, lower part one case, and no true dumbbell tumor. The tumor sizes were between 3 and 8 cm. The tumor was resected by CVTS in eight cases and VATS in one case. On histological examination, three

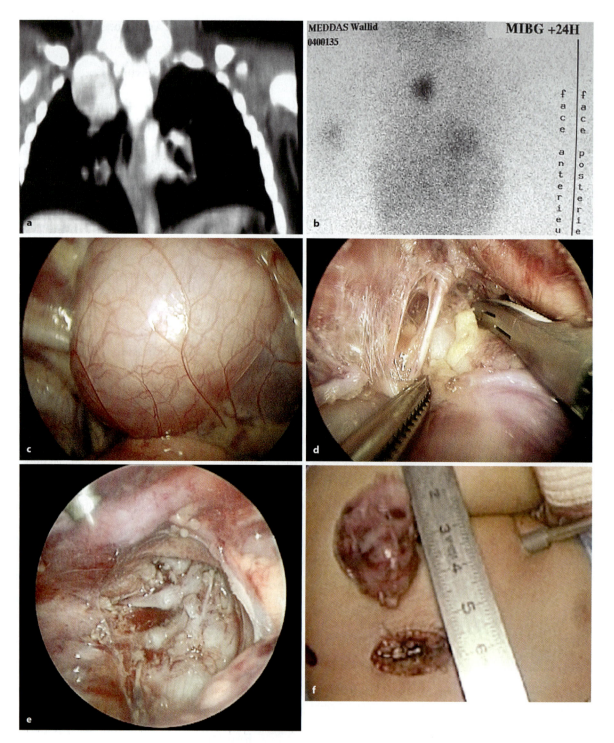

Fig. 26.5. a A CT scan of an upper mediastinal tumor on the right. Incidental finding on a chest X-ray in a 6-month-old boy. HVA and VMA slightly elevated. **b** MIBG scintiscan in the same boy. **c** Thoracoscopic view of the tumor. **d** Sympathetic chain above the tumor to be transected. **e** Operative field after tumor removal. **f** Extracted specimen

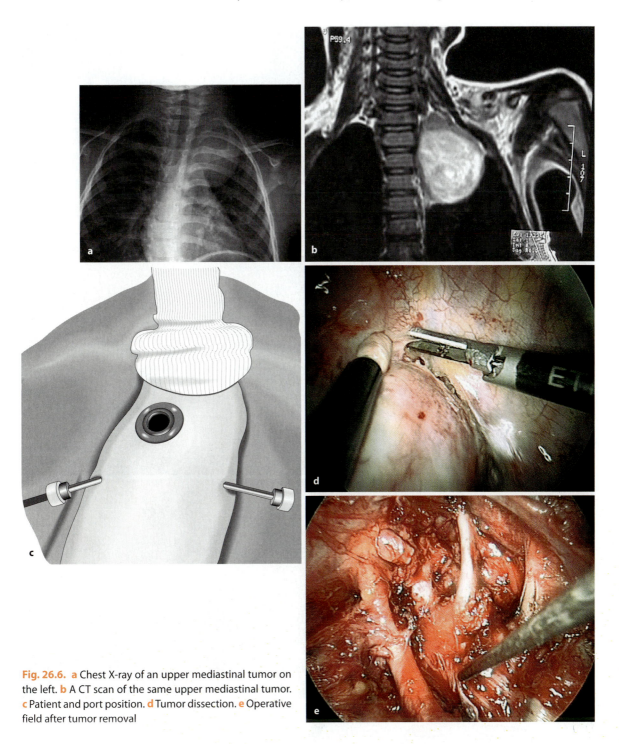

Fig. 26.6. a Chest X-ray of an upper mediastinal tumor on the left. **b** A CT scan of the same upper mediastinal tumor. **c** Patient and port position. **d** Tumor dissection. **e** Operative field after tumor removal

cases proved to be ganglioneuroma, two ganglioneuroblastoma, three neuroblastoma, and one schwannoma. Tumor resection was macroscopically complete in all cases. A drain was left in place in all cases.

There were no peroperative complications except for one injury of the dura. None of the cases were converted. Mean postoperative hospitalization was 4 days and uneventful in all cases (no chylothorax, no phrenic nerve palsy, no paraplegia).

Five patients developed a postoperative permanent Horner's syndrome, two patients suffered persistent intercostal pain and paresthesia, and the patient with peroperative dura injury had a dura diverticulum on postoperative CT scan. With a minimal follow-up of 4 years no recurrence was detected especially in case of neuroblastoma.

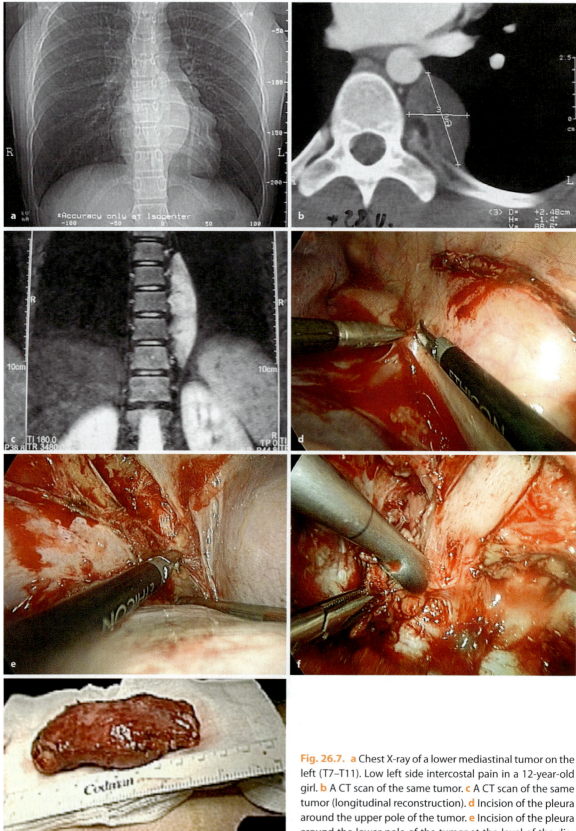

Fig. 26.7. a Chest X-ray of a lower mediastinal tumor on the left (T7–T11). Low left side intercostal pain in a 12-year-old girl. **b** A CT scan of the same tumor. **c** A CT scan of the same tumor (longitudinal reconstruction). **d** Incision of the pleura around the upper pole of the tumor. **e** Incision of the pleura around the lower pole of the tumor at the level of the diaphragm. **f** Removal of an intraforaminal extension with a curette. **g** Specimen after removal

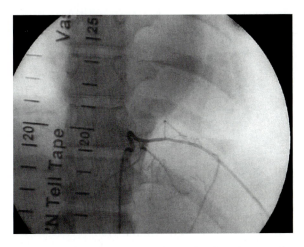

Fig. 26.8. Selective arteriography to localize the anterior spinal artery

Discussion

In the adult literature, some large series (153 cases) have been published (Liu et al. 2000). The conversion rate is quite high 10–40% (Zierold and Halow 2000), but the morbidity is limited with a good postoperative period (less pain, good cosmetic result). So in adults, the thoracoscopic approach has become the preferred method for removing neurogenic mediastinal tumors (Kumar et al. 2002; Zierold and Halow 2000), at least when benign which is the most frequent situation. Robotic surgery is being developed in this indication (Ruurda et al. 2003).

In children, more than the half of the tumors are malignant or potentially malignant. Only a few publications exist regarding the thoracoscopic approach for this indication in the pediatric literature (Patrick and Rothenberg 2001; Sandoval and Stringel 1997; Smith et al. 2002; Waldhausen et al. 2000; Warman et al. 2003). As in our experience, the number of cases is small and the follow-up short. Preliminary results, however, are very encouraging with no severe complications, less pain, and a shorter hospital stay. The conversion rate is lower than in adults. Perhaps one extra advantage of the thoracoscopic approach in small children, compared to adults, is the reduction in late postresectional disorders during growth, such as thoracic asymmetry, scapula mobility restriction, and spinal deformities including kyphosis and scoliosis. Only a prolonged orthopedic surveillance will confirm this advantage.

Conclusion

Thoracoscopy is a good technique for the removal of benign posterior mediastinal tumors in children. The complication and conversion rate is low. Postoperative recovery is smooth and hospital stay short. More experience and a longer follow-up are necessary to promote this approach for the removal of malignant tumors and to find out whether this approach really reduces the number of late sequelae.

References

Akashi A, Ohashi S, Yoden Y, et al (1997) Thoracoscopic surgery combined with a supraclavicular approach for removing superior mediastinal tumor. Surg Endosc 11:74–76

Hazelrigg SR, Boley TM, Krasna MJ, et al (1999) Thoracoscopic resection of posterior neurogenic tumor. Am Surg 65:1129–1133

Kumar A, Kumar S, Aggarwal S, et al (2002) Thoracoscopy: the preferred approach for the resection of selected posterior mediastinal tumors. J Laparoendosc Adv Surg Tech 12:345–353

Lemoine G, Montupet P (1990) Mediastinal tumors in infancy and childhood. In: Fallis JC, Filler FM, Lemoine G (eds) Pediatric Thoracic Surgery. Elsevier, Amsterdam, pp 258–272

Liu HP, Yim AP, Wan J, et al (2000) Thoracoscopic removal of intrathoracic neurogenic tumors: a combined Chinese experience. Ann Surg 232:187–190

Negri G, Puglisi A, Gerevini S, et al (2001) Thoracoscopic technique in the management of benign mediastinal dumbbell tumors. Surg Endosc 15:897–898

Patrick DA, Rothenberg SS (2001) Thoracoscopic resection of mediastinal masses in infants and children: an evaluation of technique and results. J Pediatr Surg 336:1165–1167

Pons F, Lang-Lazdunski L, Bonnet PL, et al (2003) Videothoracoscopic resection of neurogenic tumors of the superior sulcus using the harmonic scalpel. Ann Thorac Surg 75:602–604

Ruurda JP, Hanlo PW, Hennipman A, et al (2003) Robot-assisted thoracoscopic resection of a benign mediastinal neurogenic tumor: technical note. Neurosurgery 52:462–464

Sandoval C, Stringel G (1997) Video-assisted thoracoscopy for the diagnosis of mediastinal masses in children. J Soc Laparoendosc Surg 1:131–133

Smith JJ, Rothenberg SS, Brooks M, et al (2002) Thoracoscopic surgery in childhood cancer. J Pediatr Hematol Oncol 24:429–435

Waldhausen JHT, Tapper D, Sawin RS (2000) Minimally invasive surgery and clinical decision making for pediatric malignancy. Surg Endosc 14:250–253

Warman S, Fuchs J, Jesck NK, et al (2003) A prospective study of minimally techniques in pediatric surgical oncology. Med Pediatr Oncol 40:155–157

Zierold D, Halow KD (2000) Thoracoscopic resection as the preferred approach to posterior mediastinal neurogenic tumors. Surg Laparosc Endosc Percutan Tech 10:222–225

Chapter 27

The Thoracoscopic Approach to Esophageal Atresia with Distal Fistula

Klaas (N) M.A. Bax and David C. van der Zee

Introduction

Esophageal atresia has been classically approached through a posterolateral thoracotomy. The disadvantages of such a thoracotomy have been recognized for a long time, for example winged scapula, elevation or fixation of the shoulder, asymmetry of the chest wall, rib fusion, scoliosis, and breast and pectoral muscle maldevelopment (Cherup et al. 1986; Chetcuti et al. 1989; Durning et al. 1980; Emmel et al. 1996; Freeman and Walkden 1969; Jaureguizar 1985; Schier et al. 2001; Westfelt and Nordwall 1991). Moreover chronic pain after thoracic surgery, at least in adults, is a serious problem and has been reported in more than 50% of patients (Perttunen et al. 1999; Rogers and Duffy 2000). Pediatric surgeons have tried to avoid classic posterolateral thoracotomy. Brown (1952) made a vertical skin incision, detached the serratus anterior muscle, and opened the intercostal space. Soucy et al. (1991) introduced the muscle-sparing thoracotomy into pediatric surgery, while Bianchi et al. (1998) advocated transaxillary thoracotomy. More recently esophageal atresia has been approached in a thoracoscopically assisted way through a minithoracotomy (Robert and Hardy 1999), but true thoracoscopic correction was first reported in 1999 (Lobe et al. 1999). This child had an esophageal atresia without fistula. Thoracoscopic repair of an esophageal atresia with distal fistula was first reported by Rothenberg in 2000, while Bax and van der Zee published a first series of eight thoracoscopic repairs of esophageal atresia with distal fistula in 2002. In 2003 they published a series of 13 cases (van der Zee and Bax 2003). This chapter will only deal with the thoracoscopic repair of esophageal atresia with distal fistula.

Preoperative Preparation

Before Induction of General Anesthesia

The preoperative preparation is no different from the preparation for open surgery. A chest X-ray with or without a radiopaque tube in the proximal esophageal pouch as well as an abdominal X-ray will confirm the diagnosis of esophageal atresia with distal fistula. The patient should be screened for other congenital malformations belonging to the VATER or CHARGE association, and consultation by a geneticist should belong to the perioperative protocol. It would be nice to know preoperatively whether the aortic arch descends on the left or on the right in order to choose the side of the thorax to enter for the repair. If the aorta descends on the right, a left-sided approach would be preferable. A right descending aorta occurs in 1.8–2.5% of the cases (Babu et al. 2000; Bowkett et al. 1999). Ultrasound examination seems to be a poor predictor. If a right descending aortic arch is noted during thoracoscopy, it is easy to change to the opposite side. Dextroposition of the heart is not a contraindication for a right-sided thoracoscopic approach.

After Induction of General Anesthesia

General anesthesia in our hospital is usually implemented with epidural anesthesia. The child is endotracheally intubated. End-tidal CO_2 is measured continuously. An arterial line is inserted in the right radial artery for invasive blood pressure monitoring and for blood sampling. Blood gases are determined regularly. A urinary catheter is also inserted.

The 10 French Replogle tube, which has been passed through one of the nostrils into the proximal esophagus, is loosened so that the anesthesiologist can push on it when required. Amoxicillin in combination with clavulanic acid and gentamicin is given perioperatively.

Positioning

Patient

The patient is placed in a semiprone position on a short operating table with a pad underneath the right pectoral region so that the chest is tilted by about 15° to the opposite side. The table is tilted in about 15° reversed Trendelenburg (■ Fig. 27.1).

Crew, Monitors, and Equipment

The surgeon stands on the left side of the operating table with the camera operator to his or her left at the lower end of the table (■ Fig. 27.2). The scrub nurse

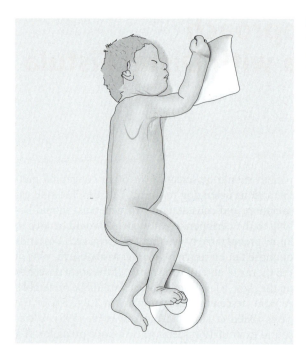

Fig. 27.1. Patient position. The patient is placed in a semi-prone position on a shortened operating table. A pad is placed underneath the right pectoral region in order to tilt the thorax over 15° to the opposite side

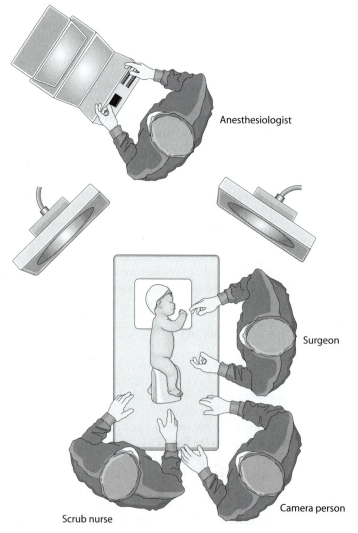

Anesthesiologist

Surgeon

Scrub nurse

Camera person

Fig. 27.2. Position of the crew and equipment. The surgeon is standing in front of the patient's abdomen with the camera operator to his or her left. Two monitors are used, one at each side of the head of the patient

Fig. 27.3. Cannulae positions. The telescope cannula is located 1 cm below the inferior tip of the scapula and slightly anteriorly. The other two cannulae are inserted more proximally, one more posteriorly and one more anteriorly

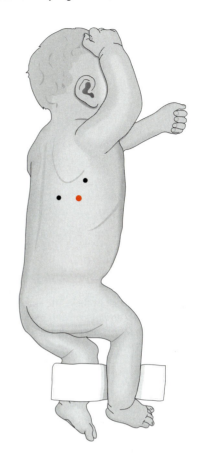

stands at the right lower end of the table. The tower stands to the right of the patient's head and the second monitor to the left.

A short (24 cm) 3.3 or 5 mm 30° telescope is used. The instruments are 20 cm long and have a 3 mm diameter.

Special Equipment

No special energy applying systems or special instruments are needed.

Technique

Cannulae

Cannula	Method of insertion	Diameter (mm)	Device	Position
1	Open	3.8 or 6	Telescope 30°, 24 cm long	1 cm below the inferior tip of the scapula and slightly more anteriorly
2	Closed	3.5	Surgeon's left-hand instrument	More posteriorly than the telescope cannula
3	Closed	3.5	Surgeon's right-hand instrument	More anteriorly and slightly more proximally than the telescope cannula

Figure 27.3 shows the positions of the cannulae. Sometimes a 2 mm cannula is inserted behind the scapula in a closed manner for a 2 mm instrument to pull on the ends of anastomotic sutures or to pull on a vessel loupe around the distal esophagus during the tying off of the fistula.

All cannulae have siliconized sleeves to fix them to the skin and underlying fascia to avoid pulling out or pushing in. It is important to put the sutures not only through the skin but also through the underlying fascia, otherwise the cannula can still be pulled out because of tenting of the skin.

Carbon Dioxide Pneumothorax

Carbon dioxide is insufflated at a pressure of 5 mmHg and a flow of 0.1 L/min. This is often not well tolerated in the beginning and close collaboration between the anesthesiologist and surgeon is needed. Increasing the ventilation rate while keeping the minute volume unchanged is helpful. Temporarily diminishing the pneumothorax pressure is also helpful. A saturation drop is counteracted by an increase in fractional intake of oxygen (FIO_2). It is most important that the surgeon is not impatient. After a few minutes, the ipsilateral lung collapses and will stay so even when almost no pneumothorax pressure is applied. From then onward, the procedure is usually much smoother than during a classic esophageal atresia repair. During thoracoscopic correction no lung retractor is required.

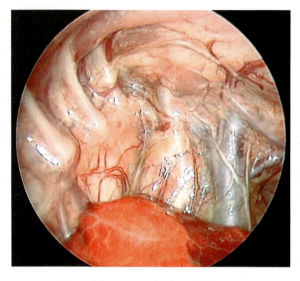

Fig. 27.4. View of the upper right chest. The lung is collapsed. The superior caval vein is seen with two phrenic nerve branches, which unite, on top. More posteriorly the vagus nerve is seen

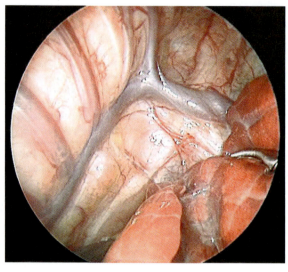

Fig. 27.5. View of the midthoracic cavity behind the lung, which is collapsed. The distal esophagus with the vagus nerve on top of it is clearly seen, as is the azygos vein

Procedure

The procedure is only started when the baby has reached a stable condition. A magnificent view of the upper chest is obtained (■ Fig. 27.4). The superior caval vein is seen anteriorly with the phrenic nerve lying on top of it. Usually two phrenic nerve branches merging from the neck are seen. More posteriorly the right vagus nerve is clearly seen lying on the trachea. The distal part of the vagus nerve lies on the distal esophagus (■ Fig. 27.5). The delicate vagal branches supplying the esophagus can be clearly seen. Some branches ascend to supply the proximal esophageal pouch as has been observed by Davies on postmortem specimens (Davies 1996). The proximal pouch is often only seen after a push by the anesthesiologist onto the Replogle tube. It lies more posteriorly against the vertebral column. The distal fistula is located at the level of the azygos vein or above it (■ Fig. 27.6). Its exact place can easily be identified as the trachea expands posteriorly at this level. The pleura above the azygos vein is opened longitudinally and the vein is freed circumferentially. The vein can then be severed between two intracorporeally placed and knotted 5×0 polyglycolic acid ligatures. Alternatively the vein can be coagulated with monopolar hook coagulation and then severed. For the same purpose the Ligasure could also be used but this requires a 6 mm cannula. With increasing experience it is often not necessary to divide the azygos vein. The distal esophagus is mobilized as close to the trachea a possible and care is taken to avoid severing of vagal branches as much as possible. After isolation of the fistula, a 10 cm-long 5×0 polyglycolic acid transfix-

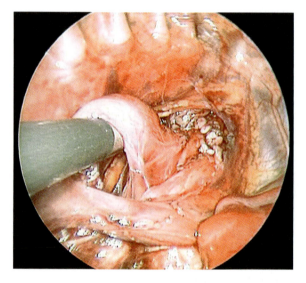

Fig. 27.6. The distal esophagus has been identified above the azygos, close to the trachea

ing suture on a round-bodied needle is applied close to the trachea and tied intracorporeally (■ Fig. 27.7). We nowadays apply the suture to the uppermost part of the fistula close to the trachea and bring the ends of the suture underneath the fistula. By doing so the ligature will stay close to the tracheal wall. In order to be able to introduce this suture through a 3.5 mm cannula, the needle has to be straightened somewhat. The distal esophagus is then transected a few millimeters distal to the transfixing suture. The end of the distal esophagus is slightly enlarged by a small cut into its dorsal rim.

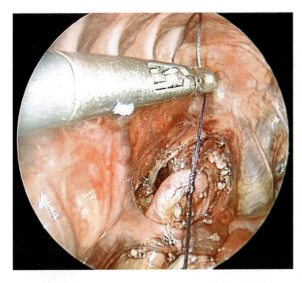

Fig. 27.7. The distal fistula is intracorporeally ligated close to the trachea

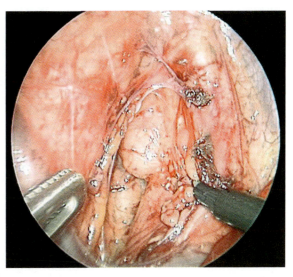

Fig. 27.8. The proximal esophageal pouch has been mobilized posteriorly

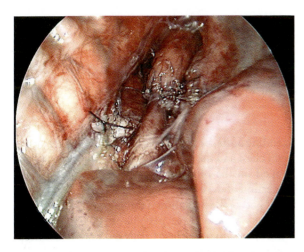

Fig. 27.9. The azygos vein has been divided between ligatures and the anastomosis has been finished

Next the proximal pouch is mobilized laterally and posteriorly (■ Fig. 27.8). No attempt is made to separate the pouch from the trachea as this interferes with its nerve supply (Davies 1996). Moreover we have the feeling that extensive mobilization does not add much length. A hole is then made through the end of the proximal pouch, using monopolar diathermy first and then hook scissors. The proximal esophagus should be well opened including the mucosa as a too small hole will result in stenosis. Because of the magnification obtained with the telescope there is a tendency to make the esophagotomy too small.

Suturing is started posteriorly in the middle of the esophagotomies. This first stitch is placed from the in-side through the proximal esophagus and back through the distal esophagus from the outside. The knot will lie in the lumen. To overcome traction, a true square knot should be made and tumbled after which the knot can be slipped in place. Finally the knot is tumbled back by pulling on its ends in a 180° fashion. The next sutures can also be placed posteriorly in the same manner in front and behind the first suture. Care should be taken to include the mucosa into the bites. Once the posterior layer has been finished, the Replogle tube is replaced with a 6 or 8 French nasogastric tube, which is passed through the anastomosis into the stomach until resistance is encountered. The tube is then pulled back a bit in order to avoid traction onto the anastomosis. The anastomosis is finished with a number of anterior sutures knotted extraluminally (■ Fig. 27.9). It may be advantageous to insert a 2 mm cannula behind the scapula into the chest for introduction of a 2 mm forceps to grab previous suture ends and to pull on them in order to turn the anastomosis a bit and to expose areas that are otherwise difficult to access. Usually about ten sutures are inserted.

After finishing the anastomosis, the operative field is irrigated, and the cannulae are removed. The anesthesiologist inflates the collapsed lung and the skin of the cannula holes are closed with adhesive tape. No chest tube is left behind.

Postoperative Care

A postoperative chest X-ray is made to evaluate lung expansion as well as the position of the endotracheal and nasogastric tube. The child remains mechanically ventilated for a few days and is then weaned from the ventilator. Feeding is started through the nasogastric tube on day 2. Oral feeding ad libitum is started when the child has been extubated and salivation has stopped. No routine contrast studies of the esophagus are performed. The child is discharged when on full oral feeding and doing well. As after open surgery, children with an esophageal atresia are regularly seen as an outpatient.

Results

So far 34 children with esophageal atresia and distal fistula have been treated thoracoscopically. Conversion was only required in one patient. This child was born after a gestation of 32 weeks with a weight of 1,230 g. It was feared that manipulation of the 6 mm cannula of the telescope in between the ribs could fracture the ribs above and below the telescope. Three patients had dextroposition of the heart but this hardly interfered with the procedure. Three patients had a right descending aorta. In one the repair was done from the right, and in the remaining two thoracoscopy on the right was ended, the children were repositioned, and the repair was done from the left. None of the patients died and operative time has come down to less than 2 h. There were four leaks, which all healed on conservative treatment. One leak was major and occurred in the second child of the series on the second day. There must have been a technical problem and an early repeat thoracoscopy might have been preferable. Twelve patients required dilation, most of them only once or twice. Four patients required an antireflux procedure and three received an aortopexy. Two patients developed a recurrent fistula and these were repaired. All these secondary procedures have been performed endoscopically as well.

Many patients had several anomalies belonging to the VATER association and two patients had anomalies in the context of the CHARGE association.

The cosmetic result of the thoracoscopic repair was excellent in all patients (Fig 27.10).

Discussion

The thoracoscopic repair of an esophageal atresia with distal fistula has the great advantage of sparing the wall of the thoracic cavity. Moreover it allows for a much better view of the anatomy. In the case of a right de-

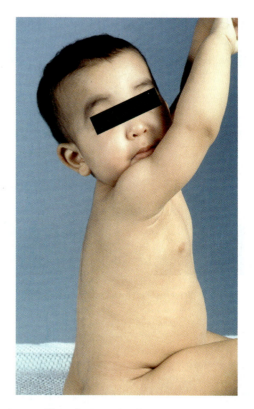

Fig. 27.10. After a few months, the scars of the portholes are hardly visible

scending aorta, not much harm is done by entering the right chest and the child can be easily repositioned and scoped on the other side. Identification and limited dissection of the esophageal ends is easy. The most difficult part of the operation is the suturing, which we do intracorporeally. Three patients in our series had a dextroposition of the heart. This did not make the operation much more difficult.

In open surgery, most corrections of esophageal atresia are done extrapleurally. There is, however, no evidence that a transpleural approach is less good.

It is often stated that the patient's own esophagus is best. We do not share this view. In esophageal atresia without fistula, most of the esophagus is usually absent. Both remaining ends can almost always be anastomosed, even thoracoscopically but this requires extensive dissection and denervation of the ends. The morbidity in these patients is high. Recently a laparoscopically assisted gastric pull-up procedure in a child with long gap esophageal atresia has been described (Ure et al. 2003).

References

Babu R, Pierro A, Spitz L et al. (2000) The management of oesophageal atresia in neonates with right-sided aortic arch. Pediatr Surg 35:56–58

Bax NMA, van der Zee DC (2002) Feasibility of thoracoscopic repair of esophageal atresia with distal fistula. J Pediatr Surg 37:192–196

Bianchi A, Sowande O, Alizai NK et al. (1998) Aesthetics and lateral thoracotomy in the neonate. J Pediatr Surg 33:1798–1800

Bowkett B, Beasley SW, Myers NA (1999) The frequency, significance, and management of a right aortic arch in association with esophageal atresia. Pediatr Surg Int 15:28–31

Browne D (1952) Patent ductus arteriosus. Proc R Soc Med 45:719–722

Cherup LL, Siewers RD, Futrell JW (1986) Breast and pectoral muscle maldevelopment after anterolateral and posterolateral thoracotomies in children. Ann Thorac Surg 41:492–497

Chetcuti P, Myers NA, Phelan PD, et al (1989) Chest wall deformity in patients with repaired esophageal atresia. J Pediatr Surg 24:244–247

Davies MR (1996) Anatomy of the extrinsic motor nerve supply to mobilized segments of the oesophagus disrupted by dissection during repair of oesophageal atresia with distal fistula. Br J Surg 83:1268–1270

Durning RP, Scoles PV, Fox OD (1980) Scoliosis after thoracotomy in tracheoesophageal fistula patients. J Bone Surg Am 62:1156–1158

Emmel M, Ulbach P, Herse B, et al (1996) Neurogenic lesions after posterolateral thoracotomy in young children. Thorac Cardiovasc Surg 44:86–91

Freeman NV, Walkden J (1969) Previously unreported shoulder deformity following right lateral thoracotomy for esophageal atresia. J Pediatr Surg 4:627–636

Jaureguizar E (1985) Morbid musculoskeletal sequelae of thoracotomy for tracheoesophageal fistula. J Pediatr Surg 20:511–514

Lobe TE, Rothenberg SS, Waldschmidt J et al. (1999) Thoracoscopic repair of esophageal atresia in an infant: a surgical first. Pediatr Endosurg Innov Tech 3:141–148

Perttunen K, Tasmuth T, Kalso E (1999) Chronic pain after thoracic surgery: a follow-up study. Acta Anaesthesiol Scand 43:563–567

Robert M, Hardy H (1999) Video-assisted repair of esophageal atresia. In: Bax NMA, et al (eds) Endoscopic Surgery in Children. Springer, Berlin Heidelberg New York, pp 130–133

Rogers ML, Duffy JP (2000) Surgical aspects of chronic post-thoracotomy pain. Eur J Cardiothorac Surg 18:711–716

Rothenberg SS (2000) Thoracoscopic repair of a tracheoesophageal fistula in a newborn infant. Pediatr Endosurg Innov Tech 4:289–294

Schier F, Korn S, Michel E (2001) Experiences of a parent support group with the long-term consequences of esophageal atresia. J Pediatr Surg 36:605–610

Soucy P, Bass J, Evans M (1991) The muscle sparing thoracotomy in infants and children. J Pediatr Surg 26:1323–1325

Ure BM, Jesch NK, Sumpelmann R et al. (2003) Laparoscopically assisted gastric pull-up for long gap esophageal atresia. J Pediatr Surg 38:1661–1662

van der Zee DC, Bax NMA (2003) Thoracoscopic repair of esophageal atresia with distal fistula: the way to go. Surg Endosc 17:1065–1067

Westfelt JN, Nordwall A (1991) Thoracotomy and scoliosis. Spine 16:1124–1125

Chapter 28

Thoracoscopic Repair of Esophageal Atresia without Fistula

Marcelo Martinez-Ferro

Introduction

Neonates without tracheoesophageal fistula represent 5–7% of all patients with esophageal atresia (EA). Depending on different authors, we classify these patients as type A or type I EA.

In most of these patients, because the esophageal segments are too far apart to allow primary anastomosis, the term "long gap" is universally accepted as a synonym for EA without fistula. Although this term represents most of the cases without fistula, occasionally in infants with EA and tracheoesophageal fistula, the upper pouch is high and the distance between upper and lower esophageal segments limits the ability to easily complete a tension-free, end-to-end esophago-esophagostomy. There is no precise definition of "long gap" because there are variations on the methods used for determining the gap length and tension. The term "long gap" should therefore be used in any type of EA in which the distance between both pouches impedes a primary anastomosis.

Although in this chapter we will only describe the thoracoscopic treatment for patients with type A EA, the displayed techniques can be used as tools for the treatment of most of the "long gap" EA cases.

Surgical Approach

The ideal surgical procedure for long gap EA remains controversial. It is difficult to obtain a consensus as to the best procedure because the individual surgeon's experience in treating this anomaly is limited. Nevertheless, it is still the opinion of most surgeons that the native esophagus is the best conduit for esophageal reconstruction. Based on this principle, several techniques have been used to internally and externally stretch one or both ends of the atretic esophagus to reduce the gap.

There are three different approaches that can be used to achieve an esophageal anastomosis, and all of them can be performed utilizing minimally invasive surgical (MIS) techniques:

1. Delayed primary anastomosis (DPA)
2. Intrathoracic esophageal elongation (IEE)
3. Extrathoracic esophageal elongation (EEE)

Management by DPA of the esophagus consists in performing an early feeding gastrostomy followed by a variable waiting period with continuous upper pouch suction and periodic assessment of the distance between the upper and lower esophageal pouches. This assessment can be done either by radiologic or combined endoscopic and radiologic examinations. During the waiting period, both pouches eventually become close enough to permit a primary esophageal anastomosis. This period can last from a minimum of 3 months to several months. Before surgery, the real distance between both pouches should be less than one vertebra to achieve a low tension anastomosis.

Regarding IEE, various innovative operative methods to manage long gap EA have been proposed. In the early 1970s, Rehbein (Rehbein and Schweder 1971) described the use of a nylon thread bridging the gap between the two ends of the esophagus attached to silver olives placed within each pouch. The olives were pushed until the two ends of the esophagus pressed together and contacted creating a fistula. Other authors used a similar technique to create a fistula between the two ends of the esophagus by simply connecting the two ends of the mobilized esophagus by a silk suture. Recently, Lee and Harrison (Lee et al. 2002) described an innovative method with thoracoscopic placement of a traction elongation device. Using this method, the two pouches are gradually coapted using traction elongation to stimulate lengthening of the pouches. Simultaneously at the National Children's Hospital "J.P.Garrahan", we developed an original thoracoscopic technique that will be described in this chapter.

The EEE was originally described by Kimura (Kimura and Soper 1994) and with this approach an extrathoracic elongation of the esophagus was used successfully in reconstructing the esophagus with an end-to-end anastomosis. The EEE has several advantages for reconstructing long gap EA. First, patients continue oral sham feedings during the staged repair, thus, preventing the development of food aversion. Second, this technique enables use of the native esophagus for reconstruction that, with time, will function as a suitable conduit for swallowing. After concluding EEE in five cases by conventional thoracotomy, we performed successful MIS esophageal anastomosis after EEE in two patients. In both, the upper pouch was elongated as

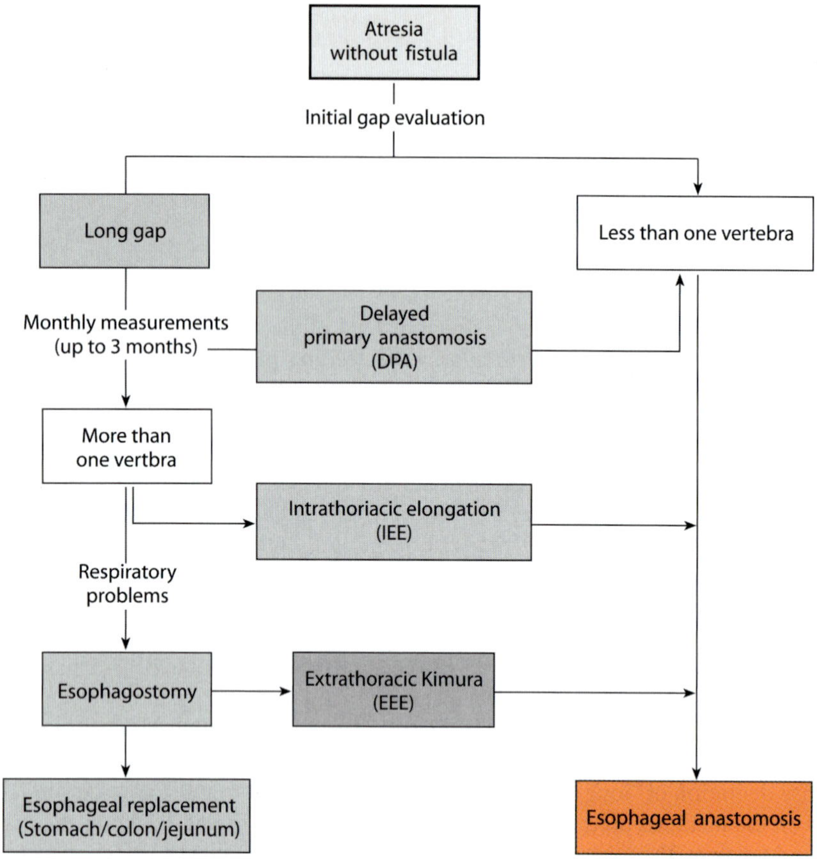

Fig. 28.1. Algorithm for the management of type A "long gap" esophageal atresia

described by Kimura and final reconstruction including upper pouch reinsertion to the thoracic cavity was performed by thoracoscopy.

In ■ Fig. 28.1 we show the algorithm used at the National Children's Hospital "J.P.Garrahan" for the management of type A long gap EA patients.

Delayed Primary Anastomosis

Preoperative Preparation

Before Induction of General Anesthesia
Gastrostomy feeding is stopped 3 h before the procedure. The upper esophageal pouch is continuously aspirated with the Replogle tube until the patient gets into the operating room.

After Induction of General Anesthesia
While still in a supine decubitus position, a radiopaque semirigid bougie is introduced under radioscopic control through the gastrostomy into the lower esophageal pouch, and securely fixed to the stoma site (■ Fig. 28.2). The end of bougie is positioned in such a way that the bougie can be manipulated during the operation in a sterile way through the draping. A softer bougie is introduced through the mouth into the upper pouch and is kept apart from the tracheal tube.

Positioning of Patient, Crew, and Monitor
The patient is positioned in three quarter left prone decubitus with a mild upward rotation of the right side. The surgeon and his assistant stand at the left side of the table facing the monitor located at the right side. The anesthesiologist stands at the head of the table and the scrub nurse at the foot (■ Fig. 28.3).

Special Equipment
No special energy applying systems are needed, but if available a 5 mm Ligasure device can be used for coagulation of the azygos vein. For the suturing 5/0 PDS on a C1 needle is used. Fluoroscopy will be used during the procedure.

Fig. 28.2. Semirigid radio-paque bougies are placed in each esophageal end in order to locate them easily during thoracoscopic surgery

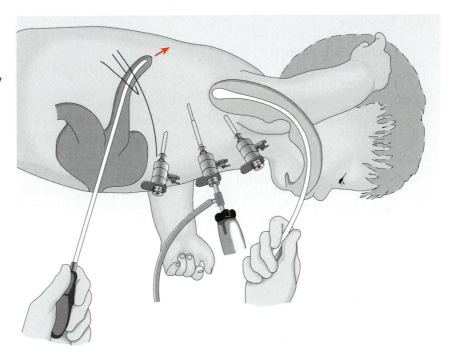

Fig. 28.3. Ceiling view of the operating room setup for the thoracoscopic correction of a EA

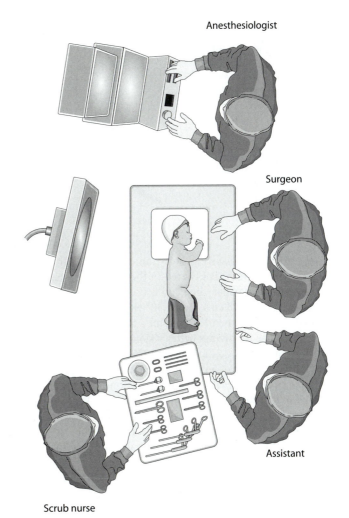

Anesthesiologist

Surgeon

Assistant

Scrub nurse

Technique

Cannulae and Position

Cannula	Diameter (mm)	Device	Accessories	Position
1	4.7	Telescope, 4 mm 30° wide angle	Rubber sealing cap, 3 mm	Sixth intercostal space, midaxillary line
2	6	Working instrument, suturing	Rubber sealing cap, 3 mm, silicone leaflet valve	Third intercostal space, inside the axilla
3	3.9	Grasping forceps	Silicone leaflet valve	Tenth intercostal space, posterior axillary line

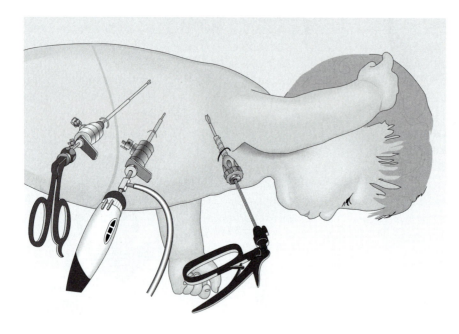

Fig. 28.4. The patient is placed in a three quarter left prone position. Three trocars are inserted as shown

Three trocars are placed as shown in ■ Fig. 28.4. The first trocar (4.7 mm) is inserted in the 6th intercostal space at the midaxillary line and is used for the insertion of a short (18 cm) 4 mm 30°telescope (arthroscope). We recommend the use of a wide angle telescope because it provides better vision in such a small working space. Through this trocar CO_2 insufflation is started. A pressure of 5 mmHg provides excellent lung retraction and is well tolerated. A second trocar is placed in the axilla at the 3rd intercostal space. We recommend the use of a 6 mm trocar with oblique outside thread for better anchorage in the thoracic wall. The trocar should have a silicone leaflet valve for easy introduction of 5/0 PDS on a C1 curved needle. This is done with a 3 mm needle holder. To prevent CO_2 leak, the trocar should have a 3 mm rubber sealing cap. The third and last trocar, a 3.9 mm one, is placed in the 9th

or 10th intercostal space at the posterior axillary line and is used for the introduction of a grasping forceps. All the trocars are fixed using the Shah-Net technique by means of a rubber suction tube and silk suture that is tied around the tube and then around the insufflation stopcock. This stabilization of the trocar avoids dislodgement and reduces the risk of CO_2 subcutaneous emphysema.

Procedure

As a first step, the azygos vein is dissected and divided with monopolar cautery or 5 mm Ligasure if available (■ Fig. 28.5). Location of the distal esophageal pouch is easily achieved by gentle moving of the bougie placed through the gastrostomy. The distal atretic end is dissected from the surrounding tissues by means of the monopolar hook, Maryland grasper, and scissors

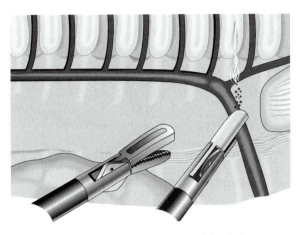

Fig. 28.5. The azygos vein is dissected and divided using monopolar cautery

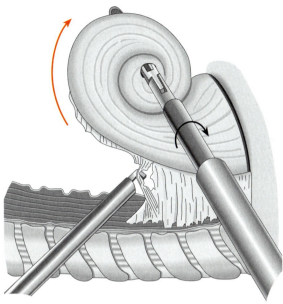

Fig. 28.7. A rolling movement, "spaghetti maneuver," is very useful for easier dissection of the upper pouch and the posterior tracheal wall

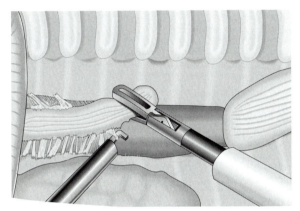

Fig. 28.6. The distal atretic esophagus is located and completely dissected from the surrounding tissues, up to the diaphragm

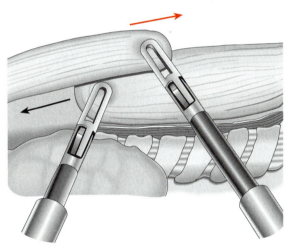

Fig. 28.8. When both esophageal ends slightly overlay, anastomosis can be performed

(■ Fig. 28.6). The upper esophageal pouch is then dissected and opened at its end. Special care must been taken when dissecting between the anterior wall of the upper pouch and the posterior wall of the trachea. At this point, deep dissection into the neck is mandatory in order to achieve enough esophageal length for performing an anastomosis. A rolling movement of the grasping forceps, "spaghetti maneuver," is of great help at this stage, thus providing an excellent view of the esophagus and the trachea (■ Fig. 28.7).

After thorough full dissection of both pouches, the feasibility of the anastomosis is checked by grasping both ends and sliding them together (■ Fig. 28.8). Next the proximal and distal ends of the esophagus are transected transversally with scissors (■ Figs. 28.9, 28.10). The anastomosis is accomplished using six to eight interrupted stitches of 5/0 PDS on a C1 needle. The first stitch of the anastomosis is placed in the midline of the posterior wall (■ Fig. 28.11). All knots are

tied extracorporeally using a Roeder knot which is pushed in place with the needle holder (■ Fig. 28.12).

Because most of the time the anastomosis is under high tension, we developed a way of avoiding all the force in one single suture thus preventing tissue tearing. The "twin traction" suture (■ Fig. 28.13) is achieved by placing two simultaneous sutures at the posterior wall. Then a Roeder knot is tied on each thread, and sequential tightening of the Roeder knot provides gentle traction with equal distribution of tension in both sutures.

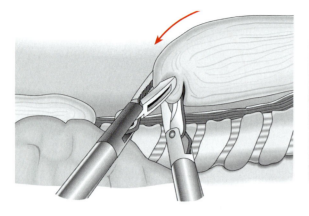

Fig. 28.9. After complete dissection of the upper pouch, its tip is completely transected transversally

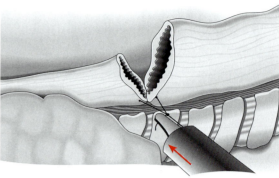

Fig. 28.12. Roeder knots are tied extracorporeally and are slid into place with the needle holder

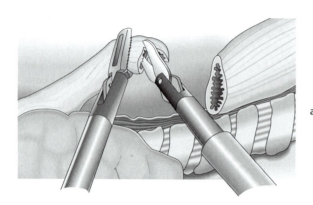

Fig. 28.10. The end of the inferior pouch is also transected transversally

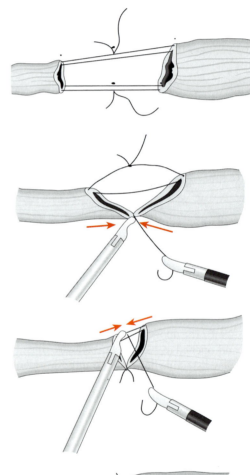

a

b

c

d

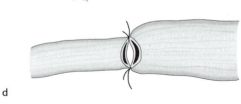

Fig. 28.11. A first stitch is placed at the midportion of the posterior wall. The knot is tied at the mucosal side

Fig. 28.13. For high-tension sutures, we developed the "twin traction" technique. Two Roeder knots are sequentially tightened. Force is distributed over both sutures thus preventing tissue tearing

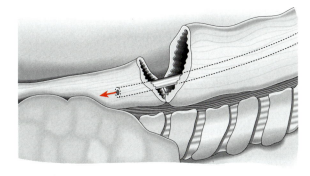

Fig. 28.14. After completion of the posterior wall, a transa-nastomotic nasogastric feeding tube is advanced into the stomach

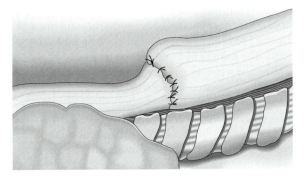

Fig. 28.15. Anastomosis completed

After completion of the posterior wall of the anastomosis, a transanastomotic Silastic tube is advanced to the stomach (■ Fig. 28.14). Once the anastomosis is concluded (■ Fig. 28.15), a 12 French chest tube is inserted through the lowermost trocar site.

Postoperative Care

Pain Control

All patients with high-tension esophageal anastomosis receive full muscle relaxation and are mechanically ventilated for at least 48 h. This allows for optimal pain management. Moreover its prevents cervical extension, which we consider an important issue, as well as profuse swallowing.

Transanastomotic Silastic Tube

Such a Silastic tube is used for three reasons. First, it serves as a tutor for the recently performed anastomosis; second it can be used for decompression of the stomach together with the gastrostomy tube; and finally it can be passed through the pylorus into the jejunum and used for feeding if a leak or any other complication occurs.

Gastrostomy

The gastrostomy, which all patients with type A EA have already had before esophageal anastomosis, is kept in place until it is no longer needed. We recom-

Fig. 28.16. Routine barium swallow performed at 5th post-operative day shows a patent anastomosis without leaks

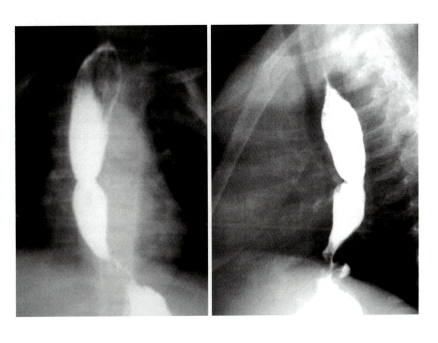

mend leaving the gastrostomy open and connected to a tube for the first 48–72 h or until feeding through the transanastomotic tube is started.

Feeding Policy

Feeding is started on the 3rd postoperative day through the transanastomotic feeding tube. On the 5th postoperative day a barium swallow is carried out (■ Fig. 28.16). If no leak is observed, oral feedings are started and the chest tube is removed.

Intrathoracic Esophageal Elongation (IEE)

Preoperative Preparation

Before Induction of General Anesthesia

Gastrostomy feeding is stopped 3 h before the procedure.

After Induction of General Anesthesia

While still in a supine decubitus position, a 14 French semirigid, hollow, radiopaque dilator is passed through the gastrostomy into the lower esophageal pouch under radioscopic control, and is strongly fixed to the stoma site. The end of the dilator is positioned in such a way that it can be manipulated during surgery in a sterile way through the drapes.

A second hollow 14 French dilator is positioned through the mouth into the upper esophageal pouch. The dilator needs to be kept apart from the tracheal tube.

Positioning of Patient, Crew, and Monitors

As for DPA.

Special Equipment

No special energy applying systems are required but if available a 5 mm Ligasure instrument can be used for electrocoagulation of the azygos vein. Fluoroscopy will be needed during the procedure. The following items should be available:

Equipment	Details
Dilator	14 French, hollow, semirigid
Injection needle	Transurethral injection needle (Bard) Catheter: 5 French, 33 cm; needle: 23 gauge, 1.3 cm
Upper sphere	Stainless steel, removable axis
Lower sphere	Stainless steel, fixed axis
Knot tier	3 mm
Thread	Prolene 5/0 and 6/0

Technique

Cannulae and Position

As for DPA.

Procedure

Dissection of both atretic esophageal ends is done in the same way as for DPA. Special care must be taken to preserve the integrity of both pouches thus avoiding accidental opening.

The whole procedure is detailed in ■ Fig. 28.17. It starts by advancing a very thin and long transurethral injection needle through the hollow dilator located in the upper pouch. The needle is used to pierce the esophageal wall. Through the inside of this needle a very thin thread of 6/0 Prolene is passed into the thorax (■ Fig. 28.17a). The tip of the thread in the thorax is grasped and pulled out through the axillary trocar. The tip of the thread is knotted around the middle of a 5/0 Prolene thread, which is then pulled backward. The middle of this 5/0 Prolene thread is placed around the removable axis of a special spherical device that will be inserted into the upper esophageal pouch (■ Fig. 28.17b).

A second 6/0 Prolene thread is inserted into the thorax through the distal hollow dilator using the same procedure (injection needle inside the hollow radiopaque dilator). The thread is grasped and exteriorized through the axillary port. This 6/0 thread is now tied to both ends of the upper pouch 5/0 thread (■ Fig. 28.17c) and used to drag it through the lower pouch and the gastrostomy.

A second stainless steel sphere with a fixed axis is now attached to the 5/0 thread (■ Fig. 28.17d) and by means of a Roeder knot and a knot tier, the sphere is advanced into the lower pouch (■ Fig. 28.17e). Gentle traction is applied in order to bring both pouches together. The whole procedure is controlled under thoracoscopic guidance (■ Fig. 28.17f).

Once the procedure is concluded, a 12 French chest tube is inserted through the lowermost trocar site. A postoperative X-ray will determine the exact position of both spheres.

Under fluoroscopic control, once a week, the knot tier is used to tighten the Roeder knot thus providing gradual approximation of both pouches (■ Fig. 28.18).

Postoperative Care

Postoperative care is similar to DPA patients.

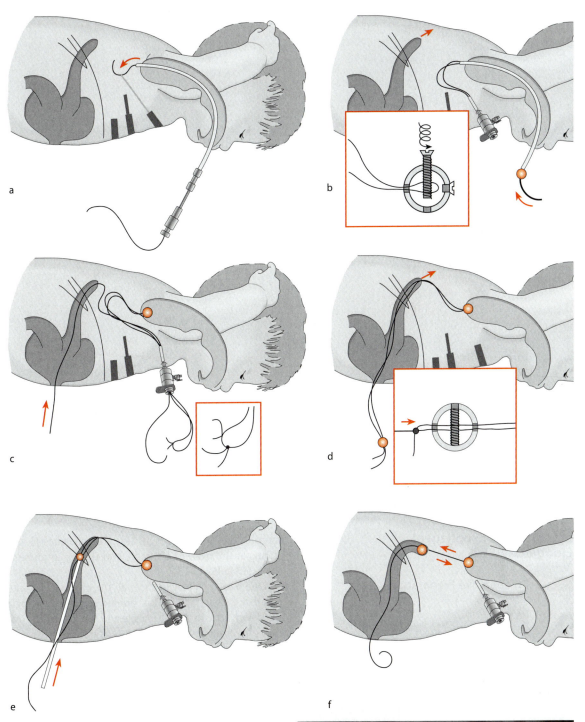

Fig. 28.17. Detailed procedure for thoracoscopic placement of a traction elongation device using two specially designed stainless steel spheres

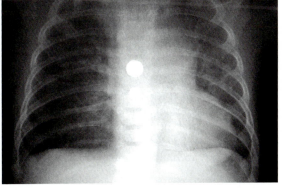

Fig. 28.18. Stainless steel spheres are almost coapting after gradual elongation of both pouches

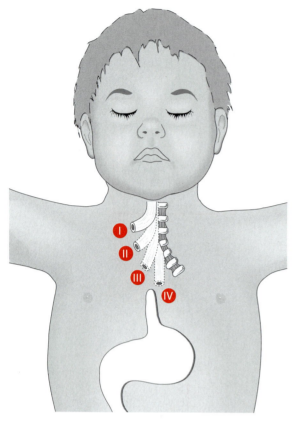

Fig. 28.19. Sequential subcutaneous extrathoracic esophageal elongation procedures have been carried out

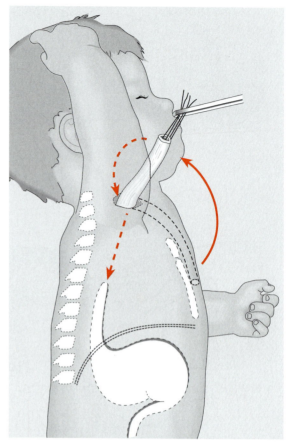

Fig. 28.20. After completed elongation, the proximal esophagus is reintroduced into the thoracic cavity

Extrathoracic Esophageal Elongation (EEE)

Preoperative Preparation

As for DPA.

Positioning of Patient
Cervical Approach

The right arm and hemithorax are fully scrubbed. Then the whole arm is foiled with a tubular gauze in order to permit its mobilization from a supine decubitus to a prone decubitus position. Initially the patient is positioned in supine decubitus so that the previously elongated esophagus (■ Fig. 28.19) can be adequately mobilized and dissected before its reinsertion to the thoracic cavity.

Thoracoscopic Approach

Holding the foiled right arm, the patient is positioned in three quarter left prone decubitus with a mild upward rotation of the right side. The surgeon and the assistant stand at the left side of the table facing the monitor located at the right side. The anesthesiologist stands at the head of the table and the scrub nurse at the foot (■ Fig. 28.3)

One bougie is placed through the gastrostomy into the distal esophagus. This bougie must be strongly fixed with tape to the stoma site and left in such a position that it can be manipulated during surgery through the sterile drapes (■ Fig. 28.2).

Special Equipment
As for DPA.

Technique

Cannulae and Position
As in DPA.

Procedure

As a first step, the azygos vein is dissected and divided with monopolar cautery or 5 mm Ligasure if available (■ Fig. 28.5). Location of the distal esophageal pouch is easily achieved by gentle moving of the bougie placed

Fig. 28.21. By blunt dissection a pathway is created in the prevertebral area, through which the upper esophagus is put into the thorax. The esophageal stay suture is pulled downward with a 3 mm grasper inserted through the lower port

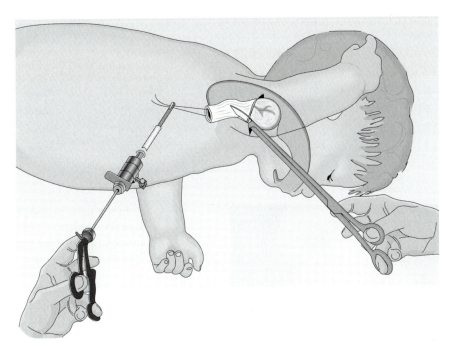

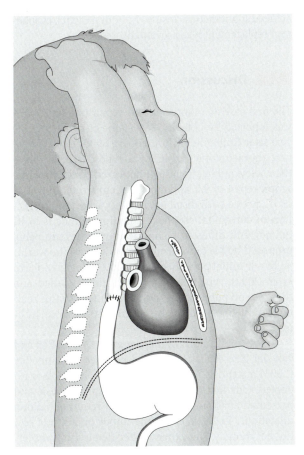

Fig. 28.22. Anastomosis is completed using the same technique as for DPA

through the gastrostomy. The distal atretic end is then dissected from the surrounding tissues by means of the monopolar hook, Maryland grasper, and scissors (■ Fig. 28.6).

Complete mobilization of the extrathoracic elongated upper esophagus is achieved by blunt dissection from the surrounding tissues. Special care must be taken not to perforate the esophagus, so it is recommended to perform two or more thoracic and cervical incisions that will provide better surgical view.

After being mobilized, the esophagus must be reinserted into the thorax (■ Fig. 28.20). With blunt dissection through the neck the surgeon creates a prevertebral pathway until the tip of a dissecting forceps is seen with the scope coming into the thorax. Two or three stay sutures are placed to the proximal mobilized pouch. Esophageal stay sutures are grabbed and pulled downward with a 3 mm grasper inserted through the lower port (■ Fig. 28.21). The proximal end of the distal esophageal pouch is transected transversally with scissors (■ Fig. 28.9). Anastomosis is accomplished using six to eight interrupted stitches of 4/0 PDS on an RB1 needle. The first stitch of the anastomosis is placed in the midline of the posterior wall (■ Fig. 28.11). All knots are tied extracorporeally using a Roeder knot and are pushed with the needle holder (■ Fig. 28.12). Once the anastomosis is concluded (■ Fig. 28.22), a 12 French chest tube is inserted through the lowermost trocar site.

Postoperative Care

Postoperative care is similar to DPA patients.

Table 28.1. Results on patients treated with delayed primary anastomosis (DPA). *Lap Nissen* Laparoscopic Nissen fundoplication

Case	Age (months)	Operative time (min)	Conversion	Intraoperative complications	Postoperative complications	Follow-up
1	4	180	No	None	None	Lap Nissen
2	4	90	No	None	None	–
3	4	100	No	None	None	Lap Nissen
4	3	120	No	None	None	Lap Nissen

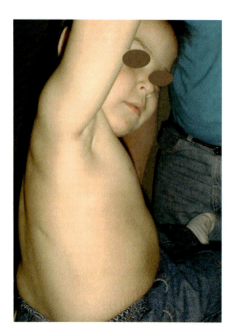

Fig. 28.23. One year after surgery. Excellent cosmetic result

Results

Four patients with EA without fistula have been treated with a DPA since March 2001 when we performed our first MIS repair of an EA with a tracheoesophageal fistula (TEF). There were no conversions. A listing of the results for each case is detailed in ■ Table 28.1. No operative complications were encountered. CO_2 insufflation in the thoracic cavity was well tolerated and provided an excellent operative field in all cases. Mean operative time was 123 min (90–180 min). No early or late postoperative complications were observed in this small series of patients. Three cases developed subsequent gastroesophageal reflux that required laparoscopic Nissen fundoplication without eventualities.

All patients show excellent cosmetic results (■ Fig. 28.23). At follow-up all patients remain without symptoms except for one patient who presents a mild tracheomalacia that requires no surgical treatment.

In the same period one patient received IEE. After 3 weeks of traction, both spheres coapted and a thoracoscopic end-to-end anastomosis was performed. Reoperation for closing a small bronchoesophageal fistula was needed 3 weeks later with good results. Because of severe gastroesophageal reflux, a Nissen fundoplication was required. The patient is now evolving uneventfully at 2 years of follow-up.

Two patients received EEE. The first case had an excellent result. The second one developed an esophageal leak that required long-term thoracic drainage to achieve spontaneous closure. In both patients, esophageal replacement was prevented.

Discussion

The first case of a thoracoscopic repair of a type A EA was reported by Lobe in 1999 (Lobe et al. 1999). One year later Rothenberg (Rothenberg 2000) reported the first thoracoscopic repair of a type C atresia. Since then, a few publications have appeared on the thoracoscopic repair of EA, and most of them are about type C or III atresia with distal fistula. Thoracoscopic correction of congenital esophageal malformations is in its infancy and different technical approaches are being proposed by the pioneering centers around the world.

In our initial published experience (Martinez-Ferro et al. 2002), type A patients were not included and there are no published series of patients with this malformation operated on by minimally invasive techniques.

In the publications of Lovorn et al. (2001), Bax and van der Zee et al. (2002), and van der Zee and Bax (2003) a stenosis rate of between 30% and 50% is reported. Our first three cases had a type C atresia and presented anastomotic stricture that required balloon dilatations. In those cases, the upper pouch was sectioned frontally. Since then we decided to cut transversally the whole tip of the upper pouch, as we used to do during open surgery (Martinez-Ferro et al. 1995). No anastomotic strictures have been observed in our four type A cases. As has been described by all authors so far, the visualization and identification of all the anatomic structures achieved thoracoscopically is far better than that found during open surgery. Also in type A atresia, it is easy to identify with precision the vagus nerve and its branches, which permits a very careful dissection avoiding damage.

Special technical maneuvers such as the "spaghetti maneuver" and the "twin traction suture" are useful tools for extensive dissection and elongation of both pouches.

Some surgeons are reluctant to dissect the lower pouch extensively because of fear of interfering with the segmental esophageal blood supply and fear of interfering with motility. Other groups advocate extensive dissection of the distal esophagus (Farkash et al. 2002), as we have for more than two decades.

All our patients tolerated well the insufflation of CO_2 at pressures between 5 and 6 mmHg. When needed, lung expansion was immediately obtained by opening one of the trocars valves. Interaction with the anesthesiologist is crucial and is facilitated by the easy visualization of the operative field and the lung status on the monitor screen.

With increasing experience operative time diminished dramatically. It is widely accepted that primary thoracoscopic repair of EA requires highly specialized skills and great experience in endosurgery of the esophagus. For acquiring such experience rapidly, Till et al. (2001) proposed the rabbit model. At our institution, most of the surgical procedures are performed by trainees. All type A atresias, however, were operated by the same surgeon, author of this chapter. Operative time could be lowered to 90 min in one case, which is similar to the 100–180 min historically needed for performing an open case.

Regarding IEE and EEE, we find that thoracoscopy adds extra technical resources that facilitate its performance. For example, the prevention of adhesions in the pleural space is an important factor in IEE patients in whom the thorax has to be reentered for the final anastomosis after gradual elongation of the esophageal pouches.

Cosmetic results where excellent in all cases. In most of the cases it was difficult to find the scars several months after the initial procedure.

In conclusion, the thoracoscopic approach to EA is feasible and relatively easy to achieve. It seems to offer important advantages over the classic open technique. As the number of cases presented here is small, further experience is needed to determine the precise role of this technique.

References

Bax KMA, van der Zee D (2002) Feasibility of thoracoscopic repair of esophageal atresia with distal fistula. J Pediatr Surg 37:192–196

Farkash U, Lazar L, Erez I, et al (2002) The distal pouch in esophageal atresia: to dissect or not to dissect, that is the question. Eur J Pediatr Surg 12:19–23

Kimura K, Soper RT (1994) Multistaged extrathoracic esophageal elongation for long gap esophageal atresia. J Pediatr Surg 29:566–568

Lee H, Farmer D, Albanese C, et al (2002) Traction elongation for treatment of long-gap esophageal atresia. Pediatr Endosurg Innov Tech 6:51–54

Lobe TE, Rothenberg SS, Waldschmidt J, et al (1999) Thoracoscopic repair of esophageal atresia in an infant: a surgical first. Pediatr Endosurg Innov Tech 3:141–148

Lovorn H, Rothenberg S, Reinberg O, et al (2001) Update on thoracoscopic repair of esophageal atresia with and without fistula. Pediatr Endosurg Innov Tech 5:135–139

Martinez-Ferro M, Rodriguez S, Aguilar D (1995) Resultados en el tratamiento de 100 recién nacidos con atresia de esófago. Rev Ci Infantil 5:104–105

Martinez-Ferro M, Elmo G, Bignon H (2002) Thoracoscopic repair of esophageal atresia with fistula: initial experience. Pediatr Endosurg Innov Tech 6:229–237

Rehbein F, Schweder N (1971) Reconstruction of the esophagus without colon transplantation in cases of atresia. J Pediatr Surg 6:746–752

Rothenberg S (2000) Thoracoscopic repair of a tracheoesophageal fistula in a newborn infant. Pediatr Endosurg Innov Tech 4:289–294

Till H, Kirlum H, Boehm R, et al (2001) Thoracoscopic correction of esophageal atresia: training in rabbits provides valuable surgical expertise and shortens the learning curve. Pediatr Endosurg Innov Tech 5:235–239

van der Zee DC, Bax NM (2003) Thoracoscopic repair of esophageal atresia with distal fistula. Surg Endosc 17:1065–1067

Chapter 29

The Thoracoscopic Approach to H Type Tracheoesophageal Fistula

Klaas (N) M.A. Bax and David C. van der Zee

Introduction

An H type tracheoesophageal fistula is usually approached through a right transverse cervical incision. When doing so the fistula is often found in a relatively distal position, which makes the procedure rather difficult. Moreover during a cervical approach the ansa cervicalis as well as the recurrent laryngeal nerves are at risk. An approach through the chest is another option but the fistula may be located in a rather high thoracic position or even in the neck. In addition a thoracotomy is major trauma and is associated with considerable morbidity, as outlined in Chapter 27. No wonder that the cervical approach has been the gold standard. With the availability of minimal access endoscopic surgical techniques one wonders whether a cervical approach is still the most appropriate one. Allal et al. (2004) published the successful thoracoscopic repair of an H type tracheoesophageal fistula in a newborn. We recently approached two such H type fistulae thoracoscopically, one in a newborn and one in a 4-year-old child.

Preoperative Preparation

Before Induction of General Anesthesia

The preoperative preparation is no different from the preparation for open surgery. The diagnosis is established either by contrast study of the esophagus and/or tracheoscopy. Using both modalities an idea can be obtained as to the localization of the fistula. Surgery should only be undertaken when the lungs are in good condition. Often there is a history of recurrent pneumonia, which should be well treated with antibiotics preoperatively. During the preoperative preparation period the patient is fed by nasogastric tube and is put onto antigastroesophageal reflux treatment.

The patient should be screened for other congenital malformations belonging to the VATER or CHARGE association, and consultation by a geneticist should be part of the perioperative diagnostic protocol.

After Induction of General Anesthesia

General anesthesia in our hospital is usually implemented with epidural anesthesia. The child is endotracheally intubated. End-tidal CO_2 is measured continuously. In newborns and young infants an arterial line should be available for invasive blood pressure monitoring and for blood gas determination.

The feeding nasogastric tube is left in situ for easy identification of the esophagus during the operation and for early postoperative feeding. The antibiotics that were preoperatively started are continued during the operation.

Positioning

Patient

The patient is placed in a left anterolateral decubitus position on a short operating table. The table is tilted in about 15° reversed Trendelenburg (Fig. 29.1). If needed the table can also be tilted to the left.

Crew, Monitors, and Equipment

The surgeon stands on the left side of the operating table with the camera operator to the surgeon's left at the lower end of the table (Fig. 29.2) and the scrub nurse at the right lower end of the table. The tower stands to the left of the patient's head and all cables come from the left and are attached to the left of the patient. None of the cables run over the patient. A second screen is placed to the right of the patient's head. A 3.3- or 5 mm 30° telescope is used. The instruments are 20 cm long and have a 3 mm diameter.

Special Equipment

No special energy applying systems or special instruments are needed.

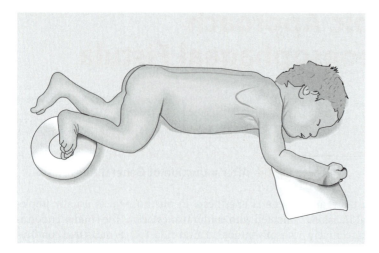

Fig. 29.1. The patient is placed in a semi-prone position on a shortened operating table. A pad is placed underneath the right pectoral regon in order to tilt the thorax over 15° to the opposite side

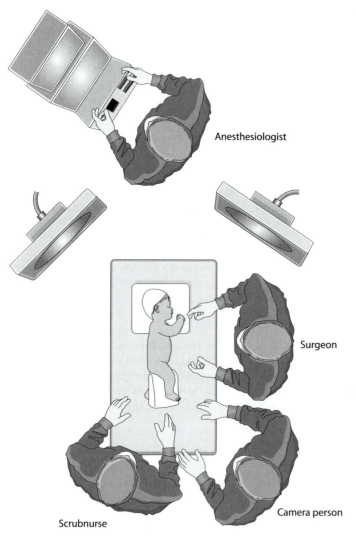

Fig. 29.2. The surgeon is standing in front of the patient's abdomen with the camera operator to the surgeon's left. Two monitors are used, one at each side of the head of the patient

Anesthesiologist

Surgeon

Scrubnurse

Camera person

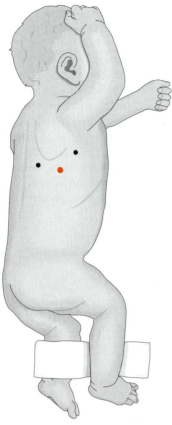

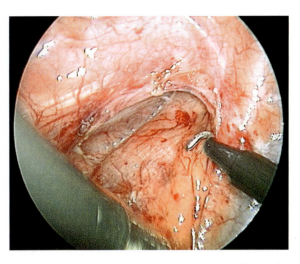

Fig. 29.4. View of the upper right chest. The head is to the *right* and the legs to the *left*. The vertebral column is in the *left upper corner*, the superior caval vein in the *right lower corner*. The mediastinal pleura has been opened between the vertebral column and the esophagus, between the azygos vein, which is not seen, and the thoracic inlet. The trachea is easy identified by its hard consistency and the place of the fistula by the bulging of the esophagus during inspiration. The esophagus has been mobilized posteriorly. The lung is collapsed and is therefore not seen. No lung retractor is used

Fig. 29.3. Cannulae positions. The telescope cannula is located 1 cm below the inferior tip of the scapula and slightly anteriorly. The other two cannulae are inserted more proximally, one more posteriorly and one more anteriorly

Technique

Cannulae

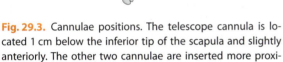

Cannula	Method of insertion	Diameter (mm)	Device	Position
1	Open	3.8 or 6	3.3 or 5 mm 30° telescope	1 cm below the inferior tip of the scapula and slightly more anteriorly
2	Closed	3.5	Surgeon's left-hand instrument	More posteriorly and slightly more proximally than the telescope cannula
3	Closed	3.5	Surgeon's right-hand instrument	More anteriorly and slightly more proximally than the telescope cannula
4 (optional)	Closed	2 mm port or directly	Grasper with ratchet	Behind the scapula, more cranially than port 2

All cannulae (■ Fig. 29.3) have siliconized sleeves to fix them to the chest to avoid pulling out or pushing in. It is important to put the sutures not only through the skin but also through the underlying fascia, otherwise the cannula can still be pulled out because of tenting of the skin.

Carbon Dioxide Pneumothorax

Carbon dioxide is insufflated at a pressure of 5 mmHg and a flow of 0.1 L/min. This is often not well tolerated by the patient in the beginning and close collaboration between the anesthesiologist and surgeon is needed.

224 Chest

Increasing the ventilation rate while keeping the minute volume unchanged is helpful. Temporarily diminishing the pneumothorax pressure is also helpful. A saturation drop is counteracted by an increase in fractional intake of oxygen (FIO_2). It is most important that the surgeon is not impatient. After a few minutes, the ipsilateral lung collapses and will stay so even when almost no pneumothorax pressure is applied. From then onward, the procedure is usually much smoother than during a classic esophageal atresia repair. During thoracoscopic correction no lung retractor is required.

Procedure

The procedure is only started when the baby has reached a stable condition. A magnificent view of the upper chest is obtained (■ Fig. 29.4). The posterior mediastinal pleura is opened longitudinally from the azygos vein all the way up. By cutting the pleura over the subclavian vessels access into the cervical area is gained. The site of the fistula is easily identified by the bulging of the esophagus at that site during each inspiration. The trachea is easily identified by its hard consistency and the overlying right vagus nerve. It is surprising to see how many small nerves run together with the fistula to the esophagus. As we are convinced that iatrogenic damage of nerves contributes to the esophageal motor disturbances after esophageal atresia repair, we try to save as many branches as possible.

We start the dissection posterior to the esophagus as there are no traversing nerve branches there. Care must be taken when the left side of the trachea is reached. The left recurrent laryngeal nerve is identified and dissected off so that the ligature of the fistula will not include the nerve.

Next the esophagus is separated from the trachea above and below the fistula (■ Fig. 29.5). All nerve branches that run together with the fistula are dissected off the fistula but left intact. After isolation of the fistula, a 10 cm-long 5×0 polyglycolic acid transfixing suture is introduced. In order to be able to introduce the needle through a 3.5 mm cannula, the needle has to be somewhat straightened. The suture is put through the uppermost part of the fistula close to the trachea, which will prevent the ligature sliding downward dur-

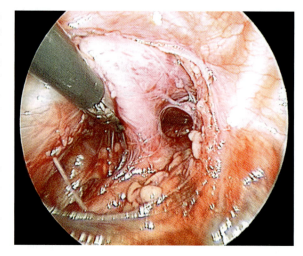

Fig. 29.5. The fistula has been dissected off the trachea superiorly and inferiorly. No nerve branches are transected

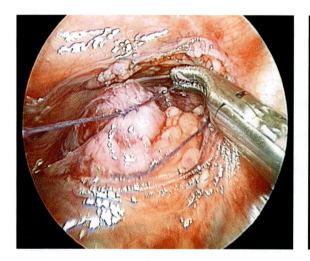

Fig. 29.6. The fistula is ligated with a 5×0 polyglycolic acid transfixing suture as close to the trachea as possible. The suture takes only the superior wall of the fistula, not the lumen. During the application of the suture and the initial tying, the esophagus is lifted up

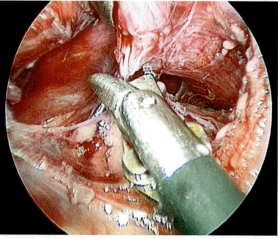

Fig. 29.7. The fistula is now divided with scissors at the esophageal side. The suture is underneath the beak of the scissors and is therefore not seen

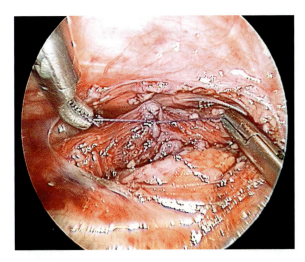

Fig. 29.8. The remaining hole in the esophagus is closed transversely with a running 5×0 polyglycolic acid running suture. No tissue is interposed between the trachea and esophagus

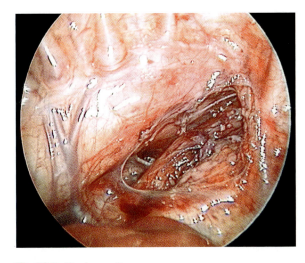

Fig. 29.9. Final operative appearance

ing tying. The needle is then cut off and removed. The long suture end is brought around the fistula but all nerve branches are kept outside the suture. During the tying, traction is carried out on the vessel loop around the proximal esophagus while the distal part of the esophagus is pulled backward with an instrument. By doing so the fistula is lifted up and the ligature can be placed close to the trachea (■ Fig. 29.6).

Next the fistula is divided distal to the ligature (■ Fig. 29.7). The remaining hole in the esophagus is closed transversally with a running 5×0 polyglycolic acid suture (■ Fig. 29.8). No tissue is interposed between the esophagus and trachea (■ Fig. 29.9).

After finishing the anastomosis, the operative field is irrigated, and the cannulae are removed. The anesthesiologist inflates the collapsed lung and the skin of the cannula holes are closed with adhesive tape. No chest tube is left behind.

Postoperative Care

The child is extubated on the operating table. Feeding can be started through the nasogastric tube immediately after surgery. Oral feeding ad libitum is given after 4 days when there are no clinical signs of leakage.

Results

So far we have treated two children with H type fistula thoracoscopically. Both fistulae were half way between the azygos vein and the thoracic inlet. Both patients have done extremely well, as did the case of Allal et al. (2004). The postoperative course was uncomplicated, and the cosmetic result was excellent.

In a neonate with membranous esophageal atresia but with a short broad fistula at the side of the membrane so that both the upper and lower esophagus were open to the trachea, the fistula appeared rather high in the neck. The dissection was done thoracoscopically but the actual closure and division of the fistula as well as resection of the esophageal membrane was done through a right cervical approach.

Discussion

With the availability of minimal access endoscopic surgical techniques for use in children and newborns, the optimal approach for dealing with an H type tracheoesophageal fistula should be reevaluated. At present we can not answer the question whether a thoracoscopic approach will be feasible in all patients with an H type fistula, but even when the fistula appears to be in too high a cervical position to be dealt with thoracoscopically, not much harm is done by doing the dissection thoracoscopically as far as possible and by continuing the dissection through a cervical approach.

References

Allal H, Montes-Tapia F, Andina G, et al (2004) Thoracoscopic repair of H-type tracheoesophageal fistula in the newborn: a technical case report. J Pediatr Surg 39:1568–1570

Abdomen

General

Chapter 30

Anesthesia for Pediatric Laparoscopy

Cindy S.T. Aun and Manoj K. Karmakar

Introduction

Recent years have seen an increasing interest in the use of laparoscopic surgery (LS) in children. Compared with conventional open surgery (OS), LS is considered minimally invasive and offers several potential benefits which include less postoperative pain, less respiratory depression, better cosmetic results, and earlier postoperative recovery. However associated physiological derangements seen during LS, which are not part of conventional OS, are challenges for the anesthesiologists caring for children undergoing LS. An appraisal of the associated physiological effects and the potential problems encountered during LS in children are essential for optimal anesthetic care. This chapter reviews the anesthetic management and perioperative care of children undergoing LS.

Preoperative Assessment and Investigation

Children for LS may present with a spectrum of scenarios. It ranges from an otherwise healthy child for simple laparoscopy to one with severe systemic disease for emergency laparoscopy. The principle of management is similar to that for any child presenting for OS. A thorough case review and a complete physical examination should be carried out to identify any medical condition that might alter the perioperative care, in particular problems such as a bleeding disorder, congenital heart disease, or pulmonary dysfunction. Medical contraindications for LS are relative. The risks and benefits should be carefully estimated. Events during laparoscopy such as high airway pressure, hypercarbia, hypothermia, and increased sympathetic stimulation are factors that increase pulmonary vascular resistance, which may result in the reversal of shunt in children with a congenital left to right intracardiac shunt. Pulmonary dysfunction may cause perioperative impairment in gas exchange. The hydration status should be carefully assessed preoperatively and corrected if necessary since the decrease in cardiac output seen after a pneumoperitoneum may be exaggerated. The need for laboratory investigations depends on the general condition of the patient and the complexity of the scheduled laparoscopic procedure. In general, healthy children do not need any special investigations. However, blood should be readily available for transfusion since major hemorrhage, although rarely seen with experienced surgeons, is a potential complication.

Premedication

Premedication to facilitate the induction of anesthesia in children presenting for LS should not be any different from that for other types of surgery. The choice depends on the anxiety level and physical status of the patient. Midazolam 0.5 mg.kg$^{\times 1}$ given orally half an hour before anesthesia facilitates the parental separation process. Parental presence is also commonly used to decrease preoperative anxiety. H_2 receptor antagonists such as cimetidine or ranitidine may be considered in patients with a high risk for pulmonary aspiration. Eutectic mixture of local anesthetics (EMLA) or amethocaine gel should be applied topically if an intravenous induction is planned.

Anesthesia

The goals of anesthesia are to provide conditions required for surgery and to rectify the physiological derangements. Although regional anesthesia (epidural or spinal), as the sole anesthetic, has been described for brief LS in adults, it is not recommended in children. General anesthesia with neuromuscular blockade, tracheal intubation, and intermittent positive pressure ventilation (IPPV) is the anesthetic technique of choice.

Induction of Anesthesia

The choice between intravenous or inhalation induction of anesthesia depends on the availability of venous access and the patient and anesthesiologist's preference. Thiopentone or propofol is recommended for intravenous induction otherwise an inhalation anesthetic such as sevoflurane or halothane may be used. It is advisable to avoid inadvertently distending the stomach during mask ventilation and to decompress the stomach routinely after endotracheal intubation in order to minimize the potential for visceral injury during trocar insertion. Rapid sequence induction with cricoid pressure should be performed in children with a risk for regurgitation and aspiration.

Endotracheal Tubes

An endotracheal tube (ETT) protects the lower airway and reduces the risk of gastric content aspiration at induction and during laparoscopy when the intra-abdominal pressure (IAP) increases. Traditionally uncuffed endotracheal tubes are used in children less than 10 years old (Cote and Tordes 1993). An appropriately sized tube should be selected so as to allow for an audible air leak around the tube at a peak inflation pressure of 20–30 cmH$_2$O. This practice allows one to use an ETT of the largest possible internal diameter, and at the same time minimize the pressure exerted on the tracheal mucosa, thereby reducing the risk for postextubation airway complications.

Recently, there has been increased interest in the use of cuffed ETT in children. Potential benefits include the avoidance of repeated laryngoscopy to change the ETT, better protection of the lower airway, less gas leak from the breathing system allowing the use of low fresh gas flows, and reduction of operating room pollution by anesthetic gases. However, the routine use of cuffed endotracheal tubes in infants and small children is controversial (Erb and Frei 2001). During LS, a cuffed ETT is particularly useful because the inflation of the cuff can be adjusted and thereby gas leak around the ETT can be reduced. This allows adequate ventilation to be maintained even though the peak airway pressure increases after creation of the pneumoperitoneum. However, the trade-off is an ETT with a smaller internal diameter when compared with an uncuffed tube. The formula that one can use to select a cuffed ETT (internal diameter in millimeters) is: [age / 4] + 3 (Khine et al. 1997). The formula for an uncuffed ETT has been: [age / 4] + 4.

Maintenance of Anesthesia and Ventilation

A balanced anesthetic technique using inhalation anesthetics, intravenous opioids, and non-depolarizing neuromuscular blocking agents is generally used for maintenance of anesthesia. However, a total intravenous anesthesia technique based on propofol and short-acting intravenous opioids such as remifentanil or alfentanil can also be used as an alternative (Manner

et al. 1998). The use of nitrous oxide (N$_2$O) during LS is controversial (Taylor et al. 1992). The concerns include its ability to cause bowel distension that might obscure the view of the surgical field (Eger and Saidman 1965), the increased risk of postoperative nausea and vomiting (Lonie and Harper 1986), and increased pressure within the ETT cuff. N$_2$O is 30 times more soluble than nitrogen. Diffusion of N$_2$O into a closed air-filled space is faster than the rate at which nitrogen can diffuse out, resulting in expansion of these gas-filled spaces in the body such as the bowels, ETT cuff, and air emboli should this happen. Studies in adults show no difference in the operating condition whether N$_2$O is used or not (Taylor et al. 1992). However, considering the pros and cons, and the relatively small size of the peritoneal cavity in children it may be preferable to omit N$_2$O.

The major difference in the anesthetic management between LS and conventional open abdominal surgery is related to the cardiopulmonary effects of the pneumoperitoneum. Raised IAP causes a cephalad displacement of the diaphragm which is further exacerbated by the head down position during surgery. Therefore the reduction in lung volumes including the functional residual capacity seen during general anesthesia can be aggravated. Pulmonary compliance is reduced (30–50%) and airway resistance is increased (20–30%), leading to an increase in peak airway pressure during mechanical ventilation (Bergesio et al. 1999; Hirvonen et al. 1995). Ventilation perfusion mismatch and alveolar dead space is also increased. Increase in the latter is generally reflected by an increase in the arterial to end-tidal P$_{CO2}$ (a-et PCO$_2$) gradient. Moreover, young infants with immature respiratory function are prone to small airway collapse during normal tidal ventilation with consequent atelectasis and hypoxemia. Ventilation should therefore be controlled for adequate oxygenation and carbon dioxide (CO$_2$) elimination. The use of positive end-expiratory pressure to reduce small airways closure during IPPV may help maintain arterial oxygenation. However, it may transiently decrease the pulmonary CO$_2$ elimination (Johnson and Breen 1999). The increase in CO$_2$ load during LS is mainly due to the absorption of the CO$_2$ insufflated, although increased metabolic production has also been suggested (Hirvonen et al. 1995). Approximately a 30% increase in minute ventilation is required to maintain normocarbia during LS (Hirvonen et al. 1995). In young children, pressure-controlled ventilation is traditionally used to circumvent the leak around the uncuffed ETT. However with a cuffed ETT, one may use the volume-controlled mode of ventilation. Airway pressure should be closely monitored and a limit for peak airway pressure set at 30 cmH$_2$O to reduce the risk of barotrauma to the lungs.

Intraoperative Fluid and Cardiovascular Function

Adequate peripheral venous access for intravenous fluid and drug administration must be secured before commencing surgery as it is extremely difficult to establish additional intravenous access later on during surgery. It is preferable to position the venous access above the diaphragm, as the pneumoperitoneum by compressing the inferior vena cava may limit the entry of administered fluids and drugs into the central circulation if the venous access were to be in the lower extremities. Central venous cannulation is indicated if peripheral venous access is impossible or when central venous pressure monitoring is required.

Several studies have evaluated the hemodynamic changes, using echocardiography, during LS in children. In children 2–6 years of age, the cardiac index decreases by 13% when the IAP is increased to 12 mmHg. The authors considered this clinically acceptable and suggested that an IAP of 12 mmHg was safe for LS in healthy children and a lower IAP be used in cases with compromised cardiovascular functions (Sakka et al. 2000). In another study where infants had a brief laparoscopy, the stroke volume index decreased (30%) and systemic vascular resistance index increased (60%) with no change in mean arterial pressure and end-tidal CO_2 (Gueugniaud et al. 1998). Decreased renal plasma flow, glomerular filtration rate, and urine output have also been reported in patients undergoing laparoscopic cholecystectomy with the IAP maintained at 12 mmHg (Iwase et al. 1993). Hemodynamic changes return to normal once the pneumoperitoneum is released. Intravenous fluid therapy is usually judged clinically based on factors such as intraoperative fluid losses and the hemodynamic changes. As a patient's position during surgery may be quite extreme, areas prone to pressure injury should be protected.

Monitoring

The level of monitoring depends on the clinical condition of the patient and the nature of the laparoscopic procedure. A routine minimum standard should include continuous electrocardiography, automated non-invasive blood pressure, pulse oximetry, temperature, and capnography. The end-tidal CO_2 generally reflects $PaCO_2$ and is used to adjust ventilatory requirements during surgery. However, end-tidal CO_2 may not consistently reflect $PaCO_2$ especially in infants. The respiratory frequency setting is usually faster and, together with increased IAP, the arterial to end-tidal (a-et) CO_2 gradient can be variable. Paradoxically a negative a-et CO_2 gradient has been reported in adults (Bures et al. 1996) and children (Laffon et al.

1998). A precordial stethoscope may help identify inadvertent endobronchial intubation should it occur. Expired tidal volume and airway pressure should be monitored to track changes in lung compliance. Invasive hemodynamic monitoring such as arterial pressure monitoring is useful in difficult and prolonged laparoscopy. It allows continuous monitoring of the arterial blood pressure and facilitates arterial blood gases sampling whenever necessary. Transesophageal echocardiography is an option for continuous cardiovascular monitoring. Core temperature should be monitored routinely. Exposure of the peritoneal cavity to a large volume of cold, non-humidified CO_2 that is continuously insufflated may contribute to the development of hypothermia, especially in small children who have a high body surface area to mass ratio and little subcutaneous fat to preserve heat. A peripheral nerve stimulator should be used to monitor the degree of neuromuscular blockade. Adequate muscle paralysis reduces muscular straining during light general anesthesia which prevents the surges in the IAP during laparoscopy. After surgery, any residual CO_2 in the abdomen should be desufflated as completely as possible to reduce CO_2 trapping that may contribute to postoperative nausea and vomiting and by irritating the undersurface of the diaphragm produce shoulder pain. Generally, in healthy children, anesthetic agents can then be discontinued, neuromuscular blockade reversed, and trachea extubated when the patient is awake. However, when compromise of postoperative ventilation is anticipated or when CO_2 load is relatively large, for example small infants who have prolonged laparoscopic procedures such as after a one-stage pull-through or Kasai procedure, it may be preferable to ventilate these children electively in the postoperative period.

Postoperative Pain

Postoperative pain after LS results from a variety of causes including the laparoscopy instrument and trocar insertion ports in the abdominal wall, distention of the peritoneum by residual CO_2, irritation of the phrenic and vagus nerve, visceral pain from the operation site, and musculoskeletal pain resulting from positioning during surgery. Currently there is a paucity of high-quality data in the literature about postoperative pain in children after LS. However, two prospective randomized single-blinded studies in children undergoing appendectomy reported that postoperative pain is maximal during the first 24 h after the laparoscopic approach (Lejus et al. 1996; Lintula et al. 2001). Pain usually presents in the abdomen but can also present in the back and shoulder. Shoulder pain, which can last for 2–29 h (Lintula et al. 2001), affects 35% of children after laparoscopic appendicectomy (Lejus et al. 1996). Children who undergo laparoscopic appendicectomy for uncomplicated appendicitis experience less pain, require fewer doses of rescue analgesics after surgery, and have a shorter hospital stay than children who undergo open appendicectomy (Lintula et al. 2001). However, if patients with complicated appendicitis (abscess formation) are also considered then there are no benefits in postoperative pain or analgesic requirements between laparoscopic or open appendicectomy (Lejus et al. 1996).

Pain after LS in children is best managed by a multimodal approach using a combination of opioids and non-steroidal antiinflammatory drugs (NSAIDs). Opioids such as morphine or pethidine (meperidine) via the intravenous route as patient-controlled analgesia (PCA) or nurse-controlled analgesia (NCA) is preferred. However, the intramuscular route may also be used in centers with lesser facility. NSAIDs can be used as an adjunct to opioid analgesics or alone in minor procedures. They may be administered rectally (diclofenac, acetaminophen) or intravenously (ketorolac) in the early postoperative period and switched to the oral route when patient can tolerate regular oral feed. Infiltration of the multiple port and trocar insertion sites in the abdominal wall with a local anesthetic agent (bupivacaine or levobupivacaine) at the end of surgery can be used empirically. There are also no data in children to support the effectiveness of instillation of local anesthetic into the peritoneal cavity or the gall bladder bed after laparoscopic cholecystectomy, as reported in adults. Further research in these areas is warranted.

References

Bergesio R, Hebre W, Lanteri C, et al (1999) Changes in respiratory mechanics during abdominal laparoscopic surgery in children. Anaesth Intensive Care 27:245–248

Bures E, Fusciardi J, Lanquetot H, et al (1996) Ventilatory effects of laparoscopic cholecystectomy. Acta Anaesthesiol Scand 40:566–573

Cote CJ, Tordes ID (1993) The pediatric airway. In: Cote CJ, Ryan JF, Todres ID, Goudsouzian NG (eds) A Practice of Anesthesia for Infants and Children, 2nd edn. Saunders, Philadelphia, pp 55–83

Eger T, Saidman LJ (1965) Hazards of nitrous oxide anesthesia in bowel obstruction and pneumothorax. Anesthesiology 26:61–66

Erb T, Frei FJ (2001) The use of cuffed endotracheal tubes in infants and small children. Anaesthetist 50:395–400

Gueugniaud PY, Abisseror M, Moussa M, et al (1998) The hemodynamic effects of pneumoperitoneum during laparoscopic surgery in healthy infants: assessment by continuous esophageal aortic blood flow echo-Doppler. Anesth Analg 86:290–293

Hirvonen EA, Nuutinen LS, Kauko M (1995) Ventilatory effects, blood gas changes, and oxygen consumption during laparoscopic hysterectomy. Anesth Analg 80:961–966

Iwase K, Takenaka H, Ishizaka T, et al (1993) Serial changes in renal function during laparoscopic cholecystectomy. Eur Surg Res 25:203–212

Johnson JL, Breen PH (1999) How does positive end-expiratory pressure decrease pulmonary CO_2 elimination in anesthetized patients? Respir Physiol 118:227–236

Khine HH, Corddry DH, Kettrick RG, et al (1997) Comparison of cuffed and uncuffed endotracheal tubes in young children during general anesthesia. Anesthesiology 86:627–631

Laffon M, Goucher A, Sitbon P, et al (1998) Difference between arterial and end tidal carbon dioxide pressures during laparoscopy in paediatric patients. Can J Anaesth 45:561–563

Lejus C, Delile L, Plattner V, et al (1996) Randomized, single-blinded trial of laparoscopic versus open appendectomy in children: effects on postoperative analgesia. Anesthesiology 84:801–806

Lintula H, Kokki H, Vanamo K (2001) Single-blind randomized clinical trial of laparoscopic versus open appendicectomy in children. Br J Surg 88:510–514

Lonie DS, Harper NJ (1986) Nitrous oxide, anaesthesia and vomiting: the effects of nitrous oxide on the incidence of vomiting in gynaecological laparoscopy. Anaesthesia 41:703–707

Manner T, Aantaa R, Alanen M (1998) Lung compliance during laparoscopic surgery in paediatric patients. Paediatr Anaesth 8:25–29

Sakka SG, Huettemann E, Petrat G, et al (2000) Transoesophageal echocardiographic assessment of haemodynamic changes during laparoscopic herniorrhaphy in small children. Br J Anaesth 84:330–334

Taylor E, Feinstein R, White PF, et al (1992) Anesthesia for laparoscopic cholecystectomy. Is nitrous oxide contraindicated? Anesthesiology 76:541–543

Chapter 31

The Basics of Laparoscopy

Mark L. Wulkan, Daniel F. Saad, and Curt S. Koontz

Introduction

Laparoscopy in children was first described in the late 1960s; however the techniques were not widely adopted into pediatric surgical practice until the mid to late 1990s (Moir 1993; Rodgers et al. 1992; Tan 1994; Waldschmidt and Schier 1991). Currently, most pediatric surgeons are practicing some form of minimally invasive laparoscopic surgery. Some of these surgeries include appendectomy, cholecystectomy, fundoplication, splenectomy, decortication of empyema, lung biopsy, and mediastinal biopsy. As surgeons become comfortable with the techniques of laparoscopic surgery, more advanced procedures are being performed. Advanced laparoscopic procedures include, portoenterostomy for biliary atresia, congenital diaphragmatic hernia repair, as well as duodenal atresia repair. Many procedures that were traditionally done open are now being performed laparoscopically. The benefits of minimally invasive surgery are covered throughout the textbook, but briefly include faster return of function, shorter hospital stay, less pain, and better cosmesis (Blucher and Lobe 1994; Leape and Ramnofsky 1980; Tan 1994).

Equipment for minimally invasive endoscopic surgery has improved tremendously since the early 1990s. The early pediatric laparoscopists were hampered by 10 mm telescopes and instruments. In addition, the video quality was inferior to what is available today. State of the art equipment includes a full complement of high-quality 5- and 3 mm instruments and trocars, and an integrated operating suite. The integrated operating suite includes flat-panel video screens, multiple high-quality video inputs, as well as computer access to other online information, such as radiographic studies and the electronic medical record. These technologic advances have allowed the development of advanced minimally invasive surgical techniques (Blucher and Lobe 1994; Wulkan and Georgeson 1998).

Anatomy and Physiology

With knowledge of the anatomic peculiarities in infants and children, laparoscopic procedures in children and even small infants can be very safe. The liver in small children is relatively large and often extends below the costal margin. The bladder is a true intra-abdominal structure. Care should be taken to avoid injury to these structures. Other anatomic differences in infants are the possibility of patent umbilical vessels, omphalenteric remnant, and urachus. The abdominal wall of infants and small children is more compliant than that of older children and adult. The small child's abdominal wall is spherical in shape, as opposed to the cylindrical adult abdomen. This allows the pediatric laparoscopist to have relatively more room at lower pressures (Waldschmidt and Schier 1991).

Positioning

Patient positioning is very important to the success of the planned operation (Bucher and Lobe 1994; Lobe 1993). For pelvic procedures, the supine position is generally sufficient. However, for procedures that require combined laparoscopic and perineal approaches, the surgeon must be more creative. In neonates, the patient can be placed across the table at the end of the bed, allowing three-sided access (Wulkan and Georgeson 1998). Trendelenburg's position is helpful to facilitate pelvic exposure and allow the small bowel and transverse colon to fall out of the way.

For upper abdominal procedures, such as fundoplication, the "French" position is often used. The surgeon stands between the patient's legs (Lobe 1993). In younger children, the legs can be "frog-legged" to avoid the use of stirrups. For upper abdominal procedures, the reverse Trendelenburg position may be helpful (Rodgers et al. 1992).

Abdominal Access

Abdominal access is most often obtained through the umbilicus. Two widely used techniques are the Veress needle technique and the Hasson technique (Moir 1993). The author prefers to use the former Veress needle technique. A technique of Veress needle insertion is as follows. Once the patient is adequately anesthetized, the stomach is suctioned and the bladder is emptied with either a catheter or a Credé maneuver. It is

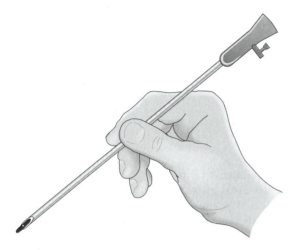

Fig. 31.1. Position for holding the Veress needle

important to note that the bladder is an intra-abdominal organ in infants and children and is susceptible to injury if not emptied (Godfrey et al. 1999). The umbilicus is anesthetized at its base. The author uses lidocaine 0.125% with epinephrine 1:400,000. Large quantities of the anesthetic can be used, which will overcome the esterase activity in the tissues and provide anesthesia for 12–18 h postoperatively. A vertical incision is made through the umbilicus at its base. The edges of the umbilical incision are elevated with forceps or a towel clip (in older children), and the Veress needle is inserted into the existing defect (you will usually find that most patients have a tiny umbilical defect). If the incision is properly positioned, the only layer that needs to be penetrated by the Veress needle will be the peritoneum. The Veress needle is directed inferiorly into the hollow of the pelvis. The Veress needle should be held like a "dart" near the tip (■ Fig. 31.1). This provides adequate control as the needle is inserted. The needle should also be directed away from any suspected adhesions or other intra-abdominal pathology. The surgeon is also cautioned that the liver in infants and children may extend below the costal margin (especially in neonates) and may be susceptible to inadvertent injury if the surgeon is not aware of its location. The surgeon will feel a "click" as the needle goes through the peritoneum. Once through the peritoneum, the needle should be advanced parallel to the abdominal wall.

The position should be verified using either the "blind man's cane" technique, or the saline drop test. The "blind man's cane" technique consists of sweeping the Veress needle under the abdominal wall to verify that it is free in the peritoneal cavity. The saline drop test is performed by placing a syringe of saline on the end of the Veress needle. First one aspirates and then removes the plunger while observing the saline. The

saline should drop freely into the abdominal cavity (■ Fig. 31.2). Once position is confirmed, the Veress needle is attached to the insufflation tubing. The surgeon may want to start insufflating with a low flow rate. The needle will generally restrict flow to 1–1.2 L/min. Note that many insufflators do not have a steady flow rate. They essentially "puff" gas into the abdomen and the higher flow rate uses bigger "puffs." This is why it is necessary to keep the flow rate low (1–2.5 L/min) in small infants during the procedure. A neonatal abdomen may be filled with as little as a few hundred cubic centimeters of carbon dioxide. In larger children you may begin with your flow at the final setting (usually about 5 L/min) and allow the needle to restrict the initial flow. If the needle is properly positioned, the abdomen should distend and can be checked by percussing the abdomen. Pressures used range from 8 mmHg for premature neonates to 12 mmHg in term infants to 15 mmHg in older children. Generally, the least pressure necessary for adequate exposure should be used (Bannister et al. 2003).

Rarely, there have been reported complications of the Veress needle technique including placement of the needle into abdominal visceral organs or vessels (Moir 1993). Bowel injury, however, is most common in patients who have had previous abdominal surgery. A complication that is unique to neonates is placement of the Veress needle into the umbilical vein, which can lead to fatal air embolism. In infants who still have an umbilical stump present, we prefer to make a transverse infraumbilical incision and aim the Veress needle inferiorly or laterally from the umbilicus. The Veress needle will need to pass through a fascial layer followed by the peritoneum. Other complications of Veress needle insertion include insufflation of the preperitoneal space. This can be determined if the insufflation pressure becomes high and the gas flow stays low shortly after initiating insufflation. If this is suspected, the Veress needle should be withdrawn and reinserted. Repeated attempts at placement, or conversion to an open access (Hasson) technique may be necessary.

Once the pneumoperitoneum is established, the primary trocar is placed. The author prefers radially expanding trocars; however any may be used. Care must be taken to avoid intra-abdominal injury. The trocar should be placed in a controlled fashion. Large deflection of the abdominal wall may lead to intra-abdominal injury. A short controlled "jab" is often the safest way to insert the first trocar, as this avoids large displacement of the abdominal wall toward viscera. However the easiest, and perhaps safest, is to use a radially expanding trocar in which a sheath over a Veress needle is placed after pneumoperitoneum is established.

The Hasson technique consists of an open "cutdown" procedure on the umbilicus (Moir 1993). Most

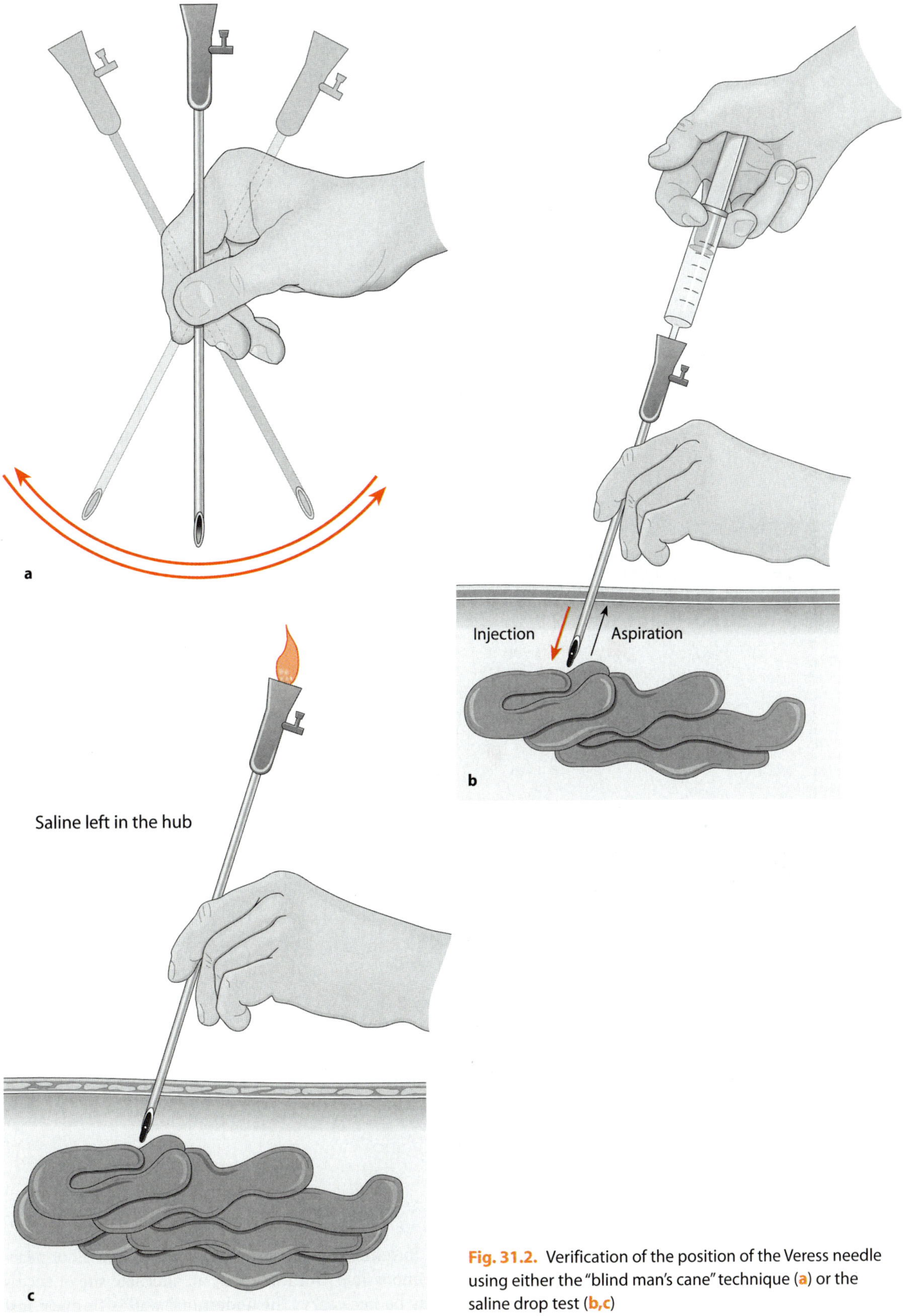

Injection   Aspiration

Saline left in the hub

Fig. 31.2. Verification of the position of the Veress needle using either the "blind man's cane" technique (**a**) or the saline drop test (**b,c**)

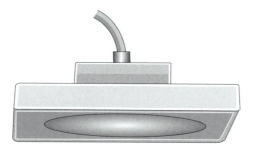

Fig. 31.3. Baseball diamond analogy to trocar placement

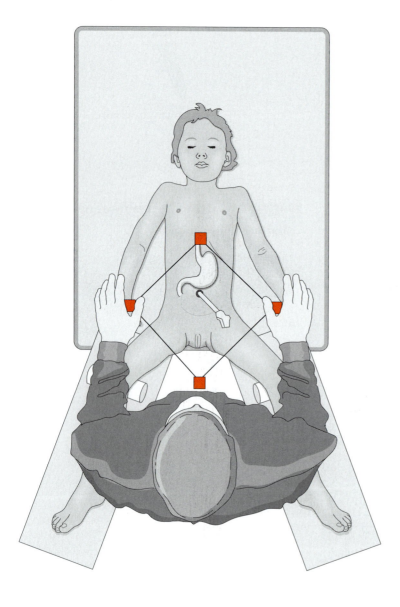

surgeons place fascial sutures on both sides of the midline. The fascia is opened between the sutures and the peritoneum is entered under direct visualization. The sutures are used to retract the fascia and to secure the trocar once it is in place.

In some patients umbilical access is difficult or nearly impossible. In these cases, an alternate site of access may be necessary. The abdominal wall is thinnest just below the costal margin. Either a Veress needle or Hasson-type technique can be used in either the right or

Fig. 31.4. Positioning of the camera scope between the surgeon's right and left hands allows better in-line view for the surgeon and is conducive to complex maneuvering

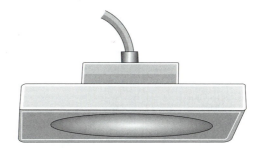

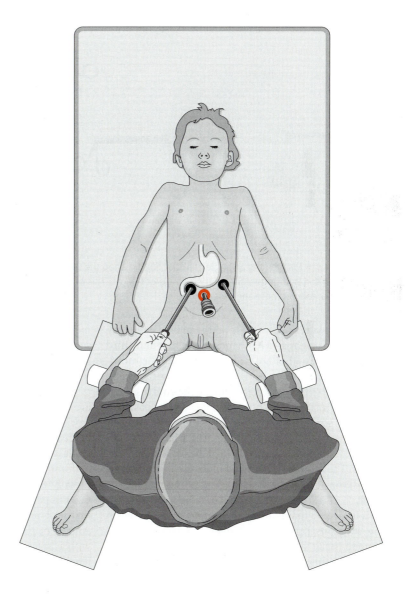

left subcostal space. The surgeon should try to aim below the liver margin on the right side. This technique may also be used when an umbilical trocar is not the best option, for example the author uses right upper quadrant access during a laparoscopic pull-through for Hirschsprung's disease (Wulkan and Georgeson 1998).

Trocar placement in laparoscopic procedures is critical. It can make the difference between a simple procedure and a difficult one. The principles of trocar and monitor placement are relatively straight forward. The concept of a baseball diamond (■ Fig. 31.3) is very useful in planning trocar placement. The surgeon

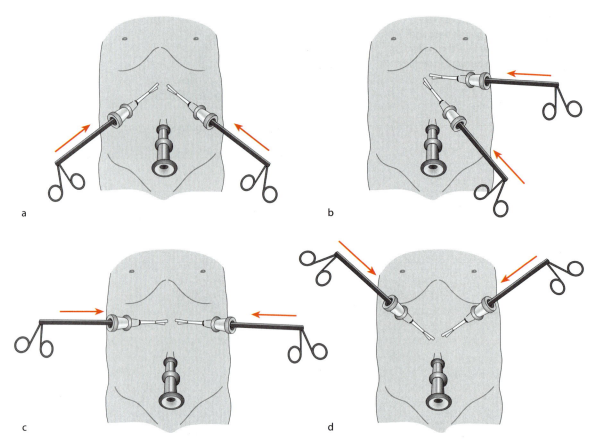

Fig. 31.5. a – d   a Maintaining an angle of about 60° between the surgeons right and left hands facilitates two-handed tissue manipulation and is important for suturing and knot tying. **b** This position is occasionally usual; however, it requires advauced skills. **c, d** Operating at these angles is difficult

is at home plate, the camera is on the pitcher's mound, the surgeon's right and left hands are at first and third bases, and the pathology is at second base. The monitor is placed in center field. This gives the surgeon an in-line view of the pathology. During the course of dissecting, suturing, and knot tying, it is always easier to keep the scope between the surgeon's right and left hands (■ Fig. 31.4). Retraction ports should, generally, be brought in outside the field of the working instruments. The monitors should be placed in an ergonomic position just below the surgeons horizontal line of sight.

It is ideal to maintain an angle of about 60° between the surgeons right and left hands to facilitate two-handed tissue manipulation. It is even more critical to maintain this angle for suturing and knot tying (■ Fig. 31.5).

Secondary trocars are placed under direct visualization after the laparoscope is introduced. Care is taken to avoid potential bleeding complications from injury to the epigastric vessels. The vessels can often be trans-illuminated through the abdominal wall with the laparoscope. An angled laparoscope directed anteriorly may be helpful. If the skin incision for trocar place-

ment is too small, there may be too much resistance for safe insertion. On the other hand, if the incision is too large, there may be a gas leak. Leaks are best managed with sutures and/or petrolatum gauze.

Standard trocar sizes range from 3 to 12 mm. There are currently several types of disposable and reusable trocars on the market. There are standard, protected-bladed trocars as well as non-bladed trocars. These include some in which you visualize the layers of the abdominal wall as you insert them. The author prefers radially expanding trocars which have several advantages in pediatrics. They tend to slip less in the abdominal wall, and the surgeon may easily increase the diameter of the trocar by replacing the inner cannula with a larger one. They are available in several different lengths including shorter trocars for small children and longer trocars for obese children.

Reusable trocars also come in many different sizes. Most have a flapper-type valve. They are available in multiple sizes from 2–3 mm to 12–15 mm. Unfortunately, there may be a size discrepancy between brands, and not every 3 mm instrument will fit through every 3 mm trocar. It is best to test your trocars with your instruments before making any purchases. Five- and

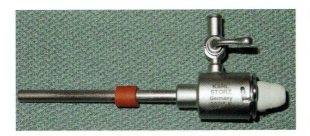

Fig. 31.6. An appropriately sized red rubber catheter placed over the trocar to make an "anti-slip" device

10 mm instruments and trocars seem to be more standardized.

Factors to consider when choosing trocars include ease and safety of insertion, stability in the tissues, slippage during the case, compatibility with existing equipment, and size of the trocar head. Very wide trocars may bump into each other restricting movement when performing minimal access procedures on smaller patients. Additionally, in small children and infants trocar slippage may become a problem. This can be solved by using a radially expanding trocar, or a reusable trocar with a "textured" shaft. There are several trocar "anti-slip" devices on the market; however it is very simple and inexpensive to place an appropriately-sized red rubber catheter over the trocar and secure this to the patient with a suture (■ Fig. 31.6).

Laparoscopic Instruments

Laparoscopic instruments are made by many different manufacturers and, as previously stated, the sizes vary. A full complement of instruments is available in 3-, 5-, and 10 mm sizes. The most commonly used instruments are 5 mm in diameter. In smaller neonates, 2- and 3 mm instruments are used. Many procedures can be performed using 3 mm instruments, even in larger children. As children approach adult size, 5 mm instruments become more useful. Before choosing instruments, one must also assess the stiffness and length of the instrument to see if it is appropriate for the procedure and the size of the patient.

Telescopes

At a minimum, the laparoscopist should have a 0° and a 30° telescope. The 30° telescope allows the surgeon to "look down" at the field. It can also be used to look around structures. Occasionally a 45° or 70° telescope is helpful to look around more acute angles. In general, the lesser angled, and the larger sized scopes provide brighter images. Telescopes are available down to 1 mm, which can be used for simple tasks such as exploration for a patent processes vaginalis. However, the smallest scopes are impractical for complex procedures.

Energy Sources

Monopolar electrocautery is the mainstay of laparoscopic procedures. It consists of a grounding electrode attached to a generator and a handpiece that is controlled with a foot pedal or a hand switch. Monopolar cautery can be used for both cutting and coagulation, and is generally safe (Carbonell et al. 2003; Moir 1993; Voyles and Tucker 1992). However, one must be careful not to cause unintended injuries. This can be avoided by making sure that your instruments are properly insulated. Electrocautery is used with cutting or coagulation current. Most generators have a "blend" setting. The electrocautery coagulates better and cuts better on a blend setting. In general, coagulation settings are for sealing vessels. The coagulation current has a larger area of tissue desiccation than cutting current. The most common instruments used to coagulate are a "hook," scissors, and grasper. Reasonably large vessels, such as the short gastric vessels, can be safely divided with hook electrocautery using coagulation current. The technique involves enough pull on the vessel with the hook to occlude the vessel, but not so much that the vessel is torn quickly. Another technique of coagulation is "pinch burning." A vessel is grasped and pinched with a dissector and burned with coagulation current. The technique of using the scissors with coagulation current as one cuts is not recommended, as this does not provide effective hemostasis.

Bipolar electrocautery is used by some laparoscopists because it is felt to be safer than monopolar electrocautery. Bipolar electrocautery consists of passing electrical current between electrodes on the instrument. These are often the opposing jaws of a grasper or scissors. The tissue injury is limited only to the area between the electrodes of the instrument.

Ultrasonic shears use ultrasonic energy to seal and coagulate vessels. This can be used on vessels up to 5 mm in diameter. There is less collateral damage compared to monopolar cautery, and burn injury is less likely.

There are several instruments which utilize computer-controlled impedance feedback bipolar technology to seal tissues. This is a bipolar device that uses impedance feedback through the tissues to change the nature of the electrical current. This is done in a way that seals vessels, and can be used on vessels up to 7 mm in diameter.

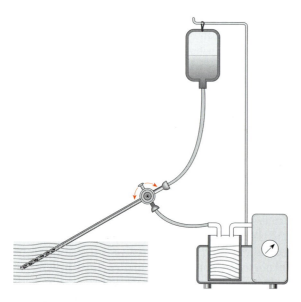

Fig. 31.7. Suction–irrigation system. Use small aliquots of fluid and, when suctioning, keep the tip of the suction device under the fluid to avoid evacuation of most of the pneumoperitoneum

Clips and Staplers

Most clips commonly used are disposable 5- and 10 mm instruments. Most of these instruments use titanium clips. There are also plastic locking clips which are applied with reusable applicators. These instruments are useful for ligating larger vessels and other structures, such as the cystic duct.

Linear cutting staplers that lay down two or three rows of staples on each side and cut between can be used for hilar vessel ligation, or bowel resection and anastomosis. The staplers may also be used to divide the appendix or Meckel's diverticulum.

Suction and Irrigation

There are several suction–irrigation systems on the market. Most provide irrigation under pressure and suction. There are both reusable and disposable systems. One of the limitations of reusable systems is that they tend to clog if not well cared for. It is generally best to avoid irrigation, if possible. Irrigation, especially with large volumes, tends to introduce fluid that may be difficult to entirely evacuate and may obscure vision. If irrigation is necessary to clean up blood or bile, small aliquots of fluid should be used. When suctioning, one should attempt to keep the tip of the suction device under the fluid to avoid evacuation of most of the pneumoperitoneum (█ Fig. 31.7). It is best to

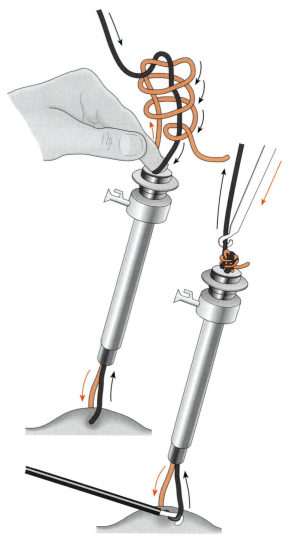

Fig. 31.8. Extracorporeal knot tying with the use of a knot pusher

avoid the need for suction or irrigation by meticulous attention to hemostasis. Blood absorbs light and may make visualization difficult.

Suturing and Knot Tying

There are several knot tying devices on the market. However, basic knot tying skills are essential for the advanced laparoscopic surgeon and can be performed either intracorporeally or extracorporeally. Facility with suturing and knot tying demonstrates advanced tissue manipulation and three-dimensional awareness, which is a must for complex laparoscopic surgery.

Extracorporeal knot tying is done with the use of a knot pusher. The sutures are left long and the throws are formed in the usual fashion and pushed down to

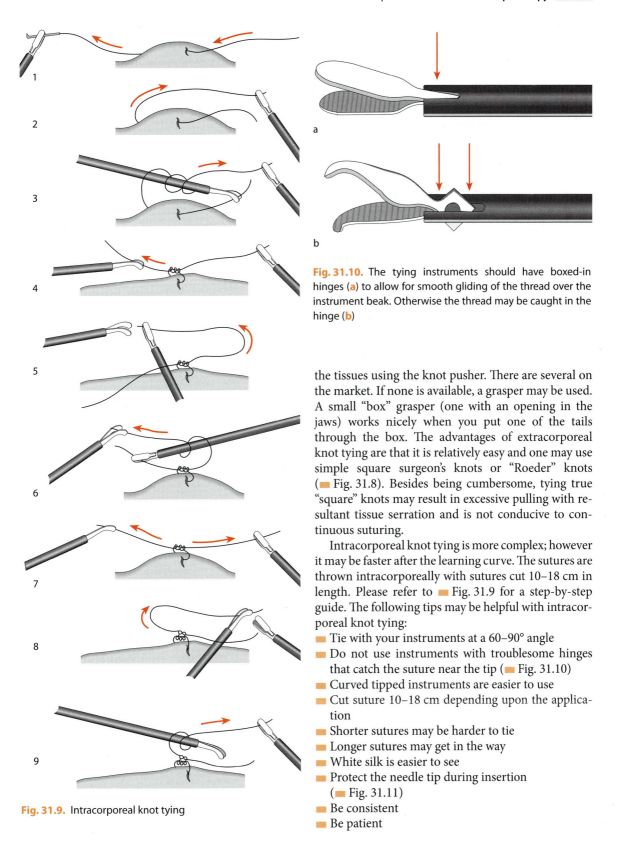

Fig. 31.9. Intracorporeal knot tying

Fig. 31.10. The tying instruments should have boxed-in hinges (**a**) to allow for smooth gliding of the thread over the instrument beak. Otherwise the thread may be caught in the hinge (**b**)

the tissues using the knot pusher. There are several on the market. If none is available, a grasper may be used. A small "box" grasper (one with an opening in the jaws) works nicely when you put one of the tails through the box. The advantages of extracorporeal knot tying are that it is relatively easy and one may use simple square surgeon's knots or "Roeder" knots (■ Fig. 31.8). Besides being cumbersome, tying true "square" knots may result in excessive pulling with resultant tissue serration and is not conducive to continuous suturing.

Intracorporeal knot tying is more complex; however it may be faster after the learning curve. The sutures are thrown intracorporeally with sutures cut 10–18 cm in length. Please refer to ■ Fig. 31.9 for a step-by-step guide. The following tips may be helpful with intracorporeal knot tying:

■ Tie with your instruments at a 60–90° angle
■ Do not use instruments with troublesome hinges that catch the suture near the tip (■ Fig. 31.10)
■ Curved tipped instruments are easier to use
■ Cut suture 10–18 cm depending upon the application
■ Shorter sutures may be harder to tie
■ Longer sutures may get in the way
■ White silk is easier to see
■ Protect the needle tip during insertion (■ Fig. 31.11)
■ Be consistent
■ Be patient

There are also pretied loop sutures that may be used for ligation of structures such as the appendix, cystic duct, or vessels (■ Fig. 31.12).

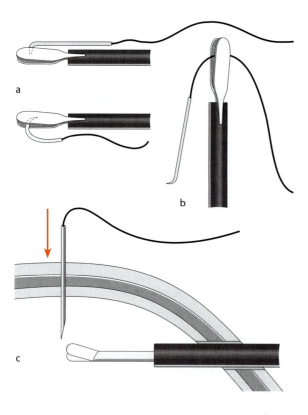

Fig. 31.11. Protect the needle tip during insertion through a cannula. This can be done in several ways (**a,b**). Alternatively, the needle can be inserted directly through the body wall (**c**)

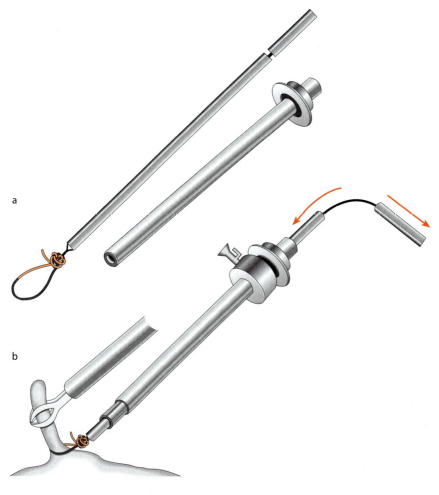

Fig. 31.12. Pretied loop sutures for ligation of appendix, cystic duct, or vessels

Hemostasis

Maintaining hemostasis is critical to any surgeon, but especially the laparoscopic surgeon. Occasionally there will be unexpected bleeding. The principles are basically the same as in open surgery. Exposure and application of a hemostatic technique is paramount. Do not forget that the laparoscopic instruments can be used to apply direct pressure to bleeding vessels. While pressure is applied, the suction device is introduced and exposure of the bleeding vessel is obtained. Once the vessel is visualized, it is grasped and coagulated, or clipped. If adequate hemostasis is not obtained in a timely manner and the patient continues to bleed, the surgeon should not hesitate to convert to a laparotomy.

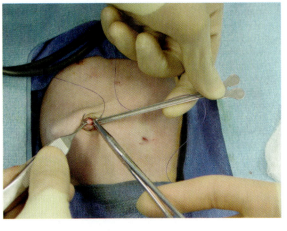

Fig. 31.13. Use of a grooved director to direct a stitch through the fascia while protecting the abdominal viscera

Closure

In general, the author chooses to close all umbilical port sites in an effort to prevent umbilical hernias. An attempt is made to reapproximate the fascia. Many larger hernias, however, will recur but will close spontaneously on their own, as in the case of most umbilical hernias. There are many different techniques for fascial closure. One technique that is very simple involves using a grooved director to direct a stitch through the fascia while protecting the abdominal viscera (■ Fig. 31.13). A half-round needle is used. In infants and small children, the fascia at 5 mm midline trocar sites is routinely closed, especially at the umbilicus. The fascia at smaller trocar sites off the midline is not routinely closed. In larger children, non-midline 5 mm trocar sites do not require fascial closure. Ten- to 12 mm trocar sites, however, should always be closed. The risk of trocar site hernia is less above the umbilicus.

Trocars should be removed under direct visualization, in order to make sure that no omentum follows the trocar out and to ensure hemostasis. Should there be significant bleeding from a trocar site, there are several ways to achieve hemostasis. The most common site of bleeding is an injured epigastric vessel. If the other trocars are still in the abdomen, the electrocautery may be used from inside the abdomen. If that does not work, a urinary balloon catheter may be placed into the trocar site and traction placed on the catheter until hemostasis is achieved (■ Fig. 31.14). An alternative is to place large transabdominal sutures around the vessel using a large needle. It is best to tie the sutures over a bolster to prevent injury to the underlying skin. Most often, the sutures or the catheter may be removed after 24–48 h.

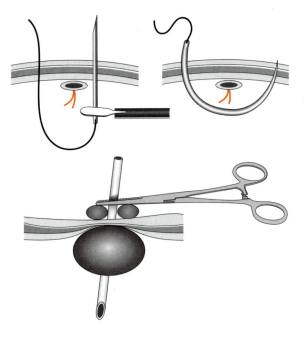

Fig. 31.14. Control of bleeding at a trocar site. *Top* Large transabdominal sutures can be tied around the vessel using a large needle. *Bottom* A urinary balloon catheter may be placed into the trocar site and traction placed on the catheter until hemostasis is achieved

References

Bannister CF, Brosius KK, Wulkan ML (2003) The effect of insufflation pressure on pulmonary mechanics in infants during laparoscopic surgical procedures. Paediatr Anaesth 13:785–789

Blucher D, Lobe TE (1994) Minimal access surgery in children: the state of the art. Int Surg 79:317–319

Carbonell AM, Joels CS, Kercher KW, et al (2003) A comparison of laparoscopic bipolar vessel sealing devices in the hemostasis of small-, medium-, and large-sized arteries. J Laparoendoscop Adv Surg Tech 13:377–380

Godfrey C, Wahle GR, Schilder JM, et al (1999) Occult bladder injury during laparoscopy: report of two cases. J Laparoendosc Adv Surg Tech A 9:341–345

Leape LL, Ramnofsky M (1980) Laparoscopy in children. Pediatrics 66:215–220

Lobe TE (1993) Laparoscopic fundoplication. Semin Pediatr Surg 2:178–181

Moir C (1993) Diagnostic laparoscopy and laparoscopic equipment. Semin Pediatr Surg 2:148–158

Rogers DA, TE Lobe, Schropp KP (1992) Evolving uses of laparoscopy in children. Surg Clin North Am 72:1299–1313

Tan H (1994) The role of laparoscopic surgery in children. Ann Chir Gynaecol 83:143–147

Voyles CR, Tucker RD (1992) Education and engineering solutions with potential problems with laparoscopic monopolar electrosurgery. Am J Surg 164:57–62

Waldschmidt J, Schier F (1991) Laparoscopical surgery in neonates and infants. Eur J Pediatr Surg 1:145–150

Wulkan ML, Georgeson KE (1998) Primary laparoscopic endorectal pull-through for Hirschsprung's disease in infants and children. Semin Pediatr Surg 5:9–13

Abdomen

Gastrointestinal Tract

Chapter 32

Esophageal Achalasia

Girolamo Mattioli, Alessio Pini Prato, Marco Castagnetti, and Vincenzo Jasonni

Introduction

Esophageal achalasia is a functional disorder of the esophagus characterized by abnormal motility of the esophageal body (non-peristaltic waves) associated with incomplete, delayed, or absent mechanical and not neurogenic relaxation of the lower esophageal sphincter (LES). The incidence of esophageal achalasia is about 0.3–11 per million per year (Podas et al. 1998). Only 5% of the patients suffering from this disease are younger than 15 years of age (Mattioli et al. 1997).

The association of childhood achalasia with alacrima and adrenal insufficiency in the triple A or Allgrove syndrome is well known (Ambrosino et al. 1986; Huebner et al. 2000; Verma et al. 1999). Associations with other diseases, such as Alport's syndrome, mongolism, Hirschsprung's disease, and megacystis-microcolon-hypoperistalsis syndrome have also been described (Al Harbi et al. 1999; Kelly et al. 1997; Leichter et al. 1988; Zarate et al. 1999). Familial cases have been reported (Kasgira et al. 1996; Nihoul-Fékété et al. 1991).

Esophageal achalasia is usually considered an acquired motility disorder. The onset of symptoms is progressive. Almost all the patients present with dysphagia for fluids, called "paroxysmal dysphagia", retention, and regurgitation of undigested food. Chest pain is described in up to 40% of patients. Pulmonary aspiration, failure to thrive, and halitosis are associated symptoms.

Many different forms of treatment have been proposed over the past decades such as calcium entry blockers, pneumatic dilatation, and botulin toxin injection. None of these are satisfactory and surgical treatment seems preferable. In 1914, Heller described a double anterior and posterior myotomy for the treatment of "cardiospasm." Later on, Zaaijer et al. proposed an anterior myotomy alone for the same purpose (Heller 1914). In children these techniques should also be associated with a fundoplication aimed at avoiding postoperative reflux and/or at protecting esophageal mucosa (Mattioli et al. 1997; Patti et al. 2001).

The technique described here is a laparoscopic anterior esophageal myotomy with partial anterior fundoplication.

Preoperative Preparation

Before Induction of General Anesthesia

Preoperative workup includes endoscopy, esophageal X-ray contrast study, and esophageal 24-h pH monitoring. After ruling out gastroesophageal reflux and organic stenosis, a manometric esophageal study is performed to confirm the diagnosis of achalasia. An esophagogram should be performed shortly before surgery, as in case of a very dilated esophagus it should be discussed whether a myotomy or segmental esophageal resection is required. This is exceedingly rare in children.

In order to reduce retention of food in the esophagus, the patient is put on clear fluids from 3 days before surgery onward. An enema is given twice, on the day before surgery and once just before surgery, in order to avoid colonic distension.

A nasogastric tube is inserted when the patient is still awake, in order to clean the dilated esophagus and hence reduce the risk of aspiration during tracheal intubation. Moreover the esophagus should be empty for intraoperative esophagoscopy and to minimize spillage of contents in the event of inadvertent perforation.

After Induction of General Anesthesia

The patient is operated on under general anesthesia. There is no need for a urinary catheter. Future port sites are infiltrated with Marcaine 1% 0.3 ml per port. Piperacillin 100 mg/kg is administered intravenously the morning before surgery and three times daily until no leakage is confirmed by X-ray contrast study, generally on postoperative day 1.

Positioning

Patient

The patient is placed in supine lithotomy position. The table is tilted in reversed Trendelenburg (■ Fig. 32.1).

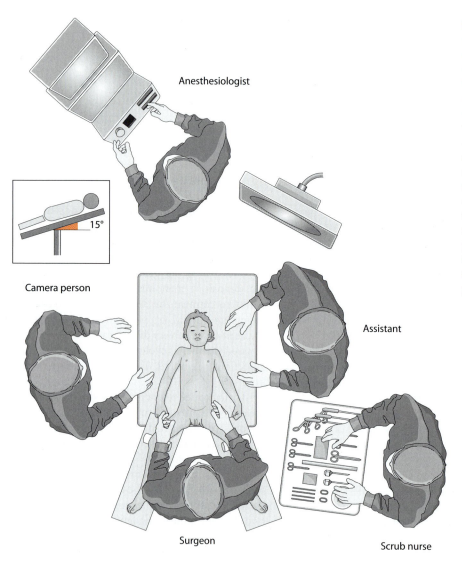

Anesthesiologist

15°

Camera person

Assistant

Surgeon

Scrub nurse

Fig. 32.1. Position of the patient, crew, and equipment. The surgeon stands in between the patient's legs. The scrub nurse with instrument table is on the right of the surgeon (left foot of the patient). The assistant stands on the left of the patient and the camera operator on the right. The anesthesiologist and his/her equipment stand at the head and right shoulder of the patient. The laparoscopic tower is near the head and left shoulder of the patient

Crew, Monitors, and Equipment

The surgeon stands in between the legs of the patient (■ Fig. 32.1). The camera operator is on the right and the assistant on the left of the child. The scrub nurse is between the assistant and the surgeon, close to the left leg of the patient.

The laparoscopy tower with monitor is positioned to the left of the head of the patient. The anesthesiologist stands at the upper end of the table in between his/her equipment, which is positioned close to the patient's right shoulder, and the laparoscopy tower. In this position he/she can help the surgeon to insert the esophagoscope to check the integrity of the esophageal mucosa after the myotomy.

Special Equipment

No special instruments or energy applying systems are required, but the esophagoscopy equipment should be on stand by.

Technique

The abdomen is prepared from the nipples down to the pubis and laterally to the posterior axillary lines. Special attention is paid to the cleaning and disinfection of the umbilicus.

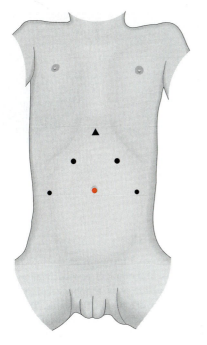

Fig. 32.2. Position of the trocars. A five-port technique is used. Only 3- and 5 mm instruments are used. The telescope is inserted through the umbilicus or alternatively through the midepigastric port. The operating ports are inserted in the left and right hypochondrium. The stomach is retracted downward by an instrument inserted through a port positioned to the left of the umbilicus. The liver is retracted upward. The position of the port for the liver retractor can be in the subxiphoidal or in the right subcostal area

A five-port technique is used. An open method is used to insert the first port, through a skin incision inside the umbilicus. In adolescents it may be better to insert this port halfway between the xiphoid process and the umbilicus in order to get a better view of the cardia. A 10–12 mmHg CO_2 pneumoperitoneum is created. All together five cannulae are inserted (■ Fig. 32.2):

1. Umbilicus or midepigastrium (5 mm), for the telescope
2. Left paraumbilical region (3 or 5 mm), for the downward retraction of the stomach during dissection
3. Subxiphoidal or in the right flank (3 or 5 mm), for retraction of the liver
4. Right hypochondrium (3 or 5 mm), working port for the grasper and dissector
5. Left hypochondrium (3 or 5 mm), working ports for dissector, hook, scissors, and needle holder

We generally prefer to use the 3 mm ports, even in older children. Two 5 mm ports are, however, required, one for a 5 mm telescope, for good-quality vision, and one for an ultrasound-activated scalpel, clip applier, or if necessary for a sponge to clean the operating field. The larger 5 mm port also allows for better irrigation and suction, which is advantageous when there is ongoing oozing during the myotomy. Lastly a larger port is more comfortable for the insertion of needles.

Cannulae

Cannula	Method of insertion	Diameter (mm)	Device	Position
1	Open	5	Telescope	Umbilicus
2	Closed	3	Working instrument	Right hypochondrium
3	Closed	5	Working instrument	Left hypochondrium
4	Closed	3	Grabbing forceps for retraction of the stomach	To the left of the umbilicus
5	Closed	3	Liver retractor	Underneath the xiphoid process or in the right flank

Procedure

The liver is retracted upward through the subxiphoidal port, and the stomach is pulled downward using an atraumatic fenestrated grasping instrument through the left paraumbilical port.

First the gastroesophageal junction is identified with a large bore indwelling catheter or an endoscopic light in situ. Next the phrenoesophageal ligament is divided, which allows the anterior esophageal wall to be freed completely. Only the anterior and lateral walls of the esophagus are dissected, without complete mobilization of the posterior wall, in order to leave the hiatus intact and to reduce the risk of posterior vagus damage and of gastroesophageal reflux. The anterior vagus nerve is identified, freed, and pushed to the right side (■ Fig. 32.3). A single anterior myotomy is performed on the left.

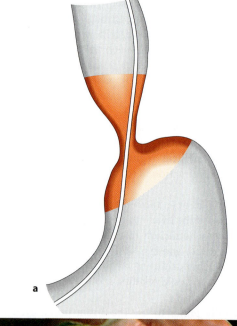

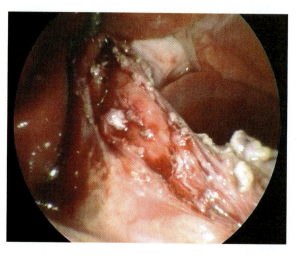

Fig. 32.4. Extramucosal myotomy of the lower esophageal sphincter. The transabdominal approach allows extensive transection or resection of the esophageal muscle layer without destroying the diaphragmatic hiatus. The esophageal muscle coat is transected longitudinally using monopolar hook electrocautery and scissors dissection. The longitudinal muscle layer is diathermized longitudinally first after which the circular muscles are divided using the hook and scissors. Once the total musculature has been divided, pulling on the transacted edges make further myotomy simple! A thin strip of muscle can be resected to increase the distance between the muscle margins. The myotomy ends when the mucosa completely herniates for a length of at least 6 cm and visual landmarks are reached. Proximally we stop when the esophagus becomes dilated and the anterior vagus nerve crosses the esophagus from left to right. Distally we finish the myotomy when the muscular fibers become vertical and the transverse esophagogastric vessels have been severed

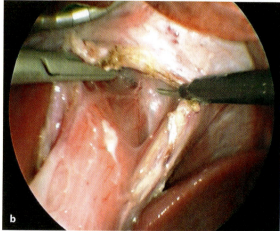

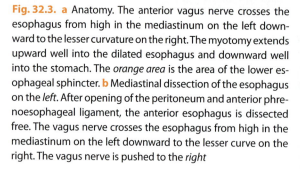

Fig. 32.3. a Anatomy. The anterior vagus nerve crosses the esophagus from high in the mediastinum on the left downward to the lesser curvature on the right. The myotomy extends upward well into the dilated esophagus and downward well into the stomach. The *orange area* is the area of the lower esophageal sphincter. **b** Mediastinal dissection of the esophagus on the *left*. After opening of the peritoneum and anterior phrenoesophageal ligament, the anterior esophagus is dissected free. The vagus nerve crosses the esophagus from high in the mediastinum on the left downward to the lesser curve on the right. The vagus nerve is pushed to the *right*

The muscular layer of the esophagus is coagulated longitudinally with a monopolar hook. Next blunt scissors dissection is used to separate the longitudinal muscular layer. The hook is then used again to pick up and to divide the circular fibers. Once the submucosal layer is reached, the mucosa is clearly seen as it herniates through the myotomy. Care must be taken to avoid

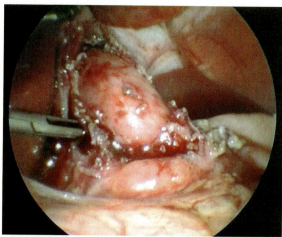

Fig. 32.5. Air is insufflated into the esophagus. The mucosa bulges into the myotomy. No leaks are visible

bleeding or mucosal perforation, particularly in the patients who have received esophageal dilations earlier. Intraoperative esophagoscopy can help to reduce the incidence of mucosal perforation. A stationary and dynamic manometric evaluation can be performed before and during dissection of the lower esophageal sphincter to help the surgeon determine the length of the myotomy. In two of our early cases muscle dissection was stopped when intraoperative manometric examination confirmed reduction of pressure to values less than 5 mmHg in the transitional high pressure zone. Later on we started to use visual landmarks only. The myotomy is stopped proximally where the esophagus is strongly dilated and where the anterior vagus nerve crosses the esophagus from the left to the right near the midanterior mediastinum (■ Fig. 32.4). Distally the myotomy is extended over the esophagogastric junction specifically at the site were a vessel crosses the hiatus from right to left and where the muscular fibers become vertical (■ Fig. 32.4). Instead of a myotomy, a thin strip of muscle can be resected to promote mucosal herniation and to allow for histological examination of the specimen. At the end of the myotomy, air is insufflated into the esophagus to check for leaks (■ Fig. 32.5).

We always perform an anterior 180° partial gastric plication in order to prevent gastroesophageal reflux and to protect the herniated mucosa by suturing the left and right esophageal muscular edges to the anterior gastric wall. Four non-absorbable 3-0 sutures, two on each side, with intracorporeal knots are used (■ Fig. 32.6 a–c).

No drains are placed, and the parietal holes are closed using absorbable cuticular suture or adhesive strips.

Postoperative Care

The nasogastric tube is removed soon after awakening. A contrast study of the esophagus is carried out on the first or second postoperative day to confirm mucosal integrity. Feeding is started after X-ray control and initiation of bowel movements. For pain relief acetaminophen is given.

Results

Since 1998 all patients with esophageal achalasia have been approached laparoscopically. Our series includes 12 children. The mean age was 10 years (range 5–14 years) and the mean weight was 45 kg (range 25–72 kg). Indication for surgery was dysphagia and respiratory symptoms, such as chronic cough or pulmonary infectious events related to microaspiration. Esopha-

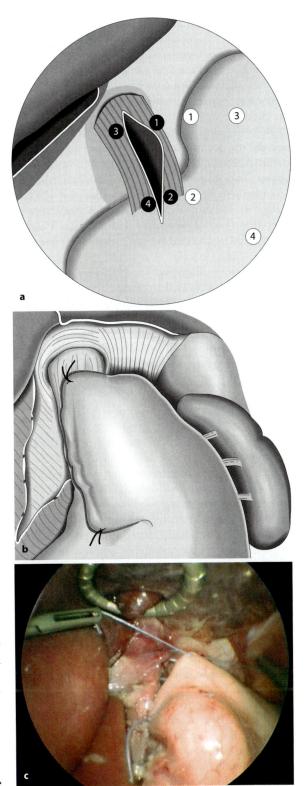

Fig. 32.6. a,b Partial, anterior 180° fundoplication. An anterior flap is created using the anterior wall of the stomach. Two non-absorbable sutures secure the anterior stomach to each side of the myotomy. This kind of procedure covers the herniated mucosa, preventing leakage and reducing the risk of reflux, without increasing the risk of dysphagia. **c** Intraoperative view

geal endoscopy and pH monitoring was normal in all the children. Esophageal manometric examination showed a characteristic esophageal motility disorder with non-propulsive low-amplitude activity of the body and delayed or incomplete esophageal sphincter relaxation. Esophagectomy was not needed in any of the children.

No conversion was necessary and mucosal perforation did not occur in any of the patients. Troublesome esophageal venous bleeding occurred in one patient but was stopped by application of a clip. No transfusion was required. The mean operative time was 125 min (range 90–180 min). No leakage was diagnosed postoperatively. Liquids were started in all on day 1 and all were on full oral feeding by day 3 when they were send home.

At a mean follow-up of 45 months (range 6–102 months), none of the patients developed gastroesophageal reflux on pH monitoring. One child developed recurrence of dysphagia 6 months after surgery. X-ray showed a stricture in the distal part of the myotomy, and dysphagia subsided after dilation. No patient needed reoperation.

Discussion

Whether the laparoscopic approach is better than the thoracoscopic one is still debated. We prefer the abdominal access for two reasons. First it allows the myotomy to be extended well onto the stomach (the lower esophageal sphincter is a subdiaphragmatic anatomical and functional structure) as recurrence of symptoms seems to be mainly related to incomplete distal myotomy. Second the abdominal approach allows for easy fundoplication.

Controversy exists as to whether a fundoplication should be performed at the same time and as to the preferred type. The decision to add a fundoplication appears to be a matter of personal preference. We think that a fundoplication reduces the risk of gastroesophageal reflux following hiatal dissection and transection of the lower esophageal sphincter. Moreover it protects the herniated mucosa from feeding injury, and therefore from postoperative perforation. We opt for an anterior partial type of fundoplication. The main disadvantage of the complete wrap (Nissen) is the creation of a high pressure zone that may cause obstruction in the poorly functioning esophagus. The anterior wrap (Dor-Thal) has the advantages of being an easier procedure and of increasing the pressure at the cardia only anteriorly, thus protecting the herniated esophageal mucosa while preventing gastroesophageal reflux. The disadvantage of a posterior fundoplication (Toupet) is the need of a complete esophageal dissection.

We underscore that we have only modified the exposure to the distal esophagus by using laparoscopic techniques. Prior to the laparoscopic era we also did a Heller extramucosal myotomy in combination with a Dor partial fundoplication. The advantages of the minimally invasive approach are well known and even more interesting in the patients requiring functional surgery of the esophagus. The complication rate is comparable with the open approach, but postoperative recovery is smoother (Mattioli et al. 2003).

In conclusion, surgery is an efficient and effective therapy for achalasia, and, in our experience, the minimally invasive approach is the current gold standard in both pediatric and adult populations.

References

Al Harbi A, Tawil K, Crankson SJ (1999) Megacystis-microcolon-intestinal hypoperistalsis syndrome associated with megaoesophagus. Pediatr Surg Int 15:272–274

Ambrosino MM, Genieser NB, Bangaru BS, et al (1986) The syndrome of achalasia of the oesophagus, ACTH insensitivity and alacrimia. Pediatr Radiol 16:328–329

Heller E (1914) Extramukose cardioplastik beim chronischen cardiospasmus mit dilatation des Ösophagus. Mitt Grenzgeb Med Chir 27:141–145

Huebner A, Yoon SJ, Ozkinay F, et al (2000) Triple A syndrome: clinical aspect and molecular genetics. Endocr Res 26:751–759

Kasgira E, Ozkinay F, Tutuncuoglu S, et al (1996) Four siblings with achalasia, alacrimia and neurological abnormalities in a consanguineous family. Clin Genet 49:296–299

Kelly JL, Mulcahy TM, O'Riordain DS, et al (1997) Coexistent Hirschsprung's disease and oesophageal achalasia in male siblings. J Pediatr Surg 32:1809–1811

Leichter HE, Vargas J, Cohen AH, et al (1988) Alport's syndrome and achalasia. Pediatr Nephrol 2:312–314

Mattioli G, Cagnazzo A, Barabino A, et al (1997) The surgical approach to oesophageal achalasia. Eur J Pediatr Surg 7:323–327

Mattioli G, Esposito C, Pini Prato A, et al (2003) Results of the laparoscopic Heller-Dor procedure for pediatric esophageal achalasia. Surg Endosc 17:1650–1652

Nihoul-Féketé C, Bawab F, Lortat Jacob J, et al (1991) Achalasia of the oesophagus in childhood. Surgical treatment in 35 cases, with special reference to familial cases and glucocorticoid deficiency association. Hepatogastroenterology 38:510–513

Patti MG, Albanese CT, Holcomb GW 3rd, et al (2001) Laparoscopic Heller myotomy and Dor fundoplication for esophageal achalasia in children. J Pediatr Surg 36:1248–1251

Podas T, Eaden J, Mayberry M, et al (1998) Achalasia: a critical review of epidemiological studies. Am J Gastroenterol 93:2345–2347

Verma S, Brown S, Dakkak M, et al (1999) Association of adult achalasia and alacrimia. Div Dis Sci 44:876–878

Zarate N, Mearin F, Gil Vernet JM, et al (1999) Achalasia and Down's syndrome: coincidental associations or something else? Am J Gastroenterol 94:1674–1677

Chapter 33

Laparoscopic Nissen Fundoplication

Philip K. Frykman and Keith E. Georgeson

Introduction

Gastroesophageal reflux disease (GERD) is a functional disorder that occurs when refluxed gastric contents produce symptoms or tissue damage. Indications for an antireflux procedure such as laparoscopic Nissen fundoplication in a child are: failure of medical therapy for GERD, dependence on aggressive or prolonged medical therapy, or high risk to develop GERD following placement of a feeding gastrostomy for nutritional support.

In 1991, Dallemagne et al. reported laparoscopic Nissen fundoplication in adults. In 1993, Georgeson and Lobe et al. separately reported laparoscopic Nissen fundoplication in children. Since then laparoscopic antireflux surgery has shown benefits to patients in reduced hospital stay and improved cosmesis, while being highly effective and performed with low morbidity and mortality (Sydorak and Albanese 2002). Although many other techniques are available for the surgical treatment of pathologic reflux in children, laparoscopic Nissen fundoplication remains the standard for correction of GERD.

Preoperative Preparation

Before Induction of General Anesthesia

The patient should be given nothing by mouth (NPO) for a minimum of 6 h and be well hydrated. There are no absolute contraindications to this technique, however relative contraindications include previous abdominal operations or cardiac or pulmonary dysfunction. The presence of a ventriculoperitoneal shunt is not a contraindication to this technique. Routine monitoring including capnography and pulse oximetry is indicated.

After Induction of General Anesthesia

An orogastric tube is placed for gastric decompression after induction of anesthesia and removed. An appropriately sized Maloney esophageal dilator is placed in the orogastric position so as to fit snugly. The bladder is emptied using the Credé maneuver in smaller children. A Foley catheter may be placed in patients where a lengthy procedure is anticipated, such as a reoperative procedure. A first generation cephalosporin may be given for prophylaxis. All access sites are injected with bupivacaine with epinephrine to provide for postoperative pain control and assist with cutaneous hemostasis.

Positioning

Patient

Infants and small children are positioned frog-legged at the foot of the operative table and secured with adhesive tape. Larger children and teenagers are positioned in dorsal lithotomy with the legs in stirrups. The operating surgeon stands between the patient's legs. The table is then placed in reversed Trendelenburg (■ Fig. 33.1).

Special Equipment

Energy Applying Systems

Electrocautery with a 3 mm hook attachment for infants and small children, and ultrasonic shears (5 mm) for larger children and teenagers are required.

Other Equipment

The liver retractor is held by a holder attached to the rail of the table on the right.

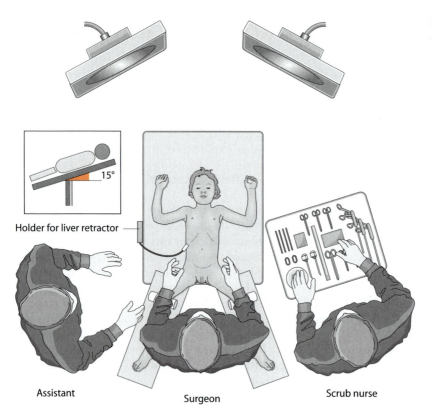

Fig. 33.1. Position of patient, crew, monitors and equipment

Holder for liver retractor

15°

Assistant

Surgeon

Scrub nurse

Technique

Cannulae

Cannula	Method of insertion	Diameter (mm)	Device	Position
1	Open	5	4- or 5 mm, 30° laparoscope, initial position	Umbilicus
2	Closed	3 or 5	Articulated liver retractor, secured with a holder	Right upper quadrant
3	Closed	4 or 5	Working instruments	Left costal margin
4	Closed	4	Laparoscope, later position	Supraumbilical, left of midline
5	Closed	3 or 4	Working instruments	Epigastric, right of midline

Procedure

The 5 mm port is placed through the umbilicus using an open technique (■ Fig. 33.2). The peritoneum is insufflated with CO_2 to 8–15 cmH$_2$O depending on the size of the patient. A 30° laparoscope is introduced in the abdomen. A 3- or 5 mm port is placed in the right anterior axillary line at the hepatic margin. An articulated retractor is placed through this port, positioned to retract the liver, and secured with a holder, thus exposing the hiatus. A 4- or 5 mm port is placed in the left anterior axillary line at the costal margin for toddlers and larger children. The position of this port is moved inferiorly (away from the costal margin) for infants to improve the working angle and allow a greater intracavity working distance. A 4 mm port is placed superior to the umbilicus and left of midline. This port will be the primary camera port for the operation. In patients where a gastrostomy will be performed in addition to Nissen fundoplication, this port site may be used as the gastrostomy site and location and should be adjusted to allow for stomach approximation to the abdominal wall. The fifth port is either 3 or 4 mm and is placed in the epigastric region either to the right of or through the falciform ligament. The surgeon operates through ports 3 and 5. The assistant holds the

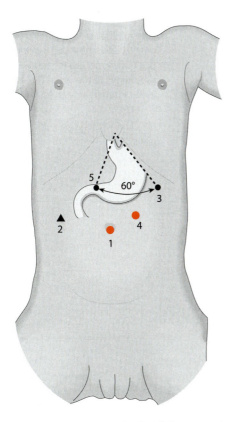

Fig. 33.2. Cannulae position and order of placement. A 5 mm port is placed in the umbilicus using an open technique and pneumoperitoneum is established (*1*). A 3- or 5 mm port is placed at the hepatic edge in the right midclavicular line for the liver retractor (*2*). A 4- or 5 mm port is placed at the left costal margin in the anterior axillary line (*3*). A 4 mm port is placed in the supraumbilical region to the left of midline (*4*). A 3- or 4 mm port is placed in the epigastric region to the right of midline either below or through the falciform ligament (*5*). Ports 3 and 5 are the primary operating ports and should be placed 60° apart in relation to the diaphragmatic hiatus

camera (port 4) and retracts using port 1. Either a mechanical holder or a second assistant may be used to hold the liver retractor.

The instruments used initially are the 3 mm grasper in the left hand and 3- to 4 mm endoshears with electrocautery attached in the right hand. The pars flaccida is incised in the avascular portion and carried superiorly using the endoshears. Small vessels traversing the superior edge are cauterized using gentle "touch" cautery with the closed endoshears and then divided. The incision is carried up to the right crus. The peritoneum is incised where the right crus meets the esophagus and, using sharp dissection, the plane between the esophagus and the right crus is developed inferiorly toward the gastroesophageal junction. Once the correct plane between the peritoneum and anterior esophagus is established, the peritoneum is elevated off the anterior esophagus to the left crus and incised. Care should be taken to identify and avoid injuring the anterior vagus nerve. The tissue plane between the esophagus and the left crus is established.

Attention is then turned to dividing the short gastric vessels. The assistant retracts the fundus to the right with a blunt grasper. The surgeon grasps the fundus near the greater curve and tents up the short gastric vessels which are divided using 3 mm hook cautery or a 5 mm ultrasonic scalpel. Once the lesser sac is opened, the division of the short gastric vessels is carried up to the superior pole of the spleen, thereby freeing the gastric fundus. The assistant retracts the cardia medially exposing the left crus. This maneuver enables the surgeon to divide the filmy attachments of the stomach to the diaphragm and develop the plane between the left crus and esophagus.

Attention is refocused on the right crus (■ Fig. 33.3). The assistant retracts the stomach to the patient's left

Fig. 33.3. Blunt dissection to develop the posterior esophageal space

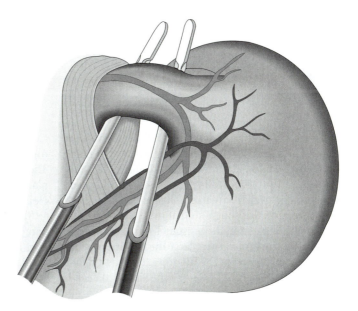

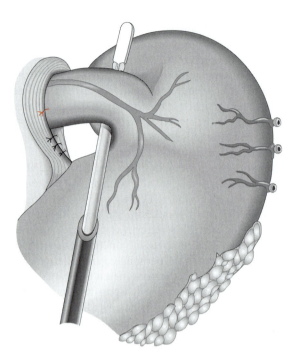

Fig. 33.4. Closure of crural defect with minimal tension. "Collar" sutures are placed at the 4 and 8 o'clock positions to secure the intra-abdominal esophagus to the crura. The 4 o'clock collar suture is hidden from view

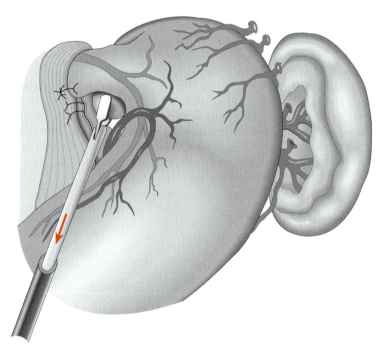

Fig. 33.5. The greater curve of the fundus is passed through the posterior esophageal window

and the surgeon sharply and bluntly dissects down the right crus to the confluence with the left crus, creating a window behind the posterior esophagus. Care is taken to identify the posterior vagal branch and avoid separating it away from the esophagus. The anesthesiologist retracts the bougie so that the tip is at the diaphragmatic hiatus and the assistant lifts the esophagus; this enables the surgeon to enlarge the posterior esophageal window to accept the fundoplication and define the crural defect (■ Fig. 33.4). The crural defect is closed using interrupted 2-0 or 3-0 (in infants) silk sutures on a ski needle and tied in intracorporeal fashion. The bougie is then advanced prior to the final suture placement to calibrate minimal tension of the crural closure.

The assistant retracts the stomach inferiorly to evaluate the length of intra-abdominal esophagus. Our goal is 2–3 cm for an infant and 3–4 cm for an older child. Further esophageal attachments can be divided to achieve the lengths mentioned above. Next, "collar"

Fig. 33.6. Order and position of suture placement for fundoplication

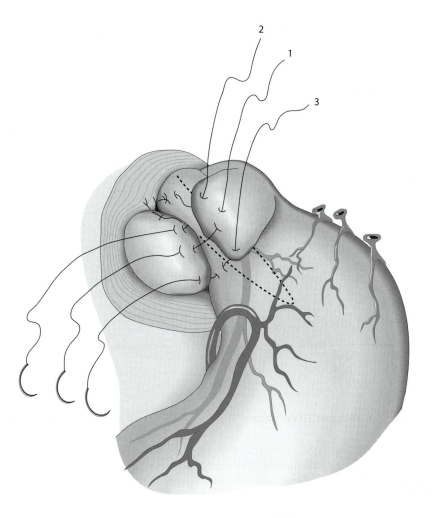

sutures of 2-0 silk are placed securing the mobilized esophagus to the right and left crus at the 8 o'clock and 4 o'clock positions, respectively. The bougie is retracted allowing the assistant to lift up the mobilized esophagus opening up the posterior esophageal window (▪ Fig. 33.5). The surgeon grasps the mobilized fundus in the right hand and passes it through the posterior esophageal window where the surgeon receives it with a grasper in the left hand and gently brings the fundus to the right side of the esophagus. Next, the surgeon performs the "shoeshine" maneuver with the fundoplication around the esophagus to ensure a loose, floppy, and symmetric fundoplication.

The assistant then grasps the leading edge of the fundoplication, and the surgeon places a single, simple interrupted 2-0 silk suture from left to right, approximating the fundus around the esophagus (▪ Fig. 33.6). A second suture is placed approximately 1 cm superior to the first suture incorporating the left portion of the fundoplication, anterior esophagus below the hiatus,

and the leading edge of the fundoplication and tied in intracorporeal fashion securing the fundoplication to the esophagus. The bougie should be advanced through the fundoplication and into the fundus. A third suture is placed approximately 1 cm inferior to the first, securing the edges of the fundoplication to the esophagus and tied. A fourth suture is placed between the middle and inferior sutures in a figure-of-eight fashion and tied (▪ Fig. 33.7). This fourth suture is placed to reinforce the sutures of the fundoplication. Care should be taken not to make the fundoplication too tight.

The bougie is removed and the liver retractor and ports are removed under direct vision with the laparoscope to ensure no port site bleeding. The fascia of the 5 mm port sites are closed with interrupted buried 2-0 or 3-0 polydioxanone suture. The umbilicus is closed using 4-0 or 5-0 fast-absorbing polyglycolic acid suture and the 3- to 4 mm port sites are closed using adhesive strips.

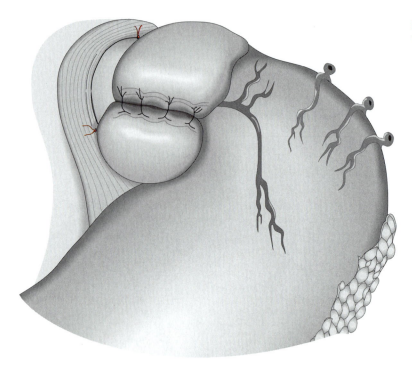

Fig. 33.7. Completed fundoplication

Postoperative Care

Patients are kept NPO overnight (without nasogastric tube) and started on liquids the morning of postoperative day 1. When patients have tolerated liquids they are advanced to a "no chunk" or puréed diet. Both patients and their parents are educated by the pediatric surgical team's dietician about the diet they must adhere to for 4 weeks following the operation.

Pain is controlled using intravenous ketorolac tromethamine (NSAID), acetaminophen (APAP, paracetamol), and judicious doses of morphine sulfate during the first 24 h. Most patients do not require narcotic analgesia at the time of discharge. Nausea is treated aggressively with intravenous ondansetron to avoid retching, as retching may cause disruption of the fundoplication. Patients are seen in follow-up about 2 weeks after surgery.

Results

There are no randomized controlled trials of open versus laparoscopic fundoplication in children, however there are some large retrospective series which form the basis of this review (Esposito et al. 2000; Georgeson 1998; Rothenberg 1998). Most patients undergoing laparoscopic fundoplication (without gastrostomy) were started on liquids by postoperative day 1, and the majority were discharged by postoperative day 2. Many of the neurologically impaired children received a

feeding gastrostomy in addition to the fundoplication, and had a longer hospitalization. The period of opiate analgesia requirement for most children after laparoscopic Nissen fundoplication is 1 day (Dick et al. 1998), and in one study 89% of patients needed only rectal and oral analgesics (Rowney and Aldridge 2000).

The complication rates of these large series are similar. The conversion rate ranged from 0.9% to 3.3%, with most occurring in the first 30 operations. The intraoperative complication rates ranged from 2.6% to 5.1% and postoperative complication rates from 3.4% to 7.3%. Intraoperative complications included esophageal and gastric perforations, and pneumothorax during hiatal dissection. Postoperative complications included dysphagia requiring esophageal dilatation, gastroparesis, pneumonia, and recurrent GERD requiring reoperation. The rate of recurrent GERD in these series ranged from 2.1% to 5%, however when physiologically studied can be as high as 14% (Tovar et al. 1998). The larger the number of children who retch postoperatively, the higher the recurrence rate.

Discussion

The recurrence rate of GERD in children undergoing open antireflux procedures is well known. The largest experience of over 7,400 patients found a recurrence rate of 7.1% (Fonkalsrud et al. 1998). When the patients are stratified, the rate was 5% for unimpaired and 15% for neurologically impaired. Patients with chronic lung disease (Taylor et al. 1994) and those under 3 months of age (Fonkalsrud et al. 1999) have higher recurrence rates. The laparoscopic antireflux procedure has a lower recurrence rate of 2.1–5%. Only as the number of these patients increases and they are followed for a longer period of time can an accurate long-term rate of recurrence be determined.

While the failure rate is low, the mechanism of fundoplication failure appears to be different between open and laparoscopic Nissen fundoplication (Graziano et al. 2003). In this study, the mechanism of failure showed increased wrap herniation and dehiscence compared to open fundoplication, where wrap slippage was the major mechanism of failure. Should the primary fundoplication fail for any reason, the reoperation can be readily performed laparoscopically.

Laparoscopic Nissen fundoplication in children can be performed safely with the advantages of a lower complication rate, quicker recovery period, and a lower failure rate than open fundoplication. The learning curve is significant because of the advanced laparoscopic skills required, but once these skills are mastered the procedure can be performed quickly and effectively.

References

Dallemagne B, Weerts JM, Jehaes C, et al (1991) Laparoscopic Nissen fundoplication: preliminary report. Surg Laparosc Endosc 1:138–143

Dick AC, Coulter P, Hainsworth AM, et al (1998) A comparative study of the analgesia requirements following laparoscopic and open fundoplication in children. J Laparoendosc Adv Surg Tech A 8:425–429

Esposito C, Montupet P, Amici G, Desruelle P (2000) Complications of laparoscopic antireflux surgery in childhood. Surg Endosc 14:622–624

Fonkalsrud EW, Ashcraft KW, Coran AG, et al (1998) Surgical treatment of gastroesophageal reflux in children: a combined hospital study of 7467 patients. Pediatrics 101:419–422

Fonkalsrud EW, Bustorff-Silva J, Perez CA, et al (1999) Antireflux surgery in children under 3 months of age. J Pediatr Surg 34:527–531

Georgeson KE (1993) Laparoscopic gastrostomy and fundoplication. Pediatr Ann 22:675–677

Georgeson KE (1998) Laparoscopic fundoplication and gastrostomy. Semin Laparosc Surg 5:25–30

Graziano K, Teitelbaum DH, McLean K, et al (2003) Recurrence after laparoscopic and open Nissen fundoplication: a comparison of the mechanism of failure. Surg Endosc 17:704–707

Lobe TE, Schropp KP, Lunsford K (1993) Laparoscopic Nissen fundoplication in childhood. J Pediatr Surg 28:358–361

Rothenberg SS (1998) Experience with 220 consecutive laparoscopic Nissen fundoplications in infants and children. J Pediatr Surg 33:274–278

Rowney DA, Aldridge LM (2000) Laparoscopic fundoplication in children: anaesthetic experience of 51 cases. Paediatr Anaesth 10:291–296

Sydorak RM, Albanese CT (2002) Laparoscopic antireflux procedures in children: evaluating the evidence. Semin Laparosc Surg 9:133–138

Taylor LA, Weiner T, Lacey SR, et al (1994) Chronic lung disease is the leading risk factor correlating with the failure (wrap disruption) of antireflux procedures in children. J Pediatr Surg 29:161–166

Tovar JA, Olivares P, Diaz M, et al (1998) Functional results of laparoscopic fundoplication in children. J Pediatr Gastroenterol Nutr 26:429–431

Chapter 34

Laparoscopic Fundoplication According to Toupet

Philippe Montupet

Introduction

André Toupet described the technique of posterior fundoplication in 1963. The technique remained in anonymity until the 1980s, when it gained popularity in the United States. We started to do Toupet fundoplications in 1976 by open approach. Since 1992, all our operations for gastroesophageal reflux disease (GERD) have been performed laparoscopically. Now, we have performed over 700 such procedures. One of the advantages of a partial fundoplication over a full one is that a partial fundoplication allows the patients to vomit and to burp. As a result the risk for developing a "gas-bloat syndrome" is lower.

Preoperative Preparation

Before Induction of General Anesthesia

Routine preoperative assessment includes an upper gastrointestinal tract (UGI) series and esophageal manometry. In this way anatomical lesions such as hiatal hernia and or esophageal dysmotility can be diagnosed. Moreover these investigations allow to compare the preoperative with the postoperative situation.

After Induction of General Anesthesia

After intubation and mechanical ventilation, a thin nasogastric tube (10–12 French) is inserted. In children weighing less than 12 kg, end-tidal P_{CO2} is measured. Ventilation is adjusted to keep end-tidal P_{CO2} within normal limits.

Fentanyl is used for intraoperative analgesia. Muscle relaxants are not systematically used. Mechanical ventilation is started at a higher frequency than normal to compensate for the CO_2 absorption. The periumbilical area is infiltrated with Marcaine. No antibiotics or urinary catheter are used.

Positioning

Patient

The child lies supine, and the operating table is tilted in head-up position. Since we use a 30° endoscope, less head-up position is required.

In patients less than 7–9 years of age, the legs are folded up at the bottom of the table. In older children the legs are extended and abducted onto leg supports so that the surgeon can stand in between them.

Crew, Monitors, and Equipment

Only one assistant is needed. A rigid arm support is anchored to the table and positioned over the left leg of the patient as a support for the assistant in order to avoid tremor and fatigue.

The video equipment is placed to the right side of the patient's head. All cables are fixed at the level of the right leg. The assistant, as well as the table of instruments, is positioned to the right of the surgeon. The surgeon stands at the bottom end of the table and faces the patient in front of him/her (■ Fig. 34.1).

Special Equipment and Instruments

No specific equipment and instruments are required. A suction and irrigation device is available but is not routinely installed. Bipolar electrocautery and a clip applier are available in the room, but are usually not used.

Two sets of instruments are available, and will be used according to age: 3 mm under 1 year of age and 5 mm if the child is older. All instruments are reusable and include a three-finger retractor, a smooth fenestrated grasper forceps, a hook, two needle holders, and scissors. A 30° telescope is preferred but a 0° is also suitable.

Non-absorbable sutures on a ski needle, 2/0 above and 4/0 under 1 year of age, are used.

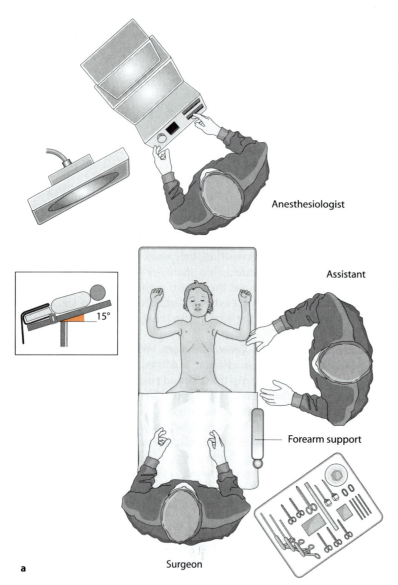

Anesthesiologist

15°

Assistant

Forearm support

Surgeon

a

Fig. 34.1. Position of the patient, crew, and equipment. **a** Children less than 7–10 years of age. Froglike position of the patient. The surgeon is at the bottom end of the table with the assistant to the left of the operating table. An armrest is attached to the table on the left and serves for stabilization of the forearm of the assistant. The assistant is always seated, and the surgeon most of the time. The screen is at the right upper end of the operating table.

Fig. 34.1. Position of the patient, crew, and equipment. **b** Children over 10 years of age. The patient is supine with the legs abducted on leg supports. The surgeon sits or stands in between the legs. The assistant is seated on the left of the operating table. An arm support is attached to the left of the operating table and serves for stabilization of the forearm of the assistant. The screen is at the right upper end of the operating table

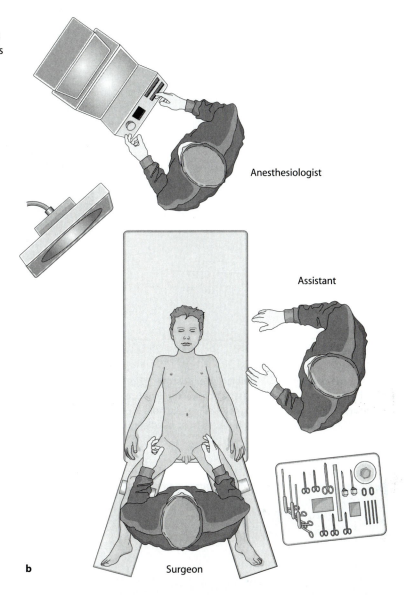

Anesthesiologist

Assistant

Surgeon

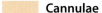
b

Technique

Cannulae

Four trocars are used: two for the surgeon's instruments and two for the assistant's instruments (scope and liver retractor) (■ Fig. 34.2). Hassan's technique is used for the insertion of the first port at the umbilicus. The three others trocars are disposable, light, and cheap. The three-finger retractor is placed through the upper port for retraction of the left lobe of the liver. The smooth grasper is introduced through the left upper quadrant port for retraction of the vault of the cardia. The electrocautery hook is introduced through the right upper quadrant port, and is used for both cutting as well as coagulation.

Pneumoperitoneum

Carbon dioxide is insufflated through the umbilical port at a pressure of 8–10 mmHg, according to the age of the child, and also according to the step of the procedure. The umbilical port is fixed with a purse-string suture that is passed through the fascia layer and is tightened in order to avoid leakage of gas. The same thread will be used at the end of the procedure to close the fascia.

Dissection

The lesser sac is widely opened unless it contains a left hepatic artery, which is saved (■ Fig. 34.3). By doing this a large and direct access to the right crus is ob-

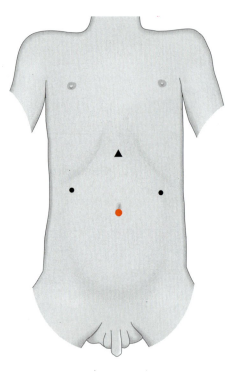

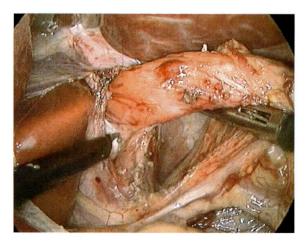

Fig. 34.4. The retroesophageal space has been developed and a good window created

Fig. 34.2. Port positions. *1* Umbilicus; endoscope (5 or 10 mm). *2* Under the xiphoid process; liver retractor (3 or 5 mm). *3* Left hypochondrium; grasping forceps, needle holder (3 or 5 mm). *4* Right hypochondrium; hook, scissors, needle holder (3 or 5 mm)

The dissection is close to the fascia of the left crus. The smooth grasper forceps is pushed toward the spleen through the gastrophrenic ligament. Then, the esophagus is retracted anteriorly and to the left by the smooth grasper forceps, and the retrocardial window is enlarged by section of the whole gastrophrenic ligament (■ Fig. 34.4).

The short gastric vessels do not need to be severed, because only the anterior wall of the fundus will be placed behind the esophagus by translation and rotation. The esophagus has to be freed on the right, anteriorly, and on the left wall, so that at least 4–5 cm of esophagus and therefore the complete lower esophageal sphincter comes to lie without tension below the hiatus (■ Fig. 34.4).

Hiatoplasty

The diaphragmatic hiatus is closed with one or two stitches of non-absorbable material. These are knotted gently and do not narrow the hiatus unless a hiatal hernia is present (■ Fig. 34.5).

Valve Positioning

The anterior wall of the fundus is pulled behind the abdominal esophagus as a wrap. The wrap initially encircles the esophagus completely and is held in place with one stitch, called a "frame" stitch, in order to keep the wrap in the abdomen during the further suturing (■ Fig. 34.5).

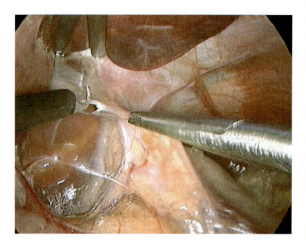

Fig. 34.3. Opening of the omentum minus

tained. The smooth grasper forceps is pushed in the angle between the right crus and the esophagus, after which the fascia is opened with the hook and the retroesophageal space entered.

The posterior vagus nerve is always identified, not only as it has to be preserved but also as it serves as a guide to find the fascia of the left crus which is found where the nerve reaches the anterior wall of the crus.

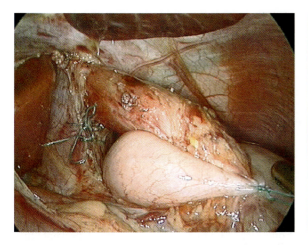

Fig. 34.5. The hiatus has been closed posteriorly to the mobilized esophagus and a frame stitch is being applied

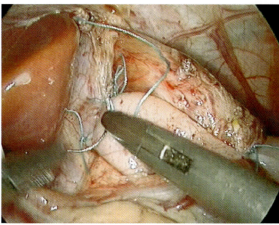

Fig. 34.6. Suturing of the right side anterior fundus to the right crus

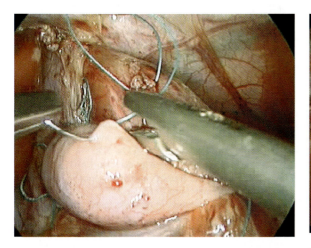

Fig. 34.7. Suturing of the right side fundus to the right anterior esophagus

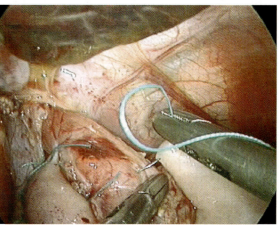

Fig. 34.8. Suturing of the left side fundus to the left anterior esophagus

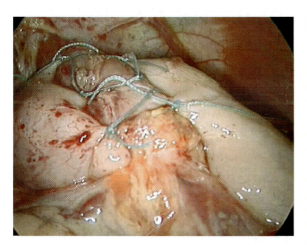

Fig. 34.9. The frame stitch has been removed and the completed fundoplication is shown

Valve Attachment

The valve is tacked to the right crus with three rows of three stitches. First, the right part of the wrap is stitched to the right crus (■ Fig. 34.6). Second the right part of the wrap is stitched to the right anterior wall of the esophagus. The middle stitch is the most important one. It fixes the right anterior esophageal wall at a suitable distance from the hiatus to the right anterior part of the fundus of the stomach without causing tension or twisting. A higher stitch, and then a lower one completes this row of sutures (■ Fig. 34.7). A final row of three stitches is placed between the gastric fundus to the left of the esophagus and the left anterior wall of the esophagus, leaving the anterior esophagus free over an angle of 90° (■ Fig. 34.8).

The frame stitch is removed completing the fundoplication (■ Fig. 34.9). The pneumoperitoneum is emptied, and the port holes are closed.

Postoperative Care

During the first 24 h, analgesia is maintained with opiates. The nasogastric tube is removed the next morning, and oral feeding is started 2 h later. All antireflux medication is discontinued, and the child is discharged after 2 or 3 days.

Follow-up is scheduled on the 10th day, to answer frequent questions about a temporary dysphagia. The follow-up is extended for 5 years, and concluded with a last UGI series.

Results

Between 1993 and 2003, 710 Toupet procedures were performed by the same surgeon. Mean patient age at surgery was 3.4 years (range 5 months to 16 years). Twenty-eight were neurologically impaired, eight had been operated for esophageal atresia, and four had previous open surgery for GERD.

No patient died, and none of procedures had to be converted to open surgery. There were no anesthesiological complications. One patient glided from the table during surgery, which could have been prevented, but had no consequences. The mean duration of the procedure was 1 h.

Some intraoperative complications occurred at the beginning of the series: four pleural perforations, four vagus nerve injuries, and five omental herniations through port holes. In two patients the nasogastric tube had been sutured in the wrap and required removal of the tacking stitch. One patient required redo fundoplication.

During the first 3 weeks, 30% of the patients transiently complained of pain or moderate dysphagia. Two needed rehospitalization and intravenous fluid administration for 2 days. One patient developed sepsis from the site of initial intravenous cannulation and stayed for an extra week in the hospital. No patients required esophageal dilatation.

Mean follow-up is over 4 years. Eleven patients needed a redo procedure, which was always performed laparoscopically and did not result in complications. The second procedure was almost the same as the primary one and we were surprised by the absence of specific difficulties. The absence of tight adhesions certainly played a role in this.

Discussion

Laparoscopic antireflux surgery has become the gold standard and three techniques, namely the Nissen, Thal, and Toupet, have proven their effectiveness. All three are not particularly difficult. The results are certainly dependent on the specific training the surgeon has had in a particular technique. A partial wrap may be preferred in terms of anatomy and of physiology. After a partial fundoplication, patients keep their ability to belch.

A failure is often related to the slipping of the valve through the hiatus. The esophageal sphincter returns into a wrong position, and GERD recurs. The technique according to Toupet, as described, prevents this from occurring.

Concerning the complications, laparoscopic antireflux surgery requires considerable training. All techniques demand a precise dissection. The fundoplication according to Toupet does not divide the short gastric vessels, and prevents too tight a wrap around the esophagus, which is probably a specific advantage.

Further Reading

Bell RCW, Hanna P, Power B, et al (1996) Clinical and manometric results of laparoscopic partial (Toupet) and complete (Rossetti) fundoplication. Surg Endosc 10:724–728

Bensoussan AL, Yasbeck S, Carceller-Blanchard A (1994) Results and complications of Toupet's partial posterior wrap: 10 years experience. J Pediatr Surg 29:1215–1217

Boix-Ochoa J (1986) Address of honored guest: the physiologic approach to the management of gastric esophageal reflux. J Pediatr Surg 21:1032–1039

Cargill G, Goutet JM, Vargas J (1983) Gastroesophageal reflux in infants and children. Manometrical analysis: possible relation with chronic bronchopulmonary disease. Gut 24:357–361

De Meester TR, Stein HJ (1992) Minimizing the side effects of antireflux surgery. World J Surg 16:335–336

Esposito C, Montupet P, Amici G, et al (2000) Complications of laparoscopic antireflux surgery in childhood. Surg Endosc 14:658–660

McKerman JB (1994) Laparoscopic repair of gastro-esophageal disease. Toupet partial fundoplication versus Nissen fundoplication. Surg Endosc 8:851–856

Montupet P (1996) Laparoscopic fundoplication in children. In: Toouli J, Gossot D, Hunter JG (eds) Endosurgery. Churchill Livingstone, Edinburgh, pp 935–940

Montupet P, Gauthier F, Valayer J (1983) Traitement chirurgical du reflux gastrooesophagien par hemivalve tubérositaire posterieure fixee. Chir Pediatr 24:122–127

Montupet P, Mendoza-Sagaon M, De Dreuzy O, et al (2001) Laparoscopic Toupet fundoplication in children. Pediatr Endosurg Innov Tech 5:305–308

Toupet A (1963) La technique d'oesophagoplastie avec phrenogastropexie appliquée dans la cure radicale des hernies hiatales. Mem Acad Chir 89:394–399

Chapter 35

Laparoscopic Thal Fundoplication in Infants and Children

David C. van der Zee and Klaas (N) M.A. Bax

Introduction

In recent years it has become more clear that the type of antireflux procedure is less relevant, as long as the three pillars of the antireflux procedure (bringing the distal esophagus into the abdominal cavity, narrowing of the hiatus, and fixation of the fundus against/around the distal esophagus and diaphragm) are properly carried out.

The Thal anterior fundoplication was originally described by Alan Thal in 1968 for patching of the distal esophagus, and later advocated by Ashcraft et al. (1978) for the treatment of gastroesophageal reflux disease. With the Thal procedure fewer complications of gas bloat, wrap disruption, and wrap displacement are described.

The principles of a laparoscopic Thal fundoplication are similar those of an open procedure (van der Zee et al. 1994).

Preoperative Preparation

Before Induction of General Anesthesia

The evening prior to the operation the patient is given an enema or a retrograde colorectal washout to avoid accumulation of feces in the colon obscuring the vision of the stomach and spleen.

After Induction of General Anesthesia

Depending on age an 8-, 9-, or 10 mm stent is placed in the esophagus to facilitate determination of the esophagus during dissection of the hiatus and prevent the hiatus from being closed too tightly.

Part of the perioperative management may be subject to local customs and personal preferences. Future porthole sites may be injected with local anesthetics.

Epidural or spinal anesthesia is subject to the personal preference of the anesthetist. If the patient is receiving analgesia by means of an epidural catheter a voiding urinary catheter is mandatory.

Positioning

Patient

The patient is placed in a supine position with the table in a 15–20° reversed Trendelenburg position. In infants and small children the legs are bent in a froglike position on a short operating table with the operation table sheet wrapped around them to prevent the child from sliding down. In older children and adolescents the legs are placed on leg holders that can be abducted to allow the surgeon to stand between the legs (■ Fig. 35.1). In children with scoliosis and/or flexion contractions alternative positioning may be pursued to allow a more or less comfortable position for the surgeon to stand (van der Zee and Bax 1996). It may sometimes be helpful to position the child with the hips over a bending point of the table and create a sort of hyperextension just above the hips to allow more space for the instruments to be maneuvered around.

Crew, Monitors, and Equipment

In infants and small children the surgeon stands at the lower side of the table with the first assistant, who holds the camera, on the surgeon's left side (■ Fig. 35.1a). It is often an advantage to have this person sitting down, thus obtaining a more stable picture. Alternatively a camera holder device can be used when not enough personnel are available. A second assistant stands or sits on the surgeon's right side to hold the liver retractor and the Babcock retracting the stomach (■ Fig. 35.1b).

The scrub nurse stands on the surgeon's left or right hand, depending on whether the surgeon is right- or left-handed, respectively.

Preferably two monitors are used on either side of the patient's head. Usually one monitor is integrated into the equipment tower. If the separate monitor is fixed to a flexible arm, the monitor is placed just over the patient's chest to obtain the optimal position for vision and handling.

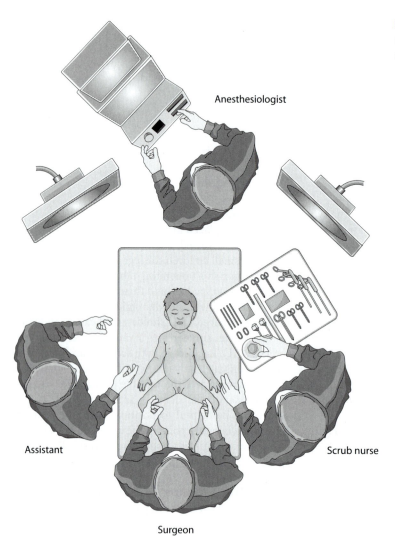

Fig. 35.1. Positioning of the patient, crew, and monitor. **a** For infants and small children

Anesthesiologist

Assistant

Scrub nurse

Surgeon

Special Equipment

No special energy applying systems are required. A reusable clipping device is at hand for clipping together the ends of the tape that is put around the intra-abdominal esophagus.

Fig. 35.1. Positioning of the patient, crew, and monitor. **b** For older children and adolescents

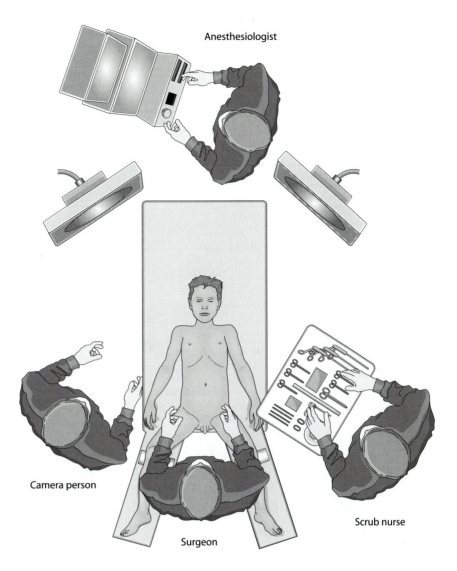

Anesthesiologist

Camera person

Surgeon

Scrub nurse

Technique

Cannulae

Cannula	Method of insertion	Diameter (mm)	Device	Position
1	Open	5	Optic/Babcock	Umbilicus
2	Closed	3/5	Optic	Halfway umbilicus/xiphoid
3	Closed	3/5	Curved grasping forceps	Right subcostal
4	Closed	3/5	Diathermy hook/scissors/suction/needle holder/clipping device	Left subcostal
5	Closed	3/5	Liver retractor	Right costal margin (Diamond Flex) or subxiphoid (Nathanson)

Figure 35.2 shows port positioning.

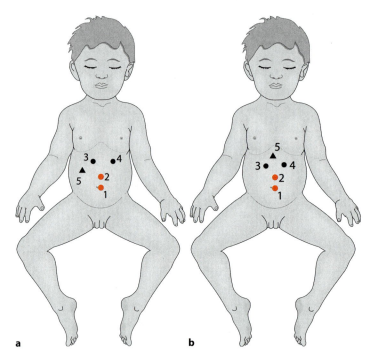

Fig. 35.2. Port positioning. The liver retractor can either be introduced subcostally on the right (**a**) or below the xyphoid (**b**). In smaller children the telescope can remain at the umbilicus. In older children is may be advantageous to insert the telescope cannula midway in the epigastrium. The umbilical canunula may then be used for traction on the stomach or vessel loop

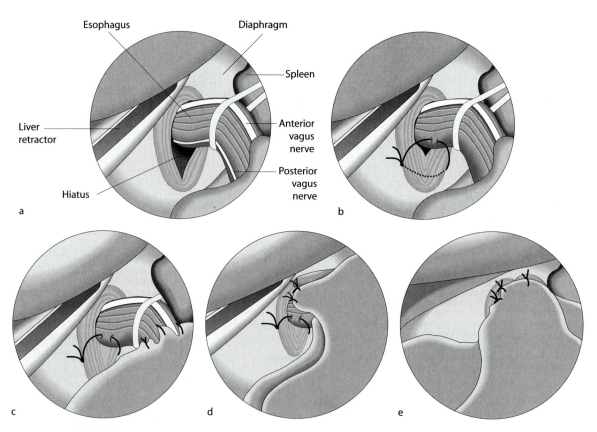

Fig. 35.3. Schematic drawing of the procedure. **a** The phrenoesophageal ligament has been cut and the esophagus has been well mobilized. **b** The hiatus is narrowed behind the esophagus with one suture that includes the posterior wall of the esophagus. An appropriately sized orogastric tube is present during the tying of the suture in order to avoid esophageal narrowing. **c** One row of three non-absorbable sutures is placed between the anterior wall of the fundus and the esophagus halfway along its intra-abdominal length. **d** A second row of three sutures fixes the anterior wall of the fundus to the uppermost part of the intra-abdominal esophagus as well as to the edge of the hiatus. **e** Completed procedure

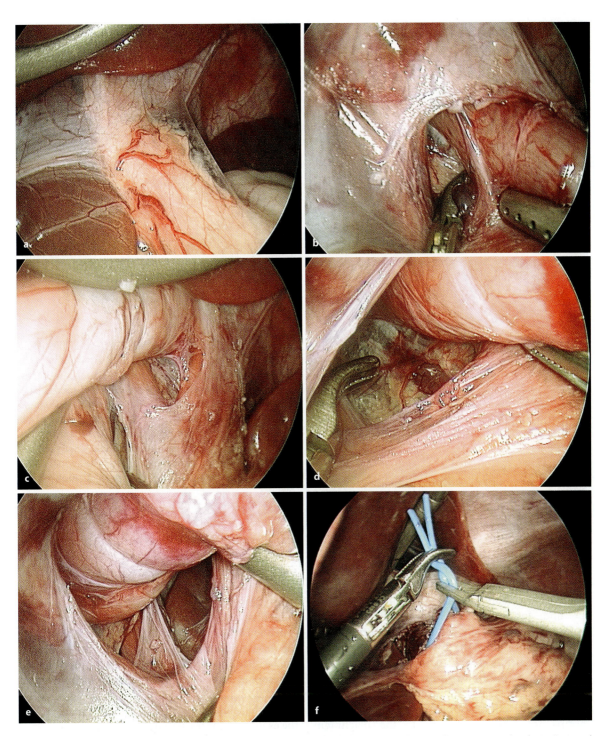

Fig. 35.4 a–f. Operative pictures of the procedure. **a** View of the hiatal area. A Nathanson liver retractor has been inserted without cannula underneath the xiphoid. The anterior vagus nerve is seen through the phrenoesophageal ligament. **b** The anterior phrenoesophageal ligament has been cut. The anterior vagus nerve is identified and saved. **c** After dissection of the left crus there is a clear entrance to the hiatus. **d** The pars flaccida of the hepatogastric ligament has been opened and the groove between the right esophageal wall and the right crus has been opened. The posterior esophageal wall is mobilized and the posterior vagus nerve identified and saved. **e** The left crus is reached and a large window between the posterior esophagus and the crura is made. **f** A vessel loop has been passed around the esophagus above the hepatic branches of the anterior vagus nerve. Both ends of the loop are clipped together with two clips. Traction on the loop is applied and the posterior dissection of the esophagus is completed.

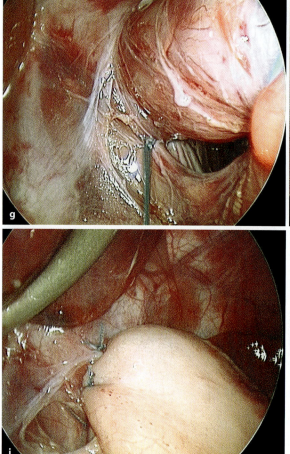

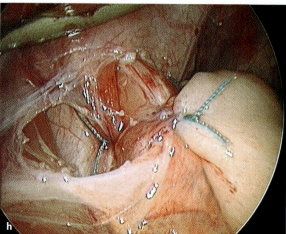

Fig. 35.4 g – i. Operative pictures of the procedure. **g** Next the hiatus is closed behind the esophagus with one non-absorbable suture that includes the posterior wall of the esophagus. During the tying of the suture an appropriately sized orogastric tube is in situ in order to avoid narrowing of the esophagus. **h** Suturing of the anterior fundus of the stomach in two rows of three sutures, first against the esophagus halfway along its intra-abdominal length and second against the uppermost part of the intra-abdominal esophagus and adjacent edge of the hiatus. **i** Completed procedure

Procedure

The procedure is schematically drawn in ▄ Fig. 35.3. The phrenoesophageal ligament is incised with the monopolar hook up to the anterior wall of the esophagus and further anteriorly over the left crus (▄ Fig. 35.4a,b). Usually a lymph node serves as a landmark above which the dissection can be started.

The dissection is continued on the left. Gentle caudal traction of the fundus with a Babcock inserted through the umbilical cannula allows the surgeon to divide the posterior gastrophrenic attachments anchoring the posterior fundus to the diaphragm (▄ Fig. 35.4c). Care should be taken not to denude the crura completely. A thin fascial layer should be left. In children it may be of benefit to divide the superior short gastric vessels up to the point that the fundus can be moved without pulling the spleen along. After completing the dissection on the left there is a clear entrance to the hiatus (▄ Fig. 35.4c).

By pulling with the Babcock on the cardia in a left caudad direction the hepatogastric ligament is put under traction. The pars flaccida is opened. The hepatic

branches of the anterior vagus nerve are preserved. The groove between the right part of the esophagus and right crus can clearly be seen and is opened. When dissection takes place in a plane directly on the esophagus there is little danger of damaging the pleura. By using blunt dissection the posterior vagus nerve can be clearly defined and retained (▄ Fig. 35.4d). By withdrawing the orogastric tube from the stomach, the esophagus can be lifted further and a window can be made behind the esophagus (▄ Fig. 35.4e). After a window is created a grasping forceps can be passed behind the esophagus to the left side and a vessel loop is pulled around the esophagus for traction during further dissection of left and right crus and of the posterior esophagus (Fig. 35.4f).

Working from the right or left side one or two 3×0 Ethibond non-resorbable sutures are used for closure of the hiatus (▄ Fig. 35.4g). The uppermost suture includes the back wall of the esophagus. During the intracorporeal tying of this suture, the orogastric tube is pushed in again into the stomach in order to avoid narrowing of the esophagus. Thereafter the orogastric tube can be removed.

The anterior valve technique according to Thal is laid in two layers. The vessel loop is left loosely in place to mark the gastroesophageal junction. For the first layer the first suture is laid halfway along the dissection line of the phrenicogastric ligament to halfway along the intra-abdominal distal esophagus on the left. The second suture is placed from the ventral part of the fundus to halfway along the ventral side of the esophagus under identification of the anterior vagus nerve (■ Fig. 35.4h). The third suture is laid from the right side of the fundus to halfway along the right side of the esophagus. As a nice gutter has now formed the vessel loop can be removed. The first suture of the second layer runs from a more distal part along the dissection line of the phrenicogastric ligament to the proximal part of the intra-abdominal esophagus and the diaphragmatic ridge (■ Fig. 35.4i). The second suture is placed on the ventral side (*cave* anterior vagus nerve!) and the third suture on the right side, thus completing the Thal anterior valve technique.

Particularly in children where approximately 50% are mentally handicapped, a concomitant gastrostomy may be placed in the same procedure, either as a percutaneous endoscopic gastrostomy (PEG) or as a formal gastrostomy. The advantage of a laparoscopically assisted PEG is that the exact location of the gastrostomy can be determined. Laparoscopically placed sutures or anchor sutures can be used to fix the stomach against the anterior abdominal wall with or without control of the gastroscope. There is no consensus on whether one of the trocar holes can be used for the gastrostomy placement.

Postoperative Care

There is no need for a nasogastric tube after the operation. In case of an indwelling gastrostomy, catheter medication can be administered through the PEG immediately after the operation. A urinary catheter is only necessary when the patient has an indwelling epidural catheter.

Feeding of the patient depends on personal preferences but may be started as soon as the patient is well awake and not feeling nauseous. When a gastrostomy has been placed feeding is usually started in smaller and more frequent portions. When these portions are well tolerated the volume can be increased to the normal quantities.

Pain relief is given either by epidural or by intravenous medication for the first day. If further medication is required, paracetamol tablets or suppositories are given. In case of postoperative nausea ondansetron 0.1 mg/kg per day is given intravenously for 12 h postoperatively.

Results

In a recently published article an overview was given over 10 years of laparoscopic Thal fundoplication in infants and children (van der Zee et al. 2002). Between 1993 and 2002, 149 children with GERD underwent 157 laparoscopic antireflux procedures; 49% were mentally handicapped. Follow-up ranged from 6 months to 9 years (median 4.5 years). Nineteen children died; all but one were not related to the antireflux procedure. Immediate relief of symptoms occurred in 120 children (80.5%). In 29 children the results were less than optimal. Eight patients underwent a laparoscopic redo procedure (5.4%). However, none of the children with a follow-up of more than 5 years show any further symptoms.

Discussion

When dissection is performed close to the esophagus, and preferably bluntly, there is little risk for pneumothorax. If pneumothorax does occur it usually has no detrimental effects on ventilation if CO_2 pressure does not exceed 5–8 mmHg. At the end of the procedure the pneumothorax can simply be drained by percutaneous thoracic puncture with an intravenous cannula. In children mediastinal emphysema is a rarely occurring and self-limiting event. Subcutaneous emphysema around the trocar site may occur when the fascia at the trocar site is not closed at the end of the procedure and CO_2 is not adequately evacuated from the abdominal cavity. Subcutaneous emphysema may be a first indication for later occurring trocar site hernia. Vagus nerve trauma can be avoided by active identification of both the anterior and posterior branches of the vagus nerve during dissection. Vagus nerve trauma may induce dysphagia or delayed gastric emptying. Symptoms will subside in due time.

Perforation of the esophagus usually occurs during dissection of the hiatus. The use of a stent in the esophagus makes it easier to determine esophageal tissue from surrounding interstitial tissue, especially when the esophagus is friable due to esophagitis (it is preferable to first treat the esophagitis before performing the antireflux procedure) or in the case of a redo procedure.

A postoperative complication is recurrent reflux, usually attributable to wrap disruption. Respiratory complications, gas bloat, and intestinal obstruction, either by intrathoracic wrap or intestinal adhesions, are only seldom seen in the Thal procedure.

The laparoscopic Thal fundoplication is a safe procedure with favorable results in the long run, irrespective of the nature of the cause, for example mental retardation.

References

Ashcraft KW, Goodwin CD, Armoury RA (1978) Thal fundoplication: a simple and safe operative treatment for gastroesophageal reflux. J Pediatr Surg 13:643–647

Thal AP (1968) A unified approach to surgical problems of the gastroesophageal junction. Ann Surg 163:542–550

Van der Zee DC, Bax NMA (1996) Laparoscopic Thal fundoplication in mentally retarded children. Surg Endosc 10:659–661

Van der Zee DC, Rövekamp MH, Pull ter Gunne AJ et al. (1994) Surgical treatment for reflux esophagitis: Nissen versus Thal procedure. Pediatr Surg Int 9:334–337

van der Zee DC, Bax NMA, Ure BM, Besselink MG et al. (2002) Long-term results after laparoscopic Thal procedure in children. Semin Laparosc Surg 9:168–171

Chapter 36

Laparoscopic Gastrostomy

Douglas C. Barnhart

Introduction

Gastrostomy is a commonly performed procedure in infants and children for a variety of diagnoses. Most often gastrostomy tubes are placed to provide either total or supplemental nutrition. Total nutrition is provided by gastrostomy in patients who have primary aspiration, dysphagia, or feeding aversion. Supplemental nutrition is provided typically for children with increased metabolic requirements such those caused by renal, cardiac, or pulmonary disorders. The technique described is versatile and straightforward. It provides clearer visualization of the site of tube placement than the percutaneous endoscopic gastrostomy technique. This technique may be combined with laparoscopic fundoplication.

Preoperative Preparation

Before Induction of General Anesthesia

Any candidate for gastrostomy should be evaluated for pathologic gastroesophageal reflux. If pathologic reflux is identified the patient should undergo a concomitant laparoscopic fundoplication. No bowel preparation is required. A dose of perioperative prophylactic antibiotics, such as second-generation cephalosporin, may be given. Routine monitoring including capnography and pulse oximetry is indicated.

After Induction of General Anesthesia

An orogastric tube should be passed for initial gastric decompression. The anesthetist should be prepared with a 60-cc syringe and clamp to insufflate the stomach during gastrostomy tube placement. The umbilicus and future gastrostomy tube site may be injected with bupivacaine with epinephrine to provide for postoperative pain control and to assist with hemostasis.

Positioning

Patient

Patients are positioned at the foot of the table (■ Fig. 36.1). In young children, the frog-leg position may be used while older children are placed in stirrups. Alternatively older children may be placed supine with the surgeon standing on the left side. The patient is secured to the table with tape.

Crew, Monitor, and Equipment

If the infant or child is position frog-legged or in dorsal lithotomy, the surgeon and the assistant stand at the foot of the bed. The monitor is at the patient's left shoulder. Alternatively in larger children, the patient may be positioned supine with the surgeon on the patient's left side and the assistant on the right.

Special Equipment

Equipment	Quantity
Monofilament suture on 40 mm half-round needle	2
4 mm, 30° laparoscope	1
Percutaneous access needle with guidewire	1
Dilators (over the wire style) 8–20 French	1
Balloon-tip gastrostomy button or gastrostomy tube	1
Access needle, guidewire, and dilators available as kit from Cook Critical Care (item C-JCDS-100-CHB)	1

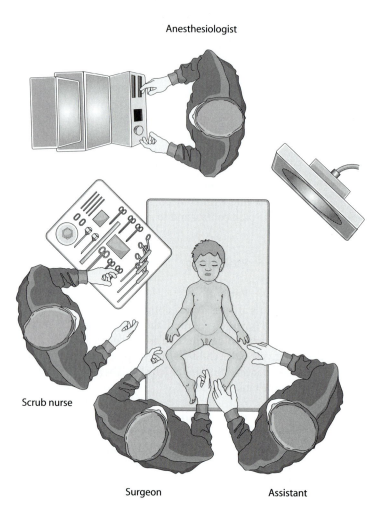

Anesthesiologist

Fig. 36.1. Position of the patient, crew, monitors and equipment

Scrub nurse

Surgeon

Assistant

Technique

Cannulae

Cannula	Method of insertion	Diameter (mm)	Device	Position
1	Open	5	4 mm, 30° laparoscope	Umbilicus
2	Closed	4	Grasper	Left upper quadrant

Port Positions

The umbilical port is inserted first using an open technique. This is subsequently used for placement of the laparoscope. The 4 mm port is placed at the site of the future gastrostomy tube placement (■ Fig. 36.2).

Procedure

Prior to port placement and insufflation of the peritoneum, the left costal margin is marked. This is helpful in eliminating the potential of placing the gastrostomy too close to the costal margin. Without this mark, it is easy to misperceive the final location of the gastrostomy tube as the relationship between the abdominal wall and costal margin changes with insufflation.

The 5 mm port is placed in the umbilicus using a blunt technique. This port is used for insufflation and

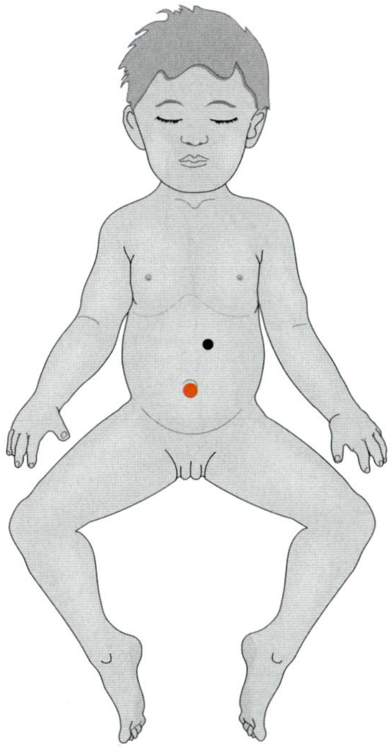

Fig. 36.2. Position of cannulae. Marking of the left costal margin is done prior to insufflation to ensure the gastrostomy is not placed too close to the costal margin

placement of the laparoscope. The 30° laparoscope is used to provide different perspectives from a single port site. If the liver obscures access to the stomach, it is retracted. This is easily accomplished by passing a monofilament suture through the abdominal wall encircling the falciform ligament and exiting the abdominal wall. This is done as an extracorporeal single stitch and tied extracorporeally to provide retraction.

A site for gastrostomy tube placement is selected. This is typically located to the left of the midline and well below the costal margin which was previously marked. Site selection should avoid the epigastric vessels. A 4 mm port may be placed or instruments may be placed directly through a stab wound in the abdominal wall. In either case entry is made with laparoscopic visualization. A 3 mm grasper is inserted and used to grasp the anterior wall of the selected portion of the stomach. For gastrostomy without fundoplication, there may be a lower rate of postoperative gastroesophageal reflux if a site along the lesser curvature is used (Seekri et al. 1991; Stringel 1990). However placing the gastrostomy tube along the greater curvature of the stomach one third of the distance from the pylorus to the fundus is preferred by the author. Placement in this location allows the stomach to easily reach the abdominal wall and generally will allow future fundoplication without gastrostomy revision if the need arises. The gastrostomy must be sufficiently distant from the

pylorus so that the gastric outlet is not obstructed by the balloon of the gastrostomy tube.

The selected portion of the stomach is then drawn to the anterior abdominal wall. Two U-stitches are placed through the abdominal wall using a large half-round needle with a monofilament suture. In infants a 27 mm needle is used while in older children a 65 mm needle may be used. These sutures incorporate 1 cm of anterior gastric wall on either side of the grasper and are placed parallel to the axis of the laparoscope (■ Fig. 36.3a). The sutures are clamped extracorporeally and will subsequently be used to apply traction to the stomach. The grasper and the 4 mm port are removed.

The stomach is insufflated through the orogastric tube by the anesthetist. This should be done until the stomach is visibly distended. The percutaneous access needle is inserted through the 4 mm port tract. The needle is inserted into the anterior wall of the stomach between the two U-stitches. In infants care must be taken to penetrate only the anterior wall of the stomach. The guidewire is advanced through the needle into the lumen of the stomach. This should advance without resistance (■ Fig. 36.3b). The needle is then removed. Traction on the U-stitches is relaxed to allow clear visualization of the guidewire entering the stomach. The tract and gastrostomy are sequentially dilated using the Seldinger technique. The tract should be dilated 4–6 French greater than the gastrostomy tube (■ Fig. 36.3c). If a gastrostomy button is to be used the length of the tract is measured so that the anterior gastric wall will be approximated against the abdominal wall. The gastrostomy tube or gastrostomy button is advanced over the guidewire into the stomach. In order to facilitate passage of the button, the smallest dilator may be placed within the button to stiffen the tube. The balloon of the gastrostomy tube is then inflated. This should provide good approximation of the gastric wall to the anterior abdominal wall. If this does not occur a shorter stemmed button must be placed. The U-stitches are secured over the flange of the tube or button (■ Fig. 36.3d). If at any point in the process, the stomach appears unstable, an additional 3 mm port may be placed in the right side of the abdomen for placement of a grasper to provide support to the stomach during dilation or tube insertion.

It is critical to verify the intraluminal location of the gastrostomy tube. Injection of air into the gastrostomy tube to demonstrate inflation and deflation of the stomach should be done routinely. The site should be inspected from various vantage points taking advantage of the 30° laparoscope. These maneuvers are typically adequate. However if there remains any doubt, an additional port should be placed to provide a different vantage point or a contrast injection should be performed.

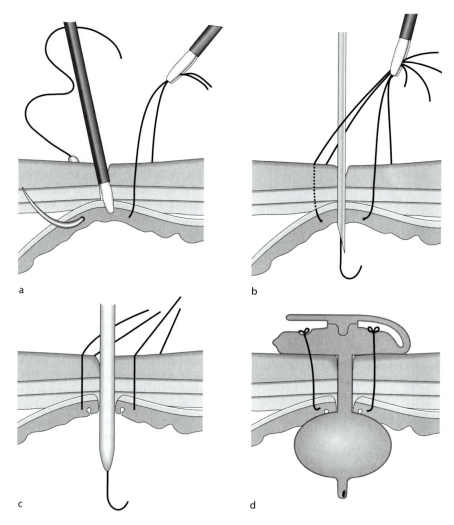

Fig. 36.3. Actual technique. **a** A large half-round needle is placed through the abdominal wall and through the stomach taking 1 cm of the stomach and then exits the abdominal wall. This is taken as a continuous single suture. Two of these traction sutures are placed in a parallel fashion. **b** The insertion needle is advanced through the access site into the lumen of the stomach after the stomach is insufflated via an oral gastric tube. The guidewire is advanced into the lumen of the stomach. **c** A Seldinger technique is used to progressively dilate the tract. **d** The gastrostomy tube is advanced into the stomach. The balloon is inflated to approximate the anterior gastric wall to the anterior abdominal wall. The traction sutures are secured over the flange of the gastrostomy tube

The insufflation is then relieved, and the umbilical port is removed. The fascia at the umbilical site is reapproximated with an absorbable suture.

Postoperative Care

Pain is typically managed with acetaminophen without the need for narcotics. The tube is maintained at dependent drainage for 24 h. Feedings may then be initiated in a graduated fashion as either a continuous infusion or as boluses. Typically full feedings can be achieved within 24–48 h. The traction sutures are removed at 48 h postoperative. A proton pump inhibitor or H$_2$ blocker may be used to decrease gastric secretions and may decrease the incidence of local site complications.

A routine gastrostomy tube change is typically performed at 6–8 weeks postoperative. At that the time the gastrostomy tract is measured and a longer button is often required.

Results

We have used this technique for gastrostomy tube placement in over 700 patients at the Children's Hospital of Alabama. Our early experience with this technique was previously reported (Collins et al. 1995; Sampson et al. 1996). The results of this procedure have been favorable. Patients, families, and referring pediatricians have appreciated the primary placement of the button-type tube. The problems encountered in longer follow-up are consistent with the early experience. The most frequent difficulty is hypertrophic granulation tissue which is easily treated with topical silver nitrate or topical steroids. Persistent gastrocutaneous fistula occurs infrequently after tube removal. Localized skin irritation is managed as an outpatient with topical skin protectants.

Discussion

The principal advantages of this technique as compared to percutaneous endoscopic gastrostomy are that it allows precise placement of the tube in relation to the pylorus and gastroesophageal junction and that it eliminates the possibility of the tube traversing the bowel. It also provides a method for primary placement of a button, which appeals to patients and families.

There are several areas which require special attention. First, it is imperative that intraluminal location of tube is assured. This is accomplished by several methods. If an additional port was placed the stomach may be inspected from multiple viewpoints. Inflation of the stomach through the gastrostomy with air can be routinely performed. In complicated cases contrast injection under fluoroscopy may be required.

In the event of early dislodgement of the tube care must be taken in replacing the tube as the stomach may not be sufficiently adhered to the anterior abdominal wall. Our practice is to replace the button with a smaller gastrostomy tube over a guidewire in such cases. It is mandatory that a contrast injection be performed after early replacement of the tube. While it may seem tempting to leave the traction sutures in place more than 48 h, this is not advisable. Early dislodgement is rare, and the extended use of these sutures increases local wound difficulties.

This technique can be more difficult in adolescents than it is in smaller children. The thickness of the abdominal wall must be accounted for and a sufficiently large taper needle must be used for the initial traction suture placement. It is critical that these sutures incorporate the gastric submucosa as well as the muscularis to provide sufficient strength for dilation and placement of the tube. In older children the additional port may be useful to help support the stomach during this phase of the operation. In any case when there is difficulty in placing the button or achieving good approximation of the gastric wall to the abdominal wall, a balloon-tip gastrostomy tube may be used instead of the button. This provides greater flexibility with regards to length and is easier to advance into the gastric lumen in difficult cases.

References

Collins JB 3rd, Georgeson KE, Vicente Y, et al (1995) Comparison of open and laparoscopic gastrostomy and fundoplication in 120 patients. J Pediatr Surg 30:1065–1070

Sampson LK, Georgeson KE, Winters DC (1996) Laparoscopic gastrostomy as an adjunctive procedure to laparoscopic fundoplication in children. Surg Endosc 10:1106–1110

Seekri IK, Rescorla FJ, Canal DF, et al (1991) Lesser curvature gastrostomy reduces the incidence of postoperative gastroesophageal reflux. J Pediatr Surg 26:982–985

Stringel G (1990) Gastrostomy with antireflux properties. J Pediatr Surg 25:1019–1021

Chapter 37

Laparoscopic Pyloromyotomy

Gordon A. MacKinlay and Douglas C. Barnhart

Introduction

Congenital hypertrophic pyloric stenosis occurs in 1 in 300–900 live births, and affects male infants up to six times more often than females. Though often called congenital, hypertrophic pyloric stenosis only very rarely has its onset of symptoms at birth and has never been described in a stillbirth. Vomiting normally commences around 2–3 weeks of age, becoming more frequent and projectile. The majority of paediatricians and surgeons believe that surgery is the treatment of choice and should be performed without delay, after correction of both dehydration and electrolyte imbalance. Globally the technique of pyloromyotomy is attributed to Wilhelm Conrad Ramstedt in respect of the procedure he undertook on 28 July 1911. However, the first record of this operation was, in fact, by Sir Harold Stiles on 3 February 1910, some 17 months earlier at the Royal Hospital for Sick Children, Edinburgh, where the original operation note can be viewed. Alain and Grousseau first undertook the operation laparoscopically in 1991. Since these initial reports the technique has gained popularity due to the obvious cosmetic benefit as well the brevity of the operation. It is a safe and appealing alternative to the traditional operation but requires attention to detail.

Preoperative Preparation

Before Induction of General Anaesthesia

Diagnosis is made by either palpation of the pyloric mass or by ultrasound examination. First the hypochloraemic alkalosis is corrected by administering 5% dextrose in 0.45% saline with added potassium chloride, if required, for associated hypokalaemia. Care must be taken if the baby is severely dehydrated and potassium (KCl at 20 meq/L) only added once urine is seen to be passed. Although the use of 0.45% saline takes twice as long to correct the deficit as normal saline would, it is safer to administer.

There are no absolute contraindications for the use of this technique. Care should be exercised in abdominal insufflation in infants with cardiac or pulmonary dysfunction. However this operation is typically brief and well tolerated.

Preanaesthetic care is similar to that of the open method with careful attention to adequate gastric irrigation and decompression prior to the administration of anaesthesia. Routine monitoring including capnography and pulse oximetry is indicated. Adjustment of ventilation or abdominal insufflation can be made to respond to changes in oxygen saturation or end-tidal CO_2, although this is rarely an issue.

After Induction of General Anaesthesia

General anaesthesia with endotracheal intubation and muscle relaxation is necessary. Port sites are infiltrated prior to incision with 0.25% bupivacaine with 1 in 200,000 adrenaline for postoperative pain relief and to minimise bleeding from small vessels. A single dose of intravenous antibiotics (e.g. first-generation cephalosporin or anti-staphylococcal penicillin) may be given for prophylaxis against an umbilical port site infection. An orogastric tube is placed for decompression and is used to help exclude mucosal perforation after completion of the pyloromyotomy. The bladder is emptied via a Credé manoeuvre.

Positioning

Patient

The baby is positioned supine at the end of the table which is preferably shortened to give access for both the surgeon and the anaesthetist (■ Fig. 37.1). Access for the surgeon may be facilitated by positioning the infant frog-legged. If preferred an across the table position may be used.

Crew, Monitors and Equipment

The surgeon stands at the end of the table, or the feet of the baby if an across the table position is selected. The assistant stands to the left of the baby and the scrub nurse to the right. The monitor is best placed across the table if a flat screen on a side arm is available. Otherwise the screen may be placed to one side of the table.

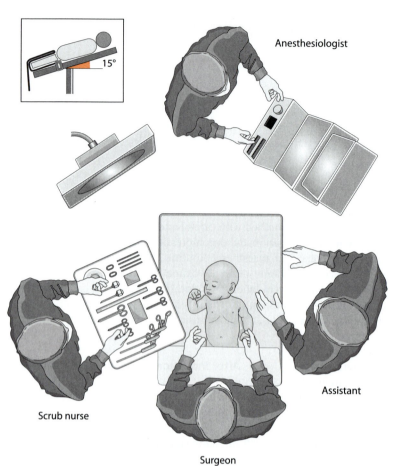

Fig. 37.1. Position of the patient and crew

Anesthesiologist

Assistant

Scrub nurse

Surgeon

Energy Applying Systems

Electrocautery with an insulated needle tip may be used but is not required.

Other Equipment

Equipment	Quantity
Disposable 3 mm sheathed arthrotomy knife	1
Laparoscopic pyloromyotomy spreaders or duodenal grasper	2
Monofilament suture on 40 mm half-round needle	1
4 mm, 30° laparoscope	1

Technique

Cannulae

Cannula	Method of insertion	Diameter	Device	Position
1	Open	5 mm port	Telescope	Umbilicus
2	Closed	3 mm incision, no port	3 mm duodenal grasper	Right upper quadrant
3	Closed	3 mm incision, no port	Arthrotomy knife, 3 mm spreader	Epigastrium

It may be helpful to use secondary ports while learning the technique but otherwise they are not necessary. There is a better cosmetic result if the 3 mm instruments are inserted without ports, and this is our preferred method.

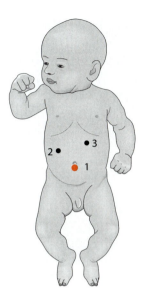

Fig. 37.2. Position of access sites. *1* Umbilicus: telescope, *2* right hypochondrium: duodenal grasping, *3* left epigastrium: incision and spreading

Port Positions

The 5 mm port is placed in the umbilicus using an open technique and pneumoperitoneum is established. Two 3 mm access sites are created without the use of ports (Fig. 37.2). The first of these sites is at the right midclavicular line approximately 1 cm below the hepatic edge. A pyloromyotomy spreader is placed through this site and used to grasp the duodenum immediately adjacent to the pylorus. The second 3 mm access site is placed directly above the pylorus. This second site is used for the electrocautery, the arthrotomy knife and the pyloromyotomy spreader.

Procedure

After infiltrating the subumbilical fold with 0.5–1 ml of 0.25% bupivacaine with 1 in 200,000 adrenaline, the 5 mm port is placed through the umbilicus using an open technique. Of necessity in small babies, only a very short length of port will be within the peritoneal cavity so care must be taken to prevent the port from slipping out. The peritoneum is insufflated to 8 cmH$_2$O pressure. A 4 mm, 30° scope is introduced, and the diagnosis is confirmed. If the infant's liver obscures access to the pylorus, it is retracted. This is easily accomplished by passing a monofilament suture through the abdominal wall, encircling the falciform ligament and exiting the abdominal wall. This is done with a 40 mm half-round needle as an extracorporeal single stitch. The suture is tied extracorporeally to provide retraction (Fig. 37.3a).

The two 3 mm access sites are varied based on the location of the pylorus and are created using the disposable arthrotomy knife. The first 3 mm access site is placed in the right midclavicular line approximately

1 cm below the margin of the liver. This site is adjusted to allow this instrument to enter the peritoneum to the right of and at the same craniocaudal level as the pylorus. Care must be taken to avoid damage to the liver which usually extends below the costal margin in neonates. A high position of the port site, however, enables the instrument inserted through it to lift the edge of the liver out of the field of view as it is advanced to gently grasp the duodenum just distal to the pylorus. A 3 mm pyloromyotomy spreader or grasper is introduced and used to grasp the duodenum immediately distal to the pylorus. For the remainder of the pyloromyotomy this grasper stabilises the pylorus. Careful attention is paid to avoid crushing or otherwise injuring the duodenum.

The second 3 mm access site is placed in the left hypochondrium closer to the midline than the other to give a more direct line of approach almost at right angles to the underlying pylorus. The electrocautery, arthrotomy knife and pyloromyotomy spreader will be sequentially introduced through this site. The gastric extent of the pylorus is palpated with the electrocautery or the knife with the blade retracted. This is done to allow clear determination of the extent of pyloromyotomy required. The electrocautery may then be used to score the serosa overlying the longitudinal incision which will be made in the pylorus. While this is not essential for haemostasis, it can be a useful adjunct for marking the intended line of incision especially in the teaching setting.

The initial incision in the muscular fibres of the pylorus is critical. This incision should be directly perpendicular to the lumen and parallel to the longitudinal fibres of the pylorus. It should reach both the gastric and duodenal extents of the pylorus. This should be made as a single smooth incision using the arthrotomy blade extended to 3 mm (Fig. 37.3b). The importance of the accuracy of this incision cannot be overemphasised. An oblique or insufficiently long incision will make subsequent spreading difficult. We find it preferable to use a disposable 3 mm arthrotomy knife, such as that made by Linvatec, as it ensures a sharp blade for each operation.

The blade of the arthrotomy knife is drawn back into the sheath. The blunt-ended sheath is placed into the incision in the centre of the pylorus. Gentle pressure is applied until it separates the underlying muscular fibres. The knife is rotated along its axis to began the separation of the muscular fibres (Fig. 37.3c). The second pyloromyotomy spreader is introduced through the left 3 mm access site. Its closed tips are introduced into the area of separation created by the sheathed knife. A slow but progressive spreading is carried out in both directions. This is accomplished by slowly spreading the instrument to full extent and then reinserting the closed spreader at the margin of the prior spreading (Fig. 37.3d). Care must be taken especial-

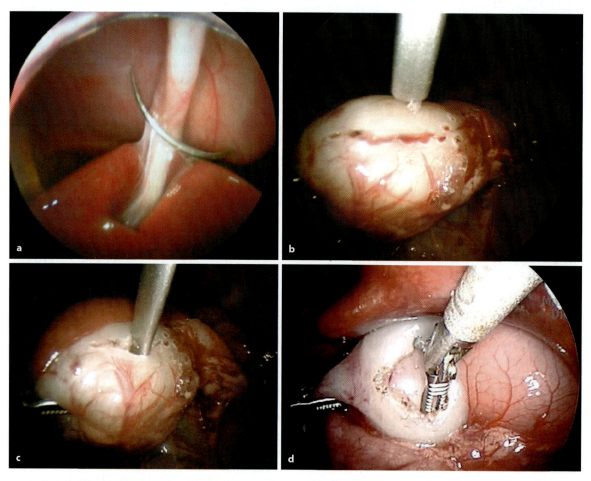

Fig. 37.3. a The liver may be retracted anteriorly by passing a 40 mm half-round needle through the abdominal wall, around the falciform ligament and back out of the abdominal wall. This monofilament suture is tied extracorporeally to retract the liver. **b** The longitudinal incision on the pylorus has been marked with the electrocautery. The arthrotomy knife is then used to incise the full length of the pylorus. **c** The blade of the arthrotomy knife has been withdrawn into the sheath. The blunt end is advanced into the centre of the incision on the pylorus with firm pressure. The knife is then rotated to begin the splitting of the muscular fibres. **d** The pyloromyotomy spreader is introduced into the gap created by the rotation of the knife. Slow progressive spreading separates the muscular fibres

ly at the duodenal end where the mucosa comes close to the surface. It is critical that both sheathed knife and the spreader enter the incision in an angle that is radial to the lumen of the pylorus. An oblique angle with either of these manoeuvres can cause a peeling of the muscular fibres rather than a precise myotomy.

Bulging of the submucosa and independent movement of the two halves of the pylorus verify complete pyloromyotomy. The pyloric margin may be verified by palpation of the gastric and duodenal edges. The mucosa is verified to be intact by careful inspection of the pyloromyotomy and this is facilitated by the magnification provided by the laparoscope. The stomach is then inflated via the orogastric tube and the pyloromyotomy inspected for air leak as evidenced by bubbles.

The upper instruments are visualised as they are withdrawn to avoid drawing omentum into the access sites. The insufflation is relieved, and the umbilical port is removed. The fascia at the umbilical site is re-approximated with an absorbable suture. The upper abdominal access sites usually require only skin closure.

Postoperative Care

The nasogastric tube is aspirated at the end of the procedure and removed. Very little analgesia is required postoperatively as the local anaesthetic instilled at the port sites offers postoperative pain relief. A paracetamol suppository at the end of the procedure may also be used and usually no further analgesia is required.

Feeding may be recommended on return to the ward. A clear feed may be given initially and the milk volume then steadily increased as tolerated.

Table 37.1. Comparison of complication rates for open and laparoscopic pyloromyotomy at the Children's Hospital of Alabama

Complication	Open ($n = 225$)	Laparoscopic ($n = 232$)	P value
Intraoperative			
Mucosal perforation	8 (3.6%)	1 (0.4%)	0.016
Duodenal injury	0	2 (0.9%)	0.16
Total (mucosal perforation and duodenal injury)	8 (3.6%)	3 (1.2%)	0.11
Postoperative			
Revision pyloromyotomy	0	5 (2.2%)	0.027
Readmission without reoperation	2 (0.9%)	3 (1.3%)	0.70
Incisional hernia	0	2 (0.9%)	0.20
Total (revision pyloromyotomy, readmission without reoperation and incisional hernia)	2 (0.9%)	10 (4.4%)	0.022
Total (intraoperative and postoperative)	10 (4.4%)	13 (5.6%)	0.57

Results

Our experiences with laparoscopic pyloromyotomy at the Royal Hospital for Sick Children and the Children's Hospital of Alabama have been recently reviewed. A retrospective study of the experience in Edinburgh was undertaken which compared the open and laparoscopic procedures for the first 18-month period after introduction of laparoscopic pyloromyotomy. A comparison was made between open and laparoscopic pyloromyotomy as two of the four consultants on the duty rota were not laparoscopic surgeons.

The number of operations during the 18-month period undertaken by laparoscopic approach was 22 and by open approach was 28. The average age and weights were comparable in the two groups. The average duration for the laparoscopic operation was 32 min (range 18–45 min). In the open group the average duration was 35 min (range 20–45 min). Only one mucosal perforation occurred in the open group and none in the laparoscopic group in this series. The laparoscopic operation was associated with statistically shorter times to first feed, first full feed and postoperative time to discharge. Lower doses of paracetamol were given to the laparoscopic group and there were fewer episodes of vomiting in this group.

The rate of wound infection for the laparoscopic group was 5% (1/22), whereas for the open group it was 18% (5/28). All wound infections resolved within a few days on oral antibiotics. In addition there was one case of wound dehiscence for the open group so the total complication rate (excluding postopera-tive vomiting) is 21% (6/28). In the laparoscopic group, however, it was necessary to repeat two of the laparoscopic procedures, due to inadequate pyloromyotomy. These numbers are small but represent the early experience in our unit.

The experience at the Children's Hospital of Alabama was recently reviewed as well (Yagmurlu et al. 2004). This experience included 232 laparoscopic pyloromyotomies over a 5-year period done by six surgeons at the Children's Hospital of Alabama. This was compared to 225 open pyloromyotomies done during the same period. All of these cases were carried out in a teaching setting with an average operative time of 24 min in the laparoscopic group. There were no deaths in the series. There was one mucosal perforation (0.4%) that was recognised and repaired immediately. There were two cases of serosal injury to the duodenum but no full-thickness injuries. Five patients (2.2%) required revision pyloromyotomy presumably due to an incomplete pyloromyotomy. Interestingly the average time to requirement for reoperation in these five patients was 24 days.

The overall complication rate was similar to our contemporaneous open series which had a higher mucosal perforation rate but no incomplete pyloromyotomies. These results are summarised in ■ Table 37.1, and are similar to those reported by the University of Michigan (Campbell et al. 2002). Bax and colleagues reported similar results with 182 cases (van der Bilt et al. 2004).

Discussion

While this technique is simple in principle, careful attention to detail is required. The accuracy of the initial incision on the pylorus is critical. If it is oblique the pyloric fibres will not spread smoothly. If it is insufficient in length, it is difficult to do additional "touch-up" work. Based on our review of the rare occurrence of incomplete pyloromyotomies at the Children's Hospital of Alabama, it seems that they failed on the gastric extent. This portion of the pyloromyotomies therefore merits particular attention. While we had no unrecognised perforations, such an occurrence could be disastrous. A careful examination of the completed pyloromyotomy to check for leaks is critical. Finally an access site hernia may occur if omentum is inadvertently drawn into the site with instrument withdrawal.

The conclusions in the recent paper by Bax and colleagues (van der Bilt et al. 2004) summarise the present experience well: "The value of laparoscopic pyloromyotomy (LP) for the treatment of hypertrophic pyloromyotomy has been proved. The LP procedure is as quick as the open procedure, has a low morbidity, and is devoid of major wound related problems. Moreover the procedure seems to be well teachable."

References

Alain JL, Grousseau D, Terrier G (1991) Extramucosal pyloromyotomy by laparoscopy. J Pediatr Surg 26:1191–1192

Campbell BT, McLean K, Barnhart DC et al. (2002) A comparison of laparoscopic and open pyloromyotomy at a teaching hospital. J Pediatr Surg 37:1068–1071

van der Bilt JD, Kramer WL, van der Zee DC, et al (2004) Laparoscopic pyloromyotomy for hypertrophic pyloric stenosis: impact of experience on the results in 182 cases. Surg Endosc 18:907–909

Yagmurlu A, Barnhart DC, Vernon A, et al (2004) Comparison of the incidence of complications in open and laparoscopic pyloromyotomy: a concurrent single institution series. J Pediatr Surg 39:292–296

Chapter 38

Laparoscopic Jejunostomy

Bryan C. Weidner

Introduction

Gastrostomy is typically preferred over jejunostomy due its easier placement and care. In addition, the patient with a gastrostomy can be bolus or drip fed while one with a jejunostomy can only be drip fed. Certain patient populations, however, are better suited for jejunostomy, such as those with gastroparesis or chronic retching. While aspiration of tube feedings is virtually eliminated with a jejunostomy, the gastroesophageal reflux of acid or bile is not. Therefore, jejunostomy is not a treatment for gastroesophageal reflux (Georgeson and Owings 1998).

There are many fine descriptions of the laparoscopically placed loop jejunostomy (Allen et al. 2002; Georgeson and Owings 1998; Rosser et al. 1999). However, the loop jejunostomy has been associated with many complications, such as leakage of enteric contents at the jejunostomy site and bowel obstruction, as well as difficulty with replacing a dislodged tube (Allen et al. 2002; Georgeson and Owings 1998). Therefore, this chapter will focus on the laparoscopic creation of a Roux-en-Y jejunostomy using a skin level device.

Preoperative Preparation

Children with failure to thrive associated with severe gastroparesis, chronic retching with intragastric feedings, or severe uncorrectable gastroesophageal reflux are candidates for a laparoscopic jejunostomy. An upper gastrointestinal series defines the anatomy and identifies any congenital abnormalities. A gastric emptying study may be of assistance in deciding whether to proceed with gastrostomy or jejunostomy.

Before Induction of General Anesthesia

Routine preparation of the patient as well as correction of any underlying volume deficit or electrolyte abnormalities is warranted.

After Induction of General Anesthesia

Port sites may be injected with 0.25% bupivacaine with or without epinephrine as per surgeon preference. A nasogastric tube is placed intraoperatively and left for postoperative gastric decompression. A urinary catheter is placed as per surgeon preference. Antibiotics may be given preoperatively as per surgeon preference.

Positioning

Patient

The patient is supine on the operating table. The patient must be securely fastened to the table in order to allow for tilting during the procedure.

Crew, Monitors, and Equipment

The surgeon and camera operator are positioned on the patient's right side. The monitor is placed on the patient's left side. The scrub nurse is on the patient's right side, near the foot of the table (■ Fig. 38.1).

Special Equipment

No special energy applying systems are required but a 12 mm endoscopic linear stapler with gastrointestinal load should be at hand.

Anesthesiologist

Fig. 38.1. Positioning of the patient, crew, and equipment

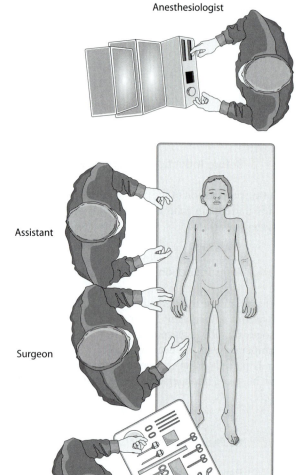

Assistant

Surgeon

Scrub nurse

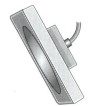

Technique

Cannulae

Cannula	Method of insertion	Diameter (mm)	Device	Position
1	Open	12	Stapler/bowel grasper	Umbilicus
2	Closed	4 or 5	Grasper	Right upper quadrant
3	Closed	4 or 5	Grasper	Mid to upper abdomen, anterior axillary line

Port Positions

Three trocars are placed in the following locations (■ Fig. 38.2). A 12 mm trocar is placed in the umbilicus and will be needed both for the stapler and to perform the jejunojejunostomy. After placement of this trocar and insufflation of the abdomen, a right upper quadrant 4- or 5 mm trocar is placed under direct visualization. This trocar is placed in the midclavicular line, at the level of the liver edge. A third 4- or 5 mm

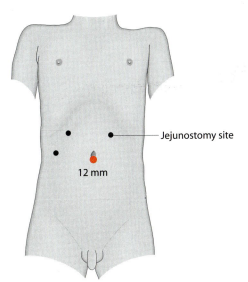

Fig. 38.2. Port positions

trocar is placed in the anterior axillary line approximately halfway between the two previously placed trocars. Tilting the table to the patient's left is helpful when placing this trocar.

Procedure

After trocar placement, the patient is placed in reverse Trendelenburg with the table tilted to the patient's right. The jejunum is identified and run in a hand-over-hand fashion to the ligament of Treitz. The site for transection is generally 10–20 cm distal to the ligament of Treitz (■ Fig. 38.3). The distal transected end will need to be free enough to reach the abdominal wall in the left midabdomen in order to create the feeding jejunostomy. Also, the proximal end will need to be long enough to be pulled out of the umbilicus for the jejunojejunostomy. The site of the jejunojejunostomy should be chosen so the Roux limb is 10–20 cm long, and so that this site can also be brought out of the umbilicus.

At this point in the operation, the feeding jejunostomy is created. The free end of the Roux-en-Y may be brought out of the abdominal wall as a permanent stoma. While this stoma does not require permanent intubation, many authors have found these stomas to be prone to leakage of intestinal contents as well as prolapse of the jejunum, and therefore recommend placement of a skin level device (Georgeson and Owings 1998; Yoshida et al. 1996). Placement of the skin level device is similar to the laparoscopic placement of a gastrostomy tube, and utilizes the U-stitch technique (Georgeson and Owings 1998). A stab wound is placed at the predetermined site in the left midabdomen, away from the costal margin. A grasper is then placed into

the abdomen, and the free end of the Roux-en-Y grasped and elevated to the abdominal wall. Two stitches are placed through the abdominal wall using a large round needle and a monofilament suture (■ Fig. 38.4). The sutures should incorporate approximately 1 cm of the jejunal wall and be parallel to the axis of the camera. The sutures are initially held with clamps, elevating the jejunal limb up to the anterior abdominal wall. A Seldinger needle is inserted through the previously placed stab wound, into the lumen of the free limb. The needle should be placed on the side of the bowel that is in full view of the camera with care being taken to position the needle into the lumen of the bowel. Moving the camera to different port sites can aid in ensuring proper needle placement. A wire is threaded through the needle into the lumen of the bowel (■ Fig. 38.5). It is often possible to see the wire moving within the lumen of the bowel, again ensuring proper placement. The needle is removed and the bowel is allowed to fall away slightly from the abdominal wall to confirm placement of the guide wire into the bowel. The tract is formed by placing progressively larger dilators over the wire and into the lumen. The tract is typically dilated to a size that is 4 French larger than the planned skin level device. The smallest dilator is placed through the button device and guided over the wire into the lumen of the bowel. The balloon is then inflated. One must watch the balloon inflate within the lumen of the free limb to ensure proper placement as well as good apposition of the bowel to the abdominal wall. An additional safety measure may be used in which air is injected through the button under direct visualization of the camera. Insufflation of the Roux limb confirms intraluminal placement of the button. The sutures are then tied over the wings of the button.

Next, the jejunojejunostomy is created. The proximal limb and the loop where the anastomosis will be placed are brought out through the umbilical port site. Care must be taken not to place too much traction on the previously placed jejunostomy. Also, the umbilical port site may need to be extended in order to perform the anastomosis in an extracorporeal fashion. An end-to-side, hand-sewn anastomosis is performed in the usual fashion, and the anastomosis is dropped back into the abdomen. ■ Figure 38.6 shows the completed operation.

The umbilical site is closed as per surgeon preference. If one chooses, the abdomen may be reinsufflated and the abdomen inspected. We have found this maneuver helpful in order to ensure proper placement of the jejunostomy as well as to ensure that no bowel or omentum is trapped in the umbilical closure. The trocars are removed under direct visualization, and the abdomen deflated. In small children, it is recommend that the anterior fascia of the other remaining port sites be closed prior to skin closure.

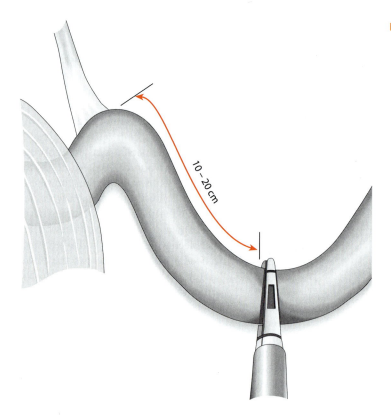

Fig. 38.3. Transection of the jejunum

10 – 20 cm

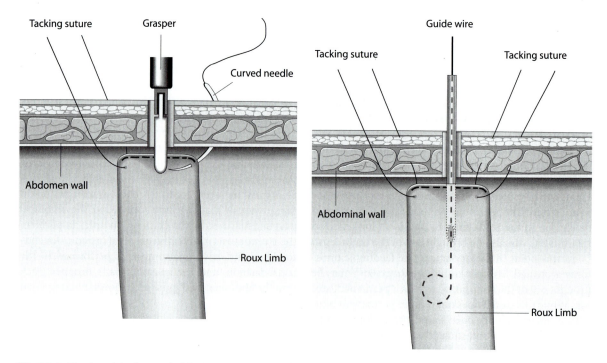

Fig. 38.4. Fixation of the free end of the Roux-en-Y to the ab-dominal wall

Fig. 38.5. Button placement using a Seldinger technique

Fig. 38.6. Jejunojejunostomy and completed operation

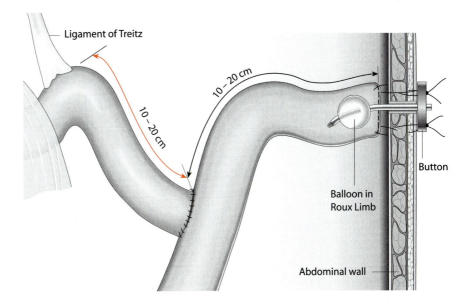

Postoperative Care

The U-stitches may be removed in 48 h. Feedings may be started once bowel function returns; however the feedings must be by drip rather than bolus. The author recommends starting at a slow rate and advancing the feedings to goal as tolerated by the patient.

Results

The placement of a laparoscopic Roux-en-Y feeding jejunostomy is a rare procedure given the preference for and versatility of gastrostomy tubes. However, several of these procedures have been performed at the author's institution without complications.

Discussion

Others have documented the utility of the Roux-en-Y jejunostomy in certain pediatric populations (Decou et al. 1993; Yoshida et al. 1996). This technique may be considered in those patients with severe gastroparesis, chronic retching, or severe, uncorrectable gastro-esophageal reflux who do not tolerate gastric feedings. The requirement for drip feedings limits the versatility of the procedure when compared to a gastrostomy. Potential complications include tube dislodgment as well as bowel obstruction due to volvulus around the Roux limb or stricture at the jejunojejunostomy.

References

Allen JW, Ali A, Wo J, et al (2002) Totally laparoscopic feeding jejunostomy. Surg Endosc 16:1802–1805

Decou JM, Shorter NA, Karl SR (1993) Feeding Roux-en-Y jejunostomy in the management of severely neurologically impaired children. J Pediatr Surg 28:1276–1280

Georgeson KE, Owings E (1998) Surgical and laparoscopic techniques for feeding tube placement. Gastrointest Endosc Clin N Am 8:581–592

Rosser JC, Rodas EB, Blancaflor J, et al (1999) A simplified technique for laparoscopic jejunostomy and gastrostomy tube placement. Am J Surg 177:61–65

Yoshida NR, Webber EM, Gillis DA, et al (1996) Roux-en-Y jejunostomy in the pediatric population. J Pediatr Surg 31:791–793

Chapter 39

Laparoscopic Treatment of Duodenal and Jejunal Atresia and Stenosis

David C. van der Zee and Klaas (N) M.A. Bax

Introduction

With the ongoing expansion of indications for endoscopic pediatric surgery and increasing experience with intracorporeal suturing, laparoscopic repair of duodenal atresia or stenosis is the challenge of the new century. In 2001 the first laparoscopic repair of a duodenal atresia was described by Bax et al. (2001), shortly followed by Rothenberg (2002) describing a series of four patients. Thereafter a few other publications have appeared (Gluer et al. 2002; Nakajima et al. 2003).

Precise anatomical knowledge is necessary to determine the distal duodenum that runs posteriorly and needs to be mobilized to perform a diamond-shaped anastomosis (Kimura et al. 1977, 1990).

Laparoscopic correction of jejunal atresia has not been described so far which is not surprising as the proximal jejunum is usually strongly dilated, which necessitates tapering.

Preoperative Preparation

Before Induction of General Anesthesia

In duodenal atresia associated anomalies including cardiac ones are frequent and about 30% of the patients have Down syndrome. These patients therefore require a thorough diagnostic workup before surgery. Most congenital cardiac anomalies, apart from duct-dependent cardiac lesions, are compatible with safe extracardiac minimal access surgery in neonates and young infants (van der Zee et al. 2003). It is important to know that associated intestinal malrotation is present in about 20% of the patients.

Timing of surgery is elective and may be delayed in case of extreme prematurity, or when cardiac surgery is warranted first. A nasogastric tube is placed to decompress the stomach.

After Induction of General Anesthesia

Part of the perioperative management may be subject to local customs and personal preferences. Future porthole sites may be injected with local anesthetics.

Epidural or spinal anesthesia is subject to the personal preference of the anesthetist. If the patient is receiving analgesia by means of an epidural catheter a voiding urinary catheter is placed and left in postoperatively for the duration of the epidural analgesia. All patients receive antibiotics perioperatively according to local customs.

Positioning

Patient

The patient is placed in a supine position with the table in a 15–20° reversed Trendelenburg position. In infants and small children the legs are bent in a froglike position on a short operating table with the operation table sheet wrapped around them to prevent the child from sliding down.

Crew, Monitors, and Equipment

In infants and small children the surgeon stands at the lower side of a short table with the assistant, who holds the camera, on the surgeon's left side (■ Fig. 39.1). It is often an advantage to have this person sitting down, thus obtaining a more stable picture. The scrub nurse stands on the surgeons' left or right hand, depending on whether the surgeon is right- or left-handed, respectively. Preferably two monitors are used on either side of the patient's head. Usually one monitor is integrated into the equipment on the endoscopy tower. If the separate monitor is fixed to a flexible arm, the monitor is placed just over the patient's chest to obtain the optimal position for vision and handling.

Special Equipment

No special instruments are required and monopolar high frequency electrocautery suffices as the energy applying system.

Fig. 39.1. Positioning of the patient, crew, and equipment

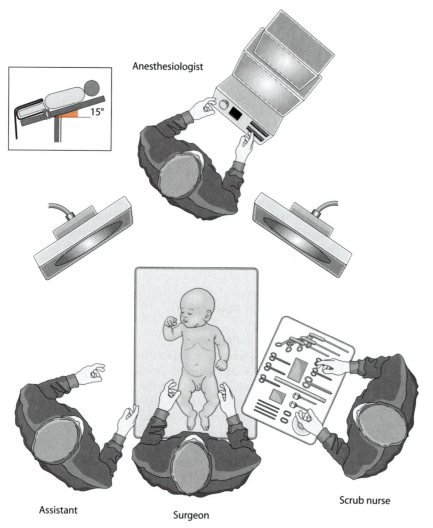

Anesthesiologist

15°

Assistant

Surgeon

Scrub nurse

Technique

Cannulae

Cannula	Method of insertion	Diameter (mm)	Device	Position
1	Open	6	Optic, 30°	Umbilicus
2	Closed	3.5	Curved grasping forceps	Right lower quadrant
3	Closed	3.5	Hook, scissors, forceps	Left hypochondrium
4, optional	Closed	3.5 or naked	Diamond Flex liver retractor	Subxiphoidal

▪ Figure 39.2 shows trocar placement.

Procedure

The first step of the procedure is to rule out the coexistence of intestinal malrotation. If there is a concomi-tant malrotation, this should be corrected first as is described in Chapter 40.

The colon is mobilized sufficiently to the left to expose the dilated bulbus and collapsed distal duodenum. The bulbus duodeni is lifted against the ventral abdominal wall with two 3 × 0 Vicryl transcutaneous stay sutures.

The proximal part of the of the distal duodenum is identified and mobilized to facilitate a diamond-shaped anastomosis (■ Figs. 39.3, 39.4). Care is taken to avoid opening of the mesentery of the colon.

The anterior wall of the distal duodenum is incised longitudinally and the anterior wall of the bulbus horizontally over a length of 1.5–2 cm. The anastomosis is made with standing Vicryl 5 × 0 sutures. The first suture is made from the corner of the incision of the distal duodenum to halfway along the lower side of the opening in the bulbus. The following sutures run from the lower side of the opening in the bulbus to left and right of the distal duodenum until the corners of the opening in the bulbus are reached. Then the ventral anastomosis is made, also with standing sutures. It is sometimes of help to make the first stitch from halfway along the upper side of the bulbus opening to the distal corner of the distal duodenum to have the distal duodenum settle itself in its position against the bulbus. A transanastomotic tube is not placed, but injection of air into the stomach by the anesthesiologist can confirm patency of the anastomosis and proximal jejunum. Finally the anastomosis can facultatively be secured with TissueCol. No drain is left behind.

In case of a duodenal web, mobilization of the duodenum is easy. As in open surgery, however, it may be difficult to determine the place where the web is exactly located. The duodenum should be pulled up against the anterior abdominal wall by means of stay sutures. Next the anterior duodenum is opened longitudinally and the web is searched for. If the web is found it should be partially excised taking care not to injure the bile duct which often opens into the edge of the opening of the web. Closure of the duodenum can be done with standing or running 5 × 0 Vicryl sutures.

As in any complex endoscopic surgical operation, there should be a low threshold for conversion. Mobilization of the duodenum prior to conversion will allow subsequent open surgery through a minilaparotomy.

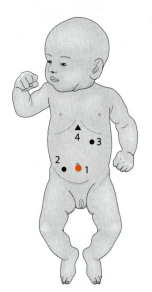

Fig. 39.2. Port positions

Postoperative Care

A nasogastric tube is left in place. Usually oral feeding can be started between day 3 and day 5 postoperatively. As at least half of the patients have Down syndrome oral feeding may be delayed. Intestinal feeding via the nasogastric tube is an alternative when the child is slow in drinking.

Fig. 39.3 a,b. Schematic drawing of the diamond-shaped anastomosis

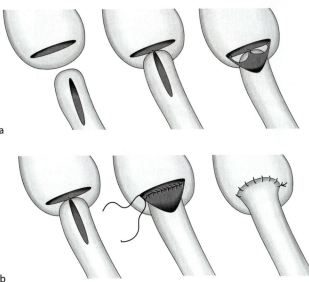

a

b

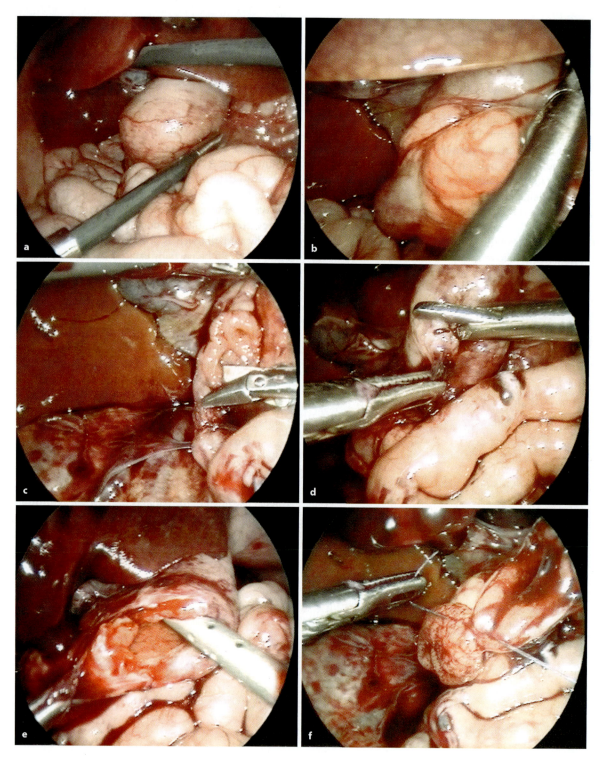

Fig. 39.4. Actual endoscopic operation. **a** The dilated bulbus is clearly seen. **b** The bulbus is pushed upward. Below the bulbus duodeni, there is a rim of pancreatic tissue. Below the pancreatic tissue the distal duodenum comes into view. **c** Longitudinal opening of the distal duodenum. **d** Transverse opening of the bulbus duodeni. **e** Suction of the bulbus duodeni through the transverse duodenotomy. **f** First stitch of the diamond-shaped anastomosis

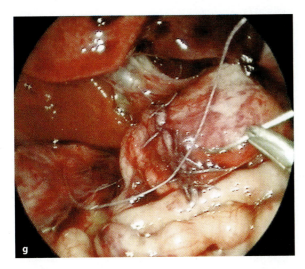

Fig. 39.4. Actual endoscopic operation. **g** Completed anastomosis

Results

In the period 2000 and 2004, 18 children with duodenal or jejunal atresia or stenosis had a laparoscopic approach. Seventeen children were operated in the neonatal period and one infant at the age of 1 year. Nine out of the 17 children with duodenal atresia or stenosis had trisomy 21. Of the 17 children with duodenal atresia or stenosis, three had stenosis and one had a web. In four the duodenal atresia was combined with malrotation. Other associated malformations were: two esophageal atresia type C, one esophageal atresia type A, one total colonic aganglionosis, two tetralogy of Fallot, one atrium-ventricular septum defect (AVDS), and one open ductus arteriosus.

Five procedures were converted (27.7%): one in the child with type A esophageal atresia as there was just not enough space to do the duodenoduodenostomy due to the hugely distend stomach and proximal duodenum, one because of the associated malrotation, one because the distal part of the web appeared difficult to find despite longitudinal duodenotomy, one for convenience, and one in the child with jejunal atresia for the tapering of the proximal bowel and subsequent anastomosis.

Thirteen procedures were laparoscopically completed, but four leaked. Two had associated esophageal atresia repaired thoracoscopically during the same general anesthesia, one had total colonic aganglionosis and iatrogenic perforation of the colon, and one has associated malrotation. In the 1-year-old child with duodenal stenosis, reoperation was required because of recurrent stenosis most likely due to overenthusiastic use of electrocautery for making the enterotomies.

We realize that we have had a high complication rate. Fortunately none of the children died. Duodenal atresia and stenosis as well as jejunal atresia is undoubtedly a difficult field to be treated by endoscopic surgery. The working space is very limited, a hand sewn anastomosis has to be made, there is often associated pathology in the gastrointestinal tract and outside, for example malrotation, esophageal atresia, and cardiac malformations, and half of the children in our series had trisomy 21. The fact that only a few publications have been published regarding this topic seems to support the difficulty of endoscopic correction (Bax and van der Zee 2001; Gluer et al. 2002; Nakajima et al. 2003; Rothenberg 2002; Steyaert et al. 2003). We have decided to do endoscopic repairs of this type of pathology only when at least two experienced endoscopic pediatric surgeons are available to do the operation together.

Discussion

Although indications for endoscopic pediatric surgery continue to expand, the laparoscopic repair of duodenal atresia/stenosis in our series has not been without complications. Therefore reflection on the consequences and complications is warranted. A low conversion threshold should be adopted.

As far as jejunal atresia is concerned, laparoscopy may be of help in determining the exact anatomy and in the correction of a concomitant malrotation, allowing for a very small laparotomy to finish the operation. For tapering of the dilated part of the jejunum and subsequent anastomosis, a laparoscopically assisted approach seems the most achievable at the present time.

References

Bax NM, Ure BM, van der Zee DC, et al (2001) Laparoscopic duodenoduodenostomy for duodenal atresia. Surg Endosc 15:217

Gluer S, Petersen C, Ure BM (2002) Simultaneous correction of duodenal atresia due to annular pancreas and malrotation by laparoscopy. Eur J Pediatr Surg 12:423–425

Kimura K, Tsugawa C, Ogawa K, et al (1977) Diamond-shaped anastomosis for congenital duodenal obstruction. Arch Surg 112:1262–1263

Kimura K, Mukohara N, Nashijima E, et al (1990) Diamond-shaped anastomosis for duodenal atresia: an experience with 44 cases over 15 years. J Pediatr Surg 25:977–978

Nakajima K, Wasa M, Soh H, et al (2003) Laparoscopically assisted surgery for congenital gastric or duodenal diaphragm in children. Surg Laparosc Endosc Percutan Tech 13:36–38

Rothenberg SS (2002) Laparoscopic duodenoduodenostomy for duodenal obstruction in infants and children. J Pediatr Surg 37:1088–1089

Steyaert H, Valla JS, Van Hoorde E (2003) Diaphragmatic duodenal atresia: laparoscopic repair. Eur J Pediatr Surg 13:414–416

van der Zee DC, Bax NMA, Sreeram N, et al (2003) Minimal access surgery in neonates with cardiac anomalies. Pediatr Endosurg Innovat Tech 7:233–236

Chapter 40

Intestinal Malrotation

Klaas (N) M.A. Bax and David C. van der Zee

Introduction

The transformation of the primitive gut from a simple straight tube into the definitive folded and fixed configuration is a complex embryonic process in which both the gut and the mesenterium play an important role. This process can be disturbed and can result in different forms of malrotation and or malfixation (Touloukian and Smith 1998). This chapter will only deal with incomplete rotation in which the duodenum together with the terminal ileum and the superior mesenteric vessels are the contents of a narrow mesenteric stalk that is not fixed to the posterior peritoneum. This configuration predisposes for volvulus of the whole small bowel and should be treated surgically as soon as the diagnosis is made.

The clinical presentation of incomplete rotation may be that of an acute high gastrointestinal obstruction or that of intermittent colicky abdominal pain. These symptoms seem to be caused by volvulus. The incidence of intestinal malrotation leading to clinical symptoms is estimated to be 1 in 6,000 live births, yet the incidence at autopsy is 0.5% and the incidence during a barium meal 0.2% (Warner 1996). This seems to indicate that there are many asymptomatic cases. Whether these cases have been truly asymptomatic remains difficult to prove.

Laparoscopy can be used either to treat symptomatic intestinal malrotation or to separate patients with doubtful intestinal malrotation on imaging into a group that is prone to volvulus and that therefore requires treatment and into a group that is not.

Preoperative Preparation

Before the Induction of General Anesthesia

The diagnosis of malrotation in symptomatic infants is usually not difficult. Abdominal cramps and bilious vomiting in the absence of abdominal distension should raise strong suspicion. An upper gastrointestinal series with careful delineation of the duodenojejunal course is the most important diagnostic tool and preferred to a contrast visualization of the colon. As a contrast medium either air (Harrisson et al. 1999) or a low-osmolar water-soluble contrast medium can be used. Complete or partial obstruction gives a spiral (whirlpool or corkscrew) appearance of the proximal jejunum (Berdon 1995). In the absence of a volvulus, the duodenum has a redundant Z-like appearance (Ablow et al. 1983). Ultrasonography can also demonstrate a dilated duodenum with tapering configuration, fixed midline bowel, and whirlpool sign (Chao et al. 2000).

Inversion of the relative position of the mesenteric vein and artery may also be an indication of intestinal malrotation. While the superior mesenteric vein normally lies to the right of the artery, in malrotation the vein lies to the left and more anteriorly. However, a high incidence of false-positives and false-negatives has been noted (Weinberger et al. 1992; Zerin and DiPiedro 1992). With ultrasound it is possible to diagnose intestinal volvulus in utero. Moreover combined with Doppler it is possible to look at the vascularization of the twisted bowel segment (Yoo et al. 1999).

Malrotation can be diagnosed using computed tomography (CT) and magnetic resonance imaging (MRI), using contrast agents (Ai et al. 1999; Marcos et al. 1999; Zissin et al. 1999). These examinations are much more expensive and CT gives a much higher exposure to X-rays. However these examinations may help in finding other diagnostic parameters, for example aplasia of the uncinate process of the pancreas (Zissin et al. 1999).

In older children the diagnosis is often much more difficult because of chronic and vague symptoms. Moreover various radiographic patterns of intestinal malrotation have been described (Long et al. 1996) while the relationship with symptoms and possible volvulus of these various forms of radiographically detected intestinal malrotation has not been clearly established. To exclude malrotation, the duodenojejunal flexure must be located to the left of the spine at the level of the duodenal bulb halfway between the lesser and greater curvature of the stomach. The question however is not whether there is intestinal malrotation or not, but whether the intestinal malrotation predisposes for volvulus or not. If the ligament of Treitz is in an equivocal position and not to the left of the spine at L1 or L2 it is important to determine the position and fixation of the cecum to assess the breadth of the mesenteric pedicle. This can accurately be done by using laparoscopy (Waldhausen and Sawin 1996).

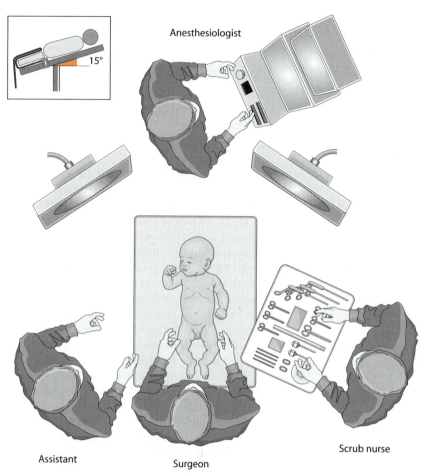

Anesthesiologist

15°

Assistant

Surgeon

Scrub nurse

Fig. 40.1. Position of the patient, crew and equipment.

In non-acute situations it is wise to washout the large bowel in order to increase the working space.

After Induction of General Anesthesia

In Utrecht often a locoregional technique is added to general anesthesia. Especially in neonates it is important to monitor respiratory gas exchange carefully. Hyperventilation resulting in hypocarbia and respiratory alkalosis should be avoided because of its negative influence on the brain.

A urinary catheter is inserted in symptomatic children and in children receiving postoperative epidural analgesia.

Positioning

Patient

The patient is positioned in a supine head up position on the operating table (■ Fig. 40.1). In infants a shortened operating table should be used. The legs can then be enveloped with the lower end of the sheet covering the table, which prevents the child from slipping down during the operation. In older children the legs can be placed on abducted leg rests. Bandaging of the legs fixes the child onto the table. Alternatively infants can be placed transversely at the lower end of the operating table.

Crew, Monitors, and Equipment

The surgeon stands at the lower end of the table or in between the legs in older children (■ Fig. 40.1). When the infant has been placed transversely, the surgeon stands at the feet of the child. The camera operator stands to the surgeon's left side and the scrub nurse to the surgeon's right side. The principal monitor stands to the right of the patient's head or opposite the infant's head when the child has been placed transversely on the table. Ideally all cables should all come from the same direction.

Special Equipment

No special energy applying systems or special instruments are needed.

Technique

Cannulae

Cannula	Method of insertion	Diameter (mm)	Device	Position
1	Open	6	Telescope 30°	Infraumbilical fold
2	Closed	3.5	Surgeon's left-hand instrument	Pararectally at umbilical level on the right
3	Closed	3.5	Surgeon's right-hand instrument	Pararectally at umbilical level on the left
4	Closed	3.5	Diamond Flex liver retractor or Kelly-type forceps	Subxiphoidal

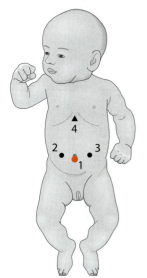

Fig. 40.2. Port position

Cannula Insertion

The first cannula is inserted in an open way through the inferior umbilical fold and will contain the telescope (5 mm, 30°). Two secondary cannulae are inserted, each one pararectally at the umbilical level (■ Fig. 40.2). These can be 3.5 mm in diameter for 3 mm instruments for children below 1 year of age, or 6 mm in diameter for 5 mm instruments for older children. In infants 20 cm-long instruments are used and in older children 30 cm-long instruments are used. It may be advantageous to insert a fourth 3.5 mm cannula just under the xiphoid process for a Diamond Flex liver retractor or for a Kelly-type forceps for the assistant.

Carbon Dioxide Pneumoperitoneum

A pressure of 8 mmHg suffices when optimal muscle relaxation is guaranteed. Flow is arbitrarily set at 2 L/min in children below 1 year of age and at 5 L/min in children beyond that age.

Procedure

Symptomatic Malrotation

It is not difficult to confirm the preoperative diagnosis. The cecum and appendix are usually in a high and rather medial position below the liver, to which they are attached by a peritoneal band. The second part of the duodenum looks long and tortuous. In symptomatic neonates, there is always a volvulus of the mesenteric stalk in a clockwise direction, which is easily recognized (■ Fig. 40.3a,b). When the bowel is not acutely ischemic, it is advantageous to leave the volvulus initially, as it retracts the bowel to the left. All peritoneal bands between the liver, retroperitoneum, and bowel are transected, and the duodenum is kocherized (■ Fig. 40.4). Next the volvulus is undone in a counterclockwise direction. The short band (anterior leaf of the mesenteric stalk) fixing the ileocecal region to the duodenum is transected (■ Fig. 40.5a,b) and the ileocecal region is displaced to the left thereby widening the mesentery anteriorly. Care should be taken not to open the mesentery of the ascending colon. To make sure that the malrotation is treated properly, the whole duodenum as well as the jejunum should lie on the right side. The easiest way to obtain this is to free the duodenum in the distal direction transecting all bands. During this dissection a ring-like peritoneal band encircling the duodenum becomes apparent and should be transected anteriorly. This band represents the end of the retroperitoneal part of the duodenum. The jejunum comes now into view. By pulling further and further on the duodenum and later on the jejunum, the whole small bowel obtains a right-sided position. A last check is made whether the anterior mesentery has been widened enough. If not, the anterior leaf of the mesentery is further incised distally and the adjacent bowel further displaced to either side.

Whether the appendix should be removed at the same time is debatable. If it is to be removed, the tip is grabbed with the forceps in the left cannula and the appendix as well as cannula are withdrawn together (■ Fig. 40.6). The appendix is then removed outside the body and its stump repositioned.

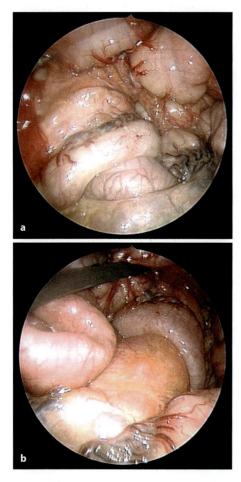

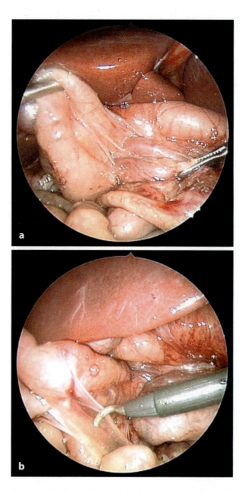

Fig. 40.3. **a** View of a volvulus of the entire small bowel. The bluish color signifies ischemia. **b** Note the edematous mesenteric stalk

Fig. 40.5 a,b. After anticlockwise detorsion, the mesenteric stalk is widened anteriorly by cutting the anterior mesenteric leaf. Veins dilated as a result of the volvulus are easily visible

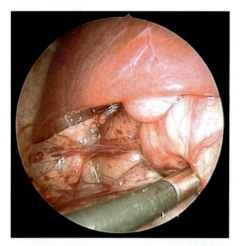

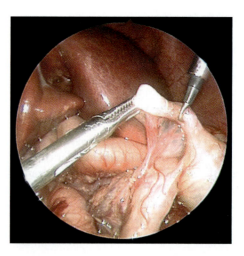

Fig. 40.4. The operation starts with the mobilization of the right colon. Adhesive bands between the right colon and the right lateral abdominal wall are divided. Next the duodenum is kocherized

Fig. 40.6. Removal of the appendix is optional. When appendectomy is planned, the appendicular vessels should be cauterized internally first, after which the appendix can be exteriorized through the left paraumbilical port

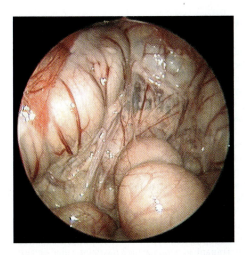

Fig. 40.7. In case of doubtful malrotation, visualization of the ligament of Treitz is of paramount importance. In this patient it can be seen that the first jejunal loop is normally suspended to the left of the vertebral column

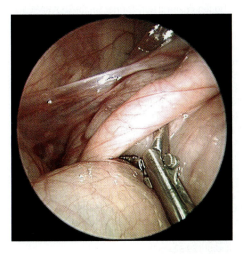

Fig. 40.8. The ileocecal region looks normal too. The appendix is attached with a band to the right lateral abdominal wall

Doubtful Malrotation

If malrotation can not be excluded on imaging, laparoscopy is an ideal tool to look at the width and fixation of the mesentery. If the mesentery is broad, the likelihood for volvulus is small and no further surgery is required. In contrast if the mesentery is narrow, the stalk should be widened.

The position of the cannulae is the same as in symptomatic malrotation. In patients without typical symptoms but with a low and rather medially placed duodenojejunal flexure, usually a normal colon is seen with normally inserted mesentery of the transverse mesocolon onto the pancreas. By lifting up the transverse colon, the duodenojejunal flexure is visualized and the broadness of the mesentery as well as its posterior fixation can easily be verified (Fig. 40.7). When there is no malrotation, one should look at the ileocecal region as well. A normally fixed ileocecal region argues against malrotation (Fig. 40.8).

Postoperative Care

In symptomatic malrotation a nasogastric tube is left behind until gastric retention has ceased. Normal feeding can then be started. The same applies for cases of doubtful malrotation in which at operation classic malrotation was proven and needed to be treated. When the diagnosis of malrotation could not be substantiated, the patient can be discharged the same day.

Results

In the period 1994–2003, 15 neonates with intestinal malrotation were approached laparoscopically. All presented with biliary vomiting since birth. Median birth weight was 3,540 g (2,210–4,390 g). Median age at operation was 7.5 days (2–34 days). At laparoscopy all proved to have volvulus but without necrosis.

Conversion was carried out in six patients, five times through a formal laparotomy, and once through a minilaparotomy. The reasons for conversion were: technical pneumoperitoneum problems, unclear anatomy, not enough progress, chylous ascites, fibrotic mesentery, and complex congenital anomalies, each in one patient.

In one patient the diagnosis of malrotation was missed at laparoscopy. At repeat but now open surgery a volvulus without necrosis was still present. Two non-converted patients presented with repeat volvulus. One patient in the converted group developed adhesive small bowel obstruction. There was no mortality.

In the same period 15 children were laparoscoped because of doubtful malrotation on upper gastrointestinal tract series made because of vomiting. Median age was 208 days (30–2,934). Two children were known to have situs inversus. In all children a broad mesenteric stalk well fixed to the posterior peritoneum was found, making a volvulus unlikely.

During the same period under study, one 5.5-year-old girl with obstruction was laparoscoped and had a paracolic hernia, which is considered a form of malrotation. Partial removal of the sac was curative.

Finally we have also laparoscoped three children, aged 13, 15.5, and 16 years, with so-called superior mesenteric artery syndrome. This has also be considered to be a form of intestinal malrotation. In all the duodenojejunal flexure was detached but the results have been disappointing.

Discussion

Treatment of symptomatic malrotation in infants is not simple. In these patients symptomatology is usually on a basis of volvulus causing edema of the mesentery and even chylous ascites. As a result the working space is very limited. Moreover the volvulus may have been present for some time and may have caused significant fibrosis of the mesentery. In one of our patients there was chylous ascites with a markedly swollen mesenteric stalk. Nevertheless we feel that infant malrotation with volvulus, but without obvious necrosis, is a good indication for a laparoscopic approach. If, however, not enough progress is made within one hour, the procedure should be converted.

Laparoscopy is an ideal tool to stratify patients with doubtful malrotation on imaging into patients who need and patients who do not need surgical treatment (Waldhausen and Sawin 1996). It has been suggested to stratify the patients on an age basis, but even above the age of 2 years there is a significant risk for volvulus (Filston and Kirks 1981; Prasil et al. 2000).

Laparoscopy is also a good tool in patients with obstruction of unknown origin. In one of our patients a paracolic hernia was found and partial resection of the sac proved to be curative. Lastly laparoscopy has been used in patients with the so-called superior mesenteric artery syndrome. We have not been able to cure three patients by taking down the duodenojejunal flexure. It may be that a laparoscopic side-to-side duodenojejunostomy should have been performed, as has been advocated. We have no experience with this procedure so far.

References

Ablow RC, Hoffer FA, Seashore JH, et al (1983) Z-shaped duodenojejunal loop: sign of mesenteric fixation anomaly and congenital bands. Am J Roentgenol 141:461–464

Ai VH, Lam WW, Cheng W et al. (1999) CT appearance of midgut volvulus with malrotation in a young infant. Clin Radiol 54:687–689

Berdon WE (1995) The diagnosis of malrotation and volvulus in the older child and adult: a trap for radiologists. Pediatr Radiol 25:101–113

Chao HC, Kong MS, Chen JY, et al (2000) Sonographic features related to volvulus in neonatal intestinal malrotation. J Ultrasound Med 19:371–376

Filston HC, Kirks DR (1981) Malrotation: the ubiquitous anomaly. J Pediatr Surg 16:614–620

Harrisson RL, Set P, Brain AJ (1999) Persistent value of air-augmented radiograph in neonatal high gastrointestinal obstruction, despite more modern techniques. Acta Paediatr 88:1284–1286

Long FR, Kramer SS, Markowitz RI et al. (1996) Radiographic patterns of intestinal malrotation in children. Radiographics 16:547–556

Marcos HB, Semelka RC, Noone TC et al. (1999) MRI of normal and abnormal duodenum using Half-Fourier Single-Shot RARE and gadolinium-enhanced spoiled gradient echo sequences. Magn Reson Imaging 17:869–880

Prasil P, Flageole H, Shaw KS et al. (2000) Should malrotation in children be treated differently according to age? J Pediatr Surg 35:756–758

Touloukian RJ, Smith EI (1998) Disorders of rotation and fixation. In: O'Neill JA, Rowe M, Grosfeld JL, et al (eds) Pediatric Surgery, 5th edn. Mosby-Year Book, St. Louis, pp 1199–1214

Waldhausen JH, Sawin RS (1996) Laparoscopic Ladd's procedure and assessment of malrotation. J Laparoendosc Surg 6(suppl 1):S103–S105

Warner BR (1996) Malrotation. In: Oldham KT, Colombani PM, Foglia RP (eds) Surgery of Infants and Children, chap 75. Lippincott-Raven, Philadelphia, pp 1229–1240

Weinberger E, Winters WD, Liddell RM, et al (1992) Sonographic diagnosis of intestinal malrotation in infants: importance of the relative positions of the superior mesenteric vein and artery. Am J Radiol 159:825–828

Yoo SJ, Park KW, Cho SY, et al (1999) Definitive diagnosis of intestinal volvulus in utero. Ultrasound Obstet Gynecol 13:200–203

Zerin JM, DiPiedro MA (1992) Superior mesenteric vascular anatomy at US in patients with surgical proved malrotation of the midgut. Radiology 183:693–694

Zissin R, Rathaus V, Oscadchy A, et al (1999) Intestinal malrotation as an incidental finding on CT in adults. Abdom Imaging 24:550–555

Chapter 41

Laparoscopic Approach in Adhesive Small Bowel Obstruction

François Becmeur

Introduction

Intestinal obstruction due to adhesions is a major healthcare problem in children (Festen 1982; Janik et al. 1981). Most adhesive obstructions occur after appendicectomy (Becmeur et al. 1997) and measures to decrease the incidence would be very welcome. Endoscopic surgery instead of classic open surgery seems to be such a measure. Reiterative surgery increases the likelihood of developing repeat obstruction but by approaching the problem of adhesive obstruction endoscopically the incidence of reiterative obstruction may well be less than after open surgery (Operative Laparoscopy Study Group 1991). Moreover the laparoscopic approach leaves less scarring and allows for a much quicker recovery.

Preoperative Preparation

Before Induction of General Anesthesia

Adhesive small bowel obstruction usually presents as an acute event and the diagnosis in most cases is not difficult. If there is no delay in diagnosis, the abdomen is very distended and electrolyte and acid-base disturbances are absent. Under such circumstances, laparoscopy should not be delayed. Alternatively, when there has been a delay in diagnosis, the child will be very sick with a distended abdomen, hypovolemia, and electrolyte and acid-base disturbances. Under such circumstances the child should be well prepared for surgery which includes gastric drainage and the correction of hypovolemia, electrolyte, and acid-base disturbances. The optimal timing for surgery is a matter of good clinical judgment. When there is suspicion of necrosis or pending necrosis, not much time should be taken for the preoperative preparation.

In small bowel obstruction there is stasis of bowel contents and it may therefore be wise to give antibiotics perioperatively.

After Induction of General Anesthesia

Especially when dilated bowel competes for the available working space, good muscle relaxation is essential. If a nasogastric tube has not been inserted before, it is done now. A urinary catheter is not needed when the child presents early and the operation is simple. When the diagnosis has been delayed, a urinary catheter is essential to monitor rehydration before and after the operation. It should be remembered that urine production during the laparoscopy itself is usually diminished. A urinary catheter is also essential in case of postoperative epidural analgesia.

Positioning

Patient

The child is put in a supine position on the operating table. The table is further tilted in whatever position (Trendelenburg, reversed Trendelenburg, tilt to the right or to the left) depending on the site of the obstruction.

Crew, Monitors, and Equipment

The site of obstruction as well as the site of the initial operation will decide where the surgical team will take position. As a general rule, the surgeon, site of interest, and monitor will be in line, and the camera operator as well as the scrub nurse stand on the same side as the surgeon and face the same monitor. The right-handed camera operator will usually stand to the left of the surgeon and the left-handed one to the right. Especially in obstruction where the exact site is not always clear peroperatively, it is advantageous to have a monitor on each side of the table so that the surgical team can move to the other side without need for moving the monitor and endoscopic tower as well. As with all endoscopic procedures it is advantageous to fix all cables together so that they can be moved en bloc.

Special Equipment

No special equipment is needed. It may be advantageous to have bipolar electrocoagulation, ultrasonic energy, or Ligasure, especially when the adhesions are dense, vascular, or extensive.

Technique

Cannulae

Cannula	Method of insertion	Diameter (mm)	Device	Position
1	Open	5	Optic	At a distance from existing scars
2	Closed	3 or 5	Forceps, scissors, bipolar, ultrasonic device, or Ligasure	At a distance from adhesions
3	Closed	3 or 5	Forceps, suction, irrigation	At a distance from adhesions

Port Placement

The first port is inserted in an open way. Preoperatively the ventral abdominal wall can be mapped ultrasonographically in order to identify places where no bowel is adherent. If the umbilicus is free, the first port can be introduced in that position.

Secondary ports are inserted in a closed way. In order to decrease the likelihood of damaging dilated bowel, muscle relaxation should be optimal and the pneumoperitoneum pressure is temporarily increased up to 15 mmHg. Secondary ports are introduced under laparoscopic guidance. They can even be placed through the scar of the previous operation provided that that part of the scar is free of adhesions and provided that the port position is at a sufficient distance from the region of trouble. During the insertion of the secondary port the trocar in the shaft is directed into the shaft of the optic. The optic itself is withdrawn into its shaft to avoid contact with the trocar. The pneumoperitoneum pressure is adjusted according to the circumstances and is negotiated with the anesthesiologist.

Procedure

At first inspection a good idea is obtained as to the site of the obstruction. This will of course match with the preoperative radiological diagnosis. Especially in early presentations, the adhesive band may be seen immediately and section of it will solve the problem. When the obstruction has been present for some time, and especially when the obstruction is rather distal, dilated loops of small bowel hide the actual site of obstruction. The best way to deal with this problem is to put the patient in the so-called appendectomy position (reversed Trendelenburg and tilt to the left) and to start with the identification of the ileocecal region. The bowel is than milked between two atraumatic forceps in a proximal direction until the site of obstruction is encountered. Adhesiolysis may be performed with scissors, monopolar hook, bipolar forceps, ultrasonic hook or scissors, or Ligasure.

After taking down the adhesion responsible for the obstruction, the remaining bowel should be searched as well. Simple adhesions can be divided but extensive adhesiolysis should not be performed as new adhesions will develop (Operative Laparoscopic Study Group 1991).

Especially when multiple dense adhesions are present and symptomatology is less acute, it may be difficult to see which adhesion is the most responsible for the symptoms. Under such circumstances extensive laparoscopic adhesiolysis may be difficult and it may be wise to convert. A conversion rate of 25% seems reasonable and should be performed under the following circumstances:

1. Poor working space as a result of dilated loops of bowel
2. Bowel necrosis requiring resection
3. Multiple adhesions without clear cut-off point of obstruction
4. Iatrogenic perforation (a small perforation can be closed laparoscopically)

In order to prevent reformation of adhesions a hyaluronate-based bioresorbable film (Becker et al. 1996; Khaitan et al. 2002) can be introduced into the abdomen. No drains are left behind. The fascia at the portholes is closed under direct vision.

Postoperative Care

Depending on the severity of the preoperative condition, the nasogastric tube is withdrawn immediately or later. When there has been no delay in diagnosis and the operation has been simple, no catheters are left in, the child may eat immediately, and is discharged the same day. Acetaminophen with or without diclofenac will be sufficient for the treatment of pain.

In complicated cases, there may be a need to leave the nasogastric tube for some time depending on the clinical picture. The same applies for the urinary catheter, which should also be left in case of postoperative epidural analgesia. One should try to avoid the use of morphinomimetics in the postoperative period because of their constipating effect.

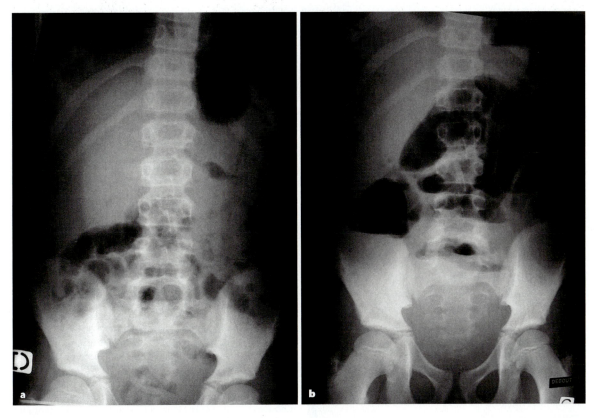

Fig. 41.1. Abdominal X-ray (a) before and (b) about 4 h after surgery

Results

Personal Results

We have operated on 30 patients with postoperative small bowel obstruction. The conversion rate has been 16%. The mean duration of laparoscopy was 45 min and postoperative stay 3 days. Patients who suffer from obstructing bands rather than from generalized adhesions will particularly benefit from the laparoscopic approach.

Literature Results

The results of laparoscopic management of acute small bowel obstructions are good in two thirds of cases in children (Figs. 41.1, 41.2) and recovery is very fast in spite of the lack of emptying of the enlarged bowel as we did by open surgery.

The conversion rate seems to be lower in pediatric series (23%) than in adult series (36%) (Chosidow et al. 2000). The success rate does not depend on the type of previous surgery. Conversions have been needed for bowel resection (25% of conversions), inability to perform the adhesiolysis (50% of conversions), bowel perforation with a trocar (15% of conversions), or bowel perforation with a forceps (10% of conversions). The reoperation rate is about 6% and is often early related failure of relief of the obstruction. The severity of the obstruction may have been misjudged and the adhesiolysis insufficient. Late recurrences may happen as well.

Discussion

Adhesive small bowel obstruction is a major healthcare problem. After laparoscopic surgery, the incidence seems to be less (Neudecker et al. 2002) and has been quoted to be almost 1% (Bailey et al. 1998). After laparoscopy 18% of the patients present with adhesions between the omentum and a trocar site. Also port site herniation may occur (Romagnolo and Magnelli 2001). Even a hole made directly through the abdominal wall by an instrument with a diameter of 2.7 mm can case omental herniation, as we experienced. It is therefore good practice to close all port sites. It is also good practice to remove the secondary ports under endoscopic vision at the end of the operation and to prevent CO_2 from escaping through these holes by finger pressure. After removal of all secondary ports, and finger occlusion of the holes, CO_2 is allow to escape through the optic port. Only then is finger pressure relieved. In

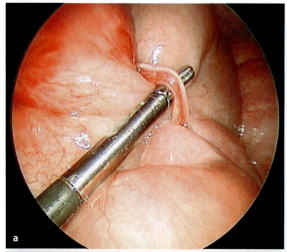

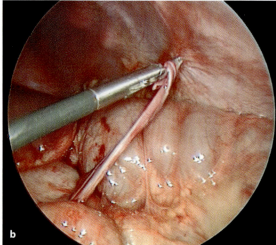

Fig. 41.2. Small bowel obstruction due to a band. **a** Obstructive band, dilated small bowel loops. **b** Situation after transection of the band

contrast to laparoscopy, 85% of the patients develop adhesions after laparotomy between bowel loops or between the laparotomy wound and bowel loops or omentum (Esposito et al. 2000). In any event a lower incidence of de novo adhesions is suspected after laparoscopic surgery for adhesive small bowel obstruction (Operative Laparoscopy Study Group 1991). The laparoscopic approach in adhesive small bowel obstruction has proven its benefit (Becmeur and Besson 1998; van der Zee and Bax 1999).

Early diagnosis and laparoscopy has the advantage that the working space is not compromised by dilated loops of bowel. As in many patients only one adhesion is present and section of the band is curative; many patients can be treated in day care! A completely different situation is encountered when diagnosis is delayed or when massive adhesions are present. Preoperative

preparation in these patients is important and the conversion threshold should be low.

When a single band is responsible for the obstruction, after resection it becomes immediately clear that that band was responsible for the obstruction and no further surgery is required. This is not always the case and in that event a further search for adhesive bands is conducted. While there is no discussion as to the place of laparoscopy in acute adhesive small bowel obstruction, there is discussion as to its place in subobstruction.

References

Bailey IS, Rhodes M, O'Rourke N et al. (1998) Laparoscopic management of acute small bowel obstruction. Br J Surg 85:84–87

Becker JM, Dayton MT, Fazio VW et al. (1996) Prevention of postoperative abdominal adhesions by a sodium hyaluronate-based bioresorbable membrane: a prospective double-blind multicenter study. J Am Coll Surg 183:297–306

Becmeur F, Besson R (1998) GECI treatment of small bowel obstruction by laparoscopy in children. Multicentric study. Eur J Pedaitr Surg 8:343–346

Becmeur F, Ringenbach P, Schwaab C et al. (1997) Occlusions sur brides en chirurgie pédiatrique. Ann Pediatr 44:463–468

Chosidow D, Johanet H, Montariol T et al. (2000) Laparoscopy for acute small-bowel obstruction secondary to adhesions. J Laparoendosc Adv Surg Tech 10:155–159

Esposito C, de Petra MR, Palazzo G et al. (2000) Is there a reduction of postoperative adhesion formation in the pediatric age group after laparoscopy compared with open surgery? Pediatr Endosurg Innov Tech 4:115–120

Festen C (1982) Postoperative small bowel obstruction in infants and children. Ann Surg 196:580–582

Janik JS, Ein SH, Filler RM et al. (1981) An assessment of surgical treatment of adhesive small bowel obstruction in infants and children. J Pediatr Surg 16:225–229

Khaitan L, Scholz S, Houston HL, Richards WO (2002) Results after laparoscopic lysis of adhesions and placement of Seprafilm for intractable abdominal pain. Surg Endosc 17:247–253

Neudecker J, Sauerland S, Neugebauer E et al. (2002) The European Association for Endoscopic Surgery clinical practice guideline on the pneumoperitoneum for laparoscopic surgery. Surg Endosc 16:1121–1143

Operative Laparoscopic Study Group (1991) Postoperative adhesion development after operative laparoscopy: evaluation at early second-look procedures. Fertil Steril 55:700–704

Romagnolo C, Minelli L (2001) Small bowel occlusion after operative laparoscopy: our experience and review of the literature. Endoscopy 33:88–90

van der Zee DC, Bax NMA (1999) Management of adhesive small bowel obstruction in children is changed by laparoscopy. Surg Endosc 13:925–927

Chapter 42

Laparoscopic Treatment of Meckel's Diverticulum

Felix Schier

Introduction

Meckel's diverticulum (MD) is suspected clinically, either upon peranal bleeding or upon inflammation. In the latter case, the preoperative diagnosis is usually appendicitis. Scintigraphy is used to prove the presence of gastric mucosa in the diverticulum. The accuracy of scintigraphy is not very good, and there is exposure to radiation involved. Using laparoscopy, however, MDs are easily seen, especially when specifically searched for, and, if found, are removed at the same time. Therefore, one could ask: why not skip scintigraphy altogether and proceed directly to laparoscopy in cases of suspected MD?

Preoperative Preparation

No special preoperative bowel preparations or other preparations are required. There are no anesthesiologic

peculiarities in laparoscopy for MD. The procedure is performed under general anesthesia with intubation. A nasogastric tube is not necessary as the stomach is out of the area of the trocars. Routine urinary catheters are unnecessary, since a distended bladder is seldom a mechanical problem to laparoscopy, but the patient should be asked to empty the bladder preoperatively. Alternatively the bladder can be emptied manually.

An antibiotic is given perioperatively as a precautionary measure in case of subsequent bowel content spillage.

Positioning of Patient, Crew, and Monitors

The patient is in a regular supine position with the head slightly down (■ Fig. 41.1). This helps to follow the small bowel in retrograde fashion, starting from the ileocecal valve. The surgeon stands on the left side

Fig. 42.1. Positioning of patient, crew, and equipment

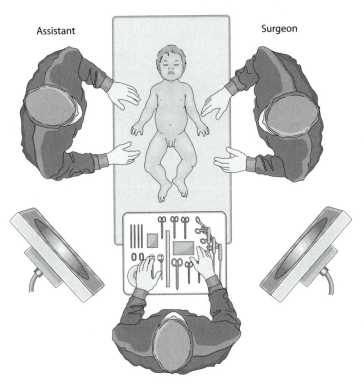

Assistant

Surgeon

Scrub nurse

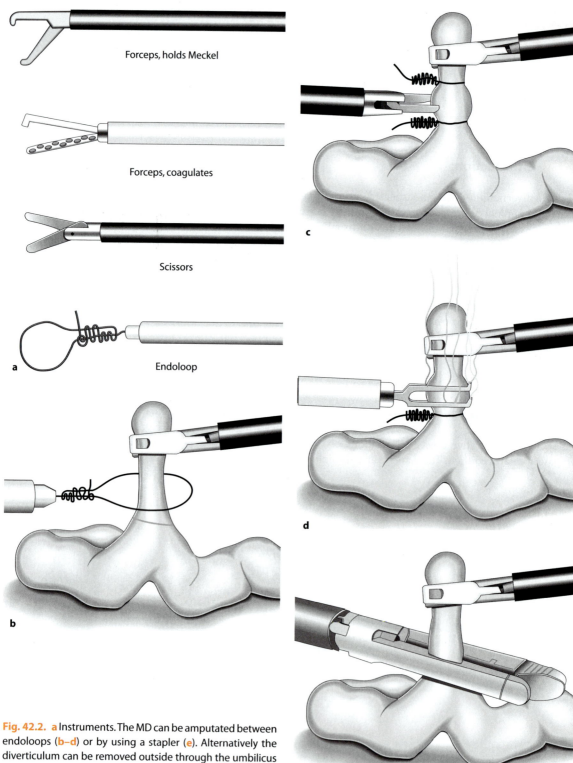

Forceps, holds Meckel

Forceps, coagulates

Scissors

Endoloop

Fig. 42.2. **a** Instruments. The MD can be amputated between endoloops (**b–d**) or by using a stapler (**e**). Alternatively the diverticulum can be removed outside through the umbilicus (not shown)

of the patient, and an assistant is opposite and holds the camera. The monitor is placed opposite the surgeon.

Special Equipment

Monopolar (a bit more risky) or bipolar cautery is used for coagulating and transecting the vessels running from the meso to the tip of the MD. Small-based MDs may be ligated with an endoloop, much like an appendix (Fig. 42.2). Endoloops can be passed through 5 mm cannulae. Care should be taken not to narrow the lumen of the remaining bowel. Broad-based MDs are resected using a stapler. Staplers require cannulae with a diameter of 12 mm. This raises the question whether the MD is not better exteriorized through an umbilical incision and resected outside in an open technique. However, this means surgery of an artificially prolapsed organ including venous congestion. When a 12 mm trocar is used for the stapler, a reducer valve is required for insertion of 5 mm instruments through the 12 mm trocar. Reducers of different manufacturers might not fit. Intracorporeally resected MD need to be retrieved in a bag or bag substitute such as the finger of a surgical glove.

Technique

Cannulae

A small transverse semicircular incision is made in a skin fold at the lower margin of the umbilicus. A Veress needle is inserted, flushed with physiologic saline, and used for insufflation of CO_2. The Veress needle is replaced, by "blind" insertion at the umbilicus, by a 5 mm trocar for the laparoscope. For this trocar we prefer a translucent model because it allows to pull the translucent cannula back as far as possible until it almost falls out. This gives extra distance to the MD which may be located just underneath.

A 2 mm (or 3 mm) trocar is inserted at the lateral margin of the left rectus sheath, below the costal margin. An instrument is introduced and the localization and the size of the MD identified. Depending on the size of the MD, either a 5 mm or a 12 mm trocar is inserted under direct vision in the left lower abdomen.

In case the MD will be exteriorized through the umbilicus and resected outside, one additional 2 mm or 3 mm trocar in the left lower abdomen suffices.

The trocars are arranged in such a way that the laparoscope at the umbilicus is located in the center and the two additional cannulae for the left and right hands in a triangle. Ergonomically the cannulae for the hands are placed so that they might be considered an extension of the forearms.

Procedure

The surgeon will decide which technique appeals most to him or her and the situation encountered. A formal wedge resection is disproportionately difficult laparoscopically. If it is considered, we would suggest enlarging the umbilical incision and performing the procedure outside the abdominal cavity.

With the laparoscopic technique, the cranial trocar for the right hand is the smaller one (2- or 3 mm) because this trocar leaves the cosmetically more prominent wound. The caudal trocar for the left hand is the bigger one. Its bigger wound will later be hidden in underwear or pubic hair. The left-hand trocar will be varied according to the procedure chosen.

Using Endoloops

The right hand uses a 2 mm or a 3 mm trocar. For the left hand a 5 mm trocar is inserted at the left lower abdominal wall. The left hand grabs the tip of the MD and exposes its vessels. The right hand coagulates and cuts the vessels step by step until the base of the MD is exposed. The endoloop is inserted through the 5 mm cannula and tightened at the base of the MD without narrowing the small bowel. A second endoloop is placed more distally and the MD is cut in between.

The author has left the stump in the past in several cases, without noticing postoperative complications. Today, with increasing expertise in suturing and knot tying, we could invert the stump and approximate the serosa on top with several stitches, although this is probably not necessary.

Using a Stapler

The right hand uses the 2 mm or 3 mm trocar. The left hand uses the 12 mm cannula with reducers to 5 mm instrument diameters. The MD vessels are ligated and transected until the anatomy is clear. The tip of the MD is held with the right hand, i.e., a 2 mm or 3 mm instrument, and a stapler is introduced via the 12 mm cannula. Care is taken not to narrow the bowel lumen (Fig. 42.3). A bag is used to remove the specimen.

We have left the cut surface open in the past, without complications. Today we place a running 4-0 slow-absorbing monofilament suture over the cut in order to invert the stapler line and in the hope that all metallic clips will be voided subsequently peranally. This suture is not easy, because the small bowel lacks fixation. It is easiest to place the suture line obliquely and start suturing in the right upper corner, running down to the left.

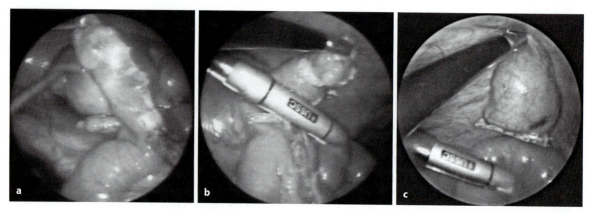

Fig. 42.3. An MD being removed with the use of a stapling device. **a** The diverticulum has been skeletonized. **b,c** Transection of the MD at its base with a stapling device

After desufflation, local anesthesia with bupivacaine is applied to all trocar insertion sites. At the 12 mm and the 5 mm trocar insertion sites the fascia is closed with 4-0 braided slow-absorbable sutures and the skin is closed with interrupted absorbable sutures. Two mm trocar sites are simply covered with a bandage.

Postoperative Care

Children are allowed regular food as soon as they are fully awake. In our practice, postoperative pain medication is given on request, not routinely. Seventy percent of children will not need any postoperative pain medication. Thirty percent will be given paracetamol as a suppository.

As soon as a regular diet is tolerated and discharge at home is acceptable to parents, the child leaves the hospital. This is usually around 3 days postoperatively.

Dressings are changed at postoperative day 4. In older children we suggest they refrain from sports for 2 weeks (with 5 mm trocars) or 4 weeks (with 12 mm trocars).

Results

Personal Results

Meckel's diverticula were removed laparoscopically in 14 patients (aged 5–14 years; median 6.2 years). Seven MDs were encountered incidentally and seven others had been suspected preoperatively because of perineal bleeding. Five had a narrow base and were ligated with endoloops. Nine were excised using a stapler. Histo-logically, ectopic gastric mucosa was demonstrated in eight patients.

There was no conversion to the open procedure. In one instance intraoperative bleeding occurred because an inadequate stapler cartridge was used. The bleeding was controlled by coagulation. The MD was identified quickly in all cases. Anesthetic times were between 25 and 65 min. The resection was complete in all patients with ectopic mucosa. No bowel stenosis developed. Some of the stapler clips were eventually evacuated with the feces.

Literature Results

Limited reference to laparoscopic treatment of MD is made in the literature. Moreover, the majority of reports consists of a few single cases (Kapischke et al. 2003; Lee et al. 2000; Martino et al. 2001; Schier et al. 1996; Teitelbaum et al. 1994; Valla et al. 1998). An exception is a report from Russia of 56 children (Dronov et al. 2002).

The laparoscopy-assisted technique is reported in 14 cases (Lee et al. 2000; Valla et al. 1998). In only one child was a complication noted, a perianastomotic abscess (Valla et al. 1998). A purely laparoscopic approach is reported in 66 children (Dronov et al. 2002; Schier et al. 1996; Teitelbaum et al. 1994; Valla et al. 1998). In about half of these children, staplers were used and in the remainder endoloops. Complications did not occur in any of the children. Finally, in only two children intracorporeal suturing was used without complications (Dronov et al. 2002). Removal of MD using a single-trocar technique has been published in two cases; the MD was exteriorized and resected in an open fashion (Martino et al. 2001).

Discussion

Scintigraphy appears almost obsolete since the advent of laparoscopy. Scintigraphy's sensitivity of approximately 60% is far below that of laparoscopy (Poulsen and Quist 2000). It is almost impossible to miss an MD during laparoscopy, even more so when specifically searched for. In scintigraphy, radiation equals three chest X-rays. Laparoscopy combines diagnosis and therapy in one single procedure.

Trocar sites are best chosen at some distance from the MD. The laparoscope advanced through the umbilicus may render an awkward view. Placing the laparoscope at the lateral abdominal wall, and the two working cannula cranially and caudally may be preferable.

The shape of the MD determines the resection technique. Long, appendix-like MDs have ectopic mucosa mostly in the tip and may be removed like an appendix using endoloops. Broad-based MDs may have ectopic mucosa anywhere (Mukai et al. 2002) and are therefore better resected together with some ileum, either by stapler or in the exteriorized fashion using open surgical techniques.

At present, probably most pediatric surgeons would use laparoscopy mainly to establish the diagnosis but remove the MD in an open technique ("laparoscopy-assisted technique"; Lee et al. 2000; Valla et al. 1998), while others would attempt to stay purely with laparoscopic techniques (Dronov et al. 2002; Schier et al. 1996; Teitelbaum et al. 1994) or they would modify the technique depending on the physical dimensions of the child or the MD: exteriorization in small children or in complicated MD, and stapler resection in older patients or clinically silent MDs (Valla et al. 1998), or use staplers mainly in MDs too broad for endoloops (Schier et al. 1996). It is not difficult to exteriorize the MD through a slightly enlarged umbilical incision. Staplers carry a risk of creating bowel stenosis. This may be prevented by placing the stapler transversely (Valla et al. 1998) or even obliquely (Schier et al. 1996; Teitelbaum et al. 1994). It is doubtful whether the "single-trocar technique" makes sense in MD (Martino 2001). The technique is complicated when it comes to dissecting a complicated MD. For merely exteriorizing an MD a regular trocar would suffice.

References

Dronov AF, Poddubnyi IV, Kotlobovskii VI et al. (2002) [Video-laparoscopic surgeries in Meckel diverticulum in children.] Khirurgiia 10:39–42

Kapischke M, Bley K, Deltz E (2003) Meckel's diverticulum. Surg Endosc 17:351

Lee KH, Yeung CK, Tam YH et al. (2000) Laparoscopy for definitive diagnosis and treatment of gastrointestinal bleeding of obscure origin in children. J Pediatr Surg 35:1291–1293

Martino A, Zamparelli M, Cobellis G et al. (2001) One-trocar surgery: a less invasive videosurgical approach in childhood. J Pediatr Surg 36:811–814

Mukai M, Takamatsu H, Noguchi H et al. (2002) Does the external appearance of a Meckel's diverticulum assist in choice of the laparoscopic procedure? Pediatr Surg Int 18:231–233

Poulsen KA, Qvist N (2000) Sodium pertechnetate scintigraphy in detection of Meckel's diverticulum: is it usable? Eur J Pediatr Surg 10:228–231

Schier F, Hoffmann K, Waldschmidt J (1996) Laparoscopic removal of Meckel's diverticula in children. Eur J Pediatr Surg 6:38–39

Teitelbaum DH, Polley TZ Jr, Obeid F (1994) Laparoscopic diagnosis and excision of Meckel's diverticulum. J Pediatr Surg 29:495–497

Valla JS, Steyaert H, Leculee R et al. (1998) Meckel's diverticulum and laparoscopy of children. What's new? Eur J Pediatr Surg 8:26–28

Chapter 43

Laparoscopic Approach to Intussusception

Felix Schier

Introduction

Many intussusceptions are reduced by enema. Some intussusceptions will reduce incompletely ("hung up in the cecum") or remain questionably reduced on radiology (▪ Figs. 43.1, 43.2). These are the ones to be treated laparoscopically. However, intussusceptions reaching into the transverse colon or further distally are almost impossible to reduce laparoscopically. Some ileoileal intussusceptions are relatively easy to reduce laparoscopically, namely the ones without a lead point.

In children with a severely distended abdomen or with peritonitis the conventional, open approach is preferable.

Preoperative Preparation

No special preoperative bowel preparations or other preparations are required. The catheter for the enema is left in place so it can be used for an intraoperative enema.

There are no anesthesiologic peculiarities in laparoscopy for intussusception. The procedure is performed under general anesthesia with intubation. A nasogastric tube is inserted routinely. Routine urinary catheters are unnecessary. An antibiotic is not given routinely.

Positioning of Patient, Crew, and Monitors

The patient is in a regular supine position with the head slightly down. The surgeon stands on the left side of the patient and an assistant is opposite and holds the camera. The monitor is placed opposite the surgeon (▪ Fig. 43.3).

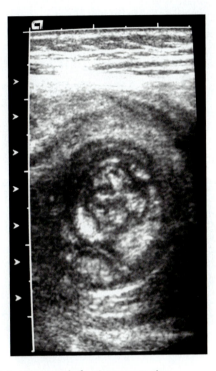

Fig. 43.1. Ultrasound of an intussusception

Special Equipment

Special energy applying systems are not required. Equipment for intraoperative enema application is kept available. Five-millimeter and 2 mm instruments are kept ready, along with the adequate trocars. In case the intussusception has reduced spontaneously, 2 mm instruments will suffice.

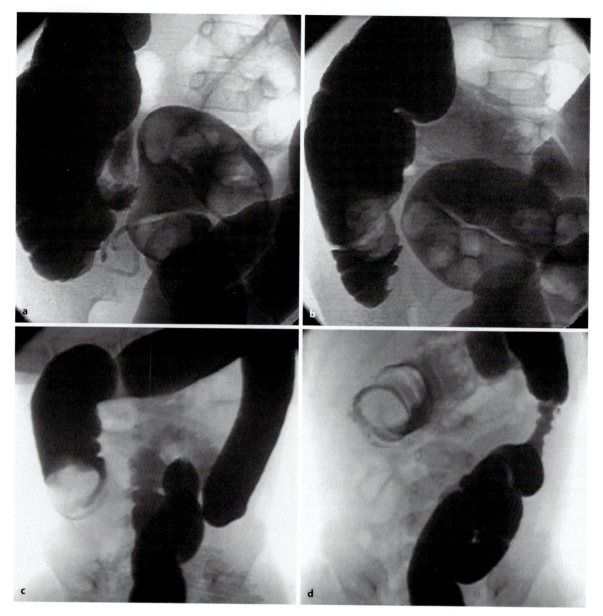

Fig. 43.2. Attempt at hydrostatic reduction under fluoroscopy. **a** Reduction complete. **b** Reduction probably complete. **c** Reduction "hangs" in the cecum. **d** Incomplete reduction

Fig. 43.3. Positioning of patient, crew, and equipment

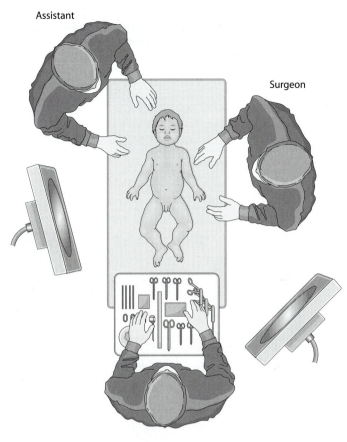

Assistant

Surgeon

Scrub nurse

Technique

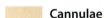

Cannulae

A small transverse semicircular incision is made in a skin fold at the lower margin of the umbilicus. A Veress needle is inserted, flushed with physiologic saline, and used for insufflation of CO_2. The Veress needle is replaced by a 5 mm trocar for the laparoscope by "blind" insertion at the umbilicus. For this trocar a transparent model is preferable because its translucent cannula shaft allows the cannula to be pulled back as far as possible until it almost falls out. This results in maximum distance and optimal overview.

Procedure

Sometimes the intussusception has reduced spontaneously in the intervening time. The anatomy is identified and the procedure terminated. If intussusception is still present, reduction is attempted using 2 mm instruments. The 2 mm instruments are unable to pull hard and they easily injure the serosal surface. Nevertheless, some intussusceptions may be reduced with 2 mm instruments. If they fail, they are replaced gradually by 5 mm instruments. If these fail as well, conversion to the open approach is undertaken.

A 2 mm (or 3 mm) trocar is inserted at the lateral margin of the left rectus sheath, in the left lower abdomen, or suprapubically. A first attempt is undertaken to pull the terminal ileum back. If successful the procedure is terminated. If unsuccessful, a second 2 mm trocar is inserted at the right lower abdomen. This cannula is used for a forceps to hold the cecum during a second attempt. If the intussusceptum reaches far into the colon (beyond the right flexure), an intraoperative enema is given under laparoscopic control. If unsuccessful, conversion to the open procedure ensues. If the intussusceptum "hangs" in the cecum, cannulae and instruments are replaced by 5 mm instruments. There is a 5 mm forceps, originally designed for bipolar coagulation, which is well suited for holding and pulling the terminal ileum (■ Fig. 43.4). The cecum tolerates forceps with teeth when used cautiously. If 5 mm instruments prove unsuccessful, conversion is added (■ Fig. 43.5). Figure 43.6 shows the algorithm for the treatment of intussusception.

After desufflation, local anesthesia with bupivacaine is applied to all trocar insertion sites. At the 12 mm and

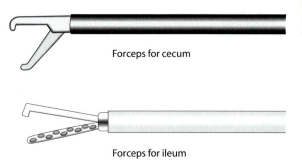

Fig. 43.4 Instruments for the reduction. A 5 mm forceps suitable for holding and pulling the terminal ileum. A forceps with teeth can be used cautiously for the cecum

Forceps for cecum

Forceps for ileum

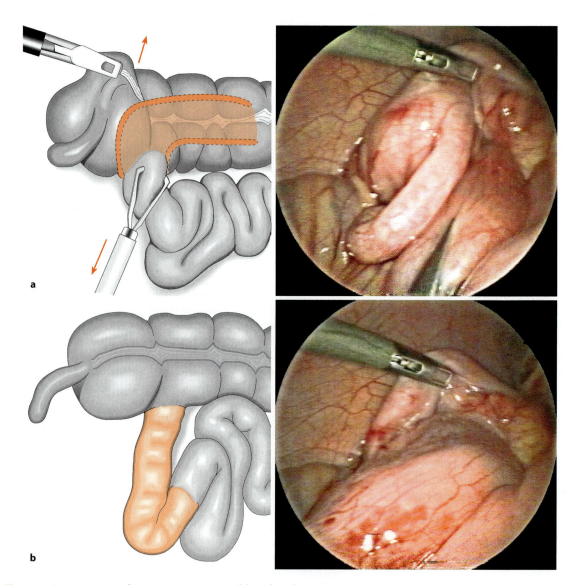

Fig. 43.5. Laparoscopic reduction. **a** Intussuscepted. **b** Reduced

Fig. 43.6. Algorithm for the treatment of intussusception

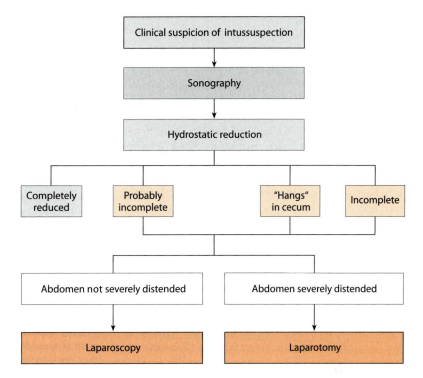

the 5 mm trocar insertion sites the fascia is closed with 4-0 braided slow-absorbable sutures and the skin is closed with interrupted absorbable sutures. Two mm trocar sites are simply covered with a bandage.

Postoperative Care

Children are allowed regular food as soon as they are fully awake. In our practice, postoperative pain medication is given on request, not routinely. Fifty percent of children will not need any postoperative pain medication and about 50% will require a paracetamol suppository. Further postoperative follow-up is identical to open surgery. Discharge home is usually around 3 days postoperatively. Dressings are changed at postoperative day 4.

Results

Personal Results

In 18 children (median age 36 months, range 1 week to 11 years) laparoscopy was performed because of suspected intussusception(s). In all but one, hydrostatic reduction was performed prior to laparoscopy. In the one child without an attempt at hydrostatic reduction a volvulus had been assumed by the radiologist. In this child the intussusceptum was identified in the transverse colon. Laparoscopic reduction was unsuccessful and conversion to open reduction was performed.

Seven laparoscopic reductions were technically easy; this group included two children with ileoileal intussusceptions. Two intussusceptions had reduced spontaneously upon laparoscopy. In two children, the diagnosis was wrong (appendicitis and inflammatory bowel disease were the correct diagnoses). In six children laparoscopic reduction was technically impossible due to dilated bowel loops, or because pulling did not work, and in one case a lymphoma at the ileocecal valve made reduction impossible. In total, in 39% of cases laparoscopic reduction was successful and in another 39% it was unsuccessful. In the remaining 21% laparoscopy prevented an unnecessary laparotomy (Schier 1997).

Literature Results

The largest series originates from Russia. Out of 98 children laparoscopy was successful in 64 patients (65%) and conversion to the open technique became necessary in 34 (34%) (Poddoubnyi et al. 1998). In an Egyptian series of 20 patients, 8 were found on laparoscopy to have reduced spontaneously. Laparoscopic reduction was not attempted in this series and the remaining 12 children underwent open surgery (Hay et al. 1999). In a series of 10 patients from The Netherlands laparoscopic reduction was successful in three children (30%). Seven of these children were older than 3 years (van der Laan et al. 2001). Finally there are two case reports of successful laparoscopic reductions, each dealing with one single patient (Cuckow et al. 1996; Galatioto et al. 1999).

Discussion

In intussusception laparoscopy has its merits even when used solely for diagnostic purposes. In an Egyptian study 20 children were subjected to laparoscopy, in whom hydrostatic reduction had been unsuccessful. In 8 of the children the intussusception was found to be in fact reduced (40%), and in 6 further children an intraoperative enema was successful (30%), leaving only 30% of children for laparotomy (Hays et al. 1999). Laparoscopic reduction was not attempted but might have been successful in a few more cases, thus leaving even fewer children for open surgery. This study also demonstrates the usefulness of intra-abdominal enema, a concept suggested earlier, not only in Western countries (Collins et al. 1989), but more so in China where vast experience with intussusception is available (up to 12 cases per night in one single hospital!). If the initial attempt is unsuccessful, a short period of waiting may be necessary in 50% of cases, followed by a repeat attempt at reduction to eventually achieve a non-surgical success rate of over 90%. In China the remaining patients undergo fluoroscopy on the operating table before operation to assess for instances of spontaneous reduction (Guo et al. 1986). Fluoroscopy might well be replaced by laparoscopy or by a repeat ultrasound. The increased intra-abdominal pressure from CO_2 insufflation might serve as an extra reducing force.

The best approach at present seems to lie somewhere in the middle between the claim that "practically every form of intussusception can be reduced laparoscopically, including the most complex forms" (Poddoubnyi et al. 1998), a position clearly too optimistic, and an attitude to generally wait in the instance of an ileoileal intussusception (Sonmez et al. 2002), a position keeping the surgical team at constant alert for some time.

In the case of failed hydrostatic reduction and the absence of a distended abdomen, a laparoscopy appears adequate, with the chance to encounter spontaneously reduced intussusception. If the intussusceptum "hangs," a first attempt is undertaken with 2 mm instruments. A repeat enema is performed on the table and 5 mm instruments are used. If both fails, conversion to the open technique ensues.

Overall, laparoscopy is probably more successful in the classic 6-month-old child with intussusception. In older children there is a higher chance of anatomic lead points, reducing the success rate of laparoscopy (van der Laan et al. 2001).

References

Collins DL, Pinckney LE, Miller KE et al. (1989) Hydrostatic reduction of ileocolic intussusception: a second attempt in the operating room with general anesthesia. J Pediatr 115:204–207

Cuckow PM, Slater RD, Najmaldin AS (1996) Intussusception treated laparoscopically after failed air enema reduction. Surg Endosc 10:671–672

Galatioto C, Angrisano C, Blois M et al. (1999) Laparoscopic treatment of appendico-cecal intussusception. Surg Laparosc Endosc Percutan Tech 9:362–364

Guo JZ, Ma XY, Zhou QH (1986) Results of air pressure enema reduction of intussusception: 6,396 cases in 13 years. J Pediatr Surg 21:1201–1203

Hay SA, Kabesh AA, Soliman HA et al. (1999) Idiopathic intussusception: the role of laparoscopy. J Pediatr Surg 34:577–578

Poddoubnyi IV, Dronov AF, Blinnikov OI et al. (1998) Laparoscopy in the treatment of intussusception in children. J Pediatr Surg 33:1194–1197

Schier F (1997) Experience with laparoscopy in the treatment of intussusception. J Pediatr Surg 32:1713–1714

Sonmez K, Turkyilmaz Z, Demirogullari B et al. (2002) Conservative treatment for small intestinal intussusception associated with Henoch-Schonlein's purpura. Surg Today 32:1031–1034

van der Laan M, Bax NM, van der Zee DC et al. (2001) The role of laparoscopy in the management of childhood intussusception. Surg Endosc 15:373–376

Laparoscopic Treatment of Enteric Duplications and Other Abdominal Cystic Masses

Henri Steyaert and Jean-Stéphane Valla

Introduction

Alimentary tract duplications and other congenital cystic abdominal masses are rare anomalies (Thompson et al. 2004). They frequently present a diagnostic challenge because they often mimic other disease entities at presentation, even after radiological investigation. Often they are discovered incidentally either prenatally or postnatally (Foley et al. 2003). Therapy continues to evolve thanks to minimally invasive surgical techniques (Schleef and Schalamon 2000). The initial aim of laparoscopy is to locate the cyst exactly and to obtain a better idea of its nature. The procedure may then be continued as a therapeutic laparoscopic procedure in which the cyst is removed.

There is a wide spectrum of cystic diseases in the abdomen. In this chapter we will consider duplications, as well as cysts of the mesentery, spleen, and pancreas, and lymphangioma.

Preoperative Preparation

An ultrasound examination is always performed shortly before the operation to make sure that the cyst is still present. No bowel preparation or prophylactic antibiotics are needed.

General anesthesia with intubation and muscle relaxation is mandatory. A nasogastric tube is placed but a urinary catheter is not required.

Positioning

Patient

The patient is placed supine on the operating table. The position of the table is adjusted according to the localization of the cyst (■ Fig. 44.1).

Crew, Monitors, and Equipment

Surgeon, pathology, and monitor are in line. A second monitor is advantageous when the position of the cyst is uncertain preoperatively. The scrub nurse usually stands to the right of the surgeon.

Equipment

Standard equipment is used. Depending on the size of the child 3- or 5 mm-diameter instruments are used. The diameter of the scope is also adapted according to the size of the child. Thirty-degree angulation of the scope is advantageous but not mandatory.

Ultrasonic dissection is of great help when dealing with large cysts. An efficiently functioning suction/irrigation system is also advantageous as hydrodissection may facilitate finding the right dissection planes. Needle holders are available for suturing in case the bowel is opened during the dissection. Endolinear staplers may sometimes be helpful.

Technique

Port Insertion and Placement

The telescope port is inserted by open umbilical approach. A purse-string suture is put around the opening to ensure an airtight seal. The suture is fixed to the sleeve of the port in order to prevent accidental removal during traction onto the port when needed. Operating ports are inserted directly through the abdominal wall but under endoscopic control. Their position is determined after endoscopic exploration of the abdominal cavity and exact localization of the pathological process (■ Fig. 44.1). Operating trocars have a diameter of 5 mm. Additional 3 mm trocars are inserted when adjuvant instruments are needed.

There is occasionally a need for several "exposing instruments" and insertion of five or six ports is not exceptional in order to accomplish a complete laparoscopic enucleation of a complex cyst. Transabdominal wall suspension of stomach or bowel by traction sutures may also be very useful in good obtaining exposure (■ Fig. 44.2e,f).

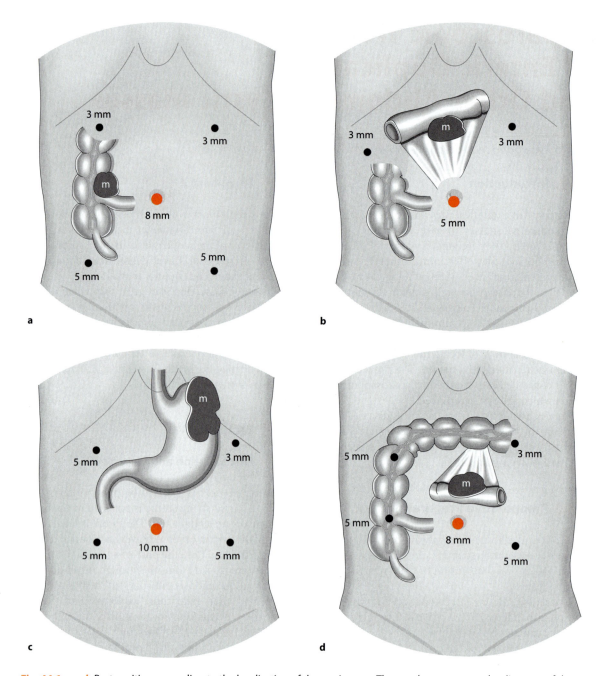

Fig. 44.1. a – d Port positions according to the localization of the cystic mass. The *numbers* represent the diameter of the trocars used. *m* Mass

Procedure

Subsequent steps of the operative procedure follow the same principles as in open surgery. Hydrodissection is an excellent tool for separation of normal from abnormal tissue. In case of a tubular duplication (which we have not encountered so far), application of an endolinear stapler may be advantageous. Most of the time an enucleation is performed. In case of a splenic or hepatic cyst partial excision with "marsupialization" is usually safer than complete excision. At the end of the procedure an omental flap may be placed in the remaining cavity. As the exact nature of the cyst is never certain before pathological examination, the cyst should always be removed in an endobag. When a limited intestinal resection is required, it is easier and faster to enlarge the umbilical opening and bring the affected loop outside the abdomen instead of doing the resection laparoscopically inside the abdomen. After outside resection and anastomosis, the anastomosed loop of bowel is repositioned into the abdomen and a laparoscopic control is performed before finishing the operation. All port holes of more than 3 mm are suture closed to avoid omental evisceration. Drainage is not necessary.

Postoperative Care

Postoperative care is very simple. There is no need for a nasogastric tube except in case of bowel resection. Feeding is started on the evening after surgery and the patient is discharged from the hospital on the first or second postoperative day depending on the level of pain control. In case of an intestinal anastomosis, feeding is started on the second postoperative day and the patient is discharged 2 or 3 days later.

An ultrasound examination is repeated 1 month and again 6 months after the operation.

Results

We have operated on 32 cases of benign cystic abdominal masses using minimally invasive techniques: 2 gastric duplications (■ Fig. 44.2), 3 duodenal duplications, 3 pancreatic duplications, 6 small bowel duplications (■ Fig. 44.3), 1 gallbladder duplication, 2 hepatic biliary cysts, 4 congenital splenic cysts, 5 pseudopapillary pancreatic cysts (Frantz's tumors), 2 posttraumatic pancreatic cysts, and 4 lymphangiomas. Enucleation has been possible in all cases of duplication and Frantz's tumor. In an ileocecal duplication, a hole in the bowel was made during the dissection but was closed endoscopically. Bowel or other organ resection was never necessary. Postoperative recovery was uneventful except in the patients who had pancreatic surgery. All these patients developed biological and sometimes clinical signs of pancreatitis lasting for 4–5 days.

Discussion

Enteric duplications and abdominal cystic masses in children are rare. There are only a few publications and these always represent case reports (Geramizadeh et al. 2002; Schleef and Schalamon 2000). There appears to be a discrete increase in the incidence of this type of pathology due to an increased detection by ultrasound, and especially by prenatal ultrasound. When a prenatal diagnosis of an intra-abdominal cyst is made, the operation is best scheduled in the second half of the first year (Foley et al. 2003). Intra-abdominal cysts should not be left in place as they can give rise to potentially lethal complications (Michael et al. 1999; Steyaert et al. 1996).

Operative management of enteric duplications and other abdominal cysts requires familiarity with this kind of pathology and may challenge even skilled surgeons (Thompson et al. 2004). A topographical diagnosis is important before deciding how to remove the lesion. Computed tomography (CT) or magnetic resonance imaging (MRI) are more helpful in determining the exact position of the lesion than in diagnosing the exact nature of it. Laparoscopy not only confirms the diagnosis but also identifies the exact localization. This diagnostic procedure may be extended into a therapeutic one according to the surgeon's experience. Depending on the localization and nature of the cyst, many surgical approaches are possible. Complete removal is of course the method of choice, but is not always possible without damaging adjacent organs. Enucleation of the cyst may endanger the blood supply of the remaining organ, which is the reason why the lesion is often resected together with adjacent bowel during open surgery. Laparoscopy, in contrast, gives a much better view of the vascularization of the lesion and adjacent organ allowing for resection of the lesion only without jeopardizing the vascularization of the remaining organ. Laparoscopic enucleation is therefore almost always possible with minimal blood loss.

In our experience of 5 cases of Frantz's tumors or papillary cystic tumor of the pancreas it was never necessary to resect part of the pancreas as has been described by others (Carricaburu et al. 2003). In case of huge cystic tumor, partial aspiration of the content may be an option before starting the dissection. However, when the tension in the cyst decreases the plane of separation is less easy to find. Mesenteric cysts and lymphangiomas are probably the most difficult to resect completely. These benign lesions may have a proliferative course (Steyaert et al. 1996). In hepatic or splenic cysts, partial excision with decapsulation is probably the least invasive and secure approach (MacKenzie et al. 2004). Sometimes, however, removal of enteric duplications or other abdominal cysts may require the closure of accidentally opened bowel, or resection of the lesion together with a piece of bowel and subsequent anastomosis. This can be done laparoscopically inside the abdomen or outside through a minilaparotomy depending on the surgeon's experience. If a laparotomy is required, a much smaller incision will suffice when compared to a laparotomy without prior laparoscopic exploration and/or dissection. Endolinear staplers may be useful but we are concerned about leaving metallic clips in a child's abdomen for a lifetime. It is probably better to try an intra-abdominal laparoscopic suture, in which case additional ports may be needed.

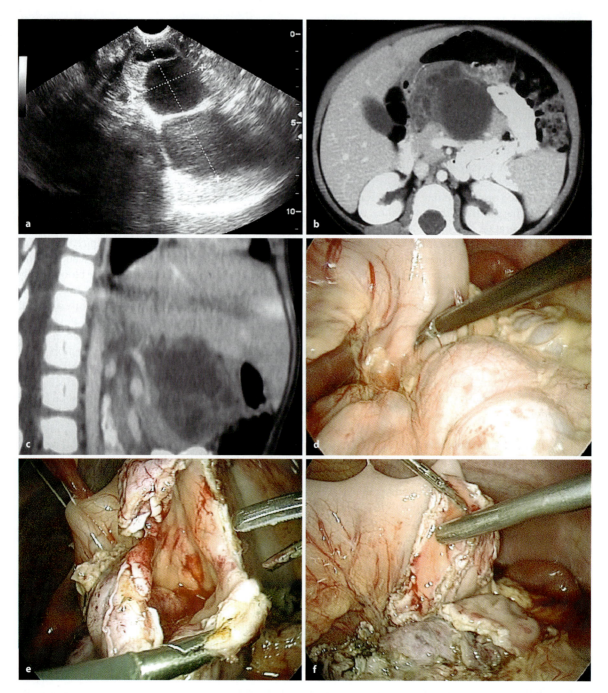

Fig. 44.2. Gastric duplication in a 2-year-old girl. **a** Transverse ultrasonography: retrogastric cystic mass. **b** CT scan. **c** MRI (sagittal). **d–e** Intraoperative views. **d** Retrogastric cyst looking like a gastric duplication. **e** Cystic mass firmly attached to the stomach. **f** Stomach and cyst are being separated (the stomach is suspended from the anterior abdominal wall by three stitches)

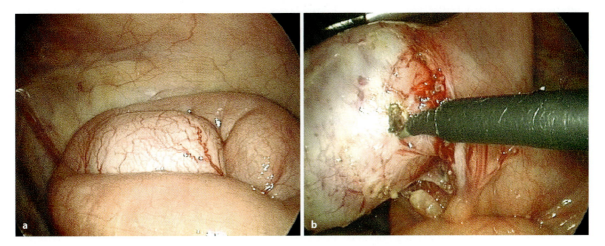

Fig. 44.3. Small bowel duplication in a 1-year-old boy. **a** Small bowel duplication. **b** Enucleation with 3 mm instruments

Conclusion

Cystic abdominal masses are increasingly detected by ultrasound both postnatally as well as antenatally. The exact nature is impossible to define without pathological examination. Preoperative ultrasound is good enough for the identification of a cyst but MRI and CT scan are necessary for topographical localization. Possible complications of such cysts demands for excision. Laparoscopy gives an exact topographical diagnosis and often allows enucleation with preservation of the remaining organ.

References

Carricaburu E, Enezian G, Bonnard A, et al (2003) Laparoscopic distal pancreatectomy for Frantz's tumor in a child. Surg Endosc 17:2028–2031

Foley PT, Sithasanan N, McEwing R, et al (2003) Enteric duplications presenting as antenatally detected abdominal cysts: is delayed resection appropriate? J Pediatr Surg 38:1810–1813

Geramizadeh B, Frootan HR, Eghbali S, et al (2002) Giant ileal duplication with extensive gastric heterotopia. J Pediatr Surg 37:114–115

MacKenzie RK, Yongson GG, Mohamed AA (2004) Laparoscopic decapsulation of congenital splenic cysts: a step forward in splenic preservation. J Pediatr Surg 39:88–90

Michael D, Cohen CR, Northover JM (1999) Adenocarcinoma within a rectal duplication cyst: case report and literature review. Ann R Coll Surg Engl 81:205–506

Schleef J, Schalamon J (2000) The role of laparoscopy in the diagnosis and treatment of intestinal duplication in childhood. A report of two cases. Surg Endosc 14:865

Steyaert H, Guitard J, Moscovici J, et al (1996) Abdominal cystic lymphangioma in children: benign lesions that can have a proliferative course. J Pediatr Surg 31:677–680

Thompson SK, Wong AL, Trevenen CL, et al (2004) Enteric duplication cyst. Am J Surg 187:316–318

Laparoscopic Continent Appendicostomy in the Management of Fecal Incontinence and Constipation

Hossein Allal

Introduction

The antegrade colonic enema (ACE) through the appendix was introduced by Malone et al. (1990) for the management of fecal incontinence. It has also been advocated for intractable constipation (Griffiths and Malone 1995; Squire et al. 1993; Wilcox and Kiely 1998). There is no doubt that ACE has dramatically changed the quality of life of many of the children with these problems. Leakage of the appendicostomy however is one of the problems and antireflux mechanisms to prevent it have been proposed. We have been creating appendicostomies with an antireflux mechanism laparoscopically with good results. The technique is presented here.

Preoperative Preparation

Before surgery the bowel is cleaned by rectal washout. General anesthesia in combination with epidural anesthesia is given. A nasogastric as well as a urinary catheter is inserted. Prophylactic antibiotics (amoxicillin + clavulanic acid) are given.

Technique

Cannulae

Cannula	Method of insertion	Diameter (mm)	Device	Position
1	Open	5 or 7	Telescope	Subumbilicus
2	Closed	3.5–5	Grasping forceps	Left iliac fossa
3	Closed	3.5–5	Scissors, hook	Left subcostal
4	Closed	3.5–5	Grasping forceps for the assistant	Right iliac fossa, at the site of the future appendicostomy

Procedure

An open approach is used for the introduction of a 5- or 7 mm telescope in the umbilicus. CO_2 is insufflated at a pressure of 8–12 mmHg depending on the age of the child. Two working ports are introduced: one in

Positioning

Patient

The patient is put in supine position on the operating table. The table is tilted in Trendelenburg and to the left so that the ileocecal region becomes more prominent.

Crew, Monitors, and Equipment

The surgeon stays to the left of the patient with the camera operator to his/her left and the scrub nurse further down. The most important monitor is positioned opposite the surgeon at the level of the patient's right hip.

Special Equipment

No special equipment is required.

the left iliac fossa and the other in the left hypochondrium. At the future site of the appendicostomy in the right iliac fossa a last trocar is inserted (Fig. 45.1).

As an antireflux mechanism around the appendix will be created by plicating the cecum, the appendix and cecum are mobilized first. Next the appendix is

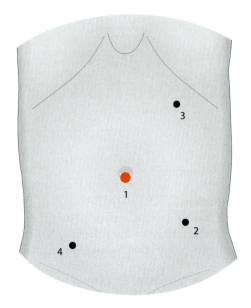

Fig. 45.1. Port positions

pushed cranially over the anterior cecal wall. This is done by the assistant with a grasping forceps introduced through the port in the right iliac fossa. The cecum is then approximated around the appendix with two to four stitches of 2/0 non-absorbable sutures. The suturing is done through the working ports in the left hypochondrium and left iliac fossa. These stitches do not include the appendiceal wall. A last stitch completes the large valve, but should not jeopardize the appendicular blood supply (■ Figs. 45.2a–f).

The appendix is then turned downward and extracted together with the port in the right iliac fossa (■ Fig. 45.3a–c.). At the same time the abdomen is desufflated to allow exteriorization of the appendix without tension. No internal fixation of the appendix is required.

The tip of the appendix is opened and may spatulate. The appendix is cannulated with a 6 French catheter. Finally the edge of the appendix is sutured to the skin (with or without a flap) with 4/0 absorbable sutures (■ Figs. 45.4a–c).

Postoperative Care

The nasogastric tube is left in place until the next morning but the urinary catheter is removed.

Results

Eighteen patients have been treated according to the described method so far. The mean operative time was 90 min (range 45–150 min). There were no peroperative or immediate postoperative complications. Mean hospital stay was 4.3 days (range 2–6 days). For the first 14 patients, we waited for the first irrigation until just before discharge on the fifth postoperative day. This has been shortened to 1 or 2 days decreasing the hospital stay accordingly.

Late complications were mainly stenosis of the stoma, which occurred in six patients. In four the stenosis was dilated daily for a month, with good results in three of them. In the long run, however, five of these patients needed a revision of the appendicostomy. Spontaneous closure occurred in one patient because the patient did not use it anymore. The indication had been intractable constipation in association with gastroesophageal reflux and failure to thrive. The appendicostomy was performed at the same time as the laparoscopic fundoplication and the percutaneous gastrostomy. Constipation disappeared because of better feeding and hydration through the gastrostomy. Leakage of the stoma occurred in one patient only. It started after an enterocystoplasty operation, 2 years after the appendicostomy. In one patient with intractable constipation, the antegrade enema failed to achieve evacuation and fecaloma formation occurred. She developed a megarectum for which she received a pull-through operation.

Evacuation takes place within 30–60 min from the beginning of the enema. The enemas are given every 3 days in 15 patients, and every 2 days in three. Four patients had transient pain for a while postoperatively during catheterization. Satisfaction expressed by patients and their families ranges from good to excellent. All feel that the antegrade colonic enema is far better than the undignified transrectal one.

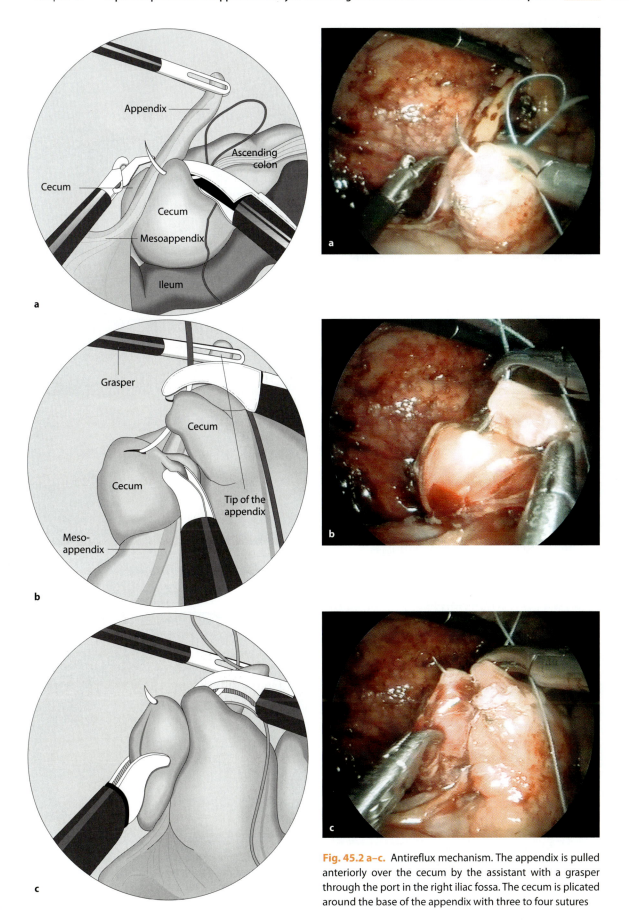

Fig. 45.2 a–c. Antireflux mechanism. The appendix is pulled anteriorly over the cecum by the assistant with a grasper through the port in the right iliac fossa. The cecum is plicated around the base of the appendix with three to four sutures

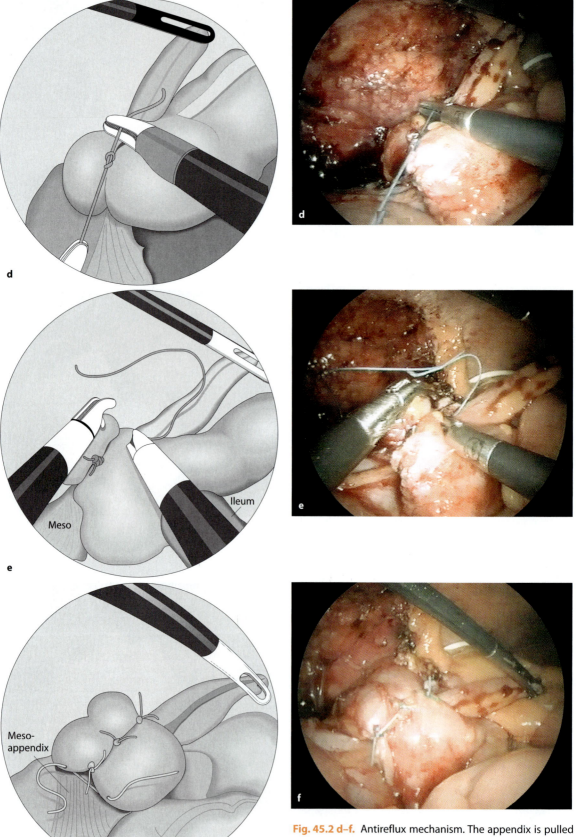

Fig. 45.2 d–f. Antireflux mechanism. The appendix is pulled anteriorly over the cecum by the assistant with a grasper through the port in the right iliac fossa. The cecum is plicated around the base of the appendix with three to four sutures

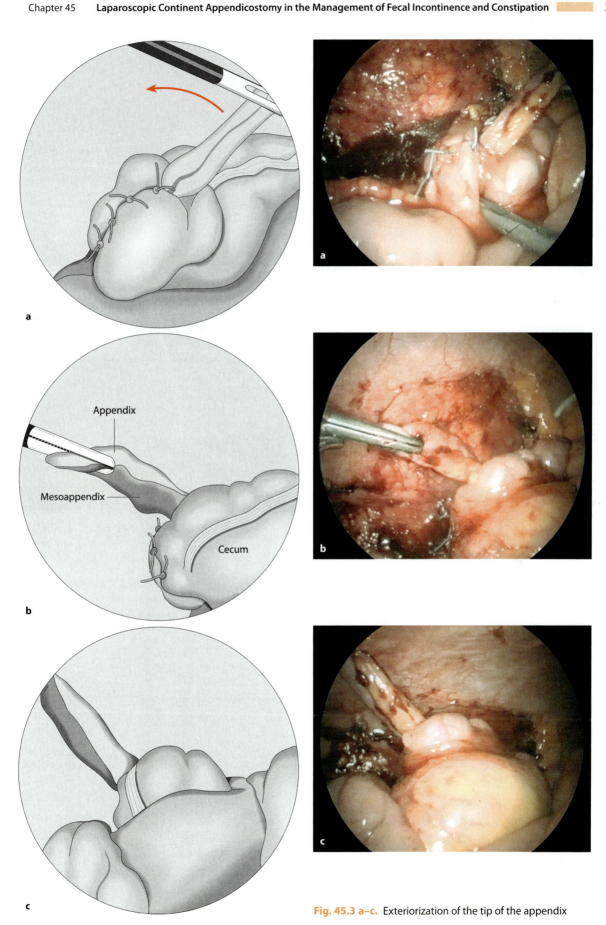

Fig. 45.3 a–c. Exteriorization of the tip of the appendix

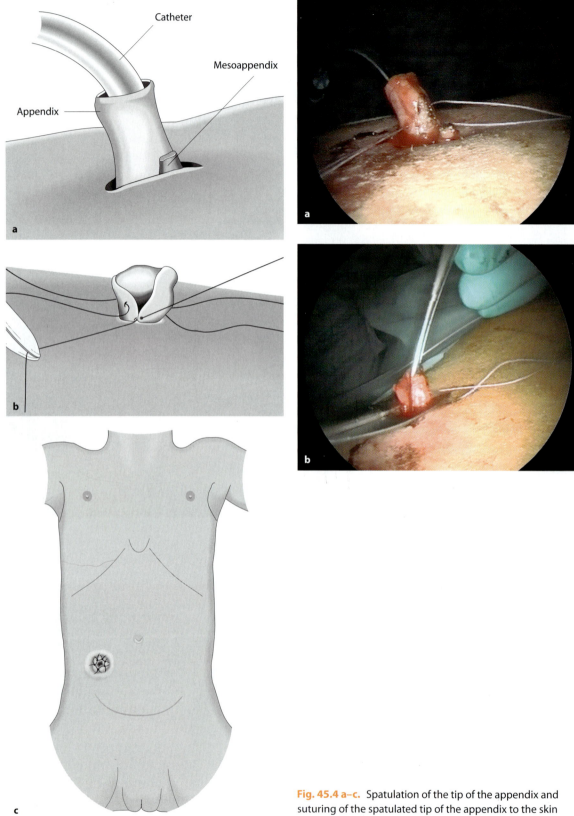

Catheter

Mesoappendix

Appendix

a

b

c

Fig. 45.4 a–c. Spatulation of the tip of the appendix and suturing of the spatulated tip of the appendix to the skin

Discussion

The antegrade colonic enema procedure was introduced by Malone et al. (1990) for the management of fecal incontinence when conservative methods have failed. At the beginning, the principal indication was fecal incontinence (Malone et al. 1990; Webb et al. 1997; Wilcox and Kiely 1998). The etiology of incontinence was: spina bifida, cerebral palsy, cloacal anomaly, sacrococcygeal teratoma, Hirschsprung's disease, anorectal malformation, and perineal trauma. Intractable constipation became an indication as well (Griffith and Malone 1995; Squire et al. 1993; Wilcox and Kiely 1998). In our series only one of three patients with constipation benefited from the appendicostomy.

Malone et al. (1990) described a method of non-refluxing appendicostomy in which the appendix is reimplanted into the cecum to create a valve. This technique has been modified by many authors (Levitt et al. 1997; Squire et al. 1993) because the reimplantation is complicated and probably unnecessary. Squire et al. (1993) described an orthotopic appendicocecostomy, with the cecum imbricated around the base of the appendix. Levitt et al. (1997) developed an antireflux procedure by laparotomy, using the cecum as a valve. We adapted this technique for laparoscopic use. We exteriorize the appendix in the right iliac fossa instead of in the umbilical region. Webb et al. (1997) described a laparoscopic appendicostomy without antireflux mechanism but did not mention the results about the leakage. In our series only one patient complained of stoma leakage. At barium enema no reflux was noticed but the conduit appeared very short. A laparoscopic appendicostomy can also be performed without difficulty after previous abdominal surgery, for example bladder reconstructive surgery or ventriculoperitoneal shunting.

Stenosis of the stoma has been reported as an almost inevitable complication irrespective of whether a circular or V-shaped stoma has been created (Griffiths and Malone 1995). Daily catheterization of the stoma for a sufficient period of time might be a preventive measure to delay the stenosis as long as possible.

A twice weekly irrigation regimen using a mixture of phosphate and normal saline seems satisfactory in most patients both in terms of time investment and in maintaining cleanliness for 48–72 h. There is no reason for delaying the start of the antegrade enemas after surgery for 10 days to a month as has been advocated (Levitt et al. 1997; Squire et al. 1993). Phosphate intoxication by using phosphate enemas has been described (McCrabe et al. 1991) but is avoided in our series as only phosphate in combination with normal saline is used in the beginning. Later we use tap water only, paying attention to the purity of the water. We have not seen complications such as stoma prolapse, retraction, or gangrene of the appendiceal stump (Ellsworth et al. 1998).

References

Ellsworth PI, Webb HW, Crump JM, et al (1998) The Malone antegrade colonic enema enhances the quality of life in children undergoing urological incontinence procedures. J Urol 155:1416–1418

Griffiths DM, Malone PS (1995) The Malone antegrade continent enema. J Pediatr Surg 30:68–71

Levitt MA, Soffer SZ, Pena A (1997) Continent appendicostomy in the bowel management of fecally incontinent children. J Pediatr Surg 32:1630–1633

Malone PS, Ransley PG, Kiely EM (1990) Preliminary report: the antegrade continent enema. Lancet 336:1217–1218

McCrabe M, Sibert JR, Routledge PA (1991) Phosphate enemas in childhood: cause for concern. BMJ 302:1074

Squire R, Kiely EM, Carr B, et al (1993) The clinical applications of the Malone antegrade colonic enema. J Pediatr Surg 28:1012–1015

Webb HW, Barraza MA, Crump JM (1997) Laparoscopic appendicostomy for management of fecal incontinence. J Pediatr Surg 32:457–458

Wilcox DT, Kiely EM (1998) The Malone (antegrade colonic enema) procedure: early experience. J Pediatr Surg 33:204–206

Chapter 46

Laparoscopic Cecostomy and Sigmoidostomy Button

Aydın Yagmurlu

Introduction

To date, the most consistently successful method of management of both constipation and encopresis has been the complete emptying of the entire colon by use of a large volume, transanal enema (Blair et al. 1992). Recently, as an alternative to the retrograde enema, Malone et al. described a continent, catheterizable appendicostomy as a conduit for the administration of prograde irrigating fluid (Malone et al. 1990). The antegrade colonic enema (ACE) program permits the possibility of continence in children for whom other methods have proved unsuccessful or unsuitable (Malone et al. 1990). Many surgical modifications have been made of the Malone procedure aiming either to simplify the surgical technique or to achieve a continent stoma that is not prone to stenosis with minimal morbidity (Cromie et al. 1996; Duel and Gonzales 1999; Shandling et al. 1996; Yeung and Lund 2000). Painful catheter insertion is a common problem causing some children and parents to abandon the procedure (Marshall et al. 2001).

Another alternative to the retrograde enema is placement of a catheter for instillation of fluid in the sigmoid colon (Gauderer et al. 2002). This procedure can be performed either percutaneously with laparoscopic control to enhance safety or in a laparoscopic fashion.

Preoperative Preparation

Before Induction of General Anesthesia

No special bowel preparation was performed for the procedure. A single dose of a broad-spectrum intravenous antibiotic was administered preoperatively and was continued for 3 days. It was changed to an oral form for a further 7 days.

After Induction of General Anesthesia

The abdomen is prepared from the nipples to the midthighs. The child is draped widely as for any abdominal operation. The patient should be securely fastened to the table to allow for tilting during the procedure.

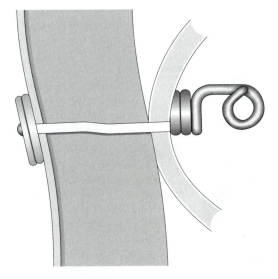

Fig. 46.1. Chait tube

Positioning

Patient

The patient is placed supine on the operating table.

Crew, Monitors, and Equipment

The surgeon and camera operator are positioned on the patient's left side. The TV monitor is placed on the right side. The scrub nurse is on the patient's right side near the foot of the table.

Special Equipment

The following are required:
- Scope 30°, 3–4 mm
- Veress needle
- Grasper, 3 mm
- U-stitch, ×2
- Needle with guidewire
- Dilator with catheter introducer
- Chait tube (Chait et al. 1997) (Fig. 46.1) or a gastrostomy button

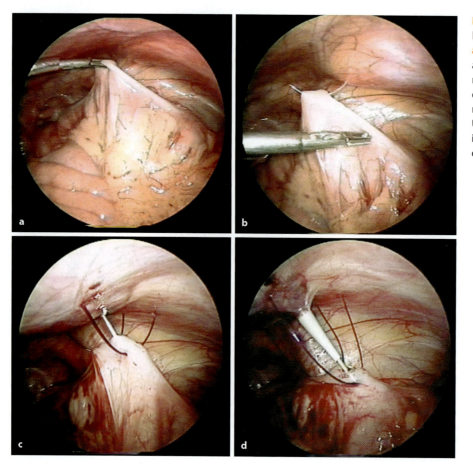

Fig. 46.2. Cecostomy button insertion. **a** Grasping of cecum at a site that would easily reach the anterior abdominal wall. **b** Placement of traction U-stitches. **c** Needle insertion. **d** Dilatation of the track

Technique

The peritoneum is accessed through the umbilicus using a Veress needle technique. The carbon dioxide pneumoperitoneum is established (10–12 cm of water pressure) and a 5 mm expandable sheath access device is inserted at the umbilicus followed by a 3- to 4 mm 0° or 30° telescope. The site chosen for cecostomy by external abdominal wall inspection is confirmed by direct laparoscopic vision, and a stab wound is made through all layers of the abdominal wall through this site with a number 11 or 15 blade. A 3 mm laparoscopic bowel grasper is passed through the stab wound into the peritoneal cavity and the underlying anterior wall of the cecum is grasped at a site that would easily reach the anterior abdominal wall and is sufficiently remote from the ileocecal valve (■ Fig. 46.2a). A large semi-circular needle attached to a monofilament suture (36.4 mm) is passed through the abdominal wall under laparoscopic visualization, through 1–2 cm of the anterior cecal wall on one side of the bowel clamp, and back through the abdominal wall (■ Fig. 46.2b). A second U-stitch is passed on the other side of the clamp grasping the cecum. The intestinal clamp is then withdrawn from the abdomen. A single-wall needle, which allows for a guidewire, is passed through the anterior abdominal wall stab wound and is introduced through the anterior wall of the cecum, in between the two polydioxanone (PDS) suspending U-stitches which provide upward traction of the cecum (■ Fig. 46.2c). A guidewire is introduced through the needle, and the needle is removed. The tract of the guidewire is widened using serial dilators from 8 French to 16–20 French (■ Fig. 46.2d). A Chait tube or an 8 French "gastrostomy" button is advanced over the guidewire into the cecum under direct laparoscopic visualization. The U-stitches are tied over the wings of the button in order to secure the cecum up to the posterior aspect of the right lower quadrant anterior abdominal wall. In the operating room, the cecostomy button is accessed using the accompanying drainage tube, which is flushed with 10 ml of saline, and connected to a bag for drainage by gravity. The umbilical access site is closed with 2-0 PDS at the fascia and 4-0 vicryl rapide at the skin. The second trocar site is closed at the skin with the same material as the umbilical access site.

For sigmoidostomy button, a 3 mm laparoscopic bowel grasper is passed through the stab wound into the peritoneal cavity and the underlying anterior wall of the sigmoid colon is grasped at a site that would easily reach the anterior abdominal wall, usually left lower quadrant. The same U-stitch technique is used for placement of a sigmoidostomy button.

Postoperative Care

The cecostomy or sigmoidostomy button is flushed with 10 ml of saline twice daily and is otherwise clamped during the hospital stay. Irrigations with 100 ml of volume once a day (90 ml of normal saline and 10 ml of glycerin) are begun 10–14 days after placement of the button, and advanced to an appropriate volume for the age and function. The external, cecal, or sigmoid tacking sutures are removed 2 weeks after the operation.

Results

Seven patients aged 4–12 years (mean±SD 7.3±1.3 years) and weighing 15–44 kg (mean±SD 24.5±4 kg) underwent laparoscopic cecostomy button placement at the University of Alabama at Birmingham. The indication in all patients was intractable fecal incontinence and constipation due to anorectal malformations in four and Hirschsprung's disease in three. All had undergone a successful retrograde enema program preoperatively. Button placement was successful in all patients with no intraoperative complications. The mean±SD operative time was 33±2 min. Hospital stay was 2–5 days (mean±SD 3.8±0.5 days).

Almost all the caregivers of all patients were satisfied with the procedure. None of the patients had accidental bowel movements with one or two daily enemas. The patients are mostly accident free unless suffering from gastroenteritis. All of the patients used one daily enema with the exception of a 6-year-old boy who required two enemas daily to remain accident free. The volume for the enema was titrated to effect (400–1,000 cc). The time for an irrigant to infuse by gravity was 10 min to 1 h (with a mode of 10 min). The time period for an enema to obtain a result was 5 min to 1 h (mode 5 min). Two patients had hypertrophic granulation tissue formation around the cecostomy button, which responded to topical silver nitrate therapy. Two unscheduled, uneventful cecostomy button changes were performed in one patient due to mechanical button malfunction.

Discussion

Placement of cecostomy tubes has previously been described using laparotomy, percutaneous, and colonoscopic techniques. The placement of a cecostomy button by laparotomy was first reported in 1996 in three patients with satisfactory results (Fukunmaga et al. 1996). Duel described similar success but cited the need for laparotomy as a disadvantage (Duel and Gonzales 1999). Shandling reported a percutaneous technique for tube cecostomy (Shandling et al. 1996). Percutaneous cecostomy is not as simple as percutaneous gastrostomy because of the variable position of the cecum and its greater mobility, which makes initial puncture more difficult and increases the chance of leakage of colon contents and the risk of peritonitis (Chait et al. 1997). Rivera et al. reported the endoscopic technique for cecostomy tube placement. The advantage of this technique is direct visualization of the cecostomy site, which avoids inadvertent placement of the cecostomy in the terminal ileum or other undesirable sites (Rivera et al. 2001). And finally Yeung and Lund (2000) presented a laparoscopic cecostomy for anterior ectopic anus with constipation in a 26-year-old woman. The laparoscopic method allows tube placement under direct vision. This technique brings with it all of the advantages seen with laparoscopic surgery: clear visualization, decreased postoperative pain, and cosmesis. Additionally this procedure is straightforward with average operative times of 32 min. The only complication observed was local granulation tissue, which was managed topically.

The laparoscopic cecostomy button creation is a simple and safe alternative to the technically more complex Malone procedure or one of its modifications. In addition, the laparoscopic cecal button procedure is applicable for those children who do not have a patent appendix, or have previously undergone an appendectomy. It has the great advantage that no stoma has to be catheterized and that it is therefore not painful. Complications of traditional surgical cecostomy or appendicostomy include stomal stenosis, stoma leakage, difficulty in intubating the stoma, and appendiceal necrosis (Malone et al. 1998). A button is a cosmetically acceptable alternative that eliminates these problems.

Inability to control bowel function may be permanent, as in patients with myelodysplasia; self-limiting, as in patients who have fecal soiling after a pull-through operation for Hirschsprung's disease; or partial, as many patients who have undergone repair of anorectal malformation (Rintala 2002). The techniques described in this chapter enable a reversible procedure, which is convenient for self-limiting and partial fecal incontinence. When the patient's continence problem resolves, the tube can be extracted easily, and the orifice will heal without the need for any other closure.

References

Blair GK, Djonlic K, Fraser GC (1992) The bowel management tube: an effective means for controlling fecal incontinence. J Pediatr Surg 27:1269–1272

Chait PG, Shandling B, Richards HM et al. (1997) Fecal incontinence in children. Treatment with percutaneous cecostomy tube placement: a prospective study. Radiology 203:621–624

Cromie WJ, Goldfischer ER, Kim JH (1996) Laparoscopic creation of a continent cecal tube for antegrade colonic irrigation. Urology 47:905–907

Duel BP, Gonzales R (1999) The button cecostomy for management of fecal incontinence. Pediatr Surg Int 15:559–561

Fukunmaga K, Kimura K, Lawrence JP et al. (1996) Button device for antegrade enema in the treatment of incontinence and constipation. J Pediatr Surg 31:1038–1039

Gauderer MWL, DeCou JM, Boyle JT (2002) Sigmoid irrigation tube for the management of chronic evacuation disorders. J Pediatr Surg 37:348–351

Malone PS, Ransley PG, Keily EM (1990) Preliminary report: the antegrade continence enema. Lancet 336:1217–1218

Malone PSJ, Curry JI, Osborne A (1998) The antegrade continence enema procedure why, when and how. World J Urol 16:274–278

Marshall J, Hutson JM, Anticich N et al. (2001) Antegrade continence enemas in the treatment of slow-transit constipation. J Pediatr Surg 36:1227–1230

Rintala RJ (2002) Fecal incontinence in anorectal malformations, neuropathy, and miscellaneous conditions. Semin Pediatr Surg 11:75–82

Rivera MT, Kugathasan S, Berger W et al. (2001) Percutaneous colonoscopic cecostomy for management of chronic constipation in children. Gastrointest Endosc 53:1–5

Shandling B, Chait PG, Richards HF (1996) Percutaneous cecostomy: a new technique in the management of fecal incontinence. Pediatr Surg 31:534–537

Yeung CK, Lund L (2000) Laparoscopic cecostomy for anterior ectopic anus with constipation: a new and technical proposal. Eur J Pediatr Surg 10:276–277

Chapter 47

Laparoscopic Appendectomy in Children

Henri Steyaert and Jean-Stéphane Valla

Introduction

Appendicitis is one of the most common pathologies in children. Laparoscopic appendectomy is now a frequently performed procedure and is probably the easiest laparoscopic therapeutic procedure to start with for training surgeons. Nevertheless its application remains controversial (Canty et al. 2000; Emil et al. 2003; Garbutt et al. 1999; Hermann and Otte 1997; Steyaert et al. 1999). The reasons for this are the good results obtained with standard open appendectomy and the fact that most appendectomies are performed during duty hours when not enough experience may be available.

Conversely laparoscopy for right iliac fossa pain has an unquestionable diagnostic benefit, particularly in girls. Preoperative ultrasonography, however, is become more and more accurate in confirming or excluding appendicitis (Dilley et al. 2001).

There are three different techniques of laparoscopic appendectomy: the "out" technique (Fig. 47.1), the "mixed in-out" technique (Fig. 47.2), and the "in" technique (Fig. 47.3). All three techniques will be described.

Preoperative Preparation

Before Induction of General Anesthesia

An ultrasound examination and plain abdominal X-ray are often done before surgery. Ultrasonography confirms the diagnosis of appendicitis and gives information as to the localization of the appendix. A plain abdominal X-ray may show a calcified fecalith and/or signs of obstruction.

After Induction of General Anesthesia

A single injection of antibiotics is given during induction of general anesthesia. A nasogastric tube is placed. A urinary catheter is not used routinely. A full bladder may be emptied by manual expression (Credé maneuver) or sterile catheterization. In case of peritonitis, and particularly in case of a pelvic abscess, a urinary catheter is inserted and usually left for the early postoperative period.

Positioning

The patient is put in a supine position with both arms alongside the body on the operating table. The surgeon stands to the left of the patient, with the assistant on the same side on the right or on the left of the surgeon depending on the technique used. The monitor is on the right side of the patient (Figs. 47.1a, 47.2a, 47.3a).

After trocar insertion the table is tilted in Trendelenburg and to the left. In this way the right colon and intestinal loops shift to the left by gravity.

Equipment

Basic equipment is used: three or four trocars (10 and 5 mm), two atraumatic forceps, a monopolar hook, scissors, an aspiration cannula, and a thin, hemostatic forceps. For the "in" technique, endoloops and endobags are useful. A specially designed needle connected to a syringe is used for the aspiration of pus through one of the cannulae for culture. This may also be done directly through the abdominal wall with the help of a Veress needle. We use a 0° 10 mm telescope. For the "out" technique a short 11 mm scope with a 5 mm operating channel is used (Fig. 47.4).

A stapler may be used in the exceptional situation of necrosis of the basis of the appendix. Drains are used as in open surgery according to the preference of the surgeon.

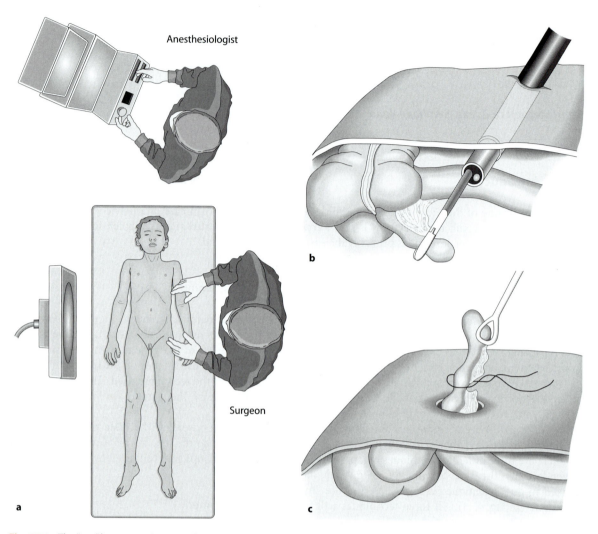

Anesthesiologist

b

Surgeon

a

c

Fig. 47.1. The "out" laparoscopic appendectomy technique. **a** Position of patient, crew, and monitor. **b,c** Schematic drawings of the procedure. The appendix has been exteriorized through the umbilicus using the operating telescope

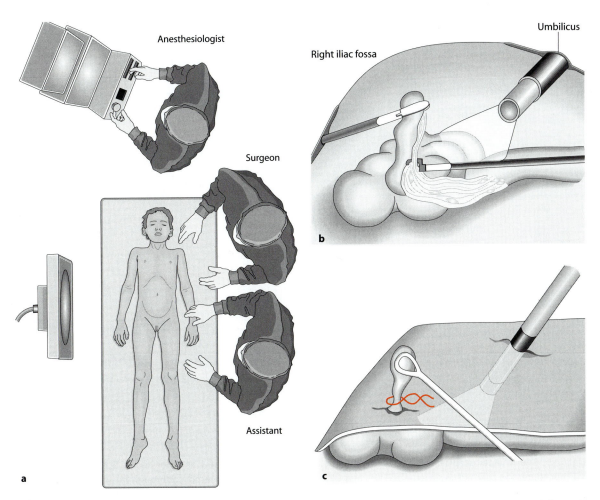

Fig. 47.2. The "mixed in-out" laparoscopic appendectomy technique. **a** Position of patient, crew, and monitor. **b,c** Schematic drawings of the procedure. The appendix is skeletonized intracorporeally but exteriorized through the port in the right iliac fossa or in the umbilicus

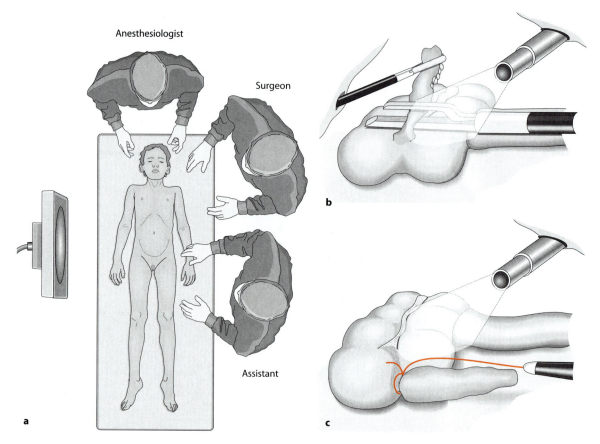

Fig. 47.3. The "in" laparoscopic appendectomy technique. **a** Position of patient, crew, and monitor. **b,c** Schematic drawings of the procedure. The appendix is skeletonized and amputated intracorporeally and removed through the umbilicus

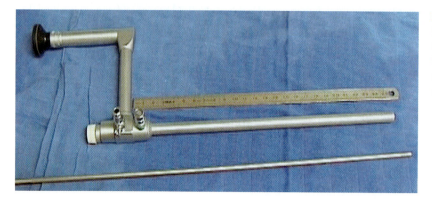

Fig. 47.4. The short operating telescope. This telescope has a total diameter of 10 mm. It contains a 5 mm channel that allows the introduction of 5 mm endoscopic instruments

Technique

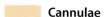
Cannulae

The first cannula is introduced by an open transumbilical technique. The umbilicus is grasped with a Kocher forceps and strongly lifted up. With an number 11 blade scalpel, handled horizontally to avoid any intra-abdominal slipping, the umbilicus is transfixed and cut. Most of the time this makes an opening directly into the peritoneal cavity in children (■ Fig. 47.5a). A curved infraumbilical incision can also be used but is a little bit more difficult particularly in obese children. The fascia and peritoneum are incised under visual control. A cannula with a blunt trocar is inserted and insufflation is started (■ Fig. 47.5b). A purse-string suture is inserted around the cannula and tied to the hub in order to avoid CO_2 leakage and to be able to pull

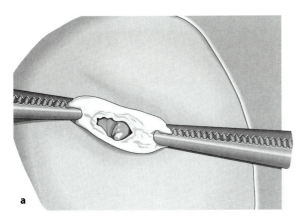
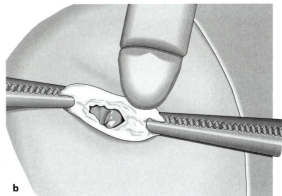

Fig. 47.5. Open transumbilical approach. **a** The umbilical scar has be incised longitudinally. **b** A cannula with blunt trocar is inserted

on the cannula to increase the working space. The number, position, and diameter of secondary cannulae is chosen according to the technique used, as well as to the position and appearance of the appendix, and the preference and experience of the surgeon (■ Fig. 47.6). In the usual three-cannulae technique two secondary 5 mm-diameter cannulae are used. Secondary cannulae are inserted under telescopic control.

Procedure

Inspection of the abdomen confirms the diagnosis. When there is no obvious appendicitis the whole abdominal cavity must be searched in a systematic way: inguinal rings, liver, gallbladder, and internal genital organs in girls. It must be completed by unfolding the distal small bowel loops in search of a possible Meckel's diverticulum. Such a search is, of course, more difficult when the "out" technique is used and under such circumstances an additional cannula may be needed. Peritoneal fluid samples are taken if necessary.

In case of peritonitis and before any mobilization of the appendix, the abdominal cavity should be rinsed with normal saline until the return becomes clear. This may be time consuming.

After rinsing, the surgeon chooses the right operative technique depending on the size, the position, and the pathological status of the appendix.

Three different techniques may be used:
1. The extra-abdominal or monotrocar or "out" laparoscopic appendectomy, also called laparoscopically assisted appendectomy
2. The "mixed" laparoscopic appendectomy
3. The intra-abdominal or "in" laparoscopic appendectomy

The three techniques are shown in the ■ Figs. 47.1, 47.2, and 47.3 and their respective features are summarized in ■ Table 47.1.

In the "out" technique the appendix is freed from adhesions with a forceps introduced through the operating channel, unrolled if necessary, and extracted trough the umbilicus. The actual appendectomy is done as in open surgery and the stump is returned to the abdominal cavity. The stump and appendicular artery ligatures are inspected once more laparoscopically before closure. In this technique the optical trocar is not fixed to the skin.

In the "mixed" technique the appendix is freed and the mesoappendix coagulated from distal to proximal and finally completely detached from the appendix. The appendix is extracted through a right iliac fossa incision or through the umbilicus after which an appendectomy is done outside the abdomen. The stump is returned to the abdominal cavity and inspected once more laparoscopically.

In the "in" technique, the appendectomy is completely performed laparoscopically inside the abdomen. In this technique the appendix is usually removed with the help of an endobag inserted either through an enlarged right iliac fossa incision or, better still, through the umbilicus.

To master all situations, the surgeon must know how to use the three different techniques. Some technical points should be clarified. When the appendix is ready to burst, manipulation has to be very gentle as rupture transforms a simple acute appendicitis into a perforated appendicitis with peritoneal contamination. To avoid rupture it is better to grasp the mesoappendix or the appendicular basis, which is often spared.

Sometimes it may be better to perform a retrograde appendectomy. This is particularly useful in case of a retrocecal perforated appendix. The operation starts

Table 47.1 Relative advantages and disadvantages of the three techniques

	Out, transumbilical	Mixed	In
Contraindications	Peritonitis, retrocecal appendicitis	Obesity	None
Efficacy	+	++	+++
Safety	+++	+	+
Speed	+++	++	+
Explorative possibilities	+	+++	+++
Esthetics	+++	+	+
Teaching value	+	++	+++
Cost	+++	++	+

close to the cecum. With the help of the monopolar or bipolar hook the basis of the appendix is freed and clipped or ligated, either with an extracorporeal or intracorporeal knotting technique. After section of the appendix between the clips or ligatures the distal appendix is freed retrogradely. In case of a retrocecal appendix it may be useful to insert a fourth trocar in the left or right hypochondrium in order to grasp the right colon and to expose the retrocecal region.

In case of an appendicular infiltrate or a localized abscess in the right iliac fossa (■ Fig. 47.7), care should be taken not to spread the pus or to injure the bowel. Most of the pus may be aspirated under telescopic vision by direct needle puncture through the abdominal wall. The abscess is then progressively freed by dividing adhesions with the suction-irrigation cannula, which is used as a hydrodissection device and which is always ready to aspirate each collection of pus as soon as it appears. Electrocoagulation is often not very effective when used on very inflamed tissue and waiting for spontaneous hemostasis is usually effective and safer.

When even the basis of the appendix is grossly inflamed it may be safer to use a stapler device for amputation of the appendix and a part of the cecum. In order to introduce such a device, one port has to be enlarged to 12 mm.

Whichever technique is used and whatever the state of the appendix, a final check is mandatory. If an "out" technique was used the umbilical cannula has to be reintroduced. Great care must been taken with this final look. Such a final look is particularly important when the basis of the appendix was subserous, as in that event the appendectomy may have been incomplete and the child may come back later with an appendicitis of the stump. In case of fecalith the surgeon must be sure that it was removed before the end of the operation (■ Fig. 47.8). If not, an abscess will form.

Drainage is carried out only in case of appendicular abscess. The umbilical fascia is closed with absorbable sutures. Port holes of 5 mm or less can be closed with adhesive skin strips only. Larger holes need to be closed with absorbable sutures in order to avoid port site herniation.

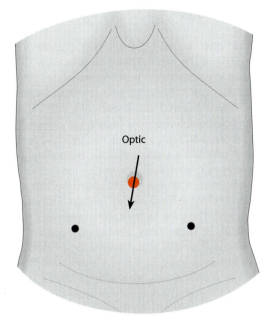

a   Position A: 36,4%

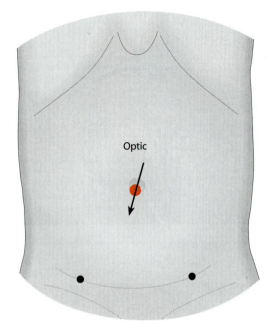

b   Position B: 22,7%

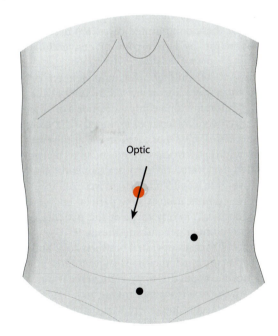

c   Position C: 40,9%

Fig. 47.6. Most often used trocar positions

Postoperative Care

Antibiotics are continued only in case of peritonitis. Under such circumstances, broad-spectrum antibiotic therapy is continued intravenously for 4–6 days according to the decrease of the inflammatory parameters in the blood. After discharge, oral antibiotics directed against aerobics and anaerobics is continued for 4–6 days (10–15 days in total) according to the hospital's protocols.

A nasogastric tube is almost never useful after the operation. A urinary catheter is only used in case of gross peritonitis and in children under 5 years of age.

Feeding is started a few hours after the operation. In case of peritonitis feeding is started after initial recovery (2–3 days in general). Pain control is best achieved by intravenous morphinomimetics for the first day or longer if needed. Some patients are nauseated and need symptomatic treatment. Any drains are usually removed after 3 days.

Discharge from the hospital is scheduled after 24 or 48 h in case of uncomplicated appendicitis and after 4–6 days in case of an appendicular abscess or peritonitis.

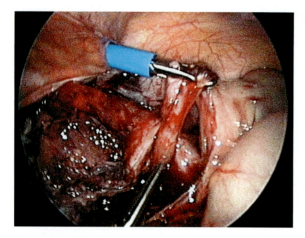

Fig. 47.7. Pelvic abscess

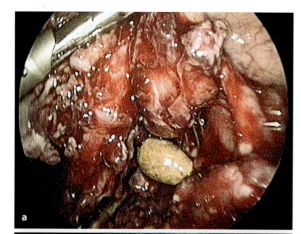

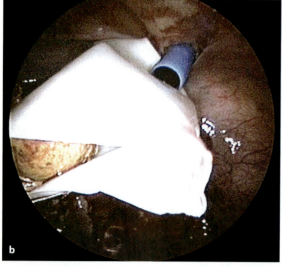

Fig. 47.8. Fecalith. **a** A fecalith is present in the pelvis. **b** Removal of the fecalith in the finger of a glove

Results

We have now carried out over 3,000 appendectomies. The charts of the first 1,379 children operated by the laparoscopic technique were reviewed in 1994 (El Ghoneimi et al. 1994); 0.9% were less than 3 years old, 2.5% were between 3 and 8 years old, and 74% were between 8 and 16 years old (mean age: 8 years). Seventy percent had acute appendicitis, 16% had peritonitis, and 14% had a macroscopically normal appendix. In case of non-complicated appendicitis (1,260 cases) the conversion rate was 0.08%, mean operative time 23 min, and mean hospital stay 1.8 days. Drainage was never used. The total complication rate was 0.6% and only 0.5% of these cases needed reoperation under general anesthesia. At initial laparoscopic evaluation of the abdomen several preoperatively undetected lesions were found. When diagnosis of appendicitis was discarded, the appendix was nevertheless removed. The conversion rate rose to 3.3%, mean operative time to 55 min, and mean hospital stay to 6.5 days in case of complicated appendicitis. Drainage was necessary in 30% of these cases. The total complication rate rose to 13.3%. Of these complicated cases, 6% needed a second operation by laparoscopy or conventional surgery.

Our first 200 children who underwent an "out" appendectomy were also reviewed in 1999 (Valla et al. 1999). Children with a clinical diagnosis of abscess or peritonitis were, of course, excluded. The technique was successful in 92% of cases. In 8% of the cases, one or two additional trocars were needed to manage unexpected perforated or retrocecal appendicitis. Mean operative time was 15 min. There were ten (5%) postoperative complications (three parietal and seven intra-abdominal). Two percent of the patients needed reoperation under general anesthesia.

Of our 400 cases operated between 2002 and 2004, 56% had acute appendicitis, 31% peritonitis, and 13% had a normal appendix. Sixty-eight percent were operated with the one trocar technique and 32% needed a three-trocar technique. There were eight (2%) complications: three umbilical granulomas, two fifth-day syndromes, and one intra-abdominal abscess were managed medically, while one omental evisceration and one bleeding needed repeat surgery. Although the peritonitis rate is higher in this last series, the total complication rate has decreased due to a better technique and a more accurate antibiotic management (decrease in intra-abdominal residual abscess rate).

Discussion

During recent decades, progress has been made in the accuracy of the diagnosis of appendicitis. Notwithstanding progress in ultrasound diagnosis, laparoscopic evaluation of the abdomen is a good tool in case of abdominal pain of unknown origin, particularly in girls (Kum et al. 1993).

The advantages of the laparoscopic approach in acute appendicitis are now obvious for more and more surgical teams (Canty et al. 2000). Many publications have reported a lower incidence of abdominal wall complications (Dilley et al. 2001; El Ghoneimi et al. 1994; Garbutt et al. 1999; Hermann and Otte 1997; Kum et al. 1993; Steyaert et al. 1999).

Intraperitoneal complications are lower with a laparoscopic approach. Appendectomy is classically the major cause of adhesive small bowel obstruction in children; 80% occur during the first year following operation. Since the era of laparoscopy the number of postoperative small bowel obstructions, even after peritonitis, has decreased considerably (Dilley et al. 2001; El Ghoneimi et al. 1994; Garbutt et al. 1999; Gilchrist et al. 1992; Hermann and Otte 1997; Kum et al. 1993; Steyaert et al. 1999). Residual abscesses, more frequent in all pioneer series of laparoscopic appendectomy, have become less of a problem because of an adapted antibiotic regimen, as shown in our recent series. But controversies remain in antibiotherapy (Nadler et al. 2003). Intraperitoneal residual abscess may be cured by medical management or may require repeat surgery, for example percutaneous, transrectal, or laparoscopic drainage (McKinlay et al. 2003).

From a technical point of view a balance must be made between several factors: safety, experience, cost, and habit. These factors apply to the type of laparoscopy, the position of cannulae, the use of different devices, and so on (Ng 2003). In our institution, nowadays, we always begin with the operating telescope, we add two more trocars when needed, we seldom use a bipolar hook, most of the time we do an anterograde appendectomy, and we use fewer and fewer endobags and exceptionally a stapler (Valla et al. 1999). But any kind of approach and use of any type of tool is possible. For example, 5 mm optics are widely used but a 2 mm scope and instruments are available as well. However, for an inflamed appendix with a diameter of more than 10 mm there is not much use for such fragile instruments.

Although we prefer an open technique for the insertion of the first trocar, insertion of this trocar using a closed technique after insufflation of the abdomen with a Veress needle may be useful in obese patients. All these techniques should be known as they may be helpful sometimes. Appendectomy is, indeed, a well-known operation that can raise some surprises.

The esthetic benefit provided by laparoscopy is difficult to quantify. It is undoubtedly superior to open surgery in case of peritonitis, in obese patients, or in patients with an ectopic appendix. When the "out" technique is used, there is barely revisible scar.

Whether laparoscopic appendectomy leads to a faster recovery and shorter hospital stay is debatable in uncomplicated appendicitis (Canty et al. 2000; Dilley et al. 2001; Eldridge et al. 2003; El Ghoneimi et al. 1994; Emil et al. 2003; Garbutt et al. 1999; Gilchrist et al. 1992; Hermann and Otte 1997; Kum et al. 1993; MacKinlay et al. 2003; Ng 2003; Steyaert et al. 1999; Valla et al. 1999). But let us not forget that laparoscopy pushed even the "traditional surgeons" to use shorter incisions, fewer drains and tubes, in a one word to be also more minimally invasive. Under such circumstances there is probably no big difference in the use of postoperative analgesics, in the start of oral feeding, and in getting up (Lejus et al. 1996).

The advantages of the laparoscopic approach become more important in case of peritonitis. The period to recover from the sepsis is the same (approximately 6 days) but after that period the child is cured. In contrast after a laparotomy, which is generally quite large for this indication, the time to recover from the parietal damage is longer (approximately 10 days).

Especially when learning the technique, one should opt for an open approach for insertion of the first trocar in order to avoid visceral or vascular injuries (Juricic et al. 1994). Laparoscopic appendectomy is an easy procedure to start training surgeons in laparoscopic surgery. The first step in this learning process is the introduction of the first trocar and exploration of the abdominal cavity. The second step is the actual appendectomy. The appendix can easily be moved away from other organs before using coagulating devices. The third step may be the use of particular devices (endoloop, endobag, endoGIA, etc.). Finally the surgeon is taught to use laparoscopic techniques in case of peritonitis without increased risk (Carasco-Prats et al. 2003).

What are today the contraindications for a laparoscopic approach? Age is no longer a limitation for the endoscopic pediatric surgical team provided that insufflation is used with care. A localized abscess and appendicitis complicated by bowel obstruction with great abdominal distension remain the only relative contraindications to laparoscopy. Controversies remain (Gibeily et al. 2003). The surgeon has to choose between immediate intervention or medical treatment with antibiotics eventually followed by ultrasound-guided or surgical drainage (Samuel et al. 2002). If the appendicitis settles, appendectomy can be performed some weeks later as has been recommended in English-speaking countries. In our institution we try to operate on all appendicitis cases without exception but ask for the parents' opinion in case of an abscess or bowel obstruction. Some parents prefer to wait, which we agree upon unless the child's temperature and inflammatory signs do not decrease substantially within the next 2 or 3 days.

Laparoscopic and conventional surgery are complementary methods in the matter of appendectomy (Newman et al. 2003). Starting the operation laparoscopically allows the surgeon and trainee to master the safety rules of the technique, to gain experience starting with the easiest cases, to evaluate thoroughly the pathological situation, and to adapt the technique even to the "out" one (Gilchrist et al. 1992). There is little doubt that the laparoscopic technique will develop naturally because of its advantages irrespective of the pathological status of the appendix. Non-complicated appendicitis poses above all a diagnostic problem: in case of a wrong clinical diagnosis, laparoscopy gives the possibility of a complete exploration of the abdominal cavity. This advantage could soon pass a major turning point if a microtelescope could be inserted under local anesthesia, in the ambulatory, into the abdomen allowing for direct visual exploration of the appendix in a child presenting with right iliac fossa pain. Then the surgeon would have a minimally invasive effective examination at his disposition to solve the daily problem of right iliac fossa pain syndrome in children.

Complicated appendicitis is not a diagnostic but a therapeutic problem, which has been classically managed with a large surgical exposure. The laparoscopic approach with its minimal access provides an unquestionable advantage in such circumstances.

Finally, even for procedures like appendectomy that do not require complex skills, further improvement in the laparoscopic equipment with the introduction of robotics may further increase the benefits (Erfanian et al. 2003). The question arises as to whether robotic surgery and telementoring are "coming in" even in appendectomy?

References

Canty TG, Collins B, Losasso B, et al (2000) Laparoscopic appendectomy for simple and perforated appendicitis in children: the procedure of choice? J Pediatr Surg 11:1582–1585

Carasco-Prats M, Soria Aledo S, Lujan-Mompean JA, et al (2003) Role of appendectomy in training for laparoscopic surgery. Surg Endosc 17:111–114

Dilley A, Wesson D, Munden M, et al (2001) The impact of ultrasound examinations on the management of children with suspected appendicitis: a 3 year analysis. J Pediatr Surg 36:303–308

Eldridge B, Kimber C, Wolfe R, et al (2003) Uptime as a measure of recovery in children postappendectomy. J Pediatr Surg 12:1822–1825

El Ghoneimi A, Valla JS, Limonne B, Valla V, et al (1994) Laparoscopic appendectomy in children: report of 1379 cases. J Pediatr Surg 29:786–789

Emil S, Laberge JM, Mikhail P, et al (2003) Appendicitis in children: a ten year update of therapeutic recommendations. J Pediatr Surg 38:236–242

Erfanian K, Luks FI, Kurkchubasche AG, et al (2003) In-line image projection accelerates task performance in laparoscopic appendectomy. J Pediatr Surg 38:1059–1062

Garbutt JM, Soper NJ, Shannon WD, et al (1999) Meta-analysis of randomized controlled trials comparing laparoscopic and open appendectomy. Surg Laparosc Endosc 9:17–26

Gibeily GJ, Ross MN, Manning DB, Wherry DC, Kao TC (2003) Late-presenting appendicitis. Surg Endosc 17:725–729

Gilchrist BF, Lobe TE, Schropp KP, et al (1992) Is there a role for laparoscopic appendectomy in pediatric surgery? J Pediatr Surg 27:209–214

Hermann BP, Otte JB (1997) Laparoscopic appendectomy: pros and cons. Literature review of 4190 cases. Acta Chir Belg 97:110–117

Juricic M, Bossavy JP, Izard P, et al (1994) Laparoscopic appendicectomy: case reports of vascular injury in two children. Eur J Pediatr Surg 4:327–328

Kum CK, Sim EK, Goh PM, et al (1993) Diagnostic laparoscopy: reducing the number of normal appendectomy. Dis Colon Rectum 36:763–766

Lejus C, Delile L, Plattner V, et al (1996) Randomized single-blinded trial of laparoscopic versus open appendicectomy in children. Anesthesiology 4:801–806

McKinlay R, Neeleman S, Klein R, et al (2003) Intraabdominal abscess following open and laparoscopic appendectomy in the pediatric population. Surg Endosc 17:730–733

Nadler E, Kimberly K, Ford H, et al (2003) Monotherapy versus multi-drug therapy for the treatment of perforated appendicitis in children. Surg Infect 4:327–333

Newman K, Ponsky T, Kittle K, et al (2003) Appendicitis 2000: variability in practice, outcomes, and resource utilization at the thirty pediatric hospitals. J Pediatr Surg 372–379

Ng WT (2003) Port placement for laparoscopic appendectomy with the best cosmesis and ergonomics. Surg Endosc 17:166–167

Samuel M, Hosie G, Holmes K (2002) Prospective evaluation of nonsurgical versus surgical management of appendiceal mass. J Pediatr Surg 37:882–886

Steyaert H, Hendrice C, Lereau L, et al (1999) Laparoscopic appendectomy in children: sense or nonsense? Acta Chir Belg 99:119–124

Valla JS, Ordorica-Flores RM, Steyaert H, et al (1999) Umbilical one puncture laparoscopic assisted appendectomy in children. Surg Endosc 13:83–85

Chapter 48

Laparoscopic Management of Crohn's Disease

Steven S. Rothenberg

Introduction

The application of minimally invasive surgical (MIS) techniques in the pediatric population has greatly expanded since the 1990s. Several advanced procedures such as laparoscopic splenectomy, fundoplication, and colon pull-through have become commonplace and in fact, in many centers, is the technique of choice. One area that has lagged behind is the MIS treatment of isolated or limited intestinal strictures associated with Crohn's disease, requiring segmental resection with anastomosis (Becmeur and Besson 1998; Hamel et al. 2001; Milsom et al. 2001). These procedures involve several obstacles not encountered in other MIS operations, the greatest of which is creating a patent and watertight anastomosis. The procedure can be broken down into three steps, mobilization, resection, and anastomosis. In a limited number of cases a stricturoplasty may be sufficient. Each of these steps provides unique challenges, and the length of intestine involved and the size of the patient may dictate the type of procedure performed. However recent advances in instrumentation and technique have made each of these situations approachable and perhaps preferable to standard open techniques.

Preoperative Preparation

Before Induction of General Anesthesia

The preoperative preparation depends somewhat on the presenting condition of the patient. If the patient presents acutely obstructed the preparation consists of intravenous hydration, nasogastric decompression, and antibiotics. Once the patient is adequately resuscitated laparoscopic exploration can be performed. If the patient presents with a more chronic history of abdominal pain and partial obstruction then they may tolerate a gentle bowel preparation with GoLYTELY or some other oral preparation. However since most of these lesions are in the terminal ileum a clear liquid diet for 2–3 days prior to surgery is usually sufficient. An upper gastrointestinal series with small bowel follow through is the most helpful preoperative study. It can usually identify the site and length of the intestinal segment involved. However the final determination is made at the time of the laparoscopic exploration. A preoperative antibiotic with a second-generation cephalosporin is usually adequate.

After Induction of General Anesthesia

A nasogastric tube should be placed with plans to leave it in for the initial postoperative period. A urinary catheter can be placed if there is a question about the patient's hydration status. A single large-bore intravenous line is placed and a central venous line is generally not necessary unless the patient is nutritionally depleted and there are plans to give postoperative hyperalimentation.

Positioning

Patient

The patient is placed in a supine position with routine padding. Occasionally it may be helpful to have the patient in a modified dorsal lithotomy position so that the surgeon can stand between the patient's legs giving better access to the upper abdomen (■ Fig. 48.1). However since most of the significant pathology tends to be in the distal small bowel this is rarely necessary.

Crews, Monitors, and Equipment

The surgeon and the assistant start on the patient's left side working toward the right lower quadrant (■ Fig. 48.1). From this position the surgeon can easily access the area of the ileocecal valve as well as the distal small bowel. The assistant may be above or below the surgeon depending on which position is more ergonomic. The scrub nurse is positioned on the right side of the table. The main monitor is placed near the right lower quadrant. A second monitor may be placed near the patient's left shoulder or hip for the scrub nurse and anesthesiologist to monitor.

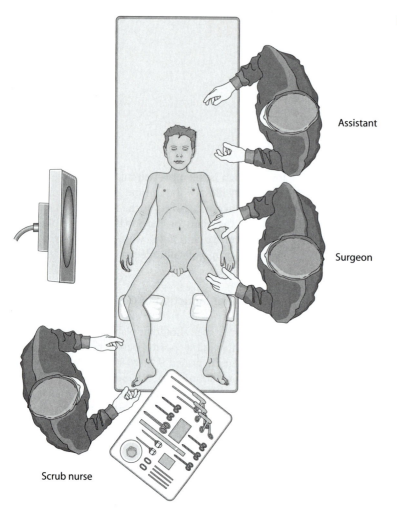

Fig. 48.1. Patient and crew position

Assistant

Surgeon

Scrub nurse

Special Equipment

It is convenient to have ultrasonic energy and/or the Ligasure at hand as well as 5 mm endoclips, staplers, and an endobag for removal of the specimen.

Technique

Cannulae

Cannula	Method of insertion	Diameter (mm)	Device	Position
1	Closed	12	30° scope 5 mm, endoscopic stapler if used, and site for specimen removal	Umbilicus
2	Closed	5	Scissors, ultrasonic shears, Ligasure, atraumatic bowel clamp	Midepigastrium
3	Closed	5	Maryland dissector, Ligasure	Suprapubic
4	Closed	5	Babcock, atraumatic clamp	Right upper quadrant

Figure 48.2 shows the positions of the trocars.

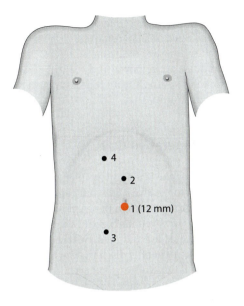

Fig. 48.2. Port placements

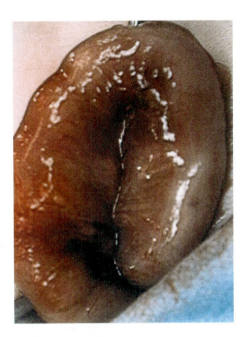

Fig. 48.3. Extracorporeal resection

Procedure

The procedure starts by insufflating the abdomen with a Veress needle through an infraumbilical incision (a Hassan technique can be used if preferred). This incision can later be extended around the rim of the umbilicus to allow for specimen removal. A 12 mm port is inserted and acts as the camera port for the majority of the procedure. This larger port is also used for later introduction of the endoscopic stapler and large specimen bag as needed.

After an initial survey the suprapubic and midepigastric ports are placed. Then with 5 mm atraumatic bowel clamps the small bowel is run from the ileocecal valve retrograde until the area or areas of affected bowel are identified. In most cases there is a single significant stricture which requires resection. Often this segment includes the ileocecal valve and requires resection of the cecum as well. As in open surgery the extent of the resection is determined by the areas which are most severely involved. With the margins of resection determined the bowel is divided at the proximal resection margin using a tissue load in the endoscopic stapler. The mesentery is divided close to the bowel wall for the extent of the resection. Depending on the surgeon's choice, the degree of inflammation and thickening of the mesentery, and the equipment available this can be accomplished with the ultrasonic shears, Endo-GIA, Ligasure, or other sealing/dividing devices. If the patient has been on steroids the tissue quality may be poor and there may be some break through bleeding no matter what method is used. Once the distal resection margin is reached the bowel is again divided with the endoscopic stapler. The resected specimen is set in the pelvis while the anastomosis is completed.

Anastomosis

At this point a decision can be made as whether or not to perform the anastomosis intracorporeally or extracorporeally. If the decision is to do the anastomosis extracorporeally then the two ends can be brought out through the extended umbilical incision or through a muscle-splitting right lower quadrant incision (■ Fig. 48.3). The resected specimen can also be brought out at this site. An end-to-end or hand sewn or stapled anastomosis is performed. The mesenteric defect is closed and the anastomosed bowel is returned to the abdomen.

If an intracorporeal anastomosis is chosen a side-to-side stapled anastomosis is usually the easiest to perform. The fourth port is placed in the right upper quadrant so that the assistant can help stabilize the bowel and follow the running suture line. The proximal and distal ends are slightly overlapped for 5–6 cm. Proximal and distal stay sutures are placed to align the bowel (■ Fig. 48.4). A small enterotomy is made at the proximal end of the alignment on the antimesenteric surface of each limb. One limb of the Endo-GIA is placed in each limb and a side-to-side anastomosis completed (■ Fig. 48.5). The resultant single enterotomy is closed with a running suture line (■ Fig. 48.6). The mesenteric defect is closed with a series of interrupted sutures. An end-to-end anastomosis can also be performed if desired. Both proximal and distal staple lines are resected and the front and back walls are closed with running sutures.

After the anastomosis is complete a large specimen bag is placed through the umbilical incision (requires removal of the cannula). Once the specimen is in the

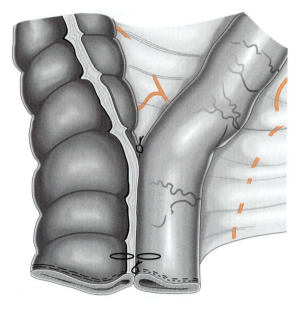

Fig. 48.4. Stay sutures for a side-to-side anastomosis

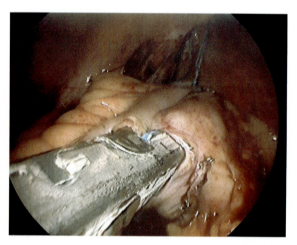

Fig. 48.5. Intracorporeal stapled side-to-side anastomosis

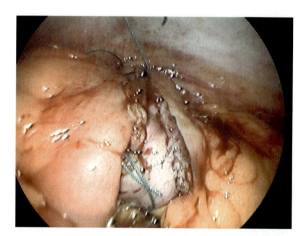

Fig. 48.6. Completed stapled anastomosis

bag the neck of the bag is brought out through the incision and the specimen is removed in a morcellated fashion to limit the size of the incision.

The cannulae are removed and the incisions closed with absorbable suture. The umbilical incision requires a good fascial closure.

Postoperative Care

The nasogastric tube is left to low intermittent suction for the first postoperative night and can usually be removed on the first or second day. Antibiotics are continued for 48 h. Intravenous narcotics are given for the first 24–48 h as needed and then switched to oral pain medication. The patient is discharged when tolerating adequate oral fluids and on oral pain medication. If the patient has been on steroids or other immunosuppressants these are weaned over the next weeks as tolerated.

Results

Laparoscopic management of inflammatory bowel disease and particularly isolated Crohn's strictures has progressed significantly since the early 1990s. The advantages of an MIS approach are numerous. First the entirety of the bowel can be examined through a few small port sites, avoiding the need for a major laparotomy. Areas of isolated stricture and significant inflammation can be identified and these areas can undergo limited resections using completely intracorporeal techniques or, depending on the circumstance and the surgeon's experience, can be mobilized and brought out through a limited muscle-sparing incision.

In the author's own experience 21 patients with intestinal strictures secondary to Crohn's disease have been treated laparoscopically. The ages ranged from 11 to 17 years. Seventeen underwent an ileocolic resection with a side-to-side ileocolic stapled anastomosis. Two had isolated ileal strictures with an end-to-end anastomosis, and two had stricturoplasty. The average operative time was 110 min. The nasogastric tube was left for 24 h in all cases and all patients were started on oral feeds on the second postoperative day. Hospital stay ranged from 3 to 7 days. There has been one anastomotic stricture requiring reresection 2 years later.

Discussion

The management of inflammatory bowel disease and specifically Crohn's disease using minimally invasive techniques is a relatively new field. The main benefits include the ability to examine the entire small bowel and then approach the diseased portion through relatively limited access. In some cases this simply facilitates mobilization of the diseased segment so that it can be removed through a relatively limited incision and an extracorporeal anastomosis performed. However improvements in instrumentation and technique have made the completion of an intracorporeal hand sewn anastomosis much more feasible. We have now accomplished this in all 21 patients in our series (Rothenberg 2002, 2003). This not only resulted in decreased surgical stress and recovery, but also a quicker return to full feeds. Performing the procedure intracorporeally seems to be associated with a shorter period of ileus. To date the patency, leak, and complication rates compare favorably with the standard open surgery. The progress since 2000 clearly indicates that more and more intestinal anastomoses will be performed using minimally invasive techniques and that the same benefits as derived in other MIS procedures are present in intestinal surgery (Tabet et al. 2001). Enabling technology such as self-knotting sutures and improved anastomotic staplers will also improve the

ease with which these procedures can be performed. It may be that the fine motor skills required to perform this anastomosis may be facilitated by robotics.

References

Becmeur F, Besson R (1998) Treatment of small-bowel obstruction by laparoscopy in children multicentric study. GECI. Eur J Pediatr Surg 8:343–346

Hamel CT, Hildebrandt U, Weiss EG, et al (2001) Laparoscopic surgery for inflammatory bowel disease. Surg Endosc 15:642–645

Milsom JW, Hammerhofer KA, Bohm B, et al (2001) Prospective, randomized trial comparing laparoscopic vs. conventional surgery for refractory ileo-colic Crohn's disease. Dis Colon Rectum 44:1–8

Rothenberg SS (2002) Laparoscopic segmental intestinal resection. Semin Pediatr Surg 11:211–216

Rothenberg SS (2003) Total intra-corporeal laparoscopic resection of Crohn's disease. J Pediatr Surg 38:593–603

Tabet J, Hong D, Kim CW, et al (2001) Laparoscopic versus open bowel resection for Crohn's disease. Can J Gastroenterol 4:237–242

Chapter 49

Total Colectomy with J Pouch

Jacqueline M. Saito

Introduction

The indications for total colectomy in the pediatric population include total colonic Hirschsprung's disease, ulcerative colitis, and familial adenomatous polyposis. Children with ulcerative colitis may require total colectomy because of disease refractory to medical management, growth arrest secondary to the disease itself, or to allow cessation of drug therapy that has adverse effects. Surgical options include total colectomy with end ileostomy, and total proctocolectomy with ileoanal anastomosis. An ileal J pouch may be used as a fecal reservoir. A diverting loop ileostomy can protect the pouch for optimal healing during recovery.

Preoperative Preparation

Before Induction of General Anesthesia

A mechanical bowel preparation may be achieved using GoLYTELY®, magnesium citrate, Fleet's phosphosoda, or castor oil. Luminal antibiotics such as erythromycin base and neomycin may also be administered. For long-segment Hirschsprung's disease, rectal washouts are often necessary to evacuate retained stool, meconium, or mucus. Intravenous antibiotics with broad activity against gram-negative bacteria, such as cefotetan, should be administered prior to initiation of the procedure.

After Induction of General Anesthesia

Gastric decompression with either a nasogastric or orogastric tube will facilitate visualization during dissection of the transverse colon and splenic flexure of the colon. A Foley catheter should be placed sterilely once the patient is prepared and draped. Decompression of the bladder facilitates maximal visualization of the rectum. Local anesthetic, either 1% lidocaine or 0.25–0.5% bupivacaine, is injected into the dermis, abdominal wall muscle, and preperitoneal space before placement of trocars.

Positioning

Patient

The patient is placed supine on the operating room table (■ Fig. 49.1). Because operating room table tilt is adjusted throughout the procedure to deflect the small bowel away from the colon, the patient must be well secured to the operating room table. Infants can be secured to the table with tape "suspenders" over the shoulders to avoid shifting on the operating room table when placed in Trendelenburg position. Infants should have the inferior chest/upper abdomen anteriorly and lower body circumferentially prepared with the legs placed in sterile stockinette. Older children will need the legs placed in stirrups and draped sterilely. Use of a beanbag may add extra stability for larger patients. Padding under the sacrum will facilitate exposure during the transanal dissection.

Crew, Monitors, and Equipment

At a minimum, two monitors are needed for easy completion of the total colectomy (■ Fig. 49.1). Due changes in position of the patient and region of colon that is dissected, the position of the surgeon and assistant surgeon will shift. Ideally, three monitors should be used to provide an adequate view with minimal strain to the surgeon and assistant. Monitors may be positioned to the right and left of the patient's upper body, and toward the feet. If only two monitors are available, one on the right toward the patient's upper body and a second monitor on the left toward the patient's feet will minimize the need to change the position of the monitors.

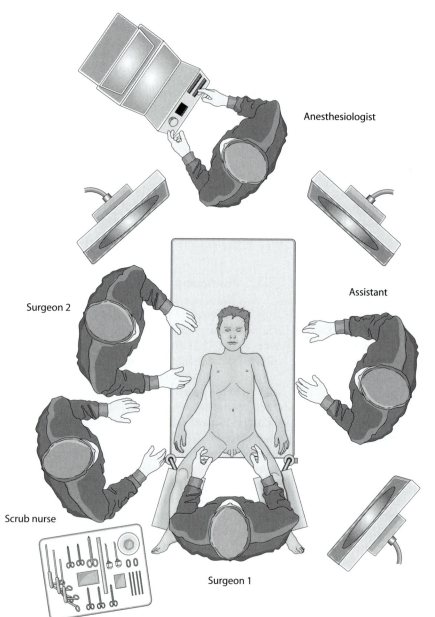

Fig. 49.1. Positioning of the patient and crew. The patient is positioned supine on the operating room table. Stirrups may be used with older children

The surgeon will primarily be positioned at the patient's feet. During the rectal dissection, the surgeon may prefer to stand on the patient's right side. The assistant surgeon generally stands on the patient's left side. The scrub nurse may stand off to the right or left toward the feet.

Special Equipment

An endoscopic stapler with tissue load for children and vascular load for infants and toddlers can be used for stapling the rectal stump and construction of an ileal J pouch. The colonic mesentery at the periphery is generally divided with electrocautery, ultrasonic scissors, or the Ligasure and scissors, but can also be ligated and divided with a vascular stapler. An optional hand-assist port may be placed through a transverse suprapubic incision in older children.

Technique

Cannulae

Cannula	Method of insertion	Diameter (mm)	Device	Position
1	Open	5, Step	Optic	Umbilicus
2	Closed	12, Step	Stapler or extracorporeal J pouch construction	Suprapubic
3	Closed	4–5, reusable or Step	Working instruments Ileostomy	Right lower quadrant
4	Closed	4–5, reusable or Step	Working instruments	Right upper quadrant
5	Closed	4–5, reusable or Step	Working instruments	Left upper quadrant

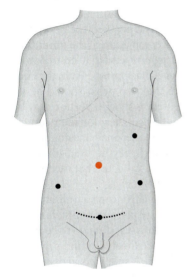

Fig. 49.2. Position of cannulae. Adapted from Georgeson (2002)

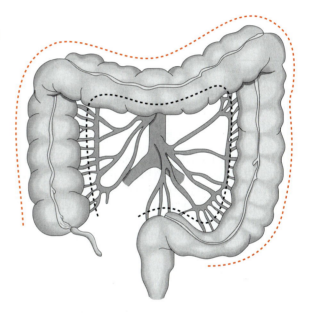

Fig. 49.3. Division of colonic peritoneal attachments and mesentery. Adapted from Georgeson (2002)

Port Positions

A total of four or five cannulae are needed to easily complete the colonic dissection (■ Fig. 49.2). Initial peritoneal access is obtained using a semiopen technique in the umbilical position, and a 5 mm trocar is placed in the umbilicus. A 12 mm port, which will accommodate an endoscopic stapler, is placed in the suprapubic position. In an older child, a hand-assisted port may be substituted. The suprapubic trocar incision may also be extended transversely for extracorporeal construction of a J pouch. Additional ports may range from 4 to 5 mm, depending on the size of the patient, and are placed in the right lower abdomen and right upper abdomen. The right lower quadrant trocar is best placed in a location that is also suitable for an ileostomy. An additional port in the left upper abdomen may facilitate completion of the colonic mobilization.

Procedure

Several principles should be followed to maximize safety and minimize the difficulty during the colonic dissection. First, stay close to the bowel when incising peritoneal attachments and dividing the mesentery (■ Fig. 49.3). This will help avoid injury to adjacent structures, such as the ureters and duodenum, and lessen the chance of bleeding from mesenteric vessels. Second, the camera and working ports should be changed as different regions of the colon are dissected. Finally, if an ileoanal anastomosis is constructed, the mesentery of the ileum should be carefully inspected to prevent twisting.

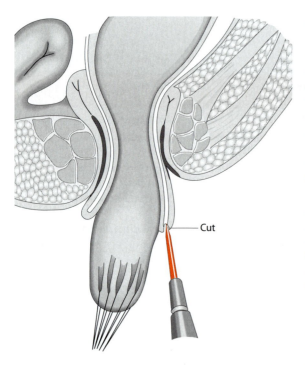

Fig. 49.4. Rectal eversion and circumferential incision of muscularis

The colonic mobilization is initiated in the sigmoid region. A window in the sigmoid mesentery is opened using electrocautery or ultrasonic scissors. The dissection is carried distally until the peritoneal reflection is reached and incised. The rectum is mobilized approximately 4 cm posteriorly and 2 cm anteriorly beyond the peritoneal reflection in an adolescent patient. The vas deferens and prostate in boys and posterior vaginal wall is girls should be identified and deflected away from the rectum.

The dissection is then carried from distal colon to proximal colon. The peritoneal reflection of the descending colon is incised sharply with scissors or the ultrasonic dissector. After a plane is generated between the mesentery and retroperitoneum, the mesentery is divided using electrocautery or the ultrasonic dissector. Dividing the mesentery close to the colon and identification of the left ureter will help prevent ureteral injury. The splenic flexure may be approached from the colon distal and proximal to this area. Opening the gastrocolic ligament provides access to the lesser sac; the transverse colon may then be followed distally toward the splenic flexure. Dividing the transverse mesocolon will complete mobilization of the colon up to the hepatic flexure.

Next, the terminal ileum and cecum are addressed. The mobility of the cecum is variable, and peritoneal attachments to the terminal ileum may be present. The peritoneal reflection of the cecum and ascending colon

is incised sharply. Reflecting the ascending colon medially, a plane should be generated between the mesocolon and retroperitoneum. The right ureter should be identified in order to avoid inadvertent injury. The duodenum is also susceptible to injury as the hepatic flexure is approached. Again, the colon mesentery should be divided close to the bowel, which will also help prevent injury to retroperitoneal structures.

Once the colon is completely mobilized with the mesentery divided, either an end ileostomy or proctectomy and ileoanal anastomosis should be constructed. With an end ileostomy, the stoma may be placed in the position of the right lower quadrant trocar. The proximal rectum is divided using an endoscopic stapler. The abdominal colon may be delivered, distal end first, through the right lower quadrant trocar site. The ileal mesentery should be inspected to ensure that it is not twisted. The distal ileum is then divided extracorporeally, and the Brooke ileostomy is constructed.

If an ileoanal anastomosis is planned, the next phase of the operation involves completion of the proctectomy, construction of an anal reservoir if desired, and completion of the ileoanal anastomosis. First, the ability of the ileum to reach the deep pelvis should be assessed. If the ileal mesentery is short, a portion may be divided to gain the length necessary for the ileum to reach into the pelvis if an ileoanal anastomosis is planned. A temporary clamp may be used to ensure adequate perfusion of the distal ileum before division of mesenteric blood vessel branches.

The proctectomy is completed using a transanal approach. Retraction stitches are placed circumferentially from the perineum to the anus just distal to the dentate line. The rectal mucosa approximately 5 mm proximal to the dentate line is incised. A submucosal dissection is carried proximally in a circumferential fashion. Once the rectum begins to evert, the peritoneal cavity may be entered posteriorly. The muscularis is incised circumferentially (Fig. 49.4). The colon may then be delivered via the anus or a suprapubic incision.

The ileal reservoir may be constructed intracorporeally or extracorporeally through a suprapubic incision. The J pouch should be 5–8 cm in length depending on the age and size of the child. Traction stitches are placed to align the ileum in the J configuration. The pouch may be stapled from the proximal end first, and completed transanally (Fig. 49.5). The J pouch or ileum, if no reservoir is constructed, is brought to the anus. Prior to performing the ileoanal anastomosis, the ileal mesentery should be checked for twists. After a small enterotomy is made at the apex of the pouch, a full thickness anastomosis is performed between the ileum and the anus using 10 to 15 interrupted stitches with absorbable suture. A protective loop ileostomy may be placed at the site of the right lower abdominal trocar.

Fig. 49.5. **a** Construction
of ileal J pouch. **b** Delivery
of J pouch to perineum.
c Transanal completion
of J pouch. Adapted from
Georgeson (2002)

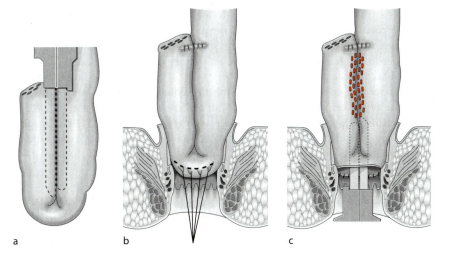

a   b   c

Postoperative Care

Postoperatively, broad-spectrum antibiotics are continued for 3 days. The bladder is decompressed with a Foley catheter for 2–3 days. Gastric decompression with a nasogastric tube may be continued briefly following surgery. An oral diet is started when the patient has ileostomy output or bowel movements. Patients who have severe diarrhea can be treated with Lomotil or loperamide, though the dose will need to be titrated. Anal dilation is avoided for 3 weeks postoperatively. Patients who undergo subtotal colectomy only may undergo completion proctectomy with ileoanal anastomosis as early as 2 months postoperatively. The protective loop ileostomy may be closed 6–8 weeks following the proctectomy.

Results

The benefits of laparoscopic total colectomy, like many minimally invasive procedures, include shorter postoperative ileus, shorter hospitalization, and superior cosmesis compared to the open approach. Multiple case series exist for laparoscopic total colectomy in the adult population. Several use historical controls in comparing outcome variables. Indications for total colectomy in the adult population include ulcerative colitis, familial adenomatous polyposis, and colonic inertia. Operative time tends to be longer with the laparoscopic compared to the open approach. Many authors have noted a "learning curve" with a trend toward shorter operative times as individual surgeons gain greater laparoscopic experience. Postoperative recovery, as reflected in return of bowel function, tolerance of an oral diet, and length of hospitalization, tends to be more rapid with the laparoscopic colectomy (Chen et al. 2000; Dunker et al. 2001; Marcello et al.

2000; Wexner et al. 2002). Functional results, such as number of bowel movements, stool consistency, soilage, and continence, are similar regardless of operative approach (Dunker et al. 2001; Milsom et al. 1997). Cosmesis as reflected in responses to a Body Image Questionnaire was superior in adults who underwent a laparoscopic-assisted colectomy with a suprapubic incision compared to colectomy via a midline laparotomy (Dunker et al. 2001). In the pediatric population, similar recovery and functional outcome have been seen following laparoscopic colectomy (Georgeson 2002; Proctor et al. 2002).

The underlying reason for a more rapid recovery following colon surgery may be related to decreased stress and physiologic disturbance with the laparoscopic technique. In Braga et al. (2002), adults were randomized to either laparoscopic or open colorectal procedures. Postoperative morbidity was comparable, though fewer infectious complications were seen in the laparoscopic group. Laparoscopic colectomy resulted in decreased impairment of immune function as reflected by recovery of lymphocyte proliferative response 2 weeks following the operation. Finally, better preservation of intraoperative bowel perfusion, as measured by gut oxygen tension, was observed during laparoscopic colon surgery.

Discussion

During total colectomy, retroperitoneal structures adjacent to the colon, such as the ureters and duodenum, are at risk for injury. Strategies to minimize the likelihood of injury include the use of blunt dissection to separate the ascending and descending colon from the retroperitoneum after sharply incising the peritoneal reflection, and division of the colonic mesentery close to its margin with the bowel. Within the pelvis, the vas deferens and prostate in boys and posterior vaginal wall in girls may also be injured during the proctectomy. Again, use of blunt dissection after sharp incision of the peritoneal reflection will help prevent injury to these adjacent structures.

Intraoperative complications can be minimized using some of the techniques described above. Mesenteric bleeding may occur even when the mesentery is ligated and divided using an endoscopic stapler. Though a greater length of mesentery is divided peripherally near the margin with the bowel, the mesenteric blood vessels are also smaller and easier to control. A crucial technical detail is the orientation of the ileum when performing an ileoanal anastomosis. An unrecognized twist of the ileum may lead to venous congestion, ischemia, and anastomotic or pouch breakdown. When using either a purely laparoscopic or a laparoscopic-assisted approach, the orientation of the ileal mesentery must be checked. Intraoperative recognition of a twisted mesentery and correction will avert a potential postoperative disaster (Milsom et al. 1997).

With ulcerative colitis, fulminant disease has been cited as a contraindication to laparoscopic colectomy. However, Bell and Seymour (2002) have reported completion of laparoscopic colectomy safely in this setting. With a more diseased colon, careful manipulation of the colon is crucial to avoid intraoperative perforation and abdominal soilage.

Reported early postoperative complications following laparoscopic-assisted total colectomy included infections and obstruction. Most case series report resolution of early bowel obstruction without operative intervention (Marcello et al. 2000; Milsom et al. 1997; Proctor et al. 2002). Infections range from local wound sepsis to deep abscesses within the abdomen and pelvis (Bell and Seymour 2002; Hasegawa et al. 2002; Marcello et al. 2000; Proctor et al. 2002). Emphasizing the need for careful patient positioning and padding, transient brachial plexus injury has been attributed to pressure on the shoulder while in Trendelenburg position in one report (Milsom et al. 1997).

Late complications are similar whether the total colectomy is performed via a laparotomy or laparoscopy (Marcello et al. 2000; Proctor et al. 2002; Rintala and Lindahl 2002). Diarrhea with dehydration and pouchitis are among the more frequent problems encountered (Dunker et al. 2001; Hasegawa et al. 2002; Marcello et al. 2000). Bowel obstruction requiring operative intervention and anastomotic stricture are also reported (Hasegawa et al. 2002). Wound hernia (Dunker et al. 2001) and Hirschsprung's disease-associated enterocolitis (Rintala and Lindahl 2002) are less common complications.

References

Bell RL, Seymour NE (2002) Laparoscopic treatment of fulminant ulcerative colitis. Surg Endosc 16:1778–1782

Braga M, Vignali A, Gianotti L, et al (2002) Laparoscopic versus open colorectal surgery: a randomized trial on short-term outcome. Ann Surg 236:759–767

Chen HH, Wexner SD, Iroatulam AJ, et al (2000) Laparoscopic colectomy compares favorably with colectomy by laparotomy for reduction of postoperative ileus. Dis Colon Rectum 43:61–65

Dunker MS, Bemelman WA, Slors JF, Van Dujivendijk P, Gouma DJ (2001) Functional outcome, quality of life, body image, and cosmesis in patients after laparoscopic-assisted and conventional restorative proctocolectomy. Dis Colon Rectum 44:1800–1807

Georgeson KE (2002) Laparoscopic-assisted total colectomy with pouch reconstruction. Semin Pediatr Surg 11:233–236

Hasegawa H, Watanabe M, Baba H, et al (2002) Laparoscopic restorative proctocolectomy for patients with ulcerative colitis. J Laparoendosc Adv Surg Tech 12:403–406

Marcello PW, Milsom JW, Wong SK, et al (2000) Laparoscopic restorative proctocolectomy: case matched comparative study with open restorative proctocolectomy. Dis Colon Rectum. 43:604–608

Milsom JW, Ludwig KA, Church JM (1997) Laparoscopic total abdominal colectomy with ileorectal anastomosis for familial adenomatous polyposis. Dis Colon Rectum 40:675–678

Proctor ML, Langer JC, Gerstle JT, et al (2002) Is laparoscopic subtotal colectomy better than open subtotal colectomy in children? J Pediatr Surg 37:706–708

Rintala RJ, Lindahl H (2002) Proctocolectomy and J-pouch ileoanal anastomosis in children. J Pediatr Surg 37:66–70

Wexner SD, Johansen OB, Nogueras JJ, et al (2002) Laparoscopic total abdominal colectomy: a prospective trial. Dis Colon Rectum 35:651–655

Chapter 50

Hand-assisted Colectomy

David C. van der Zee and Klaas (N) M.A. Bax

Introduction

Benign diseases of the colon, such as ulcerative colitis, Crohn's disease, or familial polyposis, are ideally suited for laparoscopic-assisted resection (Georgeson 2002). Hand-assisted laparoscopic surgery (HALS) represents a useful alternative to conventional laparoscopic surgery (Taragona et al. 2002). In hand-assisted laparoscopic surgery, the surgeon inserts a hand into the abdomen while pneumoperitoneum is maintained. The hand assists the laparoscopic instruments and has the advantage that it restores tactile feedback and the ability to palpate, perform blunt dissection, carry out organ retraction, and control bleeding (Romanelli et al. 2001). Also operating time is considerably reduced which is comfortable for the surgeon when an extensive reconstruction is carried out. As the wound edges are covered by a ring, there is no contamination of the wound edges by the specimen to be removed. Hand-assisted laparoscopic surgery can also be used in (living-related) donor nephrectomy and laparoscopic removal of massively enlarged spleens.

In small children the incision of 7–9 cm would not differ from a formal laparotomy. Moreover the abdominal wall in small children is too thin, causing air leakage. However, patients undergoing surgery for ulcerative colitis and Crohn's disease are usually adolescents that are approaching mature size, and in these youngsters a small Pfannenstiel incision is of great benefit compared to the large laparotomy wound.

Most surgeons (78%) prefer to insert their non-dominant hand into the abdomen, although for organ or lymph node palpation and blunt dissection sometimes the dominant hand is used.

Preoperative Preparation

Before Induction of General Anesthesia

Patients undergo an antegrade washout the day prior to the operation. Medication depends on the underlying disease (Crohn's disease, ulcerative colitis).

After Induction of General Anesthesia

Part of the perioperative management may be subject to local customs and personal preferences. Future porthole sites may be injected with local anesthetics. Epidural or spinal anesthesia is subject to the personal preference of the anesthetist. All patients receive a voiding urinary catheter and perioperative antibiotics.

Before the operation a rectal washout is undertaken to remove the last residuals and to ensure decompression of the intestine.

Positioning

Patient

The patient is placed in a supine position with the table in a 15–20° (reversed) Trendelenburg position depending on where dissection is taking place. The table may also be tilted to the right or to the left, again depending on where dissection is taking place. The legs are placed on leg holders that can be abducted to allow the surgeon to stand between the legs (■ Fig. 50.1a,b).

Crew, Monitors, and Equipment

Two monitors are used, one on each side of the patient. Through the initial Pfannenstiel laparotomy, the rectosigmoid and ileocecal regions are dissected in an open way. For the endoscopic part of the operation, the surgeon initially stands in between the legs of the patient with the camera operator on the right side of the patient and the scrub nurse opposite at the left side (■ Fig. 50.1a). For dissection of the hepatic flexure and ascending colon the surgeon stands on the patient's left side looking at the monitor on the patient's right side (■ Fig. 50.1b).

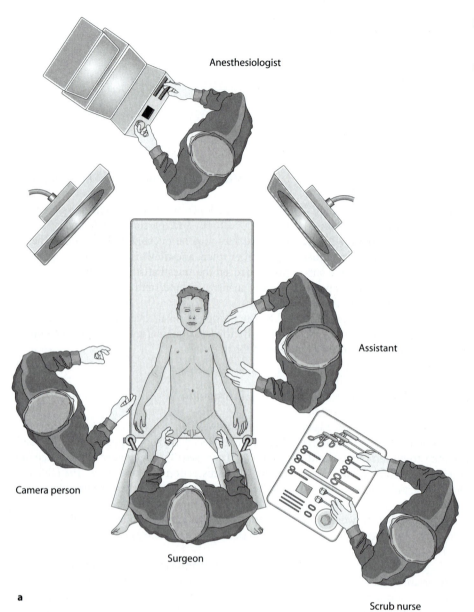

Anesthesiologist

Assistant

Camera person

Surgeon

a

Scrub nurse

Fig. 50.1. Positioning
of the patient, crew,
and equipment.
b Preparation of the hepatic
flexure and right colon

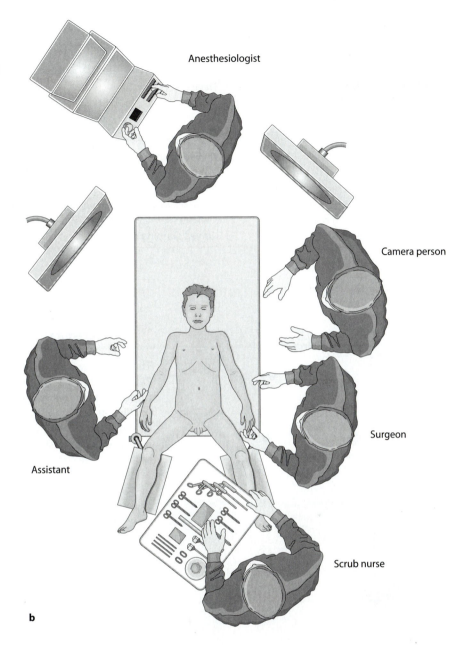

Anesthesiologist

Camera person

Surgeon

Assistant

Scrub nurse

b

Special Equipment

For this type of surgery special energy sources such as
ultrasonic energy or Ligasure or both are advantageous. Clips may be needed, and for the transection of
the bowel endostapling devices are used. Currently
four types of rings to be inserted in the laparotomy
wound are approved by the FDA: Dexterity Device, In-
tromit, Hand port, and Omniport. The Lap Disk has a
mechanism to close the port off by means of a diaphragm (■ Fig. 50.2). In the middle of the diaphragm
a regular port can be inserted.

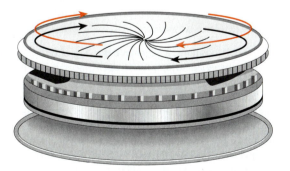

Fig. 50.2. Hand-assist device (Lap Disk). The device shown
has a diaphragm that can be opened and closed. In the closed
position it can contain a cannula in the middle

Technique

Cannulae

Cannula	Method of insertion	Diameter (mm)	Device	Position
1	Closed	6/10	Optic	Umbilicus
2	Closed	6	Curved grasping forceps/Babcock	Right upper quadrant
3	Closed	6	Curved grasping forceps/Babcock	Right lower quadrant (intended ileostomy place)
		12	Stapler	
4	Closed	6	Hook, scissors, suction, needle holder, clipping device, ultrasonic scissors	Left lower quadrant
5	Closed	6	Curved grasping forceps	Left upper quadrant

■ Figure 50.3a shows port positions.

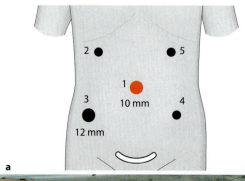

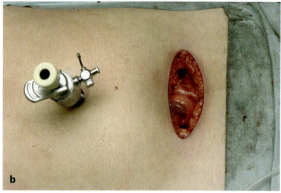

Fig. 50.3. Port positions. **a** Schematic drawing of port positions. Pfannenstiel laparotomy for: (*1*) open preparation of the rectum, sigmoid, and ileocecal region and open construction of the pouch and (*2*) the hand-assist port. Telescope (6- or 10 mm) in the umbilicus. Cannula (6 mm) in each upper quadrant. Cannula in each lower quadrant (6 mm in left lower quadrant, 12 mm in right lower quadrant for stapling device). **b** Intraoperative view of Pfannenstiel laparotomy. A 10 mm port has been inserted in the umbilicus in a closed way but under guidance through the Pfannenstiel incision

Procedure

The procedure is started with a Pfannenstiel incision of 7–9 cm that will allow the hand of the surgeon to pass through after placement of the hand-assist port (■ Fig. 50.3a). The dissection of the rectosigmoid can be started in an open way right down to the peritoneal reflection. If a one-stage procedure is planned, the dissection can be continued further down, until the point where transanal dissection from below will be needed. In some patients with abundant (steroid) adipositas and a small abdominal cavity it may be of advantage to amputate the dissected rectosigmoid using one or multiple staple cartridges. In these patients the ileocecal region is also dissected, temporarily closing the distal ileum with a stapler. Through the same incision the terminal ileum can be mobilized either to be used as an ileostomy or to be transformed into a J pouch.

After completion of the open part of the resection, the ports are inserted beginning with the umbilical port for a 5- or 10 mm 30° telescope (■ Fig. 50.3b). Next the hand-assist port is placed (■ Fig. 50.4a,b). The surgeon stands between the legs of the patient and places the non-dominant hand through the port inside the abdomen until it is comfortable. The port is then insufflated until it is airtight, and CO_2 is insufflated into the abdominal cavity. Next the secondary ports are placed, one in the left and one in the right iliac fossa. The right iliac fossa port is placed at the site of the future ileostomy. It is a 12 mm port, which will allow the use of an endolinear stapler. Later on for the dissection of the splenic and hepatic flexure additional 6 mm ports are inserted in the right and left hypochondrium.

Under direct vision the descending colon can be picked up and put under traction. In the beginning this maneuver will need some time to get accustomed to.

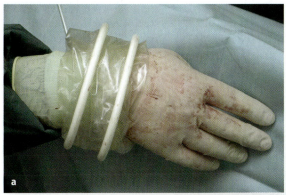
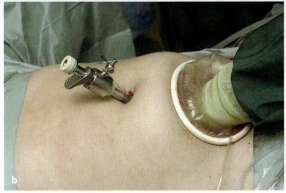

Fig. 50.4. Hand-assisted laparoscopic surgery. **a** The inflatable hand-assist port is shown around the wrist of the surgeon (this port is inserted in the laparotomy wound without the hand inside). **b** Hand in the inflated hand-assist port in the abdomen

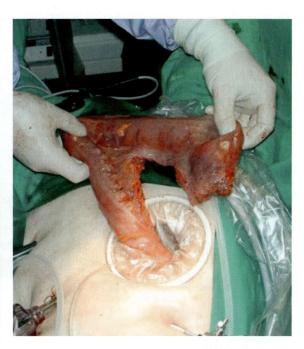

Fig. 50.5. Exteriorization of colon through the sleeve (from Omniport)

With the instruments and hand in place dissection can be started with incising the line of Toldt. Next the splenic flexure is detached using curved scissors. Then the harmonic scalpel can be introduced through the lower left trocar and the colonic mesentery can be transected toward the splenic flexure. As this is not an oncological procedure the dissection can be performed somewhat closer to the bowel, although care has to be taken not to cause a perforation as the harmonic scalpel becomes hot. When arriving at the splenic flexure the omentum needs to be prepared from the colon. It is often of help to have the assistant use a grasping forceps or Babcock from either of the other ports to present the tissue to be dissected and then stretch it with the hand feeling around the colon to make sure there is no posteriorly lying structure. After the omentum as been prepared from the colon, the transverse colon can be dissected. As most surgeons are right-handed the dissection will go anticlockwise. For dissection of the hepatic flexure the surgeon moves to the left side of the patient and uses the monitor on the right side of the patient. Be aware not to take the corner too short, or you will end up inside the colon. Sometimes the finger

fracture method may be of benefit, although the high doses of steroids make the tissue friable and it bleeds easily, troubling the view even further. Once the hepatic flexure has come free the dissection becomes easier again, and particularly when the ileocecal corner has been mobilized previously. Finally when the colon has been completely mobilized, the hand-assist port can be deflated and the colon can be retracted through the port, avoiding contamination of the wound (■ Fig. 50.5).

From this point on either a terminal ileostomy is created, or the procedure is carried on as in the open procedure for ulcerative colitis, extended Crohn's disease, or polyposis coli.

Postoperative Care

Patients may have a nasogastric tube overnight, but in patients with an ileostomy usually feeding can be started the next day. The urinary catheter remains for the time an epidural catheter is in place. Also in case of extensive pelvic dissection the urinary catheter is warranted for the first few days. Antibiotics are continued for 24 h. Usually these patients have perioperative steroids for adrenal support according to local protocol.

When patients have no epidural catheter they receive morphine intravenously for 24–48 h postoperatively. Nausea is treated with ondansetron intravenously.

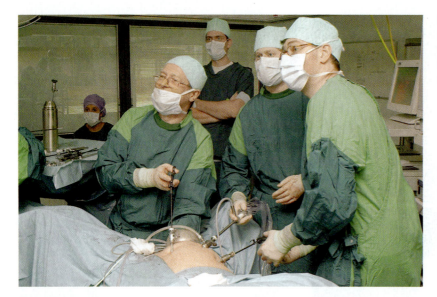

Fig. 50.6. Hand-assisted laparoscopic intervention. The left colon is being prepared. Note the poor ergonomic position of the surgeon

Results

In our own series between 1995 and 2002 ten children underwent a laparoscopic (assisted) subtotal colectomy for ulcerative colitis. As these operations initially were time consuming, from 2001 on the procedure was carried out hand-assisted with the use of an Omniport in five adolescents, reducing operating time to 1–2 h for the colectomy. In three patients a perforation occurred during dissection of the hepatic flexure, in one necessitating conversion due to contamination. Georgeson (2002) recently described a series of 18 patients undergoing laparoscopic (assisted) colectomy for ulcerative colitis with a complication rate of 25% similar to open procedures.

Discussion

Hand-assisted laparoscopic subtotal colectomy as a part of surgical treatment for ulcerative colitis in adolescents may reduce operating time considerably. Also other indications have been described (Ponski et al. 2003). Since the construction of the pouch or other technique is usually carried out through a Pfannenstiel incision, this incision can easily be used for inserting a sleeve for inserting a hand into the abdomen. However the inserted hand may be obstructive, particularly when dissecting the hepatic flexure and ascending colon, or when the abdominal cavity is small. In these cases it may be of advantage to carry out the dissection completely laparoscopically. Hand fatigue occurs in 20.6% (Litwin et al. 2000). When performing the hand-assisted procedure the surgeon usually stands in a somewhat awkward position between the legs of the patient (█ Fig. 50.6).

References

Georgeson KE (2002) Laparoscopic-assisted total colectomy with pouch reconstruction. Semin Pediatr Surg 11:233–236

Litwin DE, Darzi A, Jakimowicz J, et al (2000) Hand-assisted laparoscopic surgery (HALS) with the HandPort system: initial experience with 68 patients. Ann Surg 231:715–723

Ponsky LE, Cherullo EE, Banks KL, et al (2003) Laparoscopic radical nephrectomy: incorporating advantage hand assisted and standard laparoscopy. J Urol 169:2053–2056

Romanelli JR, Kelly JJ, Litwin DE (2001) Hand-assisted laparoscopic surgery in the United States: an overview. Semin Laparosc Surg 8:96–103

Targarona EM, Gracia E, Garriga J, et al (2002) Prospective randomized trial comparing conventional laparoscopic colectomy with hand-assisted laparoscopic colectomy: applicability, immediate clinical outcome, inflammatory response, and cost. Surg Endosc 16:234–239

Chapter 51

Endorectal Pull-through for Hirschsprung's Disease

Timothy D. Kane

Introduction

The diagnosis of Hirschsprung's disease requires biopsy-proven evidence of distal colonic aganglionosis prior to consideration for laparoscopic-assisted endorectal colon pull-through. Infants and children with Hirschsprung's disease may be considered for primary laparoscopic pull-through if there are no significant medical comorbidities or severe enterocolitis, which may contribute to the poor general health of the infant.

Preoperative Preparation

Before Induction of General Anesthesia

Decompression of the colon is achieved by frequent digital dilatation of the anorectum or colonic irrigation with saline via a rectal tube if the operation is not performed immediately after the diagnosis. Two doses of mechanical antibiotic bowel preparation (erythromycin base and neomycin) are given by mouth 14 and 8 h prior to the operation. Clear liquids are given orally for 24 h preoperatively and intravenous antibiotics (ampicillin and gentamicin) are administered on call to the operating room.

After Induction of General Anesthesia

A nasogastric tube and urinary bladder catheter are placed in older children, whereas in infants, Credé's maneuver is used to empty the bladder. Preinjection of port sites with 0.25% Marcaine (with 1:200,000 epinephrine) at 1 mL/kg total dose per patient is utilized for all incisions prior to trocar placement. Epidural or spinal anesthesia is rarely required for this procedure.

Positioning

Patient

Infants are placed transversely on the operating table in a supine position, with the surgeons standing above the patient's head and left shoulder to perform the laparoscopic portion of the procedure (■ Fig. 51.1a). Older children are placed in stirrups with the surgeon standing to the right side of the patient and the assistant surgeon on the patient's left side (■ Fig. 51.1b).

Crew, Monitors, and Equipment

Video monitors are positioned at the foot of the operating table or patient's feet (■ Fig. 51.1a,b). Infants are prepared from nipples to toes, whereas older children in stirrups are prepared from nipples to perineum.

Special Equipment

No special energy applying systems are required but bipolar high-frequency electrocoagulation may be used selectively. The harmonic scalpel and/or the Ligasure are useful in older children. A 5 mm clipping device should be available as well as an Endovascular GIA (45- and 30 mm lengths, 2.5- and 3.5 mm staple widths).

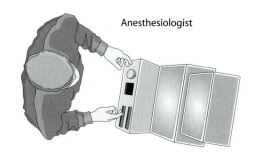

Anesthesiologist

Fig. 51.1. a Operating room setup for an infant endorectal pull-through operation

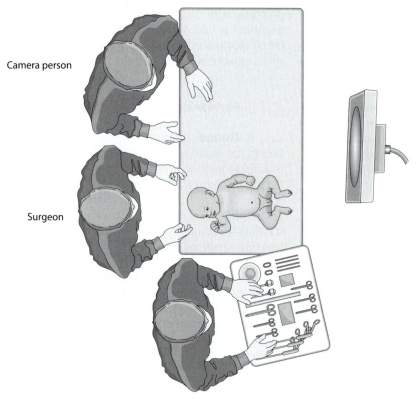

Camera person

Surgeon

Scrub nurse

Technique

Cannulae

Cannula	Method of insertion	Diameter (mm)	Device	Position
1	Open	4, reusable	Storz	Umbilicus or right upper quadrant
2	Closed	5, Step	Versastep	Right lower abdomen umbilical level
3	Closed	4, reusable	Storz	Left upper abdomen
4	Closed	4, reusable	Storz	Left lower abdomen
5	Closed	4 or 5, reusable or Step	Storz or Versastep	For additional retraction (large child)

Fig. 51.1. b Positioning for an older child for laparoscopic endorectal pull-through

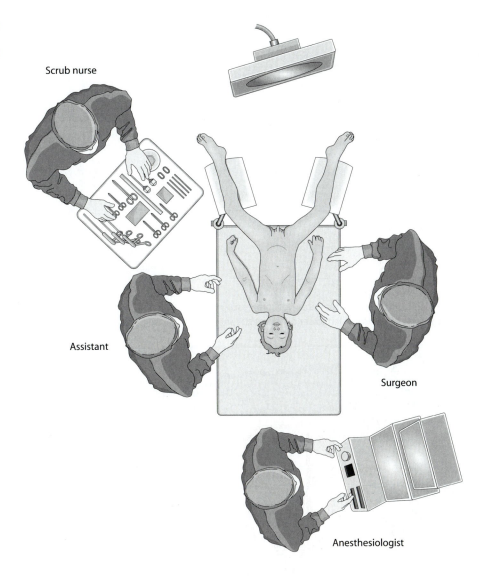

Scrub nurse

Assistant

Surgeon

Anesthesiologist

Procedure

Cannula position will depend upon the age of the patient and the general condition of the umbilicus. For many patients, pneumoperitoneum is achieved using a Veress needle through the umbilicus. Most infants will have a natural umbilical defect which allows safe open access into the abdomen. Alternatively, if the umbilical cord is still present and considered less than optimal in terms of cleanliness, the umbilicus is avoided and the initial trocar is placed in the left midabdomen at the proposed site for the left trocar using the Veress needle technique (■ Fig. 51.2). This can be done safely and avoids potential injury to the low-lying liver during access through the left upper quadrant. Depending on the size of the patient, 4- or 5 mm ports can be used. In neonates three trocars typically provide adequate access, two 4 mm and one 5 mm trocar, but a fourth trocar can be added in the suprapubic position to assist

in retraction of the colon. Pressures of $12\,cmH_2O$ are utilized for all groups. A 4 mm, 30° scope is used in infants and a 5 mm, 30° scope is used in older children.

Initially, three ports are placed to visualize the transition zone and perform seromuscular biopsies with laparoscopic scissors for histological leveling. It is best to defer further dissection until the presence of ganglion cells is confirmed histologically above the transition zone. A window is then made between the colon and superior rectal vessels using hook cautery or the ultrasonic scalpel in older children. Distal dissection of the aganglionic colon is performed circumferentially, keeping close to the colon wall and carefully preserving the mesenteric blood supply to the rectum. Blunt and sharp dissection of the avascular plane posterior to the rectum follows. Anteriorly, the rectum is dissected for about 1–2 cm below the peritoneal reflection. Care must be taken to avoid extensive lateral dissection or

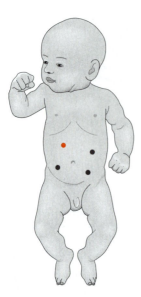

Fig. 51.2. Position of trocar sites for laparoscopic pull-through with the optional left lower quadrant site shown

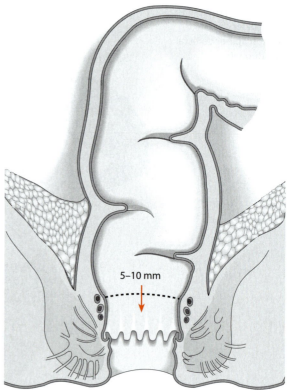

Fig. 51.4. Mucosal incision 5–10 mm above dentate line marks the beginning of the transanal dissection

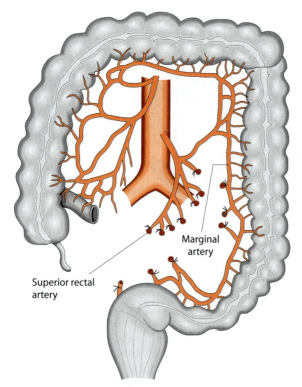

Fig. 51.3. Division of the rectal and colonic mesentery to create the colon pedicle

dissection too far anteriorly where damage to the nervi erigentes can result in secondary impotence or bladder dysfunction. By hugging the rectal wall, the circumferential dissection will join the anterior and posterior planes.

Proximal mesenteric dissection of the colon pedicle is performed using hook electrocautery or the ultrasonic scalpel with careful preservation of the marginal artery (■ Fig. 51.3). Dissection too close to the colon may cause subsequent ischemia to the pedicled colon with resultant stricture, dysfunction, or anastomotic disruption. Minimal proximal dissection is required in patients with low, rectosigmoid transition zones. Other patients will require sigmoid colon mobilization or division of the lateral colonic fusion fascia up to the splenic flexure. Periodically, the colon pedicle is assessed for its ability to reach the deep pelvis without tension. For best complete functional results, the colon pedicle should be assessed for dysganglionosis, hypo-ganglionosis, and neuronal intestinal dysplasia, conditions which often extend proximal to the aganglionic bowel in infants and children with Hirschsprung's disease.

After the endoscopic dissection of the colon and rectum has been completed, the pneumoperitoneum is released, camera and instruments are removed, and the perineal dissection is started. The trocars are left in place for subsequent visualization following the pull-through. First, six to eight 2-0 silk traction sutures are placed to evert the anus and expose the rectum. Alternatively, a Lonestar retractor may be used to evert the

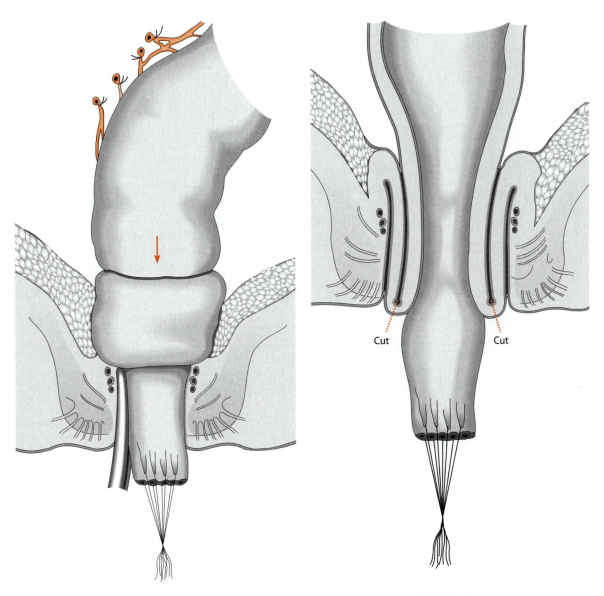

Fig. 51.5. Silk traction sutures into the rectal mucosa and development of the submucosal dissection plane with blunt dissection

Fig. 51.6. Transection of the rectal smooth muscular wall to join the intraperitoneal dissection. Transection should begin posteriorly to avoid injuring important anterior structures

anus and provide the exposure for the endorectal dissection. The mucosa is scored with electrocautery in a circular pattern 1 cm above the dentate line (■ Fig. 51.4). Three-0 silk sutures are placed into the mucosal edges to provide traction for developing a circumferential submucosal plane. The plane is relatively avascular and can be developed by both sharp and blunt dissection. The submucosal plane is developed proximally until the colorectum begins to evert or prolapse, indicating that the transanal dissection has advanced to the level of the internal perirectal dissection (■ Fig. 51.5).

A malleable retractor is placed posteriorly in between the muscular rectal sleeve and the submucosal plane of the colon. The rectal sleeve is then opened posteriorly with electrocautery to join the submucosal plane with the extramural dissection from above (■ Fig. 51.6). The perineal and laparoscopic dissection planes are connected to leave a short muscular rectal cuff. At this point, the rectal cuff is split posteriorly within 1 cm of the proposed anastomosis to allow room for the developing neorectal reservoir (■ Fig. 51.7).

Next, the colon and rectum are pulled through the anus in continuity until the proximal ganglionated

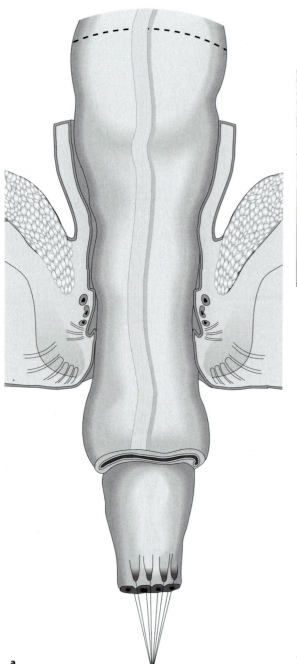

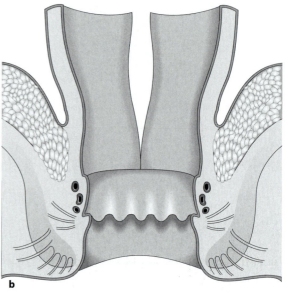

Fig. 51.7. The remaining muscular sleeve is divided posteriorly from the proximal portion down to the level of the proposed anastomosis

bowel appears at the anus. The site of the most proximal biopsy is pulled down beyond the point of the intended bowel anastomosis. The anterior one third of the colon is transected and a circumferential single-layer anastomosis is created using absorbable suture (■ Fig. 51.8). The remainder of the anastomosis is completed after transecting the posterior aspect of the pulled through colon.

Finally, reinsufflation for pneumoperitoneum is performed to inspect the colon pedicle for twisting or potential internal herniation. If necessary, interrupted sutures are used to reperitonealize the pelvis to close the potential internal hernia. The port sites are closed with fascial sutures and steristrips and the entire procedure is usually accomplished in 2–3 h.

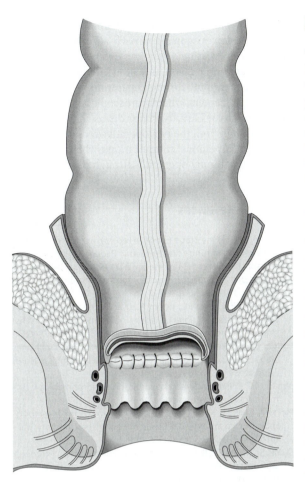

Fig. 51.8. The proximal ganglionated colon is pulled through the anus and anastomosis to the anorectal cuff performed with interrupted sutures

Postoperative Care

Nasogastric or orogastric decompression is utilized for 12–24 h postoperatively. As soon as bowel function returns, an oral diet is initiated. This will typically be on postoperative day 1 or 2. The patients remain on intravenous antibiotics for 24 h postoperatively and are discharged when they can tolerate full oral feedings.

Rectal examination or dilatation is performed 3 weeks following the surgical procedure. If necessary, parents can be taught to perform routine daily anorectal dilatations. Routine daily rectal dilations do not seem to affect anorectal compliance over the long term. Immediately following the pull-through operation, most patients will have frequent stools possibly due to the lack of a neorectal reservoir and to stretching and weakening of the internal sphincter.

Results

The first report of successful primary pull-through for Hirschsprung's disease, described by So et al. in 1980, was followed by the first report of a laparoscopic approach by Georgeson et al. in 1995. The benefits of a primary pull-through for Hirschsprung's disease have been reproduced by many authors (Bianchi 1998; Langer et al. 1999; Nmadu 1994; Pierro et al. 1997; Teitelbaum et al. 1998, 2000), and the laparoscopic approach has become highly popular for achieving this definitive treatment.

The results of the primary laparoscopic-assisted endorectal colon pull-through for Hirschsprung's disease in 80 patients from six centers were described by Georgeson et al. in 1999. Although long-term follow-up is needed, the technique has been easily applied in many centers which contributes to the broad appeal of the operation. Over 90% of patients in the series had a bowel movement within the first 24 h postoperatively (74 of 80) with an average time to tolerance of full feedings of 28 h. The mean time to discharge from the hospital was 3.7 days. The average time to perform the laparoscopic pull-through operation was 147 min, with an estimated blood loss of <10 mL, and only one patient in the series (1 of 80) required a blood transfusion. Approximately 8% (6 of 80) of patients developed postoperative enterocolitis which is below the 42% incidence reported in a series of single-stage open procedures but may be due to the lengthier follow-up and definition of enterocolitis used in the latter report.

Other early complications of the laparoscopic-assisted pull-through technique were anastomotic leak in 2 patients (2.5%), chronic diarrhea in 6 (7.5%), conversion to open technique (2.5%), bleeding (1%), and recurrent constipation (1%). Ten patients (12.5%) were readmitted following hospital discharge with 6 requiring readmission less than 3 days after discharge. Four of the ten patients requiring readmission required creation of an ostomy for anastomotic leak (2), severe enterocolitis (1), and a congenital syndrome (1).

As part of routine postoperative care, nearly half of all patients underwent routine anorectal dilations beginning 3 weeks following pull-through. Frequent stooling (greater than 6 months postoperatively) was described as problematic in 6 (7.5%). Four patients responded to dietary manipulations (lactose-free or constipating diet) whereas 2 patients (2.5%) required a secondary Duhamel procedure to establish a rectal reservoir 18 months following their initial procedure.

Overall, the multicenter experience of the laparoscopic-assisted endorectal pull-through for Hirschsprung's disease was characterized by shorter operative times, shorter postoperative recovery times, and fewer perioperative complications. Most of the patients are too young to evaluate for continence but a cohort of 18 of the older children report satisfactory continence.

Discussion

There are three distinct advantages of the minimal-access endorectal pull-through compared to the traditional open pull-through technique. First, mobilization of the colon pedicle laparoscopically minimizes peritoneal trauma. Second, the intra-abdominal colon is left intact, avoiding bacterial contamination of the peritoneal cavity. Third, transanal endorectal dissection also minimizes perineal trauma. Despite the fact that many of the benefits of the pull-through procedure can be attained by transanal pull-through alone, there are significant advantages realized by performing the laparoscopic dissection.

The most frequent early complications after laparoscopic-assisted endorectal pull-through have included enterocolitis and chronic diarrhea. These problems often respond to medical management, however, proximal diversion may rarely be necessary in extreme cases. Other less frequent problems include anastomotic leak and bleeding, which are associated with technical error.

It is critical to verify the presence of ganglion cells in the proximal colon pedicle by laparoscopic seromuscular biopsy prior to proceeding with the irreversible step of endorectal dissection. In cases of total colonic aganglionosis, a different type of pull-through operation or ostomy may be considered. In addition, laparoscopic mobilization and devascularization of the intra-abdominal aganglionic segment of the rectosigmoid colon increases the mobility of the rectum and makes the endpoint of the endorectal dissection more definitive.

By facilitating the endorectal dissection with laparoscopic mobilization of the rectosigmoid colon, there is less potential for overdilating the internal anal sphincter mechanism, thereby weakening the patient's fecal continence mechanism during the transanal dissection. In patients with longer segments of aganglionosis, the laparoscopic approach affords the needed versatility in creating a ganglionated pedicle proximal to the aganglionic colon and allows for completion of the subsequent pull-through operation.

In most centers, the laparoscopic-assisted colon pull-through for Hirschsprung's disease has resulted in a reduction in both the postoperative recovery time, as well as perioperative complications when compared with the traditional open pull-through procedures.

References

Bianchi A (1998) One-stage neonatal reconstruction without stoma for Hirschsprung's disease. Semin Pediatr Surg 7:170–173

Georgeson KE, Fuenfer MM, Hardin WD (1995) Primary laparoscopic pull-through for Hirschsprung's disease in infants and children. J Pediatr Surg 30:1–7

Georgeson KE, Cohen RD, Hebra A, et al (1999) Primary laparoscopic-assisted endorectal colon pull-through for Hirschsprung's disease: a new gold standard. Ann Surg 229:678–683

Langer JC, Minkes RK, Maziotti MV, et al (1999) Transanal one-stage Soave procedure for infants with Hirschsprung's disease. J Pediatr Surg 34:148–152

Nmadu PT (1994) Endorectal pull-through and primary anastomosis for Hirschsprung's disease. Br J Surg 81:462–464

Pierro A, Fasioli L, Kiely E (1997) Staged pull-through for rectosigmoid Hirschsprung's disease is not safer than primary pull-through. J Pediatr Surg 32:505–509

So HB, Schwartz DL, Becker M, et al (1980) Endorectal pull-through without preliminary colostomy in neonates with Hirschsprung's disease. J Pediatr Surg 15:470–471

Teitelbaum DE, Coran AG, Weitzman JJ, et al (1998) Hirschsprung's disease and related neuromuscular disorders of the intestine. In: O'Neill JA, Rowe MI, Grosfeld JL, Fonkalsrud EW, Coran AG (eds) Pediatric Surgery, 5th edn, vol 2. Mosby-Year Book, St Louis, pp 1381–1424

Teitelbaum DH, Cilley RE, Sherman NJ, et al (2000) A decade of experience with the primary pull-through for Hirschsprung's disease in the newborn period. Ann Surg 232:372–380

Chapter 52

Laparoscopic-assisted Treatment of Hirschsprung's Disease According to Duhamel

Klaas (N) M.A. Bax and David C. van der Zee

Introduction

The treatment of Hirschsprung's disease is surgical and consists of removal of all but the most distal part of the aganglionic bowel. The most distal part is conserved for continence purposes. In Utrecht we have adopted a modified Duhamel technique. The original Duhamel technique consisted of resection of the aganglionic bowel above the peritoneal reflection, retrorectal pull-through of ganglionated bowel, and an end-to-side anastomosis between the pulled through ganglionated bowel and the remaining distal aganglionic rectum (1956). In order to prevent accumulation of feces in the remaining anterior rectum, Martin and Caudill proposed the use of a clamp to divide the wall between the anterior rectum and posterior pulled through bowel (Martin and Caudill 1967). In 1968 Steichen et al. described the use of a stapler for the creation of a complete side-to-side anastomosis between the retained rectum anteriorly and the pulled through bowel posteriorly. Linear staplers, however, were large and could not be used in small infants. As a result the operation had to be postponed for about 6 months and a colostomy in ganglionic bowel was created to bypass this waiting period. When small linear staplers became available for use in endoscopic surgery in adults, it became possible to use the same small staplers transanally in small infants and even in neonates. As a result we started to do a Duhamel-Martin-Steichen procedure in infants without a preliminary colostomy (van der Zee and Bax 1996; van der Zee et al. 1993). A laparoscopic-assisted version of the technique was developed by the Utrecht group and published in 1995 (Bax and van der Zee 1994). This technique has evolved considerably over the years and it is this technique that will be presented.

Preoperative Preparation

Before Induction of General Anesthesia

Contrast studies of the colon are often performed in the initial phase of the diagnostic workup in order to exclude mechanical obstruction and to give an idea of the extent of the disease. The definitive diagnosis is made by rectal suction biopsy. Initial treatment is directed at the relief of the obstruction by rectal washouts. Once the bowel has become decompressed, there is no urgency as to the timing of the definitive operation. In Utrecht the parents are taught how to do the rectal washouts. The patient is then send home to have an elective procedure at a convenient time for both the parents and the surgical team. When the bowel cannot be decompressed satisfactorily or when the washouts pose problems, the operation is not postponed.

The day before surgery an antegrade bowel lavage is carried out.

After Induction of General Anesthesia

The patient is put under general anesthesia, but locoregional techniques are usually associated. Prophylactic antibiotics are given.

Positioning

Patient

The patient is placed in a supine position on the operating table, which is tilted in reversed Trendelenburg (Fig. 52.1). Infants may be put transversely at the end of a shortened operating table. Arm supports, placed parallel with the table can be used to extend the transverse length of the table.

The rectum is suctioned with a double lumen suction probe to make sure that the bowel is completely empty. If not bowel washout is carried out until the effluent becomes clear.

The patient is then circumferentially prepared from the xiphoid process downward to include the legs. The first sterile sheet it put underneath the patient with its adhesive strip folded upward so that this strip adheres to the lumbosacral region just above the anus. The strip is then cut at either side of the body so that the lateral parts of the adhesive strip can be unfolded and taped to the table. The feet are wrapped in small separate sheets. Finally lateral sheets are placed to start from the chest downwards underneath the buttocks and legs. Underneath the buttocks a bunch of sterile paper towels are placed, which can be removed successively when they have become stained by transanal effluent.

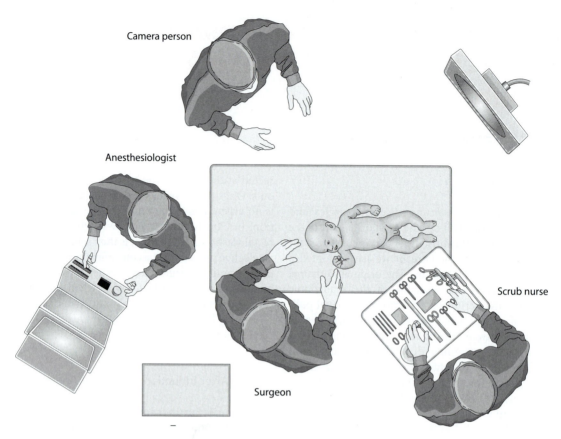

Camera person

Anesthesiologist

Scrub nurse

Surgeon

Fig. 52.1. Positioning of the patient, crew, and equipment

A urinary catheter is inserted by the surgeon. After emptying, the catheter is plugged. During the operation the bladder can be emptied again by the surgeons if needed. Usually not much urine is produced during the pneumoperitoneum and pushing the fluids by the anesthesiologist should be avoided as this will result in edema.

Crew, Monitors, and Equipment

The surgeon stands on the right side of the operating table and the camera operator on the left side. The scrub nurse stands at the right lower end of the table (■ Fig. 52.1). When the patient has been placed transversally on the operating table the surgeon stands at the patient's head with the camera operator to his left and the scrub nurse to his right.

The tower is placed behind the surgeon's back with the second monitor opposite to the surgeon. All cables are directed along the right side of the operating table.

Special Equipment

No special energy applying systems or special instruments are needed. For the side-to-side anastomosis between the anterior rectum and posterior pulled through colon an endolinear stapler with cartridges of 4.5 cm are used.

Technique

Cannulae

Cannula	Method of insertion	Diameter (mm)	Device	Position
1	Open	6	Telescope 30°	Infraumbilical fold
2	Closed	3.5/6	Surgeon's right-hand instrument	Pararectally at umbilical level in the small infant, lower down in older children
3	Closed	3.5/6	Surgeon's left-hand instrument	Middle of the epigastrium and slightly to the right in the small infant, slightly more to the right and lower down in older children
4	Closed	3.5/6	Assistant's instrument	Mirror position of cannula 2
5		10	Double lumen suction cannula	Transanally

Carbon Dioxide Pneumoperitoneum

A pressure of 8 mm Hg suffices when optimal muscle relaxation is guaranteed. Flow is arbitrarily set at 2 L/min in children below 1 year of age and at 5 L/min in children beyond that age.

Procedure

Cannula Insertion

The first cannula is inserted in an open way through the inferior umbilical fold and will contain the telescope (6 mm, 30°). Three secondary cannulae are inserted. These can be 3.5 mm in diameter for 3 mm instruments for children below 1 year of age, or 6 mm in diameter for 5 mm instruments for older children. Two secondary cannulae are inserted pararectally at the umbilical level in the newborn but lower down in older children. The right one will be used for the surgeon's right-handed instrument. The left one is used by the assistant to grasp the bowel segment to be mobilized. A last secondary cannula is inserted halfway between the xiphoid in the newborn but more to the right and lower down in older children and will be used for the surgeon's left-handed instrument (■ Fig. 52.2a,b).

Exploration and Determination of the Extent of the Disease

Usually it is immediately clear whether the patient has classic rectosigmoid or more extensive disease, confirming the preoperative contrast enema findings: the rectum is narrow while the rectosigmoid becomes progressively dilated. The bowel wall in the transitional zone between aganglionic and ganglionic bowel is thickened (■ Fig. 52.3).

The quality of the preoperative antegrade whole bowel washout is evaluated. Sometimes there may be air accumulation in the bowel just above the aganglionic colon. In rectosigmoid disease this can be emptied by transanal insertion of a double lumen suction device. The effectiveness of this procedure can be watched laparoscopically. It is advantageous to leave the suction cannula in the distal bowel for guidance.

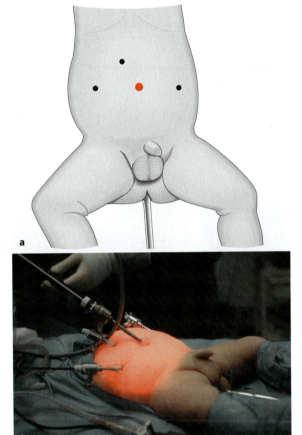

Fig. 52.2. Cannula positions. **a** Schematic drawing **b** Operative photograph

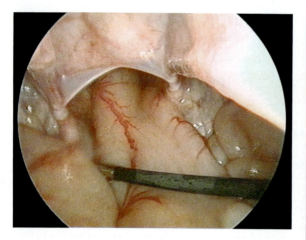

Fig. 52.3. Extent of disease. In this patient the upper rectum is dilated and has a thickened wall

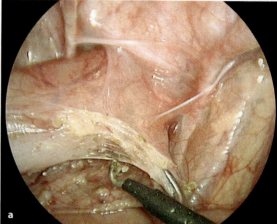

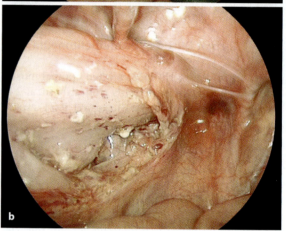

Fig. 52.5 a,b. Mobilization of the rectum above the peritoneal reflection

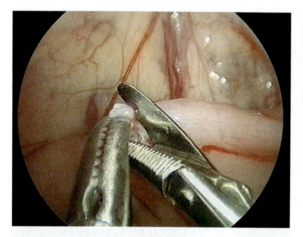

Fig. 52.4. Extramucosal biopsy taking

Both the preoperative contrast enema study as well as the intraoperative appearance may be misleading and the proximal extension of the disease has to be delineated by frozen section pathological examination of one or serial seromuscular biopsies. These biopsies are taken with a Kelly forceps in one hand and a pair of scissors in the other (■ Fig. 52.4). Usually two seromuscular biopsies suffice, one taken at the beginning of the dilatation and thickening of the bowel, confirming the diagnosis of aganglionosis, and one higher up in an area where the bowel wall looks normal, showing normal ganglion cells. If the most proximal biopsy still does not show ganglion cells a more proximal biopsy has to be taken. If inadvertently a full thickness biopsy is taken instead of a seromuscular one, the hole will not leak but should be closed with a 5 × 0 Vicryl suture. It is a good principle to put sutures over all biopsy places that are not exteriorized later on in order to prevent unrecognized leakage.

In the event of extensive aganglionosis, it may be wise to postpone further surgery until the definitive pathology report using paraffin sections and staining has become available.

Dissection of the Rectum
The Rectum Above the Peritoneal Reflection

The upper rectum is grasped and pulled up by the assistant. The mesorectum is entered from the right, close to the bowel wall, using a two-handed technique. We use a Kelly forceps in the left hand and the monopolar hook in the right hand (■ Fig. 52.5). By staying close to the bowel wall no damage is done to the surrounding structures. Moreover the vessels encountered here are relatively small and can be easily cauterized and severed with monopolar high-frequency electrocoagulation (HFE). After dividing the right leaf of the mesentery over a distance of a few centimeters, the

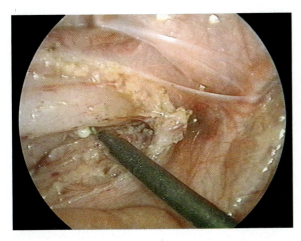

Fig. 52.6. Posterior dissection of the rectum up to the pelvic floor

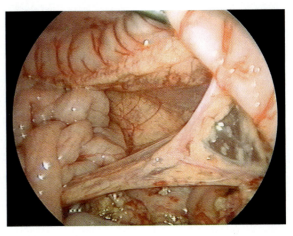

Fig. 52.7. Dissection of the colon in the cranial direction

loose areolar tissue in the middle of the mesentery is severed. Lastly, the left leaf of the mesentery is opened from the right. Once a window has been created, the dissection becomes easy as the left-sided pelvic wall is exposed through the window (■ Fig. 52.5). At the level of the peritoneal reflection, the anterior peritoneal covering of the rectum is severed as well taking care not to injure the vas or seminal vesicles.

The Rectum Below the Peritoneal Reflection

Once the peritoneal reflection is opened, the dissection is only carried further at the posterior side until the area immediately above the anus is reached. This is usually further down than expected (■ Fig. 52.6).

Dissection of the Sigmoid Colon

Next the dissection proceeds in a cranial direction (■ Fig. 52.7). If the sigmoid colon is tacked to the lateral peritoneum, Toldt's line is incised first, liberating the mesentery. The dissection of the sigmoid colon is carried out close to the bowel wall until the biopsy place with good ganglion cells is encountered. Whether more or less sigmoidal vessels or even the left colic vessels should be divided at their origin depends on the extent of the disease. Smaller vessels can be severed with monopolar HFE. Bigger vessels can be severed between ligatures, clips, or with ultrasonic energy. They can also be sealed with bipolar HFE and cut with scissors.

Subtotal Colectomy

When the aganglionosis extends proximally beyond the splenic flexure or even into the ileum, the dissection has to proceed much more proximally with transection of the middle, and even right colic vessels. The right colon and ileocecal region has then to be mobilized in order to be able to turn the right colon downward and to pull through either the right colon or even the ileum. To accomplish a subtotal colectomy, the position of the table, the monitors, and the team has to change accordingly. Many of these patients will have had a preliminary colostomy or ileostomy. Under such circumstances, the colostomy or ileostomy should be taken down at the beginning of the operation and through the ensuing minilaparotomy quite a bit of dissection can be done. The laparotomy should then be closed incorporating a cannula and the operation should be continued laparoscopically.

Removal of the Aganglionic Bowel
Transanal Eversion of the Mobilized Colon and Removal of the Aganglionic Segment

Once the proximal good biopsy place is reached and enough length for the pull-through has been created, the colon is everted through the distal rectum (■ Fig. 52.8). The eviscerated bowel is transected close to the anus in order to leave a short rectum behind (■ Fig. 52.9). The bowel is further eviscerated till the good biopsy place is reached. Here the bowel is amputated and the end closed with a running suture (■ Fig. 52.10). The mesenteric and antimesenteric edges are marked for identification so that torsion is avoided during the later retrorectal pull-through. The closed end as well as the open distal rectum are pushed back into the pelvis (■ Fig. 52.11).

Alternatively, the rectum can be closed just above the peritoneal reflection using a ligature in small children or the endolinear stapler in larger children. The disadvantage of this is that the bowel, which is often dilated, has to be pulled down through the rather small retrorectal space. Moreover the endolinear stapler requires a 12 mm-diameter port.

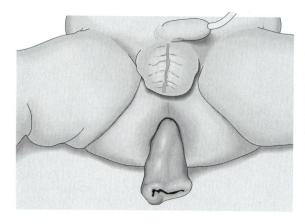

Fig. 52.8. Transanal eversion of the mobilized colon

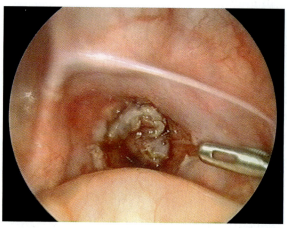

Fig. 52.11. Repositioning of the rectum and closed off colon into the abdomen

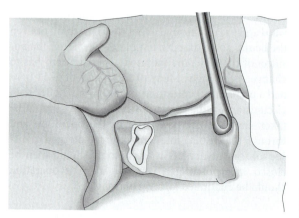

Fig. 52.9. Transection of the rectum close to the anus

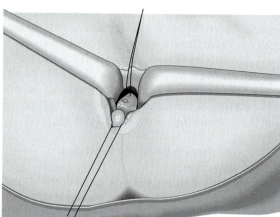

Fig. 52.12. The posterior rectum is opened about 0.5 cm above the dentate line

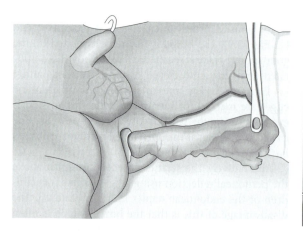

Fig. 52.10. Removal of aganglionic colon outside the body and closure of the proximal end

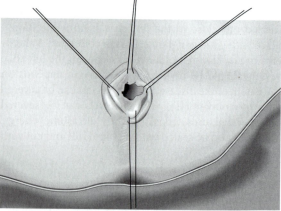

Fig. 52.13. The retrorectal space is developed from below to meet the retrorectal space that has been dissected laparoscopically

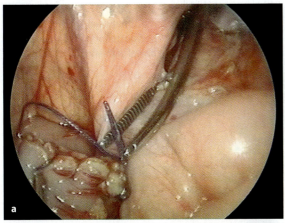

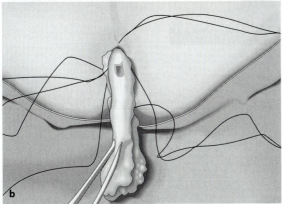

Fig. 52.14. Retrorectal pull-through. **a** Internal view. The closed off colon is grabbed through the retrorectal space and is pulled down until the good biopsy place is reached. Here the pulled through bowel is amputated. **b** External view

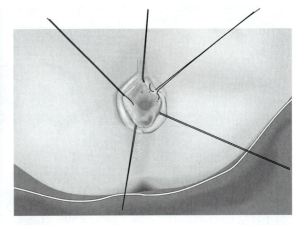

Fig. 52.15. End-to-side anastomosis between pulled through colon and the hole in the posterior rectum

bowel is grasped and pulled through under laparoscopic control in order to avoid torsion (■ Figs. 52.14). The mesentery of the pulled through bowel should be posteriorly or slightly to the right.

The pulled through bowel is opened in the ganglionic area and is anastomosed circumferentially into the hole in the distal posterior rectum (■ Fig. 52.15).

Transanal Side-to-side Anastomosis

An endoscopic linear stapler is inserted transanally with the thinner part of the beak in the rectum and the bigger part in the pulled through colon (■ Figs. 52.16, 52.17). The device should anastomose the midposterior rectum to the midanterior pulled through bowel. The intra-abdominal position of the stapling device is checked laparoscopically (■ Fig. 52.18). After firing, the anastomosis is checked for completeness. If this is not the case a second cartridge is inserted and fired.

Laparoscopic Closure of the Upper Rectum

The rectum, which is still open at its top, has to be closed. This is done laparoscopically with a running 3 × 0 Vicryl suture (■ Figs. 52.19, 52.20). The needle and suture is inserted directly through the abdominal wall.

Retrorectal Pull-through and End-to-side Anastomosis

Depending on age a transverse incision is made in the posterior rectum 0.5–1.0 cm above the dentate line (■ Figs. 52.12, 52.13). The full thickness posterior rectal wall is separated off the pelvic floor until the retrorectal space, which has been developed transabdominally, is reached.

A blunt curved forceps is inserted from below into the retrorectal space and the distal end of the proximal

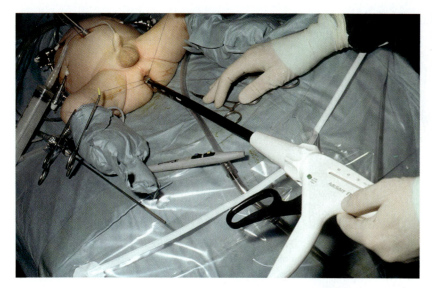

Fig. 52.16. Side-to-side anastomosis between anterior rectum and posterior pulled through bowel with endolinear stapler

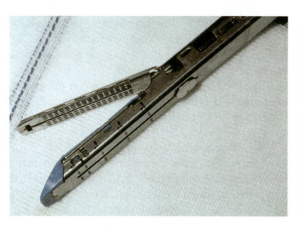

Fig. 52.17. Stapler cartridge

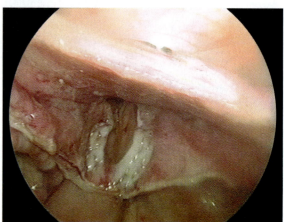

Fig. 52.19. The stapled side-to-side anastomosis is seen through the remaining opening in the rectum

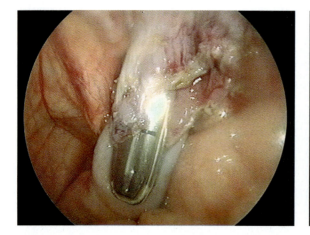

Fig. 52.18. The tip of the closed stapling device is seen intra-abdominally. One part of the beak protrudes through the anterior open rectum. The posterior part sits in the pulled through bowel

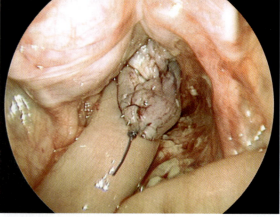

Fig. 52.20. The open rectum has been closed with a running suture

Postoperative Care

Antibiotics are given for 24 h. There is no need for a nasogastric tube. Feeding is started after evidence of functional restoration of the transit. Epidural analgesia or otherwise intravenous morphine is given for 48 h. The urinary catheter is left in place until the next morning or as long as the patient has an epidural catheter for pain relief. The patient is discharged when on full oral feeding.

Results

By September 2003 we had performed 54 laparoscopic-assisted Duhamel procedures. Median age was 67 days at diagnosis and 236 days at surgery, which means that most patients have had bowel washouts for about 5 months after the diagnosis was made. Median weight at surgery was 4,500 g. If decompression by washouts was troublesome, the operation was not postponed. The earliest laparoscopic-assisted Duhamel was done at the age of 13 days at a weight of 2,930 g, and posed no technical problems. Four patients received a colostomy or ileostomy prior to definitive surgery, all for extended disease. All these ostomies were closed at the time of the definitive procedure. The median duration of the operation was 5 h, but includes all patients, which means also the learning curve and patients with long-segment disease. At the start of our experience, we mobilized the rectum up to the pelvic floor. The rectum was amputated just above the peritoneal reflection and the proximal part was pulled through behind the rectum until the good biopsy place was encountered. After the end-to-end anastomosis of the pulled through colon, the linear endostapler was inserted and a side-to-side anastomosis between the anterior rectum and posterior pulled through bowel was made. In order to close the remaining opening in the upper rectum, the side-to-side anastomosis was pulled down with stay sutures and the open rectum was closed transanally with Vicryl sutures. By doing so no anterior pouch was left. This technique was complicated: it necessitated full mobilization of the rectum and transanal eversion of the side-to-side anastomosis. Later on we decided to perform a true Duhamel in which the rectum is only mobilized posteriorly. In order to get rid of the aganglionic bowel, the bowel is eviscerated through the rectum and is amputated outside the body. This amputation has to be performed close to the anus in order to avoid leaving too long a

rectum. The advantage of this technique is that the bowel which is sometimes bulky does not have to be divided internally. The disadvantage is that the externally closed off ganglionic bowel has to be pushed back through the remaining rectum into the abdomen, which is not ideal from the point of view of sterility. An alternative is that the rectum is closed off proximally either with a ligature in small children or with an endolinear stapler in larger children. The proximal end can then be pulled down through the opening in the lower posterior rectum. The disadvantage of this technique is that sometimes bulky bowel has to be pulled down through a rather narrow retrorectal space and posterior rectal opening. In any case the rectum is left open in this technique as well. Why is the rectum left open? If it were to be closed for example by stapler, then a complete side-to-side anastomosis is hard to achieve as the cartridges of the endolinear stapler have a fish mouth shape at the end. This end does not staple nor cut which means that always a small upper rectal pouch is left. After the side-to-side anastomosis, the upper part of the remaining rectum has to be closed which we do with a running 3×0 Vicryl suture brought in directly through the abdominal wall. This requires considerable endoscopic surgical experience.

Four patients developed leakage, one at the a biopsy site and three in the pelvis. The patient with the leaking biopsy site was treated laparoscopically while the other three were treated with a colostomy.

One patient has received an appendicostomy for soiling.

Discussion

The laparoscopic-assisted Duhamel technique, as described, has the advantage that it can be used for both rectosigmoid as well as total colonic involvement. The long interval between the diagnosis and definitive surgery in our series is related to the fact that most parents are so effective in giving rectal washouts that their children do very well during the interval. So there is no need for earlier surgery in most children. We feel that it is of great benefit that parents know how to give washouts as many children intermittently have problems with defecation despite surgery.

The cosmetic outcome of a laparoscopic-assisted Duhamel is excellent (■ Fig. 52.21). The major disadvantage of the technique is that it requires considerable endoscopic surgical expertise.

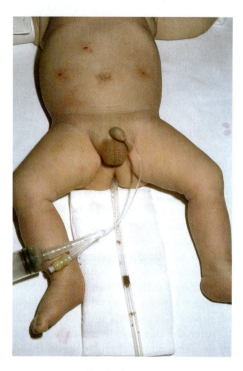

Fig. 52.21. Final look of the abdomen after withdrawal of the cannulae. Minimal scars will be left

References

Bax NMA, van der Zee DC (1994) Laparoscopic removal of the aganglionic bowel according to Duhamel-Martin in five consecutive infants. Pediatr Surg Int 10:226–228

Duhamel B (1956) Une nouvelle opération pour le mégacôlon congénitale: l'abaissement rétrorectal et trans-anal du côlon et son application possible au traitement de quelques autres malformations. Presse Med 64:2249–2250

Martin LW, Caudill DR (1967) A method for elimination of the blind rectal pouch in Duhamel operation for Hirschsprung's disease. Surgery 62:951–953

Steichen FM, Talbert JL, Ravitch MM (1968) Primary side to side anastomosis in the Duhamel operation for Hirschsprung's disease. Surgery 64:475–483

van der Zee DC, Bax NMA (1996) Duhamel-Martin procedure for Hirschsprung's disease in neonates and infants: one-stage operation. J Pediatr Surg 31:901–902

van der Zee DC, Bax NMA, Pull ter Gunne AJ, Rövekamp MH (1993) Use of EndoGIA stapling device in Duhamel Martin procedure for Hirschsprung's disease. Pediatr Surg Int 8:447–448

Chapter 53

Laparoscopic Rectopexy

David C. van der Zee, Klaas (N) M.A. Bax

Introduction

Rectal prolapse in young children is a commonly occurring event that can usually be treated conservatively. Most of these prolapses contain only mucosa. However, sometimes the prolapse is full thickness and does not respond to conservative measures, particularly in children with associated disease (Stafford 1990). In these children surgical management is indicated. Ashcraft et al. (1990) described their results with the posterior repair and suspension. The fixation of the rectum against the presacral fascia can also be approached laparoscopically. Several case-controlled and prospective randomized trials in adults have been performed, demonstrating that with the laparoscopic approach similar results can be obtained with an earlier recovery, less blood loss, less pain medication, favorable pain and mobility scores, but with a longer operating time (Kairaluoma et al. 2003; Solomon et al. 2002).

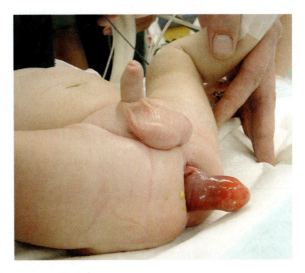

Fig. 53.1. Full thickness rectal prolapse in a baby with spina bifida

Indication

Children with full thickness prolapse in whom conservative treatment is not successful are good candidates for a laparoscopic rectopexy (█ Fig. 53.1). Rectopexy should also be part of laparoscopic-assisted pull-through for anorectal malformations in order to prevent prolapse.

Preoperative Preparation

Before Induction of General Anesthesia

The evening prior to the operation the patient is given an enema or a retrograde colorectal washout to avoid accumulation of feces in the colon.

After Induction of General Anesthesia

Part of the perioperative management may be subject to local customs and personal preferences. Future porthole sites may be injected with local anesthetics. Epidural or spinal anesthesia is subject to the personal preference of the anesthetist. If the patient is receiving analgesia by means of an epidural catheter a voiding urinary catheter is mandatory. Perioperative antibiotics are given. If necessary a repeat rectal washout can be carried out.

Positioning

Patient

The patient is placed in a supine position with the table in a 15–20° Trendelenburg position (█ Fig. 53.2a). Smaller children can be placed transversely at the lower end of the operating table (█ Fig. 53.2b,c). It usually is sufficient to have the patient empty their bladder before the operation. In small children the bladder can be emptied by suprapubic compression.

Crew, Monitors, and Equipment

In older children the surgeon stands to the right of the patient and the assistant on the left. The scrub nurse stands to the right of the surgeon. The surgeon may change to the left side of the patient when approaching the left side of the rectosigmoid (█ Fig. 53.2a). The video columns stands behind the surgeon, and the

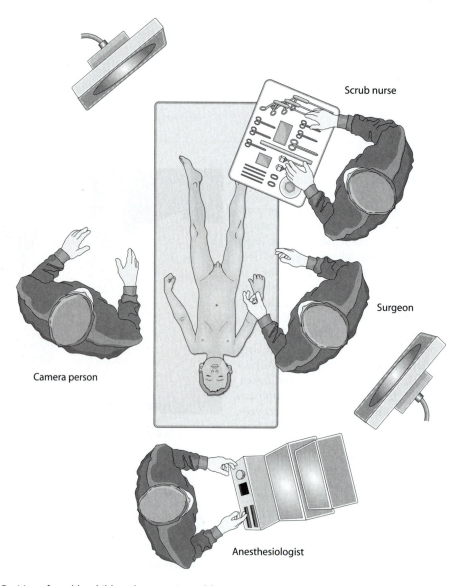

Scrub nurse

Surgeon

Camera person

Anesthesiologist

a

Fig. 53.2. a Position of an older child on the operating table.

principal monitor stands at the end of the table. In infants and small children, who lie transversely at the lower end of the table, the surgeon stands at the head of the patient, with the assistant on the left and the scrub nurse on the right (■ Fig. 53.2b). The monitor stands at the feet of the patient.

Special Equipment

No special equipment is required, but in older children ultrasonic energy and/or Ligasure may be helpful for the posterior dissection of the rectum.

Fig. 53.2. b Small children are positioned transversely and supine at the lower end of the operating table which is tilted toward the surgeon. **c** A baby placed transversely and supine at the lower end of the operating table

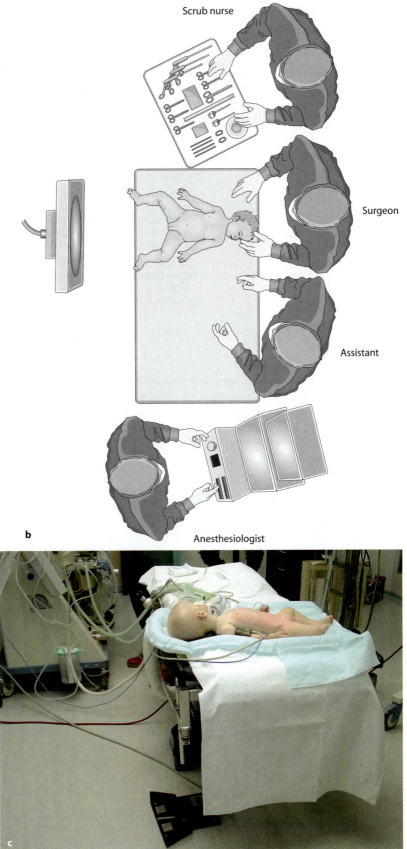

Technique

Cannulae

Cannula	Method of insertion	Diameter (mm)	Device	Position
1	Open	6	Optic	Umbilicus
2	Closed	3.5/6	Grasping forceps for retraction of the to the left when operating on the right of the rectum Surgeon´s left handed instrument when operating on the left of the rectum	Pararectally on the left at umbilical level in small children; otherwise left lower quadrant
3	Closed	3.5/6	Surgeon´s right handed instrument when operating on the right of the rectum Grasping forceps for retraction of the rectum to the right when operating on the left of the rectum	Pararectally on the right at umbilical level in small children; otherwise right lower quadrant
4	Closed	3.5/6	Surgeon´s left handed instrument during dissection/suturing on the right, surgeon´s right handed instrument during dissection/suturing on the left	In the epigastrium in small children, more to the right and lower down in older children

Procedure

Open introduction of a 6 mm cannula is through the infraumbilical fold. A cannula inserted on either side at the umbilical level in small children and lower down in the iliac fossa in older children (■ Fig. 53.3a,b). A last cannula is inserted in the epigastrium in small children, lower down and more to the right in older children. Depending on the side of the rectum to be dissected the working cannulae are changed.

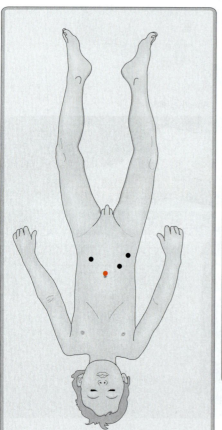

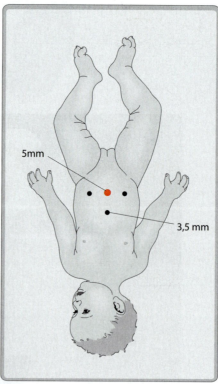

5mm

3,5 mm

Fig. 53.3. a Port positions in older children. **b** Port positions in smaller children

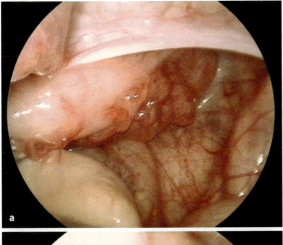

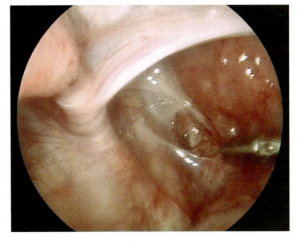

Fig. 53.6. The left pararectal space is opened

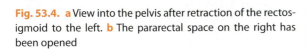

Fig. 53.4. a View into the pelvis after retraction of the rectosigmoid to the left. **b** The pararectal space on the right has been opened

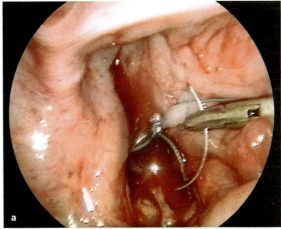

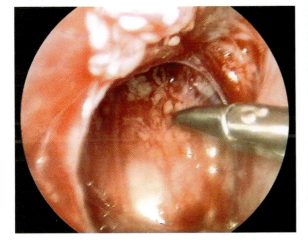

Fig. 53.5. The glistening presacral fascia is visualized

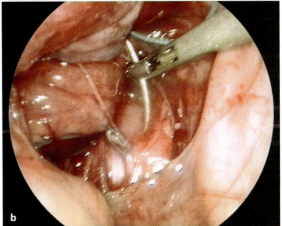

Fig. 53.7. a The left pararectal wall has been sutured to the presacral fascia. A second suture is being placed. **b** The right rectal wall is now being sutured to the presacral fascia. A left-sided suture is seen

Introduction of a Hegar dilator transanally is also helpful as it can help in pushing up the rectum to the left so that the right pararectal space can be opened, and later on to the right to enter the left pararectal space (■ Fig. 53.4a,b). The presacral fascia is visualized and dissected free from the right (■ Fig. 53.5). There is no reason to interfere with any presacral vessels or nerves. Next the left pararectal space is opened and the presacral fascia dissected free from this side (■ Fig. 53.6). A 2×0 or 3×0 non-resorbable Ethibond suture is either introduced through the trocar, or directly through the skin in infants, and a sufficient bite is taken from the presacral fascia at the level of the promontorium. The rectosigmoid is retracted maximally and moved a little to the right or the left to determine the best place for placing the suture in the colonic wall on the right side, and the knot can be tied using either the intracorporeal or extracorporeal tying technique. Principally two sutures are placed on either side of the colon (■ Fig. 53.7a,b).

Postoperative Care

There is no need for a nasogastric tube after the operation. A urinary catheter is only necessary when the patient has an epidural catheter for postoperative analgesia. Feeding of the patient may be started as soon as the patient is fully awake and not feeling nauseous.

Results

A 2-month-old child with a spina bifida developed a rectal prolapse refractory to conservative measures.

The operation was simple. No recurrence has occurred after a follow-up of 3 years. Rectopexy has become routine after laparoscopic-assisted pull-through for anorectal anomalies and is very simple as the retrorectal area has been developed during the pull-through procedure.

Discussion

Rectal prolapse necessitating surgery usually is a disease of old age (Kairaluoma et al. 2003; Solomon et al. 2002). In children mostly conservative measures are sufficiently curative (Stafford 1990). When surgical management is necessary fixation against the presacral fascia is usually curative (Ashcraft et al. 1990). The laparoscopic approach presents a minimally invasive means to reach the goal. The procedure is easy and results are equal to the open approach. Rectopexy should also be routine during the laparoscopic-assisted pull-through for anorectal anomalies.

References

Ashcraft KW, Garred JL, Holder TM (1990) Rectal prolapse: 17-year experience with the posterior repair and suspension. J Pediatr Surg 25:992–994

Kairaluoma MV, Viljakka MT, Kellokumpu IH (2003) Open vs. laparoscopic surgery for rectal prolapse: a case-controlled study assessing short-term outcome. Dis Colon Rectum 46:353–360

Solomon MJ, Young CJ, Eyers AA et al. (2002) Randomized clinical trail of laparoscopic versus open abdominal rectopexy for rectal prolapse. Br J Surg 89:35–39

Stafford PW (1990) Other disorders of the anus and rectum, anorectal function. In: O'Neill JA Jr, Rowe MI, Grosfeld JL, Fonkalsrud EW, Coran AG (eds) Pediatric Surgery, 5th edn. Mosby Year Book, St Louis, pp 1454–1455

Georgeson's Procedure: Laparoscopically Assisted Anorectoplasty for High Anorectal Malformations

Thomas H. Inge

Introduction

Minimally invasive options for correction of many surgical conditions seen in infants and children have become available and popular since the 1990s. The primary advantages seen with minimally invasive methods derive from the surgeon's ability to perform procedures within the body's major cavities with the least amount of iatrogenic injury to intervening skin, fascial, muscular, and nervous tissues (Dick et al. 1998; Kehlet and Nielsen 1998). The ability to perform reconstructive surgery with minimal trauma is especially relevant and important for the neonate with an anorectal malformation, since the intervening tissues must perform sensory and contractile functions critical for lifelong control of continence.

For many decades, the infant born with a high anorectal malformation (ARM) has represented a management challenge for pediatric surgeons and parents alike. Operative reconstruction of high ARM is a demanding and meticulous undertaking, and, despite the careful and deliberate technique of an experienced pediatric surgeon, functional outcomes are far from perfect. In the early 1990s, a minimally invasive technique for correction of high ARM was developed by Keith Georgeson – the laparoscopically assisted anorectoplasty (LAARP). His early surgical experience with LAARP was first presented at the surgical section meeting of the American Academy of Pediatrics in October of 1998 (Georgeson et al. 2000). Since that time, many other centers have gained experience with this minimally invasive technique, and have confirmed the merits of the approach to this complex and difficult malformation. This chapter will represent a current update of the technique of minimally invasive correction of high ARM.

Over the years, we have learned that muscles deep within the pelvic floor are critical to continence by virtue of their sensory as well as motor function. Before the 1950s, if reconstruction of patients with high ARM was attempted at all, it was done by way of laparotomy and a limited perineal incision (abdominoperineal pull-through). Surgeons used a blind, blunt dissection through the pelvic floor toward the perineum. It is not difficult to imagine the challenges which faced the operative team at that time, which included poor ability

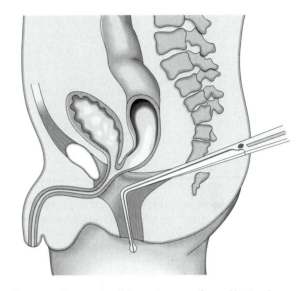

Fig. 54.1. Sacroperineal dissection as performed by Stephens

to visually inspect the depths of the infant pelvis, the real concern for eliciting hemorrhage in an area which would be difficult to easily control, and the imprecise guidance of the dissection using tactile sense. Due in part to the anterior lie of the central portion of the puborectalis sling in the patient with ARM, this critical element controlling fecal continence was often completely disrupted by blind pull-through.

Important concepts (which would contribute to modern thinking) were inspired by the work of Douglas Stephens in the premodern era (Stephens 1953). His seminal contribution, which began in the early and mid 1950s, was to recognize the importance of preservation of the integrity of the pelvic levator musculature (the puborectalis muscle in particular) and external anal sphincters. His important principles – to minimize surgical trauma and thus preserve the integrity of the muscles of continence by using alternative strategies for visualization of the pelvic floor – are still emphasized today.

Specifically, Stephens aimed to improve surgical results by improving the quality of the surgical dissection of the pelvic passage for rectal pull-through. Thus was born the sacroperineal pull-through procedure (■ Fig. 54.1), and variations thereof. With a transverse

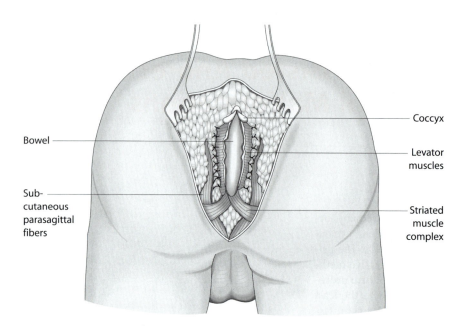

Fig. 54.2. Exposure during PSARP

Bowel

Sub-cutaneous parasagittal fibers

Coccyx

Levator muscles

Striated muscle complex

sacral incision, superoposterior to and separate from the perineal incision for anorectal anastomosis, the hope was that the surgeon could more accurately negotiate the minute and delicate pelvic floor components and place the pull-through rectum more correctly through the midline center of the levators while anterior to the central belly of the puborectalis muscle. Although surgeons of this era clearly had intended to better visualize and preserve the structures critical to continence, unfortunately, the tools and access approaches available were still unsuitable for the exacting task.

A major revolution in thinking about ARM repair came in the early 1980s when Pena and DeVries introduced an operative approach that has been considered the most important advancement in the management of the entire spectrum of ARMs (de Vries and Pena 1982). The posterior sagittal anorectoplasty (PSARP) allowed surgeons the ability to accurately place the bowel within the confines of the levator complex as well as the more distal striated muscle complex contiguous with the external anal sphincter. This technique quickly supplanted other contemporaneous operations, in large part due to its simplicity and elegance (■ Fig. 54.2). In the prelaparoscopic era, the visualization afforded to the surgeons who used this procedure was unparalleled.

Pena and others noted an improvement in functional outcome after PSARP and credit that functional improvement to the fact that the muscles of continence are not destroyed during the procedure, rather these structures are surgically separated or divided and ultimately reapproximated during reconstruction. Indeed, this operation has endured the all important test of

time, being the dominant procedure since the 1980s. There are many manuscripts and chapters devoted to every detail of this operation and a recent update of the experience with PSARP (Pena and Hong 2000). With this procedure, Pena has made a fundamental contribution to our understanding of high ARM. He showed that dissection through the external anal sphincter complex and complete surgical division of the levator muscles in the midline can be performed without destroying these important structures. Indeed, if the operation is performed well, 30–50% of patients with high ARM can be completely continent, and most of the remainder can be made socially continent. However, although the results of PSARP represent an improvement over prior operations, there remains some uncertainty as to the extent to which (1) the inherently abnormal bowel and sphincter function or (2) the dissection technique of PSARP (with division and reconstruction of the muscles critical for fecal control) contribute to the high rates of incontinence following PSARP for high ARM.

This important question provided us with the rationale to consider the possibility of accomplishing a correction of high ARM *without midsagittal division of any of the muscles of continence* (Georgeson et al. 2000). If one of the most important advances inherent in the PSARP was that of exquisite visualization of the pelvic structures of continence, Georgeson's procedure for reconstruction of high ARM provides an even greater advantage of exquisite visualization of the intrapelvic anatomy. The angled laparoscope used in Georgeson's procedure enables the surgeon to visualize in magnified detail the critical pelvic musculature. Unlike the PSARP, the vantage point for this visualization is internal, rather than external as with PSARP. Thus, with the laparoscope, the pediatric surgeon can see well within the depths of the neonatal pelvis, behind the neck of the bladder. Inspection of the pelvic floor and visualization of the individual muscles constituting the levator complex is possible. From this point of view, guidance of the dissection from perineum is precise, and any deviation from the desired path of dissection is instantaneously identified and corrected.

Preoperative Preparation

For patients who have undergone prior divided colostomy, a mechanical and antibiotic bowel preparation is indicated. In addition, through the mucus fistula, the distal rectum is irrigated with a saline solution + 100 mg/dL neomycin and erythromycin solution. If LAARP is being performed for high ARM as a primary pull-through procedure (i.e., without prior colostomy) in males, cystoscopy performed just before reconstruction enables accurate identification the level of the fistula, and detection of potentially important urologic anomalies.

Positioning

The patient is positioned supine and placed transversely across the end of the table, to allow access by the surgical team on three sides. The torso, pelvis, and lower extremities lie flat on several folded sheets to elevate the body; this allows the neck to extend and thus protects the head and endotracheal tube during laparoscopy. This positioning also allows the surgical team maximal access to the patient for both laparoscopic and perineal portions of the procedure. The bladder is next decompressed by transurethral catheterization. Catheterization prevents postoperative urinary retention and also allows for palpation of the urethra during laparoscopic dissection.

The surgeon stands above the patient's head and the assistant stands at the end of the table to the patient's left.

Technique

Access

Pneumoperitoneum is created using a Veress needle inserted into the right upper quadrant (■ Fig. 54.3). The site is infiltrated with lidocaine and a 5 mm incision is made. After 8–10 mmHg of pneumoperitoneum is established, this site is used for placement of a 5 mm radially expandable trocar (Step). Laparoscopy

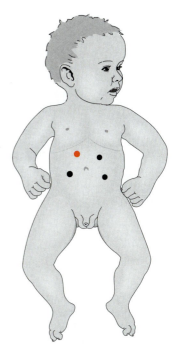

Fig. 54.3. Trocar sites for laparoscopically assisted anorectoplasty

is performed through the right upper quadrant site using a 4- or 5 mm 30° angled laparoscope. Either 5 mm or smaller 3.5 mm trocars can be placed in the left upper quadrant and left lower quadrant. Another 5 mm trocar is placed in the right lower quadrant. This site is later used for the 5 mm bipolar electrocoagulating shears, the endoloop, or the clip applier.

Procedure

Rectal Dissection

Laparoscopic rectal dissection begins at the peritoneal reflection. This dissection is facilitated by anterosuperior traction applied to the bowel wall. The most distal mesorectum is opened and divided using hook cautery or ultrasonic shears. Bipolar or ultrasonic shears are used throughout the remainder of the dissection to prevent thermal injury to the rectal wall, since viability of the pulled through segment will be dependent upon the bowel's intramural blood supply. As the rectum tapers into the fistula distally, a meticulous and deliberate dissection toward the termination of the fistula must be performed. It is most critical during this part of the dissection for the surgeon to stay close to the longitudinal layer of the bowel wall since important pelvic autonomic nerve supply to the bladder and penis pass nearby and can be injured when dissecting rectourethral fistulas. This dissection is considerably easier for rectobladder neck and rectovaginal fistulas, as compared to the slower, more meticulous dissection which is needed at the termination of a rectourethral fistula.

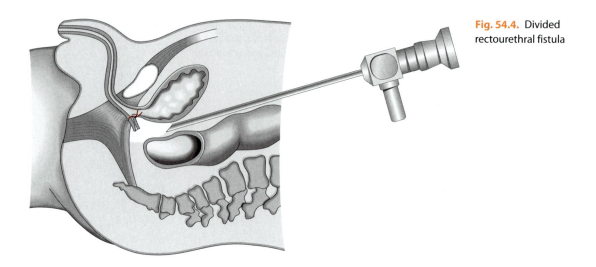

Fig. 54.4. Divided rectourethral fistula

Fistula Management

When the rectourinary or rectogenital fistula has been sufficiently cleared of surrounding tissue, it is ligated and divided (■ Fig. 54.4). This may be accomplished using an endoloop or, alternatively, the fistula can be occluded with a 5 mm titanium clip and sharply divided. The rectum is pulled up and out of the pelvis, to facilitate close inspection of the pelvic floor musculature. A 30° angled telescope is advanced just beyond the sacral prominence with the end of the lens directed upward such that the surgeon is looking beneath and around the bladder neck. In some patients, visualization of the entire pelvic diaphragm and puborectalis muscle is possible. The distal end of the divided fistula gives the surgeon clear identification of the midline (■ Fig. 54.5). Following division of the fistula, a laparoscopically placed muscle stimulator can also be used to assist in the identification of the midline of the levator muscles (Iwanaka et al. 2003; Yamataka et al. 2002; Yamataka et al. 2001).

Perineal Dissection

The legs are next elevated, the hips flexed, and the feet held together over the head to afford exposure of the perineum (■ Fig. 54.6). This position also effectively results in straightening of the vertical muscle complex to facilitate alignment of the perineal anal site, the puborectalis sling, and the sacral prominence. The muscle stimulator (Peña Muscle Stimulator; Radionics, Burlington, MA) is used to determine the anal site. A 1 cm vertical midline incision is made in the perineum at the anal dimple site identified by electrostimulation. The intrasphincteric plane is bluntly dissected with a hemostat from below for a short distance without dividing the sphincter. Ultrasonography can be used at this point to confirm midline placement of the pull-through bowel (Yamataka et al. 2002). The low profile Step Veress needle with radially expanding sheath is then placed into the perineal wound and passed through the mid-

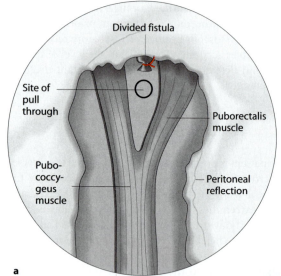

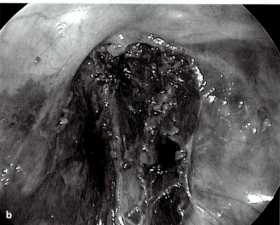

Fig. 54.5. Pelvic view after division of rectourethral fistula. **a** Schematic drawing. **b** Intraoperative view

line intrasphincteric plane and advanced between the two bellies of the pubococcygeus muscle in the midline using laparoscopic guidance. The angle of insertion should be approximately 45° from the horizontal (coronal) plane in this hip flexed position. The needle must enter the pelvis in the midline, through the levator sling, just posterior to the urethra. Due to the conical nature of the pelvic diaphragm, the sheathed needle may be deflected off the midline to either side while advancing

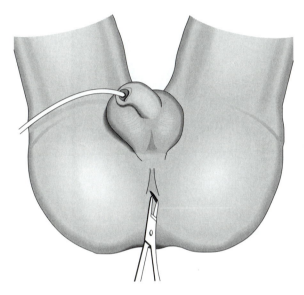

Fig. 54.6. Perineal dissection

through the muscle complex. Inadvertent deflection is readily apparent from the laparoscopic vantage point. When this occurs, the needle is removed and reintroduced until it is placed accurately within the center of the "V" of the puborectalis sling (■ Fig. 54.5). Accurate placement of the needle is only possible if the surgeon is simultaneously watching the laparoscopic image. This is the key difference between this technique and the blind techniques used in decades past. Technologic advancements in surgical laparoscopy provide the pediatric surgeon the ability to look around the pubic arch and see a magnified view of the infant pelvic floor.

The needle is next removed from the sheath, and the tract is dilated gently in a stepwise fashion to 5 mm and then to 10 mm diameter without cutting any of the critical fibers of the muscles of continence. A 10 mm Babcock clamp is inserted into the transperineal trocar and the rectum is grasped and gently guided down to the perineum, retracting it out with the trocar as a unit (■ Fig. 54.7). The anastomosis between rectum and anus is next completed with circumferential interrupted 3-0 polyglycolic acid suture. The rectum is retracted cephalad laparoscopically and secured to the presacral fascia at a convenient location using 2-0 silk sutures, in order to prevent prolapse and to provide a longer skin-lined anal canal (■ Fig. 54.8). The neoanus is sized with Hegar dilators.

Postoperatively, dilations begin at 2–3 weeks with the Hegar size noted intraoperatively. The colostomy is taken down once satisfactory healing has occurred, and an adequate orifice is present.

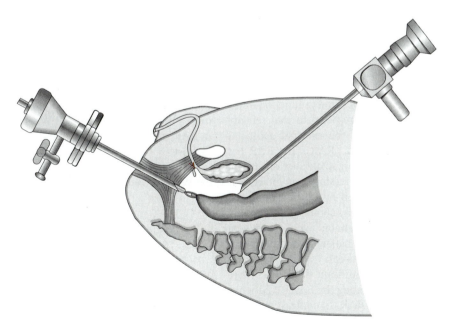

Fig. 54.7. Perineal pull-through of the distal rectum

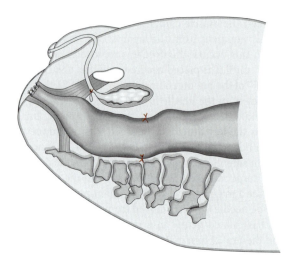

Fig. 54.8. After anorectoplasty and laparoscopic placement of anchoring sutures

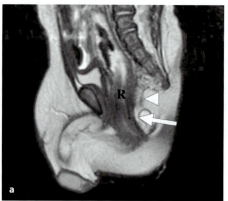

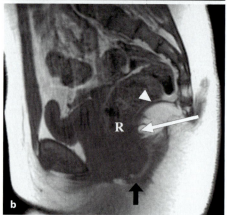

Fig. 54.9. **a** Sagittal view of the pelvis of an infant with high ARM after LAARP. *Long white arrow* posterior rectal wall at vertex of the anorectal angle, *white arrowhead* posterior elements of relatively hypoplastic pubococcygeus muscle enveloping rectum, *black arrow* relative paucity of external sphincter muscle fibers near neoanus, *R* rectum. **b** Sagittal view of normal child's pelvis for comparison. *Long white arrow* anorectal angle, *white arrowhead* well-developed posterior element of pubococcygeus muscle, *black arrow* well-developed external anal sphincter muscles near anus, *R* rectum

Physiologic Study After LAARP

Normal anorectal function is the ultimate goal of any reconstructive procedure in the patient with an ARM. Both resting anorectal tone and a rectoanal relaxation reflex can be measured and used to describe anorectal function after operation for ARM. A retrospective cohort study of patients who had undergone LAARP or PSARP between 16 and 18 months prior to the study was recently reported (Lin et al. 2003). Investigators found that 78% of LAARP patients and 54% of PSARP patients had a normal stooling pattern (one to four bowel movements per day). In these patients there was no difference in resting rectal pressure, as determined by anorectal manometry, suggesting that the groups were similarly corrected with placement of the neoanus centrally within the sphincteric muscle complex.

More intriguing was the result seen when physiologic function was examined. Distention of the rectum with an intraluminal balloon measures the integrated ability to both sense rectal distension (a function of the puborectalis muscle) and to respond to that sensory stimulus with contraction of the external sphincter complex – the rectoanal reflex (RAR). The RAR has been used as an indicator of anorectal function since it is an objective manometric expression of an intact neuromuscular reflex arc mediated by healthy perirectal sensory innervation and healthy sphincteric function. RAR was examined in 9 patients who underwent Georgeson's procedure and 13 patients who underwent PSARP. Both groups were between 1 and 2 years after operative reconstruction. Significant differences were found in the two groups. Among the LAARP patients, 8 of 9 (89%) had inducible RAR. In contrast only 4 of the 13 (31%) who had undergone PSARP demonstrated RAR. In both groups, the presence of a RAR correlated highly with a normal bowel movement frequency.

Although the numbers of patients studied were small, these data suggest that results of LAARP are more physiologic than PSARP. Whether the deficiency in RAR in patients that have undergone PSARP is indicative of a greater extent of disruption of pelvic sensory function or disability in sphincteric contraction has yet to be established.

Anatomic Study of Patients after Georgeson's Procedure

Magnetic resonance imaging (MRI) provides a good assessment of anatomic structures of the infant pelvis after LAARP, and can be used to demonstrate the relationship between the levator muscles and pulled through rectum after LAARP. As shown in sagittal view in ▓ Fig. 54.9a, there is good anatomic recreation of the

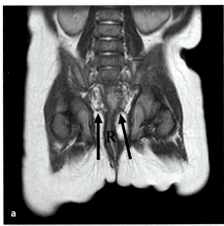

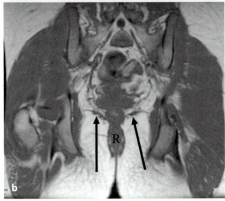

Fig. 54.10. a MRI of pelvis in a patient with high ARM in the coronal plane after LAARP. *Arrows* demonstrate the superolateral elements of the levator ani complex as well as the inferior extension of the funnel-shaped muscle to surround the pulled through bowel after LAARP. Note the relative hypoplasia of the superior aspect of the right side of the levator complex, a congenital finding in some patients with ARM. *R* Rectum. **b** MRI of pelvis in a normal child, coronal plane. *Arrows* depict the well-developed superolateral aspect of the levator ani complex. *R* Rectum

anorectal angle after LAARP. Also noted in this patient is the relative underdevelopment of the posterior aspect of the pubococcygeus muscle and paucity of external sphincter muscle more distally, as compared to a normal patient (■ Fig. 54.9b). In coronal section, MRI demonstrates the centrally placed pull-through bowel with no accompanying mesenteric fat. In this patient, there is hypoplasia of the right side of the levator ani complex, seen best at the tip of the arrow (■ Fig. 54.10a). In comparison, a normal patient has a well-developed and symmetric levator ani complex (■ Fig. 54.10b). The high ARM patient depicted in ■ Figs. 54.9a and 54.10a is now 4 years of age and is showing signs of normal bowel control. He is on no medications, can consciously recognize the urge to defecate, and the perineum is clean during the daytime without need for diapers.

Discussion

Laparoscopically assisted anorectoplasty is an anatomically sound procedure with distinct advantages. Advanced laparoscopic skills are necessary to accomplish LAARP and there is a learning curve associated with the procedure. LAARP is not necessary for patients with rectoperineal fistulae nor is it advocated for this type of low ARM. These malformations are repaired with single-staged procedures performed through the perineum. The current standard of care for repair of ARM is the PSARP and all new techniques must compare favorably to the results of this repair to justify their use.

As noted previously, the sphincteric muscles, sensory elements, and nerves responsible for fecal continence are often abnormal in patients with high ARM, and these factors, rather than the specific surgical technique used for reconstruction, are most likely the key predictors of functional outcome. In many types of malformations, traditional open repair, even when performed by experienced surgeons with excellent surgical technique, has not been highly successful in achieving fecal continence. The likelihood of being totally continent of feces with most of these malformations varies from 0% to 32%.

Laparoscopically assisted anorectoplasty accomplishes the same anatomic end result as traditional open surgery, while minimizing the risk of injury to surrounding anatomic structures, particularly the levator muscles and external anal sphincter. Nevertheless, since very few patients who have undergone this new technique have begun toilet training, and no systematic review of outcomes has been reported, we cannot yet make judgments about ultimate fecal continence. Early prognostic signs for later continence are, however, encouraging and we are hopeful that outcomes will be as good if not better than those achieved with traditional open surgery. A conclusive assessment of functional outcomes must await several more years of clinical follow-up.

References

deVries PA, Pena A (1982) Posterior sagittal anorectoplasty. J Pediatr Surg 17:638–643

Dick AC, Coulter P, Hainsworth AM, et al (1998) A comparative study of the analgesia requirements following laparoscopic and open fundoplication in children. J Laparoendosc Adv Surg Tech A 8:425–429

Georgeson KE, Inge TH, Albanese CT (2000) Laparoscopically assisted anorectal pull-through for high imperforate anus: a new technique. J Pediatr Surg 35:927–930; discussion 930–931

Iwanaka T, Arai M, Kawashima H, et al (2003) Findings of pelvic musculature and efficacy of laparoscopic muscle stimulator in laparoscopy-assisted anorectal pull-through for high imperforate anus. Surg Endosc 17:278–281

Kehlet H, Nielsen HJ (1998) Impact of laparoscopic surgery on stress responses, immunofunction, and risk of infectious complications. New Horiz 6(suppl 2):S80–S88

Lin CL, Wong KK, Lan LC et al. (2003) Earlier appearance and higher incidence of the rectoanal relaxation reflex in patients with imperforate anus repaired with laparoscopically assisted anorectoplasty. Surg Endosc 17:1646–1649

Pena A, Hong A (2000) Advances in the management of anorectal malformations. Am J Surg 180:370–376

Stephens FD (1953) Congenital imperforated rectum, recto-urethral and recto-vaginal fistulae. Aust N Z J Surg 22:161–172

Yamataka A, Segawa O, Yoshida R, et al (2001) Laparoscopic muscle electrostimulation during laparoscopy-assisted anorectal pull-through for high imperforate anus. J Pediatr Surg 36:1659–1661

Yamataka A, Yoshida R, Kobayashi H, et al (2002) Intraoperative endosonography enhances laparoscopy-assisted colon pull-through for high imperforate anus. J Pediatr Surg 37:16571660

Chapter 55

Laparoscopy in the Treatment of Female Infants with Anorectal Malformations

Maria Marcela Bailez

Introduction

In 2000 Georgeson et al. reported a laparoscopic-assisted anorectal pull-through technique for high imperforate anus. Since then isolated reports of female patients treated with this technique have been published (Ettayebi and Behamu 2001; Iwanaka et al. 2002).

In a 3-year period we used laparoscopy in the treatment of 10 girls, 10 months to 4 years of age, with anorectal anomalies. Nine had a cloacal anomaly and one a rectovaginal fistula with a high rectum. In this chapter we present our experience in an attempt to define the role of laparoscopy in the treatment of female infants with anorectal malformation (ARM).

Preoperative Preparation

Preoperatively the bowel is cleaned by means of irrigations with saline through the proximal and distal colostomy.

After induction of general anesthesia, a urinary catheter is inserted and prophylactic antibiotics are given. Future port hole sites are infiltrated with bupivacaine 0.5% up to a maximal total dose of 1.5 mg/kg.

Positioning

Patient

The patient is placed in a supine, Trendelenburg position (■ Fig. 55.1). Infants are placed obliquely or even

Fig. 55.1. Positioning of the patient, crew, and monitor. The patient is placed obliquely on the operating table. The abdomen, perineum, and lower extremities are disinfected and wrapped. The surgeon, assistant, and scrub nurse stand on the right side. The younger the patient, the more transverse their position on the table

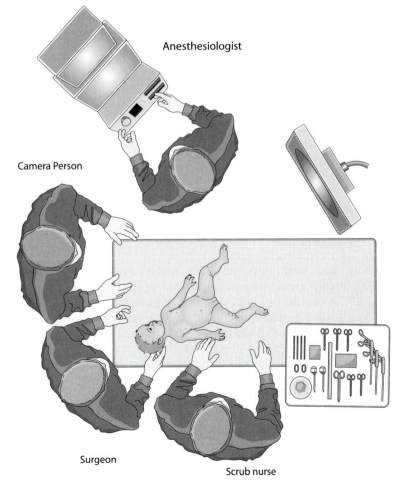

Anesthesiologist

Camera Person

Surgeon

Scrub nurse

transversely on the operating table, so that the surgeon and assistant can work from the head of the patient, either on the right or the left side of the table.

Crew, Monitors, and Equipment

Figure 55.1 shows the positions of the crew, monitors, and equipment.

Special Equipment

Ultrasonic scissors or Ligasure should be available. We prefer the latter because of its delicate tips. A transcutaneous muscle stimulator is at hand for developing the pull-through route through the pelvic floor.

Technique

Cannulae

Cannula	Method of insertion	Diameter (mm)	Device	Position
1	Closed	5[a]/4	Telescope	Right upper quadrant
2	Closed	5[a]	Working instruments	Right lower quadrant
3	Closed	3	Working instruments	Left paraumbilical region[b]

[a] With reducer cap to 4/3 mm for the 4 mm telescope and for passing sutures with a 3 mm needle holder through the right port.

[b] It is located medially or laterally to the sigmoidostomy if present.

Port Positions

We prefer to locate the port for the telescope in the right upper quadrant in infants and small children, which allows a more ergonomic dissection of the rectum and left colon. In older patients or in case a right transverse colostomy has been made, we use the umbilicus for the telescope position. The right-side operative port is located in the right lower quadrant or higher in infants. The left-side port is positioned higher than the right, next to the sigmoidostomy when present (■ Fig. 55.2).

Procedure

Group I (■ Table 55.1)

We started to use a laparoscopic approach in combination with total urogenital sinus mobilization (TUM) through a restricted posterior sagittal approach (PSARP) in two patients with cloacal malformation. Both girls had a rectum ending high between duplicated vaginas (■ Fig. 55.3 a,b). After a TUM (the urogenital sinus being either 4 or 9 cm long) through a posterior sagittal approach, the rectum was still high and its mobilization uncomfortable. So a sound was left behind in the presacral space in the path of the future descent of the rectum. The rectum was dissected out laparoscopically and the fistula transected between endosutures. The rectum was then tailored and ano-

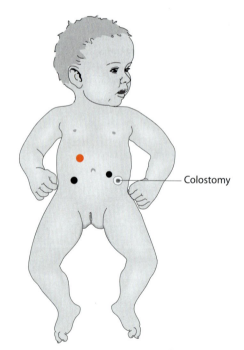

Fig. 55.2. Position of the ports

— Colostomy

rectoplasty was completed through the restricted posterior sagittal approach (RPSARP). The sequence of positions of the patients was: prone, supine, and prone again (■ Figs. 55.3 c-g).

Table 55.1 Group I patients: laparoscopic approach in combination with TUM through a restricted PSARP

	Patient 1	Patient 2
Type of ARM	Cloaca	Cloaca
Age	10 months	4 years
Length of urogenital sinus (cm)	4	9
Colostomy	Transverse	Transverse
Urinary management	Intermittent catheterization	Vesicostomy

Fig. 55.3 a – d. Group I patients.
a External appearance , **b** Preoperative contrast study showing the distal colon and duplicated vagina. R Rectum, Va vagina.
c Posterior sagittal opening of the cloacal channel. **d** A total urogenital mobilization maneuver (PSARP + TUM). Arrows indicate the mobilized urogenital sinus.

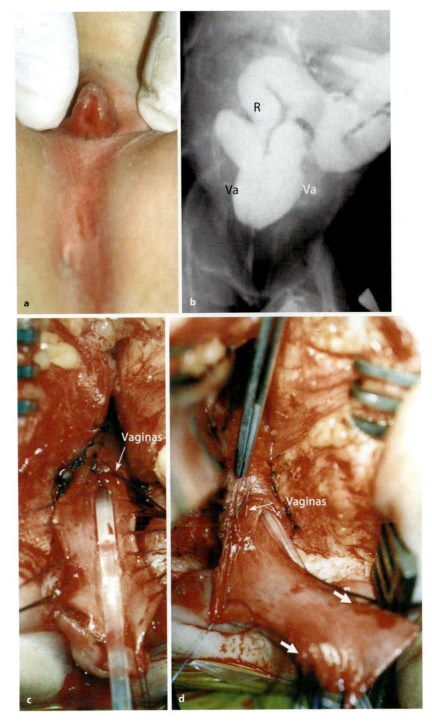

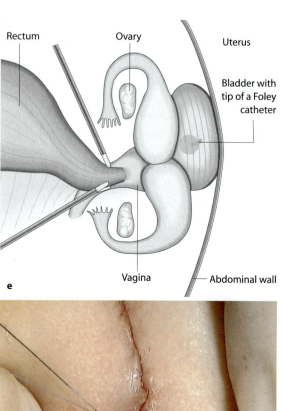
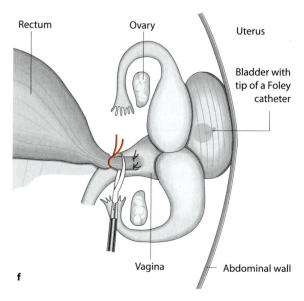

e

f

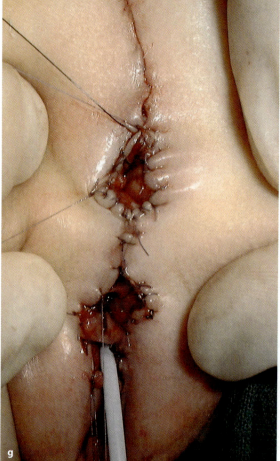

g

Fig. 55.3 e – g. e Laparoscopic identification of the rectovaginal fistula. **f**. Transection of the fistula is transected between a ligature on vaginal side and sutures on the other side. **g** Final aspect of the perineum in sagittal position

Group II (■ Table 55.2)

A laparoscopically assisted anorectal pull-through using a minimal perineal incision, as described by Georgeson et al. (2000), was used in two patients. One patient had a cloaca in combination with total vaginal agenesis (■ Fig. 55.4 a.b). Laparoscopy in this patient was very helpful. Not only did it confirm the utero-vaginal dysgenesis but it also showed that a very short distal rectosigmoid colon had been left (■ Fig. 55.4c). In this patient the following steps were taken. First the

Fig. 55.4 a – d. Patient with a cloaca (3cm channel), Müllerian remnants and vaginal agenesis. **a,b** External appearance, divided sigmoid colostomy. Short distal colon. **c** Schematic drawing of the situation before definitive surgery **d.** The distal sigmoid colostomy was taken down. The proximal 5 cm of the rectosigmoid were removed using a stapler. The proximal colostomy is also taken down and repositioned into the abdomen.

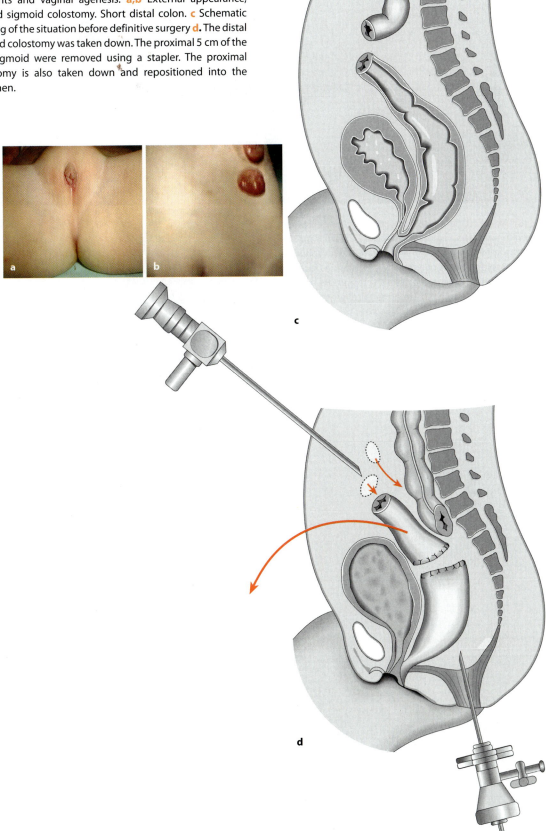

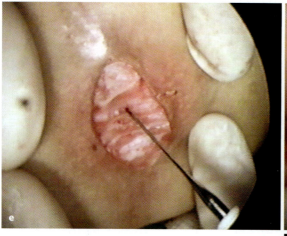

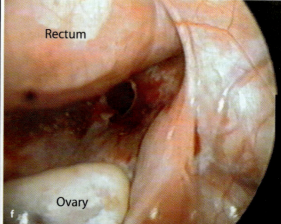

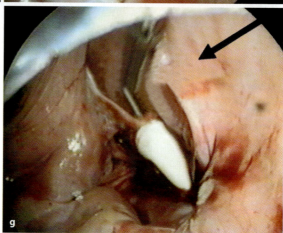

Fig. 55.4 e – h. Patient with a cloaca (3cm channel), Müllerian remnants and vaginal agenesis. **e** External incision over the sphincter and central puncture of the sphincter. **f,g** Laparoscopic views of a radially expandable trocar entering the pelvis behind the distal rectosigmoid which is left behind as a vagina. **h** Laparoscopically assisted pull through

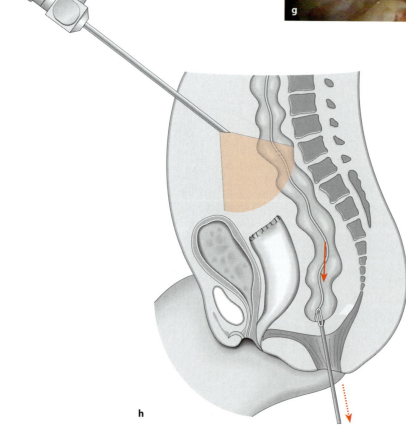

Table 55.2 Group II patients: laparoscopically assisted anorectal pull-through using a minimal perineal incision.

	Patient 1	Patient 2
Type of ARM	Müllerian remnants and absent vagina	Rectovaginal fistula
Age (years)	4	2
Length of cloacal channel (cm)	3	
Colostomy	Sigmoid colostomy	
	Short distal sigmoid colon	

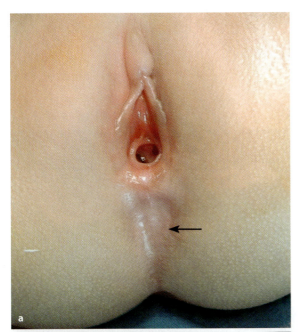
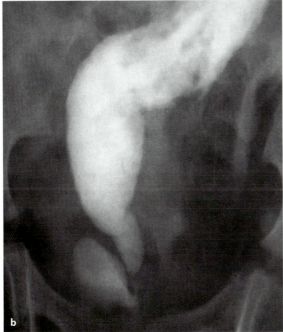

Fig. 55.5 . Patient with a rectovaginal fistula. **a** External appearance *Arrow* shows the imperforate anus. **b** Distal colonogram

distal rectosigmoid was left as a vagina. After the distal sigmoid colostomy was taken down, it was shortened by 5 cm using a stapler (■ Fig. 55.4d). Second the proximal sigmoid colostomy was taken down as well. After identification of the external sphincter area with the external muscle stimulator, a small incision was made in the midline using fine-needle monopolar electrocautery (■ Fig. 55.4e). A Veress needle with an expandable sheath was inserted through the pelvic floor under laparoscopic vision. External muscle stimulation helped in detecting the right channel for the pull-through from the inside. A 12 mm trocar was then inserted into the sheath in order to enlarge the pull-through tract (■ Fig. 55.4f-g). The proximal sigmoid colostomy was then pulled down with a 10 mm grasper and the anoplasty was completed with interrupted 5-0 absorbable sutures. Finally the cloacal channel was opened and mobilized to create a wide vaginal opening. The patient ended with neither a colostomy nor a posterior sagittal scar.

The other patient in group II had a rectovaginal fistula (■ Fig. 55.5). We used Ligasure for transection of the rectovaginal fistula but the vaginal side of the fistula was sutured closed. A probe was inserted in the vagina and was moved during the dissection to extend the posterior vaginal wall. The rectum descent was achieved using the same technique as described above.

Group III (■ Table 55.3)

Encouraged by this experience we decided to use an initial laparoscopic approach in the next six patients with cloacal anomaly. Two patients had unclear preoperative contrast studies. Laparoscopy showed a normal uterus in the midline in both patients. One had a very dilated rectosigmoid colon. A third patient had a very dilated left colon. Reconstruction was completed through a restricted sagittal approach as they were low–intermediate type. A very low dissection of the rectovaginal septum was comfortably achieved using a zoom lens and a fine needle in the patient with the non-dilated rectum which resulted in an even more restricted sagittal approach. Still laparoscopy was unnecessary in these three patients.

The next two patients appeared to be ideal candidates for a combination of laparoscopic treatment of

Table 55.3 Group III patients: initial laparoscopy to define unclear anatomy/approach.

	Patient 1	Patient 2	Patient 3	Patient 4	Patient 5	Patient 6
Type of ARM	Cloaca	Cloaca	Cloaca	Cloaca	Cloaca	Cloaca
Age	3 years	2 years	4 years	19 months	18 months	2 years
Length of urogenital sinus (cm)	1	4	5.5	3.5	3.5	7.5
Colostomy	Transverse	Sigmoid	Sigmoid	*Transverse*		Transverse
Urinary management	N	N	N			Vesicostomy
Surgery	Laparoscopy RSARP	Laparoscopy RSARP	Laparoscopy RSARP + laparotomy	Laparoscopy SARP		
Vesicostomy	Laparoscopic pull-through + TUM	Laparoscopy SARP Vesicostomy TD				

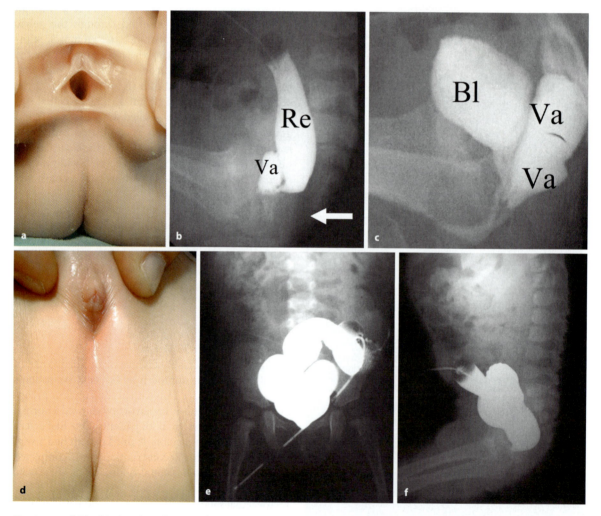

Fig. 55.6 a–f. The ideal patients for a combination of a laparoscopic pull-through together with TUM without a PSARP: a high rectum and an intermediate urogenital sinus. **a–c** Patient 4. **d–f** Patient 5. *Bl* Bladder, *RE* rectum, *Va* vagina.

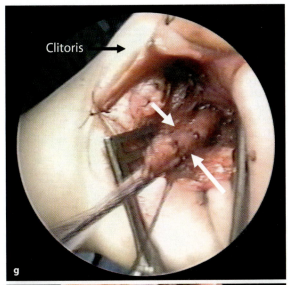

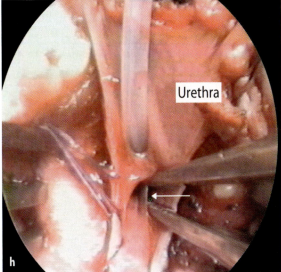

Fig. 55.6 g, h. The ideal patients for a combination of a laparoscopic pull-through together with TUM without a PSARP: a high rectum and an intermediate urogenital sinus. **g** TUM was achieved from the perineum with the patient in lithotomy position. **h** After the urethrovaginal septum reaches the perineum the vaginal septum was transected, creating a wide vaginal opening. *Arrows* show the septum

the rectum and TUM through the perineum in a lithotomy position. Both patients had a duplicated vagina and a 3.5 cm-long cloacal channel (■ Fig. 55.6 a-f ■ Table 55.3). We started with laparoscopic treatment of rectovaginal fistula as previously described. TUM was achieved from the perineum and after the urethrovaginal confluence reached the perineum the vaginal septum was transected, thus creating a wide vaginal opening (■ Fig. 55.6g-h). Disconnection of the rec-

tum from the vagina prior to dissection of the urogenital sinus made the latter easier, as there was no traction on the posterior vaginal wall.

The last patient had a 7 cm channel with two previously infected vaginas and a prolapsed vesicostomy. We started with a laparoscopic approach. The rectum was dissected and the fistula easily transected but even after a PSARP, TUM, and vesicostomy take down, the vaginas were very hard to dissect and five stones were found in their lumen. Laparoscopy only replaced laparotomy in this last case but still the sagittal approach was necessary for the very high, previously infected and fixed vaginas.

Postoperative Care

No nasogastric tube is used and feeding is started within 24 h. The urinary catheter is left in situ depending on the anomaly. Pain is controlled with a non-steroidal anti-inflammatory agent or Nubain.

Results

The age range at the time of surgery was 10 months to 4 years. Operative time ranged from 190 to 380 min. In the two ideal patients in group III operative time was 3.5 h for patient 4 and 4 h for patient 5. No adhesions or difficulties related to colostomies and vesicostomies were noted.

One patient in group I developed a postoperative rectovaginal fistula that was reoperated using a combined laparoscopic and perineal approach with no recurrence. The fistula was distal to the primary one.

Only two patients may be considered for continence at the time being: one in group I who has severe constipation and requires weekly enemas (9 cm urogenital channel) and one in group II who is completely continent (associated vaginal agenesis).

Discussion

The value of laparoscopy in treating anorectal malformations in female infants can be summarized as follows:

1. Laparoscopy replaced laparotomy in abdominal rectum treatment (group I) (classical role).
2. If the common channel was very long and the vaginal confluence high, a PSARP was required.
3. A combined endoscopic and laparoscopic assessment of the anomalies permitted a less invasive and time-consuming approach in atypical ARM (group II) (creative role).

4. Laparoscopic pull-through associated with perineal TUM is feasible in "intermediate cloacas," avoiding PSARP (group III, patient 6) (tendency role).
5. Patients with a very dilated rectum and low confluence cloacas were converted to open.

References

Ettayebi E, Behamou M (2001) Anorectal malformation: treatment by laparoscopy. Pediatr Endosurg Innov Tech 5:208–213

Georgeson KE, Inge TH, Albanese CT (2000) Laparoscopically assisted anorectal pull-through for high imperforate anus: a new technique. J Pediatr Surg 35:927–931

Iwanaka T, Arai M, Kawashima H, et al (2002) Laparoscopically assisted anorectal pull-through for rectocloacal fistula. Pediatr Endosurg Innov Tech 6:261–267

Abdomen

Liver and Biliary Tree

Chapter 56

Laparoscopic Treatment of Hydatid Disease of the Liver

Francisco J. Berchi

Introduction

Although liver tumors and cysts are in general uncommon conditions in children, in certain parts of the world, for example Spain, cystic lesions particularly those of hydatid disease are not infrequently encountered. Since April 2000 the frequency in Spain is reducing, as the Spanish Health Ministry introduced prophylactic measures both in humans and in animals against this disease.

Several procedures have been described for the treatment of hydatid liver cysts, from puncture of the cyst to liver resection or liver transplant. This chapter will deal with laparoscopic partial pericystectomy.

Preoperative Preparation

It is crucial to make an accurate diagnosis, to exclude the presence of hydatid disease elsewhere in the body, and to evaluate the patient's clinical status. It is also important to memorize the segmental anatomy of the liver.

All patients must have preoperative routine blood tests, liver function analysis, and a clotting screen. Serological tests, radioimmunology, interferon-a/b and conventional, serological study, indirect hemagglutinin, and enzyme-linked immunosorbent assay should also be carried out. Ultrasonography and computed axial tomography are the most accurate non-invasive diagnostic measures but magnetic resonance imaging (MRI) can be used as well. Informed consent is necessary and should include both the laparoscopic technique and conversion to an open procedure if and when appropriate. It is also important to inform the patient and family about the complications of surgery particularly those of perioperative intra-abdominal dissemination of hydatid fluid/scoleces and anaphylactic reaction.

Before Induction of General Anesthesia

The bowel is washed out with saline preoperatively.

After Induction of General Anesthesia

General anesthesia with full muscle relaxation is given. Future port site holes are injected with bupivacaine 0.25% with/or without adrenalin at a dose rate of 1–2 ml per port site. A nasogastric tube as well as a urinary catheter are inserted. Broad-spectrum antibiotics are administered prophylactically at the time of induction.

Positioning

Patient

The patient is positioned supine at the end of the operating table (■ Fig. 56.1). A cushion or rolled up towel under the lower thorax facilitates the laparoscopic access. The table is tilted in reversed Trendelenburg position. The patient is positioned in such a way that abdominal fluoroscopy can be used.

Crew, Monitors, and Equipment

The surgeon stands in between the legs of the patient with the assistants and scrub nurse on either side of the operating table (■ Fig. 56.1). A monitor is placed on both sides of the head of the patient. The operating table should allow for fluoroscopic imaging during the procedure when required.

Special Equipment

Ligasure and or ultrasonic energy is at hand, as is fluoroscopy. The following items should also be available: Tru-Cut or a conventional intravenous cannulae and needles (Advocat-20), a Veress needle, 10% and 20% saline solutions, a specimen retrieval bag, and a Jackson drain.

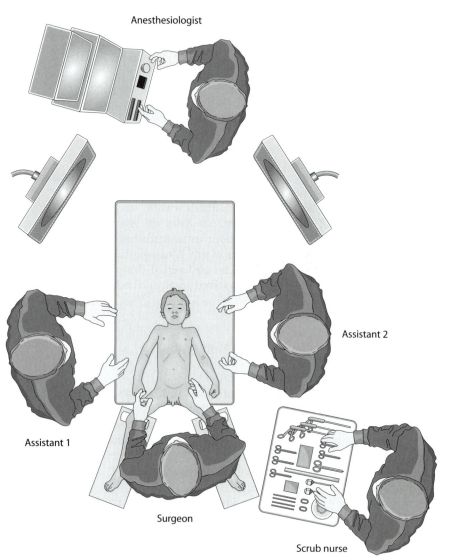

Fig. 56.1. Positioning of the patient, crew, and equipment

Anesthesiologist

Assistant 2

Assistant 1

Surgeon

Scrub nurse

Technique

Cannulae

Cannula	Method of insertion	Diameter (mm)	Device	Position
1	Open	5	5 mm 30° telescope	Umbilicus
2	Closed	3/5	Working instrument	Right upper quadrant
3	Closed	10	Working instrument, retrieval bag	Left upper quadrant

Figure 56.2 shows port positions.

Procedure

A 5 mm primary cannula is placed subumbilically using an open technique. CO_2 pneumoperitoneum is established. A second 3- or 5 mm cannula and a third 10 mm cannula are inserted in the right and left upper quadrant, respectively (■ Fig. 56.2). Occasionally a fourth cannula may be required. A 14-gauge conventional intravenous catheter or a Veress needle is introduced into the abdominal cavity for continuous irrigation of the surface of the liver and the cyst with 10% saline (■ Fig. 56.3).

After preliminary laparoscopic exploration, the liver is inspected and the cyst identified. A percutaneous transhepatic (never directly into the cyst) Tru-Cut-type needle or Advocat cannula is inserted into the cyst which is then connected to a two-way suction/irrigation device and two 20-ml syringes (■ Fig. 56.3). The cyst is aspirated with a 20-ml syringe. A sample of the aspirated contents is send for analysis (viability of the scoleces, protoscoleces, hooks, inflammatory cells, and detritus).

Twenty milliliters of hypertonic 10% or 20% saline is injected and left for 5–10 min. The contents are aspirated for a second time and a sample sent again for analysis (the viability of scoleces is checked). The procedure of injection and aspiration is repeated five times. Once the cavity is completely cleared, an incision is made directly over the cyst with diathermy and scissors or Ligasure or ultrasonic scalpel. The germinal layer of the cyst is then removed taking care to keep the germinal layer intact. A retrieval bag is used for extraction of the specimen through a cannula or via a port site (■ Fig. 56.4).

Meticulous hemostasis is essential. Bile leaks are closed by suturing with or without the use of fibrin glue. If desired an omental patch may be used to obliterate the remaining leaks. The abdominal cavity is irrigated with normal saline and every effort is made to aspirate all irrigation fluid. This maneuver is facilitated by tilting the operating table in all four directions (Trendelenburg, reversed Trendelenburg, tilt to the right, and to the left). Finally a Jackson drain is placed into the cavity through the right upper quadrant port site (■ Fig. 56.5). The pneumoperitoneum is evacuated and the fascial/muscle defects are closed with sutures.

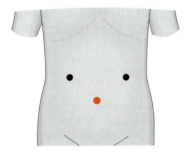

Fig. 56.2. Port site positioning

Fig. 56.3. Cyst aspiration, injection, and pericyst irrigation

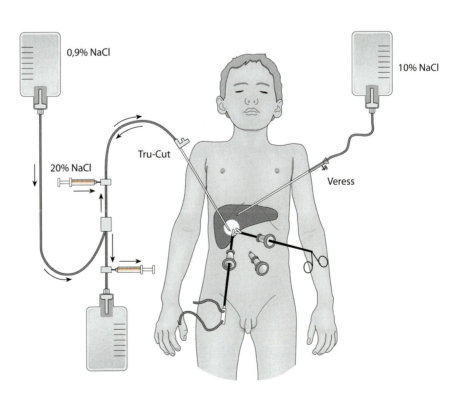

0,9% NaCl

10% NaCl

20% NaCl

Tru-Cut

Veress

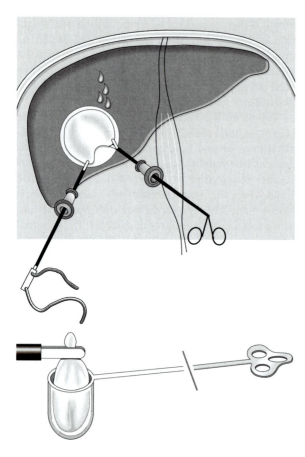

Fig. 56.4. Laparoscopic opening of the cyst with removal of the endocyst

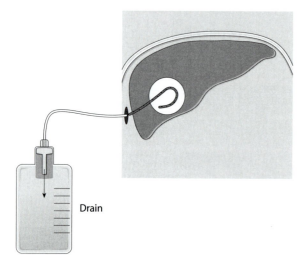

Drain

Fig. 56.5. Drainage of the remaining cavity

Postoperative Care

Preoperative and postoperative antiparasitic medication consists of albendazole for 30 days, which is repeated at 15- to 30-day intervals for 12–14 months. The drain is removed at 24–48 h and the patient is sent home within a few days. An ultrasound scan of the liver and liver function, serological, and hydatid marker tests are repeated at 6-monthly intervals.

Results

Eight children with hydatid liver cyst have been treated laparoscopically. The operation was converted to open in one child because of two separate cysts, one in segment two which was easily approached laparoscopically, but the other in segment seven posteriorly which could not be visualized laparoscopically. One patient developed a biliary leak which resolved after 18 days of drainage. There were no other complications.

Discussion

Spain has been an endemic zone of hydatid disease until few years ago. Since 1999 the incidence has decreased dramatically due to sanitary measures and other prophylactic measures in this field, which have been employed in the whole country but especially in the most endemic zone. This region called "on the flock of sheep" extends from the wide Aragon zone, through a narrow zone from Castilla La Mancha, and ends broadly in the region of Extremadura. The incidence of hydatid disease in this area in the last 5 years has been very low with just 35 new cases reported in the hospitals in Zaragoza, La Paz and 12 de Octubre both in Madrid, Badajoz, and Caceres. In the past hundreds of cases were seen in these places.

The medical treatment of hydatid disease in children has been basically albendazole, at a dose rate of 15 mg/kg per day for 28 days with a pause of 14 days. This is repeated three or more times, while controlling hepatic function closely. Albendazole seems to be superior to mebendazole (Todorov et al. 1992). Medical therapy alone, however, is relatively ineffective for hepatic cysts (Dziri et al. 2004). Preintervention and postintervention chemotherapy with albendazole offers, however, the advantage of reducing the risk of disease recurrence and intraperitoneal seeding that may develop via cyst rupture and spillage occurring spontaneously or during surgery or needle drainage (Smego and Sebanego 2005).

Surgery, in combination with albendazole, has been the mainstay of treatment of hepatic hydatid disease for many years and still is today, certainly for complicated cysts. The laparoscopic pericystectomy has proven to be safe and effective (Bickel et al. 2001; Dziri et al. 2004). We regard accessible univesicular cysts as ideal lesions for this technique. However, multivesicular cysts which are usually small, calcified, and located near the liver surface can be treated by complete laparoscopic resection using electrocautery, ultrasonic scalpel, laser, or Ligasure. As in conventional open surgery the complications of this approach include: difficult access to cysts located posteriorly or deep in the liver; bleeding from the liver either from the site of transected liver or from the wall after removal of the cyst; injury to the intrahepatic or extrahepatic bile ducts; sepsis particularly in infected cysts; and anaphylactic reaction or dissemination of disease from spillage of contents of the cyst. Unlike adult patients, children very rarely develop intraductal hydatid vesicles. When cholestasis or cholangitis are suspected ultrasound and or cholangiography will confirm the diagnosis. If disease is demonstrated, a laparoscopic choledochotomy with or without cholecystectomy and removal of the cyst may be carried out provided the surgeon has sufficient expertise. Alternatively, a preoperative or postoperative endoscopic retrograde cholangiopancreatography (ERCP) with sphincterotomy to drain the common bile duct may be performed (Dumas et al. 1999).

Puncture, aspiration, irrigation, and reaspiration of hydatid cysts, known as PAIR, was popularized by Brett et al. in 1988. Evidence is accumulating that this method of treatment is a good method in uncomplicated cysts (Dziri et al. 2004; Filice and Brunetti 1997; Goktay et al. 2005; Pelaez et al. 2000). It is certainly superior to a laparoscopic approach in cysts that are deeply located in the liver and cysts that lie posteriorly. It has been suggested that surgery should be reserved for patients with hydatid cysts refractory to PAIR or for those with difficult-to-manage cyst-biliary communication or obstruction (Smego and Sebanego 2005). Surgery and especially laparoscopic surgery in conjunction with preoperative and postoperative albendazole is certainly another option.

References

Bickel A, Loberant N, Singer-Jordan J, et al (2001) The laparoscopic approach to abdominal hydatid cysts: a prospective nonselective study using the isolated hypobaric technique. Arch Surg 136:789–795

Brett PM, Fond A, Bretagnolle M, et al (1988) Percutaneous aspiration and drainage of hydatid cysts in the liver. Radiology 168:617–620

Dumas R, Le Gall P, Hastier P, et al (1999) The role of endoscopic retrograde cholangiopancreatography in the management of hepatic hydatid disease. Endoscopy 31:242–247

Dziri C, Haouet K, Fingerhut A (2004) Treatment of hydatid cyst of the liver: where is the evidence? World J Surg 28:731–736

Filice C, Brunetti E (1997) Use of PAIR in human cystic echinococcosis. Acta Trop 64:95–107

Goktay AY, Secil M, Gulcu A, et al (2005) Percutaneous treatment of hydatid liver cysts in children as a primary treatment: long-term results. J Vasc Interv Radiol 16:831–839

Pelaez V, Kugler C, Correa D, et al (2000) PAIR as percutaneous treatment of hydatid liver cysts. Acta Trop 75:197–202

Smego RA Jr, Sebanego P (2005) Treatment options for hepatic cystic echinococcosis. Int J Infect Dis 9:69–76

Todorov T, Vutova K, Mechkov G, et al (1992) Chemotherapy of human cystic echinococcosis: comparative efficacy of mebendazole and albendazole. Ann Trop Med Parasitol 86:59–66

Chapter 57

Laparoscopic Liver Surgery

Guillaume Podevin, Marc David Leclair, Christine Grapin, Frederic Hameury, Jacques Paineau, Yves Heloury

Introduction

Unlike other areas in pediatric surgery, minimally invasive liver resection has not gained wide popularity. The reasons for this are presumably the fear for intraoperative complications such as bleeding or gas embolism. However, improvements in laparoscopic technology and increased experience in adult surgery since the first description in 1992 (Gagner et al. 1992) now authorize laparoscopic liver resections in selected pediatric patients. As in adult surgery, the first reports regarding laparoscopic liver surgery in children concerned biopsy taking (Saenz et al. 1997) and hydatid cyst management (Khoury et al. 2000). In this chapter, we report additional experience with wedge resections and with left lateral lobectomy (bisegmentectomy 2 and 3).

Indications

Despite the fact that few reports are available about laparoscopic liver surgery in children, we can postulate that many pediatric surgeons with good laparoscopic experience have already performed liver biopsies and partial resection of superficial cystic lesions. Hydatid cyst management is not discussed here. The availability of the harmonic scalpel and of tissue adhesives have greatly improved the safety of laparoscopic biopsy taking (Esposito et al. 2004). A recent case report described successful laparoscopic biopsy taking in a child with hepatic dysfunction and coagulopathy (Kimura et al. 2003). Moreover, laparoscopy allows for guided biopsy taking and is therefore more suitable when a blind percutaneous technique is not indicated or has failed.

Solid liver tumor resection by laparoscopy has not yet been assessed in pediatric surgery. To date, we have to limit the laparoscopic approach to benign lesions. Objectives should obviously be: (1) the absence of operative mortality, (2) a complication rate as well as a late outcome equal to or better than for the open approach, and (3) the absence of need for heterologous blood transfusion. Surgical experience in adults is a good help in paving the way for use in children (Berends et al. 2001; Biertho et al. 2002; Cherqui et al.

2000; Descottes et al. 2003; Gigot 2002; Kaneko et al. 1996; Lesurtel et al. 2003; Samama et al. 1998). The first key is to propose the laparoscopic approach to children and their parents from a selected group of patients with small, superficial, and peripheral lesions located in the anterior segments of the right part of the liver (anterior part of segment 4 and segments 5 and 6) or in the left lateral segments (2 and 3). Large tumors, centrally or posteriorly located tumors, and tumors close to the hepatic veins require mobilization of the liver, peroperative control of major hepatic vessels, and total vascular isolation techniques which are difficult to achieve by laparoscopy with the present state-of-the-art tools and skills. Major resections remain a tremendous and risky challenge and require scientifically relevant results from expert adult centers before starting in children (Descottes et al. 2003).

Preoperative Preparation

Radiological evaluation includes abdominal ultrasonography and/or computed tomography (CT) or both. This preoperative assessment allows for planning of the procedure according to the size and the position of the lesion. All procedures are performed after obtaining informed consent from the parents.

General anesthesia with tracheal intubation is administered with constant CO_2 level and heart rate monitoring, and nasogastric intubation. For parenchymal section, a urinary catheter and invasive blood pressure monitoring are needed. A single dose of antibiotics is given intravenously before port placement.

Positioning

The patient is placed in the supine position with the legs abducted on leg supports. The table is tilted in reverse Trendelenburg. The abdomen is draped from the sternum to the pubis and laterally to the anterior axillary lines, allowing for a good view of the whole abdomen. The surgeon stands between the patient's legs, with the camera operator on the right side and the assistant on the left side of the child (■ Fig. 57.1).

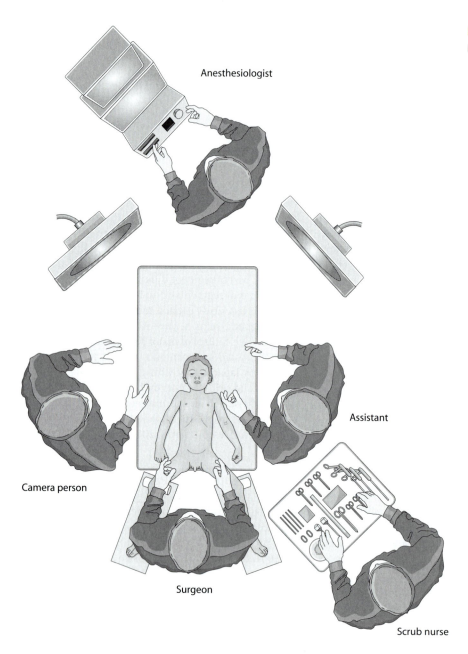

Fig. 57.1. Position of the patient, crew, and monitors

Anesthesiologist

Assistant

Camera person

Surgeon

Scrub nurse

Technique

Cannulae

Open laparoscopy is performed through a 1 cm skin incision on the left of the umbilicus. The optic port is gently inserted and a pneumoperitoneum is established with pressure monitored and maintained at less than 10 mmHg. Liver biopsy taking requires three trocars and the use of the harmonic scalpel. For large cystic lesions, wedge resections, or left lateral lobectomy (bisegmentectomy 2 and 3), a five-port technique is used (■ Fig. 57.2). Four ports, including the umbilical optic port, are inserted in a semicircular pattern from the right lower to the left upper abdominal quadrants. We use 5 mm ports, except for the working port on the left side from the umbilicus (for the surgeon's right hand), which is a 12 mm port. The particular location of the lesion may call for an adjusted approach. Tumors located in segments 6 and 7 may be approached with two trocars on the right side and one on the left side, and conversely, left lesions required two left and one right ports. The port placement is also according to patient age. The younger the child the more the ports are moved aside, in order to maintain a good working space. For example, the trocar of the right lower abdominal quadrant can be inserted through the right inguinal crease region in infants. The fifth port is inserted in a subxiphoidal position. It is advisable to use an angled scope for lesions located in the dorsal segments.

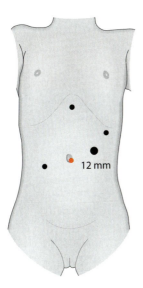

Fig. 57.2. Position of trocars for a five-port technique. Five-millimeter instruments are used, except for the 12 mm left working port

Procedure

The harmonic scalpel is useful for wedge resections. Hepatic transection is performed with a 5 mm harmonic scalpel or a 10 mm endoscopic ultrasonic dissector, which divides the tissue ultrasonically and coagulates vascular and biliary structures with a diameter of less than 2 mm. Larger-caliber structures are secured with clips, Ligasure, or a linear vascular endostapler, depending on the vessel size. A 10 mm diameter dissector can be useful for vessel dissection. In large resections, some surgeons want to be able to perform the Pringle maneuver by occluding the porta hepatis with a piece of tape introduced through a segment of Silastic tube inserted into the rightmost 10 mm port (Cherqui et al. 2000).

Surgical methods are basic for biopsies and wedge resections, consisting of parenchymal section by the harmonic scalpel, skirting around the tumor. Cystic lesions can be unroofed, with coagulation of the remaining mucosa. When the tumor is large, central, and located into the left hepatic lobe, a left lateral lobectomy (bisegmentectomy 2 and 3 according to Couinaud's classification) is performed. The first step of the procedure is the achievement of control of the left lobe vessels, underneath the implantation of the round ligament. After parenchymal dissection over a short distance, the left portal vein, the left hepatic artery, and the left biliary duct are clipped with absorbable clips or are coagulated with the Ligasure before division. A possible presence of the left hepatic artery into the lesser omentum has to be checked. The parenchymal section is then conducted. First, the planned resection is marked on the liver surface with diathermy, and follows a line on the left side of the falciform ligament from the left hepatic vein to the left porta hepatis. The actual parenchymal dissection can be carried out by meticulous step-by-step crushing of the tissue with an endoscopic clamp followed by split division of the tissue. However, this Kelly-clasty method is now usually replaced by ultrasonic dissection. The peripheral parenchyma can be easily transected with the harmonic scalpel. At the end of parenchymal section, the left hepatic vein is divided by application of a linear vascular endostapler. The left triangular ligament and the lesser omentum are divided only at the end of the procedure, just before removing the specimen from the surgical area, in order to keep the left lobe well fixed to the surroundings during parenchymal section. The specimen is extracted using a plastic retrieval bag through an enlarged trocar incision, or through a suprapubic horizontal incision for larger ones. The remaining raw surface of the liver is checked for bleeding or bile leak after rinsing, and is sealed with fibrin glue. We do not leave a drain. In the event of conversion to laparotomy, an upper transverse abdominal incision is used.

Results

From November 1995 to May 2002, seven laparoscopic liver resections were performed; ages ranged from 2 months to 7.1 years. Patient data are summarized in ■ Table 57.1.

Three young children had large cystic lesions (■ Table 57.1). A 3-month-old girl (patient 2) had an antenatal diagnosis of huge cystic lesion, which on postnatal ultrasound appeared to be connected to the anterior edge of liver segments 5 and 6. Over the next 3 months after birth the cystic lesion size decreased on ultrasound, but remained large. It was removed laparoscopically with a wedge resection which resulted in an uneventful follow-up. The other two children (patients 1 and 6), each with a large anterior hepatic cyst, had partial pericystectomy and coagulation of the remaining cyst wall with no recurrence.

Four patients had a focal nodular hyperplasia (■ Table 57.1). Diagnosis was suspected on a CT scan, which showed homogeneous lesions with peripheral enhancement following intravenous contrast associated with central scar and central artery for the two larger tumors (■ Fig. 57.3). Wedge resections were performed when technically feasible, but patient 4 underwent a left lateral lobectomy (■ Fig. 57.4) because the large tumor invaded the parenchyma close to segment 4. Operative time for these four cases was 185±22 min.

Intraoperative bleeding was minor except in patients 4 and 7, with a hemoglobin loss of 4 g/dL in these two procedures. The blood loss in these patients

Table 57.1 Patient data, final diagnosis, and surgical procedure

Patient	Date	Age (years)	Sex	Diagnosis	Size (mm)	Segments[a]	Procedure	Operative time (min)	Hospital stay (days)
1	Nov 95	0.2	M	Cystic hamartoma	46×43×35	5	Unroofing	40	4
2	Aug 99	0.3	F	Hemolymph-angioma	63×38×12	5-6	Wedge	50	2
3	Oct 99	2.5	M	Focal nodular hyperplasia	30×27×25	6	Wedge	150	5
4	Dec 01	7.1	M	Focal nodular hyperplasia	85×66×38	2-3	Left lateral lobectomy[b]	200	4
5	Feb 02	3.8	F	Focal nodular hyperplasia	43×37×25	4	Wedge	190	6
6	Mar 02	1.7	M	Cystic hamartoma	56×39×27	2	Unroofing	45	4
7	May 02	6.3	F	Focal nodular hyperplasia	54×50×32	3	Wedge	180	5

[a] Liver segments involved, according to Couinaud's classification
[b] Left lateral lobectomy is the bisegmentectomy 2 and 3

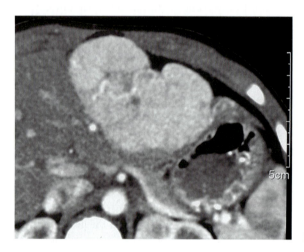

Fig. 57.3. A CT scan from a patient who had a large focal nodular hyperplasia of segments 2 and 3 (enhancement by intravenous contrast)

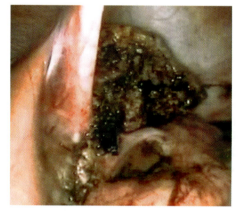

Fig. 57.4. View of the parenchymal section after a left lateral lobectomy (bisegmentectomy 2 and 3)

is explained by the necessary transection of liver parenchyma required for the resection of the large and well-vascularized tumors. No blood transfusion was required. Monitoring during the procedure did not detect any sign of gas embolism. There was no conversion to laparotomy, except for tumor extraction through a suprapubic horizontal incision in patients 4 and 7.

Postoperative Care

The postoperative anemia in the two patients who had significant peroperative blood loss was treated with oral iron and folic acid administration. There were no postoperative complications, such as bleeding, bile leak, or infection.

Oral intake was begun on the first postoperative day and patients were discharged when they no longer needed narcotics. At the first postoperative month, all the children had normal activity.

Discussion

Our preliminary experience of four peripheral solid tumor liver resections in children is encouraging as no specific difficulties during the procedure arose. The smaller working space in the case of young children did not particularly disturb the procedures. The blood loss during the resection of the two large tumors, which had a diameter greater than 5 cm, was significant but did not require blood transfusion. The laparoscopic approach could result in a more important blood loss than with the open approach, not so much because of a change in the parenchymal transection technique, which is the same in both approaches, but rather because of the increased operative time. This matter is still being debated in adult surgery, with controversial results in recent controlled studies (Lesurtel et al. 2003; Rau et al. 1998). In any case, for large resections, autologous blood transfusion should be planned.

The risk of carbon dioxide gas embolism during laparoscopic liver resection legitimately worries the surgeon. This complication has been demonstrated in animal experiments (Takagi et al. 1998) and has been reported in two procedures in adults (Croce et al. 1994; Hashizume et al. 1995). But these complications were only seen during large resections using a high-pressure pneumoperitoneum or using an argon beam coagulator. To date, pediatric practice concerns limited resections with low-pressure pneumoperitoneum. Therefore, as for surgeons working on adults (Berends et al. 2001), the role of gas embolism remains questionable in this setting.

Concerning operative indications of the tumor removal, there are more substantial differences between adult and pediatric surgery. Benign lesions are resected in adult surgery when tumors are symptomatic or of an undetermined nature (Biertho et al. 2002; Descottes et al. 2003). In our series, that only concerned the patient (patient 1) with a wrong diagnosis of cystic duodenal duplication before surgery. The other six patients had a well-assessed diagnosis by radiological evaluation and had no symptoms.

But we considered two other factors. The first one is the potential growth of focal nodular hyperplasia in a young child. Data in the literature seem to show that both resection or conservative treatment are acceptable (Reymond et al. 1995), but personal observations argue for surgical resection. Patient 7 had a 3-year follow-up before surgery, and the size of the lesion had doubled in the meantime. In another personal observation, the tumor initially in segment 4 without contact with the main vessels, led finally to a major and difficult resection through laparotomy because of its growth during the "wait and see" follow-up.

The second factor is the potential blunt liver trauma and its interaction with a large cystic or solid tumor. We know that the internal organs of a child are more susceptible to injury because of the limited amount of protective muscle and the increased flexibility and resilience of the pediatric skeleton (Inaba and Seward 1991; Takishima et al. 1996). Moreover, the most frequently injured organs in children with blunt abdominal trauma are the spleen and the liver (Gaines and Ford 2002). We therefore expected that our patients with palpable cystic or solid tumors who experienced a concurrent abdominal trauma could have a more serious liver injury. These two factors, potential growth of the tumor and possible abdominal trauma, led us to perform liver tumor resection.

We chose the laparoscopic approach in order to benefit from the expected advantages of minimally invasive surgery. Surgeons often advocate rapid recovery, lower postoperative pain, and acceptable abdominal scars. Another argument should be a diminished stress response and a greater preservation of the immune response, as demonstrated recently for laparoscopic liver resection (Burpee et al. 2002).

In conclusion, laparoscopic tumor resection of the liver requires surgeons experienced in liver surgery and in the laparoscopic approach. The recent contribution of new technologies, such as the harmonic scalpel, Ligasure, endoscopic ultrasonic dissector, and vascular endostapler, are useful and allow safe procedures without bile leak and major blood loss. Anterior and left lateral resections (segments 2–6), including left lateral lobectomy, are our present selected indications for laparoscopic pediatric liver surgery, but we can expect that virtual-reality imaging of liver disease, computer-guided surgery, and robotics are promising for future extended liver surgery.

References

Berends FJ, Meijer S, Prevoo W et al. (2001) Technical considerations in laparoscopic liver surgery. Surg Endosc 15:794–798

Biertho L, Waage A, Gagner M (2002) [Laparoscopic hepatectomy]. Ann Chir 127:164–170

Burpee SE, Kurian M, Murakame Y et al. (2002) The metabolic and immune response to laparoscopic versus open liver resection. Surg Endosc 16:899–904

Cherqui D, Husson E, Hammoud R et al. (2000) Laparoscopic liver resections: a feasibility study in 30 patients. Ann Surg 232:753–762

Croce E, Azzola M, Russo R et al. (1994) Laparoscopic liver tumour resection with the argon beam. Endosc Surg Allied Technol 2:186–188

Descottes B, Glineur D, Lachachi F et al. (2003) Laparoscopic liver resection of benign liver tumors. Surg Endosc 17:23–30

Esposito C, Damiano R, Settimi A et al. (2004) Experience with the use of tissue adhesives in pediatric endoscopic surgery. Surg Endosc 18:290–292

Gagner M, Rheault M, Dubuc J (1992) Laparoscopic partial hepatectomy for liver tumor (abstract). Surg Endosc 6:99

Gaines BA, Ford HR (2002) Abdominal and pelvic trauma in children. Crit Care Med 30(suppl 11):S416–S423

Gigot JF, Glineur D, Santiago Azagra J et al. (2002) Laparoscopic liver resection for malignant liver tumors: preliminary results of a multicenter European study. Ann Surg 236:90–97

Hashizume M, Takenaka K, Yanaga K et al. (1995) Laparoscopic hepatic resection for hepatocellular carcinoma. Surg Endosc 9:1289–1291

Inaba AS, Seward PN (1991) An approach to pediatric trauma. Unique anatomic and pathophysiologic aspects of the pediatric patient. Emerg Med Clin North Am 9:523–548

Kaneko H, Takagi S, Shiba T (1996) Laparoscopic partial hepatectomy and left lateral segmentectomy: technique and results of a clinical series. Surgery 120:468–475

Khoury G, Abiad F, Geagea T et al. (2000) Laparoscopic treatment of hydatid cysts of the liver and spleen. Surg Endosc 14:243–245

Kimura T, Nakajima K, Wasa M et al. (2003) Laparoscopic liver biopsy performed safely in a child with hepatic dysfunction: report of a case. Surg Today 33:712–713

Lesurtel M, Cherqui D, Laurent A et al. (2003) Laparoscopic versus open left lateral hepatic lobectomy: a case-control study. J Am Coll Surg 196:236–242

Rau HG, Buttler E, Meyer G et al. (1998) Laparoscopic liver resection compared with conventional partial hepatectomy: a prospective analysis. Hepatogastroenterology 45:2333–2338

Reymond D, Plaschkes J, Luthy AR et al. (1995) Focal nodular hyperplasia of the liver in children: review of follow-up and outcome. J Pediatr Surg 30:1590–1593

Saenz NC, Conlon KC, Aronson DC et al. (1997) The application of minimal access procedures in infants, children, and young adults with pediatric malignancies. J Laparoendosc Adv Surg Tech A 7:289–294

Samama G, Chiche L, Brefort JL et al. (1998) Laparoscopic anatomical hepatic resection. Report of four left lobectomies for solid tumors. Surg Endosc 12:76–78

Takagi S (1998) Hepatic and portal vein blood flow during carbon dioxide pneumoperitoneum for laparoscopic hepatectomy. Surg Endosc 12:427–431

Takishima T, Sugimoto K, Asari Y et al. (1996) Characteristics of pancreatic injury in children: a comparison with such injury in adults. J Pediatr Surg 31:896–900

Chapter 58

Laparoscopic Kasai Portoenterostomy for Biliary Atresia

C.K. Yeung and K.H. Lee

Introduction

Despite significant improvements in overall survival for infants suffering from biliary atresia over the past few decades, surgical management of this condition has remained a great challenge for paediatric surgeons. Hitherto Kasai's portoenterostomy procedure performed early in life before 8–10 weeks of age gives the best results for biliary drainage, and is widely accepted as the gold standard operation for biliary atresia. The procedure however entails a large muscle-cutting laparotomy and is associated with significant surgical trauma and postoperative pain as well as other morbidities including respiratory compromise, prolonged ileus and wound complications. Dense intra-abdominal adhesions also often ensue, imposing great difficulties and increased surgical risks should a liver transplantation later become necessary because of progressive biliary cirrhosis and end-stage hepatic failure. Substantial time has to be spent to reopening the abdomen and separating the liver and hilar structures from the surrounding adhesions during the recipient hepatectomy. This is associated with a significant increase in blood loss and risks for bowel perforation and other visceral damage. It can be envisaged that all the aforementioned morbidities could potentially be minimised with minimal access surgery. With the rapid advent of laparoscopic surgery since the early 1990s, many complex and sophisticated reconstructive procedures such as the repair of oesophageal atresia and dismembered pyeloplasty have been successfully performed in newborns and young infants using the minimally invasive surgical techniques. We describe the technique of laparoscopic Kasai portoenterostomy for infants with biliary atresia. Besides all the usual benefits of a minimal access approach, the well-illuminated and magnified laparoscopic view allows superb visibility for meticulous dissection of the hilar structures and the hepaticojejunostomy anastomosis. In addition, laparoscopic inspection with intraoperative cholangiogram also provides an accurate and reliable modality for assessment of infants with prolonged obstructive jaundice.

Preoperative Preparation

Infants with biliary atresia are jaundiced and the clotting profile may be deranged. Patients are given daily vitamin K injections preoperatively. Blood counts and clotting profiles are checked and any coagulopathy corrected. Blood is cross-matched and other blood products are reserved as required. Patients are kept fasted for 4–6 h before anaesthesia.

Before Induction of General Anaesthesia

A saline enema is given on the evening before surgery to ensure cleansing of the large bowel.

After Induction of General Anaesthesia

A nasogastric tube is inserted for bowel decompression during surgery and in the early postoperative period. A Foley catheter is inserted to monitor the urine output. Prophylactic antibiotics including ampicillin, cefuroxime and metronidazole are given on induction of anaesthesia. Further doses may be needed if the operation is prolonged.

Positioning

Patient

The patient is placed at the end of the table in a supine position with a small lumbar support, more on the right side (■ Fig. 58.1).

Crew, Monitors and Equipment

The surgeon stands at the end of the table opposite the patient's feet, with one assistant holding the camera on his/her left side, and the second assistant and the scrub nurse on his/her right (■ Fig. 58.1). The television monitor is positioned at the left upper corner. During the operation, the table may be tilted to a slightly head-up position to facilitate the dissection.

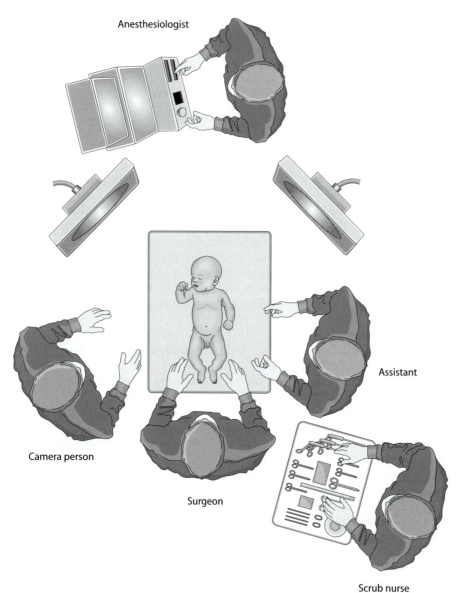

Fig. 58.1. Position of the patient, crew and equipment. A small lumbar support is placed underneath the patient (not shown)

Special Equipment

An AESOP robotic arm holds the laparoscope. The liver is retracted with a Nathanson retractor. As energy applying systems, use is made of the monopolar cautery hook. Ultrasonic energy is available as well.

Technique

Cannulae

Cannula	Method of insertion	Diameter (mm)	Device	Position
1	Closed	5, Step	Laparoscope initially, working instruments later	Supraumbilical
2	Closed	5, Step	Laparoscope later on	Right upper quadrant, midaxillary line
3	Closed	5, Step	Working instruments	Right upper quadrant, anterior axillary line
4	Closed	5, Step	Assistant's grasper, suction	Left upper quadrant
5	Closed	No cannula	Optional, Nathanson	Epigastrium

Procedure

A four-port technique is used (■ Fig. 58.2a). A 5 mm 30 laparoscope is first inserted through a 5 mm port via a supraumbilical incision. Carbon dioxide pneumoperitoneum is established at 10–12m mHg. Three more 3- to 5 mm working ports are then inserted at the right upper and left upper quadrants. Thorough laparoscopic examination and if necessary an operative cholangiogram are performed first to confirm the diagnosis of biliary atresia. Often a small, fibrotic gallbladder associated with a cirrhotic liver and an atretic extrahepatic bile duct surrounded by dilated vessels are observed to allow a definitive diagnosis without the need for an operative cholangiogram. In case of uncertainty, an operative cholangiogram is done under laparoscopic assistance to ascertain the diagnosis before proceeding to the Kasai procedure. If the liver is already cirrhotic, the liver can be sufficiently lifted upward to expose the hilar structures by passing a 0-prolene suture percutaneously round the falciform ligament just beneath the liver edge, and tying this over the abdominal wall. For infants with a less cirrhotic and hence softer and floppy liver, a Nathanson liver retractor is inserted at the epigastric region for upward retraction and stabilisation of the liver (■ Fig. 58.2b). For better and more direct visualisation of the hilar structures, the camera is now shifted to the right upper quadrant port that is sited at around the midclavicular line just beneath the lower edge of the liver.

The atretic gallbladder and the extrahepatic bile duct are now mobilised using a fine monopolar electrocautery hook needle. The gallbladder is first removed from the gallbladder fossa and the fibrous cord remnant of the extrahepatic bile duct dissected free from the portal vein and the hepatic artery (■ Figs. 58.3, 58.4). Downward retraction of the first part of duodenum by the assistant allows clear dissection of the distal end of the fibrous cord, which is transected behind the duodenum (■ Fig. 58.5). Dissection is now carried upwards towards the hepatic hilum. Tiny arterial branches and venous tributaries to the portal vein can be divided by simple electrocautery. Larger arterial branches and venous tributaries may need ligation using intracorporeal ties before division. Good countertraction and frequent suction is provided by the assistant from the left upper quadrant port. Once the base of the fibrous cone is reached and clearly defined at the posterior wall of the bifurcation of the portal vein, the fibrous cone is transected at this level flush with the liver surface with a laparoscopic knife and scissors (■ Figs. 58.6–58.8). With the superb optical magnification provided by the laparoscope, bile drainage can usually be seen from the cut ends of tiny bile ductules over the raw liver surface of the fibrous cone transection. A moist gauze roll is now temporarily packed over the raw surface, and the operation switched to preparation of the Roux-en-Y jejunal loop.

Under laparoscopic guidance the duodenal-jejunal (D-J) junction is identified, and the proximal jejunum at around 15–20 cm from the D-J junction is secured and drawn towards the umbilical port. The pneumoperitoneum is now released, and the umbilical port site is enlarged to allow the proximal jejunum to be delivered through this to outside the abdomen. A 40 cm Roux-en-Y jejunal loop is then fashioned extracorporeally using continuous 4-0 polydioxanone sutures. This Roux-en-Y loop is returned into the abdominal cavity after which the pneumoperitoneum is re-established. The correct position of the Roux loop and the rest of the intestine is checked to exclude torsion of the bowel. The Roux loop is passed through the transverse mesocolon and brought to the liver hilum in a retrocolic manner. An end-to-side hepaticoportoenterostomy is performed intracoporeally under laparoscopic magnification using 5-0 interrupted polydioxanone sutures (■ Figs. 58.9, 58.10). The mesenteric defects are also closed using 5-0 interrupted polydioxanone

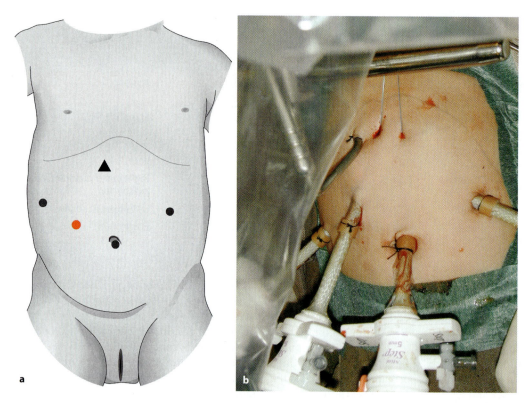

Fig. 58.2. Position of the ports. **a** Schematic drawing. *Red circle* 5 mm camera port, *black circles* 5 mm working ports, *triangle* liver retractor. **b** Intraoperative view

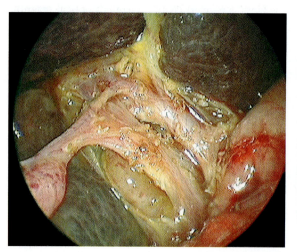

Fig. 58.3. Mobilisation of the fibrous cord from the hepatic artery

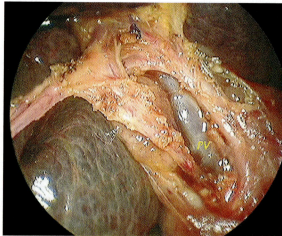

Fig. 58.4. Mobilisation of the fibrous cord from the portal vein

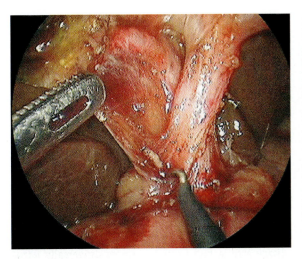

Fig. 58.5. Distal mobilisation of the fibrous cord with transection of its distal end

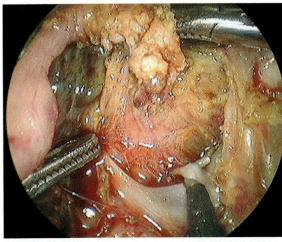

Fig. 58.6. Mobilisation of the fibrous cone down to the posterior wall of the portal vein. Portal vein tributaries are divided

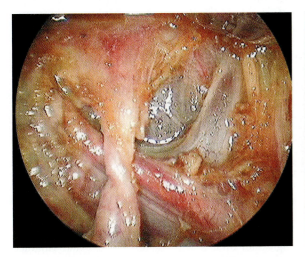

Fig. 58.7. Completed mobilisation of the fibrous cone

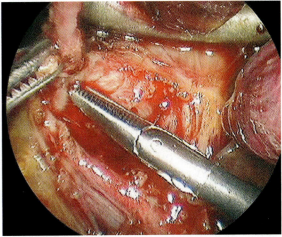

Fig. 58.8. Transection of the fibrous cone at its base

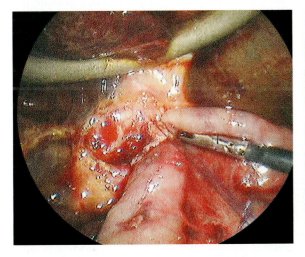

Fig. 58.9. Posterior part of the anastomosis of the hepatico-portoenterostomy

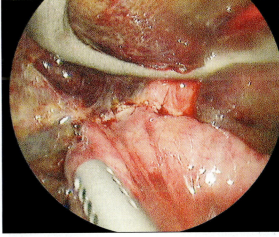

Fig. 58.10. Completed hepaticoportoenterostomy

sutures. A suction drain is placed in the subhepatic space and brought out through the right upper quadrant port at the end of the procedure. The fascial defects over the port sites are closed with absorbable sutures and the skin is closed with adhesive strips.

Postoperative Care

At the end of the operation, the port sites are infiltrated with 0.25% bupivacaine. For postoperative pain control, paracetamol suppositories and diclofenac suppositories are given round the clock for the first 48 h, and intramuscular pethidine injections are given only as required.

The nasogastric tube is left in situ and is connected to a bedside bag for free drainage and intermittent aspiration. It is removed when the intestinal ileus has resolved. The urinary catheter is kept in overnight and is removed the next day when the output is satisfactory. Feeding is commenced when there is minimal output from the nasogastric tube and when the intestinal ileus is over.

Results

Over a 3-year period, we have managed 10 patients (7 girls) with biliary atresia. The mean age at surgery was 65.5 days (range 48–89 days). The mean operative time was 278 min (range 193–435 min). An intraoperative cholangiogram was required for confirmation of diagnosis in 4 patients. The standard Kasai hepaticojejunostomy procedure was successfully performed in all 10 patients and no conversion to open surgery was required. There was no intraoperative complication encountered in any patients. Postoperatively, 5 out of 10 patients required ventilatory support in an intensive care unit for a mean of 1.2 days (0.5–2 days). Full enteral feeding was resumed at a mean of 4.2 days (2–7 days). Surgical complication was only encountered in the first patient who developed a subhepatic collection at postoperative day 7 that responded to antibiotic therapy and ultrasound-guided drainage. Bile drainage was very good in 6 patients and suboptimal in the other 4. Pulse steroid therapy for a mean of 2.5 courses (2–3 courses) was required in these 4 patients with good clinical response in 2 patients, who have both established satisfactory bile drainage subsequently.

At a mean follow-up of 21.5 months, all patients have remained alive. Good cosmetic results with inconspicuous wounds were achieved in all patients. Seven out of 10 patients (70%) became jaundice free at a mean of 2.8 months after surgery. They have all remained well and thriving except one boy who developed variceal bleeding when he was 9 months old. The varices were controlled with endoscopic injection sclerotherapy. Two patients who had remained persistently jaundiced after the Kasai operation had ongoing deterioration with multiple episodes of cholangitis. They were aggressively supported nutritionally and both have subsequently undergone successful cadaveric reduced-size liver transplantation at 9 and 12 months of age, respectively. For the last patient, the serum bilirubin dropped from 179 to 118 Ìol/l at around 4m onths after surgery (after pulse steroid therapy) and was kept on close monitoring.

Discussion

Biliary atresia had been an almost universally lethal condition until the introduction of the Kasai operation in the late 1950s and its popularisation in the late 1960s (Kasai et al. 1968). Nowadays the Kasai operation is still the mainstay of the treatment for patients with biliary atresia (Ibrahim et al. 1997; Karrer et al. 1990). An early and properly performed Kasai operation is the prerequisite in achieving a jaundice-free survival although a great proportion of patients still require liver transplantation in due course (Kasai et al. 1989). From the major reports in the literature, it has been found that both the jaundice clearance rate and the long-term outcome are related to the age at surgery (Ibrahim et al. 1997; Karrer et al. 1990; Ohi 2001). It is therefore mandatory to establish an early diagnosis so timely surgery can be performed. In addition, it has also been found that the result is much better in those centres with better experience and higher case volume (McKiernan et al. 2000).

The laparoscope has been a useful adjunct in assessing small infants with persistent neonatal jaundice (Hay et al. 2000; Senyuz et al. 2001). Both laparoscopic-guided intraoperative cholangiogram and liver biopsy can be performed safely. This helps in achieving an early and accurate diagnosis without fiddling around with the less specific investigations. This also carries the benefit of more rapid recovery when compared with conventional operative cholangiogram done via laparotomy. However, in those that prove to be biliary atresia, a formal laparotomy and conventional Kasai operation would still be needed in most centres.

With the improvement in the instrumentation and experience in laparoscopic surgery in children, more and more procedures can be performed safely nowadays (Georgeson et al. 1999; Lee et al. 2000a,b; Lobe 1998; Rothenberg et al. 1998). However, with the small abdominal cavity and hence limited working space in small infants, laparoscopic reconstructive procedures are particularly challenging. The initial success of meticulous reconstructive laparoscopic procedures such as retroperitoneoscopic pyeloplasty (Yeung et al. 2001) has prompted us to extend this technique further to hepatobiliary reconstructive surgery.

In the series, laparoscopic Kasai operation could be safely performed in all 10 patients. Although technically demanding, there was no major problem encountered during surgery. The learning curve had been very steep with the operative time decreasing dramatically from more than 7 h in the first case to just over 3 h in the last few cases. We noticed that once the logistics of the procedure was sorted out, the procedure was in fact quite straightforward. Extra precautions had been taken during the first case which explained the rather long operative time. Although the procedure is technically demanding and can be difficult, particularly for beginners, we have found that with the superb illumination and optical magnification under the laparoscope, very clear visualisation and hence meticulous dissection and access to the liver hilum are possible, thus ensuring accurate transection of the fibrous cone and a precise portoenterostomy anastomosis. This forms the cornerstone in the success of the operation. With the method described, meticulous dissection and anastomosis can be performed similar to or even superior to open surgery. We also advocate extracorporeal fashioning of the Roux-en-Y jejunostomy by enlarging the umbilical port site. This allows bowel resection and anastomosis similar to open surgery. Thus, this minimises intra-abdominal contamination and avoids the use of staples (Lee et al. 2000a).

Most of the babies had some degree of carbon dioxide retention and acidosis towards the end of the procedure and, because of their young age, most of them required a short period of ventilatory support. We had been particularly cautious for the initial few cases and this accounted for the rather long duration of ventilation and intensive care. With increase in experience, we are trying to extubate these children in the operating theatre, to minimise the duration of intensive care and to commence feeding earlier. In the series, full enteral feeding was started much earlier in the last few cases.

In the series, there were minimal surgical complications except in the first patient who developed a subhepatic collection about 1 week after surgery. This also resulted in the prolonged ileus and late resumption of feeding. It was fortunate that he responded extremely well to antibiotic therapy and percutaneous drainage. For this patient, a suction drain was not inserted at the end of the procedure and this might have accounted for the collection. Since then we have routinely left a drain there and we have not encountered any further postoperative collections in all subsequent patients.

Seven out of 10 patients (70%) had become jaundice free at 4 months after surgery. This is comparable to jaundice clearance rate ranging from 45% to 82% in the more recent large series of open Kasai in the literature (Inomata et al. 1997; Karrer et al. 1990; Kasai et al. 1989; Miyano et al. 1993). In the last patient, the serum bilirubin was on the downward trend and awaited further assessment. The procedure failed to achieve bile drainage in two patients. Both patients were closely followed up and received aggressive nutritional support and subsequently had a successful liver transplant. This combined approach definitely improves the overall survival of biliary atresia (Inomata et al. 1997). In both patients, we had found that intra-abdominal adhesions were much less severe than those after a traditional open Kasai operation. This made the subsequent recipient hepatectomy during liver transplantation much easier and morbidity-free (Polymeneas et al 2001). In those patients with a previous open Kasai operation, the procedure of recipient hepatectomy during liver transplantation is particularly difficult and this in turn contributes significantly to a higher rate of small bowel perforation and hence morbidity and even mortality. In order to minimise adhesion formation, the use of bioabsorbable membrane during conventional Kasai operation has been reported. In contrast, with the use of the laparoscope it is not necessary to make a large subcostal wound, to mobilise the liver or to expose the viscera. This might account for the lessening of intra-abdominal adhesions and hence it facilitates future liver transplantation. However, this is the observation in only two patients and of course we need more data for further evaluation.

More patient data are required to assess whether the procedure is equally safe and effective in achieving jaundice clearance as compared to the conventional Kasai operation. In addition, long-term follow-up is essential as we believe that a great proportion of patients after the laparoscopic Kasai, like the traditional counterpart, will similarly develop cirrhosis-related complications and require liver transplantation (Karrer et al. 1996; Miyano et al. 1993). With the relative short duration of follow-up, we are not certain if the laparoscopic Kasai could achieve the same long-term survival as the traditional Kasai operation although this is expected to be similar if the same initial jaundice clearance rate and postoperative complication rate could be achieved.

Conclusion

Our initial results of laparoscopic Kasai portoenterostomy are very encouraging, and we can safely conclude that the minimally invasive technique is both a good diagnostic as well as therapeutic modality for infants with biliary atresia. In experienced hands, laparoscopic Kasai portoenterostomy is effective in achieving good bile drainage although more patient data with longer follow-up are required to see if this is comparable if not superior to conventional open surgery. The learning curve is however steep but, with increase in experience, similar operative time and postoperative outcomes can be expected. The potential additional benefits of fewer intra-abdominal adhesions making a possible subsequent liver transplantation easier and safer will also warrant further evaluation.

References

Georgeson KE, Cohen RD, Hebra A, et al (1999) Primary laparoscopic-assisted endorectal colon pull-through for Hirschsprung's diseases: a new gold standard. Ann Surg 229:678–682

Hay SA, Soliman HE, Sherif HM, et al (2000) Neonatal jaundice: the role of laparoscopy. J Pediatr Surg 35:1706–1709

Ibrahim M, Miyano T, Ohi R, et al (1997) Japanese Biliary Atresia Registry, 1989 to 1994. Tohoku J Exp Med 181:85–95

Inomata Y, Oike F, Okamoto S, et al (1997) Impact of the development of a liver transplantation program on the treatment of biliary atresia in an institution in Japan. J Pediatr Surg 32:1201–1205

Karrer FM, Lilly JR, Stewart BA, et al (1990) Biliary Atresia Registry, 1976 to 1989. J Pediatr Surg 25:1076–1081

Karrer FM, Price MR, Bensard DD, et al (1996) Long-term results with the Kasai operation for biliary atresia. Arch Surg 131:493–496

Kasai M, Kimura S, Asakura Y, et al (1968) Surgical treatment of biliary atresia. J Pediatr Surg 3:665–675

Kasai M, Mochizuki I, Ohkohchi N, et al (1989) Surgical limitation for biliary atresia: indication for liver transplantation. J Pediatr Surg 24:851–854

Lee KH, Yeung CK, Tam YH, et al (2000a) Laparoscopy for definitive diagnosis and treatment of gastrointestinal bleeding of obscure origin in children. J Pediatr Surg 35:1291–1293

Lee KH, Yeung CK, Tam YH, et al (2000b) The use of laparoscopy in the management of adnexal pathologies in children. Aust N Z J Surg 70:192–195

Lobe TE (1998) Laparoscopic surgery in children. Curr Probl Surg 35:861–948

McKierna PJ, Baker AJ, Kelly DA (2000) The frequency and outcome of biliary atresia in UK and Ireland. Lancet 355:4–5

Miyano T, Fujimoto T, Ohya T, et al (1993) Current concept in the treatment of biliary atresia. World J Surg 17:332–336

Ohi R (2001) Surgery for biliary atresia. Liver 21:175–182

Polymeneas G, Theodosopoulos T, Stamatiadis A, et al (2001) A comparative study of postoperative adhesion formation after laparoscopic vs open cholecystectomy. Surg Endosc 15:41–43

Rothenberg SS, Chang JH, Bealer JF (1998) Experience with minimally invasive surgery in infants. Am J Surg 176:654–658

Senyuz OF, Yesildag E, Emir H et al. (2001) Diagnostic laparoscopy in prolonged jaundice. J Pediatr Surg 36:463–465

Yeung CK, Tam YH, Sihoe JDY, et al (2001) Retroperitoneoscopic dismembered pyeloplasty for pelvi-ureteric junction obstruction in infants and children. BJU Int 87:509–513

Chapter 59

Laparoscopic Excision of Choledochal Cyst with Hepaticojejunostomy

C.K. Yeung, K.H. Lee and Y.H. Tam

Introduction

Choledochal cyst is a common congenital biliary tract anomaly. The standard treatment of type I choledochal cyst is complete cyst excision followed by hepaticoenterostomy (Lilly 1979; Miyano et al. 1996). This minimises the risks of associated complications including biliary strictures, calculus, recurrent cholangitis and bile duct malignancy that were once prevalent when choledochal cysts were managed by internal bypass surgery without cyst excision (Todani et al. 1987). The classical approach for cyst excision and biliary reconstruction entails a laparotomy usually through a long upper abdominal transverse incision to achieve adequate surgical exposure and space for operative manipulation. This is however associated with significant postoperative pain and hence analgesia requirement, often prolonged paralytic ileus and unsightly abdominal scars. There are recent anecdotal reports of a laparoscopic approach for choledochal cysts in adults. Besides the usual benefits of minimal access surgery, a laparoscopic approach offers additional potential advantages of providing an excellently illuminated and magnified view of the porta hepatis, thereby greatly facilitating meticulous dissection of the portal structures and the subsequent hepaticoenterostomy anastomosis. We describe our technique of laparoscopic excision of choledochal cyst with hepaticoenterostomy in infants and young children.

Preoperative Preparation

Before Induction of General Anaesthesia

A saline enema is given on the evening before surgery to ensure cleansing of the large bowel.

After Induction of General Anaesthesia

A nasogastric tube is inserted for bowel decompression during and after surgery. A urinary catheter is inserted to monitor the urine output. Prophylactic antibiotics including ampicillin, cefuroxime and metronidazole are given on induction of anaesthesia. Further doses may be needed if the operation is prolonged.

Positioning

Patient

The patient is placed in a supine position with a small lumbar support, more on the right side.

Crew, Monitors and Equipment

The surgeon stands on the right side of the table, with one assistant holding the camera on the surgeon's left on the same side of the table, and the second assistant and the scrub nurse on the opposite side of the table (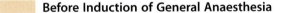 Fig. 59.1). Two television monitors are required, one positioned at the left upper corner for the surgeon, and another positioned on the right upper corner for the second assistant during subsequent dissection and hepaticojejunostomy anastomosis. During the operation, the table may be tilted to a slightly head-up position to facilitate the dissection.

Special Equipment

Intraoperative cholangiography will be performed. The laparoscope is held by an AESOP robotic arm. For liver retraction a Nathanson retractor is inserted.

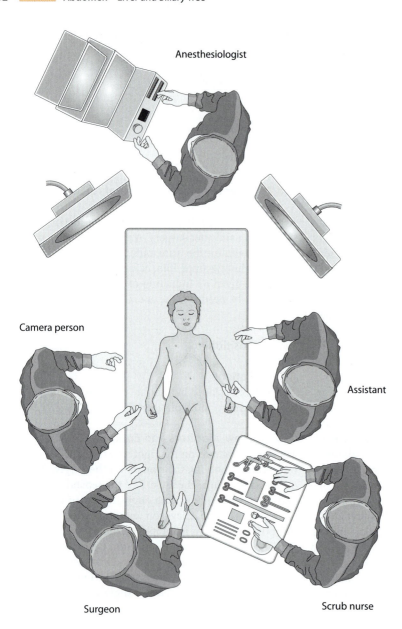

Fig. 59.1. Position of the patient, crew and equipment

Technique

Cannulae

Cannula	Method of insertion	Diameter (mm)	Device	Position
1	Closed	5, Step	Laparoscope initially, working instruments later	Supraumbilical
2	Closed	5, Step	Laparoscope later on	Right upper quadrant, midclavicular line
3	Closed	5, Step	Working instruments	Right upper quadrant
4	Closed	5, Step	Assistant's instruments	Left upper quadrant
5	Closed	No cannula	Nathanson retractor	Epigastrium

Procedure

A four-port technique is used (■ Fig. 59.2a,b). A 5 mm 30 laparoscope is first inserted through a 5 mm port via a supraumbilical incision. Carbon dioxide pneumoperitoneum is established at 10–12m mHg. Three more 3- to 5 mm working ports are then inserted at the right upper and left upper quadrants under videoscopic guidance. Thorough laparoscopic examination and if necessary an operative cholangiogram are performed first to confirm the diagnosis and delineate the anatomy especially of the pancreatic duct and the choledochopancreatic junction. A Nathanson liver retractor is inserted through a 5 mm epigastric incision (■ Fig. 59.2). In those patients without a preoperative endoscopic retrograde cholangiopancreatogram (ERCP), an intraoperative cholangiogram is performed through a needle puncturing the gallbladder (■ Fig. 59.3). After delineating the anatomy, the gallbladder is first mobilised from the liver. For better and more direct visualisation of the choledochal cyst and other hilar structures, the camera is usually shifted to the right upper quadrant port that is sited at around the midclavicular line.

The peritoneal fold over the choledochal cyst is incised. The cyst is dissected completely free from the portal vein, hepatic artery, duodenum and pancreas throughout the entire length using a combination of monopolar electrocautery with a fine needle hook and ultrasonic scalpel coagulation and dissection

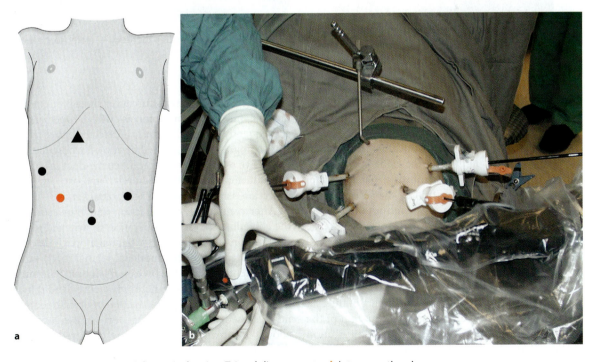

Fig. 59.2. Port position. **a** Schematic drawing. T*riangle* liver retractor. **b** Intraoperative view

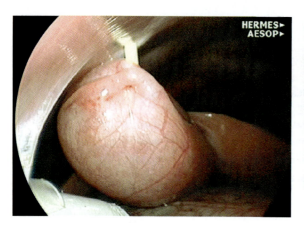

Fig. 59.3. Operative cholangiography by direct injection of contrast into the gallbladder

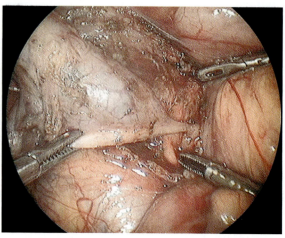

Fig. 59.5. The cyst has been completely mobilised

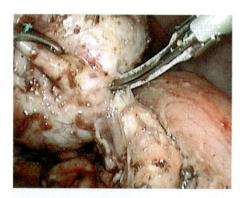

Fig. 59.4. Dissection of the distal part of the cyst from the pancreas

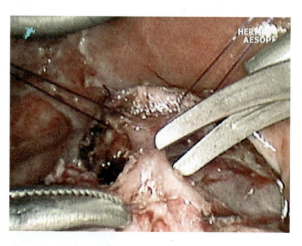

Fig. 59.6. The common hepatic duct is ready to be transected

(■ Fig. 59.4). If there is suspicion for biliary stones or any intrahepatic or extrahepatic ductal strictures, the cyst is opened and an intraoperative choledochoscopic examination is performed using a flexible choledochoscope inserted through one of the right upper quadrant ports. Downward retraction of the first part of duodenum and frequent suction by the second assistant allows clear dissection of the retroduodenal and intrapancreatic portion of the choledochal cyst. The intrapancreatic part of the cyst/duct is freed, divided and sutured without jeopardising the pancreatic duct (■ Fig. 59.5). Small arterial branches to the cyst can be divided by simple electrocautery, and larger ones by using the ultrasonic scalpel. The upper part of the cyst is then transected just above the upper margin of the cyst, usually distal to the hepatic duct bifurcation (■ Fig. 59.6). In case both the left and the right hepatic ducts are also involved, the transection will be

above the hepatic ductal bifurcation and a biductal hepaticojejunostomy anastomosis will be performed subsequently. If ductal stenosis is detected either by the cholangiogram or confirmed by choledochoscopy, the respective segment of stenosed hepatic duct is incised and a ductoplasty performed under laparoscopic magnification using fine 6-0 intracorporeal sutures.

After completion of dissection and transection of the choledochal cyst, the operation is switched to the preparation of the Roux-en-Y jejunal loop. Under laparoscopic guidance the duodenal-jejunal (D-J) junction is identified, and the proximal jejunum at around 15–20 cm from the D-J junction is secured and drawn towards the umbilical port. The pneumoperitoneum is now released, and the umbilical port site is enlarged to allow the proximal jejunum to be delivered through this to outside the abdomen. A 40 cm Roux-en-Y jejunal loop is then fashioned extracorporeally using con-

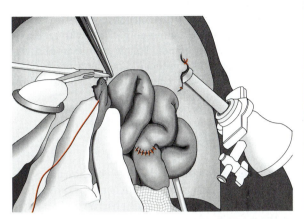

Fig. 59.7. Extracorporeal fashioning of the Roux-en-Y jejunal anastomosis

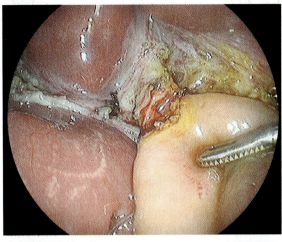

Fig. 59.9. Fashioning of the posterior part of the hepaticojejunostomy

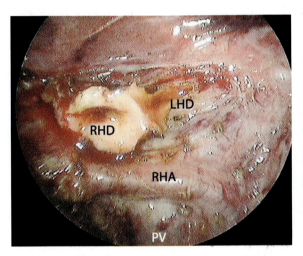

Fig. 59.8. The bile duct is prepared and ready for anastomosis. *RHD* Right hepatic duct, *LHD* left hepatic duct, *RHA* right hepatic artery

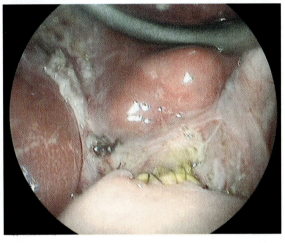

Fig. 59.10. Completed hepaticojejunostomy

tinuous 4-0 polydioxanone sutures (■ Fig. 59.7). This Roux-en-Y loop is returned into the abdominal cavity after which the pneumoperitoneum is re-established. The correct position of the Roux loop and the rest of the intestine is checked to exclude torsion of the bowel. The Roux loop is passed through the transverse mesocolon and brought to the liver hilum in a retrocolic manner. An end-to-side hepaticojejunostomy is performed intracoporeally under laparoscopic magnification using 5-0 or 6-0 interrupted polydioxanone sutures (■ Figs. 59.8–59.10). The mesenteric defects are also closed using 5-0 interrupted polydioxanone suture. A suction drain is left in the subhepatic region and brought out through the right upper quadrant port at the end of the procedure. The fascial defects over the port sites are closed with absorbable sutures and the skin is closed with adhesive strips.

Postoperative Care

At the end of the operation, the port sites are infiltrated with 0.25% bupivacaine. For postoperative pain control, paracetamol suppositories and diclofenac suppositories are given round the clock for the first 48 h, and intramuscular pethidine injections are given only as required.

The nasogastric tube is left in situ and is connected to a bedside bag for free drainage and intermittent aspiration. It is removed when the amount of back aspirate is small and when the intestinal ileus has resolved. The urinary catheter is kept in overnight and is removed the next day when the urine output is satisfactory. Feeding is commenced when there is minimal output from the nasogastric tube and when the intestinal ileus is over.

Results

Over a 3.5-year period, we had managed 22 children (13 girls) with choledochal cyst, 21 type I cysts (14 fusiform and 7 cystic) and 1 possibly type IV cyst. The mean size of cyst was 3.1 cm (range 0.9–10 cm). Laparoscopic operative cholangiogram was performed in 13 patients. Laparoscopic excision was successfully performed in 21 patients. Conversion was required in the first patient when the laparoscopic view was obscured by minor oozing. In the patient with a 10 cm cyst, this was initially punctured and aspirated before proceeding to laparoscopic excision.

In 6 patients, both the left and the right hepatic ducts were involved. The transection was therefore performed at a level above the hepatic ductal bifurcation and a biductal hepaticojejunostomy anastomosis was performed subsequently. In the other patients, the anastomosis was made at the common hepatic duct just above the upper border of the choledochal cyst. Ductal stenosis involving the hepatic duct was detected either by the cholangiogram or choledochoscopy in 3 patients; the respective segment of the stenosed hepatic duct was incised and a ductoplasty performed under laparoscopic magnification. No major intraoperative complication was encountered in all patients. The mean operative time for laparoscopic treatment was 307 min (range 228–560 min). Two patients required postoperative ventilatory support for half a day. Feeding could be started as early as the second postoperative day with a mean time to full enteral feeding of 6.6 days.

Seventeen patients had a smooth and uneventful postoperative recovery. In 4 patients, the postoperative course was complicated by subhepatic collections. Two of these responded to parenteral antibiotic treatment of which 1 patient required additional percutaneous drainage under ultrasound guidance. In another patient, there was persistent high output from the suction drain and this was later confirmed to be due to chylous ascites. This responded to total parenteral nutrition and a low fat diet. The drain was removed on postoperative day 18. One patient had a minor bile leak that was controlled by the suction drain left at the end of surgery, nil per os and total parenteral nutrition. The leakage subsequently dried up spontaneously on conservative treatment and the drain was removed. In 1 patient there was prolonged ileus and full feeding was only re-established on postoperative day 11. Three patients had minor wound problems that responded to local treatment. The mean hospital stay was 9.3 days (range 4–25 days).

On follow-up at a mean of 22 months (range 4–42 months), all patients had remained very well except 3 who had mild fat intolerance, one of whom had in addition occasional abdominal colic. The patients with fat intolerance all improved on diet manipulation. The patient with intestinal colic was admitted twice after surgery but the colic settled on conservative treatment. The wounds healed well in all patients with an excellent cosmetic appearance. Follow-up ultrasound was done in 20 patients and that did not show any hepatobiliary abnormalities. Postoperative ultrasound examination was pending in two patients.

Discussion

The current standard treatment of choledochal cyst is complete excision and hepaticoenterostomy (Lilly 1979; Miyano et al. 1996). This gives a good outcome in the majority of cases. With the advance in medical technology and surgical techniques, the application of minimally invasive surgery in children has been increasing since the 1990s. Nowadays, the laparoscopic technique is almost universally accepted as the gold standard in the management of Hirschsprung's disease, fundoplication, splenectomy, etc. (Georgeson 1998; Georgeson et al. 1995; Rothenberg 1998; Tan 1994). Its use in the management of small bowel bleeding, adnexal pathologies, etc., is also well documented (Lee et al. 2000a,b). With the increase in experience, the use of the laparoscope has extended to very sophisticated reconstructive procedures such as pyeloplasty (Yeung et al. 2001). Recently, there are sporadic case reports of laparoscopic treatment of choledochal cyst but mainly in adults (Farello et al. 1995; Shimura et al. 1998; Watanabe et al. 1999a). This is the first large series of laparoscopic excision of choledochal cyst in children.

The principle of laparoscopic surgery for choledochal cyst is similar to that of open surgery although it is much more technically demanding especially in small children in whom the peritoneal space is very limited. It is aimed to excise the cyst entirely in order to minimise the risk of future complications such as malignancy. At the beginning of the operation, it is useful to perform an intraoperative cholangiogram to give a good road map of bile ducts as well as the pancreatobiliary junction. This guides us to the level of excision and minimises the chance of damaging the pancreatic duct. In the series, we performed an intraoperative cholangiogram in the majority of cases and in particular in those without a preoperative ERCP (Miyano et al. 1996). We have found this is especially useful in those with type I fusiform cyst in which the anatomy, in particular of the pancreatobiliary junction, can be accurately delineated. Our method of intraoperative cholangiogram is relatively simple. The gallbladder is punctured after a purse-string suture is applied to the fundus. This avoids leakage during the contrast study.

The laparoscope with its magnification allows excellent visualisation of the anatomy and in turn facilitates meticulous mobilisation of the cyst from surrounding structures. By using a diathermy hook and the ultrasonic scalpel, it is possible to free the entire cyst from the surrounding structures without too much blood loss. The distal end of the cyst after separation from the duodenum and pancreas can either be ligated or clipped while the proximal end of the cyst is transacted just proximal to the upper border of the cyst. For the fashioning of the jejunal Roux loop, we advocate doing this through the enlarged umbilical wound. This enables meticulous bowel anastomosis just like open surgery and also avoids intra-abdominal contamination (Lee et al. 2000a). In addition, this also saves the cost as well as the relatively large incision for the Endo-GIA staplers used for intracorporeal bowel reconstruction (Farello et al. 1995; Shimura et al. 1998; Watanabe et al. 1999a). Moreover, with the magnification under the laparoscope, the bilioenteric anastomosis can be meticulously performed using the laparoscopic hand-suturing technique.

We have been successful in performing laparoscopic excision of choledochal cyst and reconstruction in 21 out of 22 patients (95%), the first series in the literature showing such a high success rate in children. This compares favourably with the success rate of 63% in the recent series of 8 adults with choledochal cyst (Tanaka et al. 2001). There were no major complications encountered during surgery. With the magnification under the laparoscope and the use of fine 3- and 5 mm instruments, dissection of the cyst can be done meticulously, hence minimising the risk of damaging the adjacent vital structures. In addition, with our method of extracorporeal fashioning of the Roux loop, there was no bowel-related complication in the series.

The mean operative time of 307 min also compares favourably with the 616 min in the only other large series of laparoscopic excision of choledochal cyst in 8 adults reported in the literature (Tanaka et al. 2001). The learning curve has been quite steep. The relatively long operative time is accounted for by extra precautions taken during the early cases, and in those with large cysts or those with recent infection. Once the logistics of the operation have been sorted out and the hurdle of the learning curve has been overcome, the procedure is in fact quite straightforward. In the more recent cases, the whole operation could be accomplished in just over 3.5 h.

One patient had bile leak after laparoscopic excision and reconstruction (4.5%). This also compares favourably to the leakage rate of around 7–18% in traditional open surgery (Miyano et al. 1996; Saing et al. 1997). The bile leak, like the other cases reported in the literature (Chowbey et al. 2002; Lilly 1979), settled on conservative treatment. It is valuable to place a drain be-

side the anastomosis. This helps to drain out serous collection as well as serving as a control device to contain the bile leak, if any. As in this patient, the bile leak, being contained by the abdominal drain, did not lead to generalised peritonitis. The output gradually decreased and subsequently the leak dried up.

Subhepatic collection is not a commonly reported complication after traditional open choledochal cyst excision but we had 4 patients in the series with this problem. Three of these responded to antibiotics and 1 required additional ultrasound-guided drainage. We are not certain about the exact cause for this relatively high incidence of infected collection despite the routine practice of leaving a drain there during the early postoperative days. This might be related to spillage of intestinal content during the fashioning of the hepaticojejunostomy although we had tried hard to apply frequent suction during the procedure. This is sometimes difficult especially in the small abdominal cavity of children when too much suction will eliminate the pneumoperitoneum and too little suction cannot serve the purpose. This is particularly challenging in difficult hepaticojejunostomy anastomoses.

In those patients without complications, the recovery could be very fast. As the abdomen has not been opened and hence there has been less manipulation of the bowel, bowel function actually returns quite rapidly. Feeding can be started quite early and the hospital stay can be shortened. In the series, a patient could actually tolerate full enteral feeding and be home by postoperative day 4. The overall hospital stay is longer than expected in this group of patients. This is related to extra precautions taken especially during the early part of the series. When we first introduced the new procedure, we had to make sure that the procedure was safe and everything was alright before we discharged our patients. For obvious reasons, patients would stay longer when complications occurred. With increase in experience and improvements in technique and postoperative care, we hope that the hospital stay can be dramatically shortened in most patients.

At a mean follow-up of 22 months, all patients had actually remained well except for mild fat intolerance encountered in 3 patients. They all improved on dietary manipulation. The patient with additional intestinal colic also settled on conservative treatment. The cosmetic result had been very good. The umbilical scar, the largest wound, was basically invisible in most patients. There were no biliary complications such as cholangitis, strictures or stone formation encountered in all these patients. However, regular assessment is essential as, in large series in the literature, these complications as well as biliary tract malignancy are reported on long-term follow-up (Miyano et al. 1996; Todani et al. 1995; Tsuchida et al. 2002; Watanabe et al. 1999b).

References

Chowbey PK, Katrak MP, Sharma A, et al (2002) Complete laparoscopic management of choledochal cyst: report of two cases. J Laparoendosc Adv Surg Tech 12:217–221

Farello GA, Cerofolini A, Rebonato M, et al (1995) Congenital choledochal cyst: video-guided laparoscopic treatment. Surg Laparosc Endosc Percutan Tech 5:354–358

Georgeson KE (1998) Laparoscopic fundoplication. Curr Opin Pediatr 10:318–322

Georgeson KE, Fuenfer MM, Hardin WD (1995) Primary pull-through for Hirschsprung's disease in infants and children. J Pediatr Surg 30:1017–1022

Lee KH, Yeung CK, Tam YH, et al (2000a) Laparoscopy for definitive diagnosis and treatment of gastrointestinal bleeding of obscure origin in children. J Pediatr Surg 35:1291–1293

Lee KH, Yeung CK, Tam YH, et al (2000b) The use of laparoscopy in the management of adnexal pathologies in children. Aust N Z J Surg 70:192–195

Lilly JR (1979) The surgical treatment of choledochal cyst. Surg Gynecol Obstet 149:36–42

Miyano T, Yamataka A, Kato Y, et al (1996) Hepaticoenterostomy after excision of choledochal cyst in children: a 30-year experience with 180 cases. J Pediatr Surg 31:417–421

Rothenberg SS (1998) Laparoscopic splenectomy in children. Semin Laparosc Surg 5:19–24

Saing H, Han H, Chan KL, et al (1997) Early and late results of excision of choledochal cysts. J Pediatr Surg 32:1563–1566

Shimura H, Tanaka M, Shimizu S, et al (1998) Laparoscopic treatment of congenital choledochal cyst. Surg Endosc 12:1268–1271

Tan HL (1994) The role of laparoscopic surgery in children. Ann Chir Gynaecol 83:143–147

Tanaka M, Shimizu S, Mizumoto K, et al (2001) Laparoscopically assisted resection of choledochal cyst and Roux-en-Y reconstruction. Surg Endosc 15:545–552

Todani T, Watanabe Y, Toki A, et al (1987) Carcinoma related to choledochal cysts with internal drainage. Surg Gynecol Obstet 164:61–64

Todani T, Watanabe Y, Urushihara N, et al (1995) Biliary complications after excisional procedure for choledochal cyst. J Pediatr Surg 30:478–481

Tsuchida Y, Takahashi A, Suzuki N, et al (2002) Development of intrahepatic biliary stones after excision of choledochal cysts. J Pediatr Surg 37:165–167

Watanabe Y, Sato M, Tokui K, et al (1999a) Laparoscope-assisted minimally invasive treatment for choledochal cyst. J Laparoendosc Adv Surg Tech 9:415–418

Watanabe Y, Toki A, Todani T (1999b). Bile duct cancer developed after cyst excision for choledochal cyst. J Hepatobiliary Pancreat Surg 6:207–212

Yeung CK, Tam YH, Sihoe JD, et al (2001) Retroperitoneoscopic dismembered pyeloplasty for pelvi-ureteric junction obstruction in infants and children. BJU Int 87:509–513

Chapter 60

Laparoscopic Cholecystectomy

Oliver J. Muensterer and Keith E. Georgeson

Introduction

Since its introduction by Mühe in 1985 (Litynski 1998), laparoscopic cholecystectomy has become the most widely performed laparoscopic operation worldwide. In fact, laparoscopic cholecystectomy has driven the development and acceptance of other, more complex laparoscopic procedures in adults.

Cholelithiasis and cholecystitis is much less frequent in children, and pediatric surgeons have removed relatively few gallbladders in the past. Improved imaging techniques are now detecting more gallstones in children, and the increasing availability of laparoscopic cholecystectomy is lowering the referral threshold of pediatricians.

Analgesic use is lower and hospitalization time is shorter with laparoscopic versus open cholecystectomy (Al-Salem and Nourallah 1997; Al-Salem et al. 1997; Kim et al. 1995), resulting in improved cost-effectiveness (Luks et al. 1999). Indications for laparoscopic cholecystectomy include cholelithiasis, cholecystitis, and gallbladder dyskinesia. Pigmented gallstones may result from hemolytic disorders such as sickle cell anemia, thalassemia, or spherocytosis. Nonhemolytic predisposing conditions include bowel resection, chronic total parenteral nutrition, cystic fibrosis, oral contraceptive use, pregnancy, and obesity. Calculous cholecystitis is predominantly caused by obstruction of bile flow at the gallbladder neck or cystic duct. Severe trauma, extensive burns, and prolonged sepsis are risk factors for acalculous cholecystitis. Because children under 6 years may not relate specific symptoms on questioning, we believe that finding gallstones on imaging studies in this age group is an indication for laparoscopic cholecystectomy. While the operative technique has become standardized in most pediatric surgical centers, the management of common bile duct stones and the complication of common bile duct injury remains controversial.

Preoperative Preparation

Before Induction of General Anesthesia

Abdominal ultrasound is the primary and most cost-effective imaging modality for suspected gallbladder disease, readily detecting calculi, gallbladder wall thickening, pericystic fluid, and dilation of the biliary duct system. The hepatobiliary iminodiacetic acid (HIDA) scan is highly specific for excluding acute cholecystitis and is useful to detect gallbladder dyskinesia when performed with cholecystokinin (CCK) stimulation (ejection fraction below 35%).

A cellular blood count is useful to detect the degree of anemia in patients with hemoglobinopathies or hemolysis. The conjugated bilirubin, liver enzymes, amylase, and lipase may be elevated in cases with calculous obstruction of the bile ducts. Depending on the familial background, a screen for sickle cell anemia may be indicated.

In patients with suspected common bile duct stones, preoperative endoscopic retrograde cholangiopancreatogram (ERCP) with papillotomy and retrieval of the calculi is a possible approach. Other treatment algorithms for common bile duct stones are discussed below.

To avoid complications from sickle cell anemia, affected patients are transfused to a hematocrit above 30% and a hemoglobin S fraction of less than 35%. The patients undergo aggressive hydration with 1.5 times maintenance intravenous fluids for at least 12 h before the procedure to decrease the risk of sickle cell crisis. Perioperative hypothermia, hypovolemia, and hypoxia must be avoided in these children. With meticulous attention to perioperative management, transfusion guidelines, and pulmonary care, laparoscopic surgery is safely accomplished in children with sickle cell disease (Sandoval et al. 2002).

The preoperative workup of patients planned to undergo elective laparoscopic splenectomy for hemolytic disease should include an abdominal sonogram. If concomitant gallbladder disease is found, simultaneous laparoscopic cholecystectomy is indicated.

After Induction of General Anesthesia

The patient is endotracheally intubated for the procedure. The stomach is evacuated via nasogastric suction. Routine use of preoperative antibiotics is not recommended, but may be considered in cases with cholecystitis. A bladder catheter or preoperative Credé maneuver is unnecessary, as the dissection and manipulation is performed in the right upper abdomen.

The future port site holes are injected with 1 ml of 0.25% bupivacaine. Because the vast majority of patients recover from the procedure with minimal analgesic requirements, epidural or spinal anesthesia is generally not required.

Positioning

Patient

The patient is positioned supine and is secured to the table with tape. Reverse Trendelenburg position with tilt to the left (head up, left side down) aids with intraoperative exposure of the gallbladder and bile ducts by allowing the bowel to fall away from the right upper quadrant.

Crew, Monitors, and Equipment

 Figure 60.1 shows the positions of the patient, crew, monitors, and equipment.

Fig. 60.1. Position of the patient, crew, monitors, and equipment

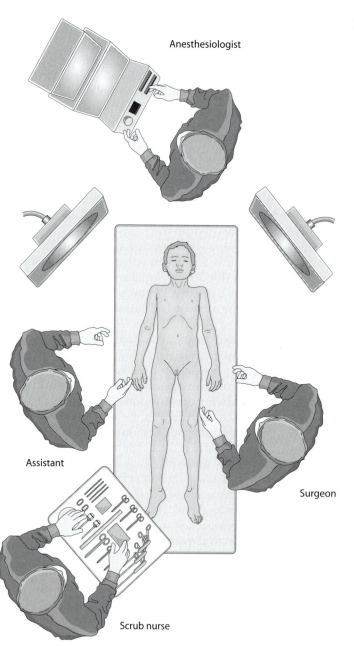

Anesthesiologist

Assistant

Surgeon

Scrub nurse

Special Equipment

No special energy applying systems are required

Other equipment	
Clips	Standard steel or self-locking plastic clips (i.e., Weck Hem-O-Lock; Weck Closure Systems, Research Triangle Park, NC, USA)
Graspers	Blunt endoscopic 3 mm graspers × 2
Dissector	Pointed-tipped curved 3 mm dissecting clamp
Scissors	Endoscopic Metzenbaum 3 mm scissors
Bag	Retrieval bag, 10 mm (i.e., USSC Endocatch; US Surgical, Norwalk, CT, USA)
X-ray	Fluoroscopy for intraoperative cholangiogram if indicated
Cholangiogram catheter	Kumar cholangioclamp with 23 g sclerotherapy needle (Holzman et al. 1994) or 6 French cholangiogram catheter (i.e., Cholangiocath; Cook Companies, Bloomington, IN, USA), if required

Port Positions

Position of the trocars depends on patient age, body habitus, relative size of the liver, location of the gallbladder, as well as surgeon preference and experience. The umbilical port is placed by a cutdown technique, the capnoperitoneum is established, and the laparoscope is inserted. The remaining ports are inserted under vision, first infiltrating the location with 0.25% bupivacaine solution, making an appropriate-sized skin incision with a number 11 blade scalpel, and then inserting the port through the fascia and peritoneum. The right lateral port is mainly used to suspend the fundus of the gallbladder anterosuperiorly. The instrument inserted through the right upper quadrant port pulls the gallbladder neck inferolaterally to open up the triangle of Calot. The dissecting instrument is inserted through the epigastric port. A 10 mm retrieval bag is introduced through the umbilical port to remove the gallbladder. ■ Figure 60.2 demonstrates the areas for port positioning of the umbilical, epigastric, right upper quadrant, and lateral ports. Generally, the younger the child, the more distant the ports should be inserted from the gallbladder to allow for adequate working space. Correspondingly, in younger children and infants, the epigastric port should be placed more laterally to increase the working space, whereas a midline position is often adequate in older children and adolescents. A 5 mm trocar is used at this location to accommodate the clip applier.

Technique

Cannulae

Cannula	Method of insertion	Diameter (mm)	Device	Position
1	Open	10, expandable trocar (i.e., Step; US Surgical, Norwalk, CT, USA)	5 mm 30° endoscope, 10 mm retrieval bag	Umbilicus
2	Closed	4, reusable (i.e., Storz trocar; Karl Storz, Tuttlingen, Germany)	Instrument for suspension of the gallbladder	Right subcostal anterior axillary line
3	Closed	4, reusable (i.e., Storz)	Working instrument	Right subcostal midclavicular line
4	Closed	5, expandable trocar (i.e., Step)	Working instrument	Mid to left epigastrium

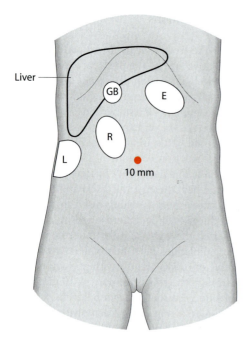

Fig. 60.2. Trocar positioning. *GB* Gallbladder, *red dot* umbilical port position (10 mm), *E* epigastric port position (5 mm), *R* right upper quadrant port position (3- to 4 mm), *L* lateral port position (3- to 4 mm)

Procedure

The abdomen of the patient is prepared and draped in a sterile fashion. The monitors, foot pedals, and other equipment are positioned to allow for a relaxed working position for both the surgeon and the assistant.

The umbilical skin is grasped and lifted upward by both lateral aspects with Adson forceps and the umbilical tissue is infiltrated with 1–2 ml 0.25% bupivacaine solution. A 10 mm vertical incision is performed through the umbilical skin with a number 11 blade scalpel and carried down through fascia and peritoneum. The Veress needle on the expanding sheath is introduced into the abdomen through the umbilical incision. A 5- or 10 mm port is introduced through the expandable sleeve after removal of the Veress needle. The abdomen is then insufflated through the umbilical port. The 5 mm 30° endoscope is introduced, and the other port sites are carefully chosen under direct endoscopic vision to allow for adequate working space and angulation. The other port sites are infiltrated with bupivacaine, a horizontal stab wound is made through the skin, and the other ports are placed, aiming toward the gallbladder.

A blunt grasping forceps is introduced from the right lateral port, grasping the fundus of the gallbladder and retracting it anterosuperiorly over the liver to expose the infundibulum and duct. A second grasper is introduced through the right upper quadrant port, pulling the gallbladder neck anteroinferiorly toward the right, thereby opening the triangle of Calot and creating a right angle between the cystic and common bile duct. This facilitates correct identification and dissection of both of these structures, preventing injury to the common bile duct (Fig. 60.3a).

Using the hook cautery and the sharp dissecting grasper, the peritoneum is stripped off the infundibulum down to the common bile duct, exposing and denuding the cystic duct and artery. Both structures are then clipped and divided with scissors. Alternatively, small arterial branches may be taken down by cautery (Fig. 60.3b–d).

The gallbladder is grasped at the neck, lifted anteriorly, and dissected off its liver bed using electrocautery. Care must be taken not to perforate the gallbladder wall, and any bleeding from the liver should be controlled. Once the gallbladder is detached, the laparoscope is changed to the 5 mm epigastric port. The 10 mm retrieval bag is introduced through the umbilical port. The gallbladder is placed inside the bag, the bag is pulled closed, and the specimen is removed through the umbilicus (Fig. 60.3e,f).

The intra-abdominal carbon dioxide is evacuated, and the umbilical fascial defect is closed with a 2-0 polydioxanone (PDS) figure-eight suture. The skin of all port sites is approximated using a simple subcuticular 4-0 poliglecaprone (i.e., Monocryl) suture, and covered with adhesive strips.

A gallbladder containing stones may be difficult to extract through the 10 mm umbilical port site. In this case, the retrieval bag is brought out through the wound and is held open by the assistant. The surgeon grasps the gallbladder with forceps, incises the wall, and extracts the stones individually until the specimen can be brought out through the incision. Large stones may be crushed into smaller fragments with a Kelly clamp to facilitate extraction.

In cases with unclear cystic duct anatomy, or to rule out common bile duct stones, an intraoperative cholangiogram may be necessary. There are two alternative techniques to accomplish this, using the Kumar cholangioclamp or by introduction of a cholangiogram catheter into the cystic duct near the gallbladder neck. In the former, the infundibulum of the gallbladder is clamped and a 23 g sclerotherapy needle is advanced through the Kumar clamp into the gallbladder neck. In the latter technique, the cholangiogram catheter is in-

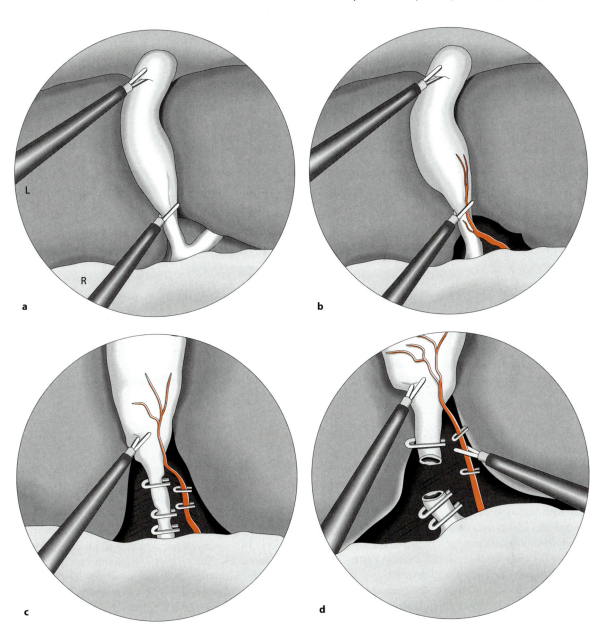

Fig. 60.3 a – d. a The grasper from the right lateral port (*L*) grasps the fundus of the gallbladder, lifts it upward and over the superior liver edge. The grasper from the right upper quadrant port (*R*) grasps the infundibulum, pulling anteriorly and toward the right, thereby opening up Calot's triangle. This creates a right angle between cystic and common bile ducts. **b** Starting from the infundibulum, the peritoneum is dissected and stripped off the cystic duct, opening up Calot's triangle. Care must be taken not to injure the cystic artery and its branches. **c** Three clips are applied onto the cystic duct, with two proximally on the side of the common bile duct. The cystic artery is clipped distally and proximally with two clips. **d** After clip application, the cystic duct and artery are divided using the Metzenbaum scissors which are introduced from the epigastric port. The right upper quadrant grasper continues to pull upward and anteriorly

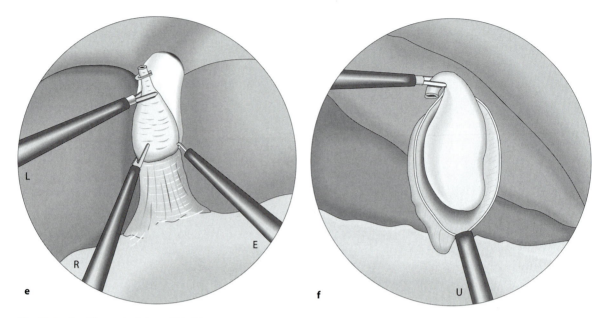

Fig. 60.3 e, f. **e** The neck of the gallbladder is grasped through the right lateral port (*L*) and lifted upward, providing traction on the junction of the gallbladder and liver. Using hook electrocautery from the epigastric port (*E*), the gallbladder is dissected off the liver bed from neck to fundus. **f** The endoscope is changed to the epigastric port, accounting for the different view. The retrieval bag is introduced through the 10 mm umbilical port (*U*). The gallbladder is placed into the bag, the bag is closed, and the gallbladder is removed through the navel

troduced through the right lateral port into the cystic duct through a small incision, and the catheter is secured in place with a clip. Regardless of the technique used, a cholangiogram is subsequently performed under fluoroscopy. Care must be taken to flush the catheter with the contrast agent before use to evacuate all air bubbles which may show up as contrast voids and falsely mimic gallstones. If normal anatomy is confirmed, the catheter is removed, and the cystic duct is clipped as described above and divided.

Laparoscopic exploration of the common bile duct, as well as choledochoscopy with stone retrieval has been described but is not routinely performed in children (Holcomb et al. 1999; Shah et al. 2001). As discussed below, other approaches to common bile duct stones have proven more efficient.

Postoperative Care

A nasogastric tube or urinary catheter is not required. The patient may be fed clear liquids when fully awake, and may advance to a regular diet as tolerated. Pain is usually controlled with a combination of oral acetaminophen and ibuprofen. Most patients are discharged on the day following the operation.

Results

In our own experience from September 1991 to October 2004, a total of 406 laparoscopic cholecystectomies were performed at our institution (mean age 10.4 years). ■ Figure 60.4 demonstrates the sharp rise in the numbers of procedures performed over the observation period. The mean conversion rate to an open procedure was 2.2%. The relative conversion rate decreased markedly with time and increased intrainstitutional experience. We performed intraoperative cholangiography in 29 cases (7.1%). Splenectomy (n=11, 2.7%), appendectomy (n=5, 1.2%), liver biopsy (n=3, 0.8%), and fundoplication (n=2, 0.5%) were the procedures most frequently performed simultaneously with laparoscopic cholecystectomy.

The most frequently reported complications from laparoscopic cholecystectomy are gallbladder perforation and biliary leak, trocar site infection, spillage of stones into the abdominal cavity, and prolonged bile leak, while major complications such as common bile duct injury are exceedingly rare (Esposito et al. 2001). Overall, the complication rate is similar to that of open cholecystectomy (Lugo-Vicente 1997a).

Fig. 60.4. Laparoscopic cholecystectomy – statistics

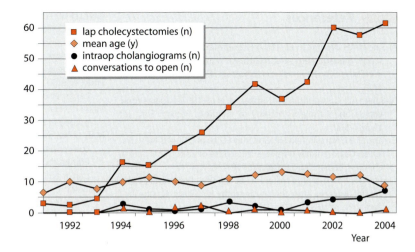

Discussion

The frequency of laparoscopic cholecystectomy in children has continuously increased since the 1990s. Whether this is due to a true rise in pediatric gallbladder pathology, a lower index of suspicion and referral threshold by pediatricians, improved diagnostic imaging, or a combination of the above remains speculative. In any case, laparoscopic cholecystectomy has become an established procedure in the treatment of children with gallbladder disease.

The management of common bile duct stones remains controversial, and several management algorithms have been proposed. Choledocholithiasis should be suspected in cases with a clinical history of jaundice or pancreatitis, laboratory findings including elevation of conjugated bilirubin, liver enzymes, amylase, or lipase, as well as preoperative sonographic evidence of common or intrahepatic bile duct dilatation, or a common bile duct stone. However, using these criteria, the reported specificity for common bile duct stones is 75%, and the sensitivity 83% (Waldhausen et al. 2001).

Some authors recommend routine preoperative ERCP with papillotomy and stone extraction before laparoscopic cholecystectomy when choledocholithiasis is suspected (Al-Salem and Nourallah 1997). The disadvantage of this approach is the need for another elaborate, expensive, and invasive procedure that requires general anesthesia in young children. Another approach is laparoscopic cholecystectomy with selective (Mah et al. 2004) or routine (Waldhausen et al. 2001) intraoperative cholangiogram, followed by ERCP, papillotomy, and stone extraction. Using intraoperative cholangiography to determine which patients require postoperative ERCP decreases the number of unnecessary endoscopic procedures. The third strategy involves performing an intraoperative cholangiogram and, if positive for common bile duct stones, proceed with either laparoscopic or open common bile duct exploration with stone retrieval.

Recently, gallbladder dyskinesia has been recognized as an etiology for chronic right upper quadrant pain in children and adolescents (Lugo-Vicente 1997b). Presenting symptoms include abdominal pain, fatty food intolerance, emesis, and diarrhea (Campbell et al. 2004). The typical diagnostic finding is delayed gallbladder emptying characterized by an ejection fraction of less than 35% on HIDA scan after intravenous administration of cholecystokinin. The majority of affected children become asymptomatic after cholecystectomy (Carney et al. 2004).

The main indications for conversion from laparoscopic cholecystectomy to an open procedure are uncontrollable bleeding and a common bile duct injury. Most other intraoperative complications can be managed laparoscopically.

The workup of postoperative jaundice and abdominal pain after laparoscopic cholecystectomy includes an abdominal ultrasound to rule out free intra-abdominal fluid, previously unrecognized choledocholithiasis, and dilated bile ducts. Laboratory evaluation comprises a cellular blood count to rule out leukocytosis and anemia, liver enzymes, fractionated bilirubin, as well as amylase and lipase levels. Bile leaks most commonly occur at the site of an inadequately clipped cystic duct stump and are managed with placement of an abdominal drain. Infrequently, an operative bile duct closure or revision is necessary.

When combination procedures such as laparoscopic splenectomy and cholecystectomy, or laparoscopic cholecystectomy and appendectomy are planned, the technically more challenging operation should predominantly dictate port placement. Therefore, in the former combination, we advocate standard port placement for splenectomy with a fifth port in the right lateral position to facilitate cholecystectomy. Conversely, an appendectomy can be performed through the port locations used for cholecystectomy as demonstrated in ■ Fig. 60.2.

References

Al-Salem AH, Nourallah H (1997) Sequential endoscopic/laparoscopic management of cholelithiasis and choledocholithiasis in children who have sickle cell disease. J Pediatr Surg 32:1432–1435

Al-Salem AH, Qaisaruddin S, Al-Abkari H, et al (1997) Laparoscopic versus open cholecystectomy in children. Pediatr Surg Int 12:587–590

Campbell BT, Narasimhan NP, Golladay ES, et al (2004) Biliary dyskinesia: a potentially unrecognized cause of abdominal pain in children. Pediatr Surg Int 20:579–581

Carney DE, Kokoska ER, Grosfeld JL, et al (2004) Predictors of successful outcome after cholecystectomy for biliary dyskinesia. J Pediatr Surg 39:813–816

Esposito C, Gonzalez Sabin MA, Corcione F, et al (2001) Results and complications of laparoscopic cholecystectomy in childhood. Surg Endosc 15:890–892

Holcomb GW 3rd, Morgan WM 3rd, Neblett WW 3rd, et al (1999) Laparoscopic cholecystectomy in children: lessons learned from the first 100 patients. J Pediatr Surg 34:1236–1240

Holzman MD, Sharp K, Holcomb GW, et al (1994) An alternative technique for laparoscopic cholangiography. Surg Endosc 8:927–930

Kim PC, Wesson D, Superina R, et al (1995) Laparoscopic cholecystectomy versus open cholecystectomy in children: which is better? J Pediatr Surg 30:971–973

Litynski GS (1998) Erich Mühe and the rejection of laparoscopic cholecystectomy (1985): a surgeon ahead of his time. J Soc Laparoendosc Surg 2:341–346

Lugo-Vicente HL (1997a) Trends in management of gallbladder disorders in children. Pediatr Surg Int 12:348–352

Lugo-Vicente HL (1997b) Gallbladder dyskinesia in children. J Soc Laparoendosc Surg 1:61–64

Luks FI, Logan J, Breuer CK, et al (1999) Cost-effectiveness of laparoscopy in children. Arch Pediatr Adolesc Med 153:965–968

Mah D, Wales P, Njere I, et al (2004) Management of suspected common bile duct stones in children: role of selective intraoperative cholangiogram and endoscopic retrograde cholangiopancreatography. J Pediatr Surg 39:808–812

Sandoval C, Stringel G, Ozkaynak MF, et al (2002) Perioperative management in children with sickle cell disease undergoing laparoscopic surgery. J Soc Laparoendosc Surg 6:29–33

Shah RS, Blakely ML, Lobe TE (2001) The role of laparoscopy in the management of common bile duct obstruction in children. Surg Endosc 15:1353–1355

Waldhausen, JHT, Graham DD, Tapper D (2001) Routine intraoperative cholangiography during laparoscopic cholecystectomy minimizes unnecessary endoscopic retrograde cholangiopancreatography in children. J Pediatr Surg 36:881–884

Abdomen

Spleen

Chapter 61

Splenectomy

Frederick J. Rescorla

Introduction

Laparoscopic splenectomy was initially reported in children in 1993 (Tulman et al. 1993) and since then has become the preferred technique at most institutions. The primary advantages cited for the laparoscopic approach include decreased postoperative pain medication requirement, less intestinal ileus, shorter postoperative hospital stay, and an improved cosmetic appearance. Operative times are usually longer with the laparoscopic approach and in addition to an initial steep learning curve the procedure may be difficult in cases of splenomegaly. Although some reports have questioned the efficacy of accessory spleen detection and potential for residual splenic function if capsular disruption occurs (Gigot et al. 1998; Targarona et al. 1998), most pediatric series have had comparable accessory spleen detection rates between open and laparoscopic cases (Minkes et al. 2000; Moores et al. 1995; Rescorla et al. 1996; Waldhausen and Tapper 1997).

Preoperative Preparation

Children with hemolytic disorders require gallbladder ultrasonography to evaluate for gallstones. Children with idiopathic thrombocytopenic purpura (ITP) can usually reach a platelet count of at least 50,000/mm with oral steroids, intravenous immunoglobulin, or Rh O(D) immunoglobulin (in Rh-positive patients). Children with sickle cell anemia are prepared with red cell transfusion to a hemoglobin level of 10 g/dL in order to prevent a crisis. Prior to splenectomy pneumococcal and *Neisseria meningitidis* vaccinations are administered. *Haemophilus influenzae* type B is part of routine immunizations and is usually not required as an additional immunization.

Before Induction of General Anesthesia

Routine NPO orders are utilized however no formal bowel preparation is necessary.

After Induction of General Anesthesia

Future port site holes are injected with 0.25% bupivacaine with 1:200,000 epinephrine (dose limit 1 ml/kg). Perioperative antibiotics are given which are continued postoperatively. A nasogastric tube and urinary catheter are in place during the procedure. A sequential compression device on the legs of adolescents is used.

Positioning

Patient

■ Figures 61.1 and 61.2 show the positions of the patient during the operation.

Crew, Monitors, and Equipment

■ Figure 61.3 shows the positions of the crew, monitors, and equipment.

Special Equipment

Ultrasonic energy should be at hand (harmonic scalpel). Other equipment is as follows:

Other equipment	
Clips	5 mm endoclips
Staplers	ETS Flex 45 Endoscopic Articulating Linear Cutter 45 mm staple line, 2.5 mm staple length (vascular thin); Ethicon EndoSurgery
Bag	Endocatch II (15 mm); Autosuture, for large spleens Endopouch (10 mm); Ethicon EndoSurgery, for small spleens

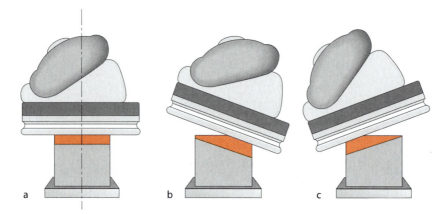

Fig. 61.1. Patient position. **a** Patient in posterolateral left at start of procedure. **b** During placement of trocars the table is tilted to the patient's left in order to achieve a typical supine position. **c** During the procedure the table is rotated to the right to achieve the lateral left position. Note the patient positioned to the right side of the table in order that instruments have full range of motion

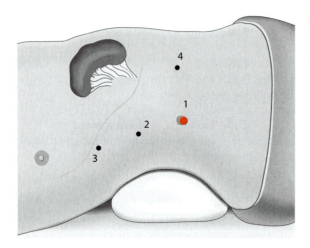

Fig. 61.2. Port positions. The patient is positioned in lateral left. A small roll is under the right side. Although not shown the left arm is draped over the head to the right side of the bed

Technique

Cannulae

Cannula	Method of insertion	Diameter (mm)	Device	Position
1	Open	15, Autosuture Versaport	Laparoscope, retrieval bag, stapler	Umbilical
2	Closed	3–5	Assistant's instrument	Midline
3	Closed	3–5	Assistant's instrument	Midline, close to the xiphoid
4	Closed	5	Harmonic scalpel	Left lower

Cannulae 2 and 3 are in the midline with cannula 3 very close to the xiphoid (■ Fig. 61.2). Cannula 4 is placed last and in adolescents may need to be placed higher in order to allow the instruments to reach to diaphragmatic attachments.

Fig. 61.3. Location of crew, monitors, and equipment

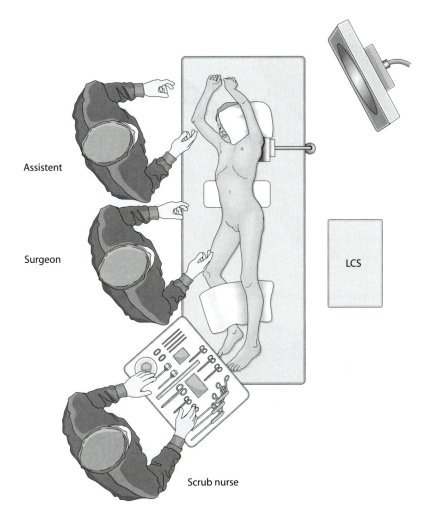

Assistent

Surgeon

LCS

Scrub nurse

Procedure

The cannulae are placed with the table rotated to the patient's left to approach the supine position (■ Fig. 61.1b). A 15 mm umbilical port is placed by the open technique in order to accommodate the 15 mm-diameter Endocatch II bag as well as the stapler. In a child with a small spleen, a 12 mm cannula is utilized since the spleen can fit in the 10 mm Endopouch. A 2-0 silk is often useful to stabilize the umbilical cannula. After insufflation to 12 mmHg and inspection of the peritoneum, the other three ports are placed by a closed technique. A 3 mm cannula can be utilized for one or both of the midline ports however these instruments need to be rather sturdy in order to lift the spleen and in many cases the 5 mm instruments will be needed. The left lower quadrant cannula is near the inguinal region in infants but may need to be higher in adolescents in order to allow the harmonic scalpel (LCS) to reach the upper splenic attachments. The table is then rotated to the right to achieve a lateral left position (■ Fig. 61.1c).

The first assistant uses primarily blunt graspers to elevate the spleen and provide traction on the various ligaments. The surgeon holds the camera (0° or 30° angled) with the left hand and the ultrasonic scalpel with the right. An initial diagnostic evaluation is performed and any accessory spleens are removed through the umbilical port. The splenocolic ligaments are divided with the LCS (■ Fig. 61.4). This device reaches high temperatures and the tips should not touch the colon. The assistant retracts the stomach to expose the lienogastric ligament and the short gastric vessels are divided working from inferior to superior with the LCS (■ Fig. 61.5). The lesser sac is inspected for the presence of accessory spleens. At the uppermost portion of the lienogastric ligament the spleen and stomach are very close and the LCS must be placed very close to the spleen in order to avoid gastric injury. At this point the first assistant gently elevates the upper pole and the diaphragmatic attachments are divided. This allows the assistant to elevate the spleen from the upper and lower poles.

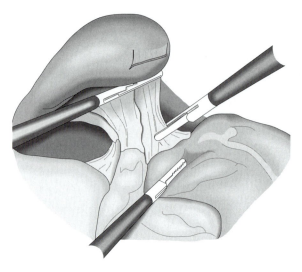

Fig. 61.4. Splenocolic ligaments divided by LCS

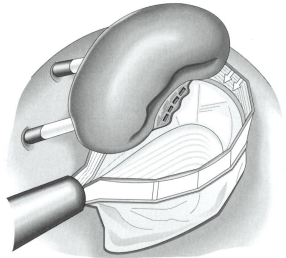

Fig. 61.7. Endocatch II bag deployed beneath spleen

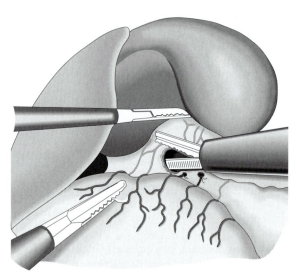

Fig. 61.5. Short gastrics divided by LCS

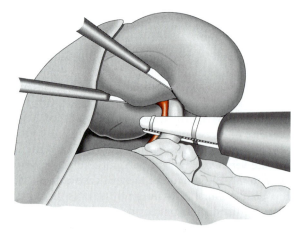

Fig. 61.6. Endoscopic stapler divides hilar vessels

If the pancreas is very close (<1 cm) to the spleen the vessels usually require individual ligation. In this situation the splenorenal ligament is left intact to allow the spleen to "hang." Small vessels are divided with the LCS and in some cases all of the vessels can be divided in this fashion. Some authors prefer the 10 mm LCS and use this on all major hilar vessels of 5- to 8 mm size (Schaarschmidt et al. 2002). Dissection around the vessels can be accomplished with the curved dolphin-nosed forceps and the 5 mm clip applier utilized with two clips placed toward the pancreas and one toward the spleen.

If the pancreas is 1 cm or greater from the pancreas the endoscopic stapler can be utilized to divide the hilar vessels. At this point the splenorenal ligament is divided with the LCS. The spleen is then completely elevated as shown in ■ Fig. 61.6 and the stapler applied. In order to accomplish this the 5 mm telescope is placed through the left lower quadrant cannula and the stapler passed through the umbilical trocar.

After the spleen is completely free it is held high in the left upper quadrant and the bag is placed through the umbilical cannula, positioned under the spleen, and deployed. The spleen is gently dropped into the open bag (■ Fig. 61.7) and with great care the surgeon "rocks" the bag back and forth to advance the spleen into the bag. Separation of the top of the bag from the metal supporting ring can be troublesome and if this occurs the first assistant must lift up on the bag with one instrument and push the spleen in with the other. The Endocatch II bag has a diameter of 13 cm and a depth of 23 cm and most spleens will fit in it.

The drawstring is pulled to separate the top of the bag from the ring and close the bag. The supporting

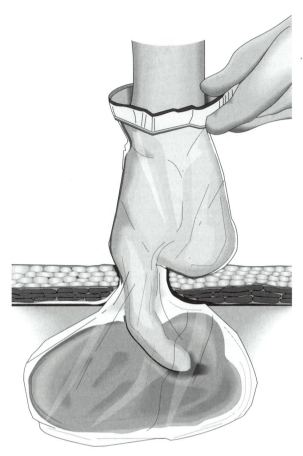

Table 61.1 Experience and results with laparoscopic splenectomy in 142 children

Operative time (min; mean and range)[a]	
Laparoscopic splenectomy	106 (45–210)
Laparoscopic splenectomy and cholecystectomy	135 (75–240)
Accessory spleens	29 (20.4%)
Length of stay (days; mean)	
Hereditary spherocytosis	1.25
Idiopathic thrombocytopenic purpura	1.15
Sickle cell anemia	2.42
Complications	
Conversion to open	4 (2.8%)
Bleeding/transfusion	2
Diaphragm perforation	1
Ileus	4
Acute chest syndrome	5
Pneumonia	1
Missed accessory spleen	1

[a] Range based on initial 127 patients

Fig. 61.8. Surgeon's finger disrupting splenic capsule and removing fragments

ring is withdrawn under direct vision and the bag is then drawn up into the cannula and the cannula removed. The neck of the bag is elevated and the surgeon's finger introduced (■ Fig. 61.8) to fracture the spleen. If a ring forceps is utilized for this step care must be taken to avoid bag disruption.

Completion laparoscopy is performed to ensure adequate hemostasis. The ports are removed and closure of the port sites performed. The fascia at the umbilical site is closed and if possible the anterior fascial layer is closed at 5 mm trocar sites. If concomitant cholecystectomy is required the lower 5 mm midline cannula is placed directly over the gallbladder and one additional trocar placed on the right side to provide retraction of the gallbladder.

Postoperative Care

The nasogastric tube and urinary catheter are removed at the end of the procedure. Pain control is achieved with an acetaminophen and codeine mixture. Intravenous non-steroidal medications (ketorolac) are given for 24 h in the absence of thrombocytopenia. Although this provides adequate pain relief for most, some may occasionally require intravenous narcotics.

A clear liquids diet is instituted upon arrival to the floor with advancement to a regular diet as tolerated. Maintenance intravenous fluids are weaned as the fluid intake advances. Most children are discharged the following day.

Results

The experience and results with laparoscopic splenectomy in 142 children at the authors institution are listed in ■ Table 61.1. The mean age was 7.3 years and weight 28.6 kg. Splenectomy was performed for spherocytosis (73), ITP (28), sickle cell anemia (26), and various other indications (15). Twenty-four underwent concomitant cholecystectomy. The postoperative hospital stay was relatively short with 103 of the children released on postoperative day 1. As noted the stay is longer in children with sickle cell anemia, a group which also had a 21% complication rate. The four conversions were for splenomegaly in 2, bleeding in 1, and adhesions from a prior procedure in 1. In one of the splenomegaly cases the spleen was completely detached laparoscopically but would not fit in the bag and therefore a left lower quadrant incision was utilized to remove the spleen.

Discussion

The data comparing laparoscopic and open splenectomy come primarily from case-controlled series rather than from prospective randomized series. Nearly every comparative series has demonstrated that laparoscopic splenectomy requires longer operating time but results in lower narcotic use and shorter length of stay in hospital (Moores et al. 1995; Rescorla et al. 1996; Waldhausen and Tapper 1997). Although operative time decreases with experience, our center's current operative times are still longer than the 83-min average with open splenectomy observed in our comparative study (Rescorla et al. 1996). Pain has generally been assessed by narcotic usage and several series have noted approximately 50% less narcotic use with the laparoscopic approach (Curran et al. 1998; Reddy et al. 2001; Rescorla et al. 1996). All comparative series in children demonstrate a shorter length of stay for laparoscopic splenectomy (Curran et al. 1998; Minkes et al. 2000; Moores et al. 1995; Rescorla et al. 1996; Waldhausen and Tapper 1997) although the length of stay for open splenectomy in children can be rather low (2.5–2.7 days) (Geiger et al. 1998; Rescorla et al. 1996).

The complication rate with laparoscopic splenectomy has been very low. A comparative evaluation of open and laparoscopic splenectomies in children between 1995 and 2002 noted no significant difference in the complication rates (Rescorla 2002). In addition there were no Clavien (Clavien et al. 1992) grade III (residual or lasting disability, iatrogenic organ resection) or grade IV (death) complications in either group. Although splenomegaly can make the laparoscopic technique difficult, most childhood spleens will fit in the Endocatch II bag. There has been concern in several series over the detection of accessory spleens (Gigot et al. 1998; Targarona et al. 1998), however most series (Moores et al. 1995; Reddy et al. 2001; Rescorla et al. 1996; Waldhausen and Tapper 1997) have had comparable rates between open and laparoscopic splenectomy.

Laparoscopic splenectomy is equal in efficacy to open splenectomy and results in less postoperative narcotic use, shorter length of stay, and an improved cosmetic appearance. Laparoscopic splenectomy requires a longer operative time than open splenectomy. A careful search must be performed for accessory spleens and the surgeon should avoid intraperitoneal splenic capsule disruption. The laparoscopic approach appears to be the preferred method for splenectomy.

References

Clavien PA, Sanabria JR, Strasberg SM (1992) Proposed classification of complications of surgery with examples of utility in cholecystectomy. Surgery 111:518–526

Curran TJ, Foley MI, Swanstrom LL, et al (1998) Laparoscopy improves outcomes for pediatric splenectomy. J Pediatr Surg 33:1498–1500

Geiger JD, Dinh VV, Teitelbaum DH, et al (1998) The lateral approach for open splenectomy. J Pediatr Surg 33:1153–1156

Gigot JF, Jamar F, Ferrant A, et al (1998) Inadequate detection of accessory spleens and splenosis with laparoscopic splenectomy: a shortcoming of the laparoscopic approach in hematologic diseases. Surg Endosc 12:101–106

Minkes RK, Lagzdins M, Langer JC (2000) Laparoscopic versus open splenectomy in children. J Pediatr Surg 35:699–701

Moores, DC, McKee MA, Wang H, et al (1995) Pediatric laparoscopic splenectomy. J Pediatr Surg 30:1201–1205

Reddy VS, Phan HH, O'Neill JA, et al (2001) Laparoscopic versus open splenectomy in the pediatric population: a contemporary single-center experience. Am Surg 67:859–863

Rescorla FJ (2002) Laparoscopic splenectomy. Semin Pediatr Surg 11:226–232

Rescorla FJ, Breitfeld PP, West KW, et al (1996) A case controlled comparison of open and laparoscopic splenectomy in children. Surgery 124:670–676

Schaarschmidt K, Kolberg-Schwerdt A, Lempe M, et al (2002) Ultrasonic shear coagulation of main hilar vessels: a 4-year experience of 23 pediatric laparoscopic splenectomies without staples. J Pediatr Surg 37:614–616

Targarona EM, Espert JJ, Balague C, et al (1998) Residual splenic function after laparoscopic splenectomy: a clinical concern. Arch Surg 133:56–60

Tulman S, Holcomb GW, Karamanoukian HL, et al (1993) Laparoscopic splenectomy. J Pediatr Surg 28:689–692

Waldhausen JHT, Tapper D (1997) Is pediatric laparoscopic splenectomy safe and cost-effective? Arch Surg 132:822–824

Chapter 62

Partial Splenectomies by Laparoscopy in Children

Olivier Reinberg

Introduction

Total splenectomy in children carries the risk of fulminant septicemia. Since the 1970s, the mortality risk by septicemia after total splenectomy has been proven to be 200 times higher than in a general pediatric population (all ages). However, it seems to be much higher below 4 years of age (8%) than above this age (3%) (Eraklis et al. 1967). In 1972, the American Association of Pediatrics (AAP) recommended for this reason not to remove the spleen before 5 years of age (Eraklis and Filler 1972). This rule is still in use today, especially in pediatric hematology.

Partial splenectomy has become feasible since a better knowledge of the vascularization of the spleen through anatomic studies of vascular moldings has been acquired (Liu et al. 1996; Revillon and Girot 1985). The splenic artery divides in the hilum or within the spleen itself into two or three intrasplenic arteries, which do not anastomose with each other and are therefore terminal branches. The veins follow the arterial distribution. This vascular arrangement divides the spleen into segments surrounded by poorly vascularized zones perpendicular to the capsula and converging to the hilum. Studying 850 splenic specimens, Liu et al. (1996) found that 86% of the spleens had two

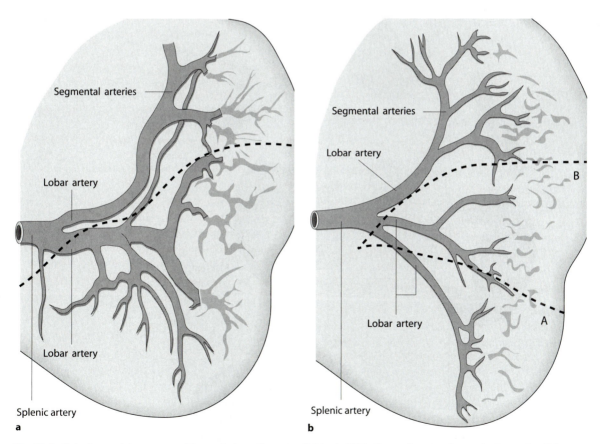

Fig. 62.1. Splenic arterial anatomy. **a** The main hepatic artery divides in 86% of cases into two intrasplenic arteries. This configuration allows for hemisplenectomy (*dotted line*). **b** The main splenic artery divides in 12% of cases into three intrasplenic arteries, allowing for a one third or two thirds partial splenectomy (*dotted lines*)

lobar arteries (■ Fig. 62.1a). Such spleens are suitable for hemisplenectomy. Three arteries were found in 12.2% of the specimens, allowing either a one third or a two thirds splenectomy (■ Fig. 62.1b). One percent of the spleens had multiple lobar arteries and only 0.8% had a unique non-divided artery. In those patients partial splenectomy is very difficult or impossible to accomplish.

On such a basis, pediatric surgeons have performed partial splenectomies mostly for hematologic or metabolic diseases (al-Salem et al. 1998; de Buys Roessingh et al. 2002; Kimber et al. 1998; Rice et al. 2003; Roth et al. 1982). In order to reduce the risk of sepsis, we never perform a total splenectomy before the age of 5 years. In our experience partial splenectomy has allowed to lower this age limit to 2.2 years thus avoiding repeat blood transfusions.

The prognosis of partial splenectomy is uncertain. In some cases the procedure is sufficient (Bowen and Gough 1994; Hayari et al. 1994; Kimber et al. 1998; Rice et al. 2003), but in others, the spleen regenerated and after a few months or years, reoperation became necessary (de Buys Roessingh et al. 2002; Rice et al. 2003). Over time, variable rates of splenic regrowth were noted, although regrowth did not necessarily correlate with recurrent hemolysis (Rice et al. 2003). However, the reoperated children had reached the age of 5 years, allowing a total splenectomy with a decreased risk of sepsis. Since 1997, we have started to perform laparoscopic partial splenectomies for onco-hematologic indications or for hamartomas.

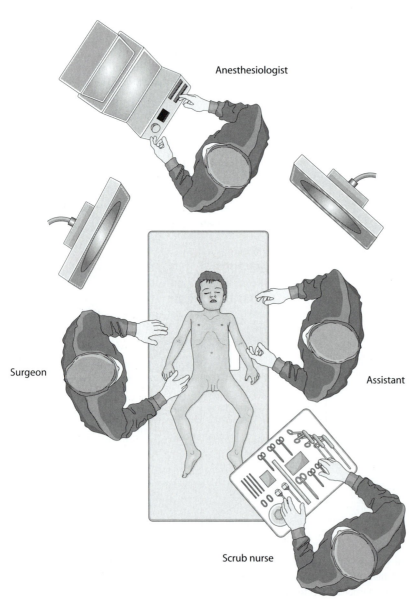

Fig. 62.2. Positioning of the patient, crew and monitors

Anesthesiologist

Surgeon

Assistant

Scrub nurse

Preoperative Preparation

All children are vaccinated against pneumococci and hemophilus at least 1 month before surgery. General anesthesia with intubation and curarization is given. A nasogastric tube is placed and kept under suction for gastric decompression. Prophylactic antibiotics are given (ampicillin or penicillin).

Positioning

The patient is placed in a supine position with the left flank slightly elevated with a bean pad. The surgeon stays to the right and the assistant to the left of the operating table. The scrub nurse also stays on the left of the table, but lower down than the assistant (■ Fig. 62.2).

Special Equipment

The availability of ultrasonic energy is a must. A Diamond-Flex circular retractor is used for elevation of the liver. This retractor can also be placed around the spleen to seize it and to easily expose the working area.

Technique

Cannulae

A Hassan-type technique is used for the insertion of the first cannula. A vertical 10 mm incision is carried out in the deepest part of the umbilicus allowing for the insertion of the telescope port. We do not refrain from making a rather large incision as this port hole will be widened later for extraction of the splenic specimen. A 7 mm with 45° beveled-end reusable trocar is inserted. A purse-string suture, which includes the peritoneum and the fascia, is inserted around the trocar, and is tied to the stopcock in order to achieve an airtight seal and to prevent the trocar from slipping out of the wound. A 7 mm-diameter, 25°, 300 mm-long telescope is set up and CO_2 insufflation started at a pressure of 10 mmHg. The use of a 7 mm or even a 10 mm telescope instead of a 4 mm one allows for the introduction of more light, which is advantageous if bleeding occurs or when the spleen is divided, as light is absorbed by the red color of blood. Next three 5 mm reusable ports are inserted, one down in the left flank (if possible 3–5 cm below the lower pole of the spleen) for instruments, one 3–5 cm right to the midline slightly above the umbilicus for instruments, and one in the right hypochondrium at the level of the liver edge for liver and/or spleen retractor (■ Fig. 62.3).

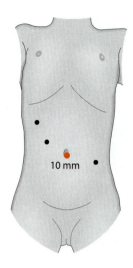

Fig. 62.3. Trocar positions for partial splenectomy

10 mm

Procedure

The spleen dissection starts at its lower pole, by dividing its epiploic and splenocolic attachments, either by coagulation and cutting, or with the use of the 5 mm-diameter harmonic scalpel, either the 14 cm short or the 36 cm long curved shears, according to the size of the patient (■ Fig. 62.4a). Next the anterior part of the splenic hilum is widely exposed and the number of segmental arteries is identified. An angulated telescope is helpful for this step as it allows a view of the whole pedicle from above (■ Fig. 62.4b). If two arteries are present a hemisplenectomy can be performed. In case of three arteries the choice will be to perform either a one third or a two thirds splenectomy. Usually the latter is preferred. The decision as to how extensive the partial resection should be is taken in the operating room together with the pediatric oncologist. As we do not know the number of arteries until we have seen them, we cannot predict preoperatively which part of the spleen can be removed.

The branches of the pedicle are dissected. We start with the lower vascular bundle for the lower segment of the spleen. Usually the artery is found first, as the vein lies behind and above it. All vascular structures are carefully dissected and freed for 1–2 cm. It is often necessary to dissect them in close touch with the splenic parenchyma in order to get sufficient and safe length. It is mandatory to avoid any laceration of the spleen as bleeding from the parenchyma is much more difficult to deal with than bleeding from a vessel. For dissection we use a monopolar hook which is not connected to the electrocautery unit, as this hook is a very convenient dissector for this purpose. Smooth short scissors or a Johann grasper can also be used (■ Fig. 62.4b). Then the vessels are separately divided to avoid any arteriovenous shunt to occur. The vascular division can be made by electrocautery or ultrasonic cautery, or by clipping (5 mm diameter). Most of the

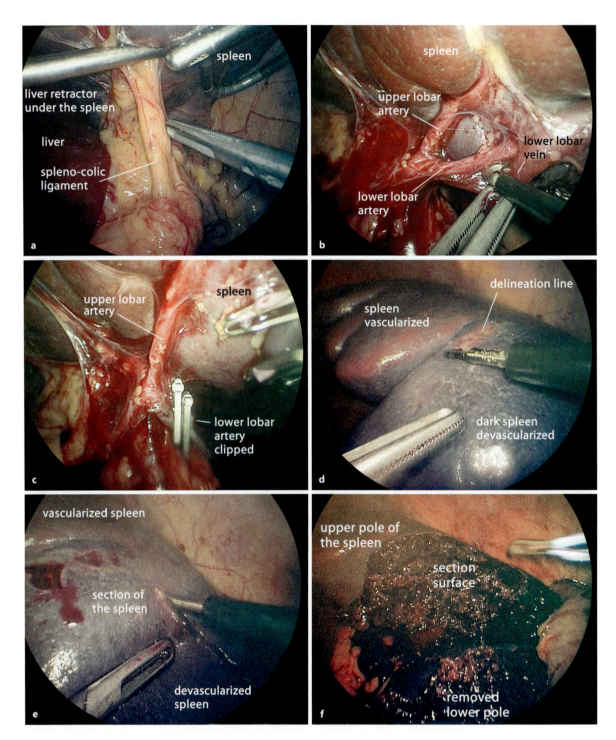

Fig. 62.4. a Division of the epiploic attachments (gastrocolic ligament) at the lower pole of the spleen. **b** View of the splenic pedicle from above and dissection of its branches. **c** Division of the lower artery. **d** Demarcation between the vascularized and ischemic parts of the spleen. **e** Transection of the spleen. **f** Partial splenectomy completed

time we clip on the proximal part of the vessel twice and transect the distal part onto the spleen either by electrocautery or ultrasonic cautery (■ Fig. 62.4c). Once the first vascular bundle is divided, the lower pole of the spleen darkens and shows a demarcation line between the vascularized and ischemic parts (■ Fig. 62.4d).

The remaining vascular branches of the hilum are dissected and divided in the same way from the lower to the upper pole of the spleen, until a sufficient amount of spleen has been devascularized. At this step the upper pole remains vascularized by one or two arterial branches from the hilum, and the short gastrosplenic vessels.

The resection line is then drawn on the surface of the devascularized spleen 1 cm from the demarcation line with an ultrasonic 5 mm-diameter sickle probe (LaparoSonic Dissecting Hook, 31 cm; Ethicon Endo-Surgery). This landmark should surround the whole spleen and is useful to avoid entering into the vascularized part of the spleen when dividing it (▪ Fig. 62.4d). The spleen is divided with the Ultracision 5 mm sickle probe. It is a time-consuming step as we set the harmonic scalpel at short wave energy (i.e., approximately 50 µm, level 2) to achieve maximal hemostasis but slow cutting. If the cutting plane remains in the devascularized part, the section is nearly bloodless (▪ Fig. 62.4e). Once the lower part has been divided, the dissection plane is rinsed and any remaining bleeding vessels can be treated by either Ultracision or bipolar coagulation (▪ Fig. 62.4f).

For division of the spleen we prefer to use the Ultracision 5 mm sickle probe instead of the curved shears, as it gives a sharp cut with no risk of loose splenic fragments. Moreover when scissors are used, grasping splenic tissue squeezes the splenic parenchyma before cutting with risk of spillage. During the division of the spleen the telescope often has to be wiped off as the Ultracision produces a foam which sticks on the lens close to the target in a narrow pediatric field.

Next, the removed spleen has to be placed into a bag. This can be a difficult and time-consuming step of the procedure. The telescope is transferred to the right inferior port to free the umbilical one (▪ Fig. 62.5). We have a second 4 mm-diameter telescope on our set but the former one can be used after widening the port incision. A self-opening bag (Endobag 10 mm in diameter, opening to 12.5 cm in diameter or Endocatch Gold 10 mm in diameter, opening to 15 cm in diameter; both by Autosuture Tyco) is introduced through the umbilicus. Alternatively a standard bag (Endobag 10 mm in diameter, opening to 10 cm in diameter; by LINA) is introduced with a grasper. Leakage of CO_2 through the umbilical wound is prevented by pulling on the purse-string suture, which was placed at the beginning of the procedure. In our opinion, this is the easiest way to place a resected spleen in its bag. The bag is closed with an atraumatic grasper or with the special string device if a self-opening bag has been used. The umbilical skin incision is widened to 2–3 cm and the midline aponeurosis to 4–5 cm with the umbilical port in place in order to avoid any tearing of the bag. Its margins are extracted through the umbilicus, and the spleen is digitally fragmented in the bag (▪ Fig. 62.6). Pieces are extracted with smooth graspers or suction.

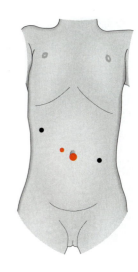

Fig. 62.5. Trocar positions for spleen extraction

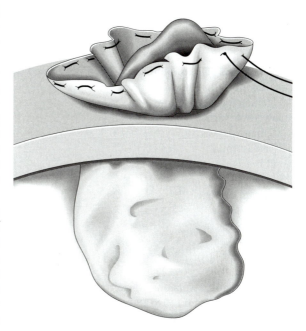

Fig. 62.6. Spleen extraction

We never use sharp instruments to avoid any damage to the bag. After splenic extraction, the bag is checked for leakage with water.

Postoperative Care

Children stay in bed for 3 days after surgery. Just before discharge an ultrasound is made to look for possible fluid collections and/or for thrombosis of the splenic vein, which did not occur in our series. Prophylactic antibiotics (ampicillin or penicillin) are given for 3 months.

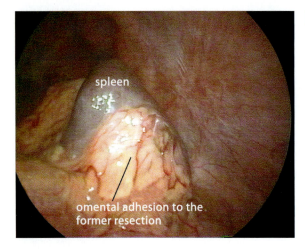

spleen

omental adhesion to the former resection

Fig. 62.7. View of the spleen at a redo procedure for total splenectomy

Results

Eleven partial splenectomies have been performed so far. The indications were:

- Hematologic conditions   9
  Pyruvate kinase deficiency   2
  Spherocystosis   5
  Thalassemia   1
  ITP   1
  (age 2.1–4.5 years)
- Benign tumors   2
  Hamartoma
  23×20×15 cm
  12×12×5 cm
  (age 8 and 11 years)

There were no conversions. Mean operating time was 140 min (limits from 110 to 180 min). We never had to convert to an open procedure. Blood loss was always below 200 ml and a blood transfusion was never required.

Our five first patients had a scintigraphy performed a few months after partial splenectomy. None showed a splenosis.

Two of the hematologic patients were reoperated for recurrent hypersplenism 1.5 and 2.1 years later, and a third patient is scheduled for total splenectomy. Total splenectomies by laparoscopy were then performed. Except for one omental adherence to the edge of the divided spleen (■ Fig. 62.7), no adhesion could be seen. In one of the patients an accessory spleen was left in situ. In case of recurrence, a third laparoscopy could be performed.

Discussion

Although only a small series has been analyzed, the results are very encouraging. Partial splenectomy allows to reduce hypersplenism in children with hematologic conditions under 5 years of age. In addition it can be performed by laparoscopy. As well as the cosmetic advantages and absence of abdominal wall trauma, it may lead to the formation of fewer adhesions. This allows for a repeat laparoscopic procedure when total splenectomy is required. It is obviously not an easy procedure, and should only be performed by trained laparoscopic pediatric surgeons.

The use of a harmonic scalpel is mandatory. In our opinion it cannot be replaced by new devices such as Ligasure for the cutting reasons mentioned above, nor by Endo-GIA. Any squeezing devices add the risk of spillage. The sickle probe allows a sharp division of the spleen, with good hemostasis. The same result has been achieved with argon beam devices, but their availability is restricted (Idowu and Hayes-Jordan 1998). We do not us either glue or hemostatic pads and do not insert drains because the introduction of foreign material increases the risk for infection if any collection should occur.

We successfully used the same technique in a case with a large (23 cm) non-parasitic splenic cyst, as has been described before (Belas et al. 1987; Hayari et al. 1994; Khan et al. 1986; Lambrecht and Weinland 1981; Moir et al. 1989; Seshadri et al. 1998; Todde et al. 1989).

The postoperative treatment regarding a lesser immunocompetence remains unclear. A significant drop in immunologic functions after open partial splenectomy has been described (Brown et al. 1989). If so, it seems wise to prevent infections by systematic vaccinations before and after surgery and by postoperative antibiotherapy for an indefinite period. Some authors, however, stop medication at 3 months postoperatively provided that the platelet count and splenic computed tomography (CT) scan are normal (Brown et al. 1989).

Recurrent hypersplenism after partial splenectomy has been documented both experimentally (Bar-Miaor et al. 1988; Hayari et al. 1994) as well as in man, even if not seen systematically (de Buys Roessingh et al. 2002; Fleshner et al. 1989). The rate of recurrence seems lower for metabolic than for hematologic disorders but higher for Gaucher's disease (de Buys Roessingh et al. 2002; Holcomb and Greene 1993; Kimber et al. 1998; Rice et al. 2003; Zimran et al. 1995). There is no reason to believe that the risk of recurrence should be otherwise when the procedure is carried out laparoscopically. Even if so, the gain of some months or years of remission without pain, without recurrent blood transfusion, and therefore allowing the child to reach an age where total splenectomy can be done with a lower risk of sepsis should be considered (Banani and Bahador 1994; Idowu and Hayes-Jordan 1998; Nouri et al. 1991).

In some diseases such partial splenectomy should not be performed. Holcomb reported a case of an 18-month-old child with Gaucher's disease who underwent an uneventful partial splenectomy. He died 4 months later after a sudden increase of the remaining spleen leading to a spontaneous rupture and massive hemorrhage (Holcomb and Greene 1993). This complication cannot be considered to be related to the laparoscopic approach but was rather to the underlying condition. Gaucher's disease could carry a higher risk of recurrence (Freud et al. 1998) and should not be considered for partial splenectomy.

References

al-Salem AH, al-Dabbous I, Bhamidibati P (1998) The role of partial splenectomy in children with thalassemia. Eur J Pediatr Surg 8:334–338

Banani SA, Bahador A (1994) Management of thalassemia major by partial splenectomy. Pediatr Surg Int 9:350–352

Bar-Miaor JA, Sweed Y, Shoshany G (1988) Does the spleen regenerate after partial splenectomy in the dog? J Pediatr Surg 23:128–129

Belas M, Audry G, Lissitzky T, et al (1987) La splénectomie partielle dans les kystes épidermoides de la rate chez l'enfant. Chir Pediatr 28:133–136

Bowen J, Gough D (1994) Splenic regeneration does not occur after sub-total splenectomy. Pediatr Surg Int 9:423–424

Brown MF, Ross AJ, Bishop HC, et al (1989) Partial splenectomy: the preferred alternative for the treatment of splenic cysts. J Pediatr Surg 24:694–696

de Buys Roessingh AS, de Lagausie P, Rohrlich P, et al (2002) Follow-up of partial splenectomy in children with hereditary spherocytosis. J Pediatr Surg 37:1459–1463

Eraklis AJ, Filler RM (1972) Splenectomy in childhood: a review of 1413 cases. J Pediatr Surg 4:382–388

Eraklis AJ, Kevy SV, Diamond LK, et al (1967) Hazard of overwhelming infection after splenectomy in childhood. N Engl J Med 276:1225–1229

Fleshner PR, Astion DJ, Ludman MD, et al (1989) Gaucher disease: fate of the splenic remnant after partial splenectomy: a case of rapid enlargement. J Pediatr Surg 24:610–612

Freud E, Cohen IJ, Mor C, et al (1998) Splenic "regeneration" after partial splenectomy for Gaucher disease: histological features. Blood Cells Mol Dis 24:309–316

Hayari L, Livne E, Bar-Maor JA (1994) Does the spleen regenerate after partial splenectomy? A morphological, biochemical, and radioautographic study in rats. Pediatr Surg Int 9:35–40

Holcomb GW III, Greene HL (1993) Fatal hemorrhage caused by disease progression after partial splenectomy for type III Gaucher's disease. J Pediatr Surg 28:1572–1574

Idowu O, Hayes-Jordan A (1998) Partial splenectomy in children under 4 years of age with hemoglobinopathy. J Pediatr Surg 33:1251–1253

Khan AH, Bensoussan AL, Ouimet A, et al (1986) Partial splenectomy for benign cystic lesion of the spleen. J Pediatr Surg 21:749–752

Kimber C, Spitz L, Drake D, et al (1998) Elective partial splenectomy in childhood. J Pediatr Surg 33:826–829

Lambrecht W, Weinland G (1981) Organerhaltende operation bel grosser epidermoidzyste de milz (Organ preserving operation in large epidermoid cyst of the spleen). Z Kinderchir 32:286–290

Liu DL, Xia S, Xu W, Fe Q, et al (1996) Anatomy of vasculature of 850 spleen specimens and its application in partial splenectomy. Surgery 19:27–33

Moir C, Guttmann S, Jequier S, Sonnino R, Youssef S (1989) Splenic cysts: aspiration, sclerosis, or resection. J Pediatr Surg 24:646–648

Nouri A, DeMontalembert M, Revillon Y, et al (1991) Partial splenectomy in sickle cell syndromes. Arch Dis Child 66:1070–1072

Revillon Y, Girot R (1985) Désartérialisation partielle de la rate et splénectomie partielle chez l'enfant. Presse Med 14:423–425

Rice HE, Oldham KT, Hillery CA, et al (2003) Clinical and hematologic benefits of partial splenectomy for congenital hemolytic anemias in children. Ann Surg 237:281–288

Roth H, Daum R, Bolkenius M (1982) Partielle milzresektion mit fibrinklebung. Eine alternativezur splenektomie und autotransplantation. Z Kinderchir 35:153–158

Seshadri PA, Poenaru D, Park A (1998) Laparoscopic splenic cystectomy: a case report. J Pediatr Surg 33:1439–1440

Todde G, Bagolan P, Fariello G, et al (1989) Kyste épidermoïde de la rate chez un nouveau-né. Diagnostic anténatal et splénectomie partielle. Chir Pediatr 30:172–174

Zimran A, Elstein D, Schiffmann R, et al (1995) Outcome of partial splenectomy for type I Gaucher disease. J Pediatr 126:596–597

Abdomen

Pancreas

Chapter 63

Laparoscopic Approaches to the Pancreas

Steven S. Rothenberg

Introduction

Diseases of the pancreas in children requiring surgical intervention are relatively rare. They include nesidioblastosis, adenomas, rare carcinomas, and pancreatic pseudocyst. While the pancreas is a retroperitoneal structure it is easily accessible using a laparoscopic approach (Bhattacharya and Ammori 2003). Access depends on the specific disease process being addressed and the portion of the pancreas involved. Surgical approaches include access through the greater sac, through mobilization of the duodenum, or transgastric. Nesidioblastosis will be discussed in a separate chapter. The approach for pancreatic pseudocyst and discrete tumors of the pancreas, which is very similar to that in open surgery, will be the primary focus of this discussion.

Preoperative Preparation

Before Induction of General Anesthesia

The most important aspect of the preoperative management is good imaging of the pancreas to help direct the surgical procedure. Abdominal imaging by ultrasound and/or computed tomography (CT) scan is of vital importance to plan the appropriate approach. CT scan can help identify the size, extent, and wall thickness of the pseudocyst as well as show evidence of a mass in the head, body, or tail of the pancreas. In some instances an endoscopic retrograde cholangiopancreatogram (ERCP) or magnetic resonance cholangiopancreatogram (MRCP) may be of benefit to identify the ductal anatomy of the pancreas. These studies can be important in trying to determine the most appropriate procedure to obtain adequate drainage of a pancreatic pseudocyst. A bowel preparation, especially a cleansing enema, may help in improving the ability to manipulate the colon out of the operative field.

After Induction of General Anesthesia

A nasogastric tube is placed and the bladder is emptied by the Credé maneuver. A preoperative dose of antibiotics, usually a second-generation cephalosporin, is given. Local anesthetic, 0.25% Marcaine, is injected at all port sites prior to making an incision.

Positioning

Patient

The patient is placed in a modified dorsal lithotomy position at the foot of the table (■ Fig. 63.1). Larger patients are placed in stirrups with the thighs extended straight out and the knees flexed at 90°. This keeps the legs from interfering with the shafts of the instruments. Smaller patients may simply be placed in a frog-leg position at the end of the table.

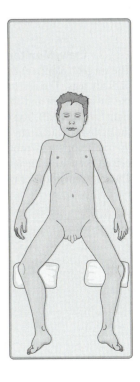

Fig. 63.1. Patient position. Modified dorsal lithotomy position

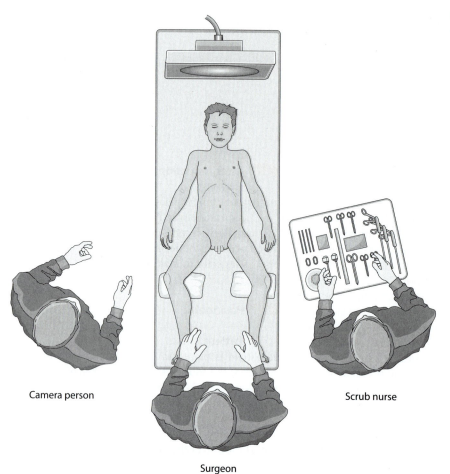

Fig. 63.2. Positioning of the crew and equipment

Camera person

Scrub nurse

Surgeon

Crew, Monitors, and Equipment

The surgeon stands at the foot of the table between the patients legs. The assistant, holding the camera, is on the surgeon's left and the scrub nurse on the surgeon's right (■ Fig. 63.2). The primary monitor is placed over the patient's head so the surgeon is working in line with the pathology and monitor. A secondary monitor is placed near the patient's left shoulder for the assistant. The instrument tower is usually on the patient's right.

Special Equipment

Ultrasonic energy and or Ligasure should be at hand. Other equipment is as follows:

Equipment	Required
Clips	Yes, 5 mm Endoclip
Staplers	Yes
Bag	Yes, for specimen removal
Intraoperative ultrasound	Yes, for adenomas

Technique

Cannulae

Cannula	Method of insertion	Diameter (mm)	Device	Position
1	Closed	3, 5, or 12	3- or 5 mm, 30° scope, endoscopic stapler if used	Umbilicus
2	Closed	5	Clip applier, scissors, ultrasonic shears	Left midquadrant
3	Closed	3 or 5	Maryland dissector	Right midquadrant
4	Closed	3 or 5	Retractor, Babcock clamp	Midepigastrium

Procedure

Pancreatico-cyst-gastrostomy

After the first three ports are placed an initial survey of the abdomen is performed (■ Fig. 63.3). The stomach is usually displaced superiorly and anteriorly by the pseudocyst. The first step is to make a gastrotomy in the anterior wall of the stomach in approximately the midportion of the stomach over the site of greatest anterior displacement. This gastrotomy can be made either sharply or with the ultrasonic shears. A long spinal needle (20 gauge), or other aspirating device, can then be placed through the anterior abdominal wall under direct vision and through the back wall of the stomach to confirm the presence of the pseudocyst. At this point the midepigastric port is placed. This site can be used to place a Babcock clamp to hold the upper rim of the gastrotomy to better expose the back wall of the stomach. Under direct vision an incision is made in the back wall of the stomach and into the pseudocyst. If the cyst wall appears to be separating from the stomach the Babcock clamp can be moved to grasp the back wall of the stomach and cyst wall together. A suction device should be in place as the back wall gastrotomy is made to limit the spillage of pseudocyst contents into the peritoneal cavity (■ Fig. 63.4).

There are two options for formalizing the communication between the stomach and pseudocyst. The simplest is to insert an Endo-GIA with a tissue load through the umbilical 12 mm port and use it to form an anastomosis between the cyst and the back wall of the stomach. One anvil of the stapler is passed through the small cyst-gastrostomy and the second is in the stomach. A single firing will create a connection of greater than 3 cm (■ Fig. 63.5a,b). The other option is to make an initial larger opening in the back wall of the stomach and suture the wall of the stomach to the pseudocyst wall. This can be done with a 2-0 absorbable suture in a running fashion. This can be challenging because the surgeon most work through the anterior gastrotomy which can hinder visualization,

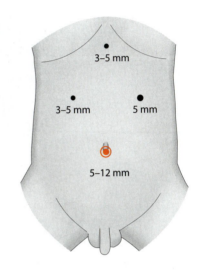

Fig. 63.3. Port positions for cyst-gastrostomy

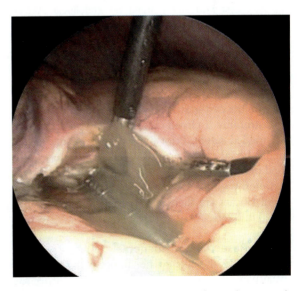

Fig. 63.4. Pancreatic pseudocyst opened into the stomach after anterior gastrotomy

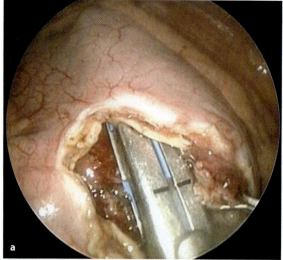

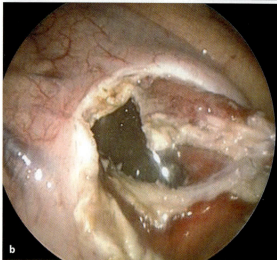

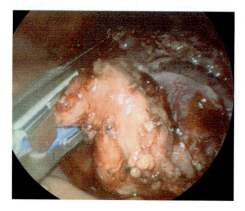

Fig. 63.6. Amputation of the distal pancreas with endolinear stapler

Fig. 63.5. Cyst-gastrostomy using an endolinear stapler. **a** Firing of the stapler. **b** Situation after stapling

especially once the cyst is decompressed. In most cases a stapled anastomosis is recommended.

Once the cyst-gastrostomy is completed the anterior gastrotomy is closed. This is done with a running 2-0 braided suture. Prior to closing the stomach care should be taken to ensure the nasogastric tube is in good position. Another option is to close the anterior gastrotomy with the stapler.

All trocars are then removed and the trocar sites closed in layers.

Resection for Adenoma

In most cases the adenoma or tumor is in the mid or distal pancreas making access through the lesser sac the preferable route. Tumors in the head of the pancreas are less amenable to an endoscopic approach. The procedure is initiated in the same fashion as with the

pseudocyst with an umbilical and two midquadrant trocars. The lesser sac is opened and the gastrocolic ligament divided to give exposure to the body and tail of the pancreas. This can be accomplished with the ultrasonic shears or Ligasure device. Stay sutures passed through the anterior abdominal wall and through the greater curve of the stomach can be used to retract the stomach anteriorly giving better exposure of the pancreas. Conversely, an epigastric port may be used for a Babcock clamp or fan retractor to hold the stomach up.

With the pancreas exposed careful examination of the body and tail should be performed to look for evidence of a discreet tumor. If none is seen intraoperative ultrasonography should be performed. The probe can be passed through the umbilical port with the camera moved to the right or left depending on the surgeon's preference. Once the tumor is identified the surgeon must decide on the extent of resection necessary. Peripheral lesions maybe enucleated using either the Ligasure or hook cautery. This should be done if the surgeon is relatively confident that the main pancreatic duct will not be injured. Fibrin glue or other tissue sealants may then be placed to help prevent the leak of any pancreatic juices. Deeper lesions or lesions confined to the distal half of the pancreas are best approached with a distal pancreatectomy.

Dissection is started at the tail of the pancreas. A stay sure maybe placed to help with retraction if necessary. The most difficult aspect of this dissection is separating the pancreas off the splenic vessels and safely sealing and dividing the branching vessels. In infants this can be done with a small hook cautery. In larger children this is most safely done with the Ligasure. As dissection approaches the midline care must be taken not to injure the superior mesenteric vessels. Once the tail of the pancreas is mobilized it can be safely divided. In infants this can be done with the Ligasure. In larger children the endoscopic stapler should be used

(■ Fig. 63.6). Again, this is passed through a 12 mm port in the umbilicus. The distal resection margin can be sealed with fibrin glue and a layer of omentum can be placed as a buttress.

A fenestrated closed drain should be left in the lesser sac to manage any possible leaks. It can be brought through the left midquadrant trocar site.

All other trocar sites are closed in layers.

Postoperative Care

A nasogastric tube is left in place and left to suction for at least 24 h following resection and for 2–3 days following pseudocyst drainage. Clear liquids may then be started and diet advanced as tolerated. In the case of resection the drain should be left in place until the child has tolerated oral feeds for 24 h. If drainage remains minimal it may then be removed. Intravenous analgesia is usually required for only the first 24–48 h.

In patients with a pseudocyst a postoperative imaging study should be obtained at 1 week and again at 1 month to ensure adequate decompression and resolution of the cyst. If pain persists or a recurrent cyst develops an ERCP may be necessary to evaluate the integrity of the main pancreatic duct.

Results

As this is a relatively rare entity in children our experience has been limited. However since 1995 all pancreatic lesions have been approached laparoscopically. There have been six children with pancreatic pseudocysts. Ages have ranged from 6 to 16 years and weight from 25 to 68 kg. Three were secondary to traumatic injury and three to chronic pancreatitis (one from gallstones). All were treated successfully with the technique described. Average operative time was 64 min and the average time to full feeds was 5 days. There were no operative or postoperative complications and there has been no recurrent pseudocyst formation.

We have only seen three adenomas all located in the tail of the pancreas. Patients' ages ranged from 2 to 7 years and weight from 15 to 46 kg. One lesion was enucleated and the other two patients had distal pancreatectomy. Average time to full feeds was 4.2 days and there were no operative complications. All patients are now symptom free.

Discussion

Disorders of the pancreas requiring surgical intervention are relatively rare but they are amenable to a laparoscopic approach. Pancreatic pseudocysts requiring drainage can be approached by a number of different modalities but a laparoscopic approach using an anterior gastrotomy has proven safe, fast, and effective (Park and Heniford 2002). Others have used an intraluminal technique by placing the trocars through the anterior gastric wall but there seems to be little advantage to this approach over a small gastrotomy (Schachter et al. 2002; Underwood and Soper 1999). The large anastomosis and minimal morbidity associated with the stapled cyst-gastrostomy would seem to be favorable to a small stent placed through the stomach and into the cyst either percutaneously or via esophagogastroduodenoscopy (EGD). Another approach not discussed here is a Roux-en-Y pancreatico-cyst-jejunostomy. This approach is through the lesser sac with a direct hand-sewn anastomosis after formation of the Roux limb. However indications for this approach in children would be exceedingly rare.

Discreet lesions of the pancreas are also amenable to a laparoscopic approach, especially in the mid or distal pancreas. The distal pancreas can be safely mobilized with minimal bleeding and the pancreatic duct can be safely sealed using devices such as the Ligasure or endoscopic stapler. The greatest difficulty can be in locating the lesion as it is often small and deep in the parenchyma of the pancreas. The inability to palpate the pancreas is the one draw back of this technique. However the laparoscopic ultrasound probe has proven to be an effective tool in identifying these lesions. Therefore a laparoscopy is an appropriate method to approach pancreatic pathology for the advanced endoscopic surgeon.

References

Bhattacharya D, Ammori B (2003) Minimally invasive approaches to the management of pancreatic pseudocysts: review of the literature. Surg Laparosc Endosc Percutan Tech 13:141–148

Park AE, Heniford BT (2002) Therapeutic laparoscopy of the pancreas. Ann Surg 236:149–158

Schachter PP, Shimonov M, Czerniak A (2002) The role of laparoscopy and laparoscopic ultrasound in the diagnosis of cystic lesions of the pancreas. Gastrointest Endosc Clin N Am 12:759–767

Underwood RA, Soper N (1999) Current status of laparoscopic surgery of the pancreas. J Hepatobiliary Pancreat Surg 6:154–164

Chapter 64

Laparoscopic Approach in Persistent Hyperinsulinemic Hypoglycemia in Infancy

Klaas (N) M.A. Bax and David C. van der Zee

Introduction

Persistent hyperinsulinemic hypoglycemia in infancy (PHHI) is a rare condition (Glaser et al. 2000). The morbidity is major despite recent advances in understanding the pathophysiology (Aynsley-Green et al. 2000). A major diagnostic problem has been the differentiation between focal and diffuse disease. In focal disease, removal of the lesion only is curative while in diffuse disease a near total pancreatectomy is the treatment of choice but the latter form of therapy invariably leads to both exocrine and endocrine pancreatic insufficiency (Cretolle et al. 2002; Dubois et al. 1995). Both forms of treatment can be carried out laparoscopically.

Preoperative Preparation

The diagnosis of PHHI is not difficult to make: high insulin blood levels despite hypoglycemia. The initial treatment is medicamentous but surgery comes into view when the child remains dependent on parenteral glucose supplementation. The question then is whether the disease is focal or diffuse. Classic imaging such as ultrasound, computed tomography (CT) or magnetic resonance (MR) is insufficient to detect focal lesions. Transhepatic portal venous sampling (Dubois et al. 1995) or selective arterial injection with calcium together with hepatic venous sampling (Abernethy et al. 1998) have been advocated but these investigations are invasive and not very reliable. More recently 18F-fluorodopa positron emission tomography (PET) scanning has been introduced with promising results (Otonkoski et al. 2003; Ribeiro et al. 2005).

A laparoscopic approach to the pancreas in babies not responding to medical treatment seems to be a good approach (Bax et al. 2003). During surgery, blood glucose is monitored meticulously.

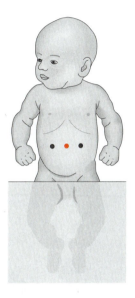

Fig. 64.1. Position of the patient on the table. The telescope sits just beneath the umbilicus and the working instruments pararectally at umbilical level

Positioning

Patient

The patient is placed in a froglike supine position at the lower end of the operating table. The table sheet is enveloped over the legs in order to avoid slipping from the table during reversed Trendelenburg (Fig. 64.1).

Crew, Monitors, and Equipment

The surgeon stand at the bottom end of the table with the camera operator to his/her left and the scrub nurse to his/her right. The stack stands to the left of the patient's head so that all cables come from the left in front of the surgeon. A second monitor stands to the right of the patient's head (Fig. 64.2).

Special Equipment

No special equipment is needed.

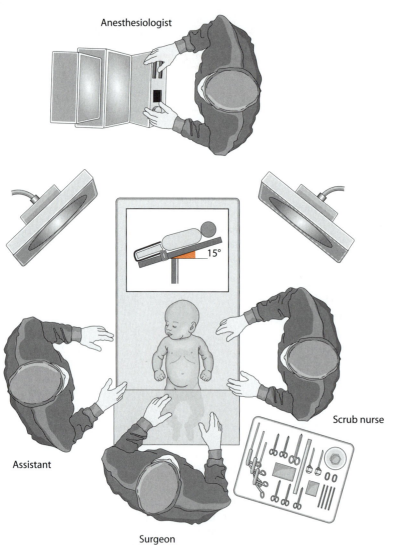

Anesthesiologist

Fig. 64.2. Positioning of the crew and monitors

15°

Scrub nurse

Assistant

Surgeon

Technique

Cannulae

Cannula	Method of insertion	Diameter (mm)	Device	Position
1	Open	6	Telescope 30°	Infraumbilical fold
2	Closed	3.5	Surgeon's right-hand instrument	Pararectally at umbilical level on the left
3	Closed	3.5	Surgeon's left-hand instrument	Pararectally at umbilical level on the right
4	Closed	3.5	Optional, Diamond-Flex ring retractor	Subcostal, anterior axillary on the right

Procedure

A 6 mm cannula is inserted through the inferior umbilical fold for a short 5 mm 30° telescope. Pararectally at the umbilical level 3.5 mm cannulae are inserted on each side for 3 mm diameter working instruments (■ Fig. 64.1). Optionally, a 3 mm cannula can be introduced subcostally on the right side in the anterior axillary line for a 3 mm Diamond Flex retractor to be put underneath the stomach after suspension of the

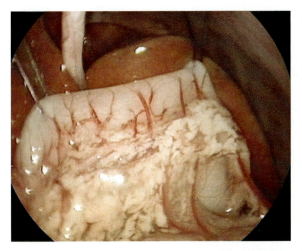

Fig. 64.3. The stomach has been suspended transabdominally

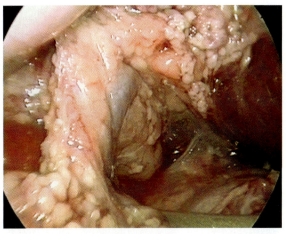

Fig. 64.5. The posterior pancreas is freed together with the splenic vein

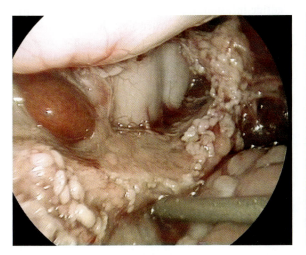

Fig. 64.4. The lesser sac has been opened. The anterior surface of the pancreas is probed with a suction cannula

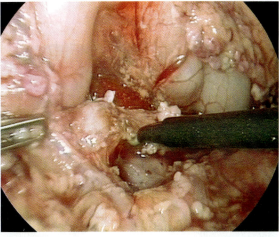

Fig. 64.6. A focal lesion has been identified in the uncinate process. The lesion feels harder than the remaining pancreas and the lobules seem larger

stomach and opening of the lesser sac. Two 3×0 stay sutures on a large, round-bodied needle are inserted through the abdominal wall and through the anterior antral and corporeal region of the stomach, respectively, and then back out again through the abdominal wall to pull the stomach up (■ Fig. 64.3). The lesser sac is opened through the gastrocolic ligament. Care is taken not to damage the gastroepiploic vessels. The splenocolic ligament is transected and the anterior side of the pancreas can now be seen. Using a 3 mm probe, for example a suction cannula, the anterior pancreatic surface can be palpated (■ Fig. 64.4). The normal pancreas looks soft. If no suspicious lesion is detected, the dissection of the pancreas is pursued. The plane underneath the tail of the pancreas is opened taking care not to open the thin mesentery of the transverse colon.

Once the inferior border of the pancreas is freed, the complete tail can easily be lifted upward together with the splenic vein (■ Fig. 64.5). Again the pancreas should be palpated with a probe. During further dissection the confluence of the splenic vein with the superior mesenteric vein is seen and the dissection can be continued until the head is seen from the posterior side. If necessary, the duodenum can be kocherized as well. Focal lesions have a distinctive macroscopic appearance. The lobules of the lesion look larger than those of the adjacent pancreatic tissue and the lesion feels hard on palpation with a probe (■ Fig. 64.6). If such a lesion is seen, its is enucleated using an electrocautery hook (■ Fig. 64.7). The cannulae are removed under telescopic control and the fascial defect at the umbilicus is closed (■ Fig. 64.8).

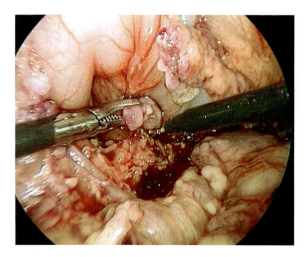

Fig. 64.7. Enucleation of the lesion

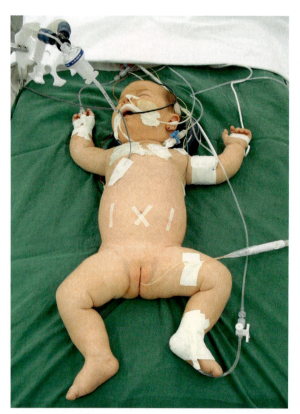

Fig. 64.8. Child at the end of the operation

If no lesion is found the tail of the pancreas up to the confluence of the superior mesenteric vein with the portal vein is freed. The splenic vessels are preserved. The distal pancreas is transected between ligatures and the specimen is removed for extensive histological examination. If the disease proves to be diffuse, medical treatment including continuous subcutaneous octreo-

tide infusion is given, but if the blood sugar can not be well controlled a near total pancreatectomy should be performed. This can also be done laparoscopically. To do so the duodenum should be extensively kocherized and the head of the pancreas including the uncinate process should be dissected free. The common bile duct should be identified and preserved. The anterior and posterior pancreaticoduodenal vessels should be preserved.

Postoperative Care

If a focal lesion has been found and removed, the postoperative course is smooth although reactive diabetes requiring insulin for a few days may occur. After distal pancreatectomy in diffuse disease, the tendency for hyperinsulinemic hypoglycemia will persist requiring further medical treatment including continuous octreotide infusion. If not successful, near total pancreatectomy is required. After near total laparoscopic pancreatectomy, the postoperative course may be smooth as well, but diabetes and exocrine pancreatic insufficiency require attention.

Results

So far we have approached four infants with PHHI laparoscopically. Three had a focal lesion. In two a lesion was found in the uncinate process. Enucleation in both was curative and postoperative complications did not occur. In the third patient preoperative 18F-fluorodopa PET scanning revealed a lesion in the corpus of the pancreas. The lesion was incompletely removed during a first laparoscopic intervention. In a second laparoscopic intervention a distal pancreatectomy including the previous operative site was curative. A focal lesion was found at the site of the initial partial removal.

The fourth patient had a generalized form of PHHI. No focal lesion was seen, even not after extensive mobilization of the pancreas. The distal pancreas was dissected off the splenic vessels up to well to the right of the mesenteric vein and close to the common bile duct. The pancreas was transected between the superior mesenteric vein and the common bile duct and the distal part was removed. Histological examination of the specimen confirmed diffuse disease. The postoperative course was smooth, but symptoms recurred despite continuous octreotide infusion. Three months after the distal pancreatectomy a near total pancreatectomy was performed laparoscopically as well. No intraoperative problems were encountered. It was amazing how little scar tissue was present and how well this could be done laparoscopically.

Discussion

There is no doubt that a laparoscopic approach to the problem of PHHI is far superior to an open approach. With a magnification of 18 times or even more, the anatomy can be beautifully seen. This amount of magnification does not only increase the likelihood of finding a focal lesion, it also allows for very fine surgery. In the event that a distal or near total pancreatectomy has to be performed, the amount of magnification makes spleen-saving surgery relatively easy (Blakely et al. 2001). A high incidence of common bile duct injury in near total pancreatectomy has been reported (McAndrew et al. 2003). There is no doubt that identification of the distal common bile duct will be easier with less likelihood of damage.

It seems that preoperative localization of focal lesions is possible now by PET scanning (Otonkoski et al. 2003, Ribeiro et al. 2005). This allows for a better preoperative planning of the operation, for example enucleation, limited resection, or extensive resection of the pancreas.

The laparoscopic approach is also advantageous in diffuse disease. It allows for a thorough inspection of the gland and removal of the tail for detailed pathological examination. If diffuse disease is confirmed, a further trial of medical treatment should be given. If the situation remains difficult to control medically, a near total pancreatectomy should be performed laparoscopically. The relative absence of scar tissue after a prior laparoscopic approach makes such a laparoscopic reintervention much simpler when compared to an open reintervention after prior open surgery.

References

Abernethy LJ, Davidson DC, Lamont GL, et al (1998) Intra-arterial calcium stimulation test in the investigation of hyperinsulinaemic hypoglycaemia. Arch Dis Child 78:359–363

Aynsley-Green A, Hussain K, Hall J, et al (2000) Medical management of hyperinsulinism in infancy. Arch Dis Child Fetal Neonatal Ed 82:F98–F107

Bax NM, Van Der Zee DC, De Vroede M, et al (2003) Laparoscopic identification and removal of focal lesions in persistent hyperinsulinemic hypoglycemia of infancy. Surg Endosc 17:833

Blakely ML, Lobe TE, Cohen J, et al (2001) Laparoscopic pancreatectomy for persistent hyperinsulinemic hypoglycemia of infancy. Surg Endosc 15:897–898

Cretolle C, Fekete CN, Jan D, et al (2002) Partial elective pancreatectomy is curative in focal form of permanent hyperinsulinaemic hypoglycaemia in infancy: a report of 45 cases from 1983 to 2000. J Pediatr Surg 37:155–158

Dubois J, Brunelle F, Touati G, et al (1995) Hyperinsulinism in children: diagnostic value of pancreatic venous sampling correlated with clinical, pathological and surgical outcome in 25 cases. Pediatr Radiol 25:512–516

Glaser B, Thornton P, Otonkoski T, et al (2000) Genetics of neonatal hyperinsulinism. Arch Dis Child Fetal Neonatal Ed 82:F79–F86

McAndrew HF, Smith V, Spitz L (2003) Surgical complications of pancreatectomy for persistent hyperinsulinaemic hypoglycaemia of infancy. Pediatr Surg 38:13–16

Otonkoski T, Veijoloa R, Huopio H, et al (2003) Diagnosis of focal persistent hyperinsulinism of infancy with 18-F-fluoro-L-DOPA PET. 42nd Annual Meeting of the European Society for Paediatric Endocrinology (ESPE), 18–21 September 2003, Ljubljana, Slovenia. Horm Res 60(suppl 2):2

Ribeiro MJ, De Lonlay P, Delzescaux T, et al (2005) Characterization of hyperinsulinism in infancy assessed with PET and 18F-fluoro-L-DOPA. J Nucl Med 46:560–566

Abdomen

Shunts and Catheters

Chapter 65

Laparoscopy and Ventriculoperitoneal Shunts

Klaas (N) M.A. Bax and David C. van der Zee

Introduction

Historically, hydrocephalus has been treated by shunting cerebrospinal fluid from the brain into many different body cavities and organs. The most commonly inserted system is the ventriculoperitoneal shunt (VPS), which consists of a silicone catheter placed inside the brain's ventricle and connected to a valve, and a longer tube which is guided subcutaneously from the head, over the neck and anterior chest wall, and into the peritoneal cavity (Grinsberg and Drake 2004). More recently endoscopic third ventriculostomy has gained popularity as a therapeutic alternative for any form of hydrocephalus that is purely obstructive in nature with one or multiple sites of obstruction between the middle third of the third ventricle and the peripontine cistern (Cinalli 2004; Punt 2004).

There are three items to be discussed in this chapter:
1. Is it safe to perform laparoscopic surgery when a VPS is present?
2. The use of laparoscopy during the insertion of a VPS.
3. Laparoscopic treatment of abdominal VPS complications.

Safety of Laparoscopic Surgery in the Presence of a VPS

Josephs et al. (1994) demonstrated in an animal model that diagnostic laparoscopy raises intracranial pressure. Since that publication concern has been raised in using laparoscopy in patients with head injury. Not only the pneumoperitoneum raises intracranial pressure but also Trendelenburg position (Rosenthal et al. 1997). No wonder that concern has been raised in applying laparoscopic surgical techniques in patients with a VPS. Meanwhile several case reports on the use of laparoscopy despite the presence of a VPS have been published without apparent negative consequences (Al-Mufarrej et al. 2005; Brown et al. 2004; Collure et al. 1995; Gaskill et al. 1998; Jackman et al. 2000; Kimura et al. 2002; Ravaoherisoa et al. 2004; Uzzo et al. 1997;

Walker and Langer 2000; Wang et al. 2003). VPS occlusion as a complication of laparoscopic surgery however has been described (Baskin et al. 1998).

The publication of Neale and Falk (1999) is reassuring, as they demonstrated in vitro that VPS can withstand high back pressures, much higher than used during laparoscopy, before they start to leak. A limitation of the study is that only one of the many available systems was tested. Moreover they warn of valve malfunction, which occurs in up to 10% of VPS problems (Kast et al. 1994). One should be aware that the VPS may be partially obstructed and that both Trendelenburg position and the pneumoperitoneum will increase intracranial pressure.

Apart from concern about intracranial hypertension there is also the concern about possible infection of the VPS. Sane et al. (1998) saw two shunt infections in a series of 23 percutaneously placed gastrostomies and advocate prophylactic antibiotic therapy. In case of simple appendicitis, the VPS can be left in place (Pumberger et al. 1998), but in case of perforated appendicitis, the drain should be externalized (Vinchon and Dhellemmes 2004).

The general conclusion to be drawn is that laparoscopic surgery in the presence of a VPS is usually safe. It is advised however to use a low pneumoperitoneum pressure, which is usually sufficient when concomitant muscle relaxation is given.

Laparoscopic-assisted Insertion of the Peritoneal Part of the Shunt

Introduction

It is logical to assume that blind placement of either the ventricular or peritoneal part of the shunt predisposes for more complications than when both parts are inserted under endoscopic control. The technique of the endoscopic insertion of the ventricular catheter is not described here but can be looked up elsewhere (Grinsberg and Drake 2004). The present chapter deals with the endoscopic insertion of the peritoneal part.

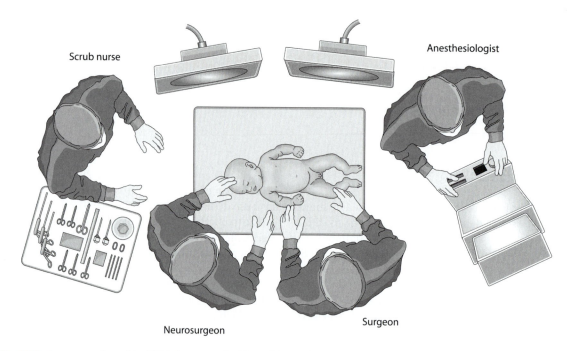

Scrub nurse

Anesthesiologist

Neurosurgeon

Surgeon

Fig. 65.1. Laparoscopic-assisted VPS placement. Position of the patient, crew, and equipment

Indications

Subgroups of patients may be particularly suited for a laparoscopic-assisted placement of the peritoneal part of the shunt, for example previous abdominal surgery or obesity (Armbruster et al. 1993; Basauri et al. 1993; Box et al. 1996; Cuatico and Vannix 1995; Khosrovi et al. 1998; Schievink et al. 1993). In patients who had previous abdominal surgery, laparoscopy will allow for placement of the catheter in an adhesion-free area. Alternatively adhesions can be divided. The advantages of such an approach are also obvious in obese patients. But even in the absence of obesity or previous abdominal surgery, a laparoscopic approach may be superior. It not only avoids a minilaparotomy with its related pain and potential complications, but also allows for an exact positioning of the catheter.

Preoperative Preparation

The indication and workup for insertion of a VPS is the responsibility of the pediatric neurosurgeon involved. In the event of previous intra-abdominal surgery, ultrasound mapping of the abdomen may be useful to determine an adhesion-free area for insertion of the first cannula. Prophylactic antibiotics (flucloxacillin, 25 mg/kg intravenously) are given after induction of general anesthesia.

Technique

The patient is positioned in such a way that both the frontal or occipital region of the head and the ab_ domen can be approached at the same time, which means a supine position of the patient with the head turned contralateral to the side to be operated upon (■ Fig. 65.1). The neurosurgeon stands next to the head of the patient on the side to be operated and looks at an opposite monitor. The laparoscopist stands at the same side of the patient next to the abdomen and looks at a second monitor in front. The neurosurgeon and pediatric surgeon assist each other. The scrub nurse stands to the left of the neurosurgeon. The anesthetist stands at the lower end of the table.

It is best to have two different camera circuits. This is not only more convenient but, more importantly, also better from the point of view of asepsis. A 3.5- or 6 mm cannula is inserted in an open way through the umbilicus, or in a different area in the event of periumbilical scarring (■ Fig. 65.2). CO_2 is insufflated at a maximal pressure of 5 mmHg and a flow of 2–5 L/min depending on the age and size of the patient.

Firstly, the inguinal region is inspected for patency of the processi vaginales. If these processi are still open, they should be closed as the likelihood of getting hydroceles and hernias is high (Grosfeld and Cooney 1974; Moazam et al. 1984). This can be done in a classic open way but can also be done laparoscopically (see Chapters 76–79). Next, a second small trocar is inserted in the right upper or right lower quadrant for a

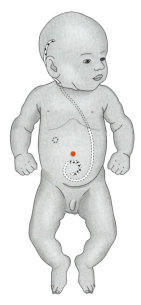

Fig. 65.2. Laparoscopic-assisted VPS placement. Position of the VP drain and cannula sites. The cannula for the scope is introduced through the inferior umbilical fold. A secondary cannula is inserted in the right hypochondrium for a grasper to position the drain in the abdomen. The peritoneal part of the drain is passed subcutaneously in a retrograde fashion through a tunneling device from the left hypochondrium to the right neck. Insertion into the abdomen is achieved with the Seldinger technique and appropriate peel a way system

grasping forceps (■ Fig. 65.2). The size of the trocar and instrument depends on the personal preference of the surgeon; 2 mm instrumentation has been described (Reardon et al. 2000). With a forceps the end of the catheter can be grasped at a later stage. Instead of two cannulae, one for the telescope and one for a working instrument, an operating laparoscope can be used (Fanelli et al. 2000).

A small incision is made in the left (or right) upper quadrant and a long tunneling device with trocar is introduced from that incision, subcutaneously along the anterior chest wall and neck up to the right (or left) frontal or occipital area, where the ventricular part of the shunt has been inserted (■ Fig. 65.2). Through the small incision in the left (or right) upper quadrant a needle is inserted into the abdomen under endoscopic control. Over a guidewire a peel a way system of appropriate size is inserted. The distal catheter of the shunt is fed into the tunneling device until its end reaches the left upper quadrant. The tunneling device is removed and the catheter inserted into the abdominal cavity via the peel a way system. The end of the catheter is now grabbed and approximately 40 cm of catheter is pulled into the abdomen to allow for growth of the patient. The distal end is nicely positioned in the lower abdomen. The peel a way system is removed and

the wound is closed with one subcuticular absorbable stitch and an adhesive strip to the skin. Meanwhile the neurosurgeon assembles the ventricular part of the shunt. Now that the shunt is complete cerebrospinal fluid runs freely into the abdominal cavity, which can be witnessed through the laparoscope. The laparoscope is withdrawn, and the fascia closed with an absorbable stitch. The skin is approximated with an adhesive strip.

If intra-abdominal adhesions are present, they can be cut, but this will usually necessitate the insertion of another cannula for an extra working instrument. Extensive adhesiolysis should be avoided as these adhesions will recur possibly sandwiching and therefore blocking the catheter.

Laparoscopic Diagnosis and Treatment of Shunt-related Intra-abdominal Complications

Introduction

The use of laparoscopy for intra-abdominal complications related to the VPS has been advocated for almost 20 years (Lemay et al. 1979; Morgan 1979; Rodgers et al. 1978). These complications can be divided as follows:
1. Infection
2. Blockage
   a. Due to omentum
   b. Due to encystation
   c. Due to disconnection or fracture
3. Bowel obstruction
4. Perforation (stomach, bowel, bladder, vagina, umbilicus, scrotum)

Contraindications

One should be aware that an increase in intra-abdominal pressure causes an increase in intracranial pressure. The lowest possible pneumoperitoneum pressure should therefore be used (see above). Trendelenburg position which also causes an increase in intracranial pressure should also be avoided as much as possible.

Technique

In General

The patient lies supine on the operating table. If the valve needs to be explored at the same time then the patient's head should face the opposite side of the region to be operated upon. When the system has been implanted into the abdomen along the patient's right side, the surgeon should stand at the patient's left side with a monitor opposite (■ Fig. 65.1). The first 3.5- or 6 mm cannula is inserted as described earlier and a classic pneumoperitoneum is created. After inspection 3.5 mm secondary cannulae are inserted as required. Alternatively a one trocar technique for insertion of an operating endoscope can be used (Esposito et al. 2003). The disadvantage of this technique is the 10 mm diameter of the operating endoscope, which requires an 11 mm cannula. During inspection the presumed problem will be identified.

In Specific Situations

Peritonitis

Laparoscopy allows to differentiate between shunt infection and other causes of peritonitis of which appendicitis is the most frequent one. In the event of peritonitis due to an infected system, material for culture is taken. One can leave the system in place and try to treat the condition with antibiotics. Alternatively, the distal end of the shunt can be exteriorized through a small hole in the abdominal wall. In a later phase, at least the distal end of the catheter will need replacement. In case of perforated appendicitis the shunt should be exteriorized as well.

Catheter Blockage

By Omentum. If the catheter is blocked by omentum, this can easily be undone laparoscopically with a grasper.

By Encystation. If encystation has taken place, this diagnosis is usually made preoperatively by ultrasound or other imaging techniques. It is important to differentiate between an infected and a non-infected cyst (Vinchon and Dhellemmes 2004). In case of infection the drain should be externalized. If not, the cyst is unroofed and the tip placed in another part of the abdomen. This can well be done laparoscopically (Brunori et al. 1998; Kim et al. 1995; Oh et al. 2001). In addition to a cannula for the laparoscope, two more cannulae for instrumentation are usually required for the actual surgery.

By Disconnection or Fracture. If shunt disconnection or fracture has occurred, the distal part of the catheter can either be removed laparoscopically or, alternatively, the peritoneal part of the shunt can be replaced in a laparoscopic-assisted way (Guzinsky 1982; Lemay et al. 1979; Pierangeli et al. 1999; Schrenk et al. 1996).

Bowel Obstruction

If a small bowel obstruction is caused by an intra-abdominal catheter, laparoscopic repositioning of the catheter and lysis of eventual adhesions will solve the problem unless the bowel is gangrenous in which case the operation should be converted (see Chapter 41).

Hollow Viscus Perforation

Perforation can occur anywhere. If a perforation occurs, the distal end of the catheter is amputated laparoscopically after which the distal end can be pulled out. Obviously the peritoneal part of the shunt needs replacement. Depending on which structure has been perforated the perforation needs closure or not.

Discussion

A VPS is not a contraindication for laparoscopic surgery. In overt peritonitis or perforation of the VPS into a hollow viscus, the drain should be exteriorized.

The combination of neuroendoscopy with laparoscopy optimizes the placement of VPS and will undoubtedly reduce complications related to shunt malpositioning. In the long term it might even reduce the frequency of shunt revisions by diminishing the incidence of distal obstruction. Moreover, by using an almost no-touch technique, the infection rate may further decline. Other advantages are the avoidance of a minilaparotomy, thus less pain, fewer adhesions, a smaller scar, and fewer wound-related complications. In shunt-related intra-abdominal problems, laparoscopy can be a very valuable tool, not only in the diagnostic but also in the therapeutic field.

Essential for this type of surgery is of course a good collaboration between the neurosurgeon, pediatric surgeon, and anesthesiologist. Endoscopic surgical techniques can also be used when the tip of the drain has to be placed in the chest (Holcomb and Smith 1995). Laparoscopic lumboperitoneal shunting has also been described (Huie et al. 1999; Johna et al. 2001).

References

Al-Mufarrej F, Nolan C, Sookhai S, et al (2005) Laparoscopic procedures in adults with ventriculoperitoneal shunts. Surg Laparosc Endosc Percutan Tech 15:28–29

Armbruster C, Blauensteiner J, Ammerer HP, et al (1993) Laparoscopically assisted implantation of ventriculoperitoneal shunts. J Laparoendosc Surg 3:191–192

Basauri L, Selman JM, Lizana C (1993) Peritoneal catheter insertion under laparoscopic guidance. Pediatr Neurosurg 19:109–110

Baskin JJ, Vishteh AG, Wesche DE, et al (1998) Ventriculoperitoneal shunt failure as a complication of laparoscopic surgery. J Soc Laparoendosc Surg 2:177–180

Box JC, Young D, Mason E, et al (1996) A retrospective analysis of laparoscopically assisted ventriculoperitoneal shunts. Surg Endosc 10:311–313

Brown JA, Medlock MD, Dahl DM (2004) Ventriculoperitoneal shunt externalization during laparoscopic prostatectomy. Urology 63:1183–1185

Brunori A, Massari A, Macarone-Palmieri R, et al (1998) Minimally invasive treatment of giant CSF pseudocyst complicating ventriculoperitoneal shunt. Minim Invasive Neurosurg 41:38–39

Cinalli G (2004) Endoscopic third ventriculostomy. In: Cinalli C, et al (eds) Pediatric Hydrocephalus, chap 25. Springer, Milano, pp 361–388

Collure DW, Bumpers HL, Luchette FA, et al (1995) Laparoscopic cholecystectomy in patients with ventriculoperitoneal (VP) shunts. Surg Endosc 9:409–410

Cuatico W, Vannix D (1995) Laparoscopically guided peritoneal insertion of ventriculoperitoneal shunts. J Laparoendosc Surg 5:309–311

Esposito C, Collela G, Settimi A, et al (2003) One-trocar laparoscopy: a valid procedure to treat abdominal complications in children with peritoneal shunt for hydrocephalus. Surg Endosc 17:828–830

Fanelli RD, Mellinger DN, Crowell RM, et al (2000) Laparoscopic ventriculoperitoneal shunt placement: a single-trocar technique. Surg Endosc 14:641–644

Gaskill SJ, Cossman RM, Hickman MS, et al (1998) Laparoscopic surgery in a patient with a ventriculoperitoneal shunt: a new technique. Pediatr Neurosurg 28:106–107

Grinsberg HJ, Drake JM (2004) Shunt hardware and shunt technique. In: Cinalli C, et al (eds) Pediatric Hydrocephalus, chap 20. Springer, Milano, pp 295–313

Grosfeld JL, Cooney DR (1974) Inguinal hernia after ventriculoperitoneal shunt for hydrocephalus. J Pediatr Surg 9:311–315

Guzinski GM, Meyer WJ, Loeser JD (1982) Laparoscopic retrieval of disconnected ventriculoperitoneal shunt catheters. Report of four cases. J Neurosurg 56:587–589

Holcomb GW 3rd, Smith HP (1995) Laparoscopic and thoracoscopic assistance with CSF shunts in children. J Pediatr Surg 30:1642–1643

Huie F, Sayad P, Usal H, et al (1999) Laparoscopic transabdominal lumboperitoneal shunt. Surg Endosc 13:161–163

Jackman SV, Weingart JD, Kinsman SL, et al (2000) Laparoscopic surgery in patients with ventriculoperitoneal shunts: safety and monitoring. J Urol 164:1352–1354

Johna S, Kirsch W, Robles A (2001) Laparoscopic-assisted lumboperitoneal shunt: a simplified technique. J Soc Laparoendosc Surg 5:305–307

Josephs LG, Este-McDonald JR, Birkett DH, et al (1994) Diagnostic laparoscopy increases intracranial pressure. J Trauma 36:815–818, see comments 818–819

Kast J, Duong D, Nowzari F, et al (1994) Time-related patterns of ventricular shunt failure. Childs Nerv Syst 10:524–528

Khosrovi H, Kaufman HH, Hrabovsky E, et al (1998) Laparoscopic-assisted distal ventriculoperitoneal shunt placement. Surg Neurol 49:127–134

Kim HB, Raghavendran K, Kleinhaus S (1995) Management of an abdominal cerebrospinal fluid pseudocyst using laparoscopic techniques. Surg Endosc 5:151–154

Kimura T, Nakajima K, Wasa M, et al (2002) Successful laparoscopic fundoplication in children with ventriculoperitoneal shunts. Surg Endosc 16:215

Lemay J-L, Dupas J-P, Capron J-P, et al (1979) Laparoscopic removal of the distal catheter of ventriculoperitoneal shunt (Ames valve). Gastrointest Endosc 25:162–163

Moazam F, Glenn JD, Kaplan BJ (1984) Inguinal hernias after ventriculoperitoneal shunt procedures in pediatric patients. Surg Gynecol Obstet 159:570–572

Morgan WW Jr (1979) The use of peritoneoscopy in the diagnosis and treatment of complications of ventriculoperitoneal shunts in children. J Pediatr Surg 14:180–181

Neale ML, Falk GL (1999) In vitro assessment of back pressure on ventriculoperitoneal shunt valves. Is laparoscopy safe? Surg Endosc 13:512–515

Oh A, Wildbrett P, Golub R, Yu LM, et al (2001) Laparoscopic repositioning of a ventriculo-peritoneal catheter tip for a sterile abdominal cerebrospinal fluid (CSF) pseudocyst. Surg Endosc 15:518

Pierangeli E, Pizzoni C, Lospalluti A, et al (1999) Laparoscopic removal of two dislocated ventriculoperitoneal catheters: case report. Minim Invasive Neurosurg 42:86–88

Pumberger W, Lobl M, Geissler W (1998) Appendicitis in children with a ventriculoperitoneal shunt. Pediatr Neurosurg 28:21–26

Punt J (2004) Third ventriculostomy in shunt malfunction. In: Cinalli C, et al (eds) Pediatric Hydrocephalus, chap 26. Springer, Milano, pp 389–396

Ravaoherisoa J, Meyer P, Afriat R, et al (2004) Laparoscopic surgery in a patient with ventriculoperitoneal shunt: monitoring of shunt function with transcranial Doppler. Br J Anaesth 92:434–437

Reardon PR, Scarborough TK, Matthews BD, et al (2000) Laparoscopically assisted ventriculoperitoneal shunt placement using 2 mm instrumentation. Surg Endosc 14:585–586

Rodgers BM, Vries JK, Talbert JL (1978) Laparoscopy in the diagnosis and treatment of malfunctioning ventriculo-peritoneal shunts in children. J Pediatr Surg 13:247–253

Rosenthal RJ, Hiatt JR, Phillips EH, et al (1997) Intracranial pressure. Effects of pneumoperitoneum in a large-animal model. Surg Endosc 11:376–380

Sane SS, Towbin A, Bergey EA, Kaye RD, Fitz CR, Albright L, Towbin RB (1998) Percutaneous gastrostomy tube placement in patients with ventriculoperitoneal shunts. Pediatr Radiol 28:521–523

Schievink WI, Wharen RE Jr, Reimer R, et al (1993) Laparoscopic placement of ventriculoperitoneal shunts: preliminary report. Mayo Clin Proc 68:1064–1066

Schrenk P, Woisetschlager R, Wayand WU, et al (1996) Laparoscopic removal of dislocated ventriculoperitoneal shunts. Report of two cases. Surg Endosc 8:1113–1114

Uzzo RG, Bilsky M, Mininberg DT, et al (1997) Laparoscopic surgery in children with ventriculoperitoneal shunts. Effects of pneumoperitoneum on intracranial pressure: preliminary experience. Urology 49:753–757

Vinchon M, Dhellemmes P (2004) Abdominal complications of peritoneal shunts. In: Cinalli C, et al (eds) Pediatric Hydrocephalus, chap 21. Springer, Milano, pp 315–327

Walker DH, Langer JC (2000) Laparoscopic surgery in children with ventriculoperitoneal shunts. J Pediatr Surg 35:1104–1105

Wang YM, Liu YC, Ye XD, et al (2003) Anesthetic management of laparoscopic surgery in a patient with a ventriculoperitoneal shunt. Acta Anaesthesiol Sin 41:85–88

Chapter 66

Endoscopic Surgery for Peritoneal Dialysis Catheters in Children

Haluk Emir

Introduction

The first reports of the use of peritoneal dialysis (PD) to treat children with renal failure were published in the late 1940s (Bloxum and Powell 1948; Swan and Gordon 1949). During the 1950s disposable nylon catheters and commercially prepared dialysis solutions became available. Thus, PD became more practical for the short-term treatment of acute renal failure (ARF). Treatment of chronic renal failure (CRF) with PD was unsuccessful until reliable peritoneal access was developed in the late 1960s. A "permanent" PD catheter was introduced by Palmer et al. in 1964, and was later modified and developed by Tenckhoff and Schecter in 1968. The second catheter is still in use today. The proportion of the children treated with PD increased after two new innovations in PD: continuous ambulatory peritoneal dialysis (CAPD) and continuous cycling peritoneal dialysis (CCPD), which were described in 1976 and 1981 respectively (Diaz-Buxo et al. 1981; Moncrief et al. 1978; Popovich et al. 1976).

Basically there are three methods for PD catheter placement:
1. Blind percutaneous techniques
2. Open surgical techniques
3. Peritoneoscopic/laparoscopic techniques

In recent years, video-assisted laparoscopy has provided new techniques for both placement and salvaging of PD catheters (Brownlee and Elkhairi 1997; Emir et al. 1997, 2000; Korten et al. 1982; Leung et al. 1998; Nijhuis et al. 1996; Owens and Brader 1995). Laparoscopic techniques have advantages: a complete intra-abdominal exploration can be performed without having a formal laparotomy, the tip of the catheter can be placed into the pelvis under direct vision, and additional surgical procedures such as adhesiolysis and omentectomy can be performed. Another important advantage, especially in pediatric patients, is that the internal inguinal orifices can be inspected and that an open processus vaginalis can closed at the same time.

Laparoscopy can also be used to rescue catheters that are dislodged or obstructed by omental wrapping and adhesions, thus increasing the life of the catheter.

This chapter mainly describes two techniques of endoscopic surgical insertion of a PD catheter. It also discusses the role of endoscopic surgical techniques and the treatment of a number of complications.

Indications for Endoscopic Surgery Related to Peritoneal Dialysis

Indications for Dialysis

Dialysis is usually necessary for treatment of ARF, CRF, and sometimes in poisoning. The generally accepted criteria for initializing acute PD in children include:
1. The treatment of metabolic disturbances unresponsive to conservative treatment, for example hyperkalemia (serum potassium >7.0 mmol/L), unrelenting metabolic acidosis, and hyperphosphatemia.
2. Fluid overload with or without severe hypertension or congestive heart failure that is not controlled with fluid restriction and diuretics.
3. Symptomatic uremia with encephalopathy and pericarditis. The rate of increase in both urea nitrogen and creatinine levels may indicate the need for dialysis.
4. Acute renal failure associated with poisoning due to dialyzable compounds

The indications for starting chronic dialysis therapy are not well defined in pediatric patients. Residual renal functions and the clinical status of the patients are the most important criteria for PD in CRF patients. Chronic dialysis therapy is usually initiated when the glomerular filtration rate declines to 5–10 ml/min per 1.73 m^2. Despite the medical therapy, the presence of complications are also considered as important criteria for initiating chronic dialysis therapy.

Preoperative Preparation for Peritoneal Dialysis Catheter Insertion

Before Induction of General Anesthesia

Special preoperative precautions are necessary for the patients with ARF or CRF. A preoperative chest X-ray is necessary to exclude silent chest infection, and to detect any significant pleural effusion or evidence of congestive heart failure associated with renal insufficiency. An electrocardiogram should be performed to look for evidence of hyperkalemia or ventricular hypertrophy. Blood analysis for electrolytes and blood gases should also be undertaken. All efforts should be made to treat metabolic conditions such as severe acidosis, hyperkalemia, or hypertension before the patient undergoes general anesthesia.

There is no absolute contraindication for laparoscopy in children with renal failure. However, for those patients with marginal cardiopulmonary function, special precautions may be necessary during the procedure. Close intraoperative monitoring of physiological changes is mandatory. An empty colon facilitates the surgical procedure and will be helpful for the proper functioning of the catheter after surgery; therefore a bowel washout is recommended before the laparoscopic procedure.

The operative procedure must be carefully planned for each patient. The catheter type, catheter size, abdominal entrance, subcutaneous tunnel course, inner cuff location, and exit site location are planned and marked before the operation (■ Fig. 66.1). If necessary the catheter is trimmed during the operation. The exit site should not be placed on skin folds or in the area where the child wears a belt. It should be easily seen and should not interfere with movements or bending. In young infants or incontinent patients the exit site should be placed high above the diaper border to minimize risk of contamination. Patients with a stoma should have the catheter exit site as far as possible from the stomal site. Presternal dialysis catheter exit may be preferable for patients with incontinence, a need for diapers, or obesity, but experience with this technique is very limited in children (Chadha et al. 2000; Warchol et al. 1998). The subcutaneous tunnel course should not be located at the possible future transplantation incision. The catheter can be inserted on either the right or left side of the abdomen according to the presence of any previous operation, catheter placement, stoma, or scar tissue, and of course according to the patient's preference. It has been suggested that the downward peristaltic waves of the descending colon may maintain the straight peritoneal catheter tip in the true pelvis, whereas a catheter tip located on the right side may be moved from the true pelvis upward

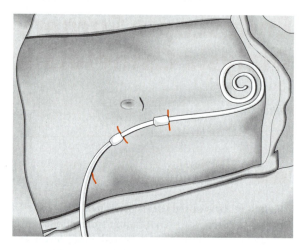

Fig. 66.1. The catheter course and localization of the cuffs are marked at the beginning of operation.

by the upward movements of the ascending colon (Cruz et al. 2001).

Prophylactic use of antibiotics, for example gentamicin, cephalosporin, or vancomycin before the operation has been reported to reduce early peritonitis and exit site infection significantly (Gadallah et al. 2000b; Verrina et al. 2000). Therefore, prophylactic use of first-generation cephalosporin is recommended unless methicillin-resistant Staphylococcus aureus is documented. Postoperative antibiotics have been recommended for 1–3 days or sometimes even more.

Intraperitoneal Configuration of the Catheter

Regarding the design of the intra-abdominal portion, there are a several types of chronic PD catheters:

1. Straight Tenckhoff catheter, with a 10 cm section containing 1 mm side-holes
2. Curled catheter, with a 20 cm section containing 1 mm side-holes
3. Straight catheter with perpendicular discs, the Toronto-Western design
4. T-fluted catheter with grooved perpendicular limbs positioned against the parietal peritoneum
5. Valli catheter (consists of a perforated Silastic balloon that protects the distal end of a standard Tenckhoff catheter)
6. Self-locating catheter (similar to a Tenckhoff catheter but includes a small 12-g tungsten cylinder at the distal end)

The straight Tenckhoff catheter, the curled catheter, and the Toronto Western (straight or curled) catheter are the most commonly used catheters in children. The use of curled catheters has increased in recent years, because of better survival and lower migration rate. Curled catheters are also reported to reduce infusion pain.

Subcutaneous Configuration of the Catheter

The creation of a long subcutaneous tunnel and the presence of single or double cuffs on the catheter help both to fix the catheter and to block the migration of microorganisms into the peritoneal cavity by the pericatheter route, thus minimizing the risk of infection. A lateral or downward direction of the catheter exit possibly minimizes the risk for infection, and an upwardly directed exit site collects debris and fluid, so possibly increasing the risk for infection.

There are two main configurations of the subcutaneous portion of the catheters for chronic PD: straight or gently curved catheters and arcuate or "swan-neck" catheters with a 150° bend. Clinical studies showed that double-cuffed catheters are better than the single-cuffed catheters and swan-neck catheters are better than the straight catheters regarding infectious complications (Harvey 2001; Lewis et al. 1997; Verrina et al. 2000). Although some pediatric series failed to demonstrate significant reduction of infectious complications with the swan-neck catheters, in most centers a downward or laterally directed catheter exit is preferred.

Type, Number, and Localization of the Cuffs

There are three options regarding the cuff: single cuff, double cuff, and disc-shaped inner cuff with silicone ball within the peritoneum. Catheters with a single cuff are usually easy to insert and to remove, and there is little risk of cuff dislodgement. They are useful for acute dialysis as they are easy to withdraw. This type of catheter is also useful for infants.

For double-cuffed catheters, the inner cuff is placed within the abdominal musculature and avoids pericatheter herniation, leakage, catheter extrusion, and exit site erosion (Ash 2002). The outer cuff is placed in a subcutaneous tunnel located, 2–2.5 cm away from the exit site, so that stratified squamous epithelium growths in over the catheter until it reaches the outer cuff (■ Fig. 66.2). This configuration provides good fixation and seal of the catheter and creates a good barrier against infection. Double-cuffed catheters seem, therefore, to have longer functioning time with lower exit site complications and a lower incidence of peritonitis when compared with single-cuffed catheters (Lewis et al. 1997). Single-cuffed catheters are also associated with a shorter time interval until the first peritonitis. Different materials have been used for the making of the cuffs, for example silver and titanium mesh (experimental), in order to reduce tunnel infection, but the superiority of these materials over Dacron has not been proved (Lewis et al. 1996; Pommer et al. 1998; Walboomers et al. 2001).

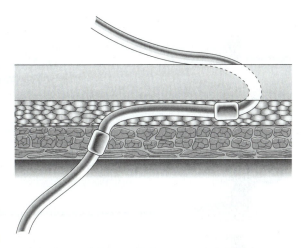

Fig. 66.2. Intracorporeal course of the catheter. The inner cuff is placed above the peritoneum, the outer cuff is in the subcutaneous tunnel, 2 cm away from the exit.

When acute dialysis is required, the peritoneal access has to be used immediately after surgery and possibly for a short time. Under such circumstances, catheters with a single cuff may be more suitable than catheters with a double cuff, and omentectomy may not be carried out. For chronic dialysis, PD catheter placement is performed electively and PD is delayed for a few days or a week, allowing the wounds to heal thus lowering the leakage risk.

After Induction of General Anesthesia

As a general principle, all laparoscopic procedures in children are performed under general anesthesia. A urinary catheter may be inserted to facilitate the operative procedure. Skin is prepared with antiseptics from the nipple to thigh level and draped to expose the abdomen from the xiphoid process to just above the pubis.

Positioning

The patient lies in a supine position. The surgeon stays on the patient's side on which PD catheter is to be inserted. For the techniques without concomitant omentectomy, the assistant stands on the other side, while the nurse and instrument table should stay on the surgeon's right side. The monitor is placed across from the surgeon near to the patient's foot.

In case of laparoscopic omentectomy, the surgeon stands on the patient's right side with the monitor placed across the table opposite to him. The assistant stands to right of the surgeon, and the scrub nurse at the opposite side of the table next to the monitor.

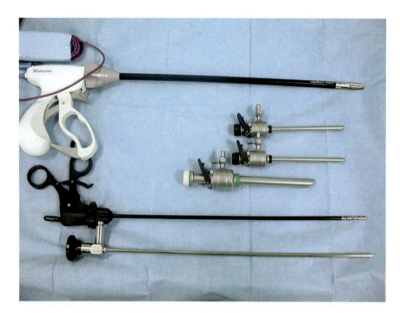

Fig. 66.3. Laparoscopic instruments for PD catheter insertion.

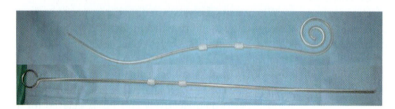

Fig. 66.4. Tenckhoff catheter with curled end which can be straightened with a steel rod put inside.

Special Equipment

No special equipment is necessary for laparoscopic PD catheter insertion other than the equipment which is used for standard laparoscopic procedures. One 10 mm and two 5 mm trocars, and one laparoscopic forceps are essential for the procedure. Bipolar electrocautery, Ligasure, or ultrasonic energy is used for laparoscopic omentectomy (■ Fig. 66.3). A long steel rod (60 cm) which can be inserted into the PD catheter should be available in case a two-cannula technique is used (■ Fig. 66.4).

Although different types of PD catheters can be used, a straight Tenckhoff catheter with a curled end may be preferred in case a two-cannula technique is used as will be described in this chapter. Different kinds of Tenckhoff catheters are available, for example 47-, 42-, 37- (pediatric) and 31 cm (neonatal) catheters with two cuffs, 37- and 31 cm (neonatal) catheters with one cuff, a 57 cm curled catheter with two cuffs, and a 39 cm (pediatric) curled catheter with one cuff. The size of the catheter and the number of the cuffs are chosen separately for each individual.

Technique

As discussed before, several types of PD catheters are available on the market and different kinds of PD catheter placement techniques have been described in the literature. Initially, this may be confusing; however, there is a general agreement at least on the basic steps of "a proper placement" of a chronic PD catheter (Ash 2002):

1. The intraperitoneal portion of catheter should be localized between the parietal and visceral peritoneum. The catheter should be directed toward the pelvis and the tip of the catheter should lie in the pouch of Douglas.
2. The inner cuff should be placed above the posterior sheath of rectus abdominis muscle.
3. The outer cuff should be located approximately 2 cm from the exit site (■ Fig. 66.2).

The direction of the catheter entrance into the abdominal cavity is also important and the more vertical the catheter is implanted, the less likely the tip will migrate out of the pouch of Douglas (Hwang et al. 1998).

Peritoneal dialysis catheter placement techniques can be categorized as follows:

1. Blind techniques using Tenckhoff's trocar or guidewire

2. Open techniques
3. Techniques using laparoscopy:
   a. Percutaneously guided technique under laparo-scopic control
   b. The Y-TEC system
   c. Laparoscopic-assisted insertion of PD catheter
   d. Laparoscopic insertion of PD catheter

In all techniques, gentle manipulation of the catheter is important and grasping the catheter with a toothed forceps should be avoided. Kinking of the catheter, which usually occurs during exteriorization of the sub-cutaneous part of the catheter, should always be pre-vented as this will lead to outflow problems.

Percutaneously Guided Technique Under Laparoscopic Control

Percutaneous insertion of the PD catheter is performed under simple peritoneoscopic visual guidance. Major organs and vessels can be seen during the procedure. However, the Veress needle is inserted blindly and there is therefore the potential risk of visceral and vas-cular injuries. Furthermore, manipulation of the cath-eter is difficult with this technique and omentectomy is not possible.

The Y-TEC System

After skin incision, the sheath of rectus abdominis muscle is exposed, and the catheter guide assembly is inserted into the abdomen. The Y-TEC scope is insert-ed into the catheter Quill guide cannula. Following initial inspection assuring intraperitoneal entry, the Y-TEC scope is removed, and pneumoperitoneum is achieved by connecting the insufflation tube to the cannula. The Y-TEC scope is reinserted and the abdo-men is inspected to identify and avoid adhesions, omentum, and bowel loops. The Y-TEC scope and the surrounding Quill guide are advanced into the largest and clearest area of intraperitoneal space and the scope is removed. The PD catheter with a stylet is inserted through the Quill guide toward the same region, and then the guide and stylet are removed. After confirm-ing the catheter is functioning well, the inner cuff of the PD catheter is inserted into the musculature with a hemostat. The catheter exit site is located and the cath-eter is tunneled through. However, the initial blind in-sertion of needle before the introduction of pneumo-peritoneum can still be associated with potential haz-ards. Furthermore the technique may not tackle intra-peritoneal adhesive bands, which can give rise to problems in the future.

Laparoscopic-assisted Insertion of Peritoneal Dialysis Catheter

A supraumbilical port is introduced into the abdomi-nal cavity by an open technique. After creating the pneumoperitoneum, the telescope is inserted and the abdominal cavity is carefully inspected. A separate 2- to 3 cm incision is made down to the peritoneum at the entry point of the PD catheter. The PD catheter is in-troduced through a small peritoneal incision and ad-vanced downward to a clear space in the pelvic cavity under direct laparoscopic vision. The peritoneal open-ing around the catheter is then closed with a purse-string suture which is passed through the base of the cuff of the Tenckhoff catheter at several points. It an-chors the catheter in position and ensures a more wa-tertight closure. Another purse-string non-absorbable suture is placed through the rectus muscle and the an-terior sheath of rectus abdominis muscle, a subcutane-ous tunnel is created, and the catheter is brought out. If adjustment of the catheter tip is necessary, another 2.5- or 3.5 mm port may be inserted with a grasping instru-ment, or a steel rod may be inserted through the cath-eter and the catheter tip placed into the pelvic cavity. An extracorporeal omentectomy can be performed through the umbilical incision.

Two-cannula Technique with Extracorporeal Omentectomy

A 1.5- to 2 cm-long supraumbilical semicircular inci-sion is made. The sheath of rectus abdominis muscle is incised transversely followed by the peritoneum and a 2-0 polyglactin purse-string suture is placed around the opening for maintaining the pneumoperitoneum subsequently. A 10 mm port with adapter for instru-ments of either 5 or 10 mm is inserted and secured by tying the purse-string suture. A CO_2 pneumoperito-neum with a pressure of 12 mmHg is created. The peri-toneal cavity, particularly the internal inguinal orifices for patency of the processus vaginalis, is inspected with a videoendoscope. In case of the presence of intra-ab-dominal adhesions or if simultaneous additional pro-cedures are needed, the technique is changed to a three-cannula technique at this stage.

A 5 mm transverse skin incision is made 4–5 cm cra-nially from the point that was marked as the future cath-eter entrance site into the abdomen through the rectus muscle. A 5 mm trocar is inserted into the abdominal cavity through the rectus muscle, after creating a 4- to 5 cm vertical straight subcutaneous tunnel over the an-terior rectus muscle sheath (Fig. 66.5a,b). The PD catheter (with a 2-0 nylon loop at the proximal end) is introduced into the abdominal cavity through the um-bilical 10 mm trocar after the telescope is switched to

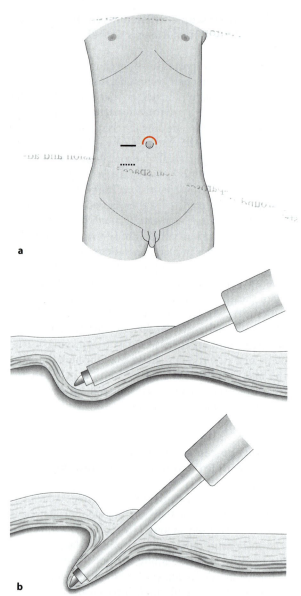

a

b

Fig. 66.5. Two-cannula insertion technique. **a** Localization of the skin incisions. *Dashed line* shows the entrance of the catheter through the rectus muscle and the peritoneum. **b** Creation of the subcutaneous tunnel with a 5 mm trocar.

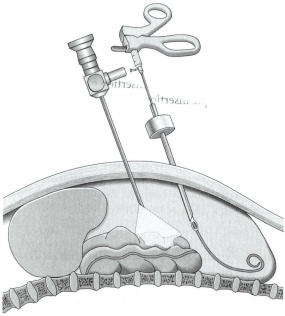

Fig. 66.6. The end of the catheter is pulled out together with the cannula through the abdominal wall and subcutaneous tunnel until the inner cuff comes to lie just above the posterior sheath of rectus abdominis muscle.

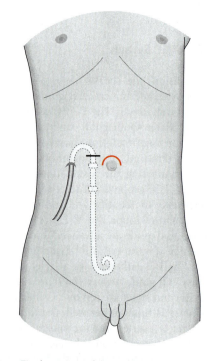

Fig. 66.7. Final position of the catheter.

the lateral 5 mm trocar. The distal end of the catheter is placed into the pelvic cavity by a grasping forceps. While the telescope is in the umbilical port, the proximal end of the catheter is grasped and pulled out through the abdominal wall and subcutaneous tunnel together with the trocar until the inner cuff is located just above the posterior sheath of rectus abdominis muscle (■ Fig. 66.6). The exact localization of the catheter tip is checked again while the abdomen is being desufflated. The distal end is repositioned with help of a steel rod inserted through the catheter, if necessary. The greater omentum is localized and the abdomen is desufflated.

The telescope is removed and the greater omentum is grasped with a laparoscopic forceps. The supraumbilical port is removed over the forceps and the greater omentum is exteriorized as much as possible through the um-

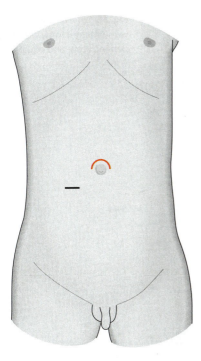

Fig. 66.8. The localization of trocars for modification of the two-cannula technique. The PD catheter is inserted into the abdomen with a steel rod through the lower abdominal trocar entrance.

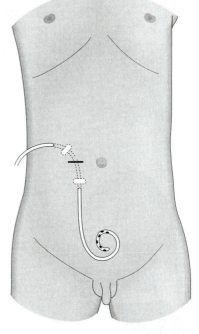

Fig. 66.9. After the distal end of the catheter is placed into the pelvis leaving the inner cuff above the peritoneum, the steel rod is pulled out and a subcutaneous tunnel is created.

bilical wound. Then a partial omentectomy is performed extracorporeally. The fascial defect at that point is closed with absorbable sutures. The subcutaneous tunnel is lengthened laterally and caudally with a slight bend and is therefore directed downward, leaving the outer cuff 2–2.5 cm from the exit site for double-cuffed catheters (■ Fig. 66.7). The catheter is flushed with dialysate and outflow is controlled followed by flushing the catheter with heparin. Finally the wound is dressed.

Alternative Technique

The same steps are followed as described above. After the abdominal cavity exploration, a 5 mm skin incision is made at the point marked as the future entrance site of the catheter through the rectus muscle into the abdomen (■ Fig. 66.8). A 5 mm trocar is introduced into the abdomen and then removed. Through this hole, the PD catheter over a long steel rod is inserted into the abdominal cavity. The steel rod is pulled back a few centimeters leaving the distal end behind. The catheter is inserted into the abdominal cavity until the inner cuff comes to lie extraperitoneally. Under laparoscopic vision, the distal end is placed into the pelvic cavity and the steel rod is pulled out. A subcutaneous tunnel is created toward caudal and lateral directions, and the catheter is passed through it (■ Fig. 66.9). Extracorporeal omentectomy and the other steps of the procedure are completed as described above.

Three-cannula Technique with Internal Omentectomy

This method of PD catheter insertion is the method of choice described by C.K. Yeung and K.F. Yip in the previous edition of this book. Abdominal exploration, near total omentectomy, and other surgical procedures such as adhesiolysis can be performed at the same time under laparoscopic vision. PD catheters for both acute and chronic dialysis can be properly placed thereby minimizing the chance of subsequent catheter occlusion and treatment failure. In order to optimize the ergonomics of surgical instruments and make efficient use of all the port sites to avoid unnecessary incision, the surgical procedure must be well planned.

The surgeon stands on the patient's right side with the monitor placed across the table just opposite to him. The assistant stands on the surgeon's right-hand side, and the scrub nurse on the opposite side of the table next to the monitor (■ Fig. 66.10). A 1.5- to 2 cm-long infraumbilical semicircular incision is made. The linea alba is incised transversely followed by the peritoneum and a 2-0 polyglactin purse-string suture is placed around the opening for maintaining the pneumoperitoneum subsequently. A 10 mm port with adapter for instruments of either 5 or 10 mm is inserted and secured by tying the purse-string suture. Pneumoperitoneum is created with CO_2 at a pressure of

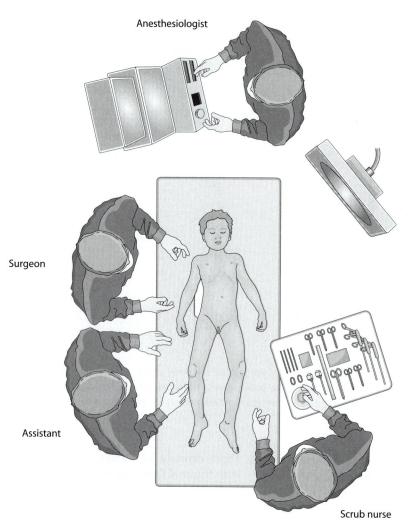

Anesthesiologist

Surgeon

Assistant

Scrub nurse

Fig. 66.10. Three cannula technique with omentectomy. Position of the patient, crew, and equipment.

12 mmHg. The peritoneal cavity is inspected with a videoendoscope. A 5 mm incision is made in the right lower quadrant of the abdominal wall. This becomes the further exit site of the Tenckhoff catheter and hence should avoid the iliac bony prominence. A 5 mm trocar is inserted under laparoscopic guidance through this incision. Another 5 mm port is inserted in the right upper quadrant under laparoscopic control (■ Fig. 66.11). A 5 mm laparoscope is inserted through the lower abdominal port. Thorough laparoscopic inspection of the peritoneal cavity is then performed. The internal inguinal orifices are inspected particularly for patent processus vaginalis. Any intra-abdominal adhesive bands can be divided and released with graspers and electrocautery. A 5 mm ultrasonic scalpel or bipolar forceps is introduced through the infraumbilical port for the surgeon's right hand, and a 5 mm grasper is inserted through the upper abdominal port for the surgeon's left hand. The omentum is grasped with the grasper, and a near total omentectomy is performed using ultrasonic scalpel or bipolar forceps thus minimizing omental blockage of the catheter

(■ Fig. 66.12). Hemostasis is achieved with the ultrasonic scalpel alone without a change of instrument, thereby shortening the operative time remarkably. After completion of the omentectomy the ultrasonic scalpel is replaced by a grasper and omental tissue can be easily removed through the infraumbilical port.

A double-cuffed PD catheter is flushed and trimmed to a suitable length if necessary. The 10 mm umbilical port and polyglactin purse-string suture are removed and the Tenckhoff catheter is introduced via the peritoneal opening which is then closed with a non-absorbable purse-string suture incorporating the base of the inner cuff. The sheath of rectus abdominis muscle is closed with interrupted non-absorbable sutures just above the top of the cuff. The catheter end is occluded with a hemostat and pneumoperitoneum is reintroduced via the air vent in the lower abdominal port. The laparoscope is now moved to the upper abdominal port and the grasper is introduced through the lower abdominal port. The catheter is manipulated with two graspers under laparoscopic guidance in such a way that the distal tip of the catheter comes to lie in the

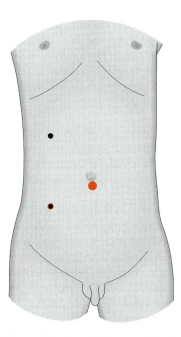

Fig. 66.11. Three cannula technique with omentectomy. Port positions.

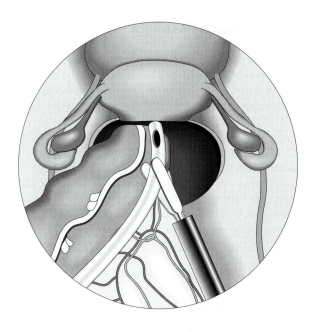

Fig. 66.13. Positioning of the tip of the catheter in front of the rectum.

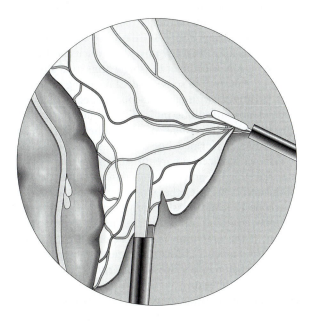

Fig. 66.12. Omentectomy.

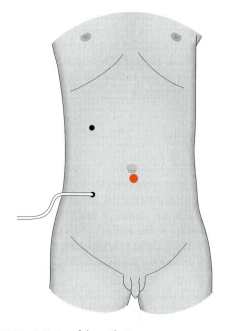

Fig. 66.14. Exit site of the catheter.

rectovaginal pouch in females and in the rectovesical pouch in males (■ Fig. 66.13).

After the procedure the abdominal ports are removed. A subcutaneous tunnel is created between the infraumbilical and lower abdominal incisions. The catheter is brought out of the lower abdominal incision with the outer cuff embedded in the subcutaneous tissue about 2.5 cm from the exit site of the catheter

(■ Fig. 66.14). The upper abdominal and infraumbilical incisions are closed with subcuticular absorbable sutures. Free two-way flow via the catheter is tested with 15–20 ml/kg of normal saline or dialysate. The catheter is then flushed with 2,000 U heparin to ensure patency. The skin incisions and catheter exit site are securely dressed. All catheter connections are also covered by sterile dressings.

Alternative Technique

The operation is started as described above and omentectomy is completed. At this stage the lower abdominal trocar is pulled out and the PD catheter over the steel rod is introduced to the abdominal cavity as described under "alternative technique for the two-cannula technique." The distal end of the catheter is located into the pelvic cavity and the steel rod is taken out. The catheter can also be manipulated with a grasper through the upper abdominal port, if necessary. The trocars are pulled out. A subcutaneous tunnel is created between the lower and upper abdominal incisions and the catheter is passed through it. The catheter exit may be directed laterally and downward by creating a new tunnel with a slight bend.

Postoperative Care

Patients who do not require extensive adhesiolysis are allowed to eat once they have regained full consciousness. Vital signs are observed overnight, and abdominal signs are monitored. If necessary, PD can be started immediately after the procedure with frequent, low-volume exchanges at 25–30% of full volume cycles, although we usually recommend waiting for 24–48 h before commencement of dialysis. Patients can be discharged home if oral diet is tolerated well and if the catheter functions properly. During the healing period, immobilization of the catheter is important to avoid catheter exit site trauma.

Flushing

Although there is no common consensus, it is believed that early flushing of the catheter with heparin solution after placement lowers the risk of catheter obstruction. For this reason, we routinely flush the catheter with heparin solution at the end of the operation and low-volume heparinized-fluid exchange is continued by the nephrology team until the fluid is clear.

Immediate or Delayed Use of the Catheter

Delayed use of the catheter could lower leakage but the infection risk may be higher in these patients.

Occurrence and Management of Complications Amenable to Endoscopic Surgical Treatment

There are many complications that can occur in conjunction with PD catheters:

1. Infection: catheter infection, peritonitis
2. Increased fluid into the peritoneal cavity: hernia, hydrocele, edema of the scrotum, hydrothorax
3. Leakage directly after insertion
4. Mechanical catheter problems: outflow problems, cuff dislodgement

For management of complications associated with a PD catheter, almost all surgical procedures can be performed laparoscopically, for example the changing or repositioning of the catheter, omentectomy, and adhesiolysis.

The most common complication of PD is infection. Excessive infection is the primary reason for PD termination in surviving patients who have not had a transplant. One peritonitis episode for each 11.5–30 catheter months is reported in different series (Bakkaloglu et al. 2005; Emir et al. 2000; Furth et al. 2000; Holtta et al. 1997; Kuizon et al. 1995; Rinaldi et al. 2004; Stone et al. 1986). The frequency of infection is greatest in the youngest patients. Refractory peritonitis, relapsing peritonitis, peritonitis associated with tunnel infection or chronic exit site infection, peritonitis associated with intra-abdominal pathology, and fungal peritonitis, either at the time of diagnosis or if there is no response to therapy within 4–7 days, are the infectious indications for catheter removal (Voinescu and Khanna 2002). A new catheter is usually reinserted after 2–4 weeks. However, in some cases of relapsing or recurrent peritonitis with staphylococcus species or presence of non-infectious indications, simultaneous removal and replacement of the catheter has been successfully performed. The principles for laparoscopic catheter replacement are the same as primary catheter placement. If previous procedures involve one side of the umbilicus, the other side should be used for the telescope to avoid possible adhesions. Any intra-abdominal adhesion can be released under laparoscopic vision. If the omentum is still present, it can be removed and a new peritoneal catheter can be placed as described before in a space in the peritoneal cavity that is free from adhesions.

The most common causes of outflow obstruction are related to the peritonitis, adhesions as a result of the surgery or previous infections, omental wrapping around the catheter, catheter dislodgment, or fibrin plaque. Blockage of the catheter can occur in 15–20% of cases in most adult series and has a much higher incidence of up to 50% in pediatric patients (Mingueala et al. 2001; Nicholson et al. 1991; Stone et al. 1986). Another important complication causing outflow problems is catheter migration. It is seen in 5–35% of patients. Migration of the catheter tip from the pouch of Douglas may cause sluggish dialysate outflow especially of the last portion of dialysate. The predisposing factors for catheter migration include improper place-

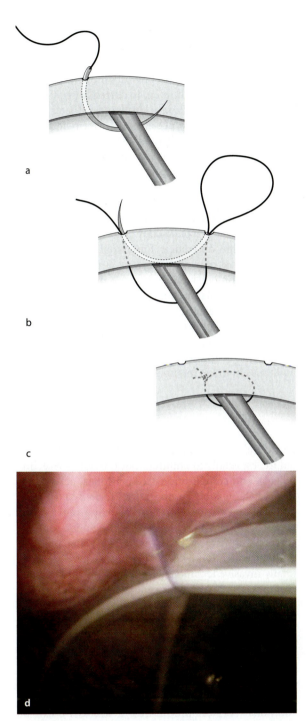

Fig. 66.15. a–c Fixation of the catheter to anterior abdominal wall. Depending on the laparoscopic technique, the catheter is pushed to the anterior abdominal wall with a forceps or steel rod inserted into the catheter. Under laparoscopic vision, a 2-0 nylon suture with a curved needle is turned around the catheter and taken out from the other side of the catheter through 1 mm skin incisions. The needle is turned back subcutaneously and tied. **d** Intraoperative view of completed fixation.

ment of the catheter, catheter type, abdominal incision, omental attachment, and the direction of the subcutaneous tunnel. The first step to avoid this problem is the correct and secure placement of the catheter. For this purpose the laparoscopic techniques have to be preferred over a percutaneous technique or a small laparotomy. The swan-neck, curled catheter is reported to have less migration risk (Gadallah et al. 2000a). Laparoscopy is ideal for the management of these obstructed catheters. Catheters with intermittent partial blockage due to malpositioning can be repositioned under laparoscopic guidance in a free peritoneal space and additional fixation of the catheter to the abdominal wall with a nylon suture may decrease further malpositioning risk (■ Fig. 66.15). As mentioned above if omentum causes catheter malfunction it can be removed laparoscopically.

Studies have reported 29–42% hernia incidence in infants and young children undergoing PD with an increased incarceration risk (Clark et al. 1992; Leblanc et al. 2001; Stone et al. 1986; Tsai et al. 1996). As a result, many surgeons have advocated routine bilateral inguinal exploration and ligation of any patent processus vaginalis at the time of PD catheter insertion (Grosfeld 1989; Matthews et al. 1990). Therefore, the internal inguinal orifices can be carefully inspected during the laparoscopy, particularly in infants and young children, and prophylactic ligation of any patent processus vaginalis can be performed.

Early or late dialysate leakage is another important complication of PD. The spectrum of dialysate leaks includes any dialysate loss from the peritoneal cavity other than via the lumen of the catheter. Early leakage most often manifests as a pericatheter leak. Late leaks tend to develop during the first year of CAPD and may present more subtly with subcutaneous swelling and edema, weight gain, peripheral or genital edema, and apparent ultrafiltration failure. The incidence of dialysate leakage is somewhat more than 5% in CAPD patients and in pediatric series it rises to 14% (Kuizon et al. 1995; Leblanc et al. 2001; Stone et al. 1986). Factors that are potentially related to dialysate leakage are those related to the technique of PD catheter insertion, the initiation of PD, and weakness of the abdominal wall, which is an important point in children (Leblanc et al. 2001). An association has been found between early leaks and immediate CAPD initiation and perhaps median catheter insertion. Therefore, leakage of dialysate could be minimized by using a peritoneal purse-string suture and by placing the catheter at the lateral edge of the rectus muscle. Endoscopic surgical placement also lowers early leakage rate (Gadallah et al. 1999).

Hydrothorax, an uncommon complication of PD (2–3%), results from the migration of dialysis fluid from the peritoneal cavity into the pleural space and occurs on the right side predominantly. The exact site of the transdiaphragmatic fluid leak remains obscure, but it is most commonly secondary to a pleuroperitoneal communication with diaphragmatic abnormalities (Gagnon and Daniels 2004; Szeto and Chow 2004). Although temporary cessation of PD remains the first-line treatment, chemical or surgical pleurodesis, and open surgical diaphragmatic plication have been reported with successful results (Kawaguchi et al. 1996). But recent studies show that video-assisted thoracoscopic pleurodesis or repair could be the treatment of choice in hydrothorax-complicated PD (Mak et al. 2002; Szeto and Chow 2004).

Results

The two-cannula technique for PD catheter insertion with some modifications has been used in 34 children with renal failure between 1996 and 2002. The mean age of the 15 female and 19 male patients was 10.2 years (range 1.5–16 years). During the mean follow-up period of 34.6 months (range 4–61 months), 9 (26.4%) patients developed 28 peritonitis episodes (one episode per 42 catheter months) and 8 (23.5%) patients needed surgical management because of catheter dysfunction and/or recurrent peritonitis. One catheter was revised because of early dialysate leakage, and another one was changed because of late dialysate leakage-related genital swelling. Comparison with the results of the 21 patients who had open surgical PD catheter placement during the same period showed a lower complication rate in the laparoscopic group. During the follow-up period, 10 secondary procedures have also been successfully performed laparoscopically such as catheter changing, catheter repositioning, and fixation of the catheter to the anterior abdominal wall. Two patients developed an umbilical hernia and one of them had a transumbilical telescope insertion during PD catheter placement. Over the time, some modifications of the technique, such as routine omentectomy, almost vertical catheter entrance into the abdomen, and avoidance of transumbilical trocar insertion, have been performed in order to reduce complications.

Discussion

During the early 1980s, laparoscopic procedures were first used in the management of PD catheter complications in adults (Kittur et al. 1991; Korten et al. 1982). With the availability of modern endoscopic techniques,

the field has been extended and laparoscopy is now for both salvage of catheter complications and insertion of the catheter with internal omentectomy even in pediatric patients. Laparoscopy provides the ability to completely explore the abdomen, to correctly position the catheter, or to reposition a displaced catheter under direct vision. It is also possible to perform additional surgical procedures such as adhesiolysis and omentectomy simultaneously without formal laparotomy. It has been reported that laparoscopic procedures for PD catheter placement lowered the early infection rate, compared to open surgery (Ates et al. 1997; Emir et al. 1997; Gadallah et al. 1999). Less tissue damage and less handling during laparoscopy may be the possible causes of this difference. Endoscopic surgical techniques are not only advantageous in terms of a lower early infection rate but also in terms of catheter blockage. Less tissue damage and handling during laparoscopy will possibly cause fewer intra-abdominal adhesion. Additionally, internal inguinal orifices can be inspected during laparoscopy and if an open processus vaginalis is diagnosed it can be fixed simultaneously and thus eliminate inguinal hernia or hydrocele risk.

Conclusions

Peritoneal dialysis is the treatment of choice for renal failure, especially in children, but it requires a secure, reliable, and complication-free peritoneal access. Unfortunately possible complications related to the peritoneal access may develop, and this may give rise to the failure of the technique. The surgical technique and the surgeon's skill are very important in placing a reliable catheter, which is the key to the success of PD. As minimally invasive techniques have gained worldwide acceptance, laparoscopic procedures have been involved in the management of PD catheters as well. In the early 1980s, salvaging of complications associated with PD catheters and then laparoscopic placement of the PD catheter were described. Nowadays laparoscopic catheter placement is a routine procedure in many centers. Complete exploration of the abdominal cavity and particularly of the internal inguinal orifices, and additional surgical procedures, if necessary, can be performed laparoscopically without the need for a formal laparotomy. More importantly proper positioning of the tip of the catheter into the pelvic cavity is easily maintained. Data from the literature as well as our experience show that laparoscopic PD catheter placement provides better catheter survival than open surgical or percutaneous catheter placement.

References

Ash RS (2002) Chronic peritoneal dialysis catheters: procedure for placement, maintenance, and removal. Semin Nephrol 22:221–236

Ates K, Ertürk S, Karatan O, et al (1997) A comparison between percutaneous and surgical placement techniques of permanent peritoneal dialysis catheters. Nephron 75:98–99

Bakkaloglu SA, Ekim M, Sever L, et al (2005) Chronic peritoneal dialysis in Turkish children: a multicenter study. Pediatr Nephrol 20:644–651

Bloxum A, Powell N (1948) The treatment of acute temporary dysfunction of the kidneys by peritoneal irrigation. Pediatrics 1:53–57

Brownlee J, Elkhairi S (1997) Laparoscopic assisted placement of peritoneal dialysis catheter: a preliminary experience. Clin Nephrol 47:122–124

Chadha V, Jones LL, Ramirez ZD, et al (2000) Chest wall peritoneal dialysis catheter placement in infants with a colostomy. Adv Perit Dial 16:318–320

Clark KR, Forsythe JL, Rigg KM, et al (1992) Surgical aspects of chronic peritoneal dialysis in neonate and infant under 1 year of age. J Pediatr Surg 27:780–783

Cruz CM, Dimkovic N, Bargman JW, et al (2001) Is catheter function influenced by the side of the body in which the peritoneal dialysis catheter is placed? Perit Dial Int 21:526

Diaz-Buxo JA, Walker PJ, Farmer CD, Chandler JT, Holt KL, Cox P (1981) Continuous cyclic peritoneal dialysis. Trans Am Soc Artif Intern Organs 27:51–54

Emir H, Söylet Y, Büyükünal C, Danismend N (1997) Laparoscopic insertion of the peritoneal dialysis catheter. Eighth Annual Meeting of European Society of Pediatric Urology, Rome, Abstract Book, p 33.

Emir H, Tekant G, Yesildag E, et al (2000) Laparoscopic insertion of Tenckhoff dialysis catheter in children: preliminary report. J Turk Pediatr Surg 14:20–24

Furth SL, Donaldson LA, Sullivan EK, et al (2000) North American Pediatric Renal Transplant Cooperative Study. Peritoneal dialysis catheter infections and peritonitis in children: a report of the North American Pediatric Renal Transplant Cooperative Study. Pediatr Nephrol 15:179–182

Gadallah MF, Pervez A, el-Shahawy MA, et al (1999) Peritoneoscopic versus surgical placement of peritoneal dialysis catheters: a prospective randomized study on outcome. Am J Kidney Dis 33:118–122

Gadallah MF, Mignone J, Torres C, et al (2000a) The role of peritoneal dialysis catheter configuration in preventing catheter tip migration. Adv Perit Dial 16:47–50

Gadallah MF, Ramdeen G, Mignone J, et al (2000b) Role of preoperative antibiotic prophylaxis in preventing postoperative peritonitis in newly placed peritoneal dialysis catheters. Am J Kidney Dis 36:1014–1019

Gagnon RF, Daniels E (2004) The persisting pneumatoenteric recess and the infracardiac bursa: possible role in the pathogenesis of right hydrothorax complicating peritoneal dialysis. Adv Perit Dial 20:132–136

Grosfeld JL (1989) Current concepts in inguinal hernia in infants and children. World J Surg 13:506–515

Harvey EA (2001) Peritoneal access in children. Perit Dial Int 21(suppl 3):S218–S222

Holtta TM, Ronnholm KA, Jalanko H, et al (1997) Peritoneal dialysis in children under 5 years of age. Perit Dial Int 17:573–580

Hwang SJ, Chang JM, Chen HC, et al (1998) Smaller insertion angle of Tenckhoff catheter increases the chance of catheter migration in CAPD patients. Perit Dial Int 18:433–435

Kawaguchi AL, Dunn JC, Fonkalsrud EW (1996) Management of peritoneal dialysis-induced hydrothorax in children. Am Surg 62:820–824

Kittur DS, Gazaway PM, Abidin MR (1991) Laparoscopic repositioning of malfunctioning peritoneal dialysis catheters. Surg Laparosc Endosc 1:179–182

Korten G, Arendt R, Brugmann E, Klein B (1982) A new procedure for the revision and reposition of functionless peritoneal dialysis catheters. Z Urol Nephrol 75:885–887

Kuizon B, Melocoton TL, Holloway M, et al (1995) Infectious and catheter-related complications in pediatric patients treated with peritoneal dialysis at a single institution. Pediatr Nephrol 9(suppl):S12–S17

Leblanc M, Ouimet D, Pichette V (2001) Dialysate leaks in peritoneal dialysis. Semin Dial 14:50–54

Leung LC, Yiu MK, Man CW, et al (1998) Laparoscopic management of Tenckhoff catheters in continuous ambulatory peritoneal dialysis. Surg Endosc 12:891–893

Lewis MA, Smith T, Roberts D (1996) Peritonitis, functional catheter loss and the siting of the Dacron cuff in chronic peritoneal dialysis catheters in children. Eur J Pediatr Surg 6:285–287

Lewis MA, Smith T, Postlethwaite RJ, et al (1997) A comparison of double-cuffed with single-cuffed Tenckhoff catheters in the prevention of infection in pediatric patients. Adv Perit Dial 13:274–276

Mak SK, Nyunt K, Wong PN, et al (2002) Long-term follow-up of thoracoscopic pleurodesis for hydrothorax complicating peritoneal dialysis. Ann Thorac Surg 74:218–221

Matthews DE, West KW, Rescorla FJ, Vane DW, et al (1990) Peritoneal dialysis in the first 60 days of life. J Pediatr Surg 25:110–115

Minguela I, Lanuza M, Ruiz de Gauna R, et al (2001) A lower malfunction rate with self-locating catheters. Perit Dial Int 21(suppl 3):S209–S212

Moncrief JW, Nolph KD, Rubin J, Popovich RP (1978) Additional experience with continuous ambulatory peritoneal dialysis (CAPD). Trans Am Soc Artif Intern Organs 24:476–483

Nicholson ML, Burton PR, Donnely PK, et al (1991) The role of omentectomy in continuous ambulatory peritoneal dialysis. Perit Dial Int 11:330–332

Nijhuis PHA, Smulders JF, Jakimowicz JJ (1996) Laparoscopic introduction of a continuous ambulatory dialysis (CAPD) catheter by a two-puncture technique. Surg Endosc 10:676–679

Owens LV, Brader AH (1995) Laparoscopic salvage of Tenckhoff catheters. Surg Endosc 9:517–518

Palmer RA, Quinton WE, Gray JF (1964) Prolonged peritoneal dialysis for chronic renal failure. Lancet 1:700–702

Pommer W, Brauner M, Westphale HJ, et al (1998) Effect of a silver device in preventing catheter-related infections in peritoneal dialysis patients: silver ring prophylaxis at the catheter exit study. Am J Kidney Dis 32:752–760

Popovich RP, Moncrief JW, Decherd JW, et al (1976) The definition of a novel wearable/portable equilibrium peritoneal dialysis technique. Trans Am Soc Artif Intern Organs 5:64

Rinaldi S, Sera F, Verrina E, et al (2004) Chronic peritoneal dialysis catheters in children: a fifteen-year experience of the Italian Registry of Pediatric Chronic Peritoneal Dialysis. Perit Dial Int 24:481–486

Stone MM, Fonkalsrud EW, Salusky IB, et al (1986) Surgical management of peritoneal dialysis catheters in children: five-year experience with 1,800 patient-month follow-up. J Pediatr Surg 21:1177–1181

Swan H, Gordon HH (1949) Peritoneal lavage in treatment of anuria in children. Pediatrics 4:586–594

Szeto CC, Chow KM (2004) Pathogenesis and management of hydrothorax complicating peritoneal dialysis. Curr Opin Pulm Med 10:315–319

Tenckhoff H, Schechter H (1968) A bacteriologically safe peritoneal access device. Trans Am Soc Artif Intern Organs 14:181–187

Tsai TC, Huang FY, Hsu JC, et al (1996) Continuous ambulatory peritoneal dialysis complicating with abdominal hernias in children. Zhonghua Min Guo Xiao Er Ke Yi Xue Hui Za Zhi 37:263–265

Verrina E, Honda M, Warady BA, et al (2000) Prevention of peritonitis in children on peritoneal dialysis. Perit Dial Int 20:625–630

Voinescu CG, Khanna R (2002) Peritonitis in peritoneal dialysis. Int J Artif Organ 25:249–260

Walboomers F, Paquay YC, Jansen JA (2001) A new titanium fiber mesh-cuffed peritoneal dialysis catheter: evaluation and comparison with a Dacron-cuffed Tenckhoff catheter in goats. Perit Dial Int 21:254–262

Warchol S, Roszkowska-Blaim M, Sieniawska M (1998) Swan neck presternal peritoneal dialysis catheter: five-year experience in children. Perit Dial Int 18:183–187

Abdomen

Abdominal Trauma

Chapter 67

Abdominal Trauma

Thomas Pranikoff

Introduction

The evaluation of acute trauma to the chest and abdomen continues to evolve. This area remains a challenge for the surgeon and may include diagnostic tests such as ultrasonography and computed tomography (CT) or laparotomy in unstable patients. Laparoscopy has only been used on a limited basis for evaluation and management of abdominal and chest trauma patients. Once injuries are identified, many will require conversion to laparotomy for definitive management. Some injuries can be managed laparoscopically depending on the magnitude of the injury and the skills of the surgeon.

Preoperative Preparation

Patients should have a nasogastric tube and Foley catheter placed to decompress the stomach and bladder. Broad-spectrum antibiotics should be administered.

Positioning

Patient

Patients should be placed in the supine position with access to all quadrants of the abdomen.

Equipment

Two monitors should be used, with one at the head of the table and one at the foot (Fig. 67.1).

Technique

Cannulae

A 5 mm expandable, disposable cannula is inserted at the umbilicus, and two aditional 5 mm cannulae are inserted at the umbilical level bilaterally.

Port Positions

Figure 67.2 shows port positions.

Procedure

Access is obtained by Veress needle or open cutdown at the umbilicus. After entering the abdomen, the lateral trocars are placed under direct vision (Fig. 67.2). Initial evaluation should include a thorough inspection of the parietal peritoneum of the anterior and lateral abdominal wall, paying particular attention to any known abdominal wall wounds. Using a 30° telescope that is rotated anteriorly will improve the view of the anterior abdominal wall (Fig. 67.3).

The upper abdomen is evaluated next. To aid in visualization of the left upper quadrant, the table can be tilted 30° to the right. The liver can be retracted by elevating the left lobe with a blunt grasper. The anterior surface of the stomach is evaluated by starting at the gastroesophageal junction and examining the anterior surface and fundus (Fig. 67.4). The spleen should be evaluated superiorly, inferiorly, and medially. The posterior and lateral aspects are more difficult to evaluate. The spleen can be retracted bluntly with a grasper to better evaluate these areas. If injury is noted and active bleeding encountered, laparotomy should be performed (Fig. 67.5). The anterior surface of the left lobe of the liver and left hemidiaphragm can be well visualized by retracting the liver posteriorly with a blunt grasper. The triangular ligaments of the liver may need to be mobilized for better exposure (Fig. 67.6). The posterior surface of the stomach can be viewed by entering the lesser sac through an avascular portion of the gastrocolic ligament. The pancreas can also be observed (Fig. 67.7).

The right upper quadrant is now evaluated. The table is placed back in a flat position or tilted 30° to the left. The right lobe of the liver is evaluated anteriorly and laterally with retraction from a grasper (Fig. 67.8). The right hemidiaphragm and right tri-

Anesthesiologist

Fig. 67.1. Position of the patient, crew and monitors

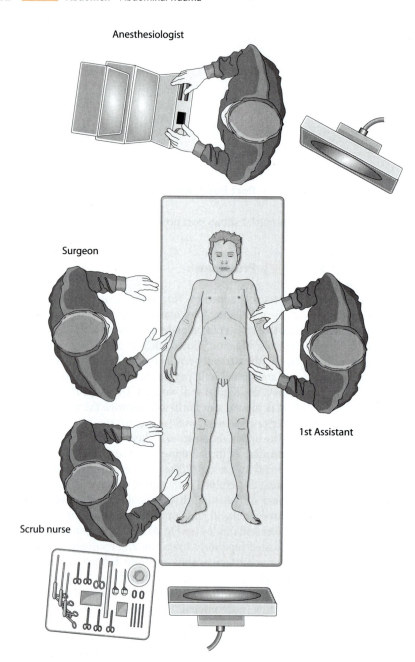

Surgeon

1st Assistant

Scrub nurse

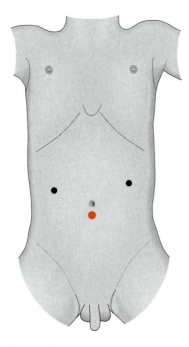

Fig. 67.2. Port positions

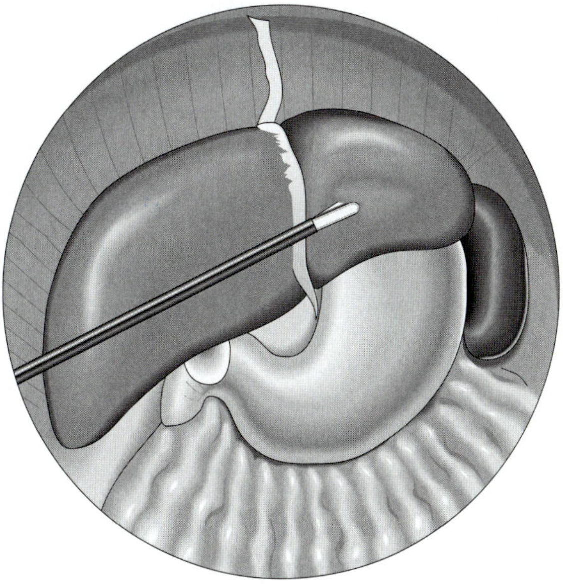

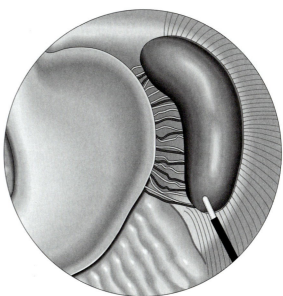

Fig. 67.4. View of the upper abdomen

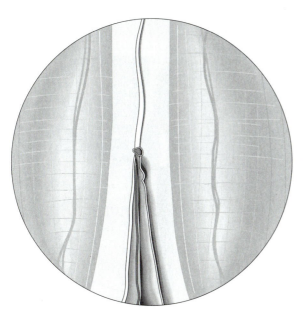

Fig. 67.3. View of the anterior abdominal wall, which is facilitated by rotation of the 30° telescope anteriorly. Note the superior and inferior epigastric vessels

Fig. 67.5. Retraction of the spleen with a grasper

angular ligament are readily visible. Liver injuries that are bleeding can be cauterized, but persistent bleeding should lead to conversion to laparotomy (■ Fig. 67.9). Injury to the diaphragm can be easily seen and can be repaired depending upon the experience of the surgeon (■ Fig. 67.10). The posterior surface of the liver is explored by elevating the right lobe with a blunt grasper.

The liver, gallbladder, and porta hepatis are seen. The duodenum and transverse colon lie inferiorly (■ Fig. 67.11). The duodenum can be evaluated anteriorly, but to adequately evaluate the second and third portions, a Kocher maneuver can be accomplished by dividing the lateral peritoneal reflection and mobilizing the duodenum medially to the inferior vena cava. The

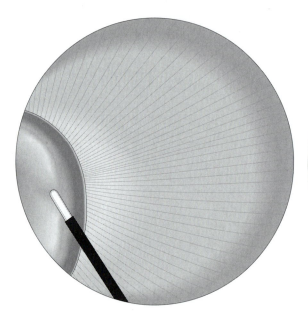

Fig. 67.6. Posterior retraction of the liver to view the anterior surface of the left lobe of the liver and left hemidiaphragm

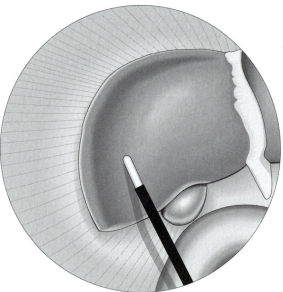

Fig. 67.8. Evaluation of right lobe of the liver

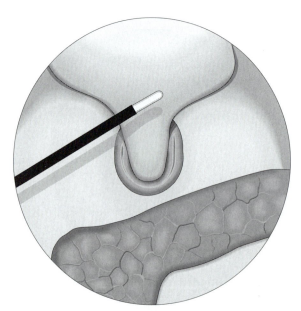

Fig. 67.7. View of the surface of the stomach and anterior surface of the pancreas

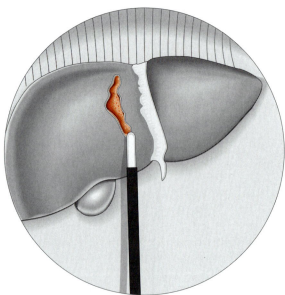

Fig. 67.9. Cauterization of a liver laceration

head of the pancreas can be seen. The duodenum is followed to the ligament of Treitz (■ Fig. 67.12).

The small bowel is evaluated by using a "hand-over-hand" technique to visualize both sides of the peritoneal surface including the mesentery until the cecum is reached. Careful examination of both surfaces including the mesentery is important (■ Fig. 67.13). The colon is then examined. The right and left colon can be

mobilized as needed for visualization of suspected injury. The right paracolic gutter is examined paying particular attention to retroperitoneal hematoma as evidence of injury. This is especially important if there is a penetrating wound overlying this area. If there is a question, the retroperitoneal attachments can be divided and the colon mobilized medially to further explore this area (■ Fig. 67.14).

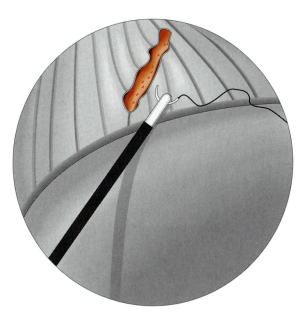

Fig. 67.10. Suture repair of an injury to the diapragm

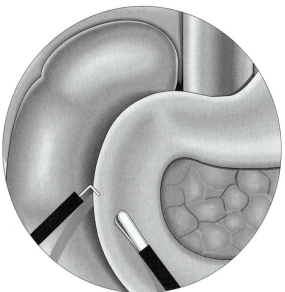

Fig. 67.12. Mobilization of the duodenum

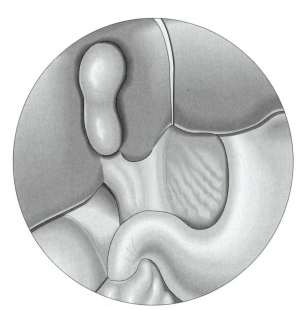

Fig. 67.11. Exploration of right upper quadrant

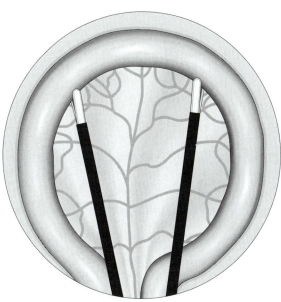

Fig. 67.13. The small bowel is evaluated by using a hand-over-hand technique

The table should be placed in Trendelenburg position and the right lower quadrant examined. The cecum, appendix, and terminal ileum can be easily seen (■ Fig. 67.15). The left paracolic gutter can be evaluated next in a similar fashion to the right paracolic gutter, taking care to evaluate for evidence of retroperitoneal injury. With the table in Trendelenburg position, the sigmoid colon can be visualized. Babcock retractors are used to examine this structure in a hand-over-

hand technique carefully observing both the anterior and posterior surfaces into the pelvis (■ Fig. 67.16).

The pelvis is visualized next. Note is made of peritoneal fluid and its character (blood, stool, bile, etc.). The rectum can be lifted out of the pelvis and examined. The pelvic organs in the female are readily seen. The urinary bladder can be seen and elevated with a grasper to evaluate for injury. The space anterior and posterior to the rectum can be well evaluated (■ Fig. 67.17).

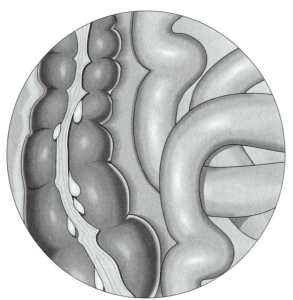

Fig. 67.14. Examination of the right colon

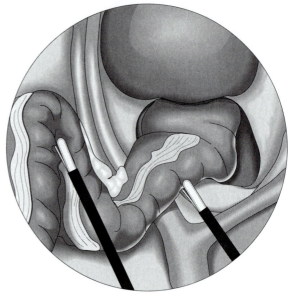

Fig. 67.16. Babcock retractors are used to examine the sigmoid colon in a hand-over-hand technique

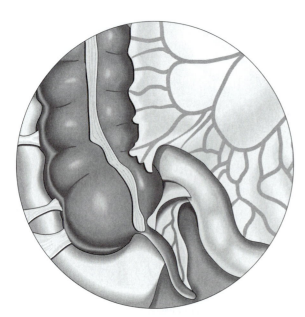

Fig. 67.15. View of the cecum, appendix, and terminal ileum in the right lower quadrant

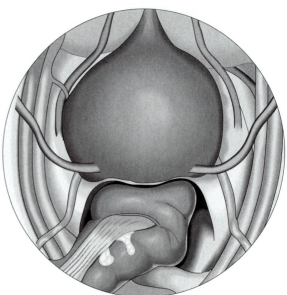

Fig. 67.17. Evaluation of the pelvis

Postoperative Care

A nasogastric tube is left in place until ileus resolves after thorough mobilization of the intestine. Feeding is begun after gastrointestinal function returns, unless contraindicated by injury.

Results

Penetrating and blunt injuries to the abdomen in stable patients pose a diagnostic dilemma, especially those that may involve the chest and injure the diaphragm. CT scanning has helped diagnose many injuries from blunt trauma, but the definitive diagnostic study remains laparotomy. The incidence of negative laparotomy is still high and has caused some surgeons to consider laparoscopy as a possible alternative for evaluation of abdominal trauma. In 1976, Gazzaniga et al. reported the use of laparoscopy for trauma in 37 out of a series of 132 consecutive patients with blunt and penetrating injuries. They noted findings of splenic injury, small intestine perforation, and minor liver lacerations. Ten patients with blunt injury had laparoscopy only, including three who had bloody peritoneal lavage. There were no false-positives and none needed further management of abdominal injuries. Eighty patients with penetrating injuries were evaluated. Four patients had laparoscopy: two had no peritoneal penetration, one had a non-bleeding omental injury, and one had a high velocity rifle injury to the chest and laparoscopy failed to reveal an injury. He subsequently developed a colonic perforation thought to be a result of cavitation effect. Sixty-seven patients with penetrating injuries underwent laparotomy without laparoscopy. Fifty-two had injuries that required surgical intervention and the remaining 15 had minimal trauma which would not have required surgical intervention. McQuay and Britt (2003) used laparoscopy in the evaluation of penetrating thoracoabdominal injuries in 80 patients. Fifty-eight (72.5%) had negative findings and were spared laparotomy. Injury to the diaphragm was found in 22 patients who all then underwent laparotomy. In 17 (77.2%) of these patients, an injury requiring surgical intervention was discovered.

Discussion

Laparoscopy for abdominal trauma in children is not utilized by many centers but is increasing in its use recently. The major indication is to evaluate for penetrating injury of the abdominal wall to confirm or rule out intra-abdominal injury. Some pediatric surgeons have managed injuries using established advanced laparoscopic techniques such as suture repair of diaphragm injury or cauterization of liver laceration. Most injuries, once identified, will require conversion to laparotomy for definitive management. (For further reading see Berci et al. 1991; Fabian et al. 1993; Ivatury et al. 1993; Mattox et al. 2000; Ochner et al. 1993; Porter and Ivatury 1999; Salvino et al. 1993; Smith et al. 1993; Sosa et al. 1992; Zantut et al. 1997)

References

Berci G, Sackier JM, Paz-Partlow M (1991) Emergency laparoscopy. Am J Surg 161:332–335

Fabian TC, Croce MA, Stewart RM, et al (1993) A prospective analysis of diagnostic laparoscopy in trauma. Ann Surg 217:557–565

Gazzaniga AB, Stanton WW, Bartlett RH (1976) Laparoscopy in the diagnosis of blunt and penetrating injuries to the abdomen. Am J Surg 131:315–318

Ivatury RR, Simon RJ, Stahl WM (1993) A critical evaluation of laparoscopy in penetrating abdominal trauma. J Trauma 34:822–828

Mattox KL, Feliciano DV, Moore EE (2000) Trauma, 4th edn. McGraw-Hill, New York, pp 588–589

McQuay N, Britt LD (2003) Laparoscopy in the evaluation of penetrating thoracoabdominal trauma. Am Surg 69:788–791

Ochner MG, Rozycki GS, Lucente F, et al (1993) Prospective evaluation of thoracoscopy for diagnosing diaphragmatic injury in thoracoabdominal trauma: a preliminary report. J Trauma 34:704–710

Porter JM, Ivatury RR (1999) Laparoscopy and thoracoscopy. In: Current Therapy of Trauma, 4th edn. Mosby, St Louis, MO, pp 155–157

Salvino CK, Esposito TJ, Marshall WS, et al (1993) The role of diagnostic laparoscopy in the management of trauma patients: a preliminary assessment. J Trauma 34:506–515

Smith RS, Fry WR, Sayers DV, et al (1993) Gasless laparoscopy and conventional instruments. The next phase of minimally invasive surgery. Arch Surg 128:1102–1107

Sosa JL, Sims D, Martin L, et al (1992) Laparoscopic evaluation of tangential abdominal gunshot wounds. Arch Surg 127:109–110

Zantut LF, Ivatury RR, Smith RS, et al (1997) Diagnostic and therapeutic laparoscopy for penetrating abdominal trauma: a multicenter experience. J Trauma 42:825–831

Abdomen

Abdominal Oncology

Chapter 68

Laparoscopy for Pediatric Abdominal Malignancies

Shawn D. St. Peter and George W. Holcomb

Introduction

Since the 1990s, minimally invasive surgery has been applied in the pediatric population for the purposes of diagnosing, staging, and treating abdominal malignancies. Although the development of these rapidly evolving techniques for the management of abdominal tumors is actively maturing in the pediatric surgery arena, its progression is overshadowed by the experience of adult surgeons. The explanation for this discrepancy is multifaceted. In terms of the nature of the disease processes, abdominal tumors are rare in children relative to adults, and these pediatric tumors are typically more amenable to systemic therapy. Anatomically, common pediatric tumors develop in surgically remote areas of the abdomen, and they are often discovered at an advanced size relative to the small size of the host which makes for arduous laparoscopic resection. In terms of technical development, many common benign indications for laparoscopic surgery exist in adults within the organs that later develop malignancy. Therefore, adult surgeons have the opportunity to refine laparoscopic operations in an organ-specific manner. A good example is the development of laparoscopic colon resection in adults which was initially employed for benign disease and later progressed to malignant conditions. In contrast, pediatric surgeons do not have a comparable opportunity to refine procedures with oncologic applications since there are few indications for laparoscopy that would facilitate the skills necessary to remove pediatric tumors such as Wilms' tumors, neuroblastomas, hepatoblastomas, and rhabdomyosarcomas. Thus, the current literature regarding laparoscopy in infants and children with malignant disease is devoid of well-defined procedures for curative resection. This chapter focuses on the broader discussion of how minimally invasive techniques can enhance the capacity to care for children with abdominal malignancies by allowing for efficacious means of diagnosis, staging, and treatment while minimizing iatrogenic injury.

Preoperative Preparation

The preoperative preparation for infants and children with cancer undergoing laparoscopic procedures does not differ significantly from patients undergoing more common operations such as fundoplication, splenectomy, cholecystectomy, and pelvic operations. It can be advantageous to have the parents give the patient an enema the night before the procedure to help evacuate the rectum for procedures in the mid to lower abdomen and pelvis. A urinary catheter is useful for bladder decompression for pelvic procedures. A nasogastric tube is inserted for upper abdominal operations. Otherwise, there is no special preparation for these patients.

Positioning

Patient

The patient is positioned supine on the operating table for most operations. For operations involving the upper abdomen, the French position may be preferable in which the surgeon stands between the patient's legs to operate. In young children, the patient can be placed frog-legged at the end of the table to achieve the same purpose. For patients requiring either a splenectomy for a malignancy or adrenalectomy, the patient is turned either into a 45° or a 90° position, respectively (■ Fig. 68.1). If the patient is undergoing a pelvic procedure, the patient can usually be placed supine on the operating table in a standard position.

Crew, Monitors, and Equipment

Positioning of the monitors is individualized according to the location of the lesion. For lesions in the right upper abdomen, positioning is similar to that for a laparoscopic cholecystectomy. For lesions in the left upper abdomen, it is similar to that for laparoscopic splenectomy. For pelvic procedures, it is best to place the monitor at the foot of the bed. If the surgeon is operating primarily on the patient's left side, then it is advantageous for he/she to stand on the patient's right side (■ Fig. 68.2). The opposite is true for a lesion on the patient's right side. For most operations, the assistant stands on the side opposite the surgeon. For procedures such as splenectomy or adrenalectomy, it may be beneficial for the assistant to stand on the same side as the surgeon (■ Fig. 68.1 a, b).

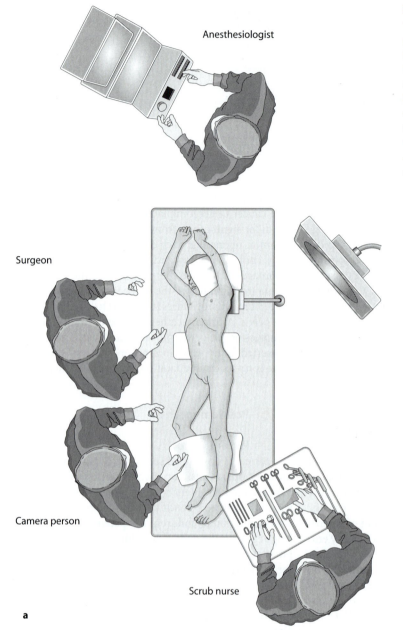

Anesthesiologist

Surgeon

Camera person

Scrub nurse

a

Fig. 68.1 a. The positioning of the patient and operative team is shown for a patient undergoing a splenectomy. We place the patient in a 45° right lateral decubitus position. The surgeon and assistant stand on the patient's left while the scrub nurse stands opposite them. The monitor is placed over the patient's left shoulder so that the surgeon and assistant are able to work in line with the spleen and the monitor.

Fig. 68.1 b. Positioning for a patient undergoing a left adrenalectomy. The patient is placed in a full 90° position. With this position, we prefer a more posterior approach to the adrenal gland and, therefore, the surgeon usually stands to the patient's back and works in line with the left adrenal gland and the monitor is over the patient's right shoulder. The assistant and scrub nurse usually stand opposite the surgeon. Thus, the assistant retracts the organ to the patient's right.

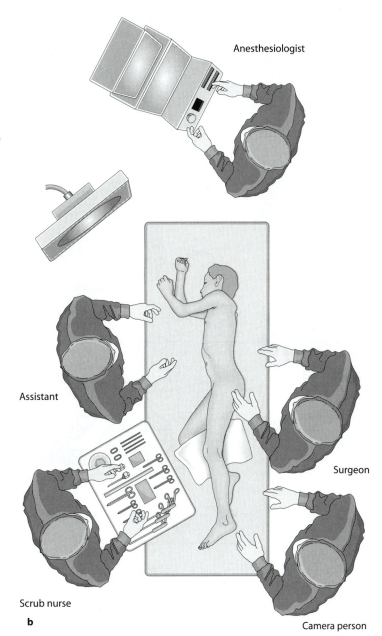

Anesthesiologist

Assistant

Surgeon

Scrub nurse

b

Camera person

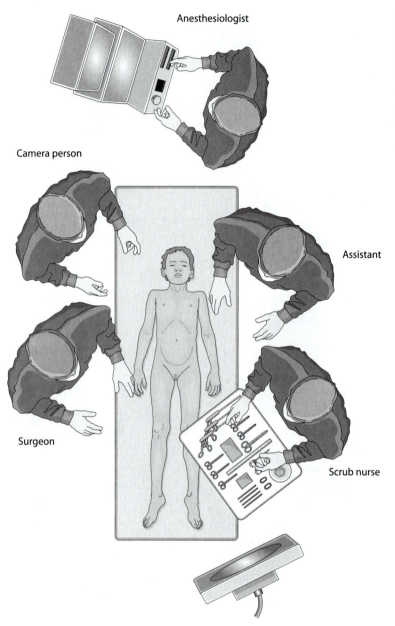

Anesthesiologist

Camera person

Assistant

Surgeon

Scrub nurse

Fig. 68.2. For a pelvic operation, whether biopsy or resection, we prefer that the surgeon stand on the side opposite the lesion. Thus, in the diagram shown, with the lesion on the patient's left side, the surgeon stands on the patient's right side. The assistant and scrub nurse stand opposite the surgeon

Special Equipment

There is usually no need for special equipment for these operations other than that used for standard laparoscopic procedures. The ultrasonic shears (LCS; Ethicon Endosurgery, Cincinnati, OH) can be advantageous in older patients for division of either the short gastric vessels or the mesentery of the small or large bowel. The Ligasure (Valley Lab, Boulder, CO) can be used for the same purpose. The Ligasure is also advantageous for ligation of hepatic parenchyma for segmentectomy or excisional biopsy of hepatic lesions.

Some surgeons prefer the use of bipolar cautery to monopolar cautery and this is certainly appropriate if desired. Endoscopic clips and staplers are part of the standard operating equipment for most laparoscopic procedures and are utilized, when needed, for operations for cancer as well. Laparoscopic ultrasound can also be beneficial if available and if one is experienced in its use. It is advised to place all specimens into an endoscopic retrieval bag to prevent port site metastases which appear to be less common now compared with the late 1990s.

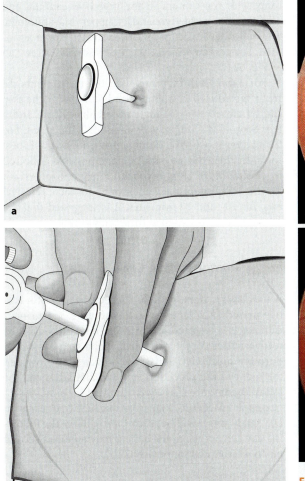

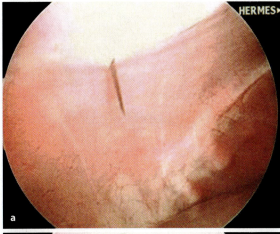

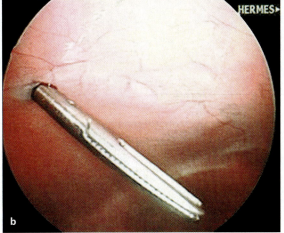

Fig. 68.4. For introduction of accessory instruments, we prefer to place the instrument directly through the abdominal wall without the use of a cannula. **a** A number 11 blade is seen to pierce the peritoneum. **b** The number 11 blade has been removed and the grasping instrument is introduced into the abdominal cavity through the stab incision

Fig. 68.3. We usually place the initial cannula in the umbilicus through a direct cutdown approach. **a** Using this approach, it is usually possible to introduce the Step expandable sheath into the abdominal cavity without the use of a Veress needle. **b** Following insertion of the expandable sheath, the cannula with blunt trocar is introduced in the abdominal cavity through the sheath. The sheath helps stabilize the cannula and the blunt trocar reduces the likelihood of injury to underlying abdominal structures

Technique

As benign and malignant lesions can be found in a variety of locations in the abdominal cavity in infants and children, one single technique does not work well for all possible operations. In general, we prefer to place a 5 mm cannula through the umbilicus using a cutdown technique. For this initial cannula, we do not utilize the Veress needle, but introduce the Step expandable sheath (US Surgical, Norwalk, CT) directly into the peritoneal cavity followed by introduction of the Step cannula with the blunt trocar (■ Fig. 68.3). In this

way, underlying viscera are not injured with the Veress needle. It is our preference to introduce instruments through the abdominal wall without the use of cannulas for most access sites (■ Fig. 68.4). Cannulas are only utilized when instruments such as the ultrasonic shears, endoscopic staplers or clips, Ligasure, or the like are needed. Location of these access sites again varies depending on the operation to be performed. For pelvic lesions, the access sites should be placed in the mid to lower abdominal wall. If the operating team prefers for the camera holder to stand on the patient's left side, then the surgeon can introduce either two instruments or cannulas in the patient's right mid-abdomen and work easily with a lesion on the patient's mid to left pelvic wall. The opposite is true for a lesion on the patient's right pelvis. For lesions in the liver, access site placement is similar to that used for cholecystec-

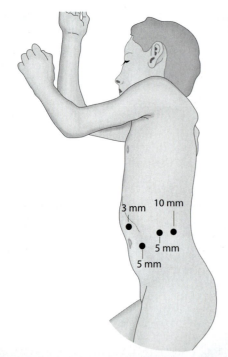

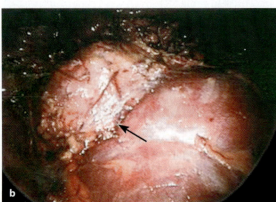

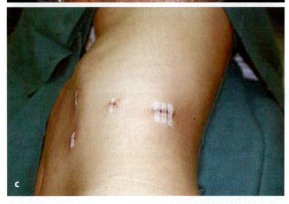

Fig. 68.5. a Location of the access sites for a laparoscopic left adrenalectomy. *Numbers* indicate diameter of site. The 10 mm incision is the one through which the specimen is usually extracted. **b** The pheochromocytoma (*arrow*) is seen lying cephalad to the left kidney. **c** Patient after excision of a left pheochromocytoma.

tomy with the camera in the umbilical cannula and working sites in the right and left upper mid-abdomen. The opposite is true for lesions in the left upper abdomen. For adrenal lesions, the access sites are shown in ■ Fig. 68.5.

For 3 mm stab incisions with the instruments directly introduced through the abdominal wall, the skin can be closed with a single absorbable suture and a SteriStrip (3M Company, St Paul, MN) is applied. For 5 mm sites in which a cannula is introduced, it is best to try to close the anterior fascia, if possible, followed by closure of the skin. Although rarely utilized except for introduction of the stapler or endoscopic retrieval bag, for 10- and 12 mm sites, it is suggested that the anterior fascia is closed at these sites as well.

Postoperative Care

A nasogastric tube is rarely needed in the postoperative period for a laparoscopic procedure. If a urinary catheter was inserted, it can either be removed in the recovery room or later in the day following the procedure. For most operations, clear liquids can be initiated the night of the procedure and the diet advanced the following day. Most patients admitted for either a second-look procedure, a laparoscopic biopsy, or excision of a small tumor will be ready for discharge the following day. On occasion, the patient may require a second postoperative day in the hospital.

Results

As outlined in the Introduction, the experience with laparoscopy for pediatric tumors cannot be described under the headings of specific operations for specific tumors, but alternatively requires a description of the results attained from institutions who have used these techniques for the general purposes of diagnosis, staging, determination of resectability, evaluation of response to treatment, and resection.

Establishing Diagnosis

At present, the most common indication for laparoscopy in a child with an abdominal malignancy is to define the histologic diagnosis in the patient presenting with a new mass (Holcomb 1999; Holcomb et al. 1995; Saenz et al. 1997; Waldhausen et al. 2000). Three major series have thus far documented their experience in utilizing minimally invasive surgery for this purpose. A multi-institutional effort in the USA conducted by the Children's Cancer Group (CCG) demonstrated remarkable efficacy of diagnostic laparoscopy as all nine patients in this series who underwent laparoscopy for suspected cancer received a definitive histologic diagnosis (Holcomb et al. 1995). Further, no conversions were reported in this series secondary to a failure to reach the goal of the operation, although two patients were converted for resection at the time of laparoscopic confirmation of a malignant condition. Similarly, a subsequent series of 15 laparoscopic operations in children with abdominal tumors described nine laparoscopies conducted for initial biopsy (Waldhausen et al. 2000). Laparoscopy adequately provided tissue to establish an accurate diagnosis in all cases. While no conversions were performed as a consequence of failure to attain tissue, two operations were converted when the frozen section analysis of the laparoscopic biopsy yielded a benign diagnosis. Yet, after conversion, no evidence of malignancy was found in either case.

LaQuaglia and his colleagues from Memorial Sloan-Kettering Cancer Center have published the largest series using laparoscopy for diagnostic purposes. They described 46 minimally invasive procedures performed in children with an abdominal malignancy, of which 39 patients underwent diagnostic laparoscopy (Seanz et al. 1997). In this series, adequate tissue to establish the diagnosis was obtained in all cases. The mean operative time in this series was 100 min with a mean hospital stay of 2 days. Conversion was required in six patients (13%) for poor visibility or limited exposure. None of the patients in this series required a delay in initiation of chemotherapy secondary to ileus or any other postoperative complication. The authors of all of these series have concluded that minimally invasive techniques allow for safe and accurate diagnosis of pediatric abdominal malignancies.

In a preliminary report from an ongoing prospective clinical trial, Warmann et al. (2003) concluded that minimally invasive surgery is an excellent approach for diagnostic interventions in patients with suspected malignancy. Although they do not distinguish between laparoscopy and thoracoscopy in their report, no conversions were required for accurate diagnosis in seven tumor biopsies. In a small study from Japan analyzing laparoscopy for neuroblastoma, six patients underwent diagnostic laparoscopy without conversion (Iwanaka et al. 2001a). Compared to nine patients who underwent open diagnostic laparotomy, laparoscopy was found to be associated with a decreased mean operative blood loss (12 ml versus 43 ml), although this difference was not significant. Those patients who underwent laparoscopy demonstrated significantly faster return to feeding and a shorter hospital stay. More importantly, these patients were able to begin systemic therapy significantly sooner than their open counterparts. Data regarding the impact of these differences on clinical outcome are not currently available.

Staging/Determination of Resectability

Despite advances in the quality of cross-sectional and three-dimensional imaging, discrepancies continue to exist between preoperative staging and the findings at the time of surgery (Yoshida et al. 2002). In a comparative study on the staging of Hodgkin's disease, surgical assessment by laparotomy was found to alter the stage in 37% compared to computed tomography and lymphography due the ability to sample the spleen and retroperitoneal lymph nodes (Baker et al. 1990). While there have been no investigations to evaluate the ability of laparoscopy to provide staging information comparable to laparotomy, inferences can be made from the scientific work conducted thus far. In pediatric solid tumors, morcellated specimens obtained at laparoscopy have been found to provide accurate histologic staging (Lobe et al. 1994; Pautler et al. 2002). Moreover, studies in the adult population with renal cell carcinoma have demonstrated that high-speed electrical morcellation did not alter the determination of histology, grade, or local invasiveness of the tumor (Landman et al. 2000; Lobe et al. 1994).

In the series reported by the CCG, four laparoscopies were performed for staging without complication. Splenectomy was performed in two of these cases (Holcomb et al. 1995). The other two series did not separately describe the results of operations performed for staging or determination of resectability.

Evaluation of Response

Exploration or reexploration to assess response to therapy is helpful in guiding clinical decision making for diseases such as neuroblastoma, rhabdomyosarcoma, germ cell tumors, or Wilms' tumors which are treated by systemic therapy in a neoadjuvant manner (■ Fig. 68.6) (Cushieri 1994; Holcomb et al. 1995; Pratt and Greene 2000; Waldhausen et al. 2000). Only two series have reported experience with this application. In a series by Waldhausen et al. (2000), six second-look operations were performed, and four were described in the CCG series (Holcomb et al. 1995). Exploration was considered successful in all ten cases as there were no conversions, and no patient subsequently displayed a clinical course that was inconsistent with the diagnosis determined by the second-look operation.

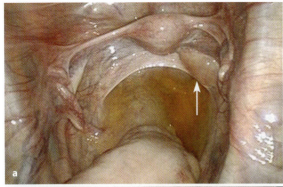
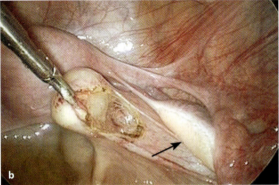

Fig. 68.6. This teenager was diagnosed with a germ cell tumor at the time of laparotomy for a pelvic mass. The operation being performed is a second-look procedure following chemotherapy. **a** Residual tumor is seen (*arrow*) below the right adnexa and along the right pelvic side wall. **b** The lesion is being excised from the peritoneum. The right ovary (*arrow*) is better visualized in this frame

Diagnosis of Metastasis/ Tumor Recurrence

Current imaging modalities, liver enzymes, and tumor markers are insensitive means for detecting malignant lesions less than 1 cm in size (Brady et al. 1991). In adults, laparoscopy has been shown to offer better detection for hepatic and peritoneal metastases than is currently possible by imaging (Watt et al. 1989). Although this is a conceptually attractive use of laparoscopy in children, very few data exist at the moment. The CCG reported on two cases in which laparoscopy was successful (Holcomb et al. 1995).

Resection

Adrenal Masses

Laparoscopic experience with tumor resection in children is largely confined to masses originating within the adrenal gland. Adrenalectomy by laparoscopy has clearly become the method of choice in adults (Liao et al. 2001; Smith et al. 1999; Thompson et al. 1997).

However, consistent with the historical evaluation of emerging techniques, the pediatric experience has trailed that of adults. Yet, laparoscopic adrenalectomy has been shown to be efficacious in the pediatric population as well (Clements et al. 1999; Miller et al. 2002; Mirallie et al. 2001; Stanford et al. 2002).

Pheochromocytoma

Among lesions with low malignant potential, some authors have opposed the notion of removing pheochromocytomas laparoscopically (Mobius et al. 1999). However, several studies have shown that safe removal of these lesions is feasible while maintaining adequate control of hemodynamic parameters in children and adults (■ Fig. 68.5) (Al-Sobhi et al. 2002; Fernandez-Cruz et al. 1996; Pretorius et al. 1998). In a study comparing measurements of fractionated catecholamines during resections, the peak rises in both epinephrine and norepinephrine during laparoscopic resection were found to be roughly half those obtained during conventional open resection (Fernandez-Cruz et al. 1996). In a recent report signifying the progression of laparoscopic skill and perhaps establishing a current boundary for the application of laparoscopy in adrenal surgery, a partial adrenalectomy was performed laparoscopically for a recurrent pheochromocytoma after the patient had undergone open bilateral partial adrenalectomy 8 years prior (Al-Sobhi et al. 2002).

Neuroblastoma

In children, neuroblastoma is the most common abdominal solid organ malignancy. While often arising in the adrenal gland, it usually presents in an advanced state which usually prohibits the possibility of laparoscopic resection. However, mass-screening in Japan has uncovered smaller lesions which may be approached laparoscopically. In a series of three patients with primary tumors in the right adrenal gland under 3 cm in greatest diameter, laparoscopic resection was successful in all cases with no recurrence at a follow-up of 17–22 months (Yamamoto et al. 1996). Subsequently, successful laparoscopic removal of a right adrenal neuroblastoma was reported in an 8-month-old infant (Nakajima et al. 1997). More recently, a case of observed neuroblastoma detected by mass-screening was found to grow from 2.7 cm at diagnosis to a maximum size of 5.1 cm during observation. This lesion was resected laparoscopically without complication (Komuro et al. 2000).

The largest and most progressive series published thus far describes five patients (mean age 5.1 years) with neuroblastoma who underwent laparoscopy for excision (Iwanaka et al. 2001b). The diameter in greatest dimension was ≥ 4 cm in four cases, with two lesions located in the right adrenal gland, two in the left adrenal gland, and one in the retroperitoneum. Exci-

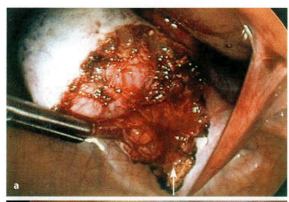
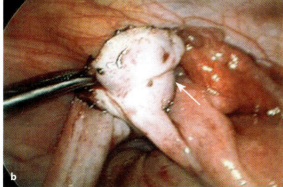

Fig. 68.7. This 12-year-old girl is undergoing resection of a left ovarian teratoma. **a** The teratoma is being dissected away from the normal ovarian tissue (*arrow*). **b** The residual ovary (*arrow*) is seen

sion was completed laparoscopically in four cases with one requiring conversion secondary to poor visualization. This tumor was a 5.3 cm, stage III lesion. Estimated blood loss was a mean 13 ml in the four successful laparoscopic excisions compared to 210 ml in the converted case.

Ovarian Masses

Ovarian tumors comprise about 2% of all tumors in children (Breen et al. 1981). The advent of laparoscopy in children, which appeared in the literature in 1973 for the evaluation of gonadal pathology, grossly preceded the contemporary acceptance of laparoscopic procedures (Gans and Berci 1973). Several subsequent publications defined laparoscopy as an effective medium for managing adnexal problems in infants and children allowing for visual inspection, detorsion, tissue biopsy, and cyst aspiration (Cohen et al. 1996; Esposito et al. 1998; Jawad and Al-Meshari 1998). In terms of tumor resection, the first laparoscopic case reported was a mature teratoma in a 3-year-old child (Liu et al. 1998). This was followed by a series of eight ovarian masses resected laparoscopically; four were determined by histologic evaluation to be mature ovarian teratomas, and all were benign (■ Fig. 68.7) (Jawad

and Al-Meshari 1998). While there is no reported laparoscopic experience with pelvic malignancy, the data produced thus far set the stage for future laparoscopic resection of these lesions.

Discussion

Diagnosis/Exploration

There are multiple advantages in conducting explorative surgery with laparoscopy. The lens on a laparoscope produces a magnified image which enhances both the detection and interpretation of small lesions. The improving resolution of cameras and visual display units further augment this advantage. In addition, the length of the telescope along with an angled view provides the capacity to see around various structures. Combining these assets with the ability to place smaller caliber laparoscopes into operative ports makes it possible to inspect peritoneal surfaces behind solid organs and in the posterior aspect of the abdominal cavity. These areas are otherwise quite difficult to expose during open operations requiring a long incision, surgical dissection, and substantial retraction. Moreover, the pivotal nature of the port allows for thorough inspection of all four quadrants in the abdomen without extending the incision or adding additional ports. In yet another dimension of exploration, the laparoscopic ultrasound probe provides the ability to precisely inspect the parenchyma of solid organs and to guide biopsy (Iwanaka et al. 1997b).

Diagnostic laparoscopy offers several physiologic advantages as well. The patient's clinical course is enhanced by a more rapid recovery which, in the presence of a malignant diagnosis, reduces the interval to initiating systemic therapy (Saenz et al. 1997; Warmann et al. 2003). Tissue trauma and systemic response to injury after an operation appears to be attenuated by laparoscopy as several studies have demonstrated decreased levels of inflammatory mediators, reactive oxygen species, and polymorphonuclear cells after minimally invasive surgery compared to the open approach (Fujimoto et al. 1999; Iwanaka et al. 1997a; Ure et al. 2002). Cell-mediated immunity is an integral component of the host defense response to malignancy. It has been clearly shown that cell-mediated immunity recovers faster after minimally invasive procedures when contrasted with comparable open operations (Da Costa et al. 1998; Vittimberga et al. 1998). Achieving preservation of immune defenses is particularly desirable when trying to establish a diagnosis or determine resectability since manipulated tumor burden remains after the operation. In these circumstances, it is theoretically sound to minimize the alteration of host defenses incurred by surgery, although clinical outcome data on this point are currently lacking. Finally, laparoscopy appears to offer better preservation of the peritoneal lining compared with open procedures and this benefit results in fewer adhesions (Pattaras et al. 2002; Takeuchi and Kinoshita 2002). This serves a tremendous advantage for operations performed in the early portion of a patient's clinical course when future procedures are likely.

Resection

The reported clinical experience with resection of primary abdominal tumors in children is small. In Japan, laparoscopic management of neuroblastomas detected by mass screening will likely continue to develop. The size and location of most abdominal tumors currently encountered in the USA makes laparoscopic resection prohibitively tenuous. However, as technical expertise and intraoperative equipment continue to evolve, this could prove to be an encroachable frontier. However, such advances must maintain the operative principles for safe cancer surgery which have historically been established by the previous generation of open resections. In adults, there appears to be no compromise in cure rates secondary to the use of laparoscopy for abdominal malignancies such as renal cell carcinoma and colon cancer, which provides an encouraging basis from which pediatric surgeons may be able forge ahead in the quest to develop curative resections by minimally invasive approaches (Chan et al. 2001; Fleshman et al. 1996; Franklin et al. 1996; Ono et al. 2001; Portis et al. 2002).

Evaluation of Response/ Second-look Procedures

At the dawn of minimally invasive surgery, previous abdominal operations were considered a contraindication to laparoscopy. While a concern with intra-abdominal adhesions in patients undergoing reexploration has been expressed by some authors, a second-look procedure was successfully completed in all ten cases where it was attempted in the two series previously mentioned (Holcomb et al. 1995; Waldhausen et al. 2000). As pediatric surgeons become more comfortable with laparoscopic techniques, the presence of adhesions or a history of prior operations will not pose such formidable apprehension. This phenomenon has already unfolded in the adult experience where a history of previous open operations no longer prevents surgeons from performing laparoscopic surgery, even when technically advanced procedures such as gastric bypass and esophagomyotomy are considered (de Csepel et al. 2001; Floch et al. 1999; Gagner et al. 2002;

Gorecki et al. 2002). Reoperative laparoscopy is now beginning to emerge in children as well (Tan and Wulkan 2002). Furthermore, as an increasing portion of tumor operations for diagnosis or determination of resectability are approached laparoscopically, surgeons will be able to enjoy an operative field with better anatomic preservation as fewer intra-abdominal adhesions can be expected.

Port Site Metastasis

Abdominal wall seeding by malignant cells is a long-feared complication of laparoscopy. Early in the experience of laparoscopy, a comprehensive survey of 409 incidental cancers found in adults during laparoscopic operations for benign conditions uncovered an alarming number of port site metastases (17%) (Whelan et al. 1997). Similarly, initial reports on laparoscopic resection for colorectal cancer described high rates of port site recurrence although these early concerns have largely been alleviated as experience has grown (Lacy et al. 1997; Larach et al. 1997). Recent data on laparoscopy for diagnosing, staging, and treating intra-abdominal malignancies in 1,650 adult patients demonstrated port site implantation in only 0.79% of these cases which was compared to open incision site recurrence after laparotomy in 0.86% of patients from the same institution (Shoup et al. 2002). The literature on laparoscopy for pediatric malignancies appears to forecast an extremely low risk for port site metastasis as no such complications have been reported in the series generated to date.

Future Direction

Extending the boundaries of laparoscopic management in pediatric abdominal malignancies will be best served by well-designed, prospective clinical trials. However, the rarity of tumors amenable to such trials requires effective patient accrual. Inadequate accrual has been exposed as the cause of failure in a nationally funded prospective pediatric surgical trial in the recent past (Ehrlich et al. 2002). Specifically, overcoming personal bias against the progression of minimally invasive surgery would promote patient referral for laparoscopic trials. The lack of universal laparoscopic skill may require centralization of these trials to institutions with the capability of performing all of the advanced laparoscopic operations. The primary goal of developing laparoscopic techniques for the management of abdominal tumors is not to demonstrate technological advancement or surgical skill, but to manage cancer in children with improved results and a better quality of life. Cooperative multi-institutional collaboration combined with comprehensive peripheral support from referral sources might provide the well-defined patient base necessary for these goals to be realized safely.

References

Al-Sobhi S, Peschel R, Zihak C, et al (2002) Laparoscopic partial adrenalectomy for recurrent pheochromocytoma after open partial adrenalectomy in von Hippel-Lindau disease. J Endourol 16:171–174

Baker LL, Parker BR, Donaldson SS, et al (1990) Staging of Hodgkin disease in children: comparison of CT and lymphography with laparotomy. Am J Roentgenol 154:1251–1255

Brady PF, Peebles M, Goldschmid S (1991) Role of laparoscopy in the evaluation of patients with suspected hepatic or peritoneal malignancy. Gastrointest Endosc 37:27–36

Breen JL, Bonamo JF, Maxson WS (1981) Genital tract tumors in children. Pediatr Clin North Am 28:355–367

Chan DY, Cadeddu JA, Jarrett TW, et al (2001) Laparoscopic radical nephrectomy: cancer control for renal cell carcinoma. J Urol 166:2095–2100

Clements RH, Goldstein RE, Holcomb GW 3rd (1999) Laparoscopic left adrenalectomy for pheochromocytoma in a child. J Pediatr Surg 34:1408–1409

Cohen Z, Shinhar D, Kopernik G, et al (1996) The laparoscopic approach to uterine adnexal torsion in childhood. J Pediatr Surg 31:1557–1559

Cushieri A (1994) Diagnosis and staging of tumors by laparoscopy. Semin Laparosc Surg 1:3–12

Da Costa ML, Redmond P, Bouchier-Hayes DJ (1998) The effect of laparotomy and laparoscopy on the establishment of spontaneous tumor metastases. Surgery 124:516–525

de Csepel J, Nahouraii R, Gagner M (2001) Laparoscopic gastric bypass as a reoperative bariatric surgery for failed open restrictive procedures. Surg Endosc 15:393–397

Ehrlich PF, Newman KD, Haase GM, et al (2002) Lessons learned from a failed multi-institutional randomized controlled study. J Pediatr Surg 37:431–436

Esposito C, Garipoli V, Di Matteo G, et al (1998) Laparoscopic management of ovarian cysts in newborns. Surg Endosc 12:1152–1154

Fernandez-Cruz L, Taura P, Saenz A, et al (1996) Laparoscopic approach to pheochromocytoma: hemodynamic changes and catecholamine secretion. World J Surg 20:762–768

Fleshman JW, Nelson H, Peters WR, et al (1996) Early results of laparoscopic surgery for colorectal cancer. Retrospective analysis of 372 patients treated by Clinical Outcomes of Surgical Therapy (COST) Study Group. Dis Colon Rectum 39(10 suppl): S53–S58

Floch NR, Hinder RA, Klingler PJ, et al (1999) Is laparoscopic reoperation for failed antireflux surgery feasible? Arch Surg 134:733–737

Franklin ME Jr, Rosenthal D, Abrego-Medina D, et al (1996) Prospective comparison of open vs. laparoscopic colon surgery for carcinoma. Five-year results. Dis Colon Rectum 39(10 suppl):S35–S46

Fujimoto T, Lane GJ, Segawa O, et al (1999) Laparoscopic extramucosal pyloromyotomy versus open pyloromyotomy for infantile hypertrophic pyloric stenosis: which is better? J Pediatr Surg 34:370–372

Gagner M, Gentileschi P, de Csepel J, et al (2002) Laparoscopic reoperative bariatric surgery: experience from 27 consecutive patients. Obes Surg 12:254–260

Gans SL, Berci G (1973) Peritoneoscopy in infants and children. J Pediatr Surg 8:399–405

Gorecki PJ, Hinder RA, Libbey JS, et al (2002) Redo laparoscopic surgery for achalasia. Surg Endosc 16:772–776

Holcomb GW 3rd (1999) Minimally invasive surgery for solid tumors. Semin Surg Oncol 16:184–192

Holcomb GW 3rd, Tomita SS, Haase GM, et al (1995) Minimally invasive surgery in children with cancer. Cancer 76:121–128

Iwanaka T, Arkovitz MS, Arya G, et al (1997a) Evaluation of operative stress and peritoneal macrophage function in minimally invasive operations. J Am Coll Surg 184:357–363

Iwanaka T, Nagabuchi E, Arkovitz MS, et al (1997b) The efficacy of diagnostic laparoscopic ultrasound. Pediatr Surg Int 12:505–508

Iwanaka T, Arai M, Ito M, et al (2001a) Challenges of laparoscopic resection of abdominal neuroblastoma with lymphadenectomy. A preliminary report. Surg Endosc 15:489–492

Iwanaka T, Arai M, Ito M, et al (2001b) Surgical treatment for abdominal neuroblastoma in the laparoscopic era. Surg Endosc 15:751–754

Jawad AJ, Al-Meshari A (1998) Laparoscopy for ovarian pathology in infancy and childhood. Pediatr Surg Int 14:62–65

Komuro H, Makino S, Tahara K (2000) Laparoscopic resection of an adrenal neuroblastoma detected by mass screening that grew in size during the observation period. Surg Endosc 14:297

Lacy A, Garcia-Valdecasas J, Delgado S, et al (1997) Postoperative complications of laparoscopic-assisted colectomy. Surg Endosc 11:119–122

Landman J, Lento P, Hassen W, et al (2000) Feasibility of pathological evaluation of morcellated kidneys after radical nephrectomy. J Urol 164:2086–2089

Larach S, Patankar S, Ferrara A, et al (1997) Complications of laparoscopic colorectal surgery: analysis and comparison of early vs. later experience. Dis Colon Rectum 40:592–596

Liao C-H, Chen J, Chueh S-C, et al (2001) Effectiveness of transperitoneal and trans-retroperitoneal laparoscopic adrenalectomy versus open adrenalectomy. J Formos Med Assoc 100:186–191

Liu YH, Wang CJ, Lee CL, et al (1998) Minimal access surgery in children: the use of laparoscopy for management of pediatric ovarian teratoma: a case report. Changgeng Yi Xue Za Zhi 21:78–81

Lobe TE, Schropp KP, Joyner R, et al (1994) The suitability of automatic tissue morcellation for the endoscopic removal of large specimens in pediatric surgery. J Pediatr Surg 29:232–234

Miller KA, Albanese C, Harrison M, et al (2002) Experience with laparoscopic adrenalectomy in pediatric patients. J Pediatr Surg 37:979–982

Mirallie E, Leclair MD, de Lagausie P, et al (2001) Laparoscopic adrenalectomy in children. Surg Endosc 15:156–160

Mobius E, Nies C, Rothmund M (1999) Surgical treatment of pheochromocytomas: laparoscopic or conventional? Surg Endosc 13:35–39

Nakajima K, Fukuzawa M, Fukui Y, et al (1997) Laparoscopic resection of mass-screened adrenal neuroblastoma in an 8-month-old infant. Surg Laparosc Endosc 7:498–500

Ono Y, Kinukawa T, Hattori R, et al (2001) The long-term outcome of laparoscopic radical nephrectomy for small renal cell carcinoma. J Urol 164:1867–1870

Pattaras JG, Moore RG, Landman J, et al (2002) Incidence of postoperative adhesion formation after transperitoneal genitourinary laparoscopic surgery. Urology 59:37–41

Pautler SE, Hewitt SM, Linehan WM, et al (2002) Specimen morcellation after laparoscopic radical nephrectomy: confirmation of histologic diagnosis using needle biopsy. J Endourol 16:89–92

Portis AJ, Yan Y, Landman J, et al (2002) Long-term follow up after laparoscopic radical nephrectomy. J Urol 167:1257–1262

Pratt BL, Greene FL (2000) Role of laparoscopy in the staging of malignant disease. Surg Clin North Am 80:1111–1126

Pretorius M, Rasmussen GE, Holcomb GW (1998) Hemodynamic and catecholamine responses to a laparoscopic adrenalectomy for pheochromocytoma in a pediatric patient. Anesth Analg 87:1268–1270

Saenz NC, Conlon KC, Aronson DC, et al (1997) The application of minimal access procedures in infants, children, and young adults with pediatric malignancies. J Laparoendosc Adv Surg Tech A 7:289–294

Shoup M, Brennan MF, Karpeh MS, et al (2002) Port site metastasis after diagnostic laparoscopy for upper gastrointestinal tract malignancies: an uncommon entity. Ann Surg Oncol 9:632–636

Smith CD, Weber CJ, Amerson JR (1999) Laparoscopic adrenalectomy: new gold standard. World J Surg 23:389–396

Stanford A, Upperman J, Nguyen N, et al (2002) Surgical management of open versus laparoscopic adrenalectomy: outcome analysis. J Pediatr Surg 37:1027–1029

Takeuchi H, Kinoshita K (2002) Evaluation of adhesion formation after laparoscopic myomectomy by systematic second-look microlaparoscopy. J Am Assoc Gynecol Laparosc 9:442–446

Tan S, Wulkan ML (2002) Minimally invasive surgical techniques in reoperative surgery for gastroesophageal reflux disease in infants and children. Am Surg 68:989–992

Thompson GB, Grant CS, Van Heerden JA, et al (1997) Laparoscopic versus open posterior adrenalectomy: a case control study of 100 patients. Surgery 122:1132–1136

Ure BM, Niewold TA, Bax NM, et al (2002) Peritoneal, systemic, and distant organ inflammatory responses are reduced by a laparoscopic approach and carbon dioxide versus air. Surg Endosc 16:836–842

Vittimberga FJ Jr, Foley DP, Meyers WC, et al (1998) Laparoscopic surgery and the systemic immune response. Ann Surg 227:326–334

Waldhausen JH, Tapper D, Sawin RS (2000) Minimally invasive surgery and clinical decision-making for pediatric malignancy. Surg Endosc 14:250–253

Warmann S, Fuchs J, Jesch NK, et al (2003) A prospective study of minimally invasive techniques in pediatric surgical oncology: preliminary report. Med Pediatr Oncol 40:155–157

Watt I, Stewart I, Anderson D, et al (1989) Laparoscopy, ultrasound and computed tomography in cancer of the oesophagus and gastric cardia: a prospective comparison for detection of intra-abdominal metastases. Br J Surg 76:1036–1039

Whelan RL, Allendorf JD, Gutt CN, et al (1998) General oncologic effects of the laparoscopic surgical approach. 1997 Frankfurt international meeting of animal laparoscopic researchers. Surg Endosc 12:1092–1109

Yamamoto H, Yoshida M, Sera Y (1996) Laparoscopic surgery for neuroblastoma identified by mass screening. J Pediatr Surg 31:385–388

Yoshida T, Matsumoto T, Morii Y, et al (2002) Staging with helical computed tomography and laparoscopy in pancreatic head cancer. Hepatogastroenterology 49:1428–1431

Abdomen

Abdominal Pain

Chapter 69

Chronic Abdominal Pain of Childhood

Perry W. Stafford

Introduction

Chronic abdominal pain of childhood occupies a significant portion of any pediatric practice. It has been estimated that one out of three children seen on a daily basis in any busy pediatric practice will have a component of abdominal pain. Fortunately, the vast majority of these children have acute pain that either resolves spontaneously or is amenable to appropriate consultation and intervention. Only a very small number of these children persist with what is known as chronic abdominal pain of childhood (CAP). This syndrome has been described quite rigorously in the pediatric gastroenterology literature as abdominal pain that persists for more than 3 months and is disabling with multiple absences from school and avoidance of normal childhood activities. A profile has been developed for a typical child with CAP. These children are generally adolescents and are predominantly female. Their pain is often aching and located periumbilically; it occasionally awakens them at night. Approximately half the children will be bothered by persistent diarrhea or constipation and very often there is a significant, usually maternal, family history of similar complaints (Silverberg 1991). Chronic abdominal pain is not only a problem of childhood, and the adult gastroenterologic and surgical literature is replete with studies discussing the appropriate evaluation and treatment of disabling abdominal pain in adults. The advent of pediatric laparoscopy has provided us with an additional means of extending our diagnostic armamentarium with a procedure that is relatively easy to perform and has a demonstrated low surgical risk. The technique is generally the same as previously described for laparoscopic appendectomy but also includes a careful and organized laparoscopic exploration of the peritoneum.

Preoperative Preparation

Since the cohort of children with CAP is large and varied, it is essential to work closely with a pediatric gastroenterologist with an interest in CAP. Often children with CAP will have undergone an extensive and often uncoordinated and repetitive evaluation prior to surgical referral that includes multiple laboratory investigations, imaging studies, and invasive gastrointestinal (GI) tests. These studies are usually normal and have only a limited negative predictive value. The preoperative evaluation can be focused and relatively limited. It should include a full laboratory evaluation (complete blood count with differential, electrolytes, liver function studies, amylase and lipase, and a urinalysis), a basic radiologic imaging series (chest and abdominal radiographs), and an ultrasound evaluation of the abdomen and pelvis. An upper GI contrast study and a barium enema can be added if indicated. Upper GI endoscopy should be done in most cases with biopsies and cultures for *Helicobacter pylori*; a lower GI endoscopic study can be added if appropriate. Computed tomography and magnetic resonance imaging are usually not needed. In the particular instance of right upper quadrant pain without gallstones on ultrasound, a CCK-PZ stimulated disHIDA scan can be helpful to identify the few children with biliary dyskinesia.

Before Induction of General Anesthesia

A formal mechanical-chemical bowel preparation is usually not necessary. Perioperative antibiotics are generally indicated; a first-generation cephalosporin [cefazolin (Ancef), 25 mg/kg] is usually sufficient. Coordination with the operative nursing team will ensure that all the needed endoscopic equipment is available and functioning.

After Induction of General Anesthesia

Nitrous oxide should be avoided to minimize intraoperative bowel distension, and epidural and spinal anesthesia are generally not needed. Preemptive local anesthesia with local infiltration in the area of planned port site insertion using a long-acting local anesthetic [bupivacaine HCl (Marcaine), 2.5 mg/kg] is recommended. It should be supplemented at the end of the procedure. An orogastric tube is generally inserted; urinary bladder catheters are not necessary if an open (Hasson) technique is utilized for the placement of the ini-

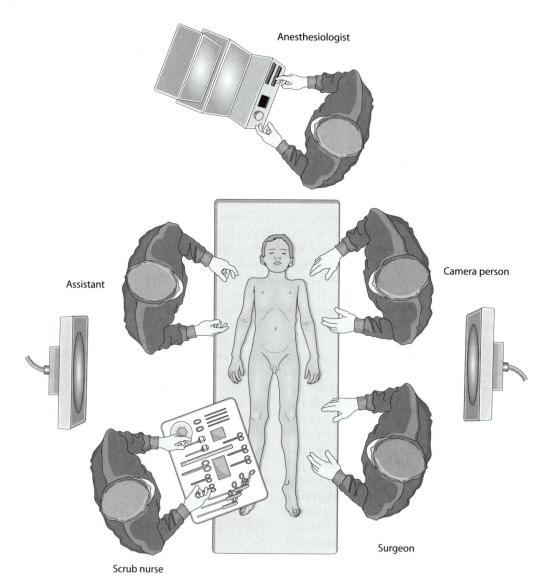

Anesthesiologist

Assistant

Camera person

Scrub nurse

Surgeon

Fig. 69.1. Operating room positioning

tial umbilical trocar and the planned operative time will be limited to 1 h or less. When inserted, both catheters are generally removed at the end of the procedure. The patient should be monitored with pulse oximetry, and end-tidal carbon dioxide tensions should be checked periodically. If the operative time is over 90 min, the insufflation pressures utilized are high, or the patient is small (less than 10 kg), the use of an arterial catheter to monitor the patient's blood pH may be appropriate since the end-tidal CO_2 may not accurately reflect the patient's acid-base status.

Positioning

The patient is identified and placed supine on the long axis of the operating table; the position of the operative team is similar to that used in most diagnostic laparoscopic procedures. Two monitors at the middle of the table are helpful to avoid malpositioning the operative team (■ Fig. 69.1). A bolster placed under the patient's midabdomen may be helpful and allow more lateral port placement. The patient should be carefully secured to the operative table to allow the use of full lateral and head-up and head-down table movement. The patient's arms should be carefully protected and tucked

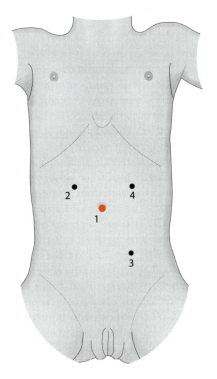

Fig. 69.2. Port positions

next to the patient's sides. After the umbilical trocar (10/12 mm) is placed by your usual technique, the remaining trocars (5 mm) are placed under direct vision. Their position can be varied according to the visualized position of the cecum, generally right upper quadrant (RUQ) and left lower quadrant (LLQ) trocars are placed initially. A third operating port can be placed in the left upper quadrant (LUQ) if the surgeon prefers an operative instrument in each hand, for example for intestinal manipulation or intracorporeal knot tying.

Special Equipment

No special equipment is needed. Bipolar high-frequency electrocoagulation (HFE) is at hand. Other energy applying systems such as ultrasonic energy and Ligasure are optional. Depending on the pathology encountered, clips or staplers may be used. In case of an acutely inflamed appendix, an endobag is used for its removal.

Technique

Cannulae

Cannula	Method of insertion	Diameter (mm)	Device	Position
1	Open/Closed	10/12	Telescope, endobag	Umbilical
2	Closed	5	Working instrument	RUQ
3	Closed	5	Working instrument	LLQ
4	Closed	5	Working instrument	LUQ (optional)

Procedure

After the initial umbilical trocar is placed and carboperitoneum is established at 12–15 cmH$_2$O, the abdomen is explored. I start in the right lower quadrant (RLQ), looking for malpositioning of the cecum and pathologic adhesions, either from the cecum to the lateral wall and/or from the terminal ileum and cecum to the iliac vessels. I then place the two primary 5 mm trocars in the RUQ and LLQ. I find the appendix and run the terminal several feet of the terminal ileum to look for a Meckel's diverticulum. During this maneuver, I assess the ileum for fat-wrapping, serositis, or thickening that might suggest inflammatory bowel disease. I then move to the RUQ and look briefly at the

liver and gallbladder for obvious inflammatory adhesions or masses. I next visualize the stomach and spleen for inflammation or abnormalities and follow the transverse colon to the sigmoid. The patient is positioned in reversed Trendelenburg (head-up) as I begin this exploration, then left side up as I look at the spleen, and into Trendelenberg (head-down) as I move to the pelvis. The pelvis is carefully examined, particularly looking for ovarian, paraovarian, and fallopian tube pathology in girls and for abdominal wall hernias in both boys and girls. The cul-de-sac is examined for peritoneal fluid collections and aspirated dry. The patient is then rolled into right side up/Trendelenburg position for the RLQ surgery. The cecum is mobilized initially, lysing abnormal adhesions if present with scissors and cautery (either "hot" scissors or hook cautery). The appendix is freed from any adhesions and removed, using your usual appendectomy technique. I prefer the use of the Endo-GIA, utilizing the GI staples for the appendix and the vascular staples for the mesentery. If the appendix appears to be acutely inflamed, an endobag is used to remove the appendix; otherwise it is brought into the umbilical trocar and removed within the barrel of the trocar. Other intraperitoneal pathology is handled in usual laparoscopic fashion as described elsewhere in this book. As mentioned, I will often place a third 5 mm trocar in the LUQ if advanced bowel techniques are needed. The entire abdomen is then lavaged with warm normal saline fluid and evaluated for hemostasis in reverse order of the initial exploration, ending with a final look at the RLQ. The lavage solution is removed as completely as possible. If needed, 10 mm Jackson-Pratt drains are placed in the pelvis and RLQ, exiting through the 5 mm port sites. The carboperitoneum is fully evacuated. The 5 mm sites are closed with absorbable suture at the skin; fascial closure is used only if the fascia is easily visualized. The umbilical port site is carefully closed both at the fascia and skin. As previously mentioned, all port sites are again infiltrated with a long-acting local anesthetic solution. I dress the wounds with SteriStrips and Telfa/Tegaderm dressings. Recently, Dermabond has been used with success.

Postoperative Care

The nasogastric or orogastric catheter is removed when the patient is ready for extubation. The urinary bladder catheter is generally removed unless extensive pelvic surgery or manipulation has been necessary. Pain control is according to the surgeon's preference; I generally prefer loading with an intravenous, non-narcotic analgesic [ketorolac tromethamine (Toradol), 0.5 mg/kg per dose, usually 30 mg in teenagers] initially at extubation and then transitioning to oral non-steroidals, the newer Cox-2 inhibitors, or codeine as soon as possible. I try to avoid the use of morphine and fentanyl intravenous or patient-controlled analgesia in order to minimize patient postoperative nausea. A clear liquid diet is started as soon as the patient is fully awake and back in their room; the diet is advanced as the patient desires. Most children are ready for discharge (pain controlled with oral analgesics and tolerating a regular diet without emesis) late on the first postoperative day; the remainder are sent home as they are ready. All children are seen in the office for a postoperative check at 2 weeks and again at 8 weeks.

Results

We have now operated on over 100 children with CAP over the last 10 years using the above protocol. The average age of the initial group of 100 children was 10.7 years and 65% were girls. The pain was predominantly in the RLQ or periumbilical and was associated with nausea and occasionally emesis, diarrhea, and constipation, and rarely weight loss. All had pain symptoms that had lasted longer than 3 months; most had a positive family history of similar pain. Thirty-five of the children had variations of abnormal-appearing adhesions from the cecum or terminal ileum that were lysed. Six children had inguinal or femoral hernias, and five had unrecognized inflammatory bowel disease. Twelve of the girls had ovarian or paraovarian cysts, and two had adhesions to the adnexa suggesting pelvic inflammatory disease. Four had a Meckel's diverticulum; three diverticula were thickened and these were removed. None appeared to be involved in the pain syndrome. All children had their appendix removed. Pathology evaluation revealed intestinal worms in three and "fibrosis" or "chronic inflammation" in nine; the remainder were "normal." No patients required conversion to an open technique. The inpatient length of stay was 2.7 days. Ninety-two percent were improved postoperatively, and most of these children were pain-free at 8-week follow-up evaluation. All of these children had returned to normal activities both at home and at school. Ten subsequently returned with pain, and five children were readmitted for persistent pain. One was found to have systemic mastocytosis, one had generalized idiopathic myositis, and three had the eventual diagnosis of regional enteritis; the other five had no diagnosis made but continued to have pain. All the children with persistent postoperative pain were referred to our Anesthesia Chronic Pain Clinic. Ten improved with medication, physical therapy, and psychological counseling. Three have persistent and intermittently recurrent pain syndromes that were poorly controlled.

Discussion

There have been many series of laparoscopic evaluation of adults with CAP published since the 1990s, but only three reports in the pediatric age group. Most adult series report that approximately 50% of the patients with CAP can be expected to have a "positive outcome," defined as operative laparoscopic findings that influence their management. The few pediatric laparoscopic series report a significantly better outcome: 73% (Schier and Waldschmidt 1994), 73% (Stylianos et al. 1996), and 92% (Stringel et al. 1999). Our experience would also support this improved outcome, but we cannot precisely explain our combined success. Certainly, our careful preoperative evaluation with both pediatric gastroenterologic and surgical input coupled with the requirement that all children have a prolonged course that exceeds 3 months excludes the more common pain etiologies that remit spontaneously in at least one third of the children. We hope that the careful and systematic laparoscopic examination of the complete abdomen, followed by repair of any discovered abnormalities and lysis of abnormal-appearing congenital adhesions and appendectomy removes many of the described lesions that may play a part in the persistent pain syndrome. Simple open appendectomy for pediatric CAP has a well-reported success rate exceeding 90% (Gorinstin et al. 1996; Latchaw et al. 1988; Schisgall 1980; Stevenson 1991), and the concept of "chronic appendicitis" has slowly been gaining popularity since the 1990s. The role of cecal adhesions has again been well reported in the adult literature, but adhesions as a cause for CAP in children has only been suggested sporadically in the endoscopic pediatric literature (Mecke et al. 1988; Mueller et al. 1995; Stringel et al. 1999). The role of inflammatory fluid in the pelvis from whatever source has also been reported to play a role in the chronic pain syndromes, and we have found a number of inflammatory mediators, including tumor necrosis factor, in the aspirated fluid. However, the precise contribution of each of these possible etiologies of CAP remains speculative. It must be emphasized that the comprehensive evaluation of a child with CAP is a team effort, and the perspective and experience of the child's pediatrician and a pediatric gastroenterologist is of paramount importance. Similarly, a chronic pain team is invaluable to assist you in treating the few non-responders with persistent postoperative pain. As is often the case in surgical science, this concept is not new, and Robert E. Gross, in the first edition of his seminal textbook *The Surgery of Infancy and Childhood* wrote in 1953, "Children with vague and recurring abdominal pain should not be subjected to hasty and lightly considered appendectomy, but in those patients who have had adequate studies to rule-out other pathologic conditions, this operation, while at times disappointing, will bring relief in a majority of instances" (Gross 1953). The contribution of diagnostic laparoscopy to the evaluation of CAP in children in the modern laparoscopic era is not speculative, and I believe that sufficient evidence now exists to add laparoscopy for CAP to the diagnostic and therapeutic armamentarium of the pediatric surgeon.

References

Gorinstin A, Serour F, Katz R, et al (1996) Appendiceal colic in children: a true clinical entity? J Am Coll Surg 182:246–250

Gross RE (1953) The Surgery of Infancy and Childhood. Saunders, Philadelphia, pp 278–279

Latchaw LA, Harris BH, Leape LL (1988) Appendectomy for chronic right lower quadrant pain in children. Contemp Surg 33:52–55

Mecke H, Semm K, Lehmann-Willenbrock E (1988) Pelvioscopic adhesiolysis. Success in the treatment of chronic abdominal pain caused by adhesions in the lower and middle abdomen. Geburtshilfe Frauenheilkd 48:155–159

Mueller MD, Tshchudi J, Herrmann U, et al (1995) An evaluation of laparoscopic adhesiolysis in patients with chronic abdominal pain. Surg Endosc 9:802–804

Schier F, Waldschmidt J (1994) Laparoscopy in children with ill-defined abdominal pain. Surg Endosc 8:97–99

Schisgall RM (1980) Appendiceal colic in childhood. The role of inspissated casts of stool within the appendix. Ann Surg 192:687–693

Silverberg M (1991) Chronic abdominal pain in adolescents. Pediatr Ann 20:179–185

Stevenson RJ (1991) Chronic right lower quadrant abdominal pain: is there a role for elective appendectomy? J Pediatr Surg 34:950–954

Stringel G, Berezin SH, Boswick HE, et al (1999) Laparoscopy in the management of children with chronic recurrent abdominal pain. J Soc Laparoendosc Surg 3:215–219

Stylianos S, Stein JE, Flanigan LM, et al (1996) Laparoscopy for diagnosis and treatment of recurrent abdominal pain in children. J Pediatr Surg 31:1158–1160

Abdomen

Sacrococcygeal Treatoma

Chapter 70

Laparoscopic Approach to Sacrococcygeal Teratomas

Klaas (N) M.A. Bax and David C. van der Zee

Introduction

Sacrococcygeal teratomas (SCT) have an incidence of 1:35,000 live born babies and are therefore the most common tumors in the newborn (Skinner 1997). Classically four anatomical types are distinguished: in type I most of the tumor is outside the body, in type II part of the tumor is outside the body but there is an important extension presacrally, in type III part of the tumor is also outside the body but the tumor extends into the abdomen, and in type IV the tumor is entirely presacral (Altman et al. 1974). There are two aspects of SCT in which a laparoscopic approach may offer a distinct advantage above classic surgery: first when the child is born with pending heart failure and/or severe coagulation disturbances, which occurs in large mainly solid SCT (Bax and van der Zee 1998; Murphy et al. 1992), and second when the tumor has a significant intrapelvic or intra-abdominal extension (Bax and van der Zee 2004), which occurs in more than 50% of the cases (Altman et al. 1974, Havranek et al. 1992).

In the first circumstance, the situation may be improved by ligation of the median sacral artery, which is the main arterial supply to the tumor. This previously required a laparotomy (Bentley 1968; Lindahl 1988; Serlo 1984), but can now easily be performed laparoscopically (Bax and van der Zee 1998). This can be done as a separate initial operation in a very unstable child or can be done as the first phase just before resection.

Ligation of the median sacral artery can also be advantageous when there is an important intrapelvic or intra-abdominal tumor component. Laparoscopy allows for a meticulous dissection of the intrapelvic or intra-abdominal part of the tumor, which is hard to achieve during open surgery.

Preoperative Preparation

In the newborn, the colon is washed out with saline. In older children and adolescents, an antegrade whole bowel lavage is carried out.

General anesthesia is used. Epidural anesthesia can be given concomitantly except in the presence of coagulation disturbances.

A nasogastric tube can be of an advantage when there is an important intra-abdominal extension of the tumor or when the upper bowel is distended. A urinary catheter is not required per se in type I tumors in which only the median sacral artery has to be interrupted. The bladder should, however, be manually emptied. In type II, III, and IV lesions, a urinary catheter should be inserted. It is advantageous to do that peroperatively after disinfection and draping. When the bladder obscures the view, the bladder can be emptied peroperatively with a syringe. Preoperatively but under general anesthesia, the rectum is aspirated with a double lumen suction device and is rinsed with saline when not empty.

Positioning of Patient, Crew, Monitors, and Equipment

Older children are placed in a supine Trendelenburg position at the lower end of the operating table. The surgeon stands on the right of the patient with the camera operator on the other side. The scrub nurse stands to the right of the surgeon. The principal monitor is at the lower end of the table.

Babies can be placed transversally at the end of the operating table (■ Fig. 70.1). The surgeon then stands at the patient's head with the camera operator to his/her left and the scrub nurse to his/her right. The principal monitor stands opposite to the surgeon at the patient's feet.

The tower is behind the surgeon and all cables come from the same direction namely along the left side of the surgeon.

The patient is prepared from the lower thorax circumferentially downward to include the legs. The feet are separately draped. Underneath the anus, small drapes are placed which are removed one by one when they become contaminated with rectal effluent.

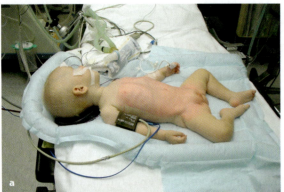

Fig. 70.1. Transverse position of the baby on the operating table

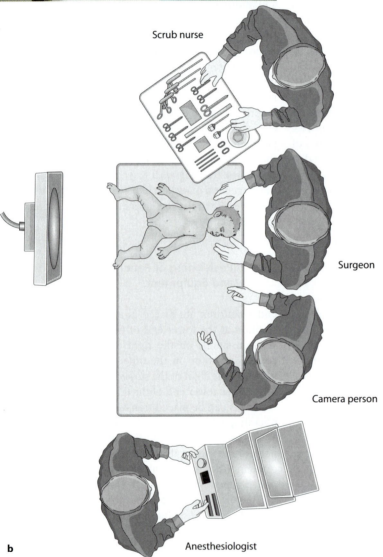

Special Equipment

Energy Applying Systems

In babies no special energy applying systems are required. In older children and adolescents, ultrasonic shears or Ligasure may be advantageous.

Other Equipment

The median sacral artery may be clipped, ligated, or coagulated with monopolar, bipolar, or Ligasure electrocoagulation or with ultrasonic energy. For the introduction of some of these devices a 6 mm cannula is required.

Technique

Cannulae

Cannula	Method of insertion	Diameter (mm)	Device	Position
1	Open	3.8–6	Telescope	Infraumbilical fold
2	Closed	3.8–6	Surgeon's right-hand instrument	Pararectally at umbilical level on the right in babies, lower down in older children
3	Closed	3.8–6	Assistant's instrument	Pararectally at umbilical level on the left in babies, lower down in older children
4	Closed	3.8–6	Surgeon's left-hand instrument	Midepigastrium in babies, lower down and more to the right in older children
5		Depending on the size of the child	Hegar dilator	Transanally

Pneumoperitoneum

Carbon dioxide is insufflated at a pressure of 8 mmHg and a flow of 2 L/min in children below 1 year of age and 5 L/min in children above 1 year of age. During the insertions of the secondary cannulae, pressure may be raised up to 10 mmHg.

Procedure

Interruption of the Median Sacral Artery in Type I Sacrococcygeal Teratoma

The uterus in the newborn girl is in the way, but can be pulled up anteriorly with a transcutaneous traction suture. For this purpose a 00 monofilament suture on a big needle is used.

The rectum is grasped and pulled to the left by the assistant. The surgeon opens the peritoneum in between the rectum and the pelvic rim on the right. The median sacral artery is immediately visible because of its large size and pulsations. The artery is easily freed from the surrounding loose areolar tissue (■ Fig. 70.2).

The artery can be interrupted in several ways, for example ligatures, clips, electrocautery, etc. (■ Fig. 70.3). Depending on the general condition of the child, the operation can be continued in a classic way or the definitive removal of the tumor can be postponed until the child is in a better condition.

Dissection of the Intrapelvic Portion of the Sacrococcygeal Teratoma

The bladder is regularly emptied by aspirating the bladder catheter. The uterus is pulled out of the way by means of a transabdominal traction suture.

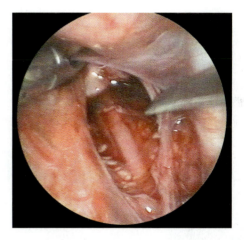

Fig. 70.2. The uterus has been suspended and the pararectal space on the right has been entered. The greatly enlarged median sacral artery has been freed

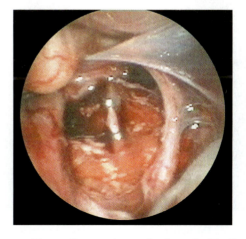

Fig. 70.3. The median sacral artery has been doubly clipped

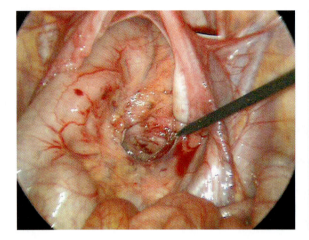

Fig. 70.4. Recurrent or incompletely resected sacrococcygeal teratoma. The uterus has been suspended and the pararectal space has been opened on the right

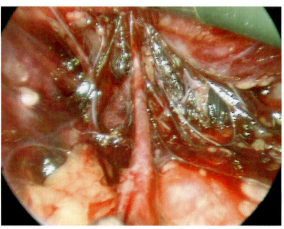

Fig. 70.7. The median sacral artery is clearly visible behind the tumor

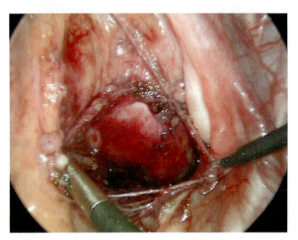

Fig. 70.5. The tumor sits in the pelvis behind the rectum

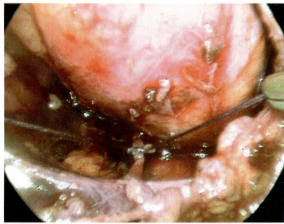

Fig. 70.8. The median sacral artery has been ligated

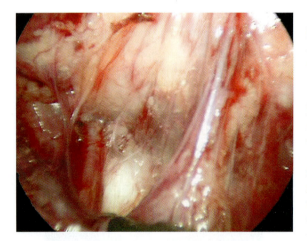

Fig. 70.6. The tumor is being dissected out posteriorly

When the intra-abdominal extension of the SCT is large and mainly cystic, more working space can be created by fine-needle aspiration of the larger cysts. Only clear cysts should be aspirated.

For right-handed surgeons, it is best to approach the SCT from the right. The assistant pulls the rectum to the left. A transanally inserted Hegar helps in pushing the rectum into the desired direction. The pelvic peritoneum is opened to the right of the mesorectum (■ Figs. 70.4, 70.5). The median sacral artery is identified and severed (■ Figs. 70.6–70.8). When the SCT is mainly cystic, the artery is not that big. The dissection of the intrapelvic portion of the tumor is relatively simple although it can be difficult to find the right plane. After complete mobilization it becomes clear that the last part of the tumor is firmly adherent to the coccyx. The laparoscopic part of the operation is now terminated and the operation continued in a classic way. Resection of the coccyx is an essential part of the operation.

Table 70.1 Details of five children with SCT treated in a laparoscopically assisted way.

Patient	Sex	Type	Cystic/solid	Age	Approach
1	F	I	Solid/cystic	1 day	Median sacral artery ligation Posterior sacrococcygeal approach
2	F	III	Cystic	3 days	Laparoscopy, conversion Posterior sacrococcygeal approach
3	F	II	Cystic	2 months	Laparoscopic mobilization Median sacral artery coagulation Posterior sacrococcygeal approach
4	F	II, recurrence	Cystic	2.5 years	Laparoscopic mobilization Median sacral artery ligation Posterior sacrococcygeal approach
5	F	IV	Solid	17.5 years	Laparoscopic mobilization Posterior sacrococcygeal approach

Postoperative Care

The postoperative care does not differ basically from the postoperative care after classic surgery.

Results

So far we have treated five children with SCT in a laparoscopically assisted way. Our experience is summarized in ■ Table 70.1 (Bax and van der Zee 2004).

Discussion

There is little doubt that prior laparoscopic interruption of the median sacral artery in hemodynamically unstable newborn babies with SCT is the treatment of choice. These babies have huge mainly solid type I SCT. The interruption of the median sacral artery in the only baby in our series with a huge type I SCT proved very easy. We have no experience at the time being with a staged operation in these babies, but a delayed second stage in the very unstable child seems logical.

In children with intrapelvic SCT, the laparoscopic approach allows for very delicate surgery, which may improve functional outcome.

References

Altman RP, Randolf JG, Lilly JR (1974) Sacrococcygeal teratoma: American Academy of Pediatrics Surgical Section Survey, 1973. J Pediatr Surg 9:389–398

Bax NMA, van der Zee DC (1998) Laparoscopic clipping of the median sacral artery in huge sacrococcygeal teratomas. Surg Endosc 12:882–883

Bax NMA, van der Zee DC (2004) The laparoscopic approach to sacrococcygeal teratomas. Surg Endosc 18:128–130

Bentley JFR (1968) Coccygeal teratoma (sacrococcygeal tumour) and other postrectal masses. In: Rob C, Smith R (eds) Operative Surgery, vol 5, part 2, 2nd edn. Butterworth, London, pp 824–829

Havranek P, Hedlund H, Rubenson A, et al (1992) Sacrococcygeal teratoma in Sweden between 1987 and 1989: long-term functional results. J Pediatr Surg 7:916–918

Lindahl H (1988) Giant sacrococcygeal teratoma: a method of simple intraoperative control of hemorrhage. J Pediatr Surg 23:1068–1069

Murphy JJ, Blair GK, Fraser GC (1992) Coagulopathy associated with large SCT. J Pediatr Surg 27:1308–1310

Serlo W (1984) Total rupture of giant sacrococcygeal teratoma. Z Kinderchir 39:405–406

Skinner MA (1997) Germ cell tumors. In: Oldham KT, Colombani PM, Foglia RP (eds) Surgery of Infants and Children. Lippincott-Raven, Philadelphia, pp 653–662

Abdomen

Obesity Surgery

Chapter 71

Laparoscopic Adjustable Gastric Banding in Adolescents

Steven R. Allen, Mark L. Wulkan and Thomas H. Inge

Introduction

Obesity in children and adolescents has increased to epidemic proportions since the late 1990s. The most recent estimates show that 16% of American children and adolescents are obese, and the prevalence is climbing. Obesity is clearly affecting the health of youngsters as well, particularly those with severe obesity. Due to the limited effectiveness of conventional weight management efforts, increased exploration of more drastic interventions has occurred, including bariatric surgical procedures. Many bariatric procedures have been developed since the 1970s including the intestinal bypass, horizontal and vertical gastroplasty, Roux-en-Y gastric bypass (RYGBP), laparoscopic adjustable gastric banding (LAGB), and most recently, electrical gastric pacing (Deitel and Shikora 2002; Livingston 2002). These operations can restrict intake, interfere with the absorption of ingested nutrients, alter physiologic satiety signals, and alter gastric motility. The goals for any weight-loss procedure are: (1) to provide durable, long-term weight reduction, (2) change eating behaviors, (3) treat obesity-related comorbidities, and (4) decrease the incidence of death attributable to obesity.

Minimally invasive options have been developed for all of the modern weight-loss procedures (O'Brien et al. 1999; Schirmer 2000). While RYGBP has been most widely used in the USA because of the excellent long-term weight loss (Pories et al. 1995), the LAGB is gaining acceptance in the USA as an effective procedure with a favorable safety profile (Ren et al. 2002). These features are important when considering surgical weight-loss options for extremely obese adolescents. The LAGB effectively allows adolescents to lose a significant amount of excess body weight and most comorbidities are reduced or resolved (Dolan et al. 2003). This chapter specifically focuses on: (1) the perioperative evaluation and preparation of the patient and family once the decision for surgery has been made, (2) the technical aspects of LAGB, (3) adolescent results of LAGB, and (4) the postoperative management of the adolescent LAGB patient.

Patient Selection in the Adolescent Population

Due to the limited information regarding long-term sequelae of bariatric interventions in adolescents, conservative indications for operation should be considered in this age group (Inge et al. 2004a). As with any surgical form of weight loss, LAGB should be a last resort after at least 6 months of organized weight-loss attempts have failed. Additionally, only those individuals with comorbidities of severe adolescent obesity should be considered for surgery.

Minimally invasive bariatric surgery is technically challenging. Surgeons planning to perform laparoscopic bariatric procedures must not underestimate the considerably increased level of difficulty which is inherent in this patient population. Having advanced laparoscopic skills is a prerequisite; in addition, one must also complete a course of study to learn the technical nuances of bariatric operations and equally importantly the discipline of bariatrics. Learning how to manage a bariatric patient in the immediate and long-term postoperative periods and becoming adept at identifying and managing a wide range of complications is critical for patient safety. Procedures should initially be proctored by an experienced laparoscopic bariatric surgeon.

Preoperative Preparation

The preoperative education of the patient, family, and referring pediatrician is critical. Patients and families should be informed of the surgical procedure, alternative operations, and the rationale for the operation to be performed. Equally as important, postoperative care including the critical return visits for band adjustment and the considerable lifestyle modifications required afterward must be conveyed verbally and in writing to the patients and caregivers during the preoperative evaluation. Also, it is critical that thorough investigations be conducted to discover unrecognized coexisting obesity-related medical conditions. A more detailed discussion of the perioperative considerations is presented elsewhere (Inge et al. 2004b).

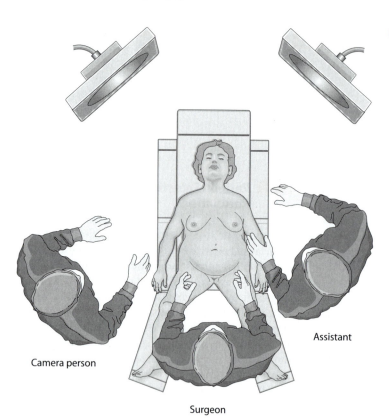

Fig. 71.1. Patient and crew position

Assistant

Camera person

Surgeon

Before Induction of General Anesthesia

Preoperative upper GI contrast studies are routinely performed, particularly when symptoms of foregut disease are present. Patients are limited to clear liquids on the day before surgery. Bowel preparation is not necessary. Preoperative medications include low molecular weight heparin for deep vein thrombosis (DVT) prophylaxis (40 mg subcutaneously and continued twice daily postoperatively while in the hospital) and a first generation cephalosporin (2 g intravenously). Additional DVT prophylaxis such as sequential compression boots must also be used intraoperatively and postoperatively. They should be applied and functioning prior to induction of anesthesia.

After Induction of General Anesthesia

General anesthesia is used for LAGB. Routine consultation with the anesthesiologist and cardiologist is recommended to assess the patient's airway, obtain the patient's and family's anesthetic history, and to determine if occult cardiovascular disease exists.

Positioning

During LAGB, the patient is placed in a modified lithotomy position, with sequential compression stockings applied. Arms can be tucked or extended. The surgeon stands between the patient's legs, the assistant stands to the patient's left, and the television monitors are positioned near the patient's left and right shoulders (■ Fig. 71.1).

Special Equipment

In general, LAGB may be performed using standard 32 cm adult instrumentation. Various manufacturers supply the equipment required and the choice of one over the other is largely the surgeon's preference. Specific instrumentation will be suggested by the band manufacturer's training course (■ Table 71.1).

Table 71.1 List of surgical instruments for laparoscopic adjustable gastric band placement

1.	Veress needle
2.	Optical system (0° or 30° laparoscope)
3.	One Nathanson liver retractor (Cook Surgical, Bloomington, IN) with articulating mechanical arm
4.	Non-traumatic grasper (5-mm) dolphin-type
5.	Non-traumatic Babcock grasper (5-mm)
6.	Coagulation hook (or harmonic scalpel)
7.	Articulating blunt dissector (e.g., Pilling Weck, part number 38-1802)
8.	Adjustable gastric band system, including closure tool and band placement tool
9.	Bioenterics balloon-tipped orogastric tube
10.	Needle driver
11.	Bipolar electrocautery forceps
12.	Five or six trocars are needed (one 15-mm, two 10-mm, and three 5-mm)
13.	Suturing material (2-0 braided permanent, e.g. Ethibond; extracorporal knot pusher; 3-0 absorbable for subcutaneous closure; 4-0 absorbable monofilament for skin closure)

Technique

Access

Due to the paucity of intra-abdominal space in many patients with morbid obesity and a large visceral obesity burden, it is of crucial importance to place the ports accurately and at the appropriate angle (in the direction of the esophageal hiatus). Pneumoperitoneum can be safely obtained using an optical trocar, a long Veress needle introduced in the left upper quadrant, or via an "open" Hassan technique in the umbilicus. The intraabdominal pressure is monitored at 15–16 mmHg. Insufflation is used through any of the 10-mm trocars except the midline trocar which contains the laparoscope. Trocar 1 (10 mm) is used for the laparoscope and is placed five fingers below the xiphoid (■ Fig. 71.2). One can avoid the fatty hepatic ligament by placing the trocar approximately 1 cm left of the linea alba at an angle that points to the left upper quadrant. The other trocars are sequentially introduced under direct vision. Trocar 2 (5 mm) is placed in the right lateral subcostal area. Trocar 3 (10 mm) is placed in the right upper quadrant (subcostal at midclavicular or on the right anterior axillary line) for an atraumatic grasping forceps and also for the band closure tool. Trocar 4 (10 or 5 mm) is placed in the left upper quadrant for the endo-Babcock or a grasping forceps (left anterior axillary line, subcostal). Trocar 5 (10 mm) is placed paramedially as shown in the figure. The site of trocar 5 will ultimately be replaced with a 15-mm trocar for introducing the band. The site marked 6 allows passage of the liver retractor.

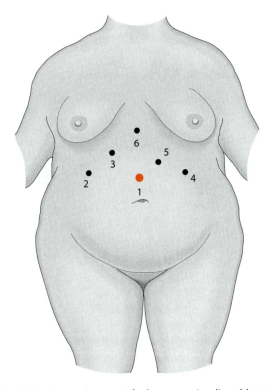

Fig. 71.2. Trocar placement for laparoscopic adjustable gastric band

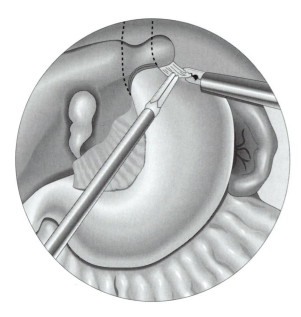

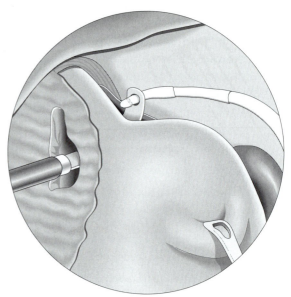

Fig. 71.3. The angle of His and lesser curve dissection. *A* Exposure of the angle of His. *B* The pars flaccida is identified

Fig. 71.5. The band is attached to the instrument

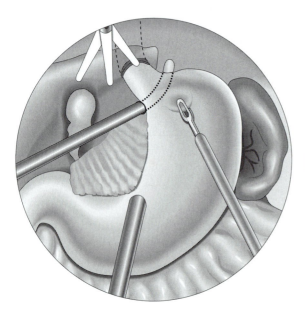

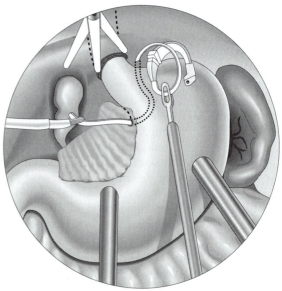

Fig. 71.4. The laparoscopic band placement (LBP) device is deployed

Fig. 71.6. The band is retracted through the retrogastric space to encircle the upper stomach

Procedure

There are 2 methods reported: (1) the pars flaccida approach and (2) the perigastric approach. We will focus on the pars flaccida technique as this technique is associated with fewer long-term complications (Ponce et al. 2005). The Nathanson retractor is deployed below the left lobe of the liver and fixed in place with the table-mounted retractor. The angle of His is then exposed by dissection of the fat pad to the left of the gastroesophageal junction (Fig. 71.3). This is most easily done by pulling the omentum away, the fundus of the stomach caudally, and the gastroesophageal (GE) junction to the right. The peritoneum is divided with electrocautery over the left crus close to the diaphragm. Next, attention is turned to the lesser curve, and the anesthesiologist is asked to pass the calibration tube with a balloon tip. Using the pars flaccida technique,

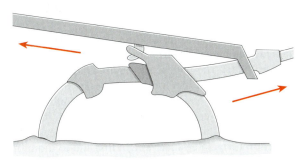

Fig. 71.7. The band is locked into place around the stomach

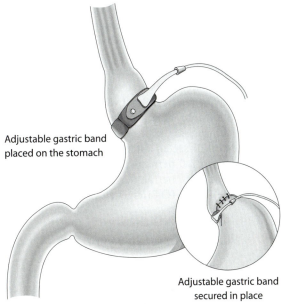

Adjustable gastric band
placed on the stomach

Adjustable gastric band
secured in place

Fig. 71.8. The adjustable gastric band in position around the stomach. *Inset* Position of sutures for the loose anterior fixation of the band to prevent prolapse and band migration. This plication is crucial to complication prevention

the surgeon dissects directly to the right of the equator of the calibration-tube balloon in the avascular space of the pars flaccida (lesser omentum). This entry into the lesser omental sac allows direct visualization of the caudate lobe of the liver. The space overlying the right crus is bluntly dissected to expose the right crus. Next, a blunt dissection beneath the esophagus from right to left is performed. There should be no resistance during this part of the procedure, and the end point of the blunt dissection is the space opened previously at the angle of His. Once this window has been created below the gastroesophageal junction, the "lap band placer" (LBP) is positioned through this opening from right to left (Fig. 71.4). The lap band is introduced into the peritoneal cavity through the 15-mm site in two moves, one to place the lap band into the abdomen and one to insert the remaining tubing. The connection tubing is slid into the LBP (approximately 2–3 inches) (Fig. 71.5) and the LBP is removed pulling the tubing around the stomach and the lap band into position. The tubing is removed from the LBP and the tubing is fed through the "buckle" of the lap band. Appropriate placement of the lap band is confirmed just distal to the pouch calibration balloon (Fig. 71.6). If there is a significant amount of fat on the lesser curve of the stomach the harmonic scalpel should be used to carefully clear this fat from the lesser curve to prevent a "tight" restriction due to the band and fat. The lap band should only be closed with the lap band closer once the lap band is optimally positioned around the stomach, just immediately below the gastroesophageal junction (Fig. 71.7).

The lap band is fixed around the stomach via an anterior plication method (Fig. 71.8). Three or four, 2-0 braided permanent sutures (15 cm long) are used. Full thickness bites are preferred. One must be sure to obtain gastrogastric sutures around the left lateral aspect of the lap band appliance, but not over the buckle. Plication over the buckle will lead to gastric wall erosion and infection.

The access port tubing is brought back into the abdominal cavity and removed through the 15-mm port site. The Nathanson retractor may now be removed. The port site is enlarged to 3–4 cm down through Scarpa's fascia. A pocket is bluntly dissected inferior to this incision. Four 2-0 Prolene sutures are placed in a square pattern into the anterior rectus sheath and threaded through the access port and tied into position. The tubing is then slid back into the abdominal cavity ensuring that the tubing is not kinked or sharply angled. The access port wound is closed.

Operative Challenges

Some patients may have significant amounts of intra-abdominal fat which makes visualization and dissection difficult. In this case, the surgeon must be gentle, making sure not to rip or tear through the fat or other underlying structures. One must also be persistent and not hesitate to add additional ports to help with retraction and dissection.

The challenge of a tight lap band may be encountered. The surgeon must always ensure the lap band is loose. A grasper should fit between the lap band and the stomach and should easily rotate. Further dissection and removal of excess fat along the lesser curve may be performed to ensure a loose closure.

A large soft liver also presents a technical challenge. A good liver retractor such as the Nathanson liver retractor is highly recommended. Again, one must be gentle and patient in the positioning of the retractor to ensure proper placement and to avoid bleeding. Once again, do not hesitate to add additional port sites in order to retract the liver; one must expect to see the diaphragm for adequate visualization.

Lastly, a patient may present with a hiatal hernia. In this case the diaphragmatic defect should be repaired first. The stomach should be reduced into the abdomen and the defect dissected anteriorly. The defect should be closed using 2-0 permanent suture in a figure-of-eight fashion. Large hernia defects may require mesh for adequate closure (O'Brien et al. 1999).

Removal of the Lap Band

Approximately 1% of patients do not tolerate the lap band and 2% of patients have complications that require removal of the lap band. Indications for removal of the lap band include prolapse of the apparatus, erosion of the lap band through the stomach, and the patient's inability to tolerate the lap band.

In the case of prolapse, the patient is positioned and the same port sites are used. Any adhesions are lysed. The old lap band is mobilized with electrocautery, divided beyond the shoulder of the device and removed. A new lap band is then placed as described above via the pars flaccida approach.

For erosion of the band into the stomach, adhesions are divided and the band is removed as above. Attention is then turned to the stomach defect. The defect is closed in a simple interrupted fashion. The gastric suture line is protected with omentum. A suture is placed at the apex of the gastric repair as a landmark should the lap band be replaced.

Postoperative Care

These patients are typically extubated in the operating room. Postoperatively, patients fast for several hours. They are cared for in a monitored, non-intensive care setting and maintenance intravenous fluids are administered based on lean body weight (usually 40–50% of actual weight). Some patients can return home the same day, but many times an overnight admission is prudent. Just as with any abdominal operation in a morbidly obese patient, complications can arise postoperatively. Signs of complication include fever, tachycardia, tachypnea, increasing oxygen requirement, oliguria, worsening abdominal pain, a feeling of anxiety, or an acute alteration in mental status. These signs require aggressive and appropriate investigation as they may signal pulmonary embolus, unappreciated bowel injury, or bleeding.

Postoperative Monitoring and Diet

Water-soluble UGI contrast study is not routinely obtained. The patient is discharged without any fluid in the lap band. The patient maintains a liquid diet for 2 weeks and a soft diet for 4 more weeks. In approximately 7 weeks, based on the patient's comfort level and ability to tolerate meals, the lap band is then inflated with 1–2 ml of sterile saline. Every 4 weeks the patient returns to evaluate weight loss and to monitor satiety and any negative side effects. If the patient demonstrates adequate weight loss and satiety, it may not be necessary to inflate the lap band any further at that time. If the patient demonstrates marginal weight loss or complains of an increased appetite the patient may be optimized by adding more saline to the lap band.

The patient should lose 1–2 pounds per week. If the patient loses less than 1 pound per week during this period then 0.3–0.5 ml should be added to the lap band. If the patient is losing 1–2 pounds per week then the physician should discuss any symptoms or appetite concerns the patient may have and make a decision on adding or removing fluid at that time.

Patients sometimes become impatient about the rate of weight loss and may request greater restriction to speed up weight loss. However, one must educate the patient that weight loss should be steady and gentle over the long-term and they should be reminded that they are on track for their long-term goal. Other long-term benefits such as improved health and better physical and social confidence should also be enforced.

Patients must be counseled on dietary intake. The single most important rule is the patient must avoid liquid calories. They must avoid high-calorie, high-sugar liquids. Patients should drink water before and after meals as water during meals increases the passage of the food, making it easier to take in more calories. Patients should also eat small portions and only eat until they feel comfortable.

It may be necessary to remove fluid at times in certain patients. Indications for the removal of fluid include: (1) signs and symptoms of obstruction, (2) pregnancy, to ensure optimization of nutritional status during this time, and (3) illness or operation, again to ensure adequate nutritional support.

Outcome

Seven LAGB studies have reported weight and BMI change on 277 patients, however the length of follow up has been short, ranging from 1.7 to 3.3 years (Abu-Abeid et al. 2003, Angrisani et.al. 2005, Fielding and Duncombe 2005, Horgan et al. 2005, Nadler et al. 2007, Silberhumer et al. 2006, Yitzhak et.al. 2006). Among 5 larger case series (Angrisani et al. 2005, Fielding and

Duncombe 2005, Nadler et al. 2007, Silberhumer et al. 2006,Yitzhak et al. 2006), a total of 262 adolescent patients age 9-19 were included. The average mean preoperative BMI was 42 to 48 kg/m2; the patients lost 37% to 70% of excess body weight during 6 months to 7 years follow up. Long term weight loss outcomes for the LAGB and standardized descriptions of comorbidies are still lacking. However, Yitzhak and coworkers (Yitzhak et al. 2006) reported that at least 80% of adolescents had sustained weight loss five years after AGB, and Fielding and Duncombe (2005) reported 30% weight reduction 3 years postoperatively in 18 patients. There was no mortality. A total of twenty-six reoperations (9.4%) were performed to correct various complications in the LAGB group. Reasons for reoperation included band slippage, intragastric migration and port/tubing problems. Band slippage was the most frequently reported LAGB complication (4.3%). LABG shows promising weight loss potential with low morbidity; however, more long term outcomes data in adolescents is needed. Other reports suggest that the younger the patient the greater the weight loss from LAGB (Busetto et al. 2002; Dixon et al. 2001).

Conclusion

There is a growing interest in laparoscopic bariatric surgery for the management of morbidly obese adolescents who have failed other means of conventional weight loss. LAGB may be an effective approach with fewer risks than gastric bypass. LAGB has been shown to be effective in reduction of weight and obesity-related comorbidities in adults in the short to intermediate term (5–7 years). LAGB also offers a reversibility that other procedures do not offer. We must prospectively evaluate the effectiveness and outcomes of LAGB in adolescents to better guide patient selection and postoperative management.

References

Abu-Abeid S, Gavert N, Klausner JM, et al (2003) Bariatric surgery in adolescence. J Pediatr Surg 38:1379-1382

Angrisani L, Favretti F, Furbetta F, et al (2005) Obese teenagers treated Lap-Band system: the Italian experience. Surgery 138:877-881.

Busetto L, Segato G, DeMarchi F, et al (2002) Outcome predictors in morbidly obese recipients of an adjustable gastric band. Obes Surg 12:83–92

Deitel M, Shikora S (2002) The development of the surgical treatment of morbid obesity. J Am Coll Nutr 21:365–371

Dixon J, Dixon M, O'Brien P (2001) Pre-operative predictors of weight loss at 1 year after LapBand surgery. Obes Surg 11:200–207

Dolan K, Fielding G (2004) A comparison of laparoscopic adjustable gastric banding in adolescents and adults. Surg Endosc 18:45–47

Dolan K, Creighton L, Hopkins G, et al (2003) Laparoscopic gastric banding in morbidly obese adolescents. Obes Surg 13:101–104

Fielding GA, Duncombe JE (2005) Laparoscopic adjustable gastric banding in severely adolescents. Surg Obes Relat Dis 1:399-405

Horgan S, Holterman MJ, Jacobsen GR, et al. (2005) Laparoscopic adjustable gastric banding for the treatment of adolescent mobid obesity in the United States: a safe alternative to gastric bypass. J Pediatr Surg 40:86-90

Inge T, Krebs N, Garcia V, et al (2004a) Bariatric surgery for severely overweight adolescents: concerns and recommendations. Pediatrics 114:217–223

Inge TH, Zeller M, Garcia V, et al (2004b) Surgical approach to adolescent severe obesity. Adolesc Med Clin 15:429–453

Livingston E (2002) Obesity and its surgical management. Am J Surg 184:103–113

Nadler EP, Youn HA, Ginsburg HB, et al; Short-term results in 53 US obese pediatric patients treated with laparoscopic adjustable gastric banding. J Pediatr Surg. 2007;42:137-141.

O'Brien P, Brown W, Smith A, et al (1999) Prospective study of a laparoscopically placed, adjustable gastric band in the treatment of morbid obesity. Br J Surg 86:113–118

Ponce J, Paynter S, Fromm R (2005) Laparoscopic adjustable gastric banding: 1,014 consecutive cases. J Am Coll Surg 201:529–535

Pories W, Swanson M, MacDonald K, et al (1995) Who would have thought it? An operation proves to be the most effective therapy for adult-onset diabetes mellitus. Ann Surg 222:339–350

Ren C, Horgan S, Ponce J (2002) US experience with the LAP-BAND system. Am J Surg 184:46S–50S

Schirmer B (2000) Laparoscopic bariatric surgery. Surg Clin North Am 80:1253–1267

Silberhumer GR, Miller K, Kriwanek S, et al (2006) Laparoscopic adjustable gastric banding in adolescents: the Austrian experience. Obes Surg 16:1062-1067

Yitzhak A, Mizrahi S, Avinoach E (2006) Laparoscopic gastric banding in adolescents.

Online resources:

General information: http://www.cincinnatichildrens.org/bariatric

Professional society link: http://www.asbs.org

Chapter 72

Laparoscopic Roux-en-Y Gastric Bypass: Principles and Procedures

Steven R. Allen and Thomas H. Inge

Introduction

Obesity has reached epidemic proportions in the pediatric and adolescent populations. As the safety and efficacy of bariatric surgery for adults has become evident, more attention has been given to consideration of bariatric surgical interventions for clinically severely obese adolescents (Inge et al. 2004a).

Minimally invasive procedures have been developed for all of the modern weight-loss procedures including the Roux-en-Y gastric bypass (RYGBP), the adjustable gastric band, the vertical banded gastroplasty (O'Brien et al. 1999; Schirmer 2000), and the biliopancreatic diversion with duodenal switch. The RYGBP has been used most widely in the USA because of its safe side effect profile, balanced with excellent long-term weight loss and maintenance (Pories et al. 1995). RYGBP effectively allows adolescents to lose one third or more of excess body weight and improves or cures most comorbidities of obesity (Inge et al. 2004b; Sugerman et al. 2003).

Minimally invasive bariatric surgery is one of the most technically difficult operations to perform. Laparoscopic skills utilized in foregut surgery are not directly transferable to bariatric surgery. Expertise in minimally invasive surgery may not confer the same level of expertise in performing minimally invasive bariatric surgery. Adequate technical training is critical prior to embarking on minimally invasive surgical treatment for adolescent severe obesity and, at a minimum, should include taking an accredited course of study in bariatric surgery (www.asmbs.org; www.sages.org) and performing procedures first proctored by an experienced laparoscopic bariatric surgeon.

Preoperative Preparation

Before Induction of General Anesthesia

The preoperative education of the patient, family, and referring pediatrician is of paramount importance but is beyond the scope of this text. The reader is referred to other sources for more complete discussion of this topic (Garcia et al. 2003).

Patients are limited to clear liquids on the day prior to RYGBP. There is no need for a bowel preparation.

Preoperative medications include low molecular weight heparin for deep vein thrombosis (DVT) prophylaxis (40 mg subcutaneously and continued twice daily postoperatively while in the hospital), and a second-generation cephalosporin (2 g intravenously). Additional DVT prophylaxis includes sequential compression boots which must be used intraoperatively and postoperatively. They should be applied and functioning prior to induction of anesthesia.

After Induction of General Anesthesia

General anesthesia is used for laparoscopic RYGBP. The airway of patients with morbid obesity can be challenging, but airway and anesthesia concerns for the morbidly obese adolescent do not differ from the morbidly obese adult. For local anesthesia, 0.25% bupivacaine with epinephrine is injected using a long spinal needle to anesthetize each trocar site from the peritoneum to the skin. No epidural or spinal block is necessary for this procedure. An orogastric tube of 34F size is placed to both decompress the stomach and act later as an internal sizing tube for creation of the "thumb-size" gastric pouch and 1- to 1.5 cm-diameter gastrojejunal anastomosis. A urinary catheter is also placed prior to operation.

Positioning

Patient

The patient can be in the flat supine position with arms abducted and legs together. The table initially should be in gentle reverse Trendelenburg position to bring the bowel inferiorly. Care should be taken to secure the thighs and lower legs, and some surgeons advocate a footplate at the end of the bed to provide plantar support for steep reverse Trendelenburg positioning.

Crew, Monitors, and Equipment

The surgeon is at the patient's right, the scrub nurse at the patient's right, and the assistant surgeon on the patient's left (■ Fig. 72.1). Given the patient's extreme girth, it is ergonomically advantageous to stand on a platform 20–40 cm above the floor. Two monitors are used and are placed near the patient's shoulders.

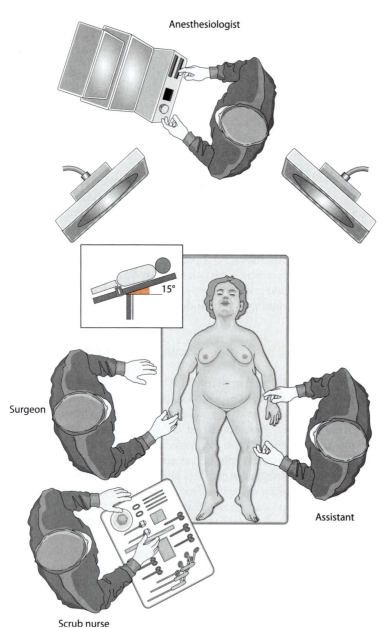

Anesthesiologist

Fig. 72.1. Operating room layout.
A Patient, *B* surgeon, *C* scrub nurse,
D assistant, *E* anesthesiologist

15°

Surgeon

Assistant

Scrub nurse

Special Equipment

In general, laparoscopic RYGBP can be performed using standard 32 cm adult instrumentation. Various manufacturers supply the equipment required and the choice of one over another is largely a matter of the surgeon's preference. Specific instrumentation used at our institution for this procedure is listed in ■ Tables 72.1 and 72.2.

Technique

For initial abdominal access, the transparent, bladeless, direct-viewing 12 mm trocar is placed through the midline, 5–10 cm above the umbilicus. Exact trocar placement is determined by laying a standard 10 mm adult laparoscopic telescope on the patient's abdomen, with the tip of the scope at the nipple level, marking a skin site at the point beside the light cord insertion point on the scope. This trocar site will provide optimal visualization of the upper and lower portions of the procedure. The three other 12 mm trocar placement sites are shown in ■ Fig. 72.2. Pneumoperitoneum to an intra-abdominal pressure of 15 mmHg is usually sufficient for adequate visualization.

Table 72.1 List of surgical instruments used at the Cincinnati Children's Hospital Medical Center for laparoscopic RYGBP

Four 10/12 mm ENDOPATH Optiview trocars (Ethicon Endosurgery)
One 0°, 32 cm laparoscope (for initial abdominal access), one 30°, 32 cm laparoscope
One Nathanson liver retractor (Cook Surgical, Bloomington, IN)
One esophageal retractor (blunt dissector; Pilling Weck, part number 38-1802)
One locking, atraumatic bowel grasper
Two non-locking atraumatic bowel graspers
One hook scissor for cutting suture
One needle driver
One bipolar electrocautery forceps (e.g., as manufactured by Wolff)
One ultrasonic dissector

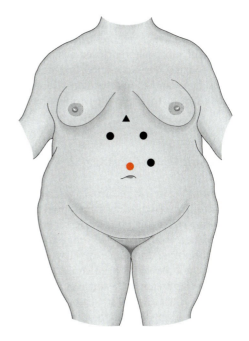

Fig. 72.2. Trocar placement for laparoscopic gastric bypass. The first trocar is placed in the midline above the umbilicus; the remainder are placed under direct laparoscopic vision. All trocars are 12 mm except for the subxiphoid site which is 5 mm

Table 72.2 Additional suggested equipment and stapling devices

1% lidocaine, 10-cc syringe, and a long (spinal) needle
One 34F orogastric tube (Kimberly Clark, part number 15034)
One ENDOPATH endoscopic linear cutter 45 mm stapler, 2.5 mm staple (white loads; Ethicon part number ATB45)
Two ENDOPATH endoscopic linear cutter 35 mm staplers, 3.5 mm staple (blue loads; Ethicon part number TSW35)
Multiple 8-inch lengths of 2-0 silk and 3-0 dyed vicryl on SH needles
One Jackson-Pratt flat drain

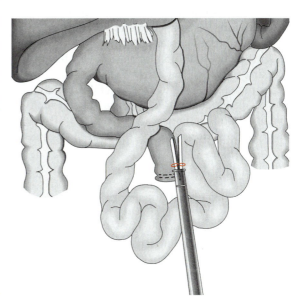

Fig. 72.3. The jejunojejunostomy is stapled with a 45 mm linear cutter and the enterotomy is then closed with a single-layer running vicryl closure

Roux Limb Construction

The omentum is raised cephalad above the colon and tucked beneath the liver edge to expose the transverse colon and proximal small intestine. The transverse mesocolon is grasped with a locking grasper just anterior to the duodenojejunal flexure and elevated anteriorly. The jejunum is divided 25–50 cm beyond the duodenojejunal flexure using the 45 mm Endo-GIA (EES, white load). Using another stapler load, a mesenteric defect is opened in continuity with this bowel transection to allow mobility of the Roux limb. Bipolar electrocautery is often needed for hemostasis.

A 100 cm Roux limb is used for most patients. At 100 cm, a single stay suture is placed to approximate the segments to be anastomosed, creating the jejunojejunostomy "Y" of the RYGBP. Opposing enterotomies are made with the harmonic scalpel or hook electrocautery. Side-to-side jejunojejunostomy is created using the 45 mm EES stapler with white load (Fig. 72.3), and the resulting enterotomy defect is closed either with a running 3-0 vicryl (SH needle) or by using another firing of the stapler. Next, the mesenteric defect is closed with a running 2-0 silk suture to avoid an internal hernia.

The Roux limb should be tunneled cephalad in a retrocolic fashion which requires a mesocolic defect to be created and subsequently closed around the Roux limb. Additionally, Petersen's defect between the small bowel mesentery and the mesocolon will need to be deliberately closed to prevent postoperative internal hernia.

Gastric Pouch Construction

The left lobe of the liver is retracted anteriorly with the liver retractor (inserted below the xiphoid) to expose the gastroesophageal junction. The lesser curve gastric pouch is created around the 34F orogastric tube. The dissection begins at the angle of His (■ Fig. 72.4). Once a sufficient plane has been created between the stomach and diaphragm at the angle of His, the esophageal retractor is used as a blunt dissector to better develop this plane along the length of the left crus.

Perigastric ultrasonic dissection along the lesser curvature approximately 8–10 cm inferior to the gastroesophageal junction (usually just below the second lesser curve vessel) begins the creation of the gastric pouch. Once the lesser sac is reached, the gastrocolic ligament is opened and the lesser sac inspected. The blunt esophageal dissector is placed into the lesser sac behind the stomach and directed through the window previously created along the lesser curve.

A "thumb-sized" lesser curve pouch is next created using the Endo-GIA 35 mm stapler with blue loads. The first transverse cut across the lesser curvature is accomplished followed by creation of the vertical transection alongside the 34F orogastric tube by multiple applications of the Endo-GIA (■ Fig. 72.5). Once the angle of His is reached, the pouch is completed (■ Fig. 72.6).

Gastrojejunal Anastomosis

There are numerous techniques for laparoscopic gastrojejunostomy including hand-sewn, the end-to-end stapled technique with anvil inserted into the pouch laparoscopically, the end-to-end stapled technique with the anvil inserted orally, and a linearly stapled technique. We have found the hand-sewn technique to be technically preferable. The remainder of this chapter will focus on details and pearls for performance of the hand-sewn technique.

The anastomosis is created by first running a posterior seromuscular 3-0 vicryl suture line to secure the antimesenteric border of the Roux limb to the inferior pouch edge. Enterotomies (1–1.5 cm) are next created in the pouch and the jejunum with the ultrasonic scalpel. Running full thickness suture lines are used to

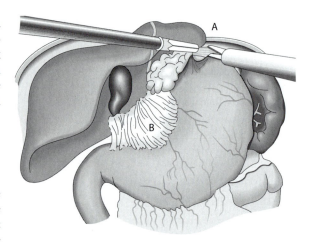

Fig. 72.4. The angle of His and lesser curve dissection. A. Minimal dissection is performed with the ultrasonic scalpel at the angle of His and subsequently this plane between the left crus and the stomach wall is further exploited safely by using the blunt esophageal retractor as a dissecting instrument (not shown). B. The lesser curve dissection is next performed close to the gastric wall, working toward the lesser sac

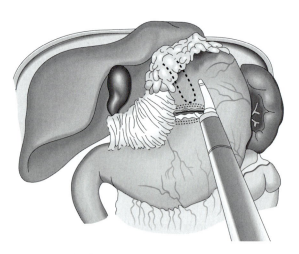

Fig. 72.5. Gastric pouch creation. The remainder of the pouch is created using the Endo-GIA along a 34F tube in the stomach (*dotted line*)

close the anastomosis over the 34F calibration tube. The final anterior seromuscular suture line is then placed. Thus, one has accomplished outer seromuscular and inner full-thickness running layers to anastomose the Roux limb to the pouch (■ Fig. 72.7). The integrity and patency of the anastomosis is assessed laparoscopically with intraluminal air insufflation under saline.

A drain to prevent fluid collection within the abdomen and for early identification of a leak is left near the anastomosis and exits via the patient's upper left trocar site. A temporary gastrostomy tube is placed in the

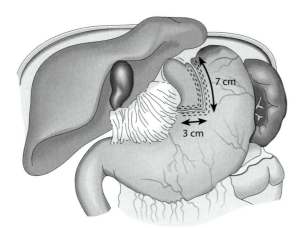

Fig. 72.6. Gastric pouch geometry

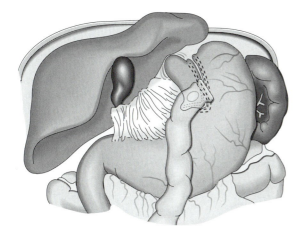

Fig. 72.7. Roux-en-Y gastric bypass

remnant stomach body if any intraoperative technical challenges are deemed significant enough to warrant deliberate decompression of the bypassed gastric remnant. With the use of the bladeless trocars the 12 mm port sites do not require fascial closure.

Postoperative Care

These patients are typically extubated in the operating room after transfer to the hospital bed. They are cared for in a monitored, non-intensive care setting, and maintenance fluids are administered based upon lean body weight (typically 40–50% of actual weight). No nasogastric tube is used. Patient-controlled analgesia with intravenous narcotics is used for the first 24–48 h. Early signs of complication include fever, tachycardia, tachypnea, increasing oxygen requirement, oliguria, hiccoughs, regurgitation, left shoulder pain, worsening abdominal pain, a feeling of anxiety, or acute alteration

in mental status. One must be vigilant as these signs warrant aggressive attention and appropriate investigation since they may signal gastrointestinal leak, pulmonary embolus, bowel obstruction, or acute dilation and impending rupture of the bypassed gastric remnant.

A water-soluble upper gastrointestinal contrast study is routinely obtained on postoperative day 1. A detailed discussion of the radiologic considerations can be found in Inge et al. (2004c). After satisfactory passage of contrast is documented without evidence of anastomotic leak, patients are begun on clear liquids and subsequently advanced to a high-protein liquid diet for the first month after operation. Patients are discharged most commonly by the second or third postoperative day.

Five basic "rules" are routinely emphasized with patients and family at each postoperative visit: (1) eat protein first (≥70 g/day); (2) drink 64–96 ounces of water or sugar-free liquids daily; (3) no snacking between meals; (4) exercise at least 30 min per day; and (5) always remember vitamin and mineral supplements.

Outcome

As of 2007, 80 patients have undergone RYGBP (2 by open laparotomy, 38 laparoscopically). Twenty-two patients have been followed for 1 year or more. Mean preoperative weight in this cohort was 361 pounds (164 kg) and body mass index (BMI) ranged from 44 to 85 kg/m^2, with a mean of 57 kg/m^2. After 1 year, the mean weight was 222 pounds (101 kg) and BMI ranged from 26 to 58 kg/m^2, with a mean of 35 kg/m^2. This represents a 39% reduction in body BMI over the year. Excess weight loss has been 63%. One patient who presented with a BMI of 85 had lost 71 kg at 1 year and has regained 6 kg at the end of his second year postoperatively. There have been no deaths due to the intervention, and no anastomotic leaks. Preoperative comorbidities of obesity have largely been reversed after gastric bypass. Three patients with type 2 diabetes and with obstructive sleep apnea have experienced complete remission and no longer require hypoglycemic medications and continuous positive airway pressure, respectively. Complications in this initial series have been similar to those observed in similar series with adult patients. One notable exception has been the sporadic observation of beriberi development after surgery in adolescence (Towbin et al. 2004) which has prompted addition of a B-complex vitamin to our regimen. More details regarding specific patient management can be obtained in the following online resource: www.cincinnatichildrens.org/bariatric. Only a few of our most extremely obese patients have required precautionary, short-term intensive care unit stays postoperatively.

References

Garcia VF, Langford L, Inge TH (2003). Application of laparoscopy for bariatric surgery in adolescents. Curr Opin Pediatr 15:248–255

Inge TH, Krebs NF, Garcia VF, et al (2004a) Bariatric surgery for severely overweight adolescents: concerns and recommendations. Pediatrics 114:217–223

Inge TH, Garcia V, Daniels S, et al (2004b). A multidisciplinary approach to the adolescent bariatric surgical patient. J Pediatr Surg 39:442–447

Inge TH, Donnelly LF, Vierra M, et al (2004c) Managing bariatric patients in a children's hospital: radiologic considerations and limitations. J Pediatr Surg 40:609–617

O'Brien PE, Brown WA, Smith A, et al (1999) Prospective study of a laparoscopically placed, adjustable gastric band in the treatment of morbid obesity. Br J Surg 86:113–118

Pories WJ, Swanson MS, MacDonald KG, et al (1995) Who would have thought it? An operation proves to be the most effective therapy for adult-onset diabetes mellitus. Ann Surg 222:339–350

Schirmer BD (2000) Laparoscopic bariatric surgery. Surg Clin North Am 80:1253–1267

Sugerman HJ, Sugerman EL, DeMaria EJ, et al (2003) Bariatric surgery for severely obese adolescents. J Gastrointest Surg 7:102–108

Towbin A, Inge TH, Garcia VF, et al (2004) Beriberi after gastric bypass surgery in adolescence. J Pediatr 145:263–267

Diaphragm

Chapter 73

Laparoscopic Treatment of Morgagni-Larrey Diaphragmatic Hernia

Mario Lima, Marcello Dòmini, and Antonio Aquino

Introduction

The Morgagni-Larrey hernia is a retrosternal or anterior diaphragmatic hernia covered with a sac. The defect is located anteromedially on either side of the junction of the septum transversum and the thoracic wall. A retrosternal defect to the right of the sternum is usually referred to as a *hernia of Morgagni*, whereas a hernia to the left of the sternum is often referred to as a *hernia of Larrey* (Becmeur et al. 2003; Lima et al. 2001a,b). Very rarely no sac is present in which case the defect extends into the pericardial space. Such defects are usually part of the pentalogy of Cantrell, and will not be considered here.

Retrosternal hernias are usually discovered in older children or in adults when they can become symptomatic (Ipek et al. 2001; Rodriguez et al. 2003) due to intestinal involvement (occlusive symptoms) or when respiratory dysfunction occurs. In pediatric patients they are mostly discovered incidentally. Surgical treatment is indicated even if asymptomatic to avoid possible complications often described in adulthood (Rodriguez et al. 2003).

Morgagni-Larrey hernias are an ideal indication for a laparoscopic repair (Becmeur et al. 2003; Georgacopulo et al. 1997; Ipek et al. 2002; Lima et al. 2001a,b; Newman et al. 1995; Rodriguez et al. 2003; van der Zee et al. 1999) and the technique is presented here.

Preoperative Preparation

Before Induction of General Anesthesia

No specific preoperative preparation is required, except a preoperative enema given in order to avoid colonic distension.

After Induction of General Anesthesia

After induction of general anesthesia including endotracheal intubation, a nasogastric tube is inserted and a prophylactic antibiotic is given.

Positioning

Patient

The child lies supine with the legs extended on abducted leg supports; younger children can be put in a frog-like position. The operation is performed with the patient in moderate anti-Trendelenburg position so that the bowel falls out of the way.

Crew, Monitors, and Equipment

The monitor is placed at the top of the table. All the cables and tubes lie on the left of the patient. The surgeon stands in between the patient's legs, with the camera operator to his/her left and the assistant to his/her right. The scrub nurse also stands to the right of the surgeon but lower down (■ Fig. 73.1).

Special Equipment

Apart from bipolar high-frequency electrocautery, no special equipment or instruments are used.

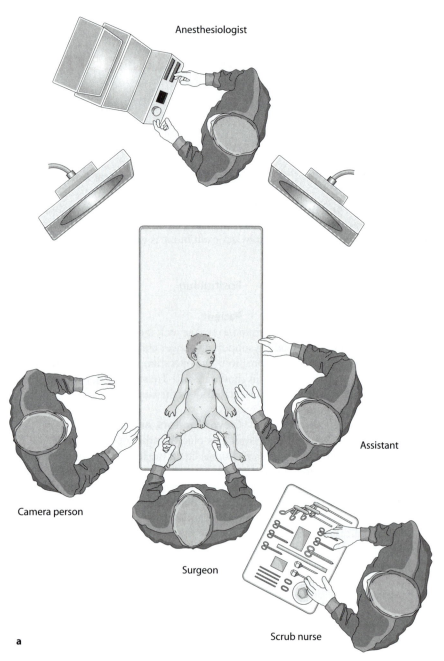

Anesthesiologist

Fig. 73.1 a. Position of a small child, crew and monitors during the operation

Assistant

Camera person

Surgeon

Scrub nurse

a

Technique

Cannulae

Cannula	Method of insertion	Diameter (mm)	Device	Position
1	Open	5 or 10	Optic 0°	Umbilical
2	Closed	3–5	Forceps and needle holder	Right hypochondrium
3	Closed	3–5	Forceps and needle holder	Left hypochondrium
4	Closed	3–5	Forceps and liver retractor	Left subcostal

Fig. 73.1 b. Position of an older child, crew and monitors

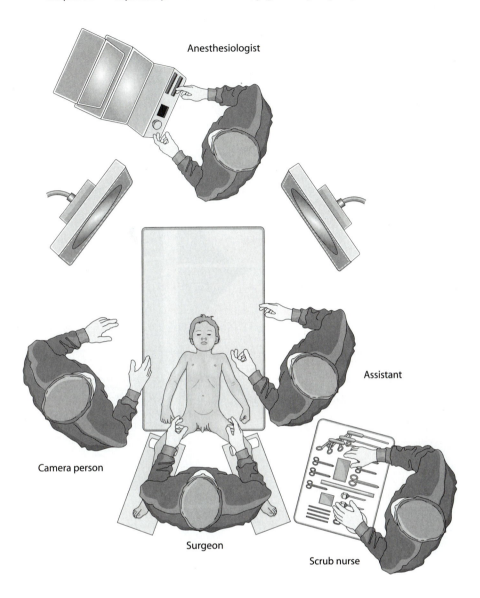

Anesthesiologist

Assistant

Camera person

Surgeon

Scrub nurse

b

Port Positions

Four ports are used. The camera port is introduced through the umbilicus by an "open" procedure, two working ports are placed in the right and left hypochondrium, and one port is in the left subcostal space (▬ Fig. 73.2).

Procedure

The first step is to bring down the herniated transverse colon or a herniated anomalous hepatic lobe. To make suturing easier, the first holding stitch is passed through the abdominal wall, through the middle of the posterior edge of the defect, and out again through the abdomi-

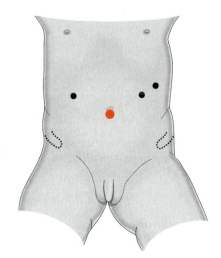

Fig. 73.2. Position of the trocars

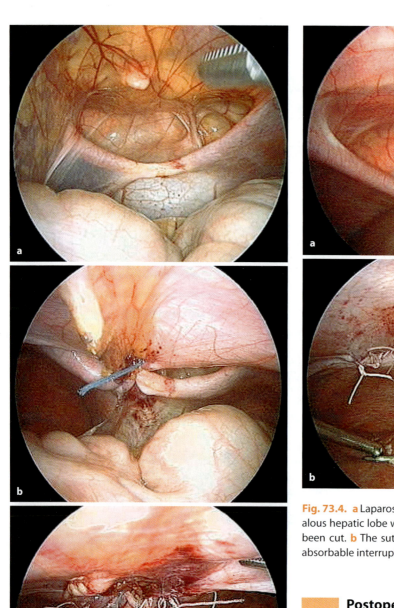

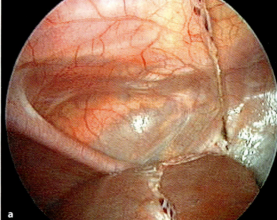

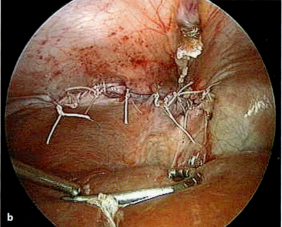

Fig. 73.4. a Laparoscopic view of a patient in which an anomalous hepatic lobe was herniated. The falciform ligament has been cut. **b** The suturing is completed with seven 2/0 non-absorbable interrupted stitches

Postoperative Care

The nasogastric tube is removed at the end of the procedure. Patients resume free oral fluid intake on the same day of laparoscopic procedure and are able to take food on the first postoperative day. Postsurgical discomfort, generally limited to the first and second day, is easily controlled by administration of non-steroidal analgesics.

Results

Three patients have been operated on for Morgagni-Larrey hernia. One of them had herniated transverse colon in the defect, and the other two had herniated liver in the defect (segments III–IV). The mean operative time was 45 min. No intraoperative problems were encountered due to the CO_2 entering the defect. All the

Fig. 73.3. a Laparoscopic view of the defect in a patient with herniation of the transverse colon. **b** Placing the first transabdominal stitch. **c** Completed repair

nal wall. Next the defect is directly sutured using 2/0 non-absorbable interrupted stitches. We prefer to perform extracorporeal knotting. In our experience it was never necessary to use patches (■ Figs. 73.3, 73.4).

children had a good postoperative recovery and all were discharged after 3 days. The follow-up period ranged from 3 months to 5 years. All patients underwent a chest radiograph 1 month after discharge and all showed disappearance of the hernia.

Discussion

We feel that all Morgagni-Larrey hernias should be repaired laparoscopically. The technique is simple and the results are good. Initial suturing may be difficult but becomes much easier when an initial transabdominal transfixing suture is used. An alternative is to put the first stitch intra-abdominally and to tie it after exerting external pressure onto the anterior epigastrium thus decreasing the anteroposterior diameter of the defect. We prefer to use interrupted non-absorbable sutures, but some authors performed a continuous suture (Becmeur et al. 2003). Patches are not usually necessary for pediatric patients, but sometimes in older children they must be employed, as happens in most instances in adulthood (Becmeur et al. 2003; Ipek et al. 2002).

It is debated in the literature whether to excise the hernial sac or not. Some authors feel that is not necessary to remove the sac and warn against the consequences of a pneumomediastinum, while others recommend removal and report no associated problems (Becmeur et al. 2003; Rodriguez et al. 2003). We leave the sac in place.

In conclusion, Morgagni-Larrey hernias in children (and adults) should be treated laparoscopically.

References

Becmeur F, Philippe P, van der Zee D, et al (2003) Laparoscopic surgery of Morgagni-Larrey hernias: a multicenter study of the Groupe d'Etude en Coeliochirurgie Infantile (GECI). Pediatr Endosurg Innov Tech 7:147–150

Georgacopulo P, Franchella A, Mandrioli G, et al (1997) Morgagni-Larrey hernia correction by laparoscopic surgery. Eur J Pediatr Surg 7:241–242

Ipek T, Altinli E, Yuceyar S, et al (2002) Laparoscopic repair of a Morgagni-Larrey hernia: report of three cases. Surg Today 32:902–905

Lima M, Lauro V, Dòmini M, et al (2001a) Laparoscopic surgery of diaphragmatic diseases in children: our experience with five cases. Eur J Pediatr Surg 11:377–381

Lima M, Ruggeri G, Dòmini M, et al (2001b) Laparoscopic treatment of Morgagni-Larrey hernia in a pediatric patient. Pediatr Endosurg Innov Tech 5:199–203

Newman L 3rd, Eubanks S, Bridges WM 2nd, et al (1995) Laparoscopic diagnosis and treatment of Morgagni hernia. Surg Laparosc Endosc 5:27–31

Rodriguez Hermosa JI, Tuca Rodriguez F, Ruiz Feliu B, et al (2003) Diaphragmatic hernia of Morgagni-Larrey in adults: analysis of 10 cases. Gastroenterol Hepatol 26:535–540

Van der Zee DC, Bax NMA, Valla JS (1999) Laparoscopic repair for diaphragmatic conditions in infants and children. In: Bax NMA, Georgeson KE, Najmaldin A, Valla JS (eds) Endoscopic Surgery in Children. Springer, Berlin, pp 323–328

Chapter 74

Thoracoscopy for Congenital Diaphragmatic Hernia

François Becmeur and Stéphane Grandadam

Introduction

In 1995 van der Zee and Bax described for the first time the closure of a posterolateral diaphragmatic hernia by laparoscopy. In 2001 we published a series of three children with a posterolateral diaphragmatic hernia successfully corrected using a thoracoscopic approach (Becmeur et al. 2001). This chapter deals with the technique of thoracoscopic repair of congenital diaphragmatic hernia.

Preoperative Preparation

Before Induction of General Anesthesia

The child should be in a stable cardiovascular and respiratory condition. Associated malformations should have been searched for. A nasogastric tube is inserted in order to decompress the stomach.

After Induction of General Anesthesia

General anesthesia can be complemented in three different ways:

1. Infiltration of the future port holes with Xylocaine 1% or Marcaine 0.25%, both diluted 50:50 with normal saline.
2. Intercostal nerve block under thoracoscopic control using the same products. The injection should be as posterior as possible in order to ensure total analgesia of parietal pleura.
3. Epidural analgesia, which has the advantage that it can be maintained in the postoperative period, except in the newborn in connection with possible coagulation problems. A single injection of morphine can be given postoperatively (30–50 γ/kg per 24 h). The risk of hemodynamic and or respiratory troubles in children with epidural analgesia is low.

One-lung ventilation is not required. The nasogastric tube is left in place. A urinary catheter is inserted in case of epidural analgesia. No antibiotics are given.

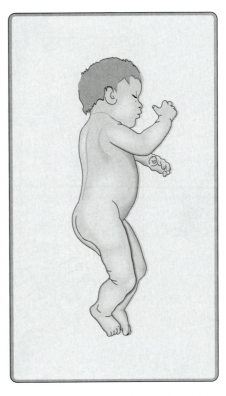

Fig. 74.1. Position of the patient for a right-sided congenital diaphragmatic defect

Positioning

Patient

The patient is placed in a lateral decubitus position as for a classic thoracotomy (■ Fig. 74.1). During surgery the table is tilted in Trendelenburg position.

Crew, Monitors, and Equipment

The surgeon stands at the ventral side of the patient with the assistant to the surgeon's left and the scrub nurse to the left of the assistant further down (■ Fig. 74.2). All three look in the same direction at the monitor, which is placed in front of the surgeon, at the level of the patient's hip or leg. Surgeon, diaphragmatic hernia, and monitor should be in line with each other.

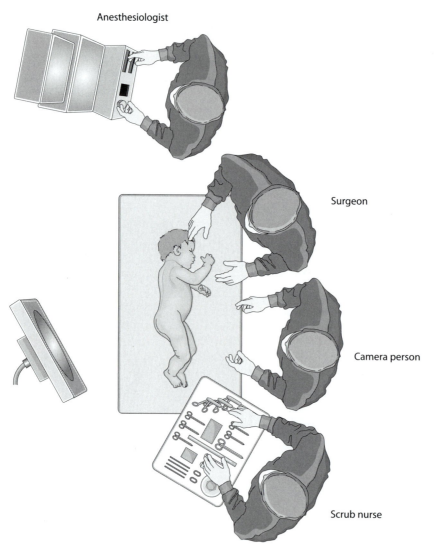

Anesthesiologist

Surgeon

Camera person

Scrub nurse

Fig. 74.2. Position of the crew and equipment for a right-sided diaphragmatic hernia

Special Equipment

Monopolar electrocautery suffices. Goretex or Mersilene mesh should be at hand when needed. As suture material Ethibond 2/0 or 3/0 is used. Short staples should be available as well.

Technique

Cannulae

Cannula	Method of insertion	Diameter (mm)	Device	Position
1	Open	5	Optic	Below the inferior tip of the scapula
2	Closed	3/5	Forceps, scissors, needle holder	Fifth intercostal space, anterior axillary line
3	Closed	3/5	Forceps	Fourth intercostal space, posteriorly

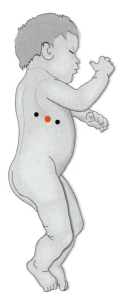

Fig. 74.3. Port positions. The telescope port is placed below the inferior tip of the scapula. The two working ports are placed at the corners of a triangle, the port for the surgeon's left-hand instrument in the 4th intercostal space on the anterior axillary line, and the port for the surgeons right-hand instrument in between the telescope port and the spine in the 5th intercostal space

Procedure

The optic is placed just below the inferior tip of the scapula (■ Fig. 74.3). The anterior insertion of the diaphragm starts at the xiphoid process and runs posteriorly along the 7th rib. The anterior port is placed in the 5th intercostal space, while the posterior port is inserted in between the optic and the spine. A too posterior or too proximal port position will hamper instrument movement.

After insertion of the port for the optic, which is done in an open way, CO_2 is insufflated at a rate of 0.1 L/min and a maximal pressure of 6–8 mmHg. As a result the lung will collapse and the herniated contents will start to reduce into the abdomen. Some problems with CO_2 insufflation, for example desaturation, have been reported, but these can be avoided by using a low flow and low maximum pressure.

The first part of the procedure consists of the reduction of the hernia contents. When a hernial sac is present, this is easily achieved within a few minutes as the thoracic insufflation will do the job (■ Fig. 74.4). When no sac is present on the left side, the reduction should be started by pushing back the herniated stomach, colon, and small intestine, to be followed by the spleen (■ Fig. 74.5). Reduction of the spleen may be difficult, especially when the defect is relatively small. To facilitate reduction, the diaphragmatic hole is kept widely open with two forceps.

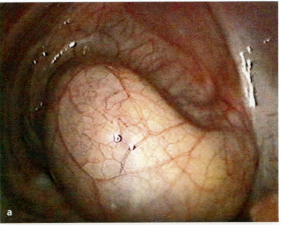

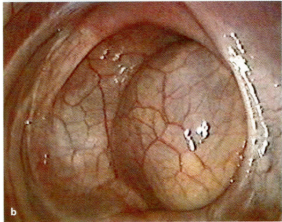

Fig. 74.4. Left-sided diaphragmatic hernia with hernial sac. **a,b** Subsequent stages of reduction by CO_2 insufflation

It is not necessary to resect the sac (■ Fig. 74.6a). Pushing the sac into the abdomen is all that is needed. Next the defect is closed. Care is taken not to interfere with the innervation and vascularization of the diaphragm.

When no sac is present, the muscular borders are not scarified. It is advantageous to free the pleuroperitoneal plate at the posterior border of the defect, close to the posterior arch of the rib. The diaphragmatic defect is closed with interrupted non-absorbable sutures (■ Fig. 74.6b). It may be necessary to use a patch, which is fixed with non-absorbable sutures or clips (■ Fig. 74.7). The same approach may be used for diaphragmatic eventration (■ Fig. 74.8).

At the end of the procedure, CO_2 is aspirated from the thorax through the stopcock of one of the ports, which will expand the lung. Chest tube drainage with a pressure of -10 to -15 mmHg favors lung expansion but may cause overstretching of a hypoplastic lung. In most instances no drain is required. A small residual CO_2 pneumothorax will disappear spontaneously.

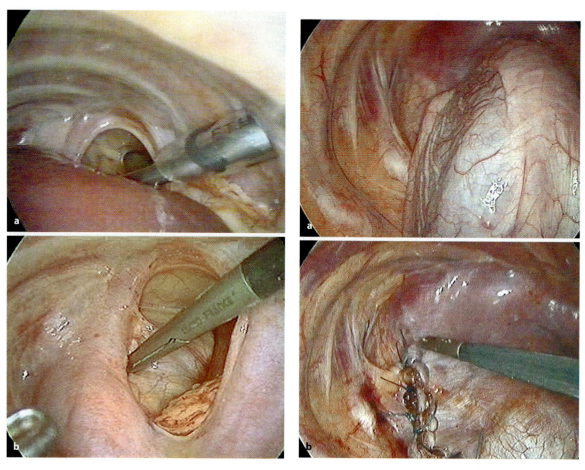

Fig. 74.5. Left-sided diaphragmatic hernia without sac. **a** Spleen in the chest. **b** After reduction

Fig. 74.6. Left-sided diaphragmatic hernia with hernial sac. **a** Before reduction. **b** After closure with interrupted sutures

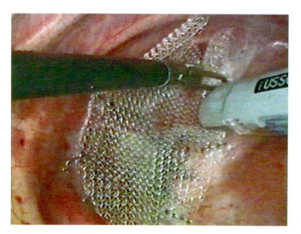

Fig. 74.7. Closure of a diaphragmatic defect using Mersilene mesh

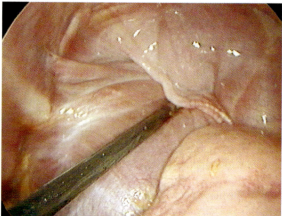

Fig. 74.8. Right-sided diaphragmatic relaxation, before plication

Postoperative Care

Epidural analgesia with morphine is maintained for 48 h. If a chest tube has been inserted, it is taken out the next day. The patient is allowed to eat within 24 h.

Results

Several reports regarding successful thoracoscopic repair of posterolateral diaphragmatic defects with or without a sac both in children as well as in adults have been published (Becmeur et al. 2001; Liem 2003; Mouroux et al. 1996; Ochoa de Castro et al. 2003; Sato et al. 1996; Silen ML et al. 1995).

Discussion

We have no experience with the thoracoscopic repair surgery of diaphragmatic defects in the neonatal period.

Carbon dioxide pneumothorax is a good way of getting the lung out of the way. Moreover it helps to reduce the herniated contents into the abdomen. Hernia reduction is not difficult, except for the spleen. Care should be taken not to injure the spleen during its reduction into the abdomen. The reduction of the herniated contents away from the optic during a thoracoscopic repair, thereby increasing the working space, is a clear advantage above a laparoscopic approach in which the herniated contents are reduced toward the optic, which obscures the view and decreases the working space.

Whether a hernial sac should be resected is debatable. Scarification of the edge of the diaphragmatic defect is not necessary. In any case one should be careful using monopolar energy onto scissors as the high temperature may injure diaphragmatic innervation and vascularization.

A disadvantage of the thoracoscopic approach is the impossibility to check for mesenteric abnormalities of the bowel, but these usually do not require treatment.

References

Becmeur F, Jamali RR, Moog R, et al (2001) Thoracoscopic treatment for delayed presentation of congenital diaphragmatic hernia in the infant. A report of three cases. Surg Endosc 15:1163–1166

Liem NT (2003) Thoracoscopic surgery for congenital diaphragmatic hernia: a report of nine cases. Asian J Surg 26:210–212

Mouroux J, Padovani B, Poirier NC, et al (1996) Technique for the repair of diaphragmatic eventration. Ann Thorac Surg 62:905–907

Ochoa de Castro A, Ramos MR, Calonge WM, et al (2003) Congenital left-sided Bochdalek diaphragmatic hernia. Thoracoscopic repair: case report. Eur J Pediatr Surg 13:407–409

Sato Y, Ishikawa S, Onizuka M, et al (1996) Thoracoscopic repair of diaphragmatic hernia. Thorac Cardiovasc Surg 44:54–55

Silen ML, Canvasser DA, Kurkchubasche AG, et al (1995) Video-assisted thoracic surgical repair of a foramen of Bochdalek hernia. Ann Thorac Surg 60:448–450

Van der Zee DC, Bax NM (1995) Laparoscopic repair of congenital diaphragmatic hernia in a 6-month-old child. Surg Endosc 9:1001–1003

Laparoscopic Repair of Diaphragmatic Defects: Congenital Diaphragmatic Hernia (of Bochdalek) and Eventration

Thane A. Blinman and Steven S. Rothenberg

Introduction

Minimally invasive surgery (MIS) is ideally suited to diagnosis and treatment of all forms of diaphragmatic defects. Obviously, the laparoscope affords accurate direct imaging of defects that have classically eluded accurate description by radiological techniques, and does so with minimal morbidity. But laparoscopy also allows repair of these defects with increased precision and vastly decreased pain compared to open techniques that rely on large incisions to give even marginal exposure (Hendrickson et al. 2003).

Here we consider the repair of Bochdalek hernias and eventrations using minimally invasive surgical (MIS) techniques in children and newborns.

The literature is littered with case reports of MIS repairs of Bochdalek hernias, but virtually all of the descriptions are of repairs in older children and adults (Harinath et al. 2002; Settembre et al. 2003; Willemse et al. 2003). Invariably, these patients had unrecognized congenital diaphragmatic hernias that were revealed during evaluation for other conditions. Alternatively, a few reports describe laparoscopy in the diagnosis or (more rarely) repair of traumatic diaphragmatic hernias (Marin-Blazquez et al. 2003; Matthews et al. 2003). Only one report describes experience with MIS repair of congenital diaphragmatic hernia (CDH) in the newborn, and here the only success came using a thoracoscopic approach (Arca et al. 2003).

Nevertheless, CDH can be repaired using MIS techniques. Recently, our institution reported 15 successful repairs of CDH (12 Bochdalek and 3 Morgagni) by laparoscopy (Hendrickson et al. 2003). Twelve of these patients were infants, and recently we successfully repaired Bochdalek CDH (B-CDH) in two additional newborns. The techniques described focus primarily on B-CDH in neonates, but the methods are similar in older children and in patients with eventration.

Preoperative Preparation

Before Induction of General Anesthesia

Babies with eventration are diagnosed by routine chest X-ray, and do not exhibit the pulmonary hypertension as seen in B-CDH. Eventration is distinguished from phrenic nerve injury by ultrasound or fluoroscopy.

Babies with B-CDH are often diagnosed *in utero* by ultrasound (or rarely by magnetic resonance imaging), but occasionally an otherwise normal baby will exhibit subtle dyspnea and a chest film will reveal air-filled loops of bowel in the chest. Over 90% of B-CDH will occur on the left. Babies with CDH will exhibit varying degrees of pulmonary hypertension and associated physiologic derangements, with some experiencing almost no cardiopulmonary compromise, and others so ill as to require extracorporeal life support (ECLS). In general, dysfunctional physiology will appear within 12 h postnatally, after a relatively benign "honeymoon," and attempting surgery during these fragile first hours has been shown to increase mortality. For this reason, immediate repair, regardless of method, has been abandoned in favor of preoperative stabilization. Babies are best repaired once FiO_2 requirement is below 50%, and positive end-expiratory pressure (PEEP) is less than 10 mmHg. Requiring pressors is not a contraindication for surgery; indeed, ongoing pressor requirement may signal a need for repair in order to restore the mediastinal structures to midline. No baby has been reported repaired by MIS while on ECLS.

After Induction of General Anesthesia

Epidural anesthesia is generally not used. Trocar sites are usually injected after the abdomen is insufflated so that ports are placed most advantageously. A Foley catheter is placed only if the overall physiologic condition warrants. All patients receive a dose of a first-generation cephalosporin unless they are already on antibiotics (many neonates will be treated with ampicillin and gentamicin for other reasons). All patients should have a sumping nasogastric tube inserted and placed to low continuous suction.

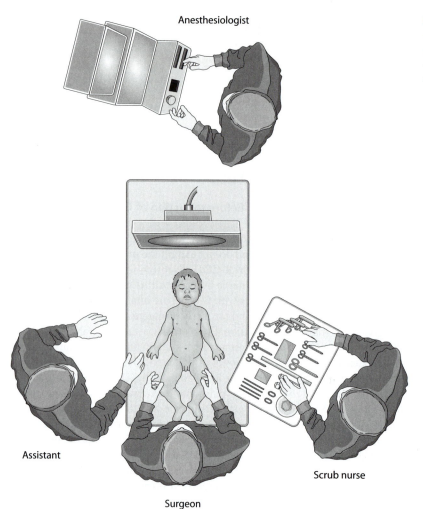

Anesthesiologist

Assistant

Surgeon

Scrub nurse

Fig. 75.1. Operating room setup. Reverse Trendelenburg positioning facilitates reduction of abdominal viscera out of the chest

Positioning

Patient

Babies are positioned supine at the foot of the table (Fig. 1). The legs are gently "frog-legged" and all extremities are carefully padded with synthetic sheepskin. A small bump may be placed beneath the abdomen if desired, but too large a bump may make closure of the diaphragm more difficult. An arterial line and two working venous lines are placed. Gentle reverse Trendelenburg position facilitates reduction of bowel out of the chest.

Crew, Monitors, and Equipment

The surgeon stands at the foot of the bed. An assistant holds the camera from the surgeon's left. Another assistant may hold a retracting instrument from the surgeon's right, standing to the left of the table. Two monitors are used. If tower-based, they should be positioned on either side of the patient's head. If located on flexible booms as part of an integrated suite, one monitor should be suspended directly above the patient's chest. Another monitor can be positioned as needed for the assistant holding the camera, typically just to the left of the patient's head (Fig. 75.1).

Special Equipment

No special energy applying systems are required. The use of Ligasure is optional. A collagen mesh should be at hand in case it is needed.

Technique

Cannulae

Cannula	Method of insertion	Diameter (mm)	Device	Position
1	Closed (Veress)	5	Camera	Umbilicus
2	Closed	5	Needle driver, scissors, cautery	Left lower quadrant
3	Closed	3	Curved dissector	Right lower quadrant
4	Closed	3	Retractor, atraumatic grasper	Right subcostal

Procedure

The following describes the method of repair of left-sided B-CDH, but the same technique is used for rare right-sided defects and for eventration. Trocar placements are shown in ■ Fig. 75.2. A 5 cm trocar is placed into the umbilicus after inflating the abdomen to 8–10 cmH$_2$0. Careful monitoring during pneumoperitoneum is essential, and the surgeon should be prepared to decrease the CO$_2$ pressure to as low as 5 cmH$_2$0 (or to convert to an open technique) if cardiovascular compromise is encountered. To date, conversion has not been needed at our institution.

Three other trocars are placed as shown. The left triangular hepatic ligament is divided sharply, and the left lobe of the liver is deflected caudally. (In cases where the left lobe is small or is already out of the way, taking down the ligament may make repair more difficult; the surgeon may elect to leave the liver in place.) For the entire case, the assistant provides exposure by maintaining gentle downward pressure on the liver and intestines. The surgeon uses non-crushing graspers to gently reduce the large and small intestine, carefully drawing the bowel all the way down to the pelvis as much as possible. Often, the spleen is in the chest as well, and this is reduced not by grabbing the spleen but by a combination of gentle blunt manipulation of the spleen and by folding the diaphragmatic rim under or over the spleen.

If there is a sac, it is excised using scissors with sparse use of electrocautery. As with open repair, complete excision of the entire sac is crucial for a lasting repair. The sac is drawn out through one of the 5 cm trocars.

The posterior rim of the diaphragm may be folded and hidden beneath loose areolar tissue. These attachments, and any adhesions to the splenic flexure of the colon, are divided sharply to fully reveal the posterior rim. Occasionally, some attachments still hold the left lobe of the liver over the medial portion of the diaphragm and these should also be divided with special care not to divide the phrenic vessels or to cut into the hepatic veins, any of which may be located more laterally than anticipated.

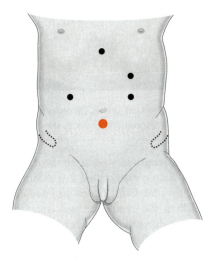

Fig. 75.2. Schematic of port placement: port sizes (mm) are indicated. Port placement is very similar to that for laparoscopic Nissen fundoplasty. The left upper quadrant port is optional, but is often helpful to retract the bowel during repair

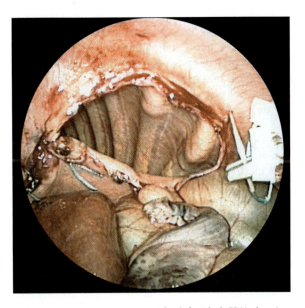

Fig. 75.3. Intraoperative view of a left-sided CDH showing the muscular rim remaining after the hernia sac has been sharply excised

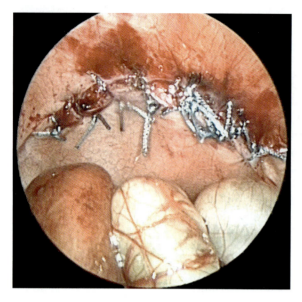

Fig. 75.4. Completed left-sided CDH repair: a series of simple interrupted 2-0 Ethibond sutures closes the defect

In most cases, primary repair of the defect is possible. Several simple interrupted 2-0 Ethibond sutures are placed from medial to lateral and tied extracorporeally. Cocking the needle far back greatly facilitates placement of sutures into the upper leaflet. Care should be used to take bites just deeply enough to provide solid closure without diminishing the amount of tissue available to cover the gap (Figs. 75.3, 75.4). Laterally, if there is no rim of diaphragmatic tissue, the anterior rim should be anchored to the ribs, avoiding the costal neurovascular bundle beneath each rib.

Occasionally, there is not enough native tissue to close the defect. In this case, as with open repair, a piece of mesh is used to bridge the gap. Although Goretex mesh has traditionally been used in open repair, and provides adequate closure, it has disadvantages, chief among these being its propensity to act more as a foreign body than as a biological scaffold. Consequently, we favor Surgisis (Cook, Bloomington, IN) mesh, a collagen-based mesh that promotes ingrowth by fibroblasts thereby allowing more "natural" healing.

A piece of mesh is cut to size extracorporeally, rolled tightly, and deployed into the abdomen by drawing it through a 5 cm port with a 3 cm instrument. It is then sutured in place using several interrupted 2-0 Ethibond sutures spaced approximately 5 mm apart. It is easier to work medial to lateral, beginning with the posterior leaflet.

For eventration, the diaphragm is plicated using several interrupted 2-0 Ethibond sutures, "closing" the slack portion of the diaphragm horizontally as with a diaphragmatic hernia. Avoid incorporating the phrenic vessels into the closure.

The left lobe of the liver should be placed directly against the repair. Directly positioning the liver prevents bowel from becoming caught above the liver, and may bolster the repair.

Chest tubes and abdominal drains are not used. Immediate postoperative chest X-ray will reveal a large pneumothorax until the CO_2 is reabsorbed and the hypotrophic lung can expand to fill the space. No attempt should be made to evacuate the pneumothorax unless the patient later develops evidence of a pulmonary air leak (usually as a consequence of ventilator-induced volutrauma/barotrauma).

The trocar sites are infiltrated with 0.25% bupivacaine and closed.

Postoperative Care

Patients invariably remain intubated immediately after repair and are weaned according to their individual physiology. Pain is controlled with ketorolac (0.5 mg/kg intravenously every 8 h for six doses) and small doses of morphine. Patients can be fed when postoperative ileus has resolved. Many patients will have gastroesophageal reflux and will require metoclopramide and an H-2 blocker for months, and a few will eventually require fundoplasty.

Results

No prospective trials have been reported, but in our series of 17 patients there were no conversions to open technique. All patients had satisfactory repair and unremarkable postoperative courses. Laparoscopic repair has not been attempted in every patient with CDH, as early attempts have been confined to the most stable patients. As experience is accumulated, we have slowly expanded the number of patients in whom MIS is attempted.

Discussion

Laparoscopic repair of CDH offers a number of advantages compared to open repair. Open repair is typically accomplished through a large subcostal incision that is obviated by MIS repair. Requirements for pain medicine are vastly diminished, possibly shortening intubation time and postoperative ileus. Cosmesis is improved. Finally, reoperation (for example, to treat gastroesophageal reflux) is facilitated by diminished postoperative adhesions invariably seen after MIS compared to open procedures.

The need for CO_2 pneumoperitoneum may present the major obstacle to accomplishing MIS repair of

CDH in patients with tenuous cardiopulmonary physiology. Still, low pressures allow adequate pneumoperitoneum for repair and minimize cardiopulmonary compromise. These considerations present no problem in eventration.

One group has advocated a thoracic approach to repair of CDH (Arca et al. 2003). This approach could have some advantages. For example, it is likely that insufflation of the chest presents some advantage to reducing the organs from the chest. But this advantage vanishes as soon as the viscera no longer totally occlude the diaphragmatic defect and CO_2 pressures equalize. It is also possible that lower insufflation pressures could be used during the repair since the ribcage does not need to be elevated like the abdominal wall. Still, if insufflation incompletely reduces the viscera, the thoracic approach offers no advantage during manual reduction of intestines or spleen, but does leave those organs relatively inaccessible in case of a problem (like an enterotomy). Finally, the thoracic approach may offer a disadvantage during placement of sutures since it is more difficult to hold bowel away from the needle and to visualize safe placement of sutures. This problem does not appear during the abdominal approach. Technical refinements to both approaches will allow pediatric surgeons to choose the approach that seems most precise and gives the soundest repair.

References

Arca MJ, Barnhart DC, Lelli JL, et al (2003) Early experience with minimally invasive repair of congenital diaphragmatic hernias: results and lessons learned. J Pediatr Surg 38:1563–1568

Harinath G, Senapati PS, Politt MJ, et al (2002) Laparoscopic reduction of an acute gastric volvulus and repair of a hernia of Bochdalek. Surg Laparosc Endosc Percutan Tech 12:180–183

Hendrickson RJ, Rothenberg SS, Partrick DA (2003) Laparoscopic repair of congenital diaphragmatic hernia. Pediatr Endosurg Innov Tech 7:97

Marin-Blazquez AA, Candel MF, Parra PA, et al (2003) Morgagni hernia: repair with a mesh using laparoscopic surgery. Hernia 8:70–72

Matthews BD, Bui H, Harold KL, et al (2003) Laparoscopic repair of traumatic diaphragmatic injuries. Surg Endosc 17:254–258

Settembre A, Cuccurullo D, Pisaniello D, et al (2003) Laparoscopic repair of congenital diaphragmatic hernia with prosthesis: a case report. Hernia 7:52–54

Willemse P, Schutte PR, Plaisier PW (2003) Thoracoscopic repair of a Bochdalek hernia in an adult. Surg Endosc 17:162

Abdominal Wall

Chapter 76

Laparoscopic Herniorrhaphy

Felix Schier

Introduction

The laparoscopic approach to inguinal hernia is more direct and more logical than the conventional open approach. The basic step of hernia repair in children is the ligation of the hernial sac's neck at the internal inguinal ring, a maneuver better performed laparoscopically than "open." At present the main hindrance to more rapid proliferation of the laparoscopic technique is missing expertise with laparoscopic techniques in general in small children, and the seemingly slightly increased recurrence rate with the laparoscopic technique.

Preoperative Preparation

Before Induction of General Anesthesia

The children are asked to empty their bladder before surgery.

After Induction of General Anesthesia

There are no anesthesiologic peculiarities in laparoscopy for inguinal hernia. The procedure is performed under general anesthesia with intubation. No nasogastric tube is needed. Routine urinary catheters are unnecessary. A distended bladder is seldom a mechanical problem to herniorrhaphy. In case the bladder is too distended during the operation, a needle is inserted under laparoscopic view through the anterior abdominal wall into the bladder and the bladder emptied. This will only be necessary in 1 out of 50 patients. It will not be necessary to empty the bladder completely.

Positioning of Patient, Crew, and Monitors

The patient is in regular supine position. The surgeon stands on the opposite side to the hernia; an assistant is opposite and holds the camera. In case of a bilateral hernia, surgeon and assistant change sides. The monitor is placed opposite the surgeon (Fig. 76.1).

Special Equipment

Energy applying systems are not required. Only two needle holders and one pair of scissors are required, preferably of 2 mm diameter. Three-millimeter diameters are more popular but leave bigger scars due to the significantly bigger 3 cm trocars (Fig. 76.2).

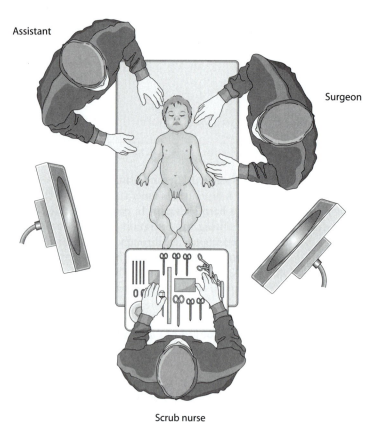

Fig. 76.1. Theater layout and trocar placement

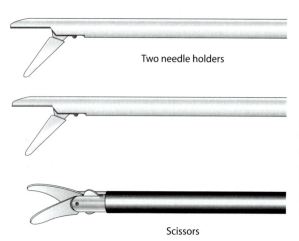

Two needle holders

Scissors

Fig. 76.2. Instruments

Technique

Cannulae

A small transverse semicircular incision is made in a skin fold at the lower margin of the umbilicus. A Veress needle is inserted, flushed with physiologic saline, and used for insufflation of CO_2. The Veress needle is re-

placed by a 5 cm trocar for the laparoscope by "blind" insertion at the umbilicus. For this trocar a transparent model is preferable, because its translucent cannula shaft allows it to be pulled back as far as possible until it almost falls out. This results in maximum distance and optimal overview.

Two 2 cm (or 3 cm) trocars are inserted at the lateral margin of the right and left rectus sheath, at about the level of the umbilicus. In small children the working trocars are inserted a bit more cranially, and in bigger infants a bit more caudally, with the intention not to arrive with the needle holders right on top of the internal inguinal ring but at some distance. This facilitates suturing.

Procedure

First, the type of hernia is identified (■ Fig. 76.3). In the laparoscopic approach, direct and femoral hernias (and combinations thereof) are found more frequently than in open surgery.

A regular suture as for open surgery is used to close the internal ring. Our preference is 4-0, absorbable or non-absorbable. The thread is shortened to approximately 8 cm (the commercially available length of 40 cm is too long to be handled inside the abdomen). The needle is inserted through the abdominal wall, and

Fig. 76.3 a – d. **a** Types of inguinal hernia. *1* Indirect hernia, *2* direct hernia, *3* femoral hernia, *1+2* "hernia en pantalon." **b** Direct hernia. **c** Femoral hernia

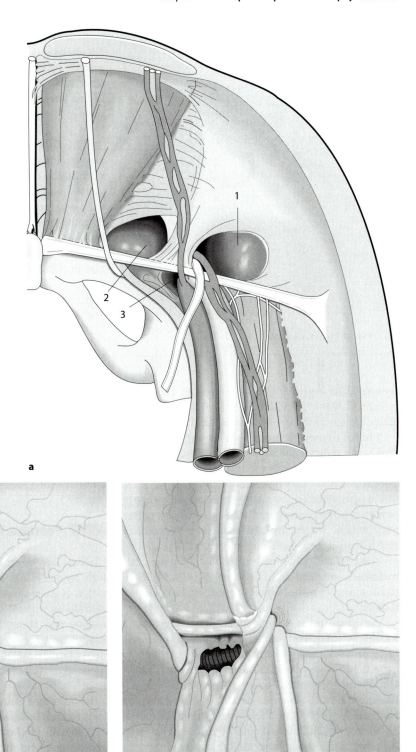

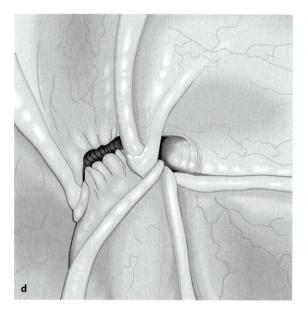

Fig. 76.3. d "Hernia en pantalon"

removed later together with a 2 cm trocar. The needle is inserted next to the internal inguinal ring in order to arrive directly at the site of suturing (■ Fig. 76.4).

If bowel or ovary is prolapsed it is first pulled back. This is not difficult since insufflation distends the abdominal cavity and pulls the internal ring open. It is astonishing how many bowel loops can prolapse. If the bowel was reduced manually prior to laparoscopy (which is not recommended with the prospect of imminent laparoscopy; manual reduction is far more rough than laparoscopic reduction, and it is a blind procedure), first the bowel is inspected for injury. Hematoma is not uncommon, but it will be seen that peristalsis moves over the hematomatous segment without difficulty.

The suture includes some underlying tissue, but not too much. There is no mechanical "repair" in children, in contrast to adult patients. Care should be taken to close the defect *medially*. All recurrences occur medially, never at the lateral aspect of the internal ring. If the suture is placed in an inverted "N"-shaped fashion, relatively loose peritoneal folds are created in order to harbor the vas and the testicular vessels (■ Fig. 76.5). Including some tissue from the other side of the epigastric vessels might serve as an extra precaution against recurrence.

In children of more than 10 years there is considerable mechanical tension on the suture. For closure of the knot it helps if the assistant applies manual pressure from outside onto the abdominal wall. Also, it is better to use two or three different sutures in these children.

Unexpected Opening on the Other Side

An opening is not equivalent to a clinical hernia. Hernias are treated surgically, not openings. Nevertheless, since it is unknown whether an opening becomes a hernia later, we treat openings like a hernia and close them.

Direct Hernia

Simple closure of the peritoneum (as in indirect hernia) might result in recurrence. The peritoneum is opened with scissors. This is easy as a small incision enlarges almost spontaneously due to the intra-abdominal pressure. The muscle and fascia margins are exposed and sutured with several sutures. Still there is a recurrence risk, and laparoscopic repair of direct hernias in children is still not perfect.

Femoral Hernia

The above applies also for femoral hernias.

Closure

After desufflation, local anesthesia with bupivacaine is applied to all trocar insertion sites. At the 5 cm trocar insertion site (at the umbilicus for the laparoscope) the fascia is closed with 4-0 braided slow-absorbable sutures and the skin is closed with interrupted absorbable sutures. Two-millimeter trocar sites are simply covered with a bandage.

Postoperative Care

Children are allowed regular food as soon as they are fully awake. In our practice, postoperative pain medication is given on request, not routinely. Fifty percent of children will not need any postoperative pain medication, and about 50% will require a paracetamol suppository. However, there is a small fraction of children who are agitated and difficult to calm down. In those cases we use an intravenous cocktail of promethazine (pethidine = 50 mg, 1/2 ampoule promethazine = 25 mg, 1 ampoule dihydroergotoxine = 0.3 mg; all three ampoules are filled into a syringe up to a total of 5 cc with physiologic saline; of this solution 0.1 cc per kilogram bodyweight is given intravenously; it is equivalent to 1 mg pethidine per kilogram bodyweight). This results in a smooth postoperative course for parents, child, and nurses.

Parents are encouraged to leave the hospital during the afternoon of surgery. However, due to our healthcare insurance system which pays non-distinctively also for an overnight stay, approximately 50% of the children stay overnight, including the mother. From a purely medical point of view, practically all children

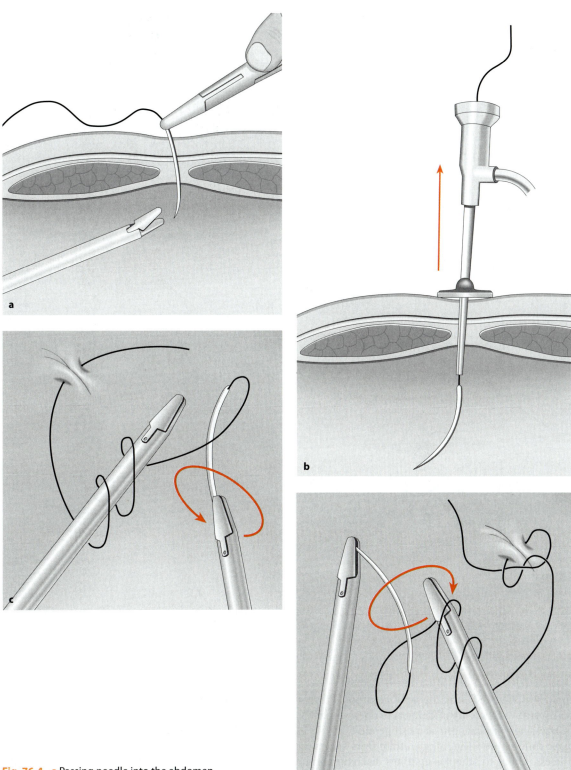

Fig. 76.4. a Passing needle into the abdomen.
b Removal of needle together with trocar. **c,d** Knot tying

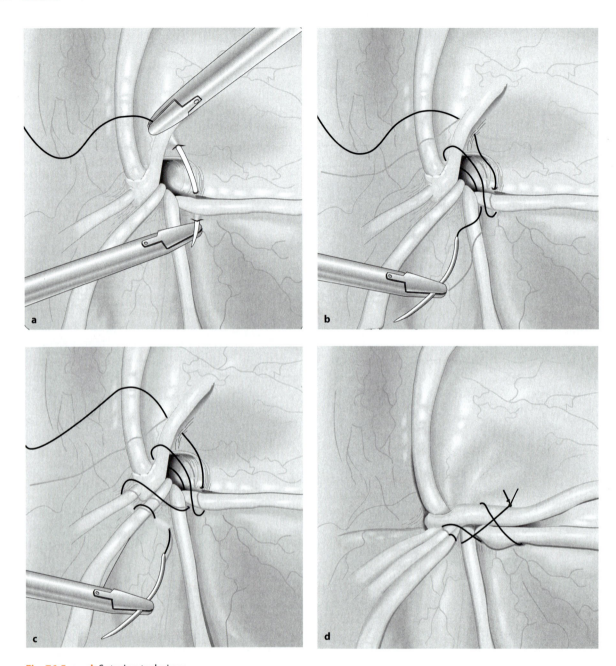

Fig. 76.5. a – d Suturing technique

could be discharged home the same afternoon. Further postoperative follow-up is identical to open surgery.

Dressings are changed at postoperative day 4. In older children we suggest they refrain from sports for 2 weeks. Going to school is up to the discretion of the family.

Results

Personal Results

Inguinal hernias have been repaired laparoscopically in 366 children: 65% were boys, the median age was 1.6 years (range 4 days to 14 years), and 505 sides were repaired. There was one conversion because of a massively dilated bowel. There were 18 (4.9%) recurrences. Postoperative hydrocele occurred in 5 (1.4%) children, 4 boys and 1 girl. There were 11 (3%) direct hernias, mostly in boys and mostly on the right side: 3 of the direct hernias were recurrences of the open technique, 1 child had 3 previous open herniotomies, and in 2 children the direct hernia was in combination with an indirect hernia ("hernia en pantaloon"). There were 5 (1.4%) femoral hernias: 3 were recurrences of open herniotomy, 2 had 3 previous open procedures, and in 1 child the femoral hernia was combined with an indirect hernia. Testicular atrophy was found in 1 (0.3%) child.

Literature Results

The largest series so far summarizes the experiences of three centers from France, Germany, and Italy. It includes 666 patients. The recurrence rate was from 2.9% to 3.5%. Hydroceles occurred in 0–1%, and direct hernias in 1.2–4% of patients. In these procedures, 2- or 3 cm instruments were used. In about half of the patients, the peritoneum was incised laterally to the internal ring. There was no difference in the recurrence rate compared to the children without peritoneal incision. The internal ring was simply closed with absorbable or non-absorbable sutures (Schier et al. 2002). In a Chinese series of 450 children, needle and thread were inserted through the abdominal wall, manipulated inside in order to carry out a partial purse-string suture, and exteriorized again. The recurrence rate was 0.9% (Lee and Liang 2002). In a study of 150 patients, operated on by the above-described technique using 2 cm instruments, there were, 1 year postoperatively, no (0%) recurrences and no complications (Shalaby and Desoky 2002). In a further study including 45 boys, operated on with 3 cm instruments, the hemicircumference of the hernia neck was incised in order to approximate the conjoined tendon with the crural arch with a non-absorbable 4-0 suture. A 3-0 absorbable purse-string suture closed the hernial sac. This resulted in a 4.4% recurrence rate (Montupet and Esposito 1999). The same technique was used in a group of 10 recurrent hernias and 3 direct hernias, all in boys, with a 0% recurrence rate (Esposito and Montupet 1998). Similarly, in a group of 6 direct hernias in boys with cryptorchidism a 0% recurrence rate was noted (Radmayr et al. 1999). There is also a group of 3 femoral hernias (a fourth patient was 17 years old), all being recurrences of open surgery. The trocars were arranged umbilical, suprapubic, and one in between, and 4 cm instruments were used. One defect was repaired by re-approximating the iliopubic tract to Cooper's ligament and overlaying a preperitoneal Teflon felt patch. The other defects were repaired using a Teflon felt plug and preperitoneal patch. All the patients also had contralateral hernias. In 2 children, the contralateral hernia was also femoral (1 was operated on in the open technique, and the other laparoscopically), and in 1 child the contralateral hernia was direct; this hernia was operated on in the open technique. There were no (0%) recurrences (Lee and DuBois 2000).

Discussion

The technique would gain wide acceptance if there was not the technical prerequisite of expertise with routine laparoscopy in small children. The technique is easy in principle and appears more logical than the open approach, which follows historical pathways. The low incidence of postoperative hydrocele is astonishing. Obviously the hernial sac can be occluded and left in situ, without resection.

Of greater concern is the recurrence rate. Open herniotomy claims a recurrence rate of 1–5%. Laparoscopic hernia repair seems to have a slightly higher recurrence rate. Initially the recurrence rate was found to be an optimistic 0% (Schier 1998). The virtual absence of recurrences is still found in the literature, not only in relatively small series (Esposito and Montupet 1998; Lee and DuBois 2000; Radmayr et al. 1999) but also in larger series (Lee and Liang 2002; Schier 1998; Shalaby and Desoky 2002). Only exceptionally, more realistic recurrence rates of more than 4% are given (Montupet and Esposito 1999). In our personal experience the recurrence rate has risen over the course of time from 0% (Schier 1998) to 0.7% (Schier 2000b) to 3.5% (Schier et al. 2002) and to almost 5% today. A sharp, and inexplicable, contrast is the recurrence rate of 0.88% in a Chinese series of 450 children (Lee and Liang 2002).

In laparoscopy, the surgeon will profit from a knowledge of how direct and femoral hernias look (Schier 2000a). They will be encountered more frequently than in open surgery, especially in recurrent cases of open surgery. Several of the children in our series were repeatedly operated on in the open technique, up to three times, each time missing either a direct or a femoral hernia. In direct and femoral hernias, the principle of simple closure of the neck of the hernia sac, as in indirect hernias, had an almost 50% recurrence rate in our series. Anatomical dissection of all structures involved and careful closure may yield better results. We would hesitate to use Teflon or other prosthetic materials in children (Lee and DuBois 2000). There is, however, insufficient accumulated knowledge about direct and femoral hernias. No individual worldwide has seen more than six such cases.

Laparoscopic hernia repair in children is certainly underrepresented in the literature. The procedure is performed by numerous non-academic institutions, and not infrequently also by non-pediatric surgeons. Its main advantages are the clear diagnostic picture, the easy exploration of the contralateral side, and the markedly reduced risk of recurrent hernia, no matter whether the previous procedure was performed in the open or the laparoscopic technique.

References

Esposito C, Montupet P (1998) Laparoscopic treatment of recurrent inguinal hernia in children. Pediatr Surg Int 14:182–184

Lee SL, DuBois JJ (2000) Laparoscopic diagnosis and repair of pediatric femoral hernia. Initial experience of four cases. Surg Endosc 14:1110–1113

Lee Y, Liang J (2002) Experience with 450 cases of micro-laparoscopic herniotomy in infants and children. Pediatr Endosurg Innov Tech 6:25–28

Montupet P, Esposito C (1999) Laparoscopic treatment of congenital inguinal hernia in children. J Pediatr Surg 34:420–423

Radmayr C, Corvin S, Studen M, Bartsch G, Janetschek G (1999) Cryptorchidism, open processus vaginalis, and associated hernia: laparoscopic approach to the internal inguinal ring. Eur Urol 36:631–634

Schier F (1998) Laparoscopic herniorrhaphy in girls. J Pediatr Surg 33:1495–1497

Schier F (2000a) Direct inguinal hernias in children: laparoscopic aspects. Pediatr Surg 16:562–564

Schier F (2000b) Laparoscopic surgery of inguinal hernias in children: initial experience. J Pediatr Surg 35:1331–1335

Schier F, Montupet P, Esposito C (2002) Laparoscopic inguinal herniorrhaphy in children: a three-center experience with 933 repairs. J Pediatr Surg 37:395–397

Shalaby R, Desoky A (2002) Needlescopic inguinal hernia repair in children. Pediatr Surg Int 18:153–156

Chapter 77

Laparoscopic Inguinal Hernia Repair

Tamir H. Keshen

Introduction

Laparoscopy has been utilized for the diagnosis and/or treatment of pediatric inguinal hernias since the 1990s. Initially described as a technique to identify the presence or absence of contralateral hernias in children (Holcomb et al. 1994; Lobe and Schropp 1992; Owings and Georgeson 2000) it has reduced the number of unnecessary contralateral inguinal explorations and the associated morbidity and complications. With the advent of innovative laparoscopic techniques and their constant evolution, pediatric inguinal hernias presently can be repaired in a safe, expeditious manner with excellent visualization, minimal tissue manipulation, and superior cosmesis. This chapter will describe, in detail, our technique of laparoscopic inguinal hernia repair and discuss several other techniques that have been developed since 1995.

Preoperative Preparation

Before Induction of General Anesthesia

Non per os prior to the operation is based on the requirements of the anesthesiologist. There is no need for a bowel preparation. A prophylactic antibiotic, such as a first-generation cephalosporin, is recommended. Routine monitoring including capnography and pulse oximetry is indicated.

After Induction of General Anesthesia

An orogastric tube is placed to decompress the stomach for the duration of the procedure. The bladder is drained via a Credé maneuver, or a Foley catheter (after preparation) for an older child. Access sites are infiltrated with bupivacaine and epinephrine for postoperative pain control and intraoperative hemostasis, respectively. There is no need for epidural or spinal anesthesia.

Positioning

Patient

The patient is placed is a supine position with the feet at the end of the bed. The legs are secured to the bed to allow for Trendelenburg positioning (■ Fig. 77.1).

Crew, Monitors, and Equipment

The surgeon is positioned on the contralateral side of the hernia, and the assistant on the ipsilateral side. The monitor is at the foot of the bed on the ipsilateral side of the hernia (■ Fig. 77.1). The surgeon and assistant will switch positions during a bilateral hernia repair.

Special Equipment

No special energy applying systems are required. Other equipment includes:
- 3-0 polydioxanone (PDS) monofilament suture with taper needle
- 30° 1.7- or 3 cm laparoscope
- Sewing needle

Technique

Cannulae

Cannula	Method of insertion	Diameter (mm)	Device	Position
1	Open	3 or 4	Laparoscope	Umbilicus
2	Closed	2 or 3	Grasper without port	Contralateral lower quadrant

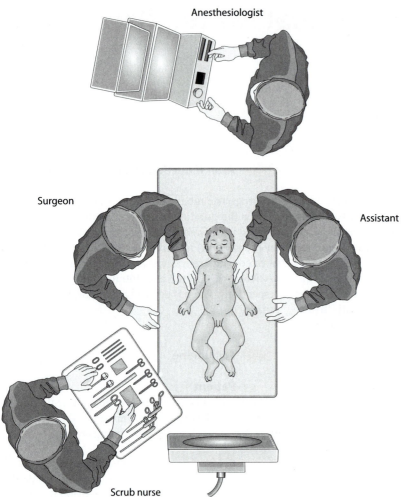

Anesthesiologist

Fig. 77.1. Positions of patient, crew, and monitors.

Surgeon

Assistant

Scrub nurse

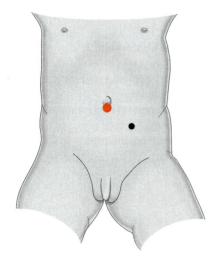

Fig. 77.2. Port positions

Figure 77.2 shows the positions of the access sites. The 3- or 4 cm umbilical trocar is used for insufflation and for the 30° 1.7- or 3 cm laparoscope. The 2- or 3 cm access site in the lower quadrant is made by a stab incision on the contralateral side, and is for the atraumatic grasper to position the peritoneum onto the needle, and to thread the suture through the eye of the sewing needle.

Procedure

The 3- or 4 cm umbilical trocar is placed via an open technique and the abdomen is insufflated to a pressure of 10 mmHg. The patient is placed in a mild to moderate Trendelenburg position to retract the viscera from the internal ring. Sometimes, the trocar needs to be anchored to the umbilical cicatrix with a suture to help prevent it from slipping out. The 30° laparoscope is advanced into the abdominal cavity (giving the surgeon a

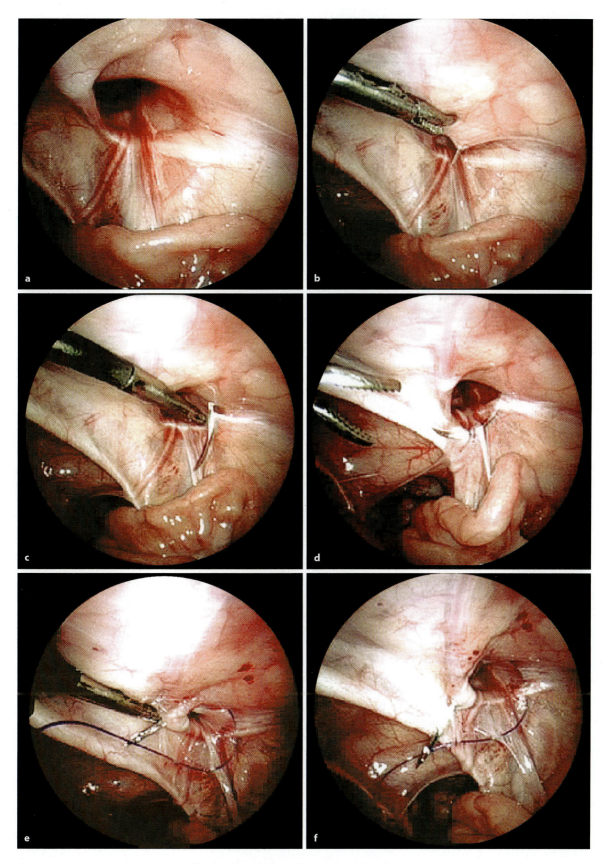

Fig. 77.3 a – f. a Intraoperative view of internal inguinal ring. **b** Insertion of needle at lateral aspect of internal ring. **c,d** Placement of purse-string suture. **e** Introduction of sewing needle. **f** Suture threaded onto sewing needle.

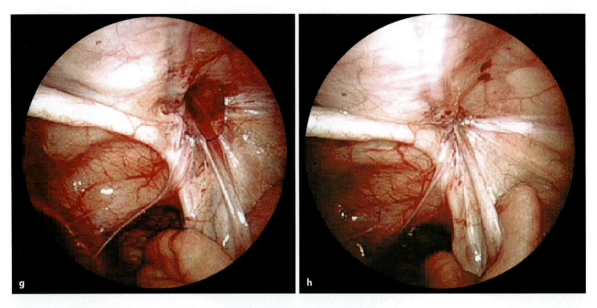

Fig. 77.3. g,h Tying the suture obliterates the defect in the internal ring

variety of angled views of the internal ring) and the internal ring is visualized (■ Fig. 77.3a). Ensure that no intra-abdominal contents are within the inguinal canal (applying pressure externally will reduce any contents). A small needle (25 or 28 gauge) is placed through the skin at the hernia site and through the superior aspect of the internal ring. This confirms where the 1 cm, transverse incision is made. The monofilament needle is grasped at the apex of the curvature. The needle is advanced through the incision and through the transversalis fascia and peritoneum at the lateral aspect of the internal ring (■ Fig. 77.3b). The needle continues its rotation medially. The peritoneum lateral to the testicular vessels is grasped by the 2- or 3 cm instrument and placed over the needle (■ Fig. 77.3c,d), followed by the peritoneum between the testicular vessels and vas deferens, and the peritoneum medial to the vas deferens. One must take great care to avoid grasping the vessels or vas when applying the peritoneum to the needle tip. Have the needle tip readily available at the site where the peritoneum will be applied, rather than grasping the peritoneum first and moving the needle toward it. The peritoneum is quite fragile, and minimal manipulation will decrease the chances of tearing it. Make every attempt, also, to minimize torque on the needle. This too will reduce the tearing of the peritoneum.

Once the peritoneum is grasped medial to the vas deferens, the needle is pushed through the abdominal wall and the suture is separated from the needle. Using the 2- or 3 cm grasper, the suture is pulled back into the abdominal cavity. Next the sewing needle is ad-

vance through the abdominal wall (at the 1 cm skin incision) and the peritoneum on the medial aspect of the internal ring (■ Fig. 77.3e). The suture is threaded through the eye of the needle with the 2- or 3 cm grasper and pulled out of the abdomen (■ Fig. 77.3f). The suture is tied with tension on the peritoneum, while visualizing the tissue with the scope, to obliterate the internal ring defect; thus, creating a high ligation of the hernia sac (■ Fig. 77.3g,h).

The 2- or 3 cm grasper is removed under direct vision (to obviate omental herniation through the stab incision). The abdomen is desufflated while withdrawing the scope and trocar. The umbilical cicatrix is approximated with a buried, absorbable suture and the skin is also closed with absorbable suture. The stab incisions are closed with Steri-Strips.

If the peritoneum is torn during the procedure, a second purse-string suture can be applied in the same manner as described above.

Postoperative Care

The orogastric tube is removed prior to extubation. The Foley catheter, if placed, is also removed prior to anesthesia reversal. Narcotics are usually unnecessary for postoperative pain control. Acetaminophen, administered in scheduled dosing for the initial 48 h postoperatively should be adequate, but can be followed by further dosing if necessary. The patient may return to normal activity at any time.

Results

We reviewed the results of 40 patients (from July 2001 to August 2003) who have undergone hernial repair by this technique. The ages ranged from 10 daysto 14 years. All cases were performed in a teaching setting and the mean operative time was 15 min. There were no recurrences or hydroceles over a 5- to 30-month follow-up. One complication of bowel obstruction occurred secondary to bowel wall incorporation in the umbilical closure. There were no injuries to the vas deferens or testicular vessels, and no evidence of testicular atrophy or high-riding testes. All patients returned to normal activity directly after the repair. Several similar techniques of laparoscopic high ligation of the sac have been described with excellent results (Lee and Liang 2002; Prasad et al. 2003; Schier et al. 2002). None of them require the removal of the hernia sac itself, with minimal to no recurrences or presence of postoperative hydroceles.

Discussion

The laparoscopic method of inguinal hernia repair has been shown in several series to be safe and simple while affording minimal complications. It provides excellent visualization of the cord and inguinal canal structures. It follows the same principles of the open technique with minimal dissection of the involved structures. There is no manipulation of the vessels or vas deferens, thus, reducing the chances for testicular injury to nil. The scope can identify a contralateral hernia in the same setting allowing for repair at the same time and conversely identifying the absence of a contralateral hernia, obviating an unnecessary contralateral exploration. The procedure also affords excellent cosmesis.

Thus far, there has been no contraindication to leaving the hernia sac in situ. Four postoperative hydroceles were reported in one of several series (Schier et al. 2002). It has been postulated that the closure of the peritoneal defect creates an ischemic response that obliterates the defect completely (Prasad et al. 2003). Regardless of the histologic response, recurrences are minimal to nil.

As described in the procedure section, care must be taken to minimize the tension on the peritoneum to prevent tearing. It is also important to incorporate the transversalis fascia laterally and conjoined tendon medially in the defect closure.

If a contralateral hernia is present, the position of the atraumatic grasper should not hinder the repair. However, it may be a little more difficult, ergonomically, when threading the suture through the eye of the sewing needle.

References

Holcomb GW, Stock JW, Morgan WM (1994) Laparoscopic evaluation for a contralateral patent processus vaginalis. J Pediatr Surg 29:970–974

Lee Y, Liang J (2002) Experience with 450 cases of micro-laparoscopic herniotomy in infants and children. Pediatr Endosurg Innov Techn 6:25–28

Lobe TE, Schropp KP (1992) Inguinal hernias in pediatrics: initial experience with laparoscopic inguinal exploration of the asymptomatic contralateral side. J Laparoendosc Surg 2:135–140

Owings EP, Georgeson KE (2000) A new technique for laparoscopic exploration to find contralateral patent processus vaginalis. Surg Endosc 14:114–116

Prasad R, Lovvorn HN III, Wadie GM, et al (2003) Early experience with needlescopic inguinal herniorrhaphy in children. J Pediatr Surg 38:1055–1058

Schier F, Montupet P, Esposito C (2002) Laparoscopic inguinal herniorrhaphy in children: a three-center experience with 933 repairs. J Pediatr Surg 37:395–397

Chapter 78

Inguinal Herniotomy: Laparoscopic-assisted Extraperitoneal Technique

C.K. Yeung and K.H. Lee

Introduction

Inguinal hernia is one of the most common surgical conditions in infants and children. Over the past few decades, inguinal exploration with clear dissection of the hernial sac off the vas deferens and spermatic vessels, and secure high ligation of the patent processus vaginalis (PPV), i.e. inguinal herniotomy, has remained the standard treatment. The procedure has stood the test of time with very low recurrence rates in experienced hands. However, there are continuing controversies regarding the management strategy for a possible contralateral patent processus vaginalis that may develop into a subsequent hernia. Routine exploration of the contralateral side, as has been adopted by some workers, may result in a significant proportion of unnecessary inguinal explorations, along with the potential complications (Wiener et al. 1996). Recently, it has become increasingly popular to examine the contralateral side laparoscopically through the open hernial sac and perform contralateral inguinal herniotomy should a patent processus vaginalis be present (Geisler et al. 2001; Holcomb et al. 1996; Miltenburg et al. 1998; Wulkan et al. 1996). However, at times the hernial sac may be too small or thin to allow passage of a laparoscope. A prominent peritoneal fold at the medial side of the contralateral deep ring may also significantly obscure the view of the laparoscope passed through the ipsilateral hernial sac. Transumbilical laparoscopy without doubt provides a better way to assess the status of the deep ring. We describe a new technique of endoscopic repair of inguinal hernia in children under the guidance of transumbilical laparoscopy. The technique is easy to learn and does not require expensive laparoscopic instruments.

Preoperative Preparation

Before Induction of General Anaesthesia

The procedure is planned as a day surgery case and no overnight hospital stay is required. No special preoperative measures are required for laparoscopic herniotomy in children. Blood taking is not indicated. Parents and patients need to be counselled that the contralateral side would only be operated on if a PPV is present on laparoscopy. As this is a relatively new procedure, the pros and cons of this technique versus conventional open herniotomy, and the possibility of conversion to open surgery will also be explained. Patients are advised to void before going to the operating theatre to avoid a full bladder during the procedure.

After Induction of General Anaesthesia

After induction of general anaesthesia the bladder is emptied by a Credé manoeuvre. No indwelling bladder catheter is required under normal circumstances. No preoperative antibiotic is necessary. Inguinal nerve blocks are not administered routinely.

Positioning

Patient

The patient should lie supine on the operating table (Fig. 78.1). The legs should be slightly separated and the perineum prepared to allow access for insertion of a urinary catheter just in case the bladder is not sufficiently emptied on laparoscopy. The scrotum in boys should also be prepared so that the assistant can apply manual pressure to expel the gas out of the scrotal sac during ligation of the PPV. The operating table can remain flat for the whole procedure if the deep ring is not obscured by the bowel. Head-down position or rotating the table can allow the bowel to fall way from the operating site if necessary.

Crew, Monitors, and Equipment

The surgeon and the assistant stand on the side opposite to the inguinal hernia while the monitor is placed on the opposite side of the table, at the same side as the hernia (Fig. 78.1).

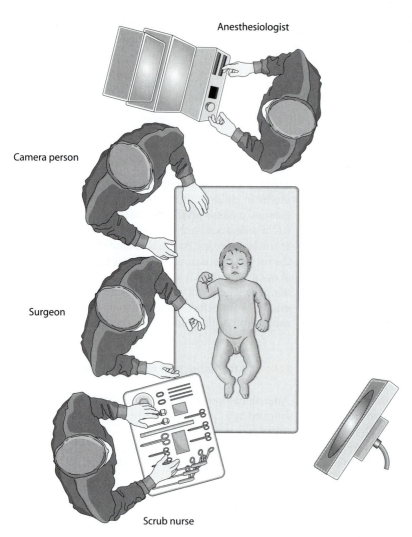

Anesthesiologist

Camera person

Surgeon

Scrub nurse

Fig. 78.1. Positioning of the patient, crew and equipment

Special Equipment

The following equipment is required:

Telescope, 3- or 5 mm	1
3 mm grasper	1
Herniotomy hook[a]	1
Beaver blade with handle	1

[a]The herniotomy hook needle takes the shape of an aneurysm needle but has a tapered and flattened tip that is specially designed to allow it to slide just beneath the peritoneal layer at the internal inguinal orifice, separating it from its surrounding structures including the vas deferens and the spermatic vessels (■ Fig. 78.2). Just behind the tip of the hook needle is an eye to carry a non-absorbable suture for ligation of the hernial sac (■ Fig. 78.3).

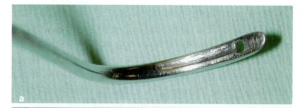

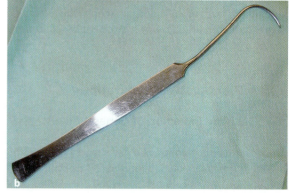

Fig. 78.2 a,b. Herniotomy hook with an "eye" at its tip

Fig. 78.3. A 2-0 suture passing through the "eye" of the hook to form a loop

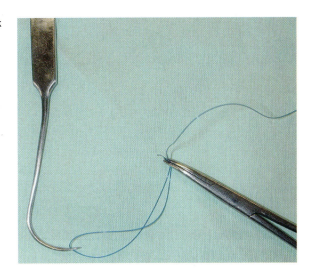

Technique

Cannulae

Cannulae	Method of insertion	Diameter (mm)	Device	Position
1	Open or closed	3 or 5	Telescope	Infraumbilical

Procedure

The operation starts with a small infraumbilical incision followed by insertion of a 3- or 5 mm cannula. Pneumoperitoneum is developed with CO_2 insufflation; a pressure of 8–10 mmHg is usually adequate.

After inspection of the peritoneal cavity and confirmation of the presence of a PPV on either side (■ Fig. 78.4), a 2- to 3 mm stab incision is made at a point that is midway between the umbilicus and the pubic tubercle, using a sharp Beaver or number 11 blade. The peritoneum should be breached under laparoscopic guidance. A 2- to 3 mm laparoscopic grasper is passed through the stab incision under laparoscopic guidance. As there is no cannula, the grasper should go through exactly the same tract made by the Beaver blade. This grasper provides important countertraction of the peritoneum during dissection of the hernial sac off the vas deferens and spermatic vessels.

The herniotomy hook is prepared by threading a doubled 3-0 polydioxanone suture through the "eye" at its tip to form a loop. A small 2 mm stab incision is made at the 12 o'clock position over the internal inguinal orifice using the sharp blade, so that the tip of the blade is just visible outside, but not penetrating through the peritoneum. The herniotomy hook carrying the suture is then passed through the stab incision until its tip can be seen stretching on the peritoneum at the level of the internal ring, but not piercing through. The hook is manipulated to dissect the peritoneum off its surrounding structures at an extraperitoneal plane, with the grasper providing countertraction from inside, circumferentially around the internal orifice (■ Fig. 78.5).

The dissection starts from anterior to posterior, and usually from lateral to medial for a right-sided hernia, and vice versa on the left side, taking particular care to avoid damage while lifting off the peritoneal layer from the vas deferens and testicular vessels in boys. After the hook has passed over the vas deferens and the spermatic vessels, its tip is rotated toward the peritoneal cavity to pierce through the peritoneum and it is brought into the abdominal cavity. Using the grasper, the double suture loop is taken out from the hook needle and brought into the abdominal cavity (■ Fig. 78.6). The hook needle now without the suture is withdrawn back along its original path in the juxta-extraperitoneal plane to the 12 o'clock position at the anterior wall of the hernial orifice, and passed round the other half of the circumference of the internal orifice just beneath the peritoneum, until the point where the suture exits into the peritoneal cavity is encountered (■ Fig. 78.7). Once circumferential dissection is completed, the tip

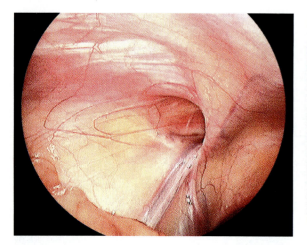

Fig. 78.4. Patent left deep ring in a case of left inguinal hernia

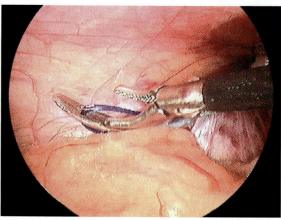

Fig. 78.6. The herniotomy hook breaches the peritoneum just lateral to the testicular vessels. The 2-0 suture loop is released with the help of the grasper

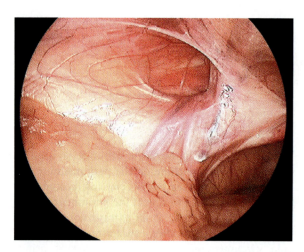

Fig. 78.5. The herniotomy hook carrying the 2-0 suture dissects around the medial hemicircumference of the left deep ring. Care must be taken to avoid catching the vas deferens and the testicular vessels

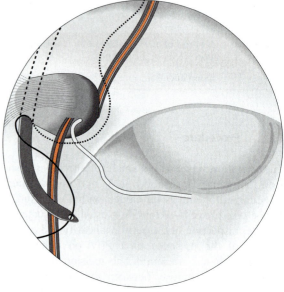

Fig. 78.7. The herniotomy hook dissects the lateral hemicircumference of the deep ring and breaches the peritoneum through the initial perforation while the 2-0 suture is surrounding the medial hemicircumference

of the herniotomy hook is manipulated through the opening through which the suture loop exits into the peritoneal cavity. Using the grasper, the end of the suture is manipulated and threaded through the eye of the herniotomy hook, and the suture is withdrawn and extracted through the initial stab incision, having finished a complete 360 extraperitoneal dissection around the circumference of the internal orifice (■ Fig. 78.8). The double suture loop now completely encircles the neck of the hernial sac, having spared the vas deferens and spermatic vessels. The sutures are tied securely after stopping the CO_2 insufflation and squeezing the air and fluid out of the sac by applying firm pressure over

the inguinal canal (■ Fig. 78.9). As the suture goes in and out through the same track, it encloses only the peritoneal layer without other intervening tissues. With gentle lifting of the abdominal wall, the cut ends of the suture becomes buried in the subcutaneous tissues. The umbilical wound is closed with fine absorbable sutures, while the two stab incisions are simply apposed with adhesive strips after infiltration of local anaesthetics at the wounds.

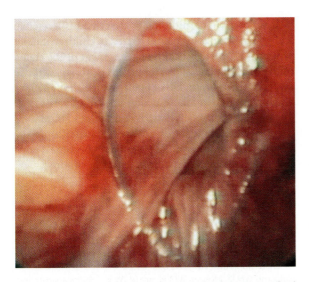

Fig. 78.8. The deep ring becomes completely circumscribed by the suture when the herniotomy hook carrying the suture is removed

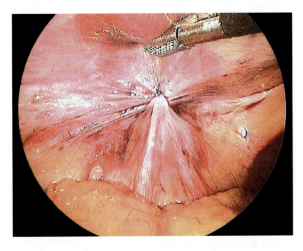

Fig. 78.9. The deep ring is closed by tying the suture

Postoperative Care

Patients can resume normal diet once they become fully awake and are usually discharged the same day with oral analgesics on an as required basis. Patients are asked to come back in a week for wound examination.

Results

We have performed laparoscopic herniotomy using this technique in 301 children (244 boys, 57 girls), with a mean age of 4.8 years (range: 1 month to 15 years). Laparoscopic inguinal herniotomy was successfully performed in 298 patients. Conversion to open surgery was required in 3 patients: a small infant with a very thin sac, an obese boy as a result of bleeding, and in another patient due to insufflation machine failure. The mean operating time in boys was 22.3 min (range: 17–46 min) for unilateral and 30.5 min (range: 25–55 min) for bilateral herniotomy while in girls was 20.5 min (12–34 min) and 27.6 min (25–39 min), respectively. All but one neonate were discharged on the same day of surgery. At 1 week follow-up, all patients remained well except in one with mild umbilical wound sepsis that responded to conservative treatment. At a mean follow-up of 21.3 months, recurrence was discovered in 2 patients (0.67%). A 15-year-old boy was found to have recurrence at 3 months after surgery when he experienced acute pain over the groin after trauma. Recurrence was also found in an infant 7 months after the laparoscopic herniotomy for huge hernia at early infancy. Open repair was performed in the 15-year-old boy while the recurrent hernia of the infant was repaired laparoscopically. There was no inguinal hernia observed in those who were found to have obliterated deep ring on laparoscopy. Good cosmetic results were universally observed.

Discussion

Transumbilical laparoscopy allows direct examination of the deep ring region and this together with the use of the grasper allows an accurate diagnosis of contralateral PPV. Transinguinal laparoscopic examination through an open sac has been widely described to evaluate for the presence of contralateral PPV. However, this method may not be feasible in those with very small or thin sacs (Geisler et al. 2001; Wulkan et al. 1996). In some cases, the overlying peritoneal fold may obscure the deep inguinal ring making transinguinal laparoscopic examination unreliable. This may lead to either false-positive or false-negative results (Liu et al. 1995). Although it is arguable that contralateral PPV might not develop into future hernia and the overall incidence of developing contralateral hernia is about 10–15% (Miltenburg et al. 1997), the closure of the PPV will definitely eliminate the risk of this and its potential complications.

Our method of using the herniotomy hook to dissect around the sac and its closure just follows the same principle as traditional open repair except avoiding the rather extensive mobilisation and its potential risk to the vas, vessels, and testes (Janik and Shandling 1982; Surana and Puri 1993). The complete and secure closure of the deep ring produced a low recurrence rate comparable to open series. Other methods of laparoscopic hernia repair have been described in children with similarly good results (Montupet and Esposito 1999; Schier 2000; Schier et al. 2002; Shalaby and

Desoky 2002). However, laparoscopic suturing is always required. The methods are technically more demanding and sometimes the tissue may be too friable to allow secure closure by suturing. The herniotomy hook is easy to use and the learning curve is usually short for those who have attained basic laparoscopic skills. But there are still several technical points worth noting:

1. The passage of the herniotomy hook through the stab incision should go perpendicularly to the skin in order to follow the right tract created by the Beaver blade.
2. The plane of dissection should be just outside the peritoneum of the deep ring where the tip of the hook should stay. Dissection should go smoothly around the circumference of the peritoneum without catching any muscle or perforating the peritoneum.
3. Countertraction with the grasper is important to spread the peritoneum which may be folded up and to facilitate lifting the peritoneum off the testicular vessels and vas.
4. Carbon dioxide insufflation should be stopped and gas accumulating into the hernia sac should be squeezed out before closure of the ring to avoid the occurrence of "pneumocele" in the distal sac.

Although there are no major complications in our series, potential risks associated with the procedure do exist. As we do not use any cannula for the 3 mm grasper, inadvertent injury to bowel may occur during its insertion through the abdominal wall. Extra care must be taken in young infants in whom the abdominal walls are usually more stretchable making the passage of the grasper more difficult. Hitting a prominent vessel is also possible when the grasper is having difficulty in getting through a stretchable peritoneum. Dissection around the deep ring should at all times stay outside the peritoneum. Damage to testicular vessels or vas can easily occur when the plane of dissection is not correct. A slight tear at some of the testicular vessels will inevitably lead to a haematoma and may preclude further safe dissection. Under those circumstances, conversion to open should be seriously considered to avoid putting the testis at risk.

Laparoscopic herniotomy as described is a reliable and safe method for repair of hernia in children if done properly. It provides accurate assessment of the status of the contralateral side. In our series, the recurrence rate is comparable to that of open repair although more data on long-term follow-up are needed to verify this. The procedure is relatively simple and does not require expensive instruments or advanced laparoscopic suturing skills. This has great potential to become a popular alternative to open hernia repair in children.

References

Geisler DP, Jegathesan S, Parmley MC, et al (2001) Laparoscopic exploration for the clinically undetected hernia in infancy and childhood. Am J Surg 182:693–696

Holcomb GW III, Morgan WM III, Brock JW III (1996) Laparoscopic evaluation for contralateral patent processus vaginalis: part II. J Pediatr Surg 31:1170–1173

Janik JS, Shandling B (1982) The vulnerability of the vas deferens (II): the case against routine bilateral inguinal exploration. J Pediatr Surg 17:585–588

Liu C, Chin T, Jan SE, et al (1995) Intraoperative laparoscopic diagnosis of contralateral patent processus vaginalis in children with unilateral inguinal hernia. Br J Surg 82:106–108

Miltenburg DM, Nuchtern JG, Jaksic T, et al (1997) Meta-analysis of the risk of metachronous hernia in infants and children. Am J Surg 174:741–744

Miltenburg DM, Nuchtern JG, Jaksic T, et al (1998) Laparoscopic evaluation of the pediatric inguinal hernia: a meta-analysis. J Pediatr Surg 33:874–879

Montupet P, Esposito C (1999) Laparoscopic treatment of congenital inguinal hernia in children. J Pediatr Surg 34:420–423

Schier F (2000) Laparoscopic surgery of inguinal hernias in children: initial experience. J Pediatr Surg 35:1331–1335

Schier F, Montupet P, Esposito C (2002) Laparoscopic inguinal herniorrhaphy in children: a three-center experience with 933 repairs. J Pediatr Surg 37:395-397

Shalaby R, Desoky A (2002) Needlescopic inguinal hernia repair in children. Pediatr Surg Int 18:153–156

Surana R, Puri P (1993) Is contralateral exploration necessary in infants with unilateral inguinal hernia? J Pediatr Surg 28:1026–1027

Wiener ES, Touloukian RJ, Rodgers BM, et al (1996) Hernia survey of the section on surgery of the American Academy of Pediatrics. J Pediatr Surg 31:1166–1169

Wulkan ML, Wiener ES, van Balen N, et al (1996) Laparoscopy through the open ipsilateral sac to evaluate presence of contralateral hernia. J Pediatr Surg 31:1174–1177

Chapter 79

Laparoscopic Contralateral Groin Exploration During Inguinal Hernia Repair

Douglas C. Barnhart

Introduction

The debate regarding the evaluation for a persistent patent processus vaginalis in infants and children presenting with a unilateral hernia has continued for decades with surgeons advocating routine bilateral exploration as early as 1955 (Rothenberg and Barnett 1955). Gans and Berci first reported the demonstration of a persistent patent processus vaginalis using laparoscopy in 1971 (Gans and Berci 1971). A large survey of North American pediatric surgeons in 1993 showed that this controversy persisted with significant variability in practice. Sixty-five percent of pediatric surgeons reported exploring the contralateral groin in boys under the age of 2 years while 84% explored the contralateral groin in girls up to the age of 4 years. Laparoscopic examination was used by only 6% of respondents and was strongly criticized by others (Wiener et al. 1996).

In 1992 Lobe and Schropp reported an initial experience with the routine use of laparoscopy for evaluation of the asymptomatic side (Lobe and Schropp 1992). Since that time laparoscopic examination of the contralateral ring has become widely accepted as a valid technique. It is a simple and brief method to assess for the presence of a persistent patent processus vaginalis. The technique eliminates the risk of injury to the vas deferens or spermatic vessels as well as local wound complications which accompany open contralateral exploration. It is preferred over observation or contralateral exploration by parents (Holcomb et al. 2004). Its widespread appeal has caused the debate to shift to the question of laparoscopic examination of the contralateral internal ring versus observation.

Two methods for the laparoscopic examination of the contralateral internal inguinal ring are described and their relative merits are discussed.

Preoperative Preparation

Before Induction of General Anesthesia

A dose of perioperative prophylactic antibiotics such as a first-generation cephalosporin may be given if one does so for routine clean cases. This is not however the practice in our institution given the very low rate of wound infection associated with inguinal herniorrhaphy in infants and children. Routine monitoring including capnography and pulse oximetry is indicated.

After Induction of General Anesthesia

Although laparoscopic contralateral examination may be performed with a laryngeal mask airway, it is my practice to routinely have the patient endotracheally intubated. This is done to reduce the possibility of aspiration during the brief period that the patient is in Trendelenburg position with the abdomen insufflated. After intubation the stomach is evacuated and the bladder emptied via a Credé maneuver.

Positioning

Patient

The patient is positioned supine and is secured to the table with tape.

Crew, Monitors, and Equipment

■ Figure 79.1 shows the position of the crew, monitors, and equipment.

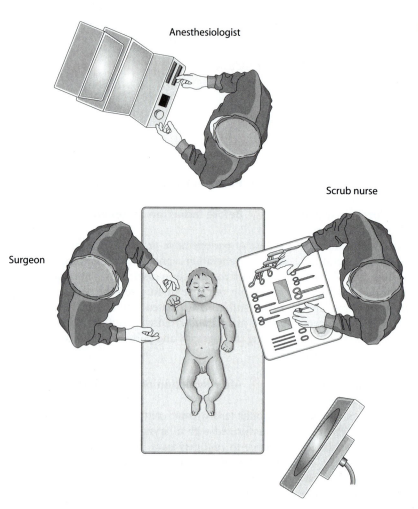

Anesthesiologist

Scrub nurse

Surgeon

Fig. 79.1. Position of the patient, crew and monitors

Special Equipment

Energy applying systems are not required. Other equipment is as follows.

Method 1: Lateral Abdominal Approach

0° 1.2 mm laparoscope	1
14-gauge intravenous catheter	2

Method 2: Symptomatic Hernia Sac Approach

70° 4 mm laparoscope	1
4 mm reusable blunt-tip laparoscopy port	1
16-gauge intravenous catheter	1
Lacrimal duct probe	1

Technique

Cannulae

Method 1: Lateral Abdominal Approach

Cannula	Method of insertion	Gauge	Device	Position
1	Cannulation of hernia sac	14	Intravenous catheter	Hernia sac
2	Closed	14	Intravenous catheter	Asymptomatic side, anterior axillary line at the level of the umbilicus

Method 2: Symptomatic Hernia Sac Approach

Cannula	Method of insertion	Size	Device	Position
1	Cannulation of hernia sac	4 mm	Blunt-tip port	Hernia sac
2 (optional)	Closed	16 gauge	Intravenous catheter	Asymptomatic side, lateral and superior to internal ring

Port Positions

For the lateral abdominal approach the initial 14-gauge intravenous catheter is placed into the peritoneal cavity through the opened hernia sac on the symptomatic side and secured with a surgical tie. This is used for insufflation. A second 14-gauge intravenous catheter is placed on the asymptomatic side at the level of the umbilicus at the anterior axillary line. This is subsequently used for placement of the 1.2 mm laparoscope (▪ Fig. 79.2a).

For the symptomatic hernia sac approach the 4 mm blunt-tip port is placed into the peritoneal cavity through the opened hernia sac on the symptomatic side and is secured with a surgical tie. This port is used for insufflation and then subsequently for the placement of the 70° laparoscope. A 16-gauge intravenous catheter is introduced under laparoscopic visualization superior and lateral to the asymptomatic internal inguinal ring if a lacrimal duct probe is needed for retraction of a peritoneal veil (▪ Fig. 79.2b).

Fig. 79.2. a Position of cannulae for the lateral abdominal approach. **b** Position of cannulae for the symptomatic hernia sac approach.

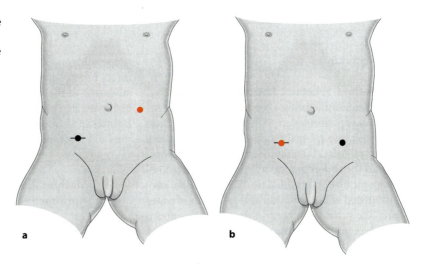

a   b

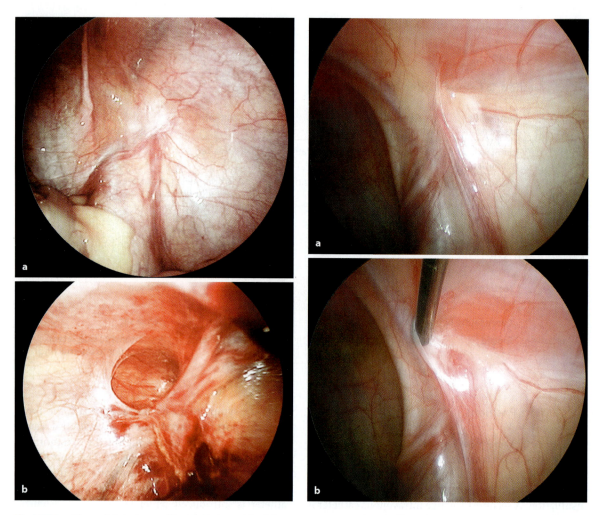

Fig. 79.3. **a** View of right internal inguinal ring with obliterated processus vaginalis. The vas deferens is observed arising medially while the spermatic vessels arise laterally. These converge at the internal ring. **b** View of left internal ring with indirect inguinal hernia. There is a widely open hernia sac anterior to the vas deferens and the spermatic vessels and lateral to the inferior epigastric vessels

Fig. 79.4. **a** View of internal ring with peritoneal veil obscuring view of internal ring. This creates the appearance of a persistent patent processus vaginalis. **b** View of same internal ring with lacrimal duct probe retracting the peritoneal veil. This demonstrates that the processus vaginalis is in fact obliterated

Procedure

Method 1: Lateral Abdominal Approach

A standard anterior approach for repair of indirect inguinal hernia is performed until the hernia sac has been dissected free. The sac is then opened and a 14-gauge plastic intravenous catheter is inserted through the hernia sac into the abdominal cavity. The hernia sac is secured about the catheter with a tie. The abdominal cavity is insufflated with carbon dioxide to 15 cm of water pressure. The patient is placed in steep Trendelenburg position. A 14-gauge intravenous catheter is introduced into the abdominal cavity at the level of the umbilicus at the anterior axillary line on the asymptomatic side. After removal of the needle stylet, the 1.2 mm laparo-

scope is advanced through this catheter. This provides a direct in-line view of the internal ring and allows measurement of the depth of the processus vaginalis. Any processus vaginalis longer than 1 cm is considered abnormal and is repaired using a standard approach (Owings and Georgeson 2000).

Method 2: Symptomatic Hernia Sac Approach

As in the first method described, the hernia sac is dissected free and opened. The 4 mm blunt-tip laparoscopy port is introduced into the abdominal cavity through the hernia sac. The sac is secured about the port with a tie and the abdomen is insufflated to 8 cm of water pressure. The 70° laparoscope is introduced through this port initially in a cephalad direction and gently swept to a lateral position. This route is used to avoid obscuring the view with the medial umbilical ligament. The vas deferens and spermatic vessels or the round ligament is identified and followed to allow clear identification of the internal ring (Chu et al. 1993). In most cases the internal ring can be adequately visualized to determine if there is a patent processus vaginalis (■ Fig. 79.3).

In some patients there is a lateral umbilical ligament, and the peritoneal fold over the inferior epigastric vessels may obscure a clear view of the internal ring. This peritoneal veil can create the false appearance of a patent processus vaginalis. A lacrimal duct probe may be introduced via a 16-gauge intravenous catheter after removal of the needle stylet. This intravenous catheter is introduced lateral and cephalad to the internal ring under laparoscopic visualization (Geiger 2000) (■ Fig. 79.4). Any patent processus vaginalis is repaired using a standard anterior approach.

Postoperative Care

Postoperative management is similar to that of a unilateral inguinal hernia repair. Pain is typically managed with either a caudal block or an inguinal nerve block. Acetaminophen is the only oral pain medicine required in most cases

Discussion

Since its introduction in 1992, laparoscopic exploration of the contralateral groin during unilateral herniorrhaphy has gained widespread acceptance in the pediatric surgery community. This relatively rapid evolution in practice is due to several factors. Primarily, it allows definitive assessment of the asymptomatic side without an accompanying risk of injury to the vas deferens and spermatic vessels. Secondly, it is a straightforward technique that can be performed using standard reusable equipment and does not require advanced laparoscopic skills. Finally, it is brief and does not add significantly to the operative time.

The results of the published experiences were evaluated in a meta-analysis (Miltenburg et al. 1998). This study analyzed 964 patients and included 13 studies with laparoscopy being performed in three different ways, the two described above and via the umbilicus. The overall sensitivity in detecting a persistent patent processus vaginalis was 99.4% while the specificity was 99.5%. The increase in operative time by the addition of laparoscopy ranged from 2 to 17 min with the aver-

age increase in operative time being under 6 min. Complications were exceedingly rare with the only complications being two wound infections for an overall complication rate of 0.002%.

The pediatric surgeons at The Children's Hospital of Alabama use both of the methods described above and recognize advantages to both. The lateral abdominal approach allows for a direct view of the contralateral internal ring. The peritoneal veil created by the lateral umbilical ligament does not confound this view and the depth of the processus can be measured. This measurement can therefore be used as the decision point for exploration. The chief limitation to this method is the requirement for a 1.2 mm laparoscope which is fragile. The symptomatic hernia sac approach uses a more durable 4 mm laparoscope but has the disadvantage of the indirect view. The problem of the peritoneal veil obscuring the view may be ameliorated by retraction with a lacrimal duct probe as described. There are no studies directly comparing these two techniques. The incidence of patency of the processus vaginalis using the lateral abdominal approach in our institution was 27.6% in infants less than 1 year of age (Owings and Georgeson 2000). Using the identical technique, another group reported that 38% of children less than 2 years had a positive laparoscopic examination (Bhatia et al. 2004). In comparison the symptomatic hernia sac approach is associated with a 47% prevalence of positive examinations in patients less than 1 year of age (Holcomb et al. 1996). With the use of selective probing as described above this rate dropped to 32% (Geiger 2000).

While the widespread acceptance of laparoscopic contralateral exploration has essentially eliminated the debate over open contralateral exploration, there remains controversy over whether unilateral repair and observation is preferable. This debate centers on the issue that the incidence of metachronous hernia is substantially lower than the incidence of patent processus vaginalis detected by laparoscopy. There are several large follow-up studies of patients who have undergone unilateral repair (Hrabovszky and Pinter 1995; Nazir and Saebo 1996). Series such as these report an incidence of metachronous contralateral hernia ranging from 5.5% to 15%. Advocates of unilateral repair and observation argue that the practice of laparoscopic examination results in exploration of the contralateral groin with its accompanying risks in many children who would not have developed a clinically apparent hernia. However, the routine use of laparoscopic exploration eliminates the need for a possible second surgery and the anesthetic risks and anxieties for the parent and child. When surveyed in a prospective and systematic fashion, 85% of parents chose laparoscopic examination over observation or open contralateral exploration (Holcomb et al. 2004). Surprisingly the majority cited the convenience of a single procedure rather than concerns over a second anesthetic as their primary motivation. It is the current practice at our institution to routinely offer laparoscopic examination and almost all parents choose this over unilateral repair and observation.

References

Bhatia AM, Gow KW, Heiss KF, et al (2004) Is the use of laparoscopy to determine the presence of contralateral patent processus vaginalis justified in children greater than 2 years of age. J Pediatr Surg 39:778–781

Chu C, Chou C, Hsu T, et al (1993) Intraoperative laparoscopy in unilateral hernia repair to detect a contralateral patent processus vaginalis. Pediatr Surg Int 8:385–388

Gans SL, Berci G (1971) Advances in endoscopy in children. J Pediatr Surg 6:199–234

Geiger JD (2000) Selective laparoscopic probing for a contralateral patent processus vaginalis reduces the need for contralateral exploration in inconclusive cases. J Pediatr Surg 35:1151–1154

Holcomb GW, Morgan WM, Brock JW (1996) Laparoscopic evaluation of the contralateral patent processus vaginalis: part II. J Pediatr Surg 31:1170–1173

Holcomb GW, Miller KA, Chaignaud BE, et al (2004) The parental perspective regarding the contralateral inguinal region in a child with a known unilateral inguinal hernia. J Pediatr Surg 39:480–482

Hrabovszky Z, Pinter AB (1995) Routine bilateral exploration for inguinal hernia in infancy and childhood. Eur J Pediatr Surg 5:152–155

Lobe TE, Schropp KP (1992) Inguinal hernias in pediatrics: initial experience with laparoscopic inguinal exploration of the asymptomatic contralateral side. J Laparoendosc Surg 2:135–140

Miltenburg DM, Nuchtern JG, Jaksic T et al. (1998) Laparoscopic evaluation of the pediatric inguinal hernia: a meta-analysis. J Pediatr Surg 33:874–879

Nazir M, Saebo A (1996) Contralateral inguinal hernial development and ipsilateral recurrence following unilateral hernial repair in infants and children. Acta Chir Belg 96:28–30

Owings EP, Georgeson KE (2000) A new technique for laparoscopic exploration of the contralateral patent processus vaginalis. Surg Endosc 14:114–116

Rothenberg RE, Barnett T (1955) Bilateral herniotomy in infants and children. Surgery 37:947–950

Wiener ES, Touloukian RJ, Rodgers BM, et al (1996). Hernia survey of the Section on Surgery of the American Academy of Pediatrics. J Pediatr Surg 31:1166–1169

Adrenal Gland

Chapter 80

Transperitoneal Adrenalectomy

D. Denison Jenkins, Karl G. Sylvester, and Craig T. Albanese

Introduction

Laparoscopic adrenalectomy was first reported in adults in 1992 (Gagner et al. 1992). As acceptance of the safety and efficacy of this minimal access approach has expanded, pediatric surgeons have begun to use this technique to remove adrenal tumors in children. The most common pediatric adrenal pathology, neuroblastoma, is generally infiltrative, large, and not well-encapsulated, and is only occasionally amenable for laparoscopic removal. Consequently, a randomized trial comparing open to laparoscopic adrenalectomy is unlikely to occur. However, numerous published reports have described successful laparoscopic removal of the adrenal gland in children, and it is now an accepted procedure to treat children with adrenal tumors (Castilho et al. 2002; Miller et al. 2002; Miralliè et al. 2001). Though the retroperitoneal approach is an alternative, this chapter will only describe transperitoneal adrenalectomy.

Preoperative Preparation

Before Induction of General Anesthesia

Bowel preparation is not necessary prior to laparoscopic removal of an adrenal tumor. Other decisions regarding preoperative preparation are based upon whether or not the mass is functional. For example, a non-functional solid adrenal tumor would not require any preoperative management, whereas a pheochromocytoma would require adrenergic blockade prior to surgery. Also, anesthetic agents that are either vagolytic or increase the arrhythmogenic effects of catecholamines should be avoided when removing a catecholamine-secreting adrenal tumor.

After Induction of General Anesthesia

After induction of general anesthesia and endotracheal intubation, an orogastric tube is placed to decrease the risk of visceral injury associated with initial access. Prophylactic antibiotics and urinary drainage are not needed. Spinal or epidural anesthesia is not used. An arterial catheter is placed prior to the extirpation of a pheochromocytoma, since hemodynamic instability is commonly seen during intubation, the establishment of pneumoperitoneum, manipulation of the adrenal mass, and after ligation of the adrenal vein (Petorius et al. 1998). Pheochromocytoma removal requires calcium channel and alpha-blockers to maintain systolic blood pressures below 150 mmHg, and short-acting beta-blockers are administered to keep the patient's heart rate less than 100 beats/min. Intraoperative use of magnesium sulfate in children to inhibit the release of catecholamines, and to directly block adrenergic receptors, has been reported (Minami et al. 2002). Fluids and alpha-agonists are used as needed to support blood pressure after the adrenal vein is ligated.

Positioning

Patient

The patient is placed in the full lateral decubitus position, with the lesion side up. This position provides optimal exposure gain through gravity. The kidney rest is raised, and the table flexed to maximize the distance between the costal margin and the iliac crest. The ipsilateral arm is supported by towels or an arm rest; all bony prominences and the axilla are padded. A molded beanbag facilitates positioning and cushioning (■ Fig. 80.1).

Crew, Monitors, and Equipment

Figure 80.1 shows the operating room setup for both right and left laparoscopic adrenalectomies.

Special Equipment

Bipolar high-frequency electrocoagulation (HFE) and ultrasonic energy and/or Ligasure are available as are clips, staplers, and a retrieval bag.

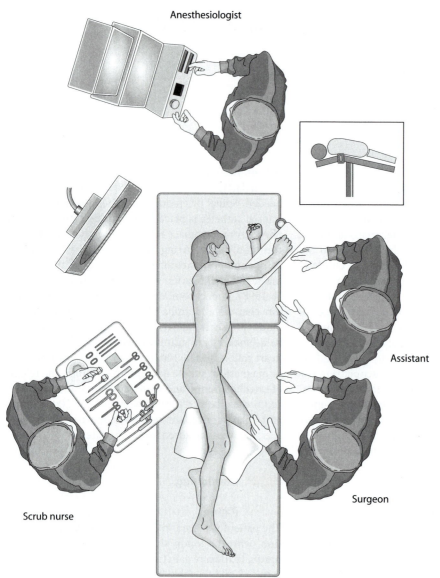

Anesthesiologist

Assistant

Surgeon

Scrub nurse

Fig. 80.1. Patient and crew position. **a**. Right laparoscopic adrenalectomy.

Fig. 80.1. Patient and crew position. **b**. Left laparoscopic adrenalectomy. Use of the full lateral decubitus position facilitates operative exposure during laparoscopic removal of an adrenal tumor

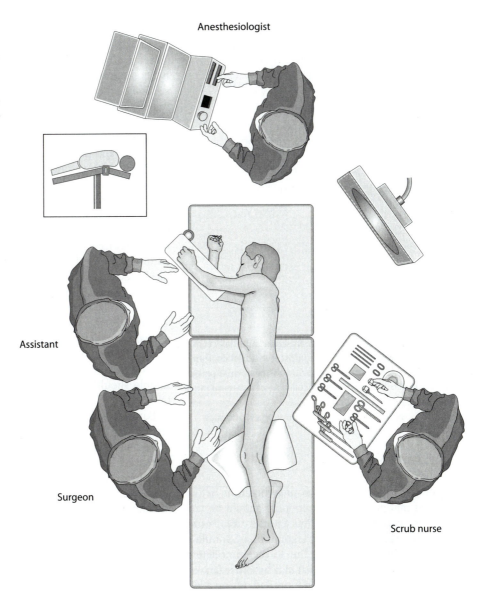

Technique

Cannulae

Cannula	Method of insertion	Diameter (mm)	Device	Position
1	Closed	3 or 5	Liver retractor	Midclavicular
2	Closed	3 or 5	Working port	Anterior axillary
3	Open or closed	5	Camera	Midaxillary
4	Closed	3 or 5	Working port	Posterior axillary

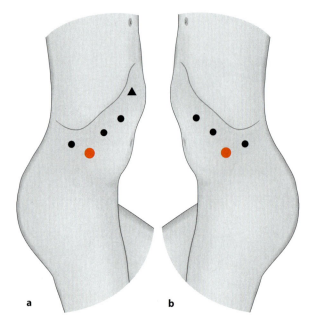

Fig. 80.2. Trocar sites **a** Right laparoscopic adrenalectomy. Triangle = liver retractor. **b.** Left laparoscopic adrenalectomy. Trocar sites are commonly placed below the costal margin between the midaxillary and midclavicular lines. Placement must be tailored to accommodate the patient's body habitus and the tumor's size in order to optimize working ergonomics

Port Positions

Trocars are usually placed two fingerbreadths below the costal margin, though positioning should be tailored to the patient's body habitus and the tumor's size in order to maximize working ergonomics. Cannula 1 is placed in the midclavicular line to accommodate a 3- or 5 mm liver retractor, which may be either fan- or diamond-shaped. This port is not needed during a left adrenalectomy. Cannula 2 is placed lateral to cannula 1, usually in the anterior axillary line. The 5 mm, 30° camera is generally placed in the midaxillary line, and the last 3- or 5 mm working port is placed in the posterior axillary line (■ Fig. 80.2).

Procedure

Trocar sites are preemptively infiltrated with local anesthetic. Pneumoperitoneum to a pressure between 12 and 15 mmHg is established. A 5 mm 30° laparoscope is inserted, and the remaining ports are placed under direct visualization. Their position is determined by the patient's body habitus, and the location of the lesion and surrounding structures, and should be individualized on a patient-specific basis.

For left-sided lesions, the descending colon is mobilized, and the lateral peritoneal attachments of the spleen are incised, freeing the spleen and the tail of the pancreas to fall away from the operating field. The dissection of the adrenal mass ultimately varies depending on the tumor size, type, and patient anatomy. Consequently, the sequence of dissection is determined on a patient-specific basis. The superior pole of the kidney is a good landmark for beginning the dissection, and identifies the lowermost extent of the adrenal gland. The dissection usually proceeds from here, and goes laterally to the abdominal wall, and then superiorly. Either endoclips or electrocautery may be used to interrupt the arterial blood supply. The adrenal vein, once mobilized, is ligated last. When removing a pheochromocytoma, the left renal and adrenal veins are ideally identified earlier in the procedure, and the main adrenal vein is clipped, stapled, or tied, depending on the vessel's size. Once the dissection is complete, a bag is placed in the abdominal cavity, and the gland removed through the 5 mm port, which may be widened in order to accommodate a large tumor. Alternatively, the lesion can be morcellated, though an adequate sample should be preserved for cytologic examination.

For right-sided lesions, an additional port is used to retract the right lobe of the liver. Once all laparoscopic instruments are in place, the right triangular ligament is incised, and the right lobe of the liver is retracted superiorly. The right colon is not generally in the operative field, though the hepatic flexure may overlie the adrenal gland and occasionally requires mobilization. Adequate exposure is usually obtained from incising the peritoneum below the liver to expose the inferior vena cava. The adrenal gland is identified, and as with left-sided lesions, the dissection depends on tumor size, type, and patient anatomy. The dissection commonly starts from the superior pole of the kidney and proceeds laterally to the abdominal wall. Once the adrenal vein is fully mobilized, it is clipped, stapled, or tied (■ Fig. 80.3). As before, if removing a pheochromocytoma, the adrenal vein is ideally identified and controlled early in the procedure. Regardless of location, excessive manipulation of a pheochromocytoma prior to ligation of the adrenal vein should be avoided to minimize systemic release of catecholamines.

Once the adrenal gland has been removed, the operative site is inspected to ensure hemostasis. Cannulae are sequentially removed under direct visualization. The fascia of each 5 mm port site is closed with a simple interrupted absorbable suture, and the skin approximated with an absorbable subcuticular stitch.

Fig. 80.3. Ideal exposure during a right laparoscopic adrenalectomy. The right lobe of the liver is retracted superiorly, exposing the adrenal gland. The right adrenal vein is fully mobilized at its confluence with the inferior vena cava prior to placement of endoscopic clips

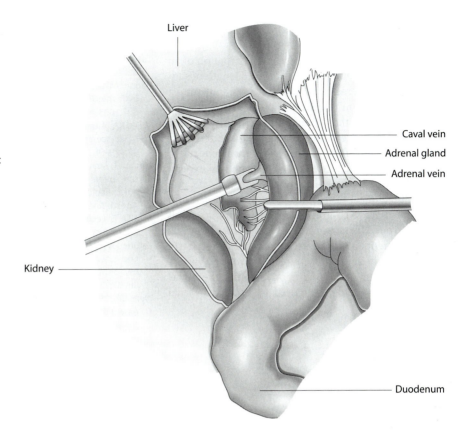

Liver

Caval vein

Adrenal gland

Adrenal vein

Kidney

Duodenum

Postoperative Care

The orogastric tube is removed at the completion of the operation. Overnight hemodynamic monitoring in an intensive care setting is recommended for functional tumors. Diet may be advanced as tolerated. Oral opioids are usually sufficient for pain control.

Results

A randomized comparison of open to laparoscopic adrenalectomy within the pediatric population has not been performed. Articles describing results are mostly case reports, though three recent papers detail institutional experience with pediatric laparoscopic adrenalectomy (Castilho et al. 2002; Miller et al. 2002; Mirallié et al. 2001). In the first study, operative time to remove a unilateral lesion laparoscopically averaged 107 min, whereas a bilateral adrenalectomy for a child with refractory Cushing's disease lasted 180 min. Pathologic examination revealed neuroblastoma in two children diagnosed preoperatively with a non-functioning adrenal tumor. Two of the 13 cases required conversion to an open procedure, one to control bleeding and the other following rupture of the adrenal gland. Mean length of stay was 5.5 days. No postoperative compli-

cations, including mortality, were reported (Castilho et al. 2002).

A second study reported a bi-institutional retrospective review of laparoscopic adrenalectomy in children. Seventeen patients underwent the procedure, with an average operating time of 120 min. Average tumor size was 4.8 cm, mean blood loss was 25 ml, and average length of hospitalization was 35 h. Follow-up averaged 29 months, with resolution of adrenal hyperfunction in every patient with either adrenocortical hyperplasia or pheochromocytoma. There were no intraoperative complications. One child with adrenocortical carcinoma required conversion to an open procedure for a renal vein tumor thrombectomy. Patients with known adrenal neuroblastomas were excluded from this study (Miller et al. 2002).

The third report detailed a 2-year experience removing adrenal tumors laparoscopically in six children, four via the transperitoneal route and two using the retroperitoneal method. Of the four lesions removed using transperitoneal laparoscopy, one required conversion to an open procedure. None of the six children died, and no postoperative complications were reported. One neuroblastoma was excised via the retroperitoneal route. All children stayed in hospital for 6 days (Mirallié et al. 2001).

Discussion

The reported benefits of laparoscopic extirpation of an adrenal mass in adults include decreased length of stay, decreased postoperative pain, and more rapid return to baseline function (Wells 1998). An improved cosmetic result is another potential benefit. Most of the recent published literature of laparoscopic adrenalectomy in children either summarizes case reports or provides a retrospective review of institutional experience. Though laparoscopic adrenalectomy is safe, one potential technical pitfall must be acknowledged and avoided. Failure to control the adrenal vein may result in uncontrolled hemorrhage, and may necessitate conversion to an open procedure. It is desirable to control this vessel early in the procedure, but given the variety of pathology and variation in body habitus, the surgical approach should be tailored to each individual case.

References

Castilho LN, Castillo OA, Dénes FT, et al (2002) Laparoscopic adrenal surgery in children. J Urol 168:221–224

Gagner M, Lacroix A, Bolte E (1992) Laparoscopic adrenalectomy in Cushing's syndrome and pheochromocytoma. N Engl J Med 327:1033

Miller KA, Albanese C, Harrison M, et al (2002) Experience with laparoscopic adrenalectomy in pediatric patients. J Ped Surg 37:979–982

Minami T, Adachi T, Fukuda K (2002) An effective use of magnesium sulfate for intraoperative management of laparoscopic adrenalectomy for pheochromocytoma in a pediatric patient. Anesth Analg 95:1243–1244

Mirallié E, Leclair MD, de Lagausie P, et al (2001) Laparoscopic adrenalectomy in children. Surg Endosc 15:156–160

Petorius M, Rasmussen GE, Holcomb GW (1998) Hemodynamic and catecholamine responses to a laparoscopic adrenalectomy for pheochromocytoma in a pediatric patient. Anesth Analg 87:1268–1270

Wells SA (1998) The role of laparoscopic surgery in adrenal disease. J Clin Endocrinol Metab 83:3041–3043

Chapter 81

Endoscopic Retroperitoneal Adrenalectomy in Children: Lateral Approach

Jean-Stéphane Valla and Henri Steyaert

Introduction

Various endoscopic surgical approaches for adrenalectomy, for example the transperitoneal or retroperitoneal approach, with various patient positions, for example supine, lateral, or prone, have been described. Choosing the best technique depends on the surgeon's preferences, the kind of disease, and the age of the patient (Zuzuki et al. 2001). Most surgeons favor a lateral transperitoneal approach (Castilho et al. 2002; De Lagausie et al. 2003; Fernandez-Crus et al. 1999; Mirallie et al. 2001). In children, we advocate a lateral retroperitoneoscopic approach because of the particular anatomy and the size of the lesions in this age group (Steyaert et al. 2003). However, as in open surgery, this technique requires a long training period and expert hands to be safe and effective. The telescope gives a magnified view of the adrenal anatomy and allows the procedure to begin with the vascular control.

Retroperitoneal endoscopic adrenalectomy can be performed with the patient positioned for either a lateral or a posterior approach (Baba et al. 1999), the former being more commonly used (Demeure et al. 1997).

Preoperative Preparation

The children are prepared for surgery as usual. No bowel preparation is required.

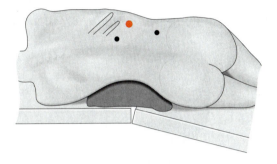

Fig 81.1 Right adrenalectomy Position of the patient

Positioning

Patient

The patient is positioned laterally on the operating table with a sand bag underneath the lumbar region and a bend in the table at the same level in order to widen the space between the 12th rib and the iliac crest (■ Fig. 81.1).

Crew, Monitor, and Equipment

The surgeon stands behind the patient. The monitor stands close to the patient's head (■ Fig. 81.2).

Special Equipment

The same equipment is used as for retroperitoneal nephrectomy (see Chapter 84 "Basic Technique: Retroperitoneoscopic Approach in the Lateral Position").

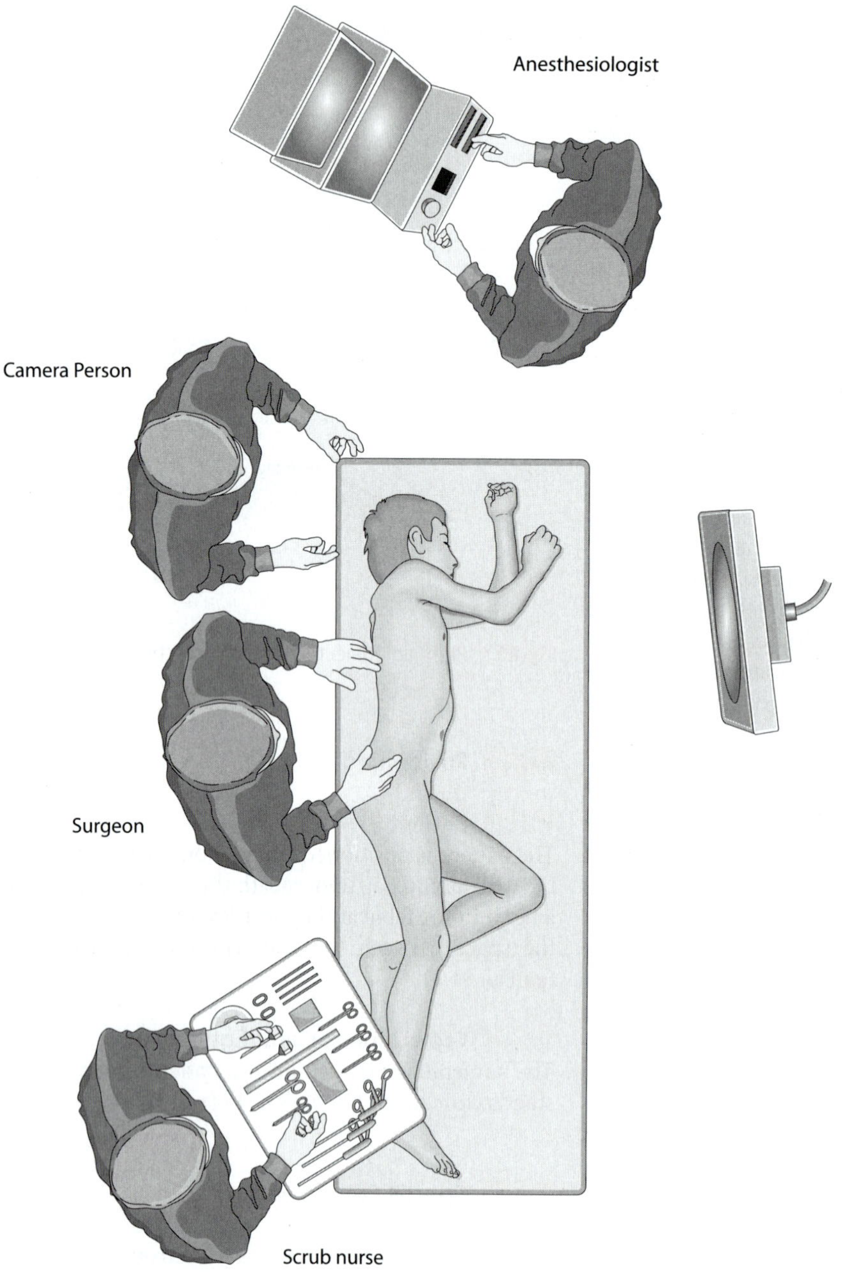

Anesthesiologist

Fig 81.2 Right adrenalectomy
Position of the crew and
equipment

Camera Person

Surgeon

Scrub nurse

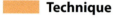

Technique

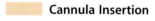

Cannula Insertion

See Chapter 84 for details of cannula insertion.

Procedure

With the help of two atraumatic instruments, palpator or peanut, the upper pole of the kidney is carefully freed. When a sufficiently large working space has been created by CO_2 insufflation and blunt pushing off of the peritoneum, a third trocar, usually a 3 mm one, may be inserted anteriorly for an instrument to retract the kidney or adrenal gland. Cephalad dissection reveals the adrenal gland.

To perform the actual adrenalectomy, the gland should not be grasped but gently pushed aside or lifted up with a blunt instrument or peanut. All manipulation should be slow, and as atraumatic as possible because the adrenal gland and its tumors are fragile and well vascularized. Any bleeding will result in a dark operative field and jeopardize high-quality endoscopic surgery.

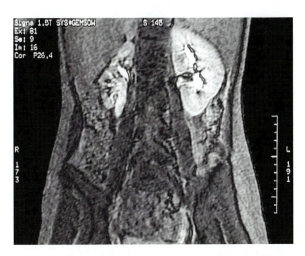

Fig 81.3 MRI of a right sided adrenal tumor sitting on a small kidney

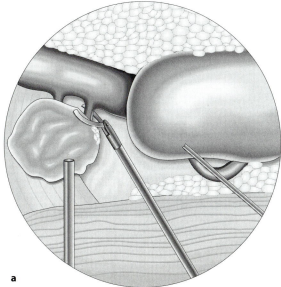

The dissection of the adrenal gland is usually started laterally but it is essential to control the vascular pedicle, and especially the main adrenal vein, first. This means that the caval vein is dissected first on the right side and the renal vein on the left side.

Right Adrenalectomy

The lower adrenal pole is dissected first, which is usually easy although multiple arterial and venous branches from the renal hilum enter the adrenal gland along its inferomedial border. The lower pole is then retracted laterally to expose the caval vein, which must be freed all along the medial border of the adrenal gland. The lower landmark is the junction with the renal vein; the right edge of the caval is freed upward until the adrenal vein is reached, which is often higher than expected. The right adrenal vein runs horizontally to the posteromedial border of the adrenal gland. Because of its rather posterior position, this vein is encountered earlier during a retroperitoneoscopic approach when compared to the left adrenal vein. The right adrenal vein is usually short, sometimes too short to put clips or intracorporeal ties on each side before transaction. If that is the case only the distal part is secured with a clip (■ Figs. 81.3, 81.4a–c). If the diameter of the vein diameter is small (2–4 mm), ultrasonic energy or high-frequency electrocoagulation can be used to sever the vein. With the Ligasure even a larger vein can be taken without problem. As a second adrenal vein may be present in about 4–10% of cases, careful dissection should be carried out until the complete medial part of the gland has been freed. The arteries are numerous but small and can be simply coagulated. The upper pole is separated from the diaphragm and the posterior part of the gland from the caval vein, representing the last delicate step of the procedure.

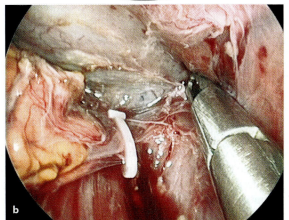

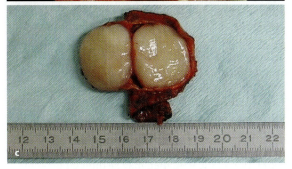

Fig 81.4 Right adrenalectomy. **a, b** Schematic drawing and intraoperative picture of the first step of the dissection: The right border of the vena cava has been freed and the adrenal vein is clipped close to it. **c** Macroscopic view of the tumor specimen, which proved to be a ganglioneuroma

Left Adrenalectomy

Unlike on the right, it may be difficult to locate the left adrenal gland and its vein. The key point is identification of the lower pole of the gland, which is in close contact with the renal vein.

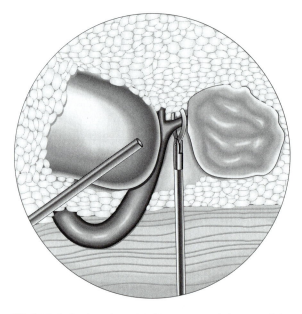

Fig 81.5 Left adrenalectomy. Dissection and division of the inferior adrenal vein

The first step is to open the avascular plane between the upper pole of the left kidney and the inferior or lateral edge of the adrenal gland. Depending on the tumor, the upper pole of the kidney is left attached to the peritoneum and retracted anteriorly or completely mobilized within Gerota's fascia and dropped posteriorly onto the psoas muscle. Anterolateral retraction of the adrenal gland facilities the next step. The dissection is continued along the medial aspect of the upper pole of the kidney toward the renal hilum until the main adrenal vein is encountered, controlled, and cut (■ Fig. 81.5). The adrenal gland is dissected along its internal border to identify and to control branches that arise from the aorta. Then the gland is mobilized along its posterior, superior, and anterior surfaces from the psoas muscle, diaphragm, and peritoneum, respectively. Small vessels arising from the inferior phrenic vessels are coagulated at that time.

Extraction of the Specimen and Closure

Extraction of the specimen may be difficult depending on the volume and the flexibility of the lumbar wall: it is easy in a case of simple hyperplasia and in infants, but harder in case of a tumor and in adolescents. The specimen is placed in a plastic bag, usually the cutoff first finger of a latex-free surgical glove, and extracted through the 10 mm incision, which is enlarged if necessary.

The telescope is reintroduced for irrigation and to check hemostasis. The fascia is closed in two layers using 2/0 absorbable sutures. The skin at each incision site is approximated with 5/0 absorbable suture in a subcuticular fashion.

Postoperative Care

Aspiration drainage is maintained for 2 days.

Results

Fourteen patients have received 16 retroperitoneal endoscopic non-renal procedures; 2 patients had bilateral disease. We carried out 14 total adrenalectomies, 1 enucleation of an adrenal tumor, and 1 removal of an extra-adrenal tumor (ganglioneuroma in the psoas muscle).

The mean diameter of the lesions was 35 mm (range 15–45 mm). The disease occurred seven times on the right side and nine times on the left. Three patients presented multiple endocrine neoplasia syndrome. The other histological diagnoses were: ganglioneuroma (4 cases) ganglioneuroblastoma (1 case), neuroblastoma (2 cases), adrenal hyperplasia (2 cases), and lipoma (2 cases).

Conversion was necessary in our first case, a 2-month-old boy, who had a small neuroblastoma on the right. There were two intraoperative complications: one diaphragmatic tear during the introduction of the posterior trocar, which was repaired at the end of the procedure, and one bleeding (100 ml) during the dissection of the left adrenal vein. There were no postoperative complications.

Mean follow-up has been 2 years (range from 6 months to 8 years). No recurrence occurred in any of the patients.

Discussion

Indications

Preoperative patient selection is of paramount importance (Valla et al. 2001). The endoscopic surgical approach should be reserved for well-defined lesions, smaller than 5 cm in diameter, and benign on clinical, radiological, and biological grounds. Complete certainty about the benign nature of the lesion can of course be difficult to define preoperatively. Good indications are cysts, pheochromocytoma, corticosurrenaloma, adenoma, hyperplasia, and ganglioneuroma. The indication can be extended to stage I non-secreting neuroblastoma in particular situations, for example tumor identified by mass screening or incidental discovery by ultrasonography before or soon after birth (De Lagausie et al. 2003).

Partial adrenalectomy is indicated in selected cases particularly in those in which there is a low possibility of malignancy, as in primary hyperaldosteronism, and those in which there is a high probability of bilateral disease, for example in MEN II and other genetic syndromes (Mirallie et al. 2001).

There seems to be no age limit for retroperitoneoscopic adrenalectomy.

Advantages and Drawbacks of Different Techniques

Open Surgery Versus Minimally Invasive Surgery

Small adrenal tumors should be removed endoscopically because they require large incisions when conventional open surgery is performed. Non-manipulative dissection and excellent magnification enable optimal resection of the adrenal gland with minimal tissue trauma. However the endoscopic retroperitoneal approach does not allow a complete intra-abdominal exploration and palpation; for example exploration of the aortic axis for extra-adrenal tumors and exploration of the contralateral adrenal gland in case of pheochromocytoma is not possible. Endoscopic surgeons are compelled to trust modern preoperative imaging techniques such as iobenguane (MIBG) scintigraphy, magnetic resonance imaging (MRI), or computed tomography (CT). The improved resolution of these imaging techniques has made surgical manual exploration of chromaffin tissue sites superfluous.

Retroperitoneal Versus Transperitoneal Approach

Most of the endoscopic surgical teams treating adults and some teams treating children (Castilho et al. 2002; De Lagausie et al. 2003) propose, at the moment, a laparoscopic transperitoneal approach in the lateral position. They criticize the retroperitoneoscopic approach for two things. The first and primary disadvantage of the retroperitoneal approach is the lack of a natural cavity: the working space needs to be created, but in children the relative absence of fat and the thin muscle layers make the retroperitoneoscopic approach very attractive. The second disadvantage of the retroperitoneal approach is that the working space is smaller than with the intraperitoneal approach. As a result, the trocars are closer to each other. However with expertise, good retroperitoneal insufflation, and good abdominal wall relaxation this obstacle can be eliminated allowing for good dissection. However if accidental injury of the caval vein occurs during right adrenalectomy, hemostasis by clamping and suturing will be very difficult.

In children, the main advantage of a retroperitoneal course is the more direct and rapid exposure without violation of the peritoneum and dissection as well as handling of intraperitoneal structures, which could be injured during these maneuvers. For a left adrenal lesion, both displacement of the spleen and downward retraction of the splenic colonic flexure are avoided; for a right adrenal lesion it is not necessary to cut the right triangular ligament and to displace the liver. However on the right side, the retroperitoneal approach requires mobilization and caudal displacement of the upper pole of the kidney before reaching the adrenal vein.

Lateral Versus Prone Position

The prone position has the advantage of being able to perform bilateral adrenalectomy without repositioning the patient (Fernandez-Crus et al. 1999; Salomon et al. 2001; Zuzuki et al. 2001). Conversion in case of a caval vein injury, however, or conversion for any other reason is much more difficult than when the patient has been put in a lateral position. So we advocate a lateral position even in cases of bilateral lesions.

Conclusion

The potential advantages of endoscopic adrenalectomy in children are similar to those reported for other applications of endoscopic surgery (small incision, decreased postoperative pain, quicker discharge). However, relatively few adrenal pathologies in children are suitable for an endoscopic approach: only small, well-encapsulated, non-invasive or infiltrative lesions, less than 6 cm in diameter, and presumed benign tumors or selected neuroblastomas are suited, and this is not usually the case in neuroblastoma, which is the most common adrenal tumor in children. Nevertheless endoscopic adrenalectomy can be performed when two rules are obeyed: rigorous selection of cases and well-trained endoscopic surgeons. Endoscopic adrenalectomy demands a meticulous technique. Joining with a specialized adult endocrine endoscopic surgeon is good practice. If these precautions are taken, this new approach is beneficial for children. Except for large adrenal lesions on the right side, the retroperitoneal approach seems a better choice for children than the transperitoneal one.

References

Baba S, Ito K, Yanaihara H, Nagata H, et al (1999) Retroperitoneoscopic adrenalectomy by a lumbodorsal approach: clinical experience with solo surgery. World J Urol 17:54–58

Castilho LN, Castilho UA, Idenes FT, et al (2002) Laparoscopic adrenal surgery in children. J Urol 168:221–224

De Lagausie P, Berrebt D, Michin J, et al (2003) Laparoscopic adrenal surgery for neuroblastoma in children. J Urol 170:932–935

Demeure MJ, Jordan M, Zeihen M, et al (1997) Endoscopic retroperitoneal right adrenalectomy with patient in lateral decubitus position. Surg Laparosc Endosc 7:307–309

Fernandez-Cruz L, Saenz A, Taura P, et al (1999) Retroperitoneal approach in laparoscopic adrenalectomy: is it advantageous? Surg Endosc 13:86–90

Mirallie E, Leclair M, De Lagausie P, et al (2001) Laparoscopic adrenalectomy in children. Surg Endosc 15:156–160

Salomon L, Soulie M, Mouly P, et al (2001) Experience with retroperitoneal laparoscopic adrenalectomy in 115 procedures. J Urol 166:38–41

Steyaert H, Juricic M, Hendrice C, et al (2003) Retroperitoneoscopic approach to the adrenal glands and retroperitoneal tumors in children: where do we stand? Eur J Pediatr Surg 13:112–115

Valla J-S, Heloury Y, Mirallie E, et al (2001) Laparoscopic adrenalectomy in children: experience of the Group d'Etude en Coelioschirurgie Infantile in 16 cases. Pediatr Endosurg Innov Tech 5:267–275

Zuzuki K, Kageyamas S, Hirano Y, et al (2001) Comparison of 3 surgical approaches to laparoscopic adrenalectomy: a non randomized background matched analysis. J Urol 66:437–443

Chapter 82

Laparoscopic Approach to Abdominal Neuroblastoma

Tadashi Iwanaka

Introduction

Neuroblastoma is one of the most common solid tumors in infants and children (Iwanaka et al. 2001c), and the indications for a laparoscopic approach to abdominal neuroblastoma are as follows:

1. Laparoscopic excision of tumor and lymph node sampling for early localized neuroblastoma (Iwanaka et al. 2001b; Nakajima et al. 1997; Yamamoto et al. 1996)
2. Laparoscopic biopsy of tumor for advanced large neuroblastoma (Iwanaka et al. 2001b)
3. Laparoscopic excision of tumor and lymphadenectomy for advanced neuroblastoma which has become very small and localized after preoperative chemotherapy (Iwanaka et al. 2001a)

In this chapter, the techniques of laparoscopic biopsy for advanced neuroblastoma and laparoscopic excision with or without lymphadenectomy for small neuroblastoma are described.

Preoperative Preparation

Before Induction of General Anesthesia

Due to the risk of injury to the right or left flexure of the colon, a glycerin enema should be given preoperatively and oral feeding should be withheld for 12–24 h before the operation. Although blood transfusions are seldom required, 10–20 ml/kg of packed red blood cells should be available.

After Induction of General Anesthesia

General anesthesia using inhalational agents and muscle relaxants without the use of nitrous oxide is recommended. Injection of a local anesthetic agent (0.5–1 ml of 1% Xylocaine) to future port sites is useful. Alternatively general anesthesia could be supplemented with regional anesthesia techniques such as epidural or spinal anesthesia. A nasogastric tube and urinary catheter are inserted. Perioperative antibiotics are not necessary.

Positioning of Patient, Crew, Monitors, and Equipment

Right Adrenal or Right Retroperitoneal Neuroblastoma

The patient is put in a 20–45 left posterolateral and 15–20 reversed Trendelenburg position on the operating table (■ Fig. 82.1a). Because intraoperative rotation of the operating table is always required, bilateral pelvic cushions and knee belts are very helpful in repositioning and stabilizing the patient.

The surgeon and camera operator stand to the left of the patient. The monitor is placed opposite to the surgeon, to the right of the patient's head. The assistant and scrub nurse stand to the right of the patient and look at the second monitor which is placed to the left of the patient's head (■ Fig. 82.1b). The high-frequency electrocautery (HFE) and ultrasonic equipment stand behind the surgeon.

Left Adrenal or Left Retroperitoneal Neuroblastoma

The positioning is a mirror image of that for right adrenal or retroperitoneal neuroblastoma (■ Fig. 82.2).

Central Retroperitoneal Neuroblastoma

The patient is placed in supine and 15–20 reversed Trendelenburg position on the operating table (■ Fig. 82.3). The surgeon stands at the feet of the patient.

Pelvic Neuroblastoma

The patient is placed in supine and 15–20 Trendelenburg position but transversely at the end of the operating table (■ Fig. 82.4). The surgeon stands at the head of the patient, while the monitor is positioned at the feet of the patient.

Special Equipment

Bipolar HFE as well as ultrasonic energy should be available. For the removal of specimens, retrieval bags are used. Fibrin glue is used for hemostasis.

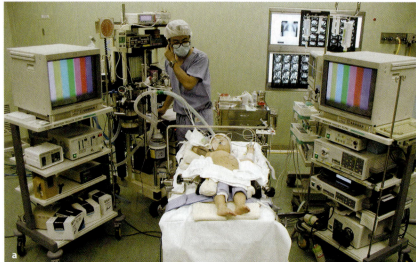

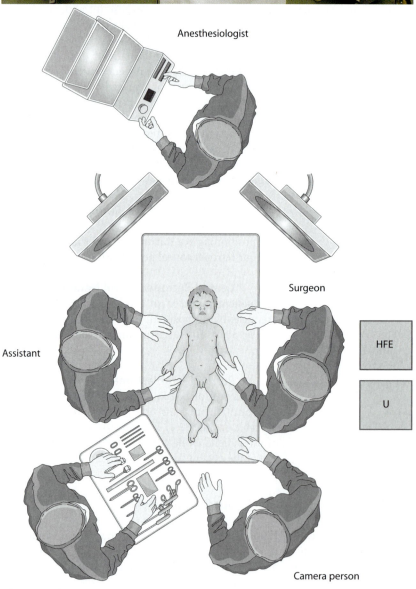

Fig. 82.1. a Position of the patient, monitors, and equipment for a right adrenal or right retroperitoneal neuroblastoma. **b** Position of the patient, crew, and equipment for a right adrenal or right retroperitoneal neuroblastoma

Fig. 82.2. Position of the patient, crew, and equipment for left adrenal or left retroperitoneal neuroblastoma

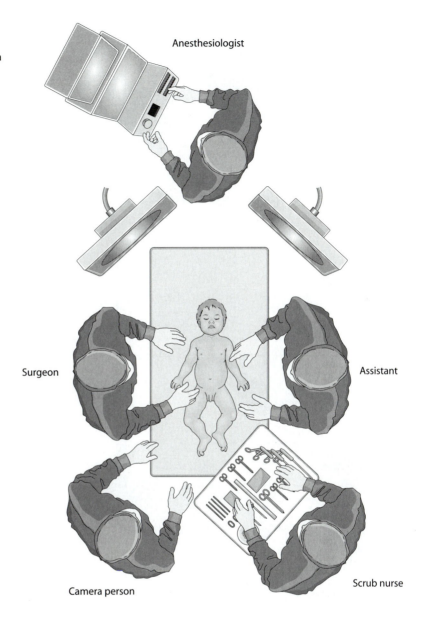

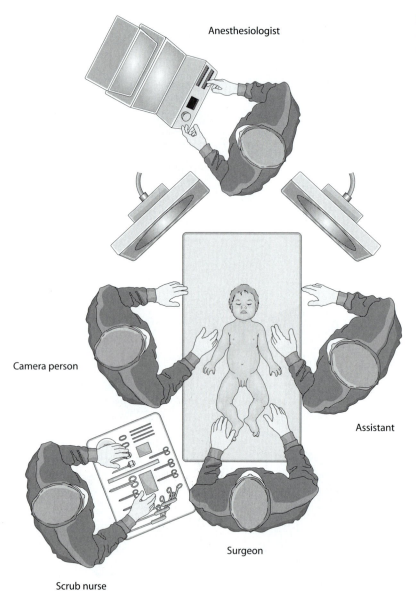

Anesthesiologist

Camera person

Assistant

Scrub nurse

Surgeon

Fig. 82.3. Position of the patient, crew, and equipment for central neuroblastoma

Fig. 82.4. Position of the patient, crew, and equipment for a pelvic neuroblastoma

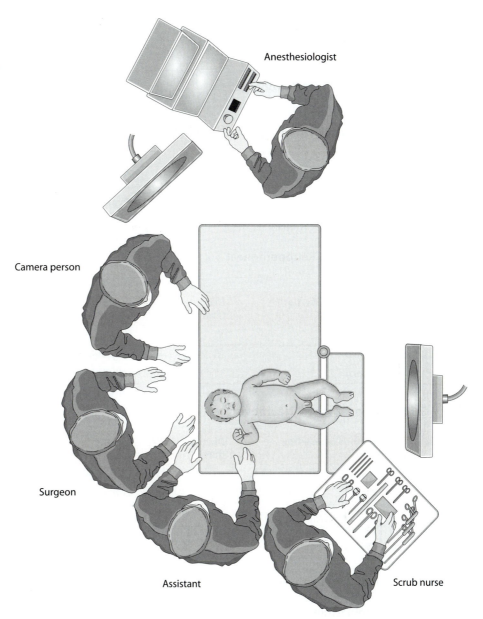

Anesthesiologist

Camera person

Surgeon

Assistant

Scrub nurse

Technique

Cannulae

Right Adrenal or Right Retroperitoneal Neuroblastoma

Cannula	Method of insertion	Diameter (mm)	Position
1	Open	12	Umbilical
2	Closed	5	Epigastrium
3	Closed	5	Right subcostal area

■ Figure 82.5 shows port locations.

Left Adrenal or Left Retroperitoneal Neuroblastoma

Cannula	Method of insertion	Diameter (mm)	Position
1	Open	12	Umbilical
2	Closed	5	Epigastrium
3	Closed	5	Left subcostal area

Central Retroperitoneal Neuroblastoma

Cannula	Method of insertion	Diameter (mm)	Position
1	Open	12	Umbilical
2	Closed	5	Left upper abdomen
3	Closed	5	Right upper abdomen
4	Closed	5	Left subcostal
5	Closed	5	Right subcostal

■ Figure 82.6 shows port locations.

Pelvic Neuroblastoma

Cannula	Method of insertion	Diameter (mm)	Position
1	Open	12	Umbilical
2	Closed	5	Left abdomen
3	Closed	5	Right abdomen

■ Figure 82.7 shows port locations.

Biopsy Taking

The procedure of biopsy taking of a right adrenal or retroperitoneal neuroblastoma is mainly described.

To create a pneumoperitoneum, the patient is placed in a supine position by rotation of the operating table. A 12 mm trocar for a 30° angled laparoscope is inserted through a small incision of the umbilicus using an open technique. The abdominal cavity is insufflated with carbon dioxide to a pressure of 8–10 mmHg and two more 5 mm working ports are inserted under endoscopic control (■ Fig. 82.5a,b). To provide good access to the right retroperitoneal space, the patient is placed in a left posterolateral and 15–20 reversed Tren-

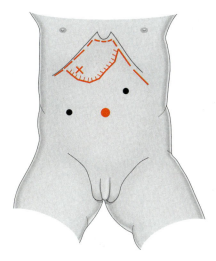

a

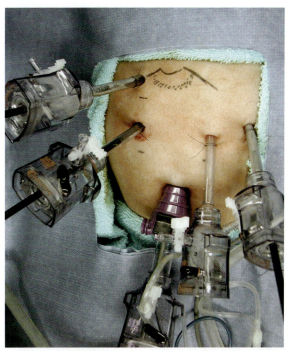

Fig. 82.6. Port location for a central neuroblastoma

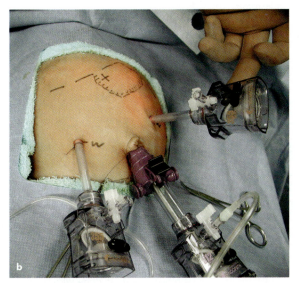

b

Fig. 82.5 a,b. Port location for right adrenal or retroperitoneal tumor

delenburg position to shift the small bowel medially and out of the upper abdominal cavity. Using a grasper the right colon is retracted medially, and the hepatic flexure is dissected using electrocautery or ultrasonic energy (■ Fig. 82.8). Care is taken not to damage the wall of the colon and gall bladder. After taking the hepatic flexure down, the duodenum is mobilized medially by sharp dissection using electrocautery and blunt dissection using a swab (■ Fig. 82.9). Large vessels, such as the inferior vena cava and renal vein, surrounding the tumor, also need to be mobilized by blunt dissection. Before taking the actual biopsy of the tumor, small arteries and veins on the surface of the tumor

should be coagulated with HFE or ultrasonic energy. The biopsy is incisional, using scissors or knife (■ Fig. 82.10). To prevent thermal damage to the specimen and to decrease exfoliation of tumor cells, HFE or ultrasonic energy are not used for taking the actual biopsy. The insufflation pressure is increased to 12 mm Hg to prevent blood loss from the surface of the incised tumor. The specimen is put into a small bag and removed from the abdominal cavity through the 12 mm umbilical port (■ Fig. 82.11). To achieve complete hemostasis, fibrin-glue is applied to the surface of the tumor. To avoid port-site recurrence, high-dose adjuvant chemotherapy is given as early as possible.

When the origin of the tumor is the right adrenal gland, additional dissection of Gerota's fascia is required. For biopsy taking of a tumor in the left retroperitoneal space or left adrenal gland, the reader is referred to the procedure on excision of the tumor in this area.

■ Figure 82.12 shows the operative findings during the procedure for biopsy taking of a tumor located in the central upper abdomen and lower central mediastinum. This procedure requires four working ports (■ Fig. 82.6) and the approach to the surface of the tumor is quite similar to the approach for fundoplication of the stomach.

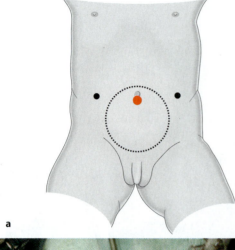

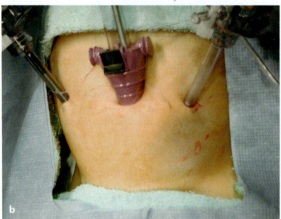

Fig. 82.7 a,b. Port location for a pelvic neuroblastoma

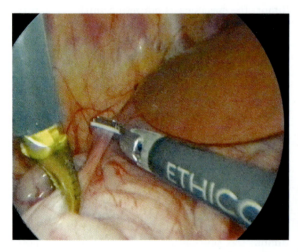

Fig. 82.8. Mobilization of the hepatic flexure of the colon

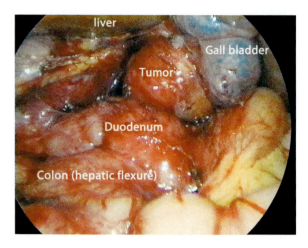

Fig. 82.9. Mobilization of the duodenum and dissection of the surface of the tumor in case of a right retroperitoneal neuroblastoma

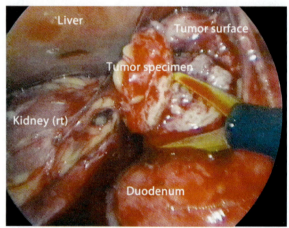

Fig. 82.10. The actual biopsy taking is done with a pair of scissors and not with an energy source in order not to damage the specimen

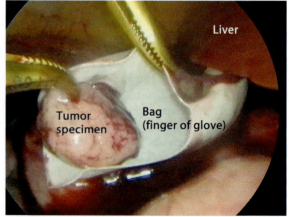

Fig. 82.11. Retrieval of the biopsy in the finger of a surgical glove

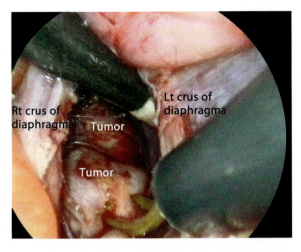

Fig. 82.12. Biopsy taking of tumor located in the upper abdomen and lower mediastinum. The approach to the tumor is similar to the approach to the esophageal hiatus during fundoplication

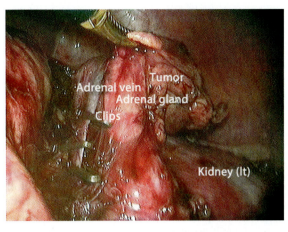

Fig. 82.14. Clipping of the left adrenal vein. This vein is always the largest one in case of the left adrenal neuroblastoma

Excision of a Left Adrenal or Left Retroperitoneal Tumor

The patient is placed in a 20 right posterolateral position. Because intraoperative rotation of the operating table is required as for biopsy of the tumor, bilateral pelvic cushions and knee belts are very useful. The surgeon stands on the abdominal side of the patient (■ Fig. 82.2). To create a pneumoperitoneum, the patient is placed in a supine position by rotation of the operating table. The insertion of the ports is the same as for laparoscopic biopsy taking of the tumor. The operating table is then rotated in a right posterolateral reversed Trendelenburg position. The splenic flexure of the colon is mobilized by incising its lateral peritoneal attachments (■ Fig. 82.13) and freeing it from the inferior pole of the spleen using ultrasonic energy. The retroperitoneal space between the spleen and kidney is bluntly dissected and opened using swabs. The spleen is retracted medially. Dissection of the retroperitoneal space reveals the left adrenal gland and neuroblastoma. The superior pole of the adrenal tumor is mobilized first, and is followed by mobilization of the medial aspect of the tumor where most of the arterial blood supply enters. Mobilization of the adrenal gland and the tumor from the aorta and control of the blood supply is accomplished using ultrasonic energy. However, clipping is recommended for the inferior adrenal vein, which is the most common drainage vein of the adrenal tumor (■ Fig. 82.14). The lateral aspect of the ad-

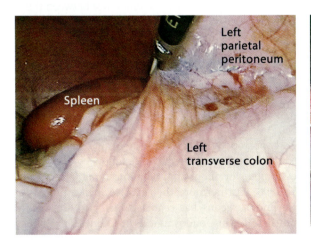

Fig. 82.13. Detachment of the splenic flexure of the colon in case of a left adrenal or retroperitoneal neuroblastoma

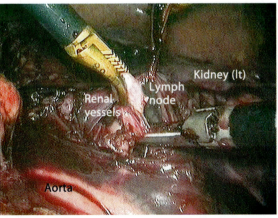

Fig. 82.15. Sampling of para-aortic lymph nodes for histopathological evaluation

renal gland is relatively avascular and ultrasonic energy or electrocautery allows for quick dissection. After the adrenal gland and its tumor are completely freed from surrounding tissues, they are placed into a retrieval bag. When the tumor is small, it can be removed from the abdominal cavity through the umbilical port. Whenever the size of tumor is bigger than 3–4 cm, an additional small incision in the lower abdomen is recommended. Breaking up of the tumor in the retrieval bag to allow removal through a small port wound is strictly prohibited to prevent tumor dissemination. Lymph node sampling is a minimum requirement of the International Neuroblastoma Staging System (INSS) for the precise staging of abdominal neuroblastomas. Even if the preoperative diagnosis of the tumor is INSS 1 , at least sampling of an attached or para-aortic lymph node should be performed. In case of advanced neuroblastoma, additional para-aortic and pararenal lymphadenectomy is required. Before starting pararenal lymphadenectomy, a third working port is placed subcostally at the midclavicular level to retract the left renal artery and vein. After dissection of the left renal vessels, a grasper via the third working port retracts these vessels with a vessel tape. Para-aortic and pararenal lymphadenectomy is performed using ultrasonic energy (■ Fig. 82.15). The retroperitoneal space is irrigated with saline solution and examined for any evidence of bleeding and lymph node swelling. Fibrin glue is applied to achieve complete hemostasis. A drain may be placed into the retroperitoneum to evacuate any fluid or blood that accumulates over the first 24–48 h postoperatively.

Excision of a Right Adrenal Gland

The technique for right adrenalectomy is similar to that for left adrenalectomy except for modifications required for differences in anatomy. However, the procedure is more difficult because of the more cephalad position of the right adrenal gland behind the liver as well as the relationship of the gland with the inferior vena cava. The adrenal vein on the right is very short and drains into the caval vein. Laparoscopic excision of a large localized right adrenal neuroblastoma is controversial.

Postoperative Care

The nasogastric tube is left in place for the first 12–48 h postoperatively depending on the extent of the surgery. The urinary catheter can be removed the same day as surgery, except when high-dose adjuvant chemotherapy is given in the immediate postoperative period or in the event of postoperative regional analgesia. Feeding starts 4–8 h after the removal of the nasogastric tube. The drain is left for a couple of days in case of excision of early neuroblastoma, and for 3–4 days in the case of lymphadenectomy.

Results

Advances in minimal access surgery and endosurgery have allowed the use of these techniques in infants and children, resulting in decreased surgical stress and improved postoperative morbidity. Since Holcomb et al. reported minimally invasive surgery for pediatric malignancies, the pros and cons of this concept have been debated (Holcomb et al. 1995).

Since November 1998, 22 biopsies for advanced neuroblastoma (4–77 months old, 4.5–19.5 kg in body weight), 6 excisions of early neuroblastoma (10–54 months old, 8.7–15.8 kg in body weight), and 3 excisions of advanced neuroblastoma with lymphadenectomy (8–71 months old, 8.7–14.6 kg in body weight) have been performed.

In our series, the time to start postoperative feeding and length of hospital stay were significantly less in the laparoscopically excised patients than in those with open tumor excisions. There was no difference between the laparoscopic versus open groups in length of operation and intraoperative blood loss. None of the patients required perioperative blood transfusions during laparoscopic tumor excision. However, one laparoscopic tumor excision for stage I neuroblastoma was converted to an open excision after a large tumor was found behind the inferior vena cava (Iwanaka et al. 2001b, 2004).

In the advanced neuroblastoma group, the time to start postoperative feeding and time to start high-dose adjuvant chemotherapy were significantly shorter in the laparoscopic biopsy cases than in the open biopsy cases. However, there was no difference between them in terms of length of operation and intraoperative blood loss and there were no patients who required intraoperative blood transfusion in spite of sharp biopsy taking (Iwanaka et al. 2001b, 2004).

Discussion

Early postoperative high-dose adjuvant chemotherapy can prevent port-site recurrence following endosurgical biopsy for abdominal neuroblastoma (Iwanaka et al. 1998). Furthermore, the Japanese Society of Pediatric Endosurgeons has reported that port-site recurrence following endosurgical procedures is an extremely rare phenomenon in the pediatric population and both laparoscopic and thoracoscopic procedures are safe and recommended for treating pediatric malignancies (Iwanaka et al. 2003).

There were no intraoperative and postoperative complications in any case of both laparoscopic biopsy and excision except one case converted to an open excision (Iwanaka et al. 2004). However, one laparoscopic tumor excision combined with para-aortic and para-renal lymphadenectomy after high-dose chemotherapy for a stage IV neuroblastoma that originated from the left adrenal gland took 164 min (Iwanaka et al. 2001a). The patient lost 15 ml of blood during the procedure. Although all pathological tumor and lymph nodes were thought to be resected, we were unable to obtain a good view of the contralateral right para-aortic lymph nodes in the small abdominal cavity. Moreover, fibrotic changes caused by preoperative chemotherapy made blunt dissection around the large vessels very difficult. Laparoscopic excision for advanced neuroblastoma remains controversial.

No patient of the biopsy group required intraoperative blood transfusion. Increasing the carbon dioxide insufflation pressure to 12–15 mmHg can prevent blood loss from the surface of incised tumor, but may result in carbon dioxide embolus if a large vein is injured. Large vessels on the surface of the tumor need to be mobilized by dissection using swabs, ultrasonic energy, or electrocautery before taking the incisional biopsy. However, if the large vessels, such as celiac artery, superior mesenteric artery, and renal vessels, are surrounded by neuroblastoma, the site and depth of biopsy must be planned with precise imaging using enhanced computed tomography and magnetic resonance angiography.

Because of the cosmetic advantage, safety, effectiveness, and all the other benefits of minimally invasive surgery, laparoscopic biopsy taking and excision of abdominal neuroblastomas is preferred above open surgery. Precise indications for laparoscopic surgery in the diagnosis and treatment of abdominal neuroblastoma should lead to a better prognosis and an improved quality of life.

References

Holcomb GW, Tomita SS, Haase GM et al. (1995) Minimally invasive surgery in children with cancer. Cancer 76:121–128

Iwanaka T, Arya G, Ziegler MM (1998) Mechanism and prevention of port-site recurrence after laparoscopy in a murine model. J Pediatr Surg 33:457–461

Iwanaka T, Arai M, Ito M et al. (2001a) Challenges of laparoscopic resection of abdominal neuroblastoma with lymphadenectomy: a preliminary report. Surg Endosc 15:489–492

Iwanaka T, Arai M, Kawashima H et al. (2001b) Surgical treatment for abdominal neuroblastoma in the laparoscopic era. Surg Endosc 15:751–754

Iwanaka T, Yamamoto K, Ogawa Y et al. (2001c) Maturation of mass-screened localized adrenal neuroblastoma. J Pediatr Surg 36:1633–1636

Iwanaka T, Arai M, Yamamoto H et al. (2003) No incidence of port-site recurrence after endosurgical procedure for pediatric malignancies. Pediatr Surg Int 19:200–203

Iwanaka T, Arai M, Kawashima H et al. (2004) Endosurgical procedures for pediatric solid tumors. Pediatr Surg Int 20:39–42

Nakajima K, Fukuzawa M, Fukui Y, Komoto Y et al. (1997) Laparoscopic resection of mass-screened adrenal neuroblastoma in an 8-month-old infant. Surg Laparosc Endosc 7:498–500

Yamamoto H, Yoshida M, Sera Y (1996) Laparoscopic surgery for neuroblastoma identified by mass screening. J Pediatr Surg 31:385–388

Urogenital Tract

Chapter 83

Introduction to Minimal Access Surgery in Pediatric Urology

Jean-Stéphane Valla

Introduction

Since the 1970s the story of pediatric urology and minimally invasive surgery has been somewhat paradoxical. The first paper about the use of laparoscopy in pediatric surgery was published in 1976 by Cortesi et al. and underlined the diagnostic interest of this procedure for intra-abdominal testes. However this "urological explorative" laparoscopy remained hidden until the end of the 1980s when the laparoscopic technique really gained impetus because of the possibility of it becoming an "operative technique." In the middle of 1990s, and in contrast to many general pediatric surgeons who definitively adopted the minimal access techniques, the majority of pediatric urologists remained reluctant because of the dramatic complications reported in an editorial in the *Journal of Urology* in 1994 by John Duckett, entitled "Pediatric laparoscopy, prudence please!" However, since about 2000, as the technique has become well mastered and safe, and as equipment specifically designed for children has become available, the use of laparoscopy in pediatric urology is gradually spreading. This is borne out by the number of publications indexed in PubMed and also by the number of chapters in this book. In the first edition in 1999 there were only 6 chapters (16%) devoted to urology, compared to 22 chapters (60%) for gastroenterology. In this new edition 34 chapters (32%) are devoted to urology, compared to 53 chapters for gastroenterology (50%).

Access to the Urogenital Tract

There are different possibilities for gaining access to the urogenital tract and each technique will be described in the following chapters.

Transperitoneal Approach

The transperitoneal approach is the approach that was used first and represents in my experience 50% of the cases. The technique is well known and easy to learn. It gives access in a natural cavity where the anatomical landmarks are obvious at first sight. This transperitoneal access allows the majority of urological procedures to be performed, not only the common procedures such as those on the gonads (testis or ovary), spermatic vessels, and kidneys, but also procedures for rare conditions such as the removal of a small ectopic kidney, Müllerian remnants, a seminal vesicle cyst, a urachal malformation, or an abdomino-scrotal hydrocele; augmentation and substitution cystoplasty; or continent urinary diversion according to Mitrofanoff's principle. The area below the bladder to the pelvic floor is perfectly seen thanks to the telescope. However this approach is not specific to urology; in classic open surgery it is less used because breaching the peritoneum carries some drawbacks. So if your philosophy is to reproduce with minimally invasive surgery (MIS) exactly the same procedure as with open surgery, you would have to imagine and settle upon another access.

Retroperitoneoscopic Approach

Durga Gaur, an Indian surgeon, is credited with the promotion of the retroperitoneoscopic approach since 1992 (Gaur 1992, 1999). This approach gives direct, fast access to the kidney, the adrenal, and the ureter. But the retroperitoneal space is a virtual space, so the surgeon must create the working space by insufflation, taking care not to injure the peritoneum. This approach represents 40% of the cases in my experience. The patient can lie in a lateral position, but a true posterior approach with the patient in prone position is also an option. The choice between a lateral and a posterior access can be adapted according to the pathology (Borzi 2001).

Another extraperitoneal access is the preperitoneal access, which gives access to the anterior part of the bladder and bladder neck. It can be useful for dissecting the urethra in order to surround it with a sling or an artificial sphincter.

Transvesicoscopic Access

The last, specifically urological, access is the transvesicoscopic access with CO_2 bladder insufflation. The trocars are introduced into the bladder through the suprapubic abdominal wall (Yeung and Borzi 2002). It gives direct access in a small, well-defined cavity for ureteral reimplantation, ureterocelectomy, bladder neck surgery, etc. This access is of a more recent date and represents only 10% of my current personal experience. It will be used more and more in the future, and will replace the Pfannenstiel incision plus anterior cystotomy.

Indications

The indications for using MIS can be classified into three categories. First it includes all diagnostic procedures, especially regarding the gonads and genital tract in girls. These procedures are widely and definitely accepted by the community of pediatric urologists. The second group comprises simple therapeutic procedures, for example simple varicocelectomy, orchidopexy, and total nephrectomy. These procedures are now practiced by an increasing number of surgeons. The third group comprises advanced techniques, for example partial nephrectomy and all reconstructive procedures such as pyeloplasty, ureteral reimplantation, ureterocelectomy, etc. These techniques are performed by only a few teams and are not yet validated, but they are challenges for the future.

Conclusions

To conclude this introduction, what have been the outstanding innovations in pediatric urology since 1980? Some are diagnostic procedures, such as ultrasound, antenatal diagnosis, magnetic resonance imaging (MRI), and mertiatide (MAG3) scintiscan, and some are therapeutic procedures, such as subureteric injection or extracorporeal shock wave lithotripsy. All these innovations have been rapidly and widely accepted. MIS is at the same time a diagnostic and therapeutic procedure but, even after more than 10 years, remains little developed. Why? Essentially because it is difficult to practice, and the number of indications is limited. However each pediatric urologist should master these new techniques. To gain expertise one should try to share this type of surgery in the same department. All members should be able to perform the simple procedures, but one surgeon must be dedicated to do advanced procedures in order to maintain sufficient skill.

References

Borzi PA (2001) A comparison of lateral and posterior retroperitoneoscopic approach for complete and partial nephrectomy in children. BJU Int 87:517–550

Cortesi N, Ferrai P, Zambarda E, et al (1976) Diagnosis of bilateral abdominal cryptorchidism by laparoscopy. Endoscopy 8:33–34

Duckett JW (1994) Laparoscopy in children: prudence please! J Urol 151:742–743

Gaur DD (1992) Laparoscopic operative retroperitoneoscopy: use of a new device. J Urol 148:1137–1139

Gaur DD (1999) The accurate placement of the balloon for retroperitoneal dissection by the percutaneous method, insuring that it expands in the right place. BJU Int 84:1095–1096

Yeung CK, Borzi PA (2002) Pneumovesicoscopic COHEN ureteric reimplantation with carbon dioxide bladder insufflations for gross VUR. BJU Int 89(suppl 2):15–86

Chapter 84

Basic Technique: Retroperitoneoscopic Approach in the Lateral Position

Jean-Stéphane Valla

Introduction

The lateral position for retroperitoneal access has been used since the early 1990s in adults and children. This access has been demonstrated as reliable for a large number of indications (Franks et al. 2003; Gaur 1999; Merrot et al. 1998; Micali et al. 2001; Ng et al. 1999; Peters 2003; Valla 1999). The lateral position is familiar to the urologist and, if an urgent open conversion is needed, the lateral position offers the best exposure to control the great vessels.

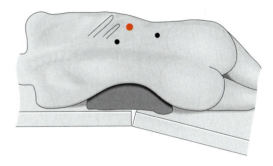

Fig. 84.1. Position of patient for renal access

Preoperative Preparation

The parents are asked to give their informed consent to the procedure. This is essential in the pediatric population because the reported benefits of a retroperitoneoscopic approach have not been firmly established. Children are prepared for surgery as usual without bowel preparation.

General anesthesia with muscular relaxation and monitoring of end-tidal CO_2 is necessary. Nitrous oxide is generally contraindicated to reduce bowel distension. A nasogastric tube is introduced for the same purpose. A bladder catheter is inserted to quantify diuresis. A preoperative antibiotic dose is given according to the etiology: it is not necessary in case of dysplastic multicystic kidney removal, but is necessary in case of a kidney destroyed by an obstructive or refluxing uropathy, pyeloplasty, or ureterotomy.

Positioning of Patient, Crew, Monitors, and Equipment

The patient is placed in a lateral kidney position with lumbar hyperflexion in order to enlarge the space between the last rib and the iliac crest (Fig. 84.1). The surgeon and assistant face the back of the patient. The video column stands on the other side, and the cables are fixed to the superior part of the operative field. If a total ureterectomy is needed at the same time, the position of the surgeon and his assistant, and the position of the video column may change during the procedure; the installation must be planned accordingly. During the renal phase of the procedure, the surgeon is placed between the assistant and the nurse and the instruments are pointed toward the diaphragmatic area (Fig. 84.2a). During ureteral phase, the surgeon stands at the head of the patient, and the instruments are pointed toward the bladder (Fig. 84.2b).

A plastic bag is fixed to the dorsal part of the patient and instruments are put away in this bag: monopolar hook, bipolar forceps, harmonic scalpel, aspiration cannula.

Special Equipment

Some devices are useful:
- A special cannula with a balloon or umbrella to avoid any dislodgment that could be frustrating, especially if it occurs during critical handling. If simple cannulas are used, they must be secured.
- An efficient suction-irrigation device is mandatory.
- The harmonic scalpel or Ligasure are useful to manage the vascular pedicle, but a simple ligature or 5 mm clips are sufficient. An endostapler has never been necessary in our experience in children.

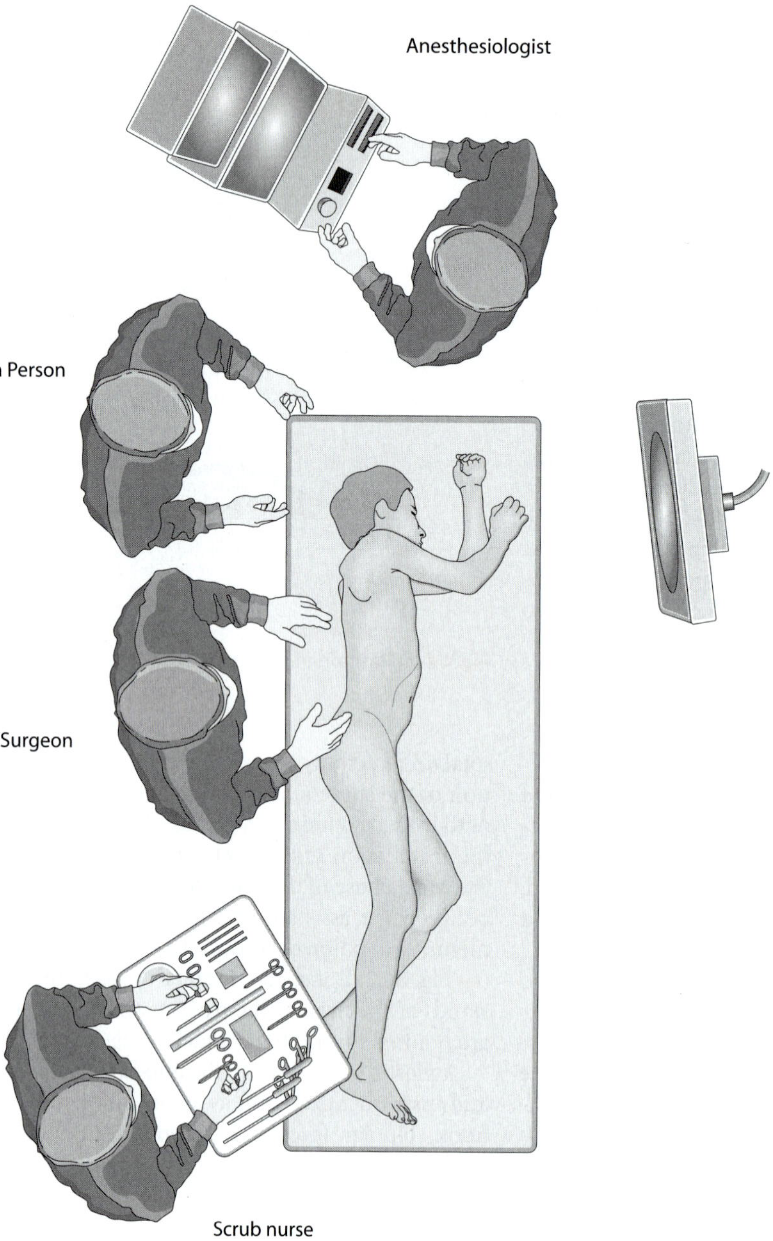

Anesthesiologist

Fig. 84.2. a Position of crew and equipment for renal access

Camera Person

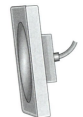

Surgeon

a   Scrub nurse

Technique

First Port Placement

We favor an open technique for primary retroperitoneal access. This is the key point of the technique because the majority of complications occur during access and the development of the working field (Peters 2003).

After sterile preparation and draping, anatomical landmarks are palpated (11th and 12th ribs, iliac crest, sacrospinalis muscle) and the surgeon mentally localizes the lateral peritoneal reflection (■ Fig. 84.3a). In children, even in adolescents, the cutaneous incision is too small to enable finger dissection of the retroperitoneal space. If the incision is oversized, resultant gas leak could be managed with large retaining sutures or large cannulas with fascial retention balloons. However to avoid a frustrating gas leak, the incision for the first cannula must be chosen carefully according to the size of the patient (0–18 years), the thickness of the abdominal wall (thin or obese child), and the disease (small or huge kidney, perinephritic adhesion or not, etc.) while thinking also of the extraction of the specimen: enlargement of the subcostal hole or inguinal incision to remove the entire ureter with the specimen. A 10 mm scope in a small child takes more room and

Fig. 84.2. b Position of crew and equipment for ureteral access

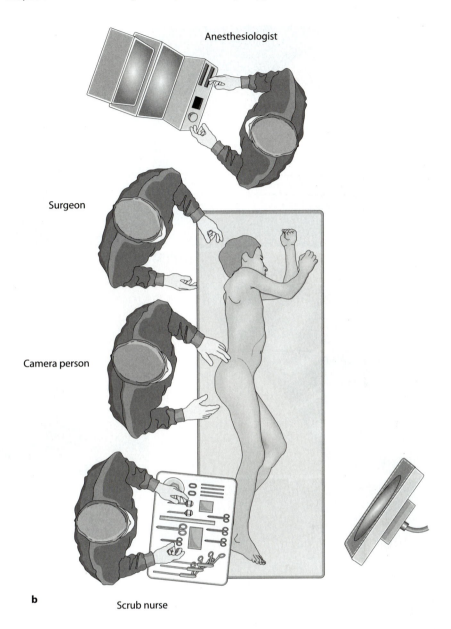

Anesthesiologist

Surgeon

Camera person

Scrub nurse

b

could impede the operating instruments. The choice must be adapted to each case: for example to remove a dysplastic multicystic kidney in a normal child less than 2 years of age, a 5 mm telescope and two 3 mm normal cannulas for operating instruments seems a good option. In contrast, in order to remove a large hydronephrotic infected kidney in an obese teenager, there is no other way for the primary access than a quite large skin incision (20 mm) and the use of a large cannula with balloon for the primary access.

In any case the skin incision (8- to 15 mm-long) is made just below the 12th rib tip at the posterior axillary line, in the area where the muscular wall is the thinnest (Fig. 84.3b). A muscle-splitting dissection is used to gain access into the retroperitoneal space; dissecting forceps, S retractors, and Metzenbaum scis-sors are usually sufficient to bluntly divide the external oblique and internal oblique muscles. After piercing the white transversalis fascia with the tip of scissors, the dissection is stopped when the yellow perirenal fat becomes visible. Two stay sutures are placed on each side of the muscular layers (2/0 short curved needle, semicircular 16 mm). In case of a large (15 mm) incision, it is sometimes possible to recognize Gerota's fascia and incise it in order to begin CO_2 insufflation directly into the perirenal space. However most often Gerota's fascia is not visible and so the working space is created in the retroperitoneal space; Gerota's fascia will be opened posteriorly in the following step.

Next, a small gauze is introduced into the retroperitoneal space and manipulated carefully to create the space (Fig. 84.3c,d). The surgeon must keep the dis-

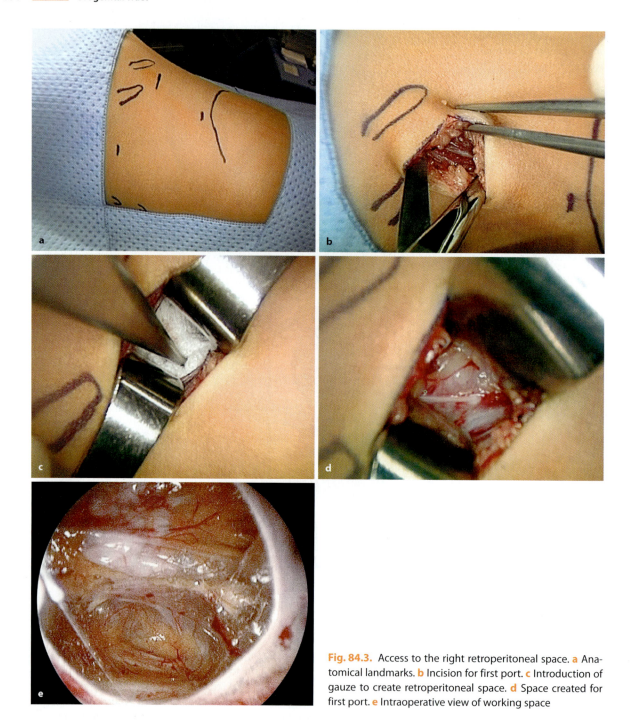

Fig. 84.3. Access to the right retroperitoneal space. **a** Anatomical landmarks. **b** Incision for first port. **c** Introduction of gauze to create retroperitoneal space. **d** Space created for first port. **e** Intraoperative view of working space

section in close touch with the posterior muscular wall to avoid peritoneal perforation. The primary blunt port (5- to 10 mm, disposable or reusable) is placed and secured to create a seal for the retropneumoperitoneum. CO_2 insufflation is started (8–10 mmHg in infants; 12–15 mmHg in children). A 0° or 30° lens is inserted. The working space, already created by the gauze, is progressively enlarged by moving the tip of the telescope, used as a palpator to free retroperitoneal fibrous tissues, behind the kidney (■ Fig. 84.3e). This allows the exposure of the anatomical landmarks: quadratus lumborum, psoas muscles, and posterior part of the kidney. The thick lateral and posterior abdominal wall, closely attached to the bony boundaries, cannot be distended by insufflation as well as the anterior abdominal wall (this explains why a good curarization is essential), so a sufficient operating space can only be achieved by pushing away peritoneum and intra-abdominal organs and by dissecting the lateral peritoneal reflection at least to the anterior axillary line.

Placement of Accessory Ports

Two additional ports (3- or 5 mm) are placed under direct vision: the posterior port is introduced first, in the costospinal angle, at the junction of the lateral border of the erector spinae muscle with the underside of the 12th rib. Before placing the inferior port just above the iliac crest, an instrument (palpator in 3 mm incision, endopeanut in 5 mm incision) is inserted through the posterior port and is gently swept medially of the lateral peritoneal reflection in the lower part of the field. Now the third inferior trocar can be introduced safely. This inferior trocar must not be placed too close to the iliac crest because the bony relief could restrict the device's mobility. This port placement allows a triangulation of ports to be achieved in order to maximize exposure and minimize instrument conflict in a small working space (■ Fig. 84.1, 84.3).

Exit

The closure of fascia is easy because of the two stay sutures placed at the beginning of the procedure. Port sites are injected with bupivacaine and lidocaine. The skin is closed with subcuticular stitches and/or adhesive strips.

Results

Our personal experience of the lateral retroperitoneoscopic approach consists of 283 cases for the following indications:

Personal experience	
Total nephrectomy	100
Varicocele	80
Pyeloplasty	40
Partial nephrectomy	35
Adrenalectomy	15
Stone	3
Retrocaval ureter	2
Biopsy	8

Operative incidents related to access involved in 71 cases (25%) of peritoneal perforation but in no case did peritoneal perforation induce a conversion. There were 9 cases of mild subcutaneous emphysema, 1 case of pelvic perforation (huge hydronephrosis), 1 case of diaphragmatic tear, and 1 case of transient abdominal wall muscle paralysis. There were no vascular injuries and no case of pneumomediastinum.

Discussion of Technical Points

As for intraperitoneal laparoscopy, the retroperitoneal approach can be performed by either a blind or an open technique. Visual control represents the best guarantee against visceral or vascular injuries, and it allows safe introduction of an atraumatic smooth trocar. But if a 5 mm port is chosen, it is difficult to see all the abdominal layers and the perirenal fat through a small hole. Capolicchio et al. (2003) have described a first port placement by blind and blunt dissection at the location of the posterior port, that is to say at the level of the costovertebral angle and not at the tip of the 12th rib as in our technique; this technique allows the introduction of a 5 mm cannula and avoids a gas leak and peritoneal entry because the peritoneal reflection is far away from this area. Blunt dissection may also be started using the Visiport system for direct vision placement of the port into the retroperitoneal space (Micali et al. 2001); but Visiport is expensive.

The creation of the working space can be carried out directly with conventional instruments or with an inflatable balloon. This last technique, described for adults by Gaur (1999), seems superfluous in children because the pediatric retroperitoneum is significantly different from the adult retroperitoneum: there is less fat and there are fewer adhesions. So we favor the creation of the working space with blunt instruments, especially endoscopic peanuts as described by Wakabayashi et al. (2003).

The consequences of CO_2 insufflation into the retroperitoneal space does not carry any specific risk. Hemodynamic changes and CO_2 diffusion were similar with intraperitoneal and retroperitoneal laparoscopic techniques as demonstrated experimentally in piglets (Diemunsch et al. 1999) and clinically in adults (Ng et al. 1999). Our results seem to confirm this as we had no deleterious effects of retroperitoneal insufflation, and no pneumothorax, pneumomediastinum, or gas embolism have been recorded.

The most common complication is peritoneal tear, particularly in smaller children where the peritoneum is thinner and less layered with fat. Accidental perforation induces pneumoperitoneum and reduces the retroperitoneal working space and visibility. In smaller children the peritoneum is permeable and intraperitoneal insufflation can occur without visible tear after prolonged operative time. The peritoneum is particularly vulnerable at the beginning of the procedure, when creating the working space, and at the end of the procedure, when dissecting the anterior part of the kidney and the lower part of the ureter. If peritoneal insufflation occurs at the beginning of the procedure, there are several potential solutions. The most elegant, but difficult, is to close the perforation with a 5/0 purse-string suture; the most simple is to desufflate the pneumoperitoneum continuously using a Veress needle. If the working space is not improved by the previous maneuvers, then Peters' advice is to open the peritoneum widely and to continue the total nephrectomy using a mixed retroperitoneal and intraperitoneal approach (Peters 2003). In our experience that has never been necessary and an unexpected peritoneal perforation has never been the sole motive for conversion.

Ten years ago at the beginning of our experience, dense perirenal adhesions due to previous nephrostomy, repeated perinephritis, or xanthogranulomatous pyelonephritis were considered as contraindications for retroperitoneoscopic nephrectomy. Now, we attempt a retroperitoneoscopic approach and most of the time we succeed (Merrot et al. 1998).

The classic open flank incision can alter the body image because of scarring and lateral abdominal wall protrusion (or posterolateral bulging), as described in adults (Yoshimura et al. 2003). Reducing the wound aggression must decrease postoperative pain, wound complications, hospital stay, and scarring. These advantages can be decisive in children expecting renal transplantation or who are on immunosuppressive therapy which delays wound healing.

Conclusion

In our mind, the lateral position for nephrectomy is considered as an established indication, even if a learning curve is necessary to reduce peritoneal tears. The lateral position is the safest option in case of conversion for vascular problems, even though this has never been necessary in our experience.

References

Capolicchio JP, Jednak R, Anidjar M, Pippi Salle JL (2003) A modified access technique for retroperitoneoscopic renal surgery in children. J Urol 170:204–206

Diemunsch P, Becmeur F, Meyer P (1999) Retroperitoneoscopy versus laparoscopy in piglets: ventilatory and thermic repercussion. J Pediatr Surg 34:1514–1517

Franks M, Schneck FX, Docimo SG (2003) Retroperitoneoscopy in children. In: Caione P, Kavoussi LR, Micali R (eds) Retroperitoneoscopy and Extraperitoneal Laparoscopy in Pediatric and Adult Urology. Springer, Berlin Heidelberg New York pp 103–118

Gaur DD (1999) The accurate placement of the balloon for retroperitoneal dissection by the percutaneous method, insuring that it expands in the right plane. BJU Int 84:1095

Merrot T, Ordorica Flores R, Steyaert H, Ginier C, Valla JS (1998) Is diffuse xanthogranulomatous pyelonephritis a contra-indication to retroperitoneoscopic nephro-ureterectomy? Surg Laparosc Endosc 8:366–369

Micali S, Caione P, Virgini G, Capozza N, Scarfini M, Micali F (2001) Retroperitoneal access in children using a direct vision technique. J Urol 165:1229–1232

Ng CS, Gill IS, Sung GT, Whalley DG, Graham R, Schweizer D (1999) Retroperitoneoscopic surgery is not associated with increased carbon dioxide absorbtion. J Urol 162:1268–1272

Peters GA (2003) Complications of retroperitoneal laparoscopy in pediatric urology: prevention, recognition and management. In: Caione P, Kavoussi LR, Micali R (eds) Retroperitoneoscopy and Extraperitoneal Laparoscopy in Pediatric and Adult Urology. Springer, Berlin Heidelberg New York pp 203–210

Valla JS (1999) Videosurgery of the retroperitoneal space in children. In: Bax KMA, Georgeson KE, Najmaldin AS, Valla JS (eds) Endoscopic Surgery in Children. Springer, Berlin Heidelberg New York pp 379–392

Wakabayashi Y, Kataoka A, Johnin K, Yoshiki T, Okada Y (2003) Simple techniques for atraumatic peritoneal dissection from the abdominal wall and for preventing peritoneal injury during trocar placement under retroperitoneoscopy. J Urol 169:256–257

Yoshimura K, Ohara H, Ichioka K, Terada N, Matsui Y, Tarai A, Arai Y (2003) Body image alteration after flank incision: relationship between the result of objective evaluation using computerized tomography and patient perception. J Urol 169:182–185

Chapter 85

Total Nephrectomy: Transperitoneal Approach

M.U. Shenoy and Duncan T. Wilcox

Introduction

Laparoscopic nephrectomy was first performed by Clayman et al. in 1990 (Clayman et al. 1991) and since then there have been numerous reports describing the success of laparoscopy in urological practice. The first paediatric laparoscopic nephrectomy was performed in 1993 (Koyle et al. 1993). The advantages with the laparoscopic approach have been a reduction in the postoperative pain, faster recovery and consequently shorter hospital stay, and improved cosmesis (Desgrandchamps et al. 1999; Erlich et al. 1994; Hamilton et al. 2000; Najmaldin 1999; Yao and Poppas 2000), although these may be less significant in the smaller patients.

Laparoscopic nephrectomy can be performed transperitoneally or via the retroperitoneal approach. The former technique is described in detail here.

Indications

These are for benign renal diseases including nonfunctioning kidneys, multicystic dysplasic kidneys and occasionally for protein-losing nephritis. There are no absolute contraindications but relative contraindications include coagulation disorders, inflammatory renal conditions, such as xanthogranulomatous pyelonephritis, and cardiopulmonary disease.

Preoperative Preparation

No specific bowel preparation is necessary. A rectal enema may be given preoperatively.

Anaesthesia

The operation is carried out under general anaesthesia. Nitrous oxide is avoided to reduce bowel distension. At the future port sites 1 ml/kg of 0.25% Marcaine is injected , ensuring that the peritoneum is infiltrated. A nasogastric tube is placed.

Positioning

Patient

The patient is placed in a lateral position with the side to be operated on uppermost. The table is broken in the standard kidney position or a ballast is placed under the patient (■ Figs. 85.1, 85.2). The patient is positioned at the edge of the table ensuring free movement of the laparoscopic instruments.

Crew, Monitors and Equipment

Figure 85.2 shows the positions of the crew and equipment.

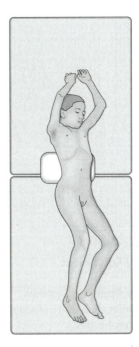

Fig. 85.1. Position for a right nephrectomy. Lateral position with a ballast placed under the right side

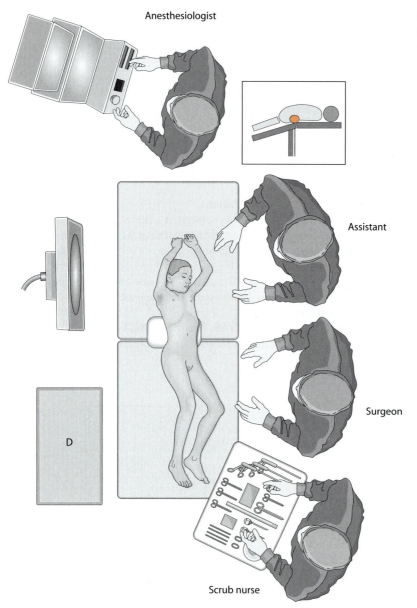

Anesthesiologist

Assistant

Surgeon

Scrub nurse

D

Fig. 85.2. Position for a right nephrectomy: crew, monitor and equipment

Special Equipment

Energy Applying Systems

Unipolar or bipolar diathermy is required, and a harmonic scalpel may be used.

Other Equipment

A clip applicator and retrieval bag are required.

Technique

Cannulae

A three-trocar technique is used (Fig. 85.3). One 10 mm umbilical port is placed by the open Hassan technique, and two 5 mm ports are placed under direct vision.

Procedure

The colon is reflected by incising the peritoneal fold laterally (Fig. 85.4) and Gerota's fascia is opened. Mobilisation of the kidney is performed using dissect-

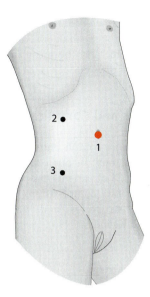

Fig. 85.3. Position of the ports: *1* umbilical, *2* and *3* in iliac fossa and right hypochondrium

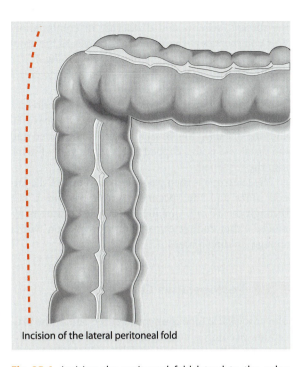

Incision of the lateral peritoneal fold

Fig. 85.4. Incising the peritoneal fold lateral to the colon (*dashed line*)

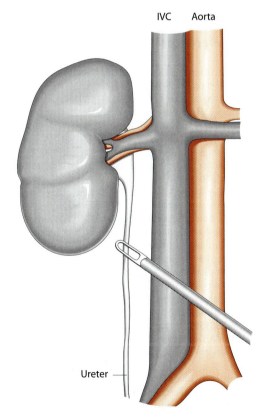

IVC   Aorta

Ureter

Fig. 85.5. Dissection of the kidney: *1* lower pole, *2* anterior surface, *3* upper pole. Ureter is held with forceps to help dissection of the renal hilum. *IVC* Inferior vena cava

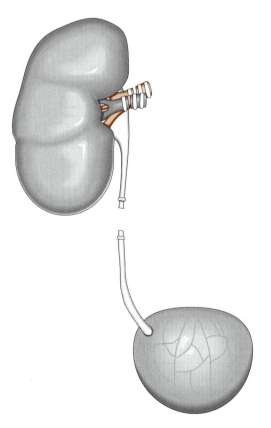

Fig. 85.6. Vessels clipped and divided between clips, two proximal and one distal

ing forceps, scissors and diathermy in combination. This commences at the lower pole, moves to the anterior surface and then to the upper pole (▬ Fig. 85.5). The ureter and/or the renal pelvis can be used to create tension allowing easier dissection.

The renal hilum is isolated and the vessels individually identified and divided between clips, two proximal and one distal (▬ Fig. 85.6). The ureter is divided and the distal end is also clipped to prevent reflux of urine into the renal bed.

The telescope is then placed through one of the lateral ports and the specimen is retrieved in a bag through the 10 mm umbilical port. The kidney is removed either completely or after morcellation with a sponge-holding forceps.

Postoperative Care

The nasogastric tube is removed at the end of the procedure. Feeding is commenced a few hours after the procedure. Analgesia is given with an opiate infusion. Oral analgesics are commenced once oral feeds are established.

Outcomes

This is a single surgeon's experience with the technique. Transperitoneal total nephrectomy was performed in 21 patients, including 12 boys and 9 girls over a 4-year period. The age at operation ranged from 9 to 184 months (mean 45.4 months) and the mean weight of the patient was 17.1 kg (range 8–64 kg). The indications for the procedure were multicystic dysplastic kidneys in 7 patients, dysplastic kidneys in 2 patients, vesicoureteral reflux (VUR) in 9 patients and pelviureteric junction (PUJ) obstruction with poorly functioning kidneys in 3 patients. The mean size of the kidneys was 5.1 cm (range 2–9 cm) and the pathology was left-sided in 14 patients and right-sided in 7 patients.

The lateral position was used in all 21 patients. The mean operating time was 97 min (range 42–250 min). Total nephrectomy was performed in 17 patients and nephroureterectomy in 4 patients with VUR. Other additional procedures were performed in 4 patients: ureteric reimplantation and Mitrofanoff formation in 1 patient (this was the patient with the operating time of 250 min), macroplastique injection into the bladder neck in 1 patient and circumcision in 2 patients.

The mean hospital stay was 1.6 days (range 1–5 days) and mean follow-up was 5.4 months (range 3–24 months). This is similar to other reports as shown in

a series of 24 patients reported by Davies and Najmaldin (1998) where the mean operative time was 85 min (range 40–160 min) and the mean hospital stay was 2 days (range 1–4 days).

Pitfalls and Complications

There were no major complications related to the laparoscopic nephrectomy in our experience. Adhesions were noted in 9.8% of patients in one series (Moore et al. 1995). Other rare complications include injury to intraperitoneal structures and port site hernias (Capelouto and Kavoussi 1993).

Conclusions

Total transperitoneal laparoscopic nephrectomy is a safe operation in experienced hands. Once the learning curve has been overcome, it can probably replace open nephrectomy procedures in most instances.

References

Capelouto CC, Kavoussi LR (1993) Complications of laparoscopic surgery. Urology 42:2–12

Clayman RV, Kavoussi LR, Soper NJ et al. (1991) Laparoscopic nephrectomy: initial case report. J Urol 146:278–282

Davies BW, Najmaldin AS (1998) Transperitoneal laparoscopic nephrectomy in children. J Endourol 12:437–440

Desgrandchamps F, Gossot D, Jabbour ME et al. (1999) A 3 trocar technique for transperitoneal laparoscopic nephrectomy. J Urol 161:1530–1532

Ehrlich RM, Gershman A, Fuchs G (1994) Laparoscopic renal surgery in children. J Urol 151:735–739

Hamilton BD, Gatti JM, Cartwright PC et al. (2000) Comparison of laparoscopic versus open nephrectomy in the pediatric population. J Urol 163:937–939

Koyle MA, Woo HH, Kavoussi LR (1993) Laparoscopic nephrectomy in the first year of life. J Pediatr Surg 28:693–695

Moore RG, Kavoussi LR, Bloom DA et al. (1995) Pediatric urology: postoperative adhesion formation after urological laparoscopy in the pediatric population. J Urol 153:792–795

Najmaldin AS (1999) Transperitoneal laparoscopic nephrectomy. In: Bax NMA, Georgeson KE, Najmaldin AS, Valla J-S (eds) Endoscopic Surgery in Children. Springer, Berlin Heidelberg New York

Yao D, Poppas DP (2000) A clinical series of laparoscopic nephrectomy, nephroureterectomy and heminephroureterectomy in the pediatric population. J Urol 163:1531–1535

Chapter 86

Total Nephrectomy: Lateral Retroperitoneoscopic Approach

Jean-Stéphane Valla and Henri Steyaert

Introduction

Retroperitoneal endoscopic surgery in the lateral position has been used since the early 1990s both in adults and in children. This access has been demonstrated to be reliable for a large number of indications particularly total ureteronephrectomy, pyeloplasty, and pyelotomy (El Ghoneimi et al. 2000; Franks et al. 2003; Hemal et al. 1999; Leclair et al. 2003; Merrot et al. 1998; Valla 1999). The lateral position is familiar to the urologist and, if urgent conversion is needed, the lateral position offers the best exposure to control the great vessels.

Preoperative Preparation

Preoperative preparation, positioning of patients, monitors, and equipment, and port placement have already been described in Chapter 84.

Positioning

Patient

The patient is positioned laterally on the operating table with a sand bag underneath the lumbar region and a bend in the table at the same level in order to widen the space between the 12th rib and the iliac crest (■ Fig. 86.1a,b). During the renal phase of the operation, the table is put in reversed Trendelenburg position, and during the ureteric phase it is in Trendelenburg.

Crew, Monitor, and Equipment

The surgeon stands behind the patient. During the renal phase of the operation, the assistant stands to surgeon's left, and during the ureteric phase at the surgeon's right (■ Fig. 86.2a,b). The monitor stands close to the patient's head during the renal phase, and near the patient's hip during the ureteric phase.

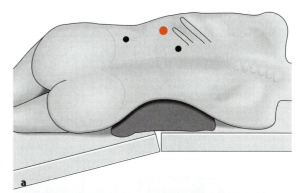

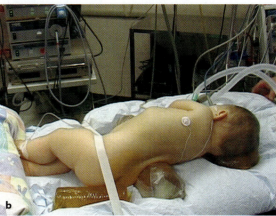

Fig. 86.1. Left lateral positioning for a left nephrectomy. **a** Older child. **b** Baby

Anesthesiologist

Fig. 86.2 Right nephrectomy. **a** Position of crew and equipment during the renal phase of the operation

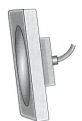

Camera Person

Surgeon

a

Scrub nurse

Technique

Cannula Insertion

Figure 86.3 shows the port positions for a left nephrectomy. See Chapter 84 for a detailed description of port insertion.

Operative Steps

Initial Dissection and Control of the Renal Hilum

After the development of the working space, the landmarks should be clearly visible, especially the posterior part of the kidney, the great vessels, and the ureter. With the help of two atraumatic instruments (probe, grasper, or peanut) Gerota's fascia is largely opened, if not already done, along the posterior part of kidney (■ Fig. 86.4).

Anterior dissection should be limited at the beginning of the procedure to prevent peritoneal injury and to prevent the kidney from dropping ventrally. When

Fig. 86.2 Right nephrectomy. **b** Position of crew and equipment during the ureteric phase of the operation

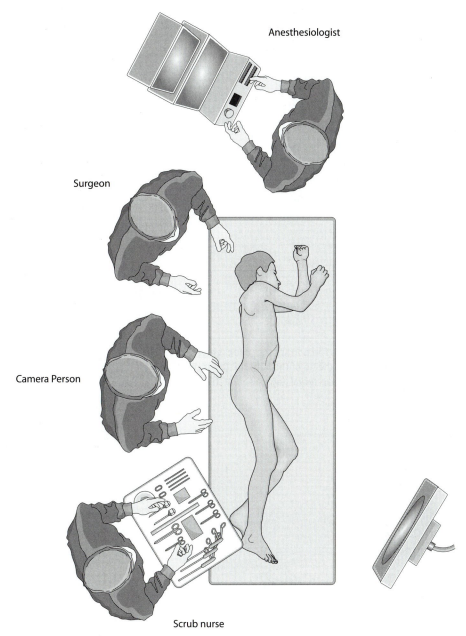

Anesthesiologist

Surgeon

Camera Person

Scrub nurse

b

the anterior peritoneal adherences are kept intact, the kidney is automatically pushed anteriorly and to the top of the operative field by the insufflation pressure, giving a good posterior access to the hilum. If this spontaneous pushing out of the operative field is not sufficiently achieved, a third operating device, usually a 3 mm one, can be introduced in the midaxillary line for retraction of the kidney into the upper part of the field.

The renal artery and vein, which appear vertically in the operative field, are cleared with a hook or scissors in the inferior part of the field where there is only one artery and one vein. When this is done close to the hilum of the kidney, where the vessels divide, several branches are encountered. The vessels do not need to be taken at their origin from the aorta or entrance into the caval vein, but an area of at least 1 cm should be exposed to allow for safe control of the vessels on each side of the intended severance. Countertraction using the non-dominant hand is useful to create a large window around the vein and artery.

If the search for the renal vessels proves difficult, the ureter may serve as a lead point; the ureter is easy to discover in the retroperitoneal space, and its dissection up to the kidney automatically leads to the renal vessels.

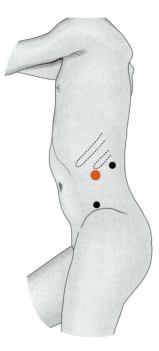

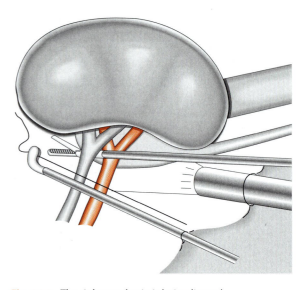

Fig. 86.5. The right renal vein is being ligated

Fig. 86.3. Port positioning. The port for the scope is inserted in an open way just below the tip of the 12th rib. The second port is inserted in the costovertebral angle and the third port above the iliac crest

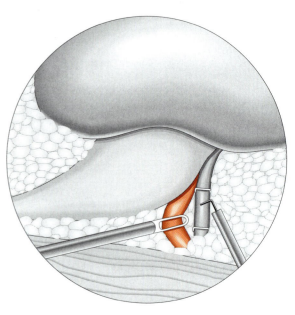

Fig. 86.6. The left renal vein has been clipped and will be severed in between the clips

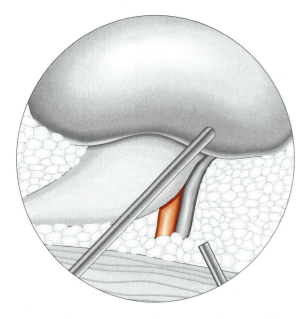

Fig. 86.4. The posterior side of the kidney is freed using blunt instruments

Vascular Control

The artery is controlled first. Many methods of hemostasis can be used depending on the anatomical situation and the diameter of the vessel. Monopolar coagulation with the hook suffices in case of tiny vessels, bi-

polar coagulation, ultrasonic severance, or Ligasure in case of middle-sized vessels, and extracorporeal ligature or clips in case of large vessels (Figs. 86.5, 86.6).

Specimen Dissection

Dissection using electrocautery or ultrasonic scissors continues from caudal to cranial. Polar vessels may be encountered. Careful dissection allows them to be recognized and to be dealt with according to their size. The upper pole dissection separates the kidney from the adrenal gland in an avascular plane (Fig. 86.7).

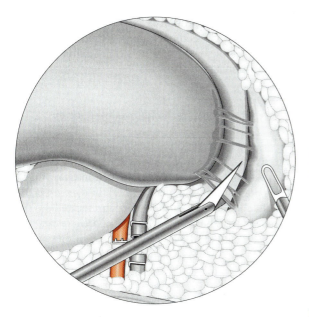

Fig. 86.7. Renal artery and vein have been divided. The upper pole is now freed

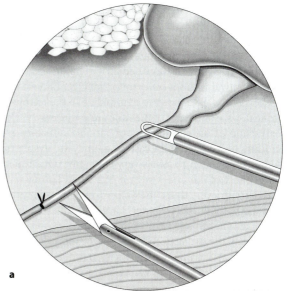

a

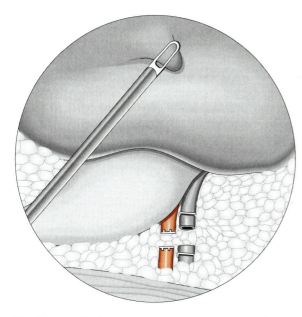

Fig. 86.8. Finally the anterior surface of the kidney is released from the peritoneum

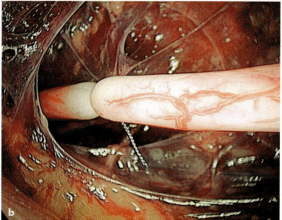

b

Fig. 86.9 a,b. The ureter has been distally ligated and will be severed

Lastly the anterior part of the kidney is freed and now the kidney is totally disconnected (■ Fig. 86.8).

▌ Management of the Ureter
Non-refluxing Ureter
Ureterectomy can be limited to the lumbar part and a ligature is not necessary; it can just be cut (■ Fig. 86.9a,b).

Refluxing or Dilated Ureter
Here total ureterectomy is essential to avoid postoperative complications related to the stump. In children less than 5 or 6 years of age it is possible to remove the lower part of the ureter retroperitoneoscopically. After changing the position of the team and monitor, the ureteral dissection is carried out down to the bladder, taking care not to injure the peritoneum (which sticks around the ureter) or the gonadal vessels. The smaller the child, the easier it is to reach the bladder. In boys the vas is seen crossing the ureter, which marks the inferior level of resection. The ureteral ligature is made by using a pretied ligature or by an extracorporeal ligature. In children over 5 or 6 years of age, and particularly in girls with a very dilated low ectopic ureter, it seems preferable to remove the lower part of the ureter in an open manner through a low inguinal incision. This short incision allows resection of the ureter close

to the bladder or vagina and extraction of the ureter together with the kidney through this incision.

Specimen Removal

The benign nature of most pediatric renal diseases enables removal without concern for spillage. Endoscopic retrieval bags are difficult to manipulate in the retroperitoneal space and most of the time are unnecessary. The extraction of the specimen is of variable difficulty according to its volume. In case of multicystic dysplastic kidney, extraction becomes very easy after puncture of all or most of the cysts. In case of a small kidney or a kidney with a very thin cortex, the extraction can be performed without morcellation. Large specimens can be extracted after enlargement of the 10 mm port hole, with or without the use of an endobag and/or morcellation. If a low inguinal or Pfannenstiel incision is needed for another purpose, the kidney can be extracted through it.

Removal of the Ports

After extraction of the specimen, the primary port with telescope is reintroduced to check the hemostasis at low insufflation pressure particularly near the hilum. If needed a drain is introduced through the inferior cannula. Ports are removed under direct vision.

Postoperative Care

In case of drainage, the drain is removed at day 1 or day 2 postoperatively. An ultrasound is performed after 1 week and 1 month to check the lumbar area. Annual controls focus on the remaining kidney.

Special Circumstances

Dense Perirenal Adhesions

At the beginning of our experience, about ten years ago, dense perirenal adhesions as a result of a previous nephrostomy, repeated perinephritis, or xanthogranulomatous pyelonephritis were considered to be a contraindication for retroperitoneoscopic nephrectomy. Under these circumstances nowadays we try a retroperitoneoscopic approach and in most instances we succeed (Merrot et al. 1998).

Horseshoe/Ectopic Kidney

We and others (Leclair et al. 2003) have performed nephrectomy for horseshoe or ectopic sigmoid kidney using the same lateral approach or a modified 45° flank position. Aberrant vascular anatomy is common in these cases and careful dissection with clamping of the vessels before transection is mandatory especially in case of a sigmoid ectopic kidney. Ultrasonic scissors are very useful for cutting between healthy and destroyed parenchyma.

The Preoperatively Invisible Kidney

Sometimes a kidney is not visible preoperatively. If the non-visible kidney it is suspected to be located in the lower part of the abdomen, a transperitoneal approach seems preferable (Yeung et al. 1999). In contrast if the "invisible" kidney is suspected to be located in the normal place, the retroperitoneal approach can still be successfully used as we experienced in one of our cases.

Pretransplant Bilateral Nephrectomies

Pretransplant bilateral nephrectomies can be performed endoscopically using a bilateral retroperitoneal approach (El Ghoneimi et al. 2000).

Giant Hydronephrosis

Destroyed kidneys with giant hydronephrosis are usually under low pressure. A careful open insertion of the primary port will avoid entering the renal cortex or pelvis. After having dissected the posterior part, decompression of the renal pelvis by needle aspiration under visual control creates a large working space and therefore good exposure.

Personal Results

From 1993 to 2003 a total of 100 total nephrectomies have been performed for the following indications:

Multicystic dysplastic kidney	26
Kidney destroyed by reflux	35
Kidney destroyed by obstructive uropathy	28
Small kidney with hypertension	5
Small invisible kidney "with incontinence"	5
Xanthogranulomatous pyelonephritis	1

There were no conversions, no major complications, and no significant blood loss (no transfusions were given). Mean operative time was 95 min. In 25 cases the peritoneum was accidentally opened, but in none of the patients was conversion required. There were 4 cases of mild subcutaneous emphysema, but a pneumomediastinum or pneumothorax did not occur. Three mild postoperative complications occurred: one paralytic ileus, one wound infection, and one hematoma in the operative area. All disappeared within 1 week and without reoperation. In 32 cases a small suction drain was left for 24 h.

Pain medication requirement was minimal and no patient needed pain medication after 48 h. One day after surgery the patients were allowed to take solid food. All children returned to unrestricted activities within 6 days. A clinical and ultrasonic check-up was performed 1 week and 1 month after surgery. Mean total follow-up has been 4.8 years (range 6 months to 10 years).

Discussion

The results of six main pediatric retroperitoneoscopy series have been analyzed by Franks et al. in 2003. The results of these series are similar to ours (El Ghoneimi et al. 1998). Unfortunately there is a lack of large series and of prospective comparative studies to confirm the potential advantages. It is, however, logical to assume that less body wall trauma gives less postoperative pain, fewer wound complications, a shorter hospital stay, and a better cosmetic result. These advantages can be decisive in children who will need a renal transplantation or in children on immunosuppressive therapy which impairs wound healing (El Ghoneimi et al. 2000).

Borer et al. (1999) have shown that total nephrectomy is feasible using 2 mm instruments. May be a more important point of their publication is the fact that they have been using a prone patient position. Borzi has analyzed the pros and cons of using a lateral versus a prone patient (Borzi 2001): the lateral position creates more space, gives better access to an ectopic kidney, and achieves complete ureterectomy in almost all cases, but peritoneal tears are more common.

Conclusion

The advantages and drawbacks of a retroperitoneal versus a transperitoneal approach for nephrectomy have been already discussed (Chapter 83). Concerning total nephrectomy, the immediate access to the renal hilum during retroperitoneoscopy is a key advantage. We consider the lateral retroperitoneoscopic approach to be an established method, even when there is a learning curve for decreasing the incidence of peritoneal tears. The lateral position is the safest one in case conversion for vascular problems is required.

References

Borer JG, Cisek LJ, Atala A, et al (1999) Pediatric retroperitoneoscopic nephrectomy using 2mm instrumentation. J Urol 162:1725–1729

Borzi PA (2001) A comparison of lateral and posterior retroperitoneoscopic approach for complete and partial nephroureterectomy in children. BJU Int 87:517–520

El Ghoneimi A, Valla JS, Steyaert H, et al (1998) Laparoscopic renal surgery via a retroperitoneal approach in children. J Urol 160:1138–1141

El Ghoneimi A, Sauty L, Maintenant J, et al (2000) Laparoscopic retroperitoneal nephrectomy in high risk children. J Urol 164:1076–1079

Franks M, Schneck FX, Docimo SG (2003) Retroperitoneoscopy in children. In: Caione P, Kavoussi LR, Micali R (eds) Retroperitoneoscopy and Extraperitoneal Laparoscopy in Pediatric and Adult Urology. Springer, Berlin Heidelberg New York, pp 103–118

Hemal AK, Gupta NP, Wadha SN (1999) Modified minimal cost retroperitoneoscopic nephrectomy, nephrectomy with isthmusectomy and nephroureterectomy in children: a pilot study. BJU Int 83:823–827

Leclair MD, Camby C, Capito C, et al (2003) Retroperitoneoscopic nephrectomy of a horseshoe kidney in a child. Surg Endosc 17:1156

Merrot T, Ordorica Flores R, Steyaert H, et al (1998) Is diffuse xanthogranulomatous pyelonephritis a contra-indication to retroperitoneoscopic nephro-ureterectomy? Surg Laparosc Endosc 8:366–369

Valla JS (1999) Videosurgery of the retroperitoneal space in children. In: Bax NMA, Georgeson KE, Najmaldin AS, Valla JS (eds) Endoscopic Surgery in Children. Springer, Berlin Heidelberg New York, pp 379–392

Yeung CK, Liu KW, Ng WT, et al (1999) Laparoscopy as the investigation and treatment of choice for urinary incontinence caused by small "invisible" dysplastic kidney with infrasphincteric ureteric ectopia. BJU Int 84:324–328

Chapter 87

Total Nephrectomy: Prone Retroperitoneoscopic Approach

Craig A. Peters

Introduction

Nephrectomy is indicated in conditions with complete or near-complete absence of renal function, and is usually performed to prevent infection due to urinary stasis or to limit the risk of hypertension resulting from renal damage due to the associated condition. While malignancies are a clear indication for nephrectomy, these applications have not been conducted in children using laparoscopic techniques in any relevant numbers to date. Pretransplantation nephrectomy is indicated for a variety of reasons, including infection, hypertension, and size of the patient. The most frequent indications for nephrectomy or nephroureterectomy (■ Table 87.1) are vesicoureteral reflux and obstruction with non-function of the kidney. The latter is usually due to severe ureteropelvic junction obstruction or primary megaureter, but may also be due to an obstructing ectopic ureter or ureterocele. A single-system ectopic ureter that drains into the vagina or perineum and causes incontinence is a very satisfying indication for nephrectomy in that these patients become dry after surgery. The challenge is in making that diagnosis (Borer et al. 1998). Other possible indications include severe, unreconstructable ureteral strictures and poor renal function, or any cause of renal functional loss associated with ureteral obstruction distal to the midureter.

Selection criteria and the pathophysiology of these various conditions are detailed elsewhere, but, in general, there is little benefit to reconstructing a renal unit with less than 10% of total function on a radionuclide renal scan. There are no data to indicate the "correct" cutoff below which nephrectomy should be performed, but it should be recognized that in most cases associated with a congenital condition, function less than 10–15% will seldom increase despite successful surgery (McAleer and Kaplan 1999). The actual threshold used varies widely and is largely a matter of individual preference.

The complete absence of function on a renal scan is a good indication that it is reasonable to remove the affected unit. If it is more practical to simply achieve urinary drainage or absence of reflux, then removal is not considered essential. The long-term risks of leaving a poorly functioning renal unit remain incompletely defined and for this reason some surgeons elect to remove the affected renal unit. The concept of whether an affected unit would be able to prevent dialysis if the contralateral unit were lost is used by some, and while this may be excessively stringent, it is generally felt that 30% function is required to prevent dialysis. Perhaps optimistically, our practice has been to use a level of 10% of total uptake as the cutoff for renal salvage versus removal. It must be recognized that this is in fact an arbitrary distinction that is not based on any outcome data.

Table 87.1 Indications for nephrectomy and nephroureterectomy

Vesicoureteral reflux
Ureterovesical junction obstruction
Ectopic ureter (single system)
Reflux and obstruction associated with posterior urethral valves, neurogenic bladder
Ureteropelvic junction obstruction
Multicystic dysplasia
Pretransplantation nephrectomy

Preoperative Evaluation

In most cases the decision to perform a nephrectomy or nephroureterectomy is made on the basis of a thorough evaluation, however, occasionally it is clear that renal removal is needed, yet the functional status of the urinary tract has not been defined. The particular questions that should be answered include the status of the contralateral kidney, the presence or absence of reflux, and the location of the affected, poorly functioning kidney. These are usually evident as long as there has been a functional test such as an intravenous pyelogram (IVP) or succimer (DMSA) scan performed, a cystogram, and an ultrasound to document the location and presence of the kidney. On occasion, the kidney is so small as to make imaging difficult and some supportive evidence that the kidney is present should be sought. Computed tomography (CT) can be used in very small kidneys (Borer et al. 1998). With this information, subsequent surgical decisions can be made with confidence.

There are probably no absolute contraindications to retroperitoneal nephrectomy. Relative contraindications include multiple prior renal surgeries and uncontrolled infection or undrained abscess. The latter might be amenable to retroperitoneal nephrectomy, but this is an individual decision. As laparoscopic experience has evolved, the contraindications to laparoscopic removal of the kidney have diminished. Patients with coagulopathies due to renal failure have undergone safe laparoscopic nephrectomy (El-Ghoneimi et al. 2000).

The selection of performing the nephrectomy or nephroureterectomy using transperitoneal versus retroperitoneal approaches has also evolved in recent years. Our approach is that nephrectomy or nephroureterectomy should be performed retroperitoneally unless there are specific reasons to perform it transperitoneally. These indications would include the need to remove all of the ureter, down to the bladder. Such cases include refluxing or obstructed systems, as seen in ectopic ureters. If a contralateral open surgical ureteral reimplantation is planned, this permits open removal of the distal ureteral stump and permits retroperitoneal nephroureterectomy.

Preoperative Preparation

Patients are placed on a low residue diet the day before surgery and a single rectal suppository to reduce stool bulk. A blood clot is sent to the blood bank if needed, but no blood is prepared for transfusion as this is a rare occurrence. Parents are counseled as to the potential need for conversion to open technique in the event of inadequate control or development of any increased risk factors during the procedure.

Instruments

Instrument size can be tailored to patient size. We have used a variety of port sizes, from 2 to 10 mm (Borer et al. 1999), but in general for small children, neonates to early teens, the 3.5 mm instrument systems have been appropriate. Since clip appliers are needed for vascular control in most cases, a 5 mm port is necessary. These have reducers to permit use of the 3.5 mm instruments without an air leak. Working instruments include a scissor with electrocautery, an optional hook cautery device, a delicate grasping and dissecting instrument, preferably curved, and a larger grasping instrument for retraction. An irrigating and aspirating device is needed. The harmonic scalpel can be used in nephrectomy or nephroureterectomy, but it is most useful in partial nephrectomy. There are several retracting devices that spread out intracorporeally, but these are not often needed if the field is set up appropriately.

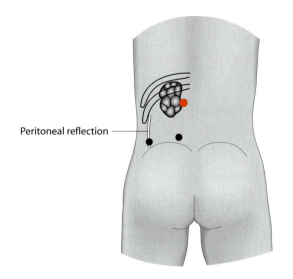

Peritoneal reflection

Fig. 87.1. Port placement for prone retroperitoneal nephrectomy. Initial port at costovertebral angle is used for specimen extraction. Usually this is a 5 mm port, while the secondary ports are 3 mm

Positioning

Patient

For retroperitoneal renal access two basic approaches are used, lateral and prone. Each has its advantages and disadvantages. The prone approach is favored by this author for all nephrectomy, but is less useful for nephroureterectomy when the entire ureter must be removed (Borer and Peters 2000). Leaving a small stump is usual with the prone approach, but in general this is not of any consequence, unless there is an impairment of ureteral drainage, as in refluxing ectopic ureters. In such a case, the lateral retroperitoneal approach or a transperitoneal technique would be recommended as it permits complete ureteral resection. The prone approach will be described in this section (Borer et al. 1999; Borzi 2001).

The prone approach (■ Fig. 87.1) is performed in the true prone position and the first port is at the costovertebral angle. Secondary ports are placed above the iliac crest lateral to the sacrospinalis muscle and at the posterior axillary line. The approach permits direct access to the renal hilum without needing to retract the kidney, and has a lesser chance of peritoneal injury. About two thirds of the ureter may be removed easily from this access.

Care is taken to provide adequate padding and support. If the operating table is to be moved during the procedure this movement should be tested before the patient is draped to make sure that new pressure points are not produced. A bladder catheter is placed in all cases.

Fig. 87.2. Positioning for left nephrectomy in the prone position.
a Staff position in older patient
with surgeon at side and assistant.
b Staff position for infant where
surgeon stands at feet of patient

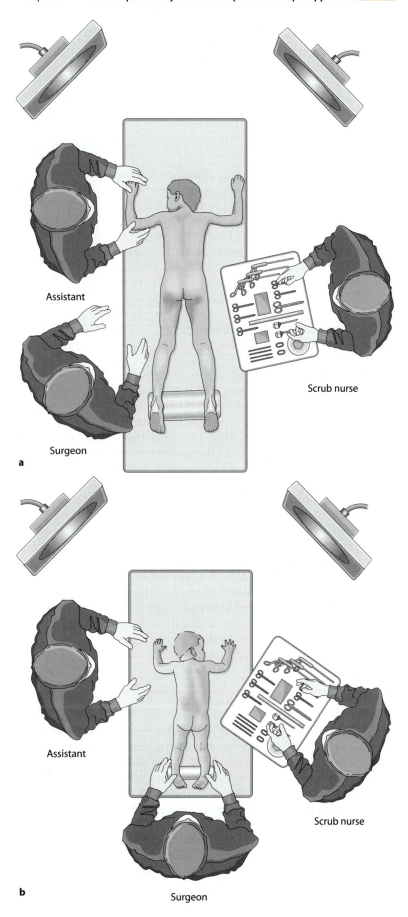

Surgical Team Positioning

Proper positioning of the surgeon and assistants is critical and is shown in ■ Fig. 87.2.

Technique

Port Placement

Figure 87.1 shows the basic port placement for the prone and lateral retroperitoneal approaches to the kidney. Attention must be paid to avoiding placing the ports too close together, which will restrict movement, particularly if ports with larger heads are in use. Placing the port too far from the retroperitoneal working area runs the risk of injury to the peritoneum. Secondary ports are placed under direct vision.

Establishing the Operative Space in the Retroperitoneum

Establishing the retroperitoneal working space is critical for all subsequent steps with this procedure. For prone access, the initial port placed at the costovertebral angle is slightly larger to permit blunt dissection to the level of Gerota's fascia. After sequential blunt spreading without muscle incision, the slightly brownish perinephric fat can be seen to bulge upward. This is the indication that Gerota's space has been entered. A dissecting balloon, made from a finger of a size 8 glove and tied to a 10 French stiff catheter with two 2-0 silk ties and lubricated, is inserted into the space. It is inflated with warm saline, up to 200 cc. The position of the bulge should be symmetric and spread throughout the area of surgery. Once the balloon is fully inflated, it is left in place for 3–5 min for hemostasis. The balloon is removed and the cannula with the endoscope is inserted. A fascial box stitch is placed to seal the insertion, retain the cannula, and close the wound at completion, as with the working ports (see below).

Developing the Working Space

With the endoscope in place, the retroperitoneum is visualized, and usually the kidney is readily apparent in a slightly superior position (■ Fig. 87.3). The endoscope is then used to bluntly expand the working space medially and inferiorly. Occasionally it is helpful at this time to expand the space superiorly, but this is usually done after the secondary ports are placed. Care must be taken to prevent peritoneal injury during this maneuver, as the edge of the peritoneum is medial to the working space and may be delicate. If the working space does not develop well, it is best to place the me-

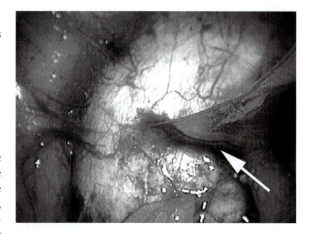

Fig. 87.3. Appearance of the posterior aspect of the left kidney with prone retroperitoneal exposure. The hilum is indicated by the *arrow*

dial port above the iliac crest and at the edge of the paraspinus muscles and then to use a blunt dissector to facilitate sweeping the peritoneum medially.

Secondary Port Placement

Two secondary ports are placed above the iliac crest at the edge of the paraspinous muscles and at the posterior axillary line. These should be placed under direct vision, but the actual entry site may not be visible in the tight working space, so the anticipated trajectory should be closely monitored. The radially expanding port system is used by this author, with Veress needle-type port introduction. This works well, but other methods are perfectly adequate. We place fascial closure stitches for all ports over 3 mm in size, and try to do so before starting the procedure to permit rapid closure at completion (Poppas et al. 1999). Once the secondary ports are placed, dissection of the kidney may begin.

Renal Exposure

It is important to develop enough renal exposure to provide orientation to the position of the kidney. This will permit directed dissection toward the hilum. Because of magnification and the inability to gauge size, locating the hilum without seeing much of the posterior surface of the kidney may be difficult. This degree of exposure should be readily accomplished with blunt dissection. The location of the hilum is usually evident once the lower pole of the kidney has been identified, but it is useful to expose the superior aspects as well to make sure the entire hilum is being exposed. With the prone retroperitoneal approach, the kidney tends to fall laterally and down from the surgeon's perspective,

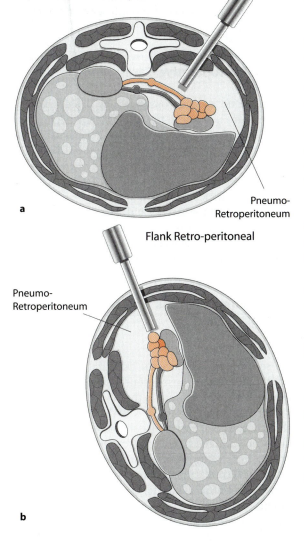

Prone Retro-peritoneal

Pneumo-
Retroperitoneum

a

Flank Retro-peritoneal

Pneumo-
Retroperitoneum

b

Fig. 87.4. Diagram of comparative exposure of the renal hilum in prone and lateral retroperitoneal renal access. From Peters CA (2000) Laparoendoscopic renal surgery in children. J Endourol 14:841–848

which stretches the hilar vessels and facilitates exposure (■ Fig. 87.4). In the lateral retroperitoneal approach however, the kidney tends to fall toward the hilum and may obscure the vessels. In this approach, it is important to approach the hilum before the lateral renal attachments have been taken down. These lateral attachments serve to provide passive lateral retraction and facilitate hilar dissection.

Control of the Renal Hilum

The critical step in any nephrectomy/nephroureterectomy is renal vascular control. With the prone approach this is facilitated by the position of the kidney, which tends to fall forward, which will reveal and stretch the renal vessels. They are exposed by a combination of blunt and sharp dissection. Small amounts of bleeding are not of great concern and can be fulgurated. Anticipation of possible anomalous vessels should be borne in mind, both at the lower and upper poles. Blunt dissection just away from the renal hilum will usually reveal the posterior artery rapidly, followed by the vein. The artery is isolated and divided first, using Ligaclips. Some authors will divide and ligate small arteries with cautery, but this is not our preference. Two clips are placed on the side that is to remain and one on the specimen side. Branches of the main renal artery must be sought, as often the dissection is closer into the hilum than usually performed with open dissection. Once the artery is taken, the vein may be controlled in a similar fashion.

Ureteral Control (Alternative)

In the setting of a more fibrotic perinephric tissue, identifying the ureter first, especially if it is going to be part of the resection, is useful. Once the ureter, usually at the lower pole is identified, it can serve as an excellent handle by which the kidney may be exposed very well. This facilitates identification of the hilum as it provides traction and exposure of the renal vessels. Dissecting toward the hilum is then undertaken with subsequent control of the vessels as described above.

Mobilizing the Kidney

Once the vessels have been controlled, the remainder of the kidney is mobilized, usually starting at the lower and medial aspect, moving medially, and then over the upper pole. If the upper pole mobilization is not moving steadily, it is best to complete the lateral and anterior mobilization, which then permits retraction on the kidney to facilitate upper pole exposure. A combination of sharp and blunt dissection is used with cautery applied generously throughout the mobilization. Care should be exercised during the mobilization to look for accessory renal vessels that may not have been controlled. This is more often seen in dysplastic or malpositioned kidneys.

During mobilization it is best to leave a hydronephrotic kidney or large cysts intact to facilitate blunt dissection. Near the completion of the process these can be decompressed by needle aspiration or incision and drainage. This may be needed earlier to permit grasping the kidney for traction.

Upper Pole Mobilization

The adrenal gland will be visualized during upper pole mobilization and should be left intact. Avoiding injury to the adrenal vessels is helpful. Sharp dissection close to the renal capsule of the upper pole will limit this risk. There are a few small vessels between the upper pole and the perinephric fat of the upper pole.

Ureteral Dissection (for Nephroureterectomy)

It is most efficient to transect the ureter below the level of the lower pole of the kidney to perform the ureteral dissection. This permits better mobility. Dissection is performed with traction on the ureter with a grasping instrument and use of the scissors to perform blunt and sharp dissection with cautery at sites of ureteral vasculature. From the prone approach it is possible to remove the ureter to about 2 cm below the iliac vessels. At the point of maximal dissection, the ureter is transected. In the case of a refluxing ureter, it must be ligated with suture. Clips are less effective and can be dislodged from the ureter due to its thick muscular wall. Either a suture ligature or free tie is appropriate. If there is no reflux, the ureter is transected and fulgurated for hemostasis. If there is uncertainty as to the presence of reflux, it is best to ligate it. An obstructed ureter, however, should not be ligated.

Specimen Removal

Once the ureter is transected, it is removed directly through the port containing the grasping instrument. The kidney is then removed through the largest port, usually 5 mm, using a heavy, locking grasping instrument with teeth. The kidney should be grasped at a pole and the entire instrument and port are brought out. The kidney is then grasped extracorporeally with a heavy Allis clamp or Kelly clamp. In some cases the decompressed kidney is easily removed, but in some situations, it must be pulled forcefully. Twisting will often help. In very large kidneys, the port site may need to be enlarged to permit removal. We have occasionally used scissor morcellation for larger organs.

Closure

All port sites are closed with the preplaced fascial sutures as noted. A dose of long-acting local anesthetic (bupivacaine 0.25%) is injected into the abdominal wall, and the subcutaneous tissues are closed with Vicryl and the skin with a subcuticular monofilament suture. The bladder catheter is left in place only if there is concern about bladder closure with a nephroureterectomy.

Postoperative Care

There are no special considerations postoperatively. Patients are encouraged to take fluids and begin a diet if comfortable. They may ambulate on the same day and some are discharged later in the day. In general, most will stay overnight and are discharged home on limited activity for 5 days with low-level analgesics. Follow-up is dependent upon the conditions for which they underwent the surgery and associated conditions. If there are no other issues, patients having had a simple nephrectomy will usually return only for a wound check 4–8 weeks postoperatively.

Complications

Access

All access methods have the potential for complications, particularly transperitoneal approaches. This is usually inadvertent injury to the bowel, either through a suture for fascial fixation or with the Veress needle. In all such cases, the occurrence should be recognized on inspection and the small injury can be closed with one or two imbricating sutures and the procedure completed. If secondary ports are placed under direct vision, there is little chance for bowel or vascular injury. In retroperitoneal techniques, perforation of the peritoneum is not uncommon and may create a pneumoperitoneum that obscures development of the retroperitoneal operative space. This can be managed by venting the peritoneum with an angiocatheter, or by opening the peritoneum widely from the retroperitoneal position. This still provides the positioning advantages of the retroperitoneal approach, although it becomes a transperitoneal procedure. We have not seen adverse events with this maneuver.

Vascular Control

Gaining vascular control is critical and the most frequent complication is missing small branches of the main hilar vessels. These can be torn with subsequent renal mobilization. Careful dissection and inspection in the hilar region is needed to prevent this.

Injury to the vein during mobilization can occur and may not always be immediately evident due to the pressure of the insufflating gas. Temporary pressure with a blunt instrument to limit bleeding followed by clearing the field with irrigation and suction permits an assessment of the situation. If a further port is needed to gain safe control, it should be placed. Otherwise, the vein can be lifted to limit bleeding and its dissection completed and a clip applied to control the bleeding and permit ligation. If the bleeding site cannot be identified, random clip placement is not wise. A concerted effort to place pressure on the area of bleeding, exposing the field, and searching for the site should be made for a limited period of time. If this does not permit control, consideration for conversion to an open procedure should be given.

When working in the hilum, particularly with the prone retroperitoneal approach on the right, exposure can be so good that the renal vein and the vena cava are exposed. If the camera is not oriented properly, the cava may appear to be the main renal vein, and the actual vein an inferior branch. The cava is smaller than normal due to the insufflating pressure. Before any clips are applied, careful inspection and reinspection are warranted.

Renal Mobilization

Mobilizing the kidney is not usually associated with high risk of injury. It should be borne in mind where the adrenal vessels are, and where the duodenum is on the right side. On the left the tail of the pancreas may be fairly close to the medial upper pole.

Peritoneal Perforation

While peritoneal perforation during early retroperitoneal mobilization is usually readily noted, during subsequent dissection, this may not be evident except as a gradually diminishing operative field. This is due to insufflation of the peritoneum in an almost "tension pneumoperitoneum" manner that closes down the retroperitoneal field. If this occurs and gas is flowing into the surgical field, look for peritoneal insufflation. Measures to deal with this were discussed above.

Ureteral Mobilization

Complications associated with ureteral mobilization are those due to injury to the many structures adjacent to the ureter in the deep pelvis, particularly the iliac vessels, the vas deferens in boys and the uterine vessels in girls. The gonadal vessels can usually be preserved, but may cause substantial bleeding if injured. Caution should be exercised in the deep pelvis to avoid bowel injury if the rectum is not well decompressed.

References

Borer JG, Peters CA (2000) Pediatric retroperitoneoscopic nephrectomy. J Endourol 14:413–416; discussion 417

Borer JG, Bauer SB, Peters CA, et al (1998) A single-system ectopic ureter draining an ectopic dysplastic kidney: delayed diagnosis in the young female with continuous urinary incontinence. Br J Urol 81:474–478

Borer JG, Cisek LJ, Atala A, et al (1999) Pediatric retroperitoneoscopic nephrectomy using 2 mm instrumentation. J Urol 162:1725–1729; discussion 1730

Borzi PA (2001) A comparison of the lateral and posterior retroperitoneoscopic approach for complete and partial nephroureterectomy in children. BJU Int 87:517–520

El-Ghoneimi A, Sauty L, Maintenant J, et al (2000) Laparoscopic retroperitoneal nephrectomy in high risk children. J Urol 164:1076–1079

McAleer IM, Kaplan GW (1999) Renal function before and after pyeloplasty: does it improve? J Urol 162:1041–1044

Poppas DP, Bleustein CP, Peters CA (1999) Box stitch modification of Hasson technique for pediatric laparoscopy. J Endourol 13:447–450

Chapter 88

Laparoscopic Heminephrectomy

CK Yeung, Holger Till and Peter Borzi

Introduction

The surgical management of children with renal duplication depends on a variety of factors such as parenchymal function of each moiety and the presence or absence of other associated pathologies such as ectopic ureterocele or vesicoureteral reflux. The prime objectives of any treatment must include controlling infection, protecting normal ipsilateral and contralateral kidney function and maintaining continence. In cases of poorly functioning or non-functioning moieties, a heminephrectomy (HN) may be considered and with the continued development of minimally invasive urology, this procedure can now be safely performed laparoscopically. Various routes for surgical access to the diseased kidney have been published such as a posterior retroperitoneal, a lateral retroperitoneal and a transperitoneal approach (Borzi and Yeung 2004; Saggar et al. 2004; Wang et al. 2004). The authors advocate a selective approach for surgical access according to the complexity of the procedure. Basically, a posterior retroperitoneal approach is suitable for isolated heminephrectomy without the need for extensive mobilisation and excision of a dilated megaureter in younger children (<5 years). Since this indication is rarely encountered, it will not be dealt with in detail in this chapter. In comparison, a lateral retroperitoneal approach (RHN) allows greater working space and more flexibility for extensive distal ureteral manipulation. Hence, heminephrectomy in older children, heminephroureterectomy or excision of low-lying kidneys can be tackled by LHN. Finally, for duplex systems with non-functioning moieties and complicated ureteroceles, a one-stage heminephrectomy with extravesical ureterocelectomy, reimplantation of the lower moiety ureter and bladder base repair would be best dealt with by a transperitoneal route (THN) (Borzi and Yeung 2004). The latter two techniques shall be described in this following chapter.

Preoperative Preparation

Before surgery a thorough understanding of the underlying renal pathology must be attained. Preoperative examinations should focus on the anatomical malformations of the whole urinary tract and their functional implications. Investigation may include ultrasonography, succimer (DMSA) scintiscan, MCU, intravenous pyelography (IVP) or even a magnetic resonance (MR) urogram. In most cases cystoscopy should be performed.

Before surgery parents are counselled for the minimally invasive procedure and the option for open surgery.

Before Induction of General Anaesthesia

The child is given a preoperative enema the night before surgery. Preoperative antibiotic prophylaxis should be administered either with a broad-spectrum medication or according to the child's specific urine testing.

After Induction of General Anaesthesia

Before final positioning, a preinterventional cystoscopy can be performed. In cases in which ureterocelectomy and lower urinary tract reconstruction are required, complete cystoscopic de-roofing of the ureterocele and catheterisation of the normal orthotopic lower moiety ureter may be performed before laparoscopy. In case of any doubt, an intraoperative retrograde urogram should be performed to define the upper urinary system.

Positioning

Patient

For THN the patient should be placed in a semilateral position close to the edge of the operating table (■ Fig. 88.1a) with the ipsilateral side elevated. This approach utilises gravity for retraction of the colon, allows clear dissection of the ureters even down to the bladder level and facilitates a safe access to the renal pedicle. For RHN the patient is positioned in lateral decubitus (■ Fig. 88.1b).

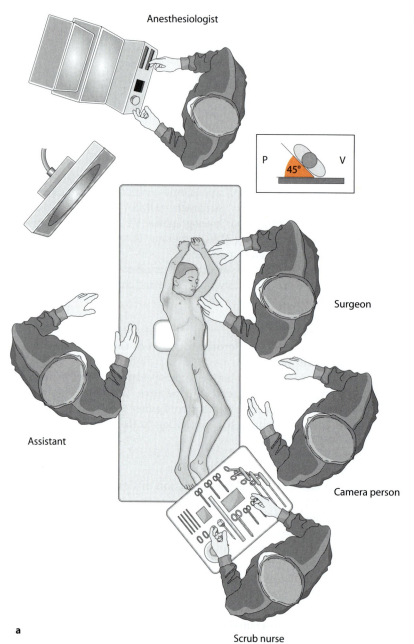

Anesthesiologist

Surgeon

Assistant

Camera person

Scrub nurse

a

P   45°   V

Fig. 88.1 a. Semilateral patient position in transperitoneal heminephrectomy (THN). Crew operating from the front of the patient

Crew, Monitors and Equipment

For THN the surgeon and assistant stand on the contralateral side, facing the pathology and the monitor in a straight line. When RHN is planned, the surgeon and assistant stand on the diseased side. Usually both procedures require only one assistant and a second monitor is not essential (■ Fig. 88.1a, b).

Special Equipment

Energy Applying Systems

Equipment	Requirement
Bipolar high-frequency electrocoagulation (HFE)	Yes
Ultrasonic energy	Yes
Ligasure	No
Argon	No
Laser	Maybe (Ogan et al. 2003)
Other	Maybe (Bishoff et al. 2003)

Other Equipment

Clips and a retrieval bag are available, as is fluoroscopy.

Fig. 88.1 b. Lateral patient position in retroperitoneal herminephrectomy (RHN). Crew operating from the back of the patient

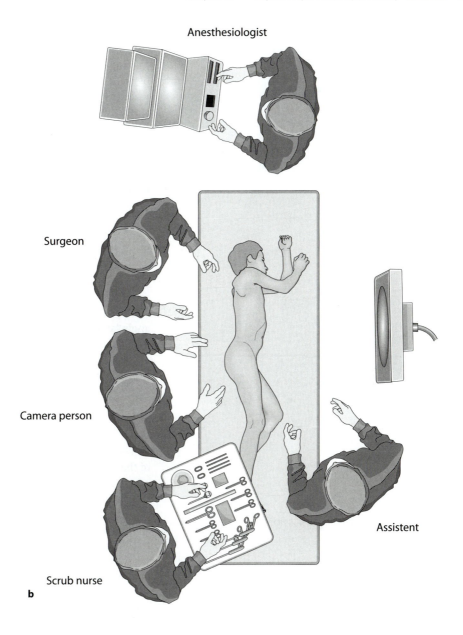

b

Technique

Cannulae

Cannula	Method of insertion	Diameter (mm)	Device	Position for RHN	Position for THN
1	Open	5	Step	One to two fingerbreadths below the 12th rib	Periumbilical
2	Closed	5	Step	Below the costovertebral angle	Upper quadrant, ipsilateral
3	Closed	5	Step	One to two fingerbreadths above the iliac crest at the level of the midaxillary to anterior axillary line	Lower quadrant ipsilateral
4	Closed	5	Step	As needed, but rarely indicated	As needed, rarely

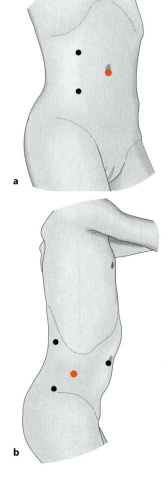

Fig. 88.2. Port position. **a**: THN, **b**: RHN

Port Placement

Careful planning of the definite port positions is crucial and should follow basic ergonomic principles.

For THN an umbilical visualisation port is introduced (5 mm, 30° scope) (Fig. 88.2a). A pneumoperitoneum is installed at a pressure of 10–12 mmHg with a CO_2 flow rate of 1–3 L/min. Two additional 5 mm instrument ports are introduced under direct vision, one in the anterior axillary line of the ipsilateral upper quadrant and the other in the anterior axillary line of the ipsilateral lower quadrant. This may later serve for specimen removal.

For RHN, initial access to the retroperitoneum is achieved with an open technique through a 1 cm incision one to two fingerbreadths below the border of the 12th rib (Fig. 88.2b). The incision is deepened by muscle splitting and blunt dissection down to the lumbodorsal fascia. The dissection must be directed close to the posterior wall to avoid inadvertent entry into the

peritoneal cavity. The retroperitoneal space is entered and developed using a glove balloon fashioned from the finger of a powder-free surgical glove as described by Gaur (Gaur 1992). The makeshift balloon dissector, which is tied to the end of a 10F feeding tube, is inserted into the retroperitoneal space and inflated. Inflation is maintained for 3 min. A 5 mm trocar is inserted and fixed with purse-string sutures to the skin to maintain an airtight seal. The pneumoretroperitoneum is maintained at a pressure of 10–12 mmHg with a CO_2 flow rate of 1–3 L/min. Videoretroperitoneoscopy is performed using a 0° or 30° laparoscope. The retroperitoneal space is further enlarged with sweeping motions with the laparoscope to free retroperitoneal fibrous tissue. The peritoneum is swept medially to prevent entry into the peritoneum. Once adequate space is achieved, two additional 3- to 5 mm working ports are inserted under direct videoendoscopic guidance. The second port is inserted below the costovertebral angle lateral to the paraspinal muscles while the third port is inserted around one to two fingerbreadths above the iliac crest at the level of the midaxillary to anterior axillary line. A fourth port is rarely indicated.

Procedure

In THN the affected kidney is exposed by mobilisation of the colon, using the electrocautery hook. Because of gravity, the colon usually falls away medially without employing an additional retractor. In RHN the kidney is easily identified after entering the retroperitoneal space due to the paucity of perirenal and retroperitoneal fat in infants and children.

Both methods continue, depending on the surgeon's preference, to start the dissection at either the renal pelvis or the ureter. However, in children with ureteroceles and a dilated upper pole ureter, it may be easier to identify both ureters first and then start the separation. The lower pole ureter probably has a normal calibre and lies posterolateral. Using the electrocautery hook or blunt dissection, the dilated ureter is followed towards the renal pedicle. Once it is confirmed that it definitely drains the upper pole, it may be divided inferiorly to the renal pedicle, employing clips or the harmonic scalpel. While developing the plane between the renal vessels and pelvis, care must be taken to avoid vascular damage. During the identification it may be helpful to place vessel loops (secured with clips). Once the supply to the upper pole has been defined, each vessel may be ligated either with clips or sutures (4-0 Vicryl).

The upper pole ureter can then be passed underneath the renal pedicle to assist with further traction. Appreciating the line of demarcation, the renal capsule is incised with the electrocautery hook. Separation of both moieties is continued with the harmonic scalpel or electrocautery. Significant bleeders must be sutured. Finally interrupted sutures (4-0 polyglactin) should seal the cut surface to avoid blood loss and possible urinary leakage. Experimental studies also suggest the use of fibrin sealant of laser tissue soldering to prevent leakage (Bishoff et al. 2003; Ogan et al. 2003)

The remaining portion of the upper pole ureter is followed down to the level of the pelvic inlet and dissected. In a refluxing unit it must be ligated with clips or ablated with the harmonic scalpel. Finally the specimen should be extracted in a bag through the inferior port. If the volume is too big, either the port site must be enlarged or the tissue can be morcellated within the bag.

Postoperative Care

The child may be started on a regular diet on day 1 postoperatively and progressed accordingly. A Foley catheter may be kept in place for a few days to monitor urine output. Postoperative analgesia is given until the patient feels fit for discharge. The schedule for postoperative investigations depends on associated urological pathologies and may include ultrasonography and a mertiatide (MAG3) diuretic renogram.

Results

Only a few series are presently available about the outcome of laparoscopic heminephrectomy in children (Janetschek et al. 1997; Jordan and Winslow 1993). In 1993 Jordan reported the case of a 14-year-old girl with bilateral renal duplication. He performed laparoendoscopic right upper pole partial nephrectomy with ureterectomy and experienced an uncomplicated postoperative course. Janetschek et al. (1997) published a series of 14 laparoscopic heminephroureterectomies of upper renal poles for ectopic refluxing megaureter and obstructive ureterocele or lower poles for reflux nephropathy. In 2 patients he combined the laparoscopic upper pole heminephroureterectomy with open ureteric reimplantation of the refluxing lower pole ureter. In summary he encountered no intraoperative or postoperative complications, but a significantly longer operating time. Wang et al. (2004) reported the results from 3 patients following transperitoneal upper pole heminephrectomy. Mean operative time was 198 min. One patient developed a urinary leak, which resolved after superselective renal arterial embolisation. All patients were well at 5.3 months follow-up.

The authors recently reported a large combined series of transperitoneal (TP) and retroperitoneal (RP) endoscopic complete and partial nephroureterecto-

mies in children. During a 5-year period 63 partial nephroureterectomies for duplex (52 upper, 8 lower) or singleton polar disease (xanthogranulomatous pyelonephritis 1, cyst 2) were performed and 8 of these patients required additional ureterectomy, bladder repair and lower moiety reimplantation. The operating time reflected the complexity of the excision and lower urinary reconstruction [lateral and posterior RP: 25–145 min (mean 92 min), TP with ureterocelectomy and bladder neck repair: 105–355 min (mean 153 min)]. Hospital stay for RP and simple TP was 1–4 days (mean 1.5 days) and for complicated TP 2–8 days (mean 3.5 days).

Discussion

Ehrlich et al. (1992) reported the first laparoscopic partial nephrectomy in a child. Subsequent reports showed that laparoscopic nephrectomy (Figenshau et al. 1994), nephroureterectomy (Janetschek et al. 1993), and heminephroureterectomy (Janetschek et al. 1997; Jordan and Winslow 1993) could be performed with minimal morbidity in infants. Heminephroureterectomy is a technically demanding procedure especially in paediatric urology and the basic approach to the non-functioning moiety, laparoscopic versus retroperitoneoscopic, is still a matter of ongoing discussion.

The retroperitoneoscopic approach excludes the intraperitoneal organs from the operative field. The posterior approach gives a rapid exposure to the renal pedicle and allows clear definition of the duplex polar vascular anatomy. Our previously published experiences showed that in children younger than 5 years, the majority of the ureteral length can be excised by this approach. The need for lower urinary tract surgery after duplex upper or lower pole heminephrectomy is around 15% (Cain et al. 1998; Plaire et al. 1997) and we contend that retroperitoneoscopic hemiuretronephrectomy is an appropriate first-line treatment. Simultaneous reconstruction, such as lower moiety reimplantation or bladder neck repair, requires a transperitoneal access. It allows the entire procedure to be achieved in one position through unchanged ports.

Both techniques similarly imply the benefits of shorter postoperative hospital stay when compared with open surgery, small portal sites that heal rapidly and superior cosmetic results compared to the scar of open surgery.

In summary laparoscopic heminephrectomy is a safe and advantageous alternative to conventional surgery. The lateral retroperitoneal approach avoids exposure of intraperitoneal structures and allows complete ureterectomy. The transperitoneal route is recommended when complete moiety excision with lower urinary reconstruction is anticipated.

References

Bishoff JT, Cornum RL, Perahia B, et al (2003) Laparoscopic hem-inephrectomy using a new fibrin sealant powder. Urology 62:1139–1143

Borzi PA, Yeung CK (2004) Selective approach for transperitoneal and extraperitoneal endoscopic nephrectomy in children. J Urol 171:814–816

Cain MP, Pope CJ, Casale AJ, et al (1998) Natural history of reflux-ing distal ureteral stumps after nephrectomy and partial ne-phrectomy for vesicoureteral reflux. J Urol 160:1026–1027

Ehrlich RM, Gershman A, Fuchs G (1992) Laparoscopic nephrec-tomy in a child. Expanding horizons for laparoscopy in pediat-ric urology. J Endourol 6:463

Figenshau RS, Clayman RV, Kerbl K, et al (1994) Laparoscopic ne-phroureterectomy in the child. Initial case report. J Urol 151:740

Gaur D (1992) Laparoscopic operative retroperitoneoscopy: use of a new device. J Urol 156:1120–1124

Janetschek G, Reissigl A, Peschel R, et al (1993) Laparoscopic ne-phroureterectomy in infants. J Endourol Suppl 4:236

Janetschek G, Seibold J, Radmayer C, et al (1997) Laparoscopic heminephroureterectomy in pediatric patients. J Urol 158:1928–1930

Jordan GH, Winslow BH (1993) Laparoendoscopic upper pole par-tial nephrectomy with ureterectomy. J Urol 150:1940–1943

Ogan K, Jacomides L, Saboorian H, et al (2003) Sutureless laparo-scopic heminephrectomy using laser tissue soldering. J En-dourol 17:295–300

Plaire JC, Pope JC, Kropp BP, et al (1997) Management of ectopic ureters: experience with the upper tract approach. J Urol 158:1245–1247

Saggar VR, Singh K, Sarangi R (2004) Retroperitoneoscopic hem-inephrectomy of a horseshoe kidney for calculi disease. Surg Laparosc Endosc Percutan Tech 14:172–174

Wang DS, Bird VG, Cooper CS, et al (2004) Laparoscopic upper pole heminephrectomy for ectopic ureter: initial experience. Can J Urol 11:2141–2145

Laparoscopic Dismembered Pyeloplasty for Ureteropelvic Junction Obstruction: Transperitoneal Approach

Felix Schier

Introduction

Indications for the procedure are identical to the open approach. Also, the basic surgical steps are identical to open surgery. In adult patients, all types of repairs have been performed laparoscopically: Anderson-Hynes dismembered pyeloplasty, Y-V plasty, Heineke-Mikulicz pyloroplasty, and Davis intubated ureterotomy (Jarrett et al. 2002). There is no reason why this should not be possible in children as well.

A main disadvantage of the minimally invasive approach is the comparatively high operating room time of more than 1.5 h, up to 7 h (Peters et al. 1995; Schier 1998; Tan 1999). Suturing skills are the limiting factor for the operative time and also for the postoperative result, to an extent as in no other pediatric laparoscopic procedure.

Preoperative Preparation

Before Induction of General Anesthesia

No special preparations are required. An antibiotic (cephalosporin) may be given if a stent is used. A stent is recommended, especially in the first cases, and can be either a double-J stent or a nephrostomy catheter (Rüsch, 71394 Kernen, Germany) (■ Fig. 89.1).

In case the resected ureteropelvic junction (UPJ) can not be exteriorized through a cannula (the technique will be described below), a small endobag will be needed for the specimen. A cut off finger of a rubber glove will do as well.

There is an illuminated catheter which is inserted cystoscopically and makes the ureter easily visible (Cook, Spencer, Indiana, USA) (■ Fig. 89.2). This might help in older children. In small children the ureter is rather easy to identify.

Complete sets of 2 mm instruments are available (Storz, Tuttlingen, Germany) (■ Fig. 89.3). Three-millimeter or even 5 mm instruments may be used as well. The instruments needed are a hook for incising the peritoneum, forceps and scissors for dissecting the UPJ, and a pair of needle holders for suturing.

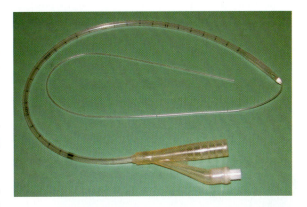

Fig. 89.1. Transanastomotic percutaneous nephrostomy catheter (Rüsch, 71394 Kernen, Germany)

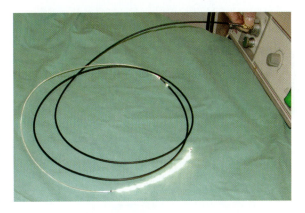

Fig. 89.2. Illuminated catheter (Cook, Spencer, Indiana, USA)

Either monofilamentous or braided 6-0 or 7-0 sutures are used. Monofilamentous threads are available in a translucent variety, without color. It is strenuous for the eye of the surgeon to use non-colored threads. Monofilament threads have a more pronounced "memory"; braided threads will not keep their spatial configuration as well as monofilament ones. Braided threads also tend to stick to neighboring anatomical structures and need to be picked up more often (probably a capillary effect). Therefore colored monofilament threads appear better suited for laparoscopic pyeloplasty.

The laparoscope has a 5 mm diameter and has a side view of 30°. Smaller laparoscopes exist of course, but they make suturing and knotting more difficult. Laparoscopists overcome absent two-dimensionality by using monocular clues such as parallax, color, and shade differences, relative size changes, focusing, and other indirect evidence of spatial relations during endoscopic surgery. These cues do not work well with small-diameter laparoscopes. Thirty-degree laparoscopes are more demanding for the camera operator than 0° laparoscopes. Also the camera operator's position is tiring and so camera operator problems are best overcome with a camera-holding device (■ Fig. 89.4).

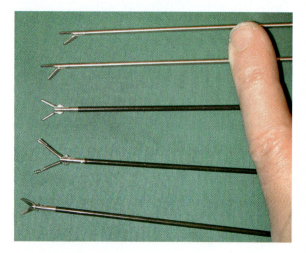

Fig. 89.3. Set of 2 mm instruments

After Induction of General Anesthesia

There are no anesthesiologic peculiarities in the transperitoneal technique for UPJ obstruction. The procedure is performed under general anesthesia with intubation. A neutral electrode is placed for high-frequency coagulation. If a double-J stent is to be used, cystoscopy is performed and the stent is inserted. Later, during laparoscopy, the stent will be shining through the retroperitoneum, thereby facilitating identification of the ureter. An antibiotic is given (cephalosporin) as long as the stent remains in place.

Positioning of Patient, Crew, and Monitors

The author has tried several patient positions, from a flat supine position to the 90° lateral position. The flat supine position is acceptable for processes at the anterior surface of the kidney. Otherwise it is the least desirable position for pediatric urology.

In contrast, the 90° lateral position is exaggerated (■ Fig. 89.5a). The bowel tends to fall onto the laparoscope when inserted at the umbilicus. Also, Veress needle insertion through the umbilicus is more difficult, i.e., risky, in the 90° lateral position. In the 90° lateral position the procedure takes place "at the ceiling," i.e., the instruments come from below. If the child is positioned at the center of the table, instrument movement may be restricted physically by the table surface. Therefore the child is placed at the margin of

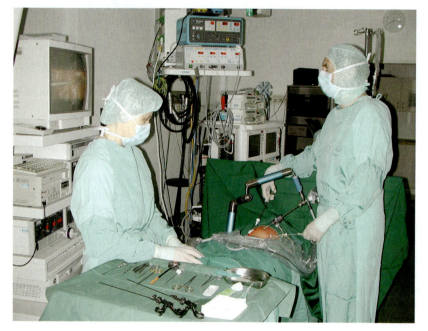

Fig. 89.4. Camera-holding device

Fig. 89.5. **a** The 90° lateral position, **b** the 30–45° position

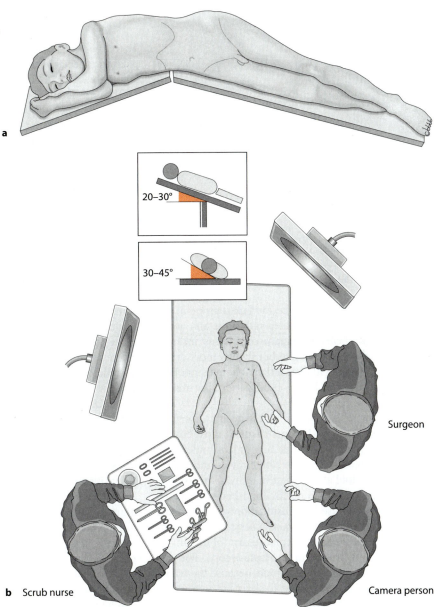

20–30°

30–45°

a

Surgeon

b   Scrub nurse

Camera person

the table. Also, patients positioned 90° laterally often have the thighs bent, resulting in subsequent mechanical obstruction of the instruments. The thigh of the patient may restrict the caudal instrument, when the hip joint is bent too much. The thigh of the affected side should therefore be extended.

A good compromise is the 30–45° lateral position (■ Fig. 89.5b). It allows for safe Veress needle access through the umbilicus and also good visualization. If required, the table may be tilted in order to increase the lateral position. This position is preferable for pyeloplasty.

The surgeon stands in front of the child with the camera operator to the surgeon's left and the scrub nurse opposite. Two monitors are used; the most important one is opposite to the surgeon.

Special Equipment

There is no need for special energy applying systems. The peritoneum is opened with regular hook cautery. Except for the stents (at the discretion of the surgeon) and perhaps a small endobag (again at the discretion of the surgeon) no further equipment is needed. An irrigation/suction device is kept ready in case urine spills upon opening the dilated pelvis.

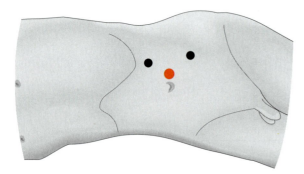

Fig. 89.6. Trocar placement

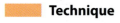

Technique

Cannulae

When inserting the trocar for the laparoscope at the umbilicus, the kidney is located rather distant, at the level of the lowest ribs. The laparoscope is best inserted *not* at the level of the umbilicus but slightly more cranially (■ Fig. 89.6). It will then arrive right in front of the kidney. This provides better visualization, but results in less favorable cosmesis.

The umbilicus is used for Veress needle insertion. Direct access to the abdominal cavity is most easy at this point as there is the least amount of underlying anatomy. A small transverse semicircular incision is made in a skin fold at the lower margin of the umbilicus. The Veress needle is inserted, flushed with physiologic saline, and used for insufflation of CO_2. If the trocar for the laparoscope is also inserted at the umbilicus, the Veress needle is replaced, by "blind" insertion, by a 5 mm trocar for the laparoscope. For this trocar we prefer the Ethicon model because the translucent cannula can be pulled back as far as possible until it almost falls out. This gives extra distance in a small abdominal cavity. If the laparoscope is not inserted at the umbilicus but more laterally, it is inserted at the lateral margin of the rectus sheath. There are no vessels to be injured here.

Two 2 mm trocars (or 3 mm) are inserted at the lateral margin of the rectus sheath. The trocars are arranged in such a way that the laparoscope is located in the center and, together with the two additional cannulae for the left and right hand, eventually forms a triangle. Ergonometrically the cannulae for the hands are placed so that they might be considered an extension of the forearms.

Procedure

There is no big difference technically between a pyeloplasty on the left versus the right side. Still, the left side is slightly easier to be operated upon.

The peritoneum is opened with a hook (■ Fig. 89.7). If the pelvis is distended, it might be possible to approach it through the mesentery of the colon. Otherwise, the peritoneum is incised laterally to the colon until it falls down by gravity. The pelvis and ureter are exposed as far as necessary (■ Fig. 89.8). Two stay sutures will each hold the cranial pelvis and the ureter (■ Fig. 89.9). These are regular 4-0 sutures (of any material) for "open" surgery with a long needle. The needle is bent open until it almost is straightened, inserted directly through the abdominal wall, grabbed from inside with a needle holder, passed through the wall of the cranial pelvis and exited reversely through the abdominal wall in order to be grabbed from outside and clamped with a forceps. Passing the needle from the outside to the inside is easy. Passing the needle from the inside to the outside is more difficult. Therefore the needle needs to be of the "cutting" variety and it has to be sufficiently long. The site for insertion of the suture is determined by the topographics of the kidney and pelvis. Usually it is at the posterior axillary line and close to the lowest rib. The liver may be lifted up a bit by the stay suture. Similarly, a stay suture is placed at the ureter a few centimeters caudal to the expected anastomosis. These two stay sutures will align the anastomosis and facilitate tissue approximation and suturing.

There are special, long-branched scissors for trimming of the pelvis and spatulation of the ureter (■ Fig. 89.10). Also, there are new delicate forceps for suturing. They are available as 2 mm or 3 mm "Babcocks" (Storz, Tuttlingen, Germany). Most other laparoscopic instruments appear too rough for handling the mucosa while suturing the anastomosis.

When using solely 2 mm trocars it may appear difficult to exteriorize the resected specimen. The specimen is pushed, in retrograde fashion, "into the face" of the camera operator, into the 5 mm trocar for the laparoscope while the laparoscope is pulled back until the specimen is visible from outside. It is then taken with an instrument within the trocar and removed.

The anastomotic suture material is identical to open surgery, 6-0 or 7-0. Colorless or translucent sutures are difficult to see laparoscopically, especially when blood stained. Colored threads are more comfortable for the laparoscopist's eye, and 6-0 and 7-0 threads have needles to be inserted through commercially available 2 mm trocars. The needles will scratch along the cannula but arrive unharmed intra-abdominally. Needles are removed later through the same trocar. All suturing is completed with intracorporeal knotting (■ Figs. 89.11).

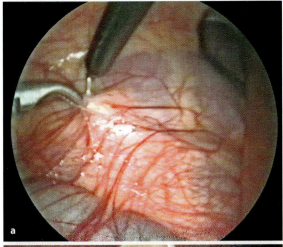

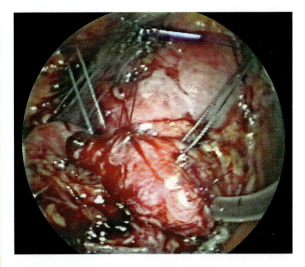

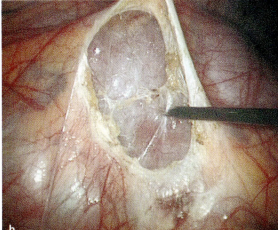

Fig. 89. 9. Stay sutures at the pelvis and the ureter

Fig. 89.7 a,b. Opening the peritoneum

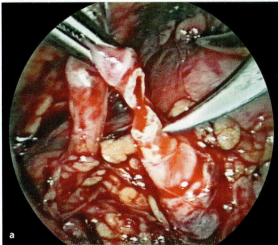

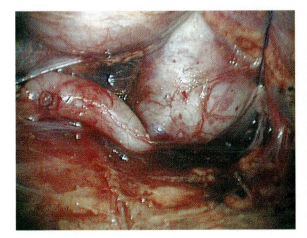

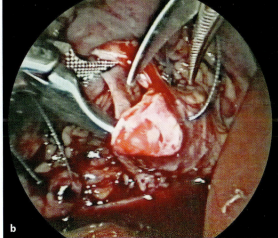

Fig. 89.8. Ureteropelvic junction

Fig. 89.10 a,b. Resection of the UPJ and trimming of the pelvis

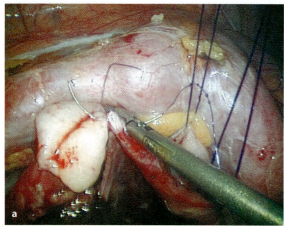

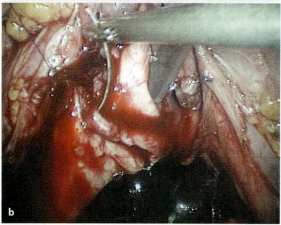

Fig. 89.11. **a** Suturing the back wall, **b** Suturing the anterior wall

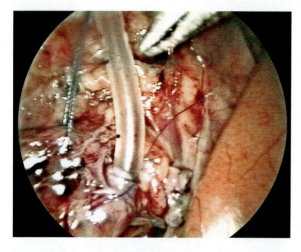

Fig. 89.12. The stent is exited through the pelvis and secured by a purse-string suture

As a safety measure, stents are advisable in the initial cases of a series (▪ Fig. 89.12). Nephrostomy catheters (Rüsch, 71394 Kernen, Germany) are placed transanastomotically and exited through a separate stab incision in the cranial pelvis, secured there by a purse-string suture, and exteriorized through the abdominal wall. It is suggested to consider covering the completed anastomosis with fibrin glue. Fibrin glue dissolves within a few days and will have disappeared after the risk of a urinoma has subsided. Another option is placement of a drain near the anastomosis.

After desufflation, local anesthesia with bupivacaine is applied to all trocar insertion sites. At the 5 mm trocar insertion site the fascia is closed with 4-0 braided slow-absorbable sutures and the skin is closed with interrupted absorbable sutures. Two-millimeter trocar sites are simply covered with a bandage.

Postoperative Care

Children are offered regular food as soon as they wish. In our practice, postoperative pain medication is given on request, not routinely. Sixty percent of children will not need any postoperative pain medication, and about 40% will be given paracetamol as a suppository. Pain perception, however, is different in different societies.

With a double-J catheter the children would leave the hospital as soon as they and the parents feel comfortable. This is usually around 3 days postoperatively. The double-J catheter is removed around 10 days postoperatively. A transanastomotic nephrostomy catheter is left until the 7th postoperative day. Starting with the 8th postoperative day, the nephrostomy catheter is intermittently clamped for a few hours. If there are no colics after clamping it is removed. If there are colics, the clamp is reopened and the catheter left for another few days. In some countries, the children remain in hospital with a nephrostomy catheter. In other countries parents will take the child home with the nephrostomy catheter in place, and they may even remove the catheter themselves.

Dressings are changed at postoperative day 4. In older children we suggest to refrain from sports for 2–4 weeks. This suggestion is not based on scientific data.

Results

Personal Results

Seventeen patients, aged from 3 months to 15 years (median 5.5 years) have been operated on. Operating room time ranged from 2.0 to 7.2 h (median 2.8 h). Nine nephrostomy catheters and eight double-J stents were placed. Stents were left for 7–11 days. There have been two complications: two urinomata (one in the very first patient, where no stent had been placed initially, and one in the 13th patient, despite a double-J stent being placed). Five-millimeter instruments were used for the first six cases, and for the following cases 2 mm instruments were used. The laparoscope was always of 5 mm diameter, and in the last six cases was of the 30° variety.

Literature Results

One publication reports of one patient, age 7 years, where the operating room time was 5 h and no complication occurred (Peters et al. 1995). A second publication reports of 18 patients, aged 3 months to 15 years (mean 17 months). Three children had had previous surgery. There were four complications: one trocar hematoma, one misplaced stent, and two complete obstructions of the anastomosis in two children of 3 months of age (both children were reoperated laparoscopically later) (Tan 1999). Except for a third publication by the author, containing the results detailed in the previous section, there are no further publications dealing with transperitoneal dismembering pyeloplasty in children.

Discussion

In adult patients, numerous laparoscopic pyeloplasties are reported in the literature (Jarrett et al. 2002). In children, reports are still rare (Peters 1995; Schier 1998; Tan 1999). Essentially there are only two series, one of 17 patients and one of 18 patients. Two publications by one author contain the same patients (Tan 1999, 2001).

Most reservations against the transperitoneal approach are based on the assumption that it would create postoperative intra-abdominal adhesions and that it permits urine to spread within the abdominal cavity in case of urinoma. There is no proof that intra-abdominal adhesions really do occur to a significant extent after transabdominal interventions. This is indirectly supported by studies demonstrating that previous intra-abdominal surgery does not interfere with subsequent laparoscopic urologic interventions. Most likely the colon will fall back after finishing the procedure and seal off the kidney within a few hours. Intra-abdominal urinary leakage is only a problem when massive. Most leakages are, however, small and close spontaneously. Stents, either placed transanastomotically or next to the anastomosis, will not completely abolish the likelihood of urinoma. In the author's series, one urinoma occurred with a nephrostomy catheter and one with a double-J stent, so neither seems to provide absolute safety. Transanastomotic stents are possibly used more liberally in the minimally invasive technique because most initial cases are difficult and surgeons therefore use stents as a safety measure. In one of the author's cases the catheter was dislocated from the pelvis around the 5th postoperative day, possibly by bowel peristalsis or by movements of the patient who was ambulating at the time. Urine drainage continued, but there was no free fluid found intra-abdominally on sonography. Two days later the catheter was removed without complications. A similar event was reported earlier (Tan 1999).

Technically, other researchers also prefer 5 mm laparoscopes. In addition, breaking the table and using a stay suture at the ureter are considered unnecessary (Tan 2001). In contrast, the author's point of view is that refraining from a stay suture carries the risk of a disappearing ureter as soon as it is transected. This is prevented by dissecting the ureter at some length (Tan 2001); this again may jeopardize blood supply to the anastomotic area.

The transperitoneal access appears more straightforward to most pediatric surgeons. The anatomic exposure is obvious. However, trained urologists prefer to stay retroperitoneally. In order to compare, the author has repeatedly witnessed retroperitoneal interventions performed by experienced surgeons. Balancing the retroperitoneal against the transperitoneal approach, he feels that there is more space available and better accessibility given via the transperitoneal route. The only difficulty in the transperitoneal technique is when the pelvis is hidden deep in the parenchyma. When this occurs the pelvis needs to be exposed by additional stay sutures.

The statement that "laparoscopic pyeloplasty should not be performed under the age of 6 months" (Tan 1999) may be based on two individual cases of obstruction after stent removal in 3-month-old children. The author's personal experience includes four children of that age, with only one leakage in one child. Thus, the statement appears too harsh, but it has not been revoked so far (Tan 2001). It has also been stated that right-sided procedures are a bit more difficult due to physical hindrance of the suturing trocar by the liver (Tan 1999, 2001). In the author's experience this is in fact the case, but not to a major degree.

In summary, given sufficient expertise with laparoscopic suturing, laparoscopic pyeloplasty will be as effective as the "open" procedures, with decreased postoperative morbidity.

References

Jarrett TW, Chan DY, Charambura TC, et al (2002) Laparoscopic pyeloplasty: the first 100 cases. J Urol 167:1253–1256

Peters CA, Schlussel RN, Retik AB (1995) Pediatric laparoscopic dismembered pyeloplasty. J Urol 153:1962–1965

Schier F (1998) Laparoscopic Anderson-Hynes pyeloplasty in children. Pediatr Surg Int 13:497–500

Tan HL (1999) Laparoscopic Anderson-Hynes dismembered pyeloplasty in children. J Urol 162:1045–1047

Tan HL (2001) Laparoscopic Anderson-Hynes dismembered pyeloplasty in children using needlescopic instrumentation. Urol Clin North Am 28:43–51

Chapter 90

Retroperitoneoscopic Dismembered Pyeloplasty

C.K. Yeung and N. Magsanoc

Introduction

Laparoscopic pyeloplasty was first described as a minimally invasive surgical technique by Schuessler et al. in 1993. Since then, several centres have adapted the approach and have published large series reports with extended follow-up with note of a greater than 90% success rate. These results surpass the outcome observed in endoscopic incisional procedures in correcting pelviureteric junction obstruction (PUJO), and are comparable with the outcome of open pyeloplasty which remains the reference standard for correcting PUJ obstruction in children.

Initially described as a transperitoneal approach, it is gradually gaining popularity through an extraperitoneal or retroperitoneal approach since its description by Kavousi and Peters in 1993. Since 80–90% of renal surgery may be best approached through a retroperitoneal route, it was logical to develop this route (Valla 1999). The reported experiences of a few centres in the procedure to date show that it is safe and effective. However, long-term outcome studies are still needed.

Preoperative Preparation

Patients for surgery must have prior documented evidence of PUJ obstruction. Documentation includes ultrasonography, radiological demonstration of obstruction by excretory urography, retrograde or antegrade pyelography, or hold up or significant delay in drainage on isotope renography.

Before Induction of General Anaesthesia

The patient is given a preoperative enema the night before surgery. Preoperative cystoscopy and ureteral catheterisation are not necessary.

After Induction of General Anaesthesia

The patient is given a broad-spectrum antibiotic as prophylaxis. An age-appropriate Foley catheter is inserted. A nasogastric tube is inserted for decompression.

Positioning of Patient, Crew and Equipment

Correct patient positioning is an essential part of the operation. From our experience, we adhere to two principles that will dictate the position of the patient, which in turn will facilitate a more efficient operation. The first principle is to approach the kidney posteriorly. The posterior approach is more advantageous since there is early identification of the renal pelvis with minimal dissection. The second principle is to suture the pelviureteric anastomosis with your dominant arm at all times. The description of the technique in the text that follows is described for a right-handed surgeon. The same will be true for the left-handed surgeon but will be just the opposite.

The surgeon stands at the right side of the bed for both left and right pyeloplasty. We employ this position to facilitate suturing of the pelviureteric anastomosis with the right hand (in a right-handed surgeon) beginning from the most dependent part of the renal pelvis. Attempting to anastomose the pelvis to the ureter using the non-dominant arm only sacrifices the quality of the operation.

For a right-sided pyeloplasty, the patient is placed in a left anterolateral position (■ Fig. 90.1) close to the right edge of the operating table. This position places the posteriorly oriented kidney in a more vertical position thereby facilitating a more direct access to the renal pelvis. Lumbar padding is placed to further open and extend the costal angle.

For a left-sided pyeloplasty, the patient is placed in a semiprone position close to the right edge of the operating table (■ Fig. 90.2). The surgeon and the camera operator both stay on the right side of the operating table with the monitor across from them, while an assistant stands at the other side of the table (■ Figs. 90.3, 90.4).

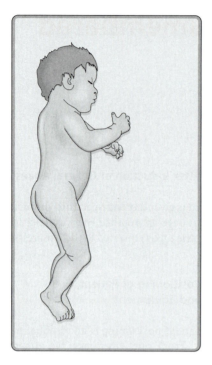

Fig. 90.1. Position for a right pyeloplasty

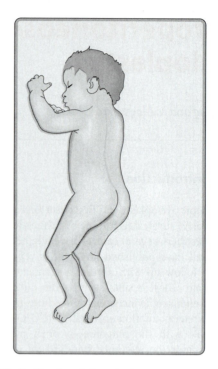

Fig. 90.2. Position for a left pyeloplasty

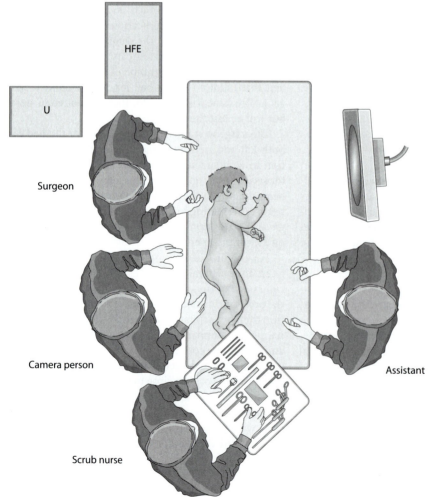

Fig. 90.3. Patient, crew and equipment positioning in a right pyeloplasty. *HFE* high-frequency electro-coagulation, *U* ultrasonic energy

Fig. 90.4. Patient, crew and equipment positioning in a left pyeloplasty. *HFE* high-frequency electrocoagulation, *U* ultrasonic energy

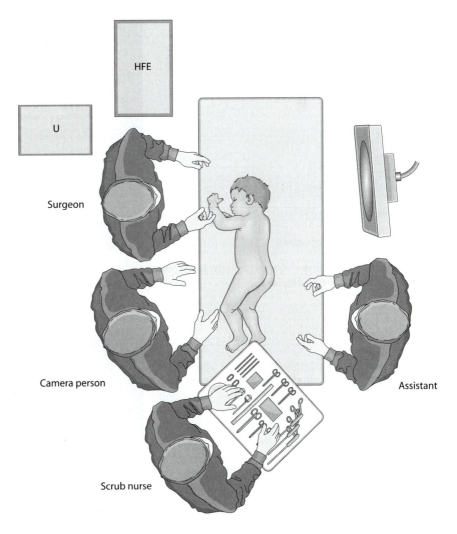

Instruments and Equipment

The following equipment is required:
- 5 mm 30° or 0° laparoscope
- 2 × 3- to 5 mm working ports
- 3 mm atraumatic grasping forceps
- 3 mm diathermy hook
- 3 mm needle holder
- 6F infant feeding tube
- 18-gauge venous cannula
- 4F or 5F double pigtail stent
- 6-0 polydioxanone sutures
- Bipolar electrocautery

Technique

Cannulae

Cannula	Method of insertion	Diameter (mm)	Device	Position
1	Open	5	Step, 0° or 30° telescope	One to two fingerbreadths below the 12th rib
2	Closed	5	Step, working instruments	Below the costovertebral angle
3	Closed	5	Step, working instruments	One to two fingerbreadths above the iliac crest at the level of the midaxillary to anterior axillary line
4	Closed	5	Step	As needed, but rarely indicated

- Figure 90.5 shows port placement.

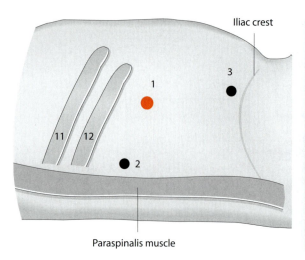

Fig. 90.5. Port placement in a right pyeloplasty. Same port placement is used for a left pyeloplasty

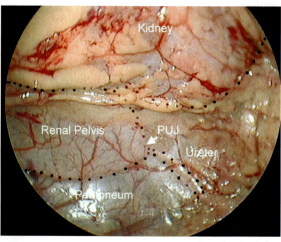

Fig. 90.6. Orientation of structures in a right pyeloplasty where the renal pelvis is inferior to the kidney

Procedure

The procedure is started by marking out the anatomical landmarks, which include the 12th rib, iliac crest, and the paraspinal muscles, to facilitate port placement (■ Fig. 90.5). Initial access to the retroperitoneum is achieved with an open technique through a 1 cm incision one to two fingerbreadths below border of the 12th rib at the posterior axillary line for larger children or at the midaxillary line for smaller children. The incision is deepened by muscle splitting and blunt dissection down to the lumbodorsal fascia. The dissection must be directed close to the posterior wall to avoid inadvertent entry into the peritoneal cavity. The retroperitoneal space is entered and developed using a glove balloon fashioned from the finger of a powder-free surgical glove as described by Gaur in 1992. The makeshift balloon dissector, which is tied to the end of a 10F feeding tube, is inserted in the retroperitoneal space and inflated. Inflation is maintained for 3 min. A 5 mm trocar is inserted and fixed with purse-string sutures to the skin to maintain an airtight seal. The pneumoretroperitoneum is maintained at a pressure of 10–12 mmHg with a CO_2 flow rate of 1–3 L/min. Videoretroperitoneoscopy is performed using a 0° or 30° laparoscope. The retroperitoneal space is further enlarged with sweeping motions with the laparoscope to free retroperitoneal fibrous tissue. The peritoneum is swept medially to prevent entry into the peritoneum. Once adequate space is achieved, two additional 3- to 5 mm working ports are inserted under direct videoendoscopic guidance. The second port is inserted below the costovertebral angle lateral to the paraspinal muscles while the third port is inserted around one to two fingerbreadths above the iliac crest at the level of the midaxillary to anterior axillary line. A fourth port is rarely indicated.

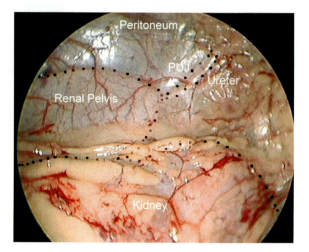

Fig. 90.7. Orientation of structures in a left pyeloplasty where the renal pelvis is superior to the kidney

At this point, the kidney, renal pelvis and the PUJ junction may be easily identified due to the paucity of perirenal and retroperitoneal fat in infants and children. However the orientation of the structures for a right pyeloplasty will be different from a left pyeloplasty as a result of the patient position. In a right pyeloplasty where the patient is in a right anterolateral position, the renal pelvis will be seen inferior to the kidney (■ Fig. 90.6). In contrast, in a left pyeloplasty where the patient is in a semiprone position, the renal pelvis will be seen superior to the kidney (■ Fig. 90.7).

The lower pole of the kidney and the renal pelvis are exposed. The PUJ is identified. Care must be taken in preserving the periureteric vasculature during dissection. The anterior surface of the kidney is not dissected off the peritoneum so that the kidney remains natu-

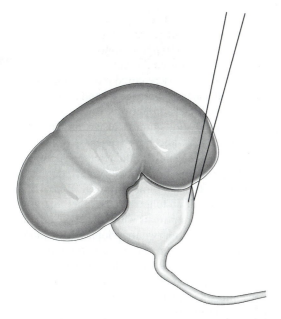

Fig. 90.8. A hitch stitch is placed through the renal pelvis

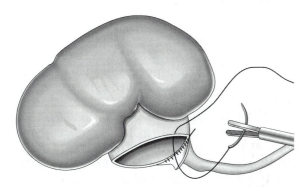

Fig. 90.9. Anastomosis of the anterior wall of the reduced renal pelvis using running 6-0 polydioxanone sutures

rally retracted medially without the need for individual kidney retraction (El-Ghoneimi et al. 2003). At this point, possible causes of PUJ obstruction may be identified such as crossing blood vessels or a fibrotic band. Any fibrotic band identified kinking the ureter is divided.

Once adequate mobilisation is achieved, the line of incision for pelvic reduction is planned. A 4-0 polydioxanone suture on a straight needle is passed percutaneously in the abdominal wall and through the renal pelvis, and passed back through the abdominal wall at the same entry point. This stitch serves to mark the upper limit of the line of the pyeloplasty during pelviureteric anastomosis. But more importantly, it serves as a hitch stitch to present and stabilise the pelvis to facilitate intracorporeal suturing during anastomosis (■ Fig. 90.8). It is important to leave a long external length of suture

to enable intraoperative adjustment of the tension as needed.

The renal pelvis is partly dismembered above the area of pathology using fine scissors at the most dependent portion. The pelvis is incompletely dismembered to maintain stability and to decrease tension on the suture line. The ureter is divided and spatulated medially. Should a concomitant intrarenal calculus be present, intervention at this point is ideal using a flexible scope. If a crossing vessel is present, the ureter and the renal pelvis are transposed to the opposite side.

A short segment (approximately 2–3 cm) of a 6F feeding tube is inserted through a working port and into the open end of the spatulated ureter to separate the anterior and posterior walls which will allow more accurate suture placement.

Anastomosis of the most dependent portion of the reduced renal pelvis is performed using 6-0 polydioxanone sutures on a 3/8th round-bodied needle. The first suture is placed at the most dependent portion of the renal pelvis to the apex of the spatulated ureter. An intracorporeal technique is used to tie the knots. Suturing is started at the anterior wall of the reduced pelvis using running sutures (■ Fig. 90.9).

After completion of the anterior wall, a transanastomotic double pigtail stent is passed through the pelvis down to the bladder. Insertion of the stent is facilitated by passing an 18-gauge venous cannula through the abdominal wall. A flexible guidewire is inserted through the cannula and manipulated into the ureter and advanced to the bladder. The venous cannula is withdrawn and a 4F or 5F double pigtail catheter is passed over the guidewire into the bladder. Position of the stent may be confirmed by fluoroscopy. Should fluoroscopy not be available, methylene blue may be infused into the bladder through the Foley catheter. Position is confirmed when there is note of backflow of the methylene blue into the pigtail stent. The posterior wall of the renal pelvis is then sutured in a similar running fashion to the upper corner (■ Fig. 90.10).

The remaining pelvis still attached is trimmed off and dismembered. The suture from the anterior wall is then tied intracorporeally to the suture from the posterior wall. Additional interrupted sutures may be placed in the area of the pelvis not closed by the initial suturing. The hitch stitch is released and the upper ureter is inspected to ensure a good tension-free anastomosis and that no kinking has occurred.

The retroperitoneal cavity is desufflated and haemostasis is ascertained. Insertion of a drain is usually not necessary. The ports are then withdrawn. The 5 mm port sites are repaired by interrupted absorbable sutures. There is no need to repair the 2- to 3 mm port sites.

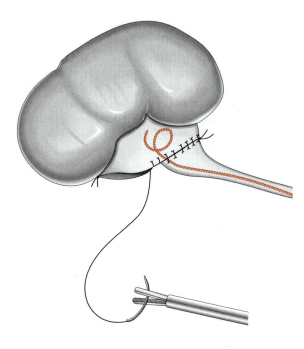

Fig. 90.10. The posterior wall of the renal pelvis is sutured in a similar fashion

Postoperative Care

The patient is started on a normal diet as tolerated on day 1 postoperatively and progressed accordingly. The Foley catheter is maintained for 2 days. Postoperative analgesia is given until the patient is discharged. The prophylactic antibiotic is resumed. The double pigtail stent is removed after 4–6 weeks. Follow-up ultrasonography and mertiatide (MAG3) diuretic renography is done 3 months after removal of the stent.

Results

Over a 4-year period, retroperitoneoscopic dismembered pyeloplasty performed for PUJO was performed for a total of 44 patients (29 boys, 15 girls). The mean age at the time of surgery was 34 months (range 3 months to 14.1 years). Retroperitoneoscopic dismembered pyeloplasty was successfully performed in 42 patients. Open conversion was required in two cases in the early part of the series: one in a 3-month-old infant with huge hydronephrosis due to limitation of space, and the other due to previous nephrostomy drainage for pyonephrosis resulting in dense perinephric adhesions. The mean operation time was 139 min (range 95–430 min). All patients made a rapid and uneventful initial recovery, with no anastomotic leak. The patients were followed up at 3 months postoperatively

with an ultrasound scan and at 6 months with an ultrasound and diuretic isotope renography. At a mean follow-up of 22 months (range 5 months to 3.8 years) all have remained asymptomatic and well except for 2 patients who subsequently required redo pyeloplasty because of unsatisfactory drainage secondary to kinking of an otherwise intact anastomosis. Both patients were young infants at 5 and 6 months of age, respectively, at the time of surgery, and both had massive hydronephrosis with a renal pelvic diameter of 50 mm and 73 mm, respectively. Both underwent redo laparoscopic pyeloplasty via a transperitoneal approach and have remained well on follow-up. Another infant who had massive hydronephrosis with a renal pelvic diameter of 50 mm and underwent pyeloplasty at 4 months of age developed recurrent urinary tract infection postoperatively with persistent hydronephrosis. This settled after a period of percutaneous nephrostomy drainage and subsequent follow-up investigations revealed satisfactory drainage with no decrease in differential renal function, and the patient has also remained asymptomatic and well.

Discussion

The reporting of retroperitoneoscopic dismembered pyeloplasty in infants and children in the literature is quite limited and long-term results still have not been established. Our initial experience in our centre has a greater than 90% success rate with a mean operative time of 143 min (range 103–235 min). Most of the reported failures occurred within the first 2 years of doing the procedure. One problem we encountered is when a retroperitoneoscopic approach is adapted for very young infants with very large hydronephrotic renal pelvis. This is due to the limited operative space combined with difficulty in orientation. As a result, a transperitoneal approach is recommended for infants with a grossly hydronephrotic renal pelvis (transverse pelvic diameter greater than 50 mm). Another problem encountered is poor visualisation in the retroperitoneal space due to peritoneal perforation resulting in difficulty in maintaining the pneumoretroperitoneum. This problem may be remedied by repairing the peritoneal perforation or by insertion of a Veress needle in the peritoneal cavity if the perforation is small, or by liberally enlarging the perforation to convert the retroperitoneal and intraperitoneal space into a single cavity.

There are several complications associated with the procedure which may occur intraoperatively or postoperatively. These include urine leak or urinoma formation due to an anastomosis that is not watertight or due to distal obstruction caused by improper placement or kinking of the pigtail stent. Trauma to the vesicoureteric junction sustained during a difficult insertion of the double pigtail stent may be a cause of obstruction. Decompression of the renal pelvis with a percutaneous tube may be needed if the aetiology of the leak is obstruction. However, the effects of urine leak are only confined to the retroperitoneum as compared to a more disastrous effect if urine leaks within the peritoneum in a transperitoneal approach. Bowel injury may also occur during dissection because of the close proximity of the peritoneum to the kidney. Pyelonephritis may likewise occur. This is treated medically, however an obstructive aetiology must always be ruled out.

References

El-Ghoneimi A, Farhat W, Bolduc S, et al (2003) Laparoscopic dismembered pyeloplasty by a retroperitoneal approach in children. BJU Int 92:104–108

Gaur D (1992) Laparoscopic operative retroperitoneoscopy: use of a new device. J Urol 156:1120–1124

Kavoussi LR, Peters CA (1993) Laparoscopic pyeloplasty. J Urol 150:1891–1894

Schuessler WW, Grune MT, Tecuanhuey LV, Preminger GM, et al (1993) Laparoscopic dismembered pyeloplasty. J Urol 150:1795–1799

Valla J-S (1999) Videosurgery of the retroperitoneal space in children. In: Bax NMA, Georgeson KE, Najmaldin A, Valla J-S (eds) Endoscopic Surgery in Children. Springer, Berlin Heidelberg New York, pp 379

Chapter 91

Minimally Invasive Surgery and Management of Urinary Tract Stone in Children

Jean-Stéphane Valla, CK Yeung, and Henri Steyaert

Introduction

Urinary stone disease is rare in childhood but its incidence is increasing even in developed countries. In the early 1970s there was only one treatment: removal by open surgery. Today there are several "minimally invasive" technical solutions available: extracorporeal shock wave lithotripsy (ESWL), ureteroscopy (USC), percutaneous nephrolithotomy (PCNL), and minimally invasive surgery (MIS) by the transperitoneal or retroperitoneal approach (Bellman and Smith 1994; Gaur et al. 1994).

The advent of minimally invasive modalities has transformed the management of stone disease in adults and has reduced the place of open surgery to less than 2%. Its impact has been more limited in pediatric practice where open stone surgery is still performed in 15–50% of the cases (Zargooshi 2001). MIS is emerging today in that field and competes not only with the "old open surgery" but also with other minimally invasive techniques.

Minimally invasive surgery allows all the classical open procedures to be reproduced: cystotomy (Baltislam et al. 1997; Segarra et al. 2001; Van Savage et al. 1996), ureterotomy (Feyaerts et al. 2001; Goel and Hemal 2001; Keeley et al. 1999; Skrepetis et al. 2001), pyelotomy, and nephrotomy (Jordan et al. 1997; Micali et al. 1997; Miller et al. 2002; Ramakumar and Segura 2000). Surprisingly MIS was not mentioned at all in the recent paper of Jayanthi et al. (1999), which is unfortunate and misleading.

Proper patient selection remains the most important factor in the successful treatment of pediatric patients with urolithiasis. The goal is to render the patient stone free with the least possible morbidity, risk, and cost.

Preoperative Preparation

Preoperative investigation includes renal ultrasonography, intravenous urography, and succimer (DMSA) scintiscan to localize stones and to check the urinary tract for abnormalities. The high rate of metabolic abnormalities in children with urinary calculi suggest that all should undergo metabolic evaluation, even at first presentation. Such evaluation can be performed before or after stone management.

Before surgery, the urinary tract should be free from infection. Bowel preparation is optional, but unnecessary when a retroperitoneal approach is used. A broad-spectrum intravenous antibiotic should be given at the beginning of the procedure.

Equipment

- Telescope 5 or 10 mm in diameter, 0° or 30°.
- A balloon for developing the retroperitoneal working space is useful in case of peripyelic or periureteral inflammatory changes.
- A good suction-irrigation apparatus is needed for flushing out debris and for removal of this debris from the pelvis or the retroperitoneum.
- Loops or Babcock forceps to suspend the ureter and to avoid stone migration.
- Retractable endoscopic knife (as used for pyloromyotomy).
- Sharp scissors (3 mm) to open the urinary tract. It is better to avoid the use of diathermy to open the ureter.
- Endoscopic grasper with wide opening or spoon forceps.
- Small plastic bag.
- Two needle holders (3 mm) for suturing.
- Ultrasonic scissors in case a diverticulum has to be resected or in case a nephrotomy for a staghorn calculus has to be performed.

Special Equipment

- Pediatric cystoscope for ureteral catheterization in case of an upper urinary tract stone. At the beginning of the procedure, a simple ureteral catheter is placed below the stone for X-ray control and for flushing the urinary tract from inside after stone removal. This extended catheter must be secured to the urethral catheter and must be accessible to the nurse. At the end of the procedure, cystoscopy is often necessary to place a double-J stent.

- Intraoperative fluoroscopy is important for localizing the stone and for confirmation of its complete removal. The operating table should be adapted for doing fluoroscopy.
- An intraoperative laparoscopic steerable ultrasound-color Doppler device is not necessary for ureteric or pelvic stone stones as such stones are easily detected as they cause bulging. In contrast such a device is very useful for identification of stones in the kidney and for identification of the major parenchymal vessels in case of nephrotomy.
- A flexible cystoscope or "nephroscope" with a variety of flat-wire baskets is useful to explore the intrarenal cavity [in case of pyeloureteral junction (PUJ) obstruction most stones are mobile, and are well away from the obstruction either in the calices or in the redundant part of renal pelvis]. If peroperative flexible nephroscopy is used, two cameras and two video towers are necessary.
- Small caliber dye or holmium:YAG laser can be useful for fragmentation or vaporization of large stones.

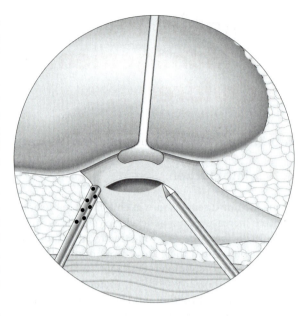

Fig. 91.1. Posterior transverse pyelolithotomy for stone in the right renal pelvis

Technique

We will describe pyelolithotomy, nephrolithotomy, and ureterolithotomy by the retroperitoneal approach, because this approach is the logical way for access of the upper urinary tract. For the distal ureter, the transperitoneal way is the best suited. Finally, we will describe cystolithotomy by the suprapubic approach for bladder stones.

Pyelolithotomy

The same approach and port placement as for nephrectomy is used (see Chapters 84 and 86). The posterior part of renal pelvis is freed from adjacent structures via blunt and sharp dissection. It can be useful to retract the renal parenchyma with a 5 mm Lowe retractor, introduced directly through the abdominal wall. This retractor lifts up the kidney, which exposes the posterior part of the pelvis and caliceal necks after dissection of the renal hilum. A transverse pyelotomy is then made above the ureteropelvic junction with a cold knife and/or scissors (■ Fig. 91.1). To avoid multiple manipulation of the pelvic wall with graspers, the lower part of the pelvis is anchored to the psoas muscle with a stitch (■ Fig. 91.2a). By doing so, the pelvis is kept open. Renal stones are visualized and extracted

through the pyelotomy incision with a rigid grasping forceps or a flat-wire basket (■ Fig. 91.2b). The removal of stones from the pelvis is continuously followed with the telescope. Rigid instruments can be used to remove stones from the upper and middle calices, but for stones in the lower calices the flexible cystoscope introduced through the anterior port allows extraction of the stones under visual control.

Stones too large to be passed through the trocar are placed in a small laparoscopic bag (usually the finger of a glove), which is removed at the end of the procedure. Smaller stone debris in the calices or pelvis is flushed out and then aspirated using the laparoscopic suction-irrigation apparatus. The pyelotomy is closed using a 4/0 polyglycolic acid running suture (■ Fig. 91.3). Methylene blue-stained saline is flushed through the ureteral catheter to check that the suture is watertight. An open-ended catheter is placed outside the pelvis for gravity drainage.

When performing stone removal in a patient who will also undergo a pyeloplasty (Ramakumar et al. 2002), the pyelotomy incision should be placed in such a way that it will be incorporated later on into the final usually dismembered pyeloplasty. It is important however not to transect the ureter before removing the stone. Again the PUJ is anchored to the psoas muscle to stabilize the pelvis outside the renal hilum.

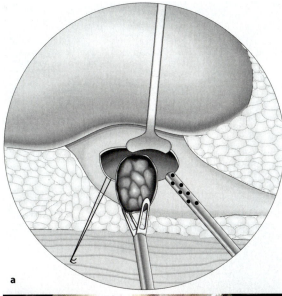

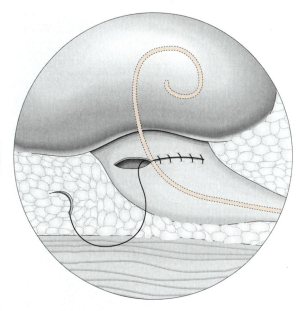

Fig. 91.3. Closure of the lithotomy with a running suture. After completion of the anastomosis the ureteral catheter is flushed with methylene blue-stained saline to check that the suture is watertight

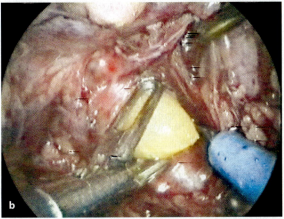

Fig. 91.2. Removal of stone from the renal pelvis after pyelolithotomy. **a** Schematic drawing. Note the anchoring of the renal pelvis to the psoas muscle with a stitch. **b** Intraoperative view

Nephrolithotomy

Before performing a nephrotomy, the artery and vein must be dissected free, as for a nephrectomy, in case there is a necessity to clamp the vascular pedicle (with a laparoscopic bulldog clamp or vessel loop).

An ultrasonic Doppler probe is useful to avoid injury of the main parenchymal vessels and to localize the stones. If not available, stones can be identified by direct puncture. The thinnest part of the cortex is incised using ultrasonic scissors and the stones are extracted. As the renal cortex is fragile a watertight closure is not possible. This is not a problem and the nephrotomy can be left open as long as the urinary tract is drained.

In case of renal caliceal diverticula (Miller et al. 2002; Ramakumar and Segura 2000; Ruckle and Se-

gura 1994), the nephrolithotomy is combined with diverticulectomy or marsupialization. Biological fibrin glue can be helpful to prevent leakage (■ Figs. 91.4, 91.5).

Ureterolithotomy

For proximal and midureteral calculi we favor the retroperitoneoscopic approach. Before performing the ureterolithotomy, it is safer, but not mandatory, to place a guidewire or a catheter past the stone up into the renal pelvis. This is done preoperatively under general anesthesia with the patient in lithotomy position. The ureteral catheter is introduced and fixed to a Foley catheter below it. The patient is then placed in the lateral position on the radiolucent operating table.

The ureter is identified, anterior to the psoas muscle, which is simple due to the bulging effect of the calculus. Dissection down to the calculus is carried out with a Babcock forceps introduced through the anterior cannula and a hook through the posterior cannula. A loop or a Babcock forceps is placed around the ureter, proximal to the stone, to prevent migration. Dissection may be somewhat difficult due to the inflammatory changes. A 5- or 3 mm retractable endoscopic knife (the same as for pyloromyotomy) is inserted through the anterior cannula and incises the ureter longitudinally (to avoid interference with the ureteral blood supply) over the stone. The calculus is then grasped with a forceps and removed directly, if small, or in a

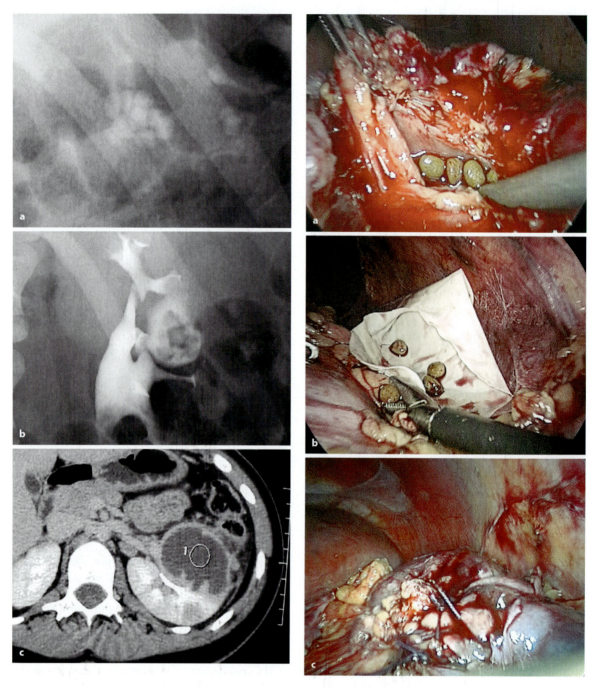

Fig. 91.4. Imaging of stones in a caliceal diverticulum. **a** Plain abdominal X-ray showing stones in the left upper pole diverticulum. **b** Intravenous pyelography showing the caliceal diverticulum with opacities. **c** CT scan showing the anterior localization of the diverticulum

Fig. 91.5. Intraoperative views of the removal of the caliceal stones. **a** Opening of the anterior caliceal wall and localization of the stones. **b** The stones are collected in a bag. **c** Closure of the nephrotomy

bag if large. The ureteral incision is sutured with several 5/0 or 4/0 interrupted polyglycolic acid sutures with an intracorporeal knotting technique. We attempt to obtain a tight closure, taking care not to induce a stricture. If there is no stricture no ureteral drainage is left behind but in particular situations it is safer to leave a simple ureteral stent or to insert a double-J stent. Such a stent is advanced beyond the ureterotomy into the renal pelvis under retroperitoneoscopic vision. Alternatively the patient is placed back into lithotomy position at the end of the operation and a double-J stent is introduced under fluoroscopic guid-

least three trocars are needed: one 5 mm trocar in the umbilicus for the camera and two (3- or 5 mm) trocars in a triangular pattern on the side of the stone. The video column is on the side of the stone, and the surgical team opposite. An additional trocar may be placed for operative assistance or for suction-irrigation. After incision of the peritoneum, the same steps are carried out as during a retroperitoneal approach. We advise to close the peritoneum at the end of the procedure.

Cystolithotomy

If possible a cystoscope is introduced first through the urethra or Mitrofanoff conduit in order to fill the bladder with the usual fluid or with CO_2 and to allow for visual control when introducing the suprapubic port. The diameter of this port is chosen according to the size of calculi, but a 10 mm one usually suffices (■ Fig. 91.7).

If no urethra or Mitrofanoff conduit is available, the bladder is filled through a suprapubic cystostomy with a 22-gauge needle until it is easily palpable. A small suprapubic incision is made to introduce a 3- or 5 mm trocar and telescope. The second suprapubic port is introduced under visual control. It is also possible to use only one trocar (11 mm) for the 10 mm operating channel telescope. The thickness of rectus abdominis muscle and bladder wall must be estimated in order to avoid injury to the posterior bladder wall. Gentle dilatation of the port hole is useful before introducing a cannula with blunt trocar. In patients who previously had an augmentation intestinocystoplasty, the incision should be made as low as possible to avoid violation of the peritoneum.

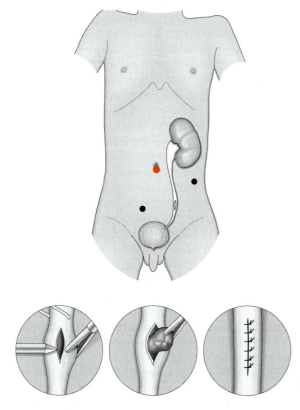

Fig. 91.6. Removal of a stone in the distal left ureter

ance. The Foley catheter and drain are typically removed on postoperative day 2, and the ureteral stent after 4–8 weeks.

For distal ureteral calculi we favor the transperitoneal approach (■ Fig. 91.6). The patient is positioned in dorsal decubitus with moderate lateral rotation. At

Fig. 91.7. Suprapubic cystolithotomy with cystoscopic control

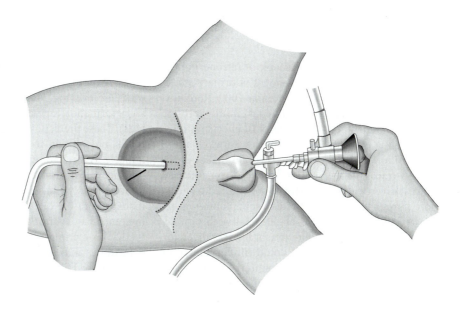

The way for stone extraction varies according to their size. The goal is to remove all the stones and not to leave any small fragments behind, which could serve as a nidus for further stone formation, especially in an abnormal bladder as after intestinocystoplasty. In case of calculi that are less than 8 mm in diameter, suction with a tube is the easiest way. In case of calculi around 10 mm in diameter, a grasping forceps should be used, taking care not to break the stone into pieces. Stones larger than 15 mm in diameter can be managed by laser lithotripsy and aspiration. They can also be placed in a bag (piece of glove) and extracted after mechanical lithotripsy with the help of one or two 3 mm devices. Stones larger than 30 mm are best managed by open cystolithotomy.

At the end of the procedure a visual check is mandatory. If residual stones are suspected, an X-ray is performed and fluoroscopy is carried out. The port hole is sutured and a catheter is placed for straight drainage for 2–5 days depending on the status of the bladder.

Results

We have operated on 16 cases as follows:
- Nephrotomy   2
- Pyelotomy   3
- Ureterotomy   4
- Cystotomy   7

Our results are the following:
- Conversion rate   1/16
- Stone clearance   15/16
- Complications   0/16

Discussion

Indications

The indications for the laparoscopic or retroperitoneoscopic approach in the management of urinary stones in children remain debatable (Kumar 2002; Rofeim et al. 2001). Many factors should be taken into account: size of the patient, clinical symptoms, effects on renal parenchyma, size and location of the stone, chemical composition of the stone, associated anomalies of the urinary tract (such as solitary kidney, ectopic kidney, caliceal diverticulum, congenital or acquired obstruction, fibrotic meatus after ureteral reimplantation, reconstructed or augmented bladder, possibility of access through urethra, neourethra, or bladder diversion such as Mitrofanoff) which could hinder the stone management or require correction in the same operative session, personal experience and training of the surgeon, technical possibilities in and around the insti-

tution, ability to achieve success with the least number of procedures, and safety concerns for the patient.

Extracorporeal shock wave lithotripsy is considered to be the gold standard for first-line treatment even in toddlers and infants, and even in staghorn calculus. Its use however is debated in case of stones located in distal ureter or bladder, in case of hemostatic anomalies or cystinuria, or in case of stones of infective origin. Half of the pediatric stones have an infectious origin. They are bulky, have a soft matrix, and are not suitable for ESWL. They often need several sessions under general anesthesia for their removal.

Since the emergence of new small ureteroscopes, ureterocystoscopy is now possible even in small children (2 or 3 years old) but with the risk of intraoperative ureteral injury and postoperative reflux or stenosis. The young male urethra may be damaged by the insertion of large cystoscopes required for ureteral catheter and stent insertion. In these patients it may be better to introduce the ureteroscope by the suprapubic approach though a 3- or 5 mm trocar and to guide it cystoscopically. Laparoscopy is also a way of protecting the young male urethra.

In the same manner, percutaneous techniques, even the newer minipercutaneous one, are not always easy to use in small children and special training is needed. Laparoscopy offers peroperative visual guidance for insertion of a PCNL in case of particular anatomical situations such as ectopic or horseshoe kidney (Holman and Toth 1998; Ramakumar and Segura 2000).

But all these techniques need special expensive equipment that is usually available only in big "stone centers." On the contrary, laparoscopic equipment today is an integral part of the basic equipment in each operating theatre and the majority of pediatric surgeons are now familiar with this technique. A clear advantage of the endoscopic surgical approach is the single-session clearance rather than the repetitive endourological or lithotripsy sessions. Parents frequently request definitive stone management in one single general anesthesia (Zargooshi 2001).

Urinary tract calculi are often observed in children with pre-existing abnormalities that predispose to stone formation (urine stasis, infections, foreign materials). These predisposing urological abnormalities are reflux, obstruction by PUJ stenosis, megaureter, ureterocele, valves, stump of ectopic ureter, urogenital sinus, neurological bladder, reconstructed bladder (enterocystoplasty). In selected cases it is advantageous to manage both the calculi and the anatomical defect simultaneously, avoiding multiple procedures and anesthetics. Sometimes patients with severe orthopedic deformities may not be amenable to endourological treatment or ESWL.

Finally it would be logical to distinguish two situations. First, there are cases that should be selectively considered for MIS as the first-choice therapy. These cases can be managed by a "basic" pediatric urology team with a well-trained surgeon in laparoscopy. Such indications are the following:

- Impacted ureteral stones that cause obstruction and are located at a distance from the kidney and the bladder
- Coexisting anatomical abnormalities which can be corrected by MIS
- Single pelvic large cystinic calculus
- Destroyed kidney that needs a nephrectomy
- A stone in the bladder

Second, there are complex cases that necessitate a stone center where all special equipment is available and where the pediatric urologist, adult urologist, nephrologist, and interventional radiologist collaborate. Such centers offer a broad multimodal minimally invasive approach to urinary stones. The perceived benefits of a such approach must, however, not be outweighed by the potential morbidity inherent to repeated interventions, particularly those requiring general anesthesia in small children. In such cases MIS is used as salvage procedure after failure of other minimally invasive techniques. It does not replace other minimally invasive techniques but rather complements them.

Relative contraindications for a retroperitoneoscopic approach include previous open or retroperitoneoscopic surgery or failed percutaneous nephrolithotomy with its attendant perirenal adhesions. In these cases, the transperitoneal route remains open.

Technique

Upper urinary tract calculi have been traditionally removed through an open extraperitoneal lumbotomy. Since the availability of MIS, the discussion about the transperitoneal or retroperitoneal approach for nephrectomy and adrenalectomy has been reopened with pro and con arguments. Each surgeon should choose the method with which he or she feels comfortable. Theoretically a transperitoneal approach is a disadvantage because of the potential of urinary leak or spillage of stone debris. However, in case of a diverticulum located in the anterior part of the kidney, the transperitoneal approach seems more logical. As for open surgery, ureteral catheterization, careful dissection, and suturing techniques are all that are required for successful laparoscopic lithotomy.

Concerning stones in the bladder, percutaneous vesicolithotomy provides a minimally invasive means of extracting vesical calculi, especially in patients with an absent or small caliber, sensitive or reconstructed urethra (Van Savage et al. 1996). It avoids any damage of the urethra and reduces trauma to the bladder. It is a very simple procedure with practically no learning curve. The smaller the calculus, the easier the procedure. A follow-up protocol with frequent bladder imaging in patients with a known predisposition of vesicolithiasis is of utmost importance. A potential disadvantage of the procedure is extraperitoneal fluid extravasation.

Results

Since the first cases, 10 years ago (Bellman and Smith 1994; Gaur et al. 1994; Ruckle and Segura 1994), several studies of laparoscopic/retroperitoneoscopic stone management have been published in adults with good results: 15 cases by Holman and Toth (1998), 17 cases by Micali et al. (1997), 19 cases by Ramakumar and Segura (2000), 24 cases by Feyaerts et al. (2001), and 31 cases by Hemal et al. (2003). Two comparatives studies in adults reveal distinct benefits of MIS when compared to open surgery (Goel and Hemal 2001). Very few cases have been published in children (Jordan et al. 1997; Valla et al. 1997), so it is too early to draw definitive conclusions in children.

Conclusion

Minimally invasive surgery allows stones to be retrieved out of the body in a single session and to manage, at the same time, urinary tract anomalies such as PUJ obstruction. It should be considered as a first-choice therapy in selected cases and as a salvage or second-choice therapy for stone removal regardless of its location or presence of anatomical variants after failure of other mini-invasive treatment. MIS should always be considered before open surgery. Laparoscopic equipment nowadays is available in every modern hospital and will replace open surgery for urinary stones in the near future.

References

Baltislam E, Germiyanoglu C, Karabulut A, et al (1997) A new application of laparoscopic instruments in percutaneous bladder stone removal. J Laparoendosc Adv Surg Tech 7:241–244

Bellman GC, Smith AD (1994) Special considerations in the technique of laparoscopic ureterolithotomy. J Urol 151:146–149

Feyaerts A, Rietbergen J, Navarra S, et al (2001) Laparoscopic ureterolithotomy for ureteral calculi. Eur Urol 40:609–613

Gaur DD, Agarwal DK, Purohit KC, et al (1994) Retroperitoneal laparoscopic ureterolithotomy for multiple upper mild ureteral calculi. J Urol 151:1001–1002

Goel A, Hemal AK (2001) Upper and mid-ureteric stones: a prospective unrandomized comparison of retroperitoneoscopic and open ureterolithotomy. BJU Int 88:679–682

Hemal AK, Goel A, Goel R (2003) Minimally invasive retroperitoneoscopic ureterolithotomy. J Urol 169:480–482

Holman E, Toth C (1998) Laparoscopically assisted percutaneous transperitoneal nephrolithotomy in pelvic dystopic kidney: experience in 15 successful cases. J Laparoendosc Adv Surg Tech 8:431–435

Jayanthi VR, Arnold PM, Koff SA (1999) Strategies for managing upper tract calculi in young children. J Urol 162:1234–1237

Jordan GH, McCammon KA, Robey EL (1997) Laparoscopic pyelolithotomy. Urology 49:131–134

Keeley FX, Gialas I, Pillai M, et al (1999) Laparoscopic ureterolithotomy: the Edinburgh experience. BJU Int 84:765–769

Kumar U (2002) Laparoscopic management of urolithiasis: is this an option? Dialog Paediatr Urol 25:7

Micali S, Morre RG, Averch TD, et al (1997) The role of laparoscopy in the treatment of renal and ureteral calculi. J Urol 157:463–466

Miller SD, Ng CS, Streem SB, et al (2002) Laparoscopic management of caliceal diverticular calculi. J Urol 167:1248–1252

Ramakumar S, Segura JW (2000) Laparoscopic surgery for renal urolithiasis: pyelolithotomy caliceal diverticulectomy and treatment of stones in a pelvic kidney. J Endourol 14:829–832

Ramakumar S, Lancini V, Chan DY, et al (2002) Laparoscopic pyeloplasty with concomitant pyelolithotomy. J Urol 167:1378–1380

Rofeim D, Yohannes P, Badlani GH (2001) Does laparoscopic ureterolithotomy replace shock-wave lithotripsy or ureteroscopy for ureteral stones? Curr Opin Urol 11:287–291

Ruckle HC, Segura JW (1994) Laparoscopic treatment of a stone filled, caliceal diverticulum: a definitive minimally invasive therapeutic option. J Urol 151:122–124

Segarra J, Palou J, Montleo P, et al (2001) Hasson's laparoscopic trocar in percutaneous bladder stone lithotripsy. Int Urol Nephrol 33:625–626

Skrepetis K, Doumas K, Siafakas I et al. (2001) Laparoscopic versus open ureterolithotomy. Eur Urol 40:32–37

Valla JS, Heloury H, Steyaert H, et al (1997) Retroperitoneoscopic approach for pyelo and ureterolithotomy in children. Eighth Annual Meeting of ESPU, Ome 3–7 April

Van Savage JG, Khoury A, McLorie G, et al (1996) Percutaneous vacuum vesicolithotomy under direct vision: a new technique. J Urol 156:706–708

Zargooshi J (2001) Open stone surgery in children: is it justified in the era of minimally invasive therapies? BJU Int 88:928–931

Chapter 92

Retroperitoneoscopic Treatment of Retrocaval Ureter

Jean-Stéphane Valla and Alaa El Ghoneimi

Introduction

Retrocaval ureter is a rare congenital anomaly, resulting from an abnormal development of the inferior vena cava (IVC). Sometimes it produces obstruction because of kinking at the level of its retrocaval course. In patients suffering from recurrent infection, obstruction, and flank pain, surgical treatment is indicated.

A procedure similar to a dismembered pyeloplasty is utilized to correct this anomaly. It can be approached by a transperitoneal or retroperitoneal approach but, as for a pyeloureteric junction (PUJ) obstruction, we favor the retroperitoneal one (■ Fig. 92.1).

Preoperative Preparation

Preoperative evaluation and preparation for retroperitoneoscopic reconstruction of the retrocaval ureter is identical to that for retroperitoneoscopic dismembered pyeloplasty (Chapter 90; ■ Figs. 92.2, 92.3).

After induction of general anesthesia, cystoscopy is carried out to cannulate the right ureteral orifice and to pass, under fluoroscopic guidance, a ureteral catheter (simple external ureteral stent or double pigtail). A guidewire is often needed to overcome the reverse "S" shaped deformity of the retrocaval ureter (■ Fig. 92.4).

The patient, crew, monitor, and equipment are positioned as for a retroperitoneal dismembered pyeloplasty (■ Fig. 92.5).

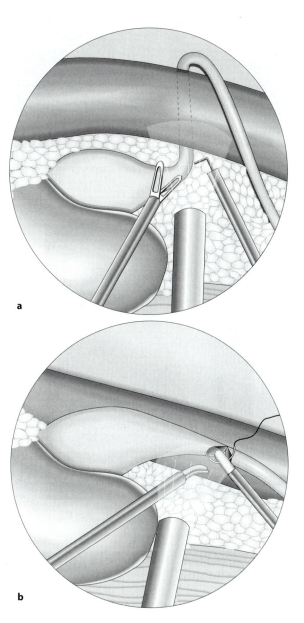

Fig. 92.1. Schematic representation of the retroperitoneal approach for a retrocaval ureter. *Top* Initial step, dissection of the retrocaval part of the ureter. *Bottom* After sectioning and uncrossing of the ureter, the ureter is reanastomosed without tension

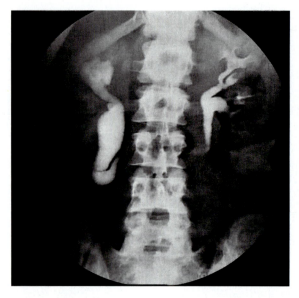

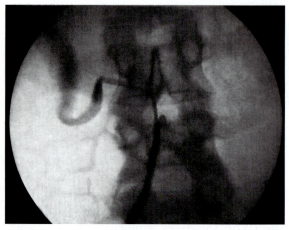

Fig. 92.4. Retrograde pyelography of a retrocaval ureter

Fig. 92.2. Anteroposterior intravenous pyelogram (IVP) of a retrocaval ureter

the ureter. The lower part of the ureter is usually adherent to the anterior part of the IVC and iliac vein. Using blunt and sharp dissection the ureter is freed from its surrounding tissue for a distance of 3 cm above and below the IVC crossing. The ureter is mobilized behind the vena cava until a "shoe shine" maneuver is possible (■ Fig. 92.6).

The ureter is transected above the IVC crossing and the stent is partially withdrawn. The distal ureter is uncrossed and repositioned to lie anterior to the vena cava. Usually a segment of redundant fibrotic stenotic ureter is excised proximally. The distal ureteral stump is spatulated and the stent advanced into the renal pelvis. A tension-free anastomosis is then created with interrupted or running absorbable suture, intracorporeally knotted (■ Fig. 92.7).

The retroperitoneal area is drained with a closed suction drain.

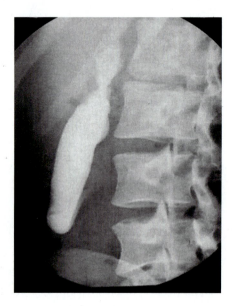

Fig. 92.3. Lateral IVP of a retrocaval ureter

Postoperative Care

Postoperative care and complications are also the same as described in the chapter on retroperitoneoscopic pyeloplasty (Chapter 90).

Technique

Trocar insertion and position is the same as for retroperitoneal dismembered pyeloplasty.

The proximal dilated ureter is identified first. It is located more medially than usual, close to the IVC. At the level of the third lumbar vertebra, the upper portion of the ureter passes under the IVC. The telescope is then turned toward the lower part of the operative field in order to identify and dissect the lower part of

Results

Our experience is limited to three cases, two boys aged 10 and 17 years and one girl aged 11 years. The girl had been diagnosed prenatally to have hydronephrosis, but at long-term follow-up the hydronephrosis had remained stable for a long time and only increased lately. In one patient, the retrocaval fibrotic portion of the ureter was was wrongly left in situ. As aresult a reoperation in this patient was needed a year later.

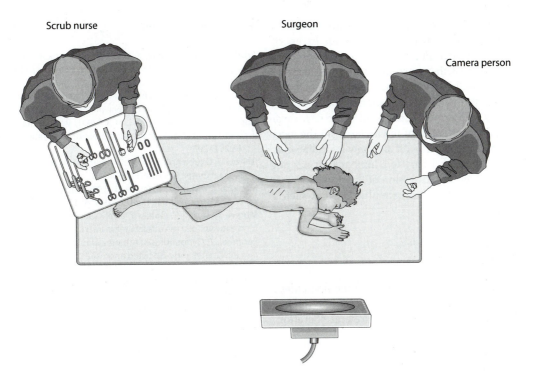

Scrub nurse

Surgeon

Camera person

Fig. 92.5. Position of patient, crew and monitor

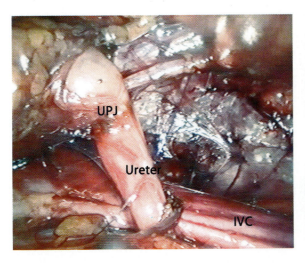

Fig. 92.6. Intraoperative view of the dissected retrocaval ureter

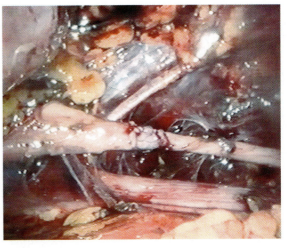

Fig. 92.7. Intraoperative view after sectioning of the ureter and reconstruction

Discussion

Preoperatively other associated congenital anomalies, such as horseshoe kidney and double IVC, that may complicate the procedure and the choice of the approach have to be diagnosed or ruled out by imaging studies (Perimenis et al. 2002).

A systematic preoperative retrograde pyelography allows to confirm the diagnosis and to avoid surprises during the retroperitoneoscopic approach, for example

PUJ obstruction as was the case in one of our patients.

In the literature the transperitoneal approach (Amalingam and Selverajan 2003; Ameda et al. 2001; Ishitoya et al. 1996; Matsuda et al. 1996; Polascik and Chen 1998; Salomon et al. 1999) has been used more often than the retroperitoneal one (Gupta et al. 2001; Mugiya et al. 1999; Salomon et al. 1999). The choice depends on the surgeon's preference.

Surprisingly, the treatment of retrocaval ureter is easier than PUJ reconstruction because the excess of length of the retrocaval ureter causes no tension during the creation of the anastomosis and because the lower position of the anastomosis site allows for a more ergonomic position, i.e. triangulation of the two operating devices. The only delicate point is the retrocaval dissection, but separation of the ureter from the vena cava is not technically difficult and only few adhesions are present. Although injury to a lumbar vein has not been reported yet, the dissection of the posterior wall of the IVC should be done carefully to avoid such a complication.

Conclusion

Minimally invasive surgery should be the first choice for correction of a retrocaval ureter. A retroperitoneoscopic approach is well suited for ureteral liberation, transection, and reanastomosis.

References

Amalingam M, Selverajan K (2003) Laparoscopic transperitoneal repair of retrocaval ureter: report of two cases. J Endourol 17:85–87

Ameda K, Kakizaki H, Jarabayashi T, et al (2001) Laparoscopic ureteroureterostomy for retrocaval ureter. Int J Urol 8:71–74

Gupta NH, Hemal AK, Singh I, et al (2001) Retroperitoneoscopic ureterolysis and reconstruction of retrocaval ureter. J Endourol 15:291–293

Ishitoya S, Okubo K, Arai Y (1996) Laparoscopic ureterolysis for retrocaval ureter. Br J Urol 77:162–163

Matsuda T, Yasumoto R, Tsujino T (1996) Laparoscopic treatment of a retrocaval ureter. Eur Urol 29:115–118

Mugiya S, Suzuki K, Ohhira T, et al (1999) Retroperitoneoscopic treatment of a retrocaval ureter. Int J Urol 6:419–422

Perimenis P, Gyffopoulos K, Athanasopoulos A, et al (2002) Retrocaval ureter and associated anomalies. Int Urol Nephrol 33:19–22

Polascik TJ, Chen RN (1998) Laparoscopic ureteroureterostomy for retrocaval ureter. J Urol 160:121–122

Salomon L, Hozneck A, Balian C, et al (1999) Retroperitoneal laparoscopy of a retrocaval ureter. BJU Int 84:181–182

Complicated Ureteroceles with Non-functioning Renal Moieties in Duplex Kidneys: One-stage Radical Laparoscopic Treatment

C.K. Yeung, S.K. Chowdhary and J.D. Sihoe

Introduction

The optimal management of large ectopic extravesical ureteroceles that are associated with a non-functioning renal moiety in a duplex system has remained a challenging problem and the focus of continuing controversies. Traditional surgical management strategy for this condition usually consists of a two-stage open approach. The first stage entails removal of the non-functioning renal moiety, usually the upper pole of the kidney, and excision of the dilated upper moiety ureter, via a muscle-cutting flank incision. The second stage involves the excision of the lower end of the dilated ureter together with the ectopic ureterocele, reconstruction of the resulting defect in the bladder base and bladder neck, and reimplantation of the normal lower moiety orthotopic ureter to prevent subsequent vesicoureteric reflux. Excellent long-term results have been reported by various workers using this approach. However such management strategy necessitates two major abdominal operations via large open incisions, usually during two separate hospital admissions in quick succession.

The magnitude of the surgery and the potential morbidity associated with such a staged open surgical approach led to the development of a simpler, more conservative approach commencing with either cystoscopic incision of the ureterocele or upper pole heminephrectomy, followed by observation and waiting (Coplen and Duckett 1995). Despite reports of initial favourable short-term results from some centres, more recently there have been increasing reports regarding unsatisfactory long-term outcome, with a significant proportion of patients returning with symptoms which necessitated definitive surgery (Cooper et al. 2000). Furthermore, surgery at the lower urinary tract after repeated attacks of urinary tract infections often becomes more difficult due to more dense adhesions, resulting in an increased risk of operative morbidity. Hence the more simplistic approach with either cystoscopic incision of ureterocele or heminephrectomy alone may not necessarily be the best approach for large complicated caecoureteroceles associated with a non-functioning renal moiety in the long term. The pendulum has swung back and more experts have now considered that more radical and definitive surgery with removal of the non-functioning renal moiety together with excision of the caecoureteroceles, followed by complete lower urinary tract reconstruction, should be the treatment of choice (Ade Ajayi et al. 2001; Hagg et al. 2000).

The transperitoneal laparoscopic approach allows all the components of surgery, including removal of diseased areas (upper pole heminephrectomy, ureterectomy and extravesical excision of caecoureteroceles) together with reconstruction of the lower urinary tract (repair of bladder base defect and extravesical reimplantation of the lower moiety ureter), to be performed in one stage in a single operative session. This is made possible by the ability of the laparoscope to access all quadrants of the abdominal and pelvic cavity down to the pelvic floor. By simply swinging the direction of vision of the telescope and planning the instrument ports appropriately, surgery to both the upper as well as the lower urinary tract can be easily undertaken. The remarkable optical magnification provided by the endoscope also facilitates precise surgical dissection and meticulous reconstruction deep down in the pelvis. We have been using this one-stage approach in the management of complex caecoureteroceles associated with non-functioning renal moieties over the past few years, with very satisfactory results (Borzi and Yeung 2004).

The operative procedure consists of three different parts performed in the following sequence:

1. Transurethral cystoscopic de-roofing and resection of intravesical and urethral elements of caecoureteroceles, and retrograde insertion of ureteric catheter to lower (normal) moiety ureter
2. Transperitoneal laparoscopic heminephroureterectomy
3. Laparoscopic excision of ureterocele, repair of bladder base/bladder neck and extravesical reimplantation of lower moiety ureter

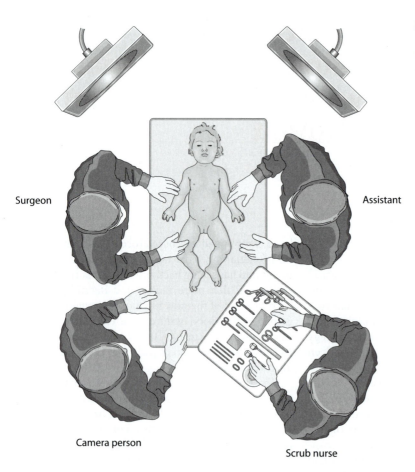

Fig. 93.1. Operating room setting for laparoscopic left heminephrectomy

Surgeon

Assistant

Camera person

Scrub nurse

The operative techniques of the different parts of this one-stage laparoscopic management will be described in this chapter.

Preoperative Preparation

The patient is admitted the day before surgery for preoperative evaluation. For patients who have undergone an initial cystoscopic incision of ureterocele in early infancy, usually because of infective complications, our general policy is to wait until the child is about one year of age before considering for definitive surgery. Preoperative imaging including ultrasound, micturating cystourethrogram and isotope renal scans are reviewed. Detailed counselling of the parents is given regarding the techniques used for the various parts of the one-stage laparoscopic surgery, possible technical difficulties and complications, and the possibility for the need of intraoperative open conversion, and informed consent for surgery is obtained. The side of surgery is marked with indelible ink. Bowel preparation with a fleet enema is usually given the evening before to ensure that no excessive faecal loading occurs.

Induction of Anaesthesia

The patient is prepared for general anaesthesia with endotracheal intubation and muscle relaxation as usual. The use of nitrous oxide should be avoided to minimise bowel distension. A nasogastric tube is inserted especially if the lesion is on the left side. A broad-spectrum antibiotic is routinely given intravenously for prophylaxis on induction of anaesthesia.

Positioning of Patient, Crew, Monitors and Equipment

Cystoscopic Resection of Ureterocele and Retrograde Catheterisation of Lower Moiety Ureter

The patient is placed in a supine and slightly Trendelenburg position on a radiolucent table that allows fluoroscopy. The patient's legs are separated to allow access to the urethral orifice for cystoscopy and retrograde ureteric catheterisation. The surgeon stands between the patient's legs at the end of the table, with the video column placed usually on one side and the fluoroscope on the other.

Fig. 93.2. Operating room setting for laparoscopic excision of ureterocele and ureteric reimplantation

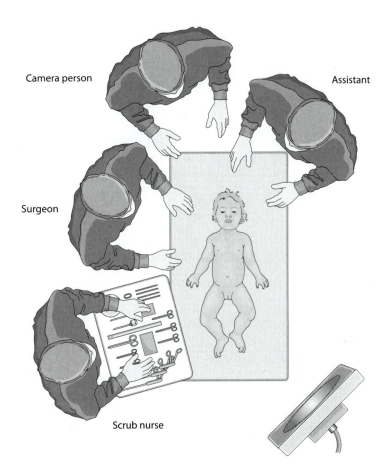

Camera person

Assistant

Surgeon

Scrub nurse

Laparoscopic Upper Pole Heminephrectomy and Ureterectomy

After the cystoscopic de-roofing of the ureterocele and retrograde ureteric catheterisation, the patient is placed in a semilateral position close to the edge of the operating table, with the ipsilateral side of the pathology elevated. Silicone gel pads are used to support all the pressure points. Shoulder hyperabduction is avoided while resting the extended forearm to prevent brachial plexus injury. The patient should be secured to the table by adhesive straps. During the procedure, the table can be rotated so that gravitational force can be maximised for retraction of the colon and the small bowel away from the operative field. The surgeon and the camera person stand on the contralateral side of the pathology facing the patient (■ Fig. 93.1). The monitor is placed across the table in a straight line with the surgeon. As usually only one assistant is required a second monitor is not essential.

Laparoscopic Excision of Ureterocele, Repair of Bladder Base/Bladder Neck and Reimplantation of Lower Moiety Ureter

After completion of the laparoscopic upper pole heminephrectomy and ureterectomy down to the pelvic brim, the table is de-rotated so that the patient is in a more supine position. The focus of the procedure now shifts from the abdominal to the pelvic cavity. The surgeon and the assistant face downwards towards the pelvis, and the video column and monitor are also shifted to be placed towards the end of the table (■ Fig. 93.2).

Technique

Cystoscopic Resection of Ureterocele and Retrograde Catheterisation of Lower Moiety Ureter

Transurethral cystoscopy is first carried out to delineate the anatomy and extent of the caecoureterocele, and the location of its ectopic orifice. Cystoscopic assessment is also made regarding the size and extent of the detrusor defect in the hemitrigone and bladder neck as a result of the ureterocele. The position of the

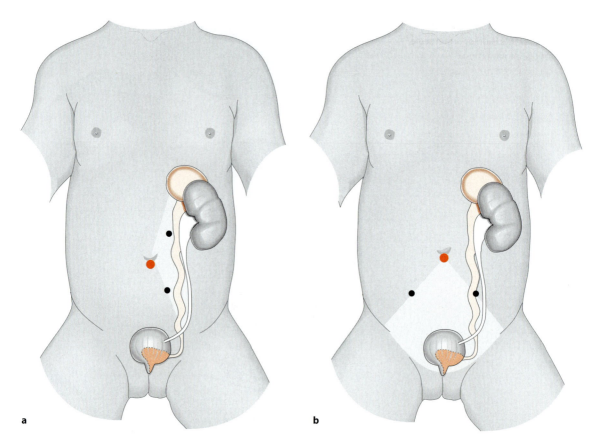

Fig. 93.3. Ports, laparoscope and instrument positions during (a) laparoscopic upper pole heminephrectomy and ureterectomy and (b) laparoscopic excision of ureterocele, repair of bladder base/bladder neck and reimplantation of lower moiety ureter

normal (usually lower) moiety ureteric orifice is also identified. All intravesical and infravesical/urethral elements of the caecoureterocele are then fulgurated and removed as completely as possible with electrocautery using a resectoscope. Particular caution is taken to ensure that no infravesical elements of the caecoureterocele remain that may constitute a flap-valve urethral obstruction in future.

After complete de-roofing and resection of the intravesical and urethral elements of the caecoureterocele is achieved, the lower (normal) moiety ureter orifice is cannulated and a 3F or 4F ureteric catheter is inserted under fluoroscopic control to the lower renal moiety. This acts as a ureteric stent to protect the normal ureter during subsequent extravesical excision of the ureterocele and ureteric reimplantation.

Laparoscopic Upper Pole Heminephrectomy and Ureterectomy

This is performed via a transperitoneal route. After positioning of the patient, skin preparation is made from the nipples down to mid thighs. Transperitoneal lapa-

roscopy is started using a 5 mm 30° lens via a 5 mm supraumbilical port inserted by open Hasson technique (■ Fig. 93.3a). Carbon dioxide pneumoperitoneum is maintained at a pressure of 10–12 mmHg. Two more 3- to 5 mm instrument ports are then inserted on the side of pathology under videoendoscopic guidance, along the anterior axillary line at the upper and lower quadrants. These two ports will provide instrument access during the upper pole heminephrectomy and ureterectomy. A fourth port may sometimes be required on the contralateral upper quadrant particularly when the lesion is on the right side to support the liver.

Upper pole heminephrectomy is started by first exposing the affected kidney with mobilisation of the overlying colon. This can be quickly done by using the electrocautery hook. Because of gravity, the colon usually will fall away medially if adequately mobilised, without the need to employ an additional retractor during the rest of the procedure. The renal vascular pedicle is exposed and carefully dissected so that the vascular supply to the upper and lower moieties can be accurately delineated. The upper pole of the kidney is mobilised from the surrounding tissues which are of-

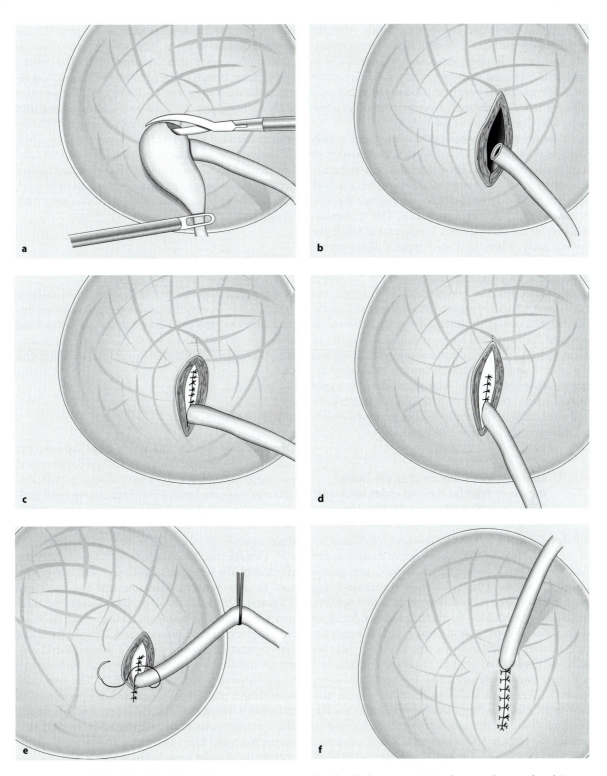

Fig. 93.4. a Laparoscopic upper pole nephroureterectomy completed and telescope pointing downwards towards pelvic cavity. Ureterocele everted by traction on the dilated upper pole ureter. **b** Defect over bladder base revealed after excision of ureterocele. **c** Bladder mucosal defect closed using interrupted sutures. Incision made over upper end of detrusor muscle defect. **d** Bladder muscle over the upper end of defect is split and gently pushed sideways until the underlying bladder mucosa is exposed to extend the trough along the posterior bladder wall in preparation for subsequent ureteral reimplantation. **e** Laparoscopic extravesical reimplantation of the lower moiety ureter in a Lich-Gregoir fashion started by approximating bladder muscle on both sides of the trough over the ureter with interrupted absorbable sutures. **f** Bladder base repair and extravesical reimplantation of lower moiety ureter completed

ten adherent due to previous pyelonephritis. After the upper moiety has been cleared all around from its cranial and lateral borders, dissection is undertaken to further identify each of the polar vessels. These are then individually isolated and divided either between clips but more often simply with the help of an ultrasonic scalpel as they are of small size.

Attention is now turned to the dilated and usually tortuous upper moiety ureter, which is mobilised from its retroperitoneal attachment down to the pelvic brim, and upwards until the renal vascular pedicle is reached. Special care is given to identify and safeguard the lower moiety ureter during this process. This is often facilitated by the presence of a ureteric stent inside the lower moiety. When the dilated upper moiety ureter is mobilised up to the renal vascular pedicle, the ureter is divided and its proximal part attached to the upper moiety renal pelvis is passed from behind the renal vessels and retrieved from above. With traction on the divided megaureter, the interpelvic plane between the pelvis of the upper and lower moieties can usually be identified. Dissection is deepened along this plane and the intervening renal parenchyma can be divided using an ultrasonic scalpel. After removal of the upper moiety, careful haemostasis to the raw surface is done and any breach of the renal pelvis of the lower moiety is repaired using fine monofilament sutures.

Laparoscopic Excision of Ureterocele, Repair of Bladder Base/Bladder Neck and Reimplantation of Lower Moiety Ureter

Further dissection is then continued with mobilisation of the distal part of the dilated upper moiety ureter down in the pelvic cavity. An additional 5-mm port is inserted over the iliac fossa on the ipsilateral side (Fig. 93.3b). The dilated ureter is dissected down to the base of the bladder. By hitching the bladder up to the anterior abdominal wall using a monofilament suture inserted percutaneously, the posterior bladder wall and bladder base can be inspected and accessed with ease using the laparoscope. The upper and lower moiety ureters are carefully separated down to the ureterovesical junction. With traction applied to the upper moiety ureter, the ureterocele can be everted to outside the bladder and completely excised extravesically (Fig. 93.4a,b). The resulting defect in the bladder base and bladder neck is repaired in two layers using interrupted intracorporeal absorbable sutures, starting first with the mucosal defect (Fig. 93.4c). The lower moiety normal ureter usually lies on the medial side of the defect and can be conveniently reimplanted extravesically by incorporating it into the subsequent muscular closure. After the mucosal defect is closed, the muscle layer of the bladder wall from the superior end of the defect is incised to expose the underlying bladder mucosa. This incision is then extended along the course of the lower pole ureter to create a comfortable trough in preparation for extravesical reimplantation of the ureter (Fig. 93.4d). The detrusor is then closed over the lower pole normal ureter with interrupted fine absorbable sutures to complete the reconstruction (Fig. 93.4e,f).

The surgical specimens including the excised nonfunctioning upper renal moiety, the dilated ureter and ureterocele are retrieved through the umbilical port. This is followed by closure of the port sites after infiltration with 0.25% bupivacaine.

Postoperative Care

Postoperatively, the patient is kept on Foley catheter drainage for 3–4 days. Normal oral diet is resumed immediately after the procedure day and antibiotics and analgesics are continued for 48 h. The patient is usually discharged by the fourth or fifth postoperative day.

Results

Over the past 5 years this single-stage laparoscopic treatment has become our preferred standard surgical treatment for complex and large prolapsing caecoureteroceles associated with a non-functioning renal moiety that are complicated by recurrent urinary infections. Nineteen children have undergone this single-stage laparoscopic excision of ureterocele combined with bladder base reconstruction and ureteric reimplantation. The series includes 12 girls and 7 boys with ages ranging between 9 months and 9 years (mean 3.3 years). This however does not include caecoureteroceles associated with functioning renal moieties, for which excision of ureterocele followed by bladder base reconstruction and usually a double-barrel ureteric reimplantation via an intravesical pneumovesicoscopic approach will be performed. The one-stage laparoscopic procedure was successfully performed in all children with none converted to an open operation. The operative time ranged between 165 and 355 min (mean 208 min). Like other complex endoscopic procedures there was a steep learning curve, with the operative time decreasing sharply as experience accumulated. Hospital stay ranged from 3 to 8 days, with a mean stay of 4.8 days. All patients were followed up regularly and remained asymptomatic and well with a mean follow-up period of 28.3 months (range 8 months to 5.8 years).

Discussion

This novel laparoscopic technique has been developed in the background of extensive experience with open reconstructive surgery for complex ureteroceles using a "staged approach" strategy in earlier years. Traditionally, complex ureteroceles have been managed in a stepwise manner with a few major surgical procedures, usually comprising open transvesical excision of ureterocele together with reconstruction of the detrusor defect and reimplantation of the ipsilateral lower pole ureter, and an upper pole partial nephrectomy and total ureterectomy through a separate flank incision. As most ureteroceles present in early infancy, aggressive radical surgery with total reconstruction in the lower urinary tract in this young age group will also pose additional technical challenges. Notwithstanding this, the alternative more conservative approach commencing with either cystoscopic incision of the ureterocele or upper pole heminephrectomy followed by observation and waiting has not been able to withstand the test of time in the management of complex caecoureteroceles, as many recent reports have revealed an increasing frequency of children requiring second-stage definitive surgery (Casale et al. 2005; Gran et al. 2005).

The rapid development of minimally invasive surgical techniques in paediatric patients with good results has led to more complex urological procedures being performed laparoscopically (Fingenshau et al. 1994; Janetschek et al. 1997). As a retroperitoneoscopic approach for the upper pole heminephrectomy would not allow complex surgery to be done for the lower urinary tract at the same setting, a transperitoneal laparoscopic approach has been adopted to allow surgery on pathologies in the upper as well as the lower urinary tract to be undertaken during a single operation. The pelvic part of this procedure is a combination of an extravesical excision of the everted large ectopic ureterocele, together with repair of the resulting bladder base and bladder neck defect, followed by a Lich-Gregoir type of ureteric reimplantation of the normal lower moiety ureter. The ureteric reimplantation can be conveniently incorporated into the bladder base repair, as described earlier in the methodology section. With accumulation of experience, the whole procedure can be routinely completed in less than 3 h, with minimal postoperative pain and discomfort.

The single-stage laparoscopic surgery for this complex anomaly allows the completion of all necessary surgical procedures in one stage. The remarkable optical magnification provided by the laparoscope further facilitates very precise dissection and meticulous reconstruction of the bladder base and bladder neck region. In light of the minimal invasiveness to the patient, as well as the greatly enhanced cost-effectiveness, this laparoscopic one-stage radical approach has the potential to become the treatment of choice for such complex cases in the near future.

References

Ade Ajayi N, Wilcox DT, Duffy PG, et al (2001) Upper pole heminephroureterectomy: is ureterectomy necessary? BJU Int 88:77–79

Borzi P, Yeung CK (2004) Selective approach for transperitoneal and extraperitoneal endoscopic nephrectomy in children. J Urol 171:814–816

Casale P, Grady RW, Lee RS, et al (2005) Symptomatic refluxing distal ureteral stumps after nephroureterectomy and heminephroureterectomy: what should we do? J Urol 173:204–206

Cooper CS, Passerini Glazel G, Hutcheson JC, et al (2000) Long term follow-up of endoscopic incision of ureteroceles: intravesical versus extravesical. J Urol 164:1097–1099

Coplen DE, Duckett JW (1995) The modern approach to ureteroceles. J Urol 153:166–168

Fingenshau RS, Clayman RV, Kerbl K, et al (1994) Laparoscopic nephroureterectomy in the child: initial case report. J Urol 151:740–741

Gran CD, Kropp BD, Cheng EY et al. (2005) Primary lower urinary tract reconstruction for non-functioning renal moieties associated with obstructed ureteroceles. J Urol 173:198–201

Hagg MJ, Mourachov PV, Snyder HM, et al (2000) The modern endoscopic approach to ureterocele. J Urol 163:940–943

Janetschek G, Siebold J, Radmeyer C, et al (1997) Laparoscopic hemi-nephroureterectomy in pediatric patients. J Urol 158:1928–1930

Valla S, Breeaud J, Carfagna L, et al (2003) Treatment of ureterocele on duplex ureter: upper pole nephrectomy by retroperitoneoscopy in children based on a series of 24 cases. Eur Urol 43:426–429

Chapter 94

Urachal Abnormalities

John F. Bealer and Steven S. Rothenberg

Introduction

Laparoscopic excision of urachal cysts and sinuses takes full advantage of minimally invasive surgery offering superb visualization of both the urachus and the urinary bladder (Groot-Wassink et al. 2000; Khurana and Borzi 2002; Yohannes et al. 2003). These advantages facilitate an accurate and complete excision of the urachus with a secure closure of the bladder's dome. Laparoscopy also offers the opportunity to evaluate cases in which the diagnosis is not clear by clinical presentation or imaging studies, without committing to a larger exploration.

Preoperative Preparation

Before Induction of General Anesthesia

The diagnosis is initially suspected by persistent umbilical drainage and usually confirmed by ultrasonography (McCollum et al. 2003; Ueno et al. 2003). The authors prefer to treat abscessed urachal cysts in a staged fashion by being first incised and drained. The ongoing infection is then treated for several weeks (typically 2–4 weeks) with antibiotics prior to complete excision.

Patients are generally admitted to the hospital on the day of surgery and have undergone an appropriate period of fasting. For children smaller than 5 kg in weight, one or two glycerin suppositories the night prior to surgery can be helpful in decompressing the rectum and sigmoid colon.

After Induction of General Anesthesia

Following the induction of general anesthesia, patients are placed supine while a nasogastric tube and a Foley catheter are inserted. There are three major reasons for inserting a urinary catheter. First, the urinary catheter decompresses the bladder to make entry into the abdomen safer. Second, the catheter can be used to distend the bladder during surgery to help define the bladder dome and to conveniently position it for closure. Finally, bladder distention may be used to test the security of bladder closure. Postoperatively, in cases where a large bladder defect was closed, the catheter may be desirable for bladder decompression. Standard prophylactic antibiotics are routinely administered.

Positioning of Patient, Crew, Monitors, and Equipment

The patient is placed supine on the operating table. After trocars are placed into the abdomen, the table is tilted into a 20–30° Trendelenburg position. This head-down position helps expose the pelvis by allowing the small bowel to fall cranially. In infants, the child is usually placed perpendicular to the table axis, allowing the surgeon to stand at the patient's head with the video monitor directly across the table from the surgeon at the baby's feet. In larger children, the monitor is still placed at the patient's feet but the surgeon will stand at the patient's side facing caudally. As in all laparoscopic procedures, boom-mounted monitors greatly facilitate equipment setup and positioning (■ Fig. 94.1a,b).

Special Equipment

No special equipment or energy applying systems are required.

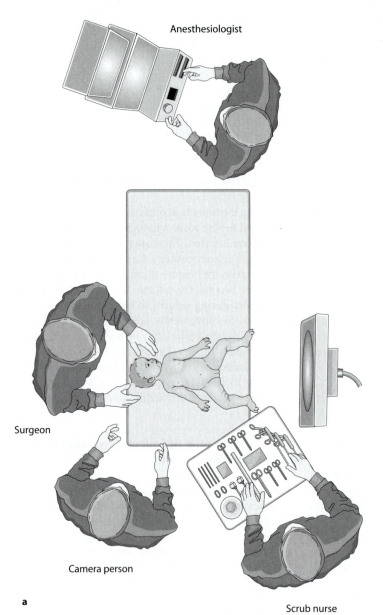

Anesthesiologist

Surgeon

Camera person

Scrub nurse

a

Fig. 94.1 Patient and crew postioning.
a Infant

Technique

Cannulae

Cannula	Method of insertion	Diameter (mm)	Device	Position
1	Closed	5	Optic	Epigastrium or left upper quadrant
2	Closed	3 or 5	Needle holder, scissors, hook	Right upper quadrant or epigastrium
3	Closed	3	Curved forceps	Left upper quadrant or left lower quadrant

Fig. 94.1 Patient and crew postioning. **b** Older child

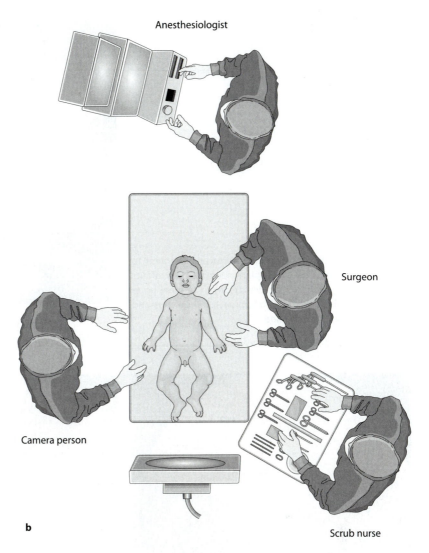

Anesthesiologist

Surgeon

Camera person

Scrub nurse

b

Procedure

Three trocars are usually used for this procedure and their positioning is based on patient size. In babies, a 5 mm trocar is initially placed in the epigastrium. The authors routinely place all trocars using a "closed" technique but this is a matter of preference. After placement of the initial trocar, the abdomen is insufflated with carbon dioxide to maintain a constant intra-abdominal pressure of 15 mmHg. Through this initial trocar a 4- or 5 mm, preferably 30°, laparoscope is placed into the abdomen. The two additional "working" trocars are placed in the right and left upper abdominal quadrants (Fig. 94.2).

In larger children, the pelvis may be a significant distance from the epigastrium. This distance makes the procedure more difficult to visualize and challenging to perform with the trocars all in the upper abdomen. In the older, larger, child an alternate trocar arrangement may be preferable. This alternate arrangement is

rotated toward the patient's left-hand side. The 5 mm trocar placed for the laparoscope is positioned in the patient's left upper quadrant while the two working trocars are placed in the epigastrium and left lower quadrant. The lower quadrant trocar is positioned lower than the umbilicus, approximately halfway between umbilicus and pubis, lateral to the nipple line (Fig. 94.2).

Once in the abdomen the urachal structure, either cyst or sinus, should be identified and mobilized from its insertion into the umbilicus (Fig. 94.3). Maintaining traction on the freed umbilical end, the entire structure is mobilized caudally from its peritoneal attachments down to the dome of the urinary bladder (Fig. 94.4). The two lateral umbilical ligaments define the lateral borders of the urachal structure being excised. During the dissection, instilling sterile saline into the bladder via the indwelling Foley catheter can help distinguish bladder dome from the urachal structure. The dissection is performed using electrocautery

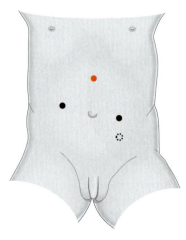

Fig. 94.2. Schematic representation of trocar placement to excise urachal cyst or sinus. Port placements for both infants and children are depicted. In older children, the three ports left of the umbilicus are used to approach the urachus and bladder from the left lateral side

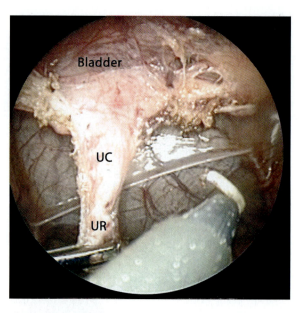

Fig. 94.4 Intraoperative view of urachal structures being mobilized from the umbilicus toward the bladder

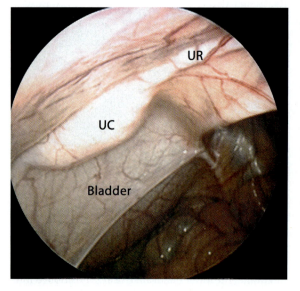

Fig. 94.3. Intraoperative view of urachal cyst. *UR* Urachus, *UC* urachal cyst

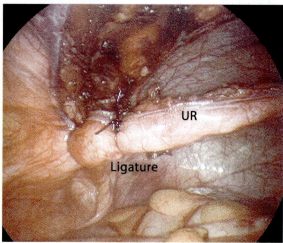

Fig. 94.5. Intraoperative view of urachal ligation

delivered via scissors or endosurgical hook. Once the urachal structure has been mobilized to the level of the urinary bladder it must be divided and the bladder closed. Urachal structures with a narrow connection to the bladder may be divided and secured by a simple suture tie, a suture ligature, or an endosurgical clip (■ Fig. 94.5). Wider-based structures will require a one- or two-layered closure of the bladder dome using 3-0 Vicryl or polydioxanone (PDS) suture. Alterna-

tively, the larger urachal structure may be excised and the bladder closed using an endostapler. Stapling, while providing a very secure bladder closure, has the distinct size disadvantage of requiring a 12 mm trocar. In most cases, once the urachal structure is excised it may be removed through a 5 mm trocar. In cases of large urachal cysts, the 5 mm trocar maybe too small and an intraumbilical incision may be the most cosmetic means to remove the specimen.

Postoperative Care

In cases of small cysts and simple sinuses, patients are revived from anesthesia, taken to the recovery room, and then discharged from the hospital. In cases where a significant closure of the bladder was performed, the urinary catheter is left to decompress the bladder and the patient is admitted to the hospital. During this period of decompression the patient is maintained on prophylactic antibiotics.

Results

In the author's experience, we have excised two urachal cysts and eight urachal sinuses. The cysts both presented initially as abscesses and were drained prior to definitive resection. The two patients with cysts remained in the hospital for 2–4 days following excision while all of the sinus patients were managed as outpatients. A single complication occurred in a cyst patient. That patient had a chronic indolent subcutaneous infection at the umbilicus where the specimen was removed. This infection responded promptly to local wound debridement and oral antibiotics.

Discussion

The natural progression of surgical advancement has always moved from performance, to refinement, to mastery of a technology or technique. Mastery is prob-ably best demonstrated by adapting a technology or technique to many different problems. Endosurgery for babies and children is crossing the refinement stage for common surgical problems and now adapting itself to manage uncommon conditions. Our personal series and that reported by other authors confirm that endo-surgical excision of urachal structures can be performed safely and effectively (Groot-Wassink et al. 2000; Khurana and Borzi 2002; Yohannes et al. 2003). Laparoscopy also adds a valuable tool in the initial evaluation in cases where the diagnosis is unclear. While the reported complication rate for these procedures is remarkably low, pitfalls do exist. These potential problems have primarily revolved around gaining peritoneal access and the security of bladder closure.

References

Groot-Wassink T, Deo H, Charfare H, et al (2000) Laparoscopic excision of the urachus. Surg Endosc 14:680–681

Khurana S, Borzi PA (2002) Laparoscopic management of complicated urachal disease in children. J Urol 168:1526–1528

McCollum MO, Macneily AE, Blair GK (2003) Surgical implications of urachal remnants: presentation and management. J Pediatr Surg 38:798–803

Ueno T, Hashimoto H, Yokoyama H, et al (2003) Urachal anomalies: ultrasonography and management. J Pediatr Surg 38:1203–1207

Yohannes P, Bruno T, Pathan M, et al (2003) Laparoscopic radical excision of urachal sinus. J Endourol 17:475–479; discussion 479

Chapter 95

Minimally Invasive Techniques for Lower Urinary Tract Reconstruction

Steven G. Docimo and Rajen Butani

Introduction

Several techniques for bladder reconstruction have been devised using open and minimally invasive techniques. The first laparoscopic bladder augmentation was carried out using stomach, and in 1994 was a long and technically difficult procedure (Docimo et al. 1995). Since then, several small series of laparoscopic bladder augmentation, including autoaugmentation have been described, but these techniques have not had widespread acceptance (Braren and Bishop 1998; Gill et al. 2000). In this chapter, laparoscopic-assisted techniques will be described. In this paradigm, the operative steps of access, mobilization and dissection, and harvest of substrate materials for reconstruction are all accomplished laparoscopically. The more technically demanding portions of the procedure, including bladder neck reconstruction, ureteral reimplantation, and assembly of augmentation, stoma, and buttressing materials can be performed using usual open techniques through a remarkably small lower abdominal incision.

Preoperative Preparation

Before Induction of General Anesthesia

- Thorough urodynamic assessment to define reconstructive goals and needs.
- Assessment of fecal continence and bowel management, without which urinary continence is somewhat pointless.
- Bowel preparation, mechanical and antibiotic.

After Induction of General Anesthesia

- General anesthesia is most suited to these procedures
- Epidural anesthesia may be used adjunctively if the patient does not have spinal dysraphism, and may be helpful in preventing bladder pain in the immediate postoperative period.

- Spinal anesthesia has not been used, except in an attempt to prevent autonomic dysreflexia in patients with cervical spinal cord injury and quadriplegia.
- A nasogastric tube is sometimes left in the patient postoperatively, thus is more practical than an orogastric tube.
- A urinary catheter is placed in the sterile field after the patient is prepared if any urethral or bladder neck reconstruction is contemplated. Otherwise it may be placed prior to the start of the procedure.
- Antibiotics are administered, including anaerobic coverage if large intestine use is anticipated.

Positioning

Patient

The patient is placed supine taking care to pad all pressure points with foam or gel to prevent decubitus ulceration (Fig. 95.1). Girls may need to be in a frog-legged position if urethral or introital reconstruction is anticipated. The patient must be well secured to the operating table to allow deep Trendelenburg and table rotation. Exceptions for the supine position would include nephrectomy in preparation for ureterocystoplasty, in which case the shoulders and flank would be elevated on a cushion ipsilaterally, leaving the pelvis flat.

Crew, Monitors, and Equipment

The operation begins and ends with the surgeon and the assistant on opposite sides of the table (Fig. 95.1). This might not be the case during certain laparoscopic maneuvers, depending on the procedure being performed.

Special Equipment

Coagulating scissors are used, and the harmonic scalpel may be helpful. A 5 mm clip applier is available as well as staplers with gastrointestinal and vascular cartridges.

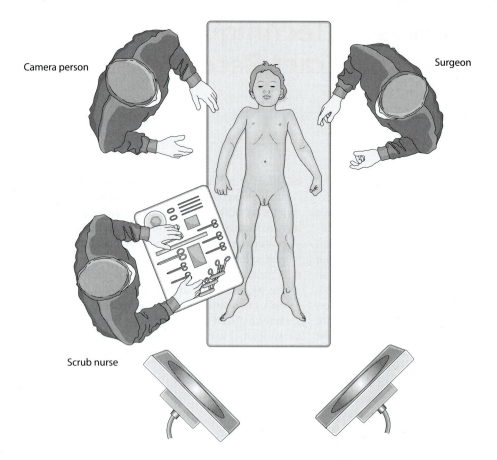

Camera person

Surgeon

Scrub nurse

Fig. 95.1. Patient and crew positioning. The patient is generally positioned supine and well secured to the table to allow changes in positioning. For a ureterocystoplasty, the patient is placed in a 45° flank position, with the kidney to be removed up. The operation begins and ends with surgeon and assistant on opposite sides of the table. This might not be the case during certain laparoscopic maneuvers, depending on the procedure being performed

Technique

Cannulae

Cannula	Method of insertion	Diameter (mm)	Device	Position
1	Open	10	Step	Umbilical
2	Closed	5 or 10	Any	Along line of proposed open incision or at site of secondary stoma
3	Closed	2, 3, or 5	Any	Midepigastrium

■ Figure 95.2 shows port positions.

Procedure

Each of these operations is unique and is based on the anatomy and needs of the patient at hand. Therefore, the steps of the procedure will be generalized. First, access must be obtained to the abdomen. If an umbilical stoma is to be created, the procedure is started by de-

veloping a U-shaped flap of the lower umbilicus, as has been described for creation of a concealed umbilical stoma (Ben-Chaim et al. 1995; Glassman and Docimo 2001). Construction of the stoma, though it occurs last, is one of the most important steps of the operation, both from a functional and cosmetic standpoint. Therefore, the initial umbilical incision must be com-

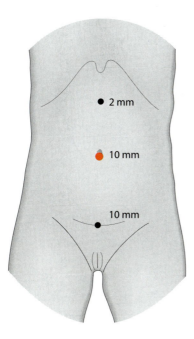

Fig. 95.2. Port placement and usual open incision. The Pfannenstiel incision can be quite small for these procedures, often no more than 4–5 cm

patible with the expected finished product. As the umbilical flap is raised using a stay suture, the midline umbilical fascia is opened sharply, and the peritoneum can be entered using a hemostat. A radially dilating 10- or 12 mm trocar sleeve is introduced under direct vision and then dilated (Cuellar et al. 2000). This gives a large enough aperture to deliver the stoma at the end of the procedure, but radial dilation avoids a defect large enough to increase risk of peristomal herniation. The abdomen is then insufflated, and pressure is determined by the size of the child.

Accessory ports are now placed based on the expected procedure. For example, if the child is to have a continent appendicovesicostomy and bladder augmentation via a small Pfannenstiel incision, the second port can be placed along the proposed incision line, and a third 2- or 3 mm port can be placed in the midepigastrium (■ Fig. 95.2). If two stomas are planned, one for the bladder and the other for a Malone antegrade continence enema (MACE) stoma, the second port is placed in the expected stoma site, after developing a U-shaped flap as described for the umbilicus (Hedican et al. 1999). If a nephrectomy is planned, port placement will be optimized for that procedure based on side and patient size. For harvest of stomach, two lateral ports at the anterior axillary line at the level of the umbilicus have been used (Docimo et al. 1995). All ports are secured to the skin with suture to prevent inadvertent removal during the case.

At this point, the expected procedure will dictate the steps to be followed. For use of the appendix, the right colon can be mobilized as extensively as needed such that the base of the appendix can be easily reached through a low incision. Alternatively, the appendix can be harvested by creating a window at the base of the mesoappendix and dividing the appendicocecal junction with Endo-GIA. Take care to avoid injury to an exposed ventriculoperitoneal shunt, often seen in these patients. The shunt requires no special anesthetic or surgical precautions during laparoscopy (Jackman et al. 2000), but great care should be used to avoid contamination during intestinal work. If small bowel is to be used for augmentation, usually no dissection is required as this can be readily harvested through a small Pfannenstiel incision. If the sigmoid is going to be used, sometimes it is floppy and requires no dissection, and other times the lateral peritoneal line can be taken down to facilitate later manipulation. If one plans a ureterocystoplasty, laparoscopic nephrectomy is carried out in the usual fashion, but the adventitia around the ureter, possibly but not always including the gonadal vessels, is carefully preserved (■ Fig. 95.3). If division of the bladder neck is anticipated, for example for a child with bladder exstrophy, an omental flap can be readily harvested and available for the end of the reconstruction. Larger omental vessels can be divided using clips, cautery, or the harmonic scalpel with equal effectiveness. When using cautery, remember that the flap being developed is on a pedicle; take care not to let the pedicle act as the sole conduit of electrical current during cautery or the viability of the flap may be compromised. Bipolar cautery might be advantageous here, but is not necessary.

When all of the components for the planned reconstruction are easily available through the planned lower abdominal incision, the laparoscopic portion of the procedure is finished. This can take a few minutes, if it is obvious that the procedure can be done without any laparoscopic mobilization, or can take several hours if there are extensive adhesions and/or difficult anatomy. The lower abdominal incision is now created. These procedures can often be done through incisions of 4–5 cm, since the substrates for reconstruction should all be in easy reach. Prior to entering the peritoneum, all bladder work can be accomplished extraperitoneally. This decreases the exposure of the intra-abdominal contents, as well as risk of ileus. Along these lines, we are careful never to use packing, deep retractors, or any unnecessary manipulation of the bowel. Bladder procedures might include bladder neck reconstruction, bladder neck division, ureteral reimplantation, removal of bladder calculi, etc. When the bladder is prepared, the peritoneum is opened on either side of the bladder, and the urachus is divided. The appendix, if used, is brought into the field, separated from the cecum using

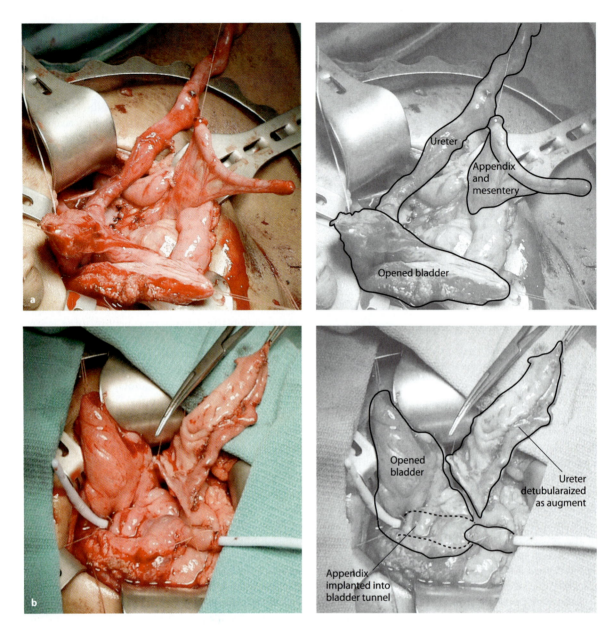

Fig. 95.3. An example of the open portion of reconstruction through a small Pfannenstiel incision. A laparoscopic nephrectomy has been performed on the right, preserving blood supply to the ureter. The ureter is detubularized and used as an augment without detaching from the bladder. The appendix is harvested laparoscopically or open, and implanted into the bladder as a stoma

the technique of choice, opened, and irrigated. A catheterizable lumen is confirmed. If appendicovesicostomy is the only procedure to be done, this is usually accomplished completely laparoscopically. Otherwise, a decision is made whether to implant the appendix into the anterior bladder wall, posterior bladder wall, or into a bladder flap, depending on the length needed to reach the umbilicus. Alternatives to appendix would also be considered at this time, including ileal or sigmoid Monti tubes, bladder tubes, and others (Cain et al. 1999).

If bladder augmentation is to be performed, the tissue of choice is isolated. This can be ileum, sigmoid, ureter, or stomach. Bowel harvesting and reanastomosis is performed using standard open techniques, with the length needed based on patient age and size, as well as type of segment used. Drainage of the reconstructed bladder usually consists of a suprapubic catheter, which can be brought out through the second port site if only one stoma is created. A 10 French Foley catheter is generally left through the stoma, and sutured to the skin to prevent traction of the balloon on the continence mechanism, which can lead to failure. When these details have been attended to, the omental flap, if needed, can be sutured into place into the bladder neck defect as a buttressing layer to prevent fistula.

If a MACE stoma is to be constructed, there are a few options. The appendix can be separated from the cecum, reversed, tunneled into a taenia, and then brought to the skin. It can be left in situ on the cecum and plication sutures used to create a continence mechanism, or it can be brought directly to the skin with no reconfiguration with a good likelihood of continence. Both the bladder and fecal stomas are matured to the skin after they are shortened to prevent catheterization difficulties due to redundancy. The bladder stoma is spatulated on the ventral side, and the previously created U-shaped skin flaps are incorporated to give a concealed appearance, and decrease the risk of stenosis (Glassman and Docimo 2001). The wound is closed in standard fashion, and the skin is closed with subcuticular sutures, to enhance the cosmetic result. Whether suction drains are used depends on surgeon preference, as well as the procedure performed.

Postoperative Care

- A nasogastric tube may be used if a small bowel or gastric anastomosis has been created.
- The bladder may be drained via a suprapubic catheter, stoma catheter, urethral catheter, or a combination of the above. Adequate urinary drainage is necessary after bladder reconstruction, and time should be taken at the end of the procedure to make sure that drainage is effective. This is difficult to deal with postoperatively, and occasionally requires a return to the operating room to reposition catheters.
- Resumption of normal diet is generally faster after laparoscopic-assisted procedures than open procedures, but timing of oral intake must be based on the specific procedure done, as well as the clinical appearance of the patient.
- For pain control while in the hospital, either a continuous epidural infusion or patient-controlled analgesia (PCA) consisting of controlled intravenous injection of narcotic medications may be very effective. By discharge, oral pain medication should be adequate, whether narcotic or non-steroidal anti-inflammatory agents. We have a low threshold for the use of ketorolac, even immediately postoperatively in the patient with normal renal function. The risk of bleeding is minimal, and this is a very effective agent for bladder pain and spasm.

Results

In the largest reported series (Chung et al. 2004), 30 patients successfully underwent primary laparoscopic-assisted reconstruction without intraoperative complications. Twenty-five patients had a history of prior abdominal surgery, including 16 with ventriculoperitoneal shunts. No patients required blood transfusions. Median hospital stay was 6 days including a day for bowel preparation.

Thirty-nine catheterizable stomas were created in 29 patients. These included 26 Mitrofanoff stomas (17 appendix, 5 sigmoid, 3 ileum, 1 bladder) with (13) or without (13) concurrent augmentation cystoplasty and 13 antegrade continence enema (ACE) stomas (12 appendix, 1 ileum). One gastrocystoplasty takedown with appendiceal Mitrofanoff and ileal augmentation and 2 laparoscopic-assisted nephrectomies and ureteral augmentations with 1 undergoing appendiceal Mitrofanoff were performed. Simultaneous ACE (9 appendix, 1 ileum) and Mitrofanoff (4 appendix, 3 ileum, 2 sigmoid, and 1 tubularized bladder) procedures were performed in 10 patients (■ Table 95.1). Twenty-three Pfannenstiel, 6 lower midline, and 1 small midline incisions were made. Concurrent procedures in 19 patients included bladder neck reconstruction (7), fascial sling (3), revision of epispadias (2), ureteral reimplantations (1), redo orchidopexy (1), and previously mentioned bladder augmentations (4 sigmoid, 9 ileum, and 2 ureter).

After mean follow-up of nearly 3 years (range 3–57 months), 94.8% of the stomas were continent of urine and/or stool and easily catheterizable. Stomal revisions were required in 7.7% of the stomas after mean 19 months (range 8–36 months) follow-up. Indications for revision included urinary incontinence per appendicovesicostomy necessitating channel modification (1), incontinence per sigmoid vesicostomy requiring revision at 3 years (1), and difficult catheterization of ACE requiring respatulation (1). The stomal stenosis rate was 5.1%. Minor procedures were required in 25.6% of the stomas consisting of indwelling catheterization, dilation, collagen injection, and cystoscopy. All augmented bladders maintained good capacity and compliance.

Complications occurred in 5 patients. One patient had a partial small bowel obstruction immediately postoperatively. Another had late traumatic bladder perforation after falling on a ball in the playground. A patient with quadriplegia had delayed ileus but recovered without intervention. Additional complications included deep venous thrombosis and wound infection.

The cosmetic result is difficult to measure objectively. Often, complex reconstruction can be performed with no outward sign with the patient in a bikini or

Table 95.1 Results of simultaneous ACE and Mitrofanoff procedures in 10 patients. *MI-ACE* Monti ileum antegrade continence enema stoma, *AV* appendicovesicostomy, *ACE* appendiceal antegrade continence enema, *SV* tubularized sigmoid vesicostomy, *TIV* tubularized ileal vesicostomy, *MIV* Monti ileal vesicostomy, *DVT* deep venous thrombosis, *TB* tubularized bladder stoma

Stomas	Patients	Stomal revisions	Minor procedures	Complications	Continent stomas
MI-ACE, AV	1	0	1	Small bowel obstruction knuckled ileum, dilatation MI-ACE	2
ACE, AV	3	0	1	Complete stenosis ACE, lower extremity DVT, catheter ACE	5
ACE, SV	2	1[a]	1	Revision SV, takedown SV, catheter ACE	3
ACE, TIV	2	1	1	Respatulation ACE, cystoscopy TIV	4
ACE, MIV	1	0	1	Wound infection, catheter placement ACE	2
ACE, TB	1	0	0	None	2
Total	10	2 (10%)	5 (25%)		18 (90%)

[a] Revised twice

racing bathing suit. Subjectively, the patients and their parents have been pleased with the results, especially when they are acquainted with those who had traditional incisions.

Discussion

Most patients who require reconstructive surgery for urinary and fecal incontinence can expect a successful outcome, as measured by improved continence. It is now feasible to focus on other measures of outcome, including cosmetic appearance and self-esteem. Scars on the torso affect body image, and it is expected that the potential for this effect will be greater in pediatric patients (Sarwer et al. 1998). Children who have other reasons for impaired body image, such as spina bifida or bladder exstrophy, might be expected to benefit the most from improved cosmetic appearance. The initial goal, however, has to be a functional result that is equivalent or better than standard open approaches before cosmetic appearance is a worthwhile outcome.

Why not do these reconstructions entirely laparoscopically? Since we performed the first laparoscopic gastrointestinal bladder augmentation (Docimo et al. 1995) several cases or small series have been reported (Gill et al. 2000). These are difficult procedures that are not yet generally applicable. The most technically demanding aspects of reconstruction, such as ureteral reimplantation, bladder neck reconstruction, or creation of a Mitrofanoff stoma, have infrequently been performed laparoscopically. Until endoscopic techniques "catch up," perhaps with the aid of robotics, it is our feeling that laparoscopic-assisted reconstruction, which allows for the performance of technically demanding reconstruction through a small open incision, represents the state-of-the-art in minimally invasive lower urinary tract reconstruction.

When a midline incision is used for lower tract reconstruction, often the upper half is only necessary to mobilize a high cecum (Brown 1975), a non-redundant sigmoid colon, harvest stomach tissue, perform nephrectomy to obtain ureter for augmentation, or harvest omentum to buttress a bladder neck closure. All of these procedures can be performed laparoscopically in most patients. This is true even in patients with prior abdominal surgery, as was the case in the majority of the patients reported here.

An ideal stoma site with low risk of herniation or stomal stenosis is created during open access with a radially dilating trocar in the umbilicus, using a posterior umbilical flap to conceal the stoma (Cuellar et al. 2000). We have had good success with the stoma sites in this series, and in fact all of the umbilical stomas revised for stenosis in our previously reported umbilical stoma experience were created without laparoscopic assistance (Glassman and Docimo 2001).

Two of 26 urinary stomas were revised for leakage (7.7%) in our reported series. This compares favorably with patients undergoing traditional open reconstruction (Cain et al. 1999). The revision rate of 7.7% (1 of 13) of the MACE stomas is as good as or better than previously reported open procedures (Curry et al. 1999; Sugarman et al. 1998).

When one considers the lifelong implications of abdominal reconstructive surgery, there is significant potential for morbidity related to adhesions and bowel obstruction. It is well established that laparoscopic techniques decrease the likelihood of adhesion formation, and our experience thus far with laparoscopic-assisted surgery has suggested a similar benefit (Moore et al. 1994; Schafer et al. 1998).

Laparoscopic-assisted lower urinary tract reconstruction is applicable to most children and adults who require upper abdominal access, allowing shorter recovery time and the potential for decreased adhesion formation. Functional outcomes are equal to or better than those of traditional open approaches, and laparoscopic-assisted reconstruction remains our approach of choice to these complex procedures. With advances in technology, total laparoscopic approaches may become more reasonable, but until then, these procedures will be the only easily available minimally invasive procedures for bladder reconstruction.

Unfortunately, to date we have no objective data concerning cosmetic appearance and affects on body image and self-esteem. In the patients with exstrophy, spina bifida, and other disorders commonly requiring reconstruction, there are many issues affecting body image other than abdominal scars. Subjectively, patients and their families have been delighted with the cosmetic results, as have their healthcare providers. This may be the most important reason to continue to pursue minimally invasive forms of lower urinary tract reconstruction.

References

Ben-Chaim J, Rodriguez R, Docimo SG (1995) Concealed umbilical stoma: description of a modified technique. J Urol 154:1169–1170

Braren V, Bishop MR (1998) Laparoscopic bladder autoaugmentation in children. Urol Clin North Am 25:533–540

Brown SF (1975) Congenital malformations associated with myelomeningocele. J Iowa Med Soc 65:101–104

Cain MP, Casale AJ, King AJ, et al (1999) Appendicovesicostomy and newer alternatives for the Mitrofanoff procedure: results in the last 100 patients at Riley Children's Hospital. J Urol 162:1749–1752

Chung SY, Meldrum K, Docimo SG, et al (2004) Laparoscopic-assisted reconstructive surgery: a seven year experience. J Urol 171:372–375

Cuellar DC, Kavoussi PK, Baker LA, et al (2000) Open laparoscopic access using a radially dilating trocar: experience and indications in 50 consecutive cases. J Endourol 14:755–756

Curry JI, Osborne A, Malone PS (1999) The MACE procedure: experience in the United Kingdom. J Pediatr Surg 34:338–340

Docimo SG, Moore RG, Kavoussi LR (1995) Laparoscopic bladder augmentation using stomach. Urology 46:565–569

Gill IS, Rackley RR, Meraney AM, et al (2000) Laparoscopic enterocystoplasty. Urology 55:178–181

Glassman DT, Docimo SG (2001) Concealed umbilical stoma: long-term evaluation of stomal stenosis. J Urol 166:1028–1030

Hedican SP, Schulam PG, Docimo SG, et al (1999) Laparoscopic assisted reconstructive surgery. J Urol 161:267–270

Jackman SV, Weingart JD, Kinsman SL, et al (2000) Laparoscopic surgery in patients with ventriculoperitoneal shunts: safety and monitoring. J Urol 164:1352–1354

Moore RG, Kavoussi LR, Bloom DA, et al (1994) Postoperative adhesion formation after urological laparoscopy in the pediatric population. J Urol 153:792–795

Sarwer DB, Whitaker LA, Pertschuk MJ, et al (1998) Body image concerns of reconstructive surgery patients: an under recognized problem. Ann Plast Surg 40:403–407

Schafer M, Krahenbuhl L, et al (1998) Comparison of adhesion formation in open and laparoscopic surgery. Dig Surg 15:148–152

Sugarman ID, Malone PS, Terry TR, et al (1998) Transversely tubularized ileal segments for the Mitrofanoff or Malone antegrade colonic enema procedures: the Monti principle. Br J Urol 81:253–256

Chapter 96

Laparoscopic Bladder Neck Reconstruction

C.K. Yeung and J.D. Sihoe

Introduction

Urinary incontinence due to bladder neck incompetence is a common condition presented to paediatric urologists. The most frequent situation is incontinence in children suffering from spina bifida and neuropathic bladder-sphincteric dysfunction. Urinary incontinence in these patients poses not only a medical but also a significant psychological and social problem. The associated low self-esteem, stigmatisation by the society and adverse influence in school performance all render it a serious health issue with multiple negative effects on a child's development. The medical obligation to treat this condition with an aim for protection of the upper urinary tract and achieving a socially acceptable degree of continence can never be denied. However, successful management remains a technical challenge to the paediatric urologists. The introduction of the concepts of continent diversion and clean intermittent catheterisation, in combination with augmentation cystoplasty for bladders with poor compliance and reduced capacity, and bladder neck surgery for bladders with outlet incompetence, has allowed many of these children to become dry. Although different surgical options exists in current literature for bladder neck reconstruction, a consensus has yet to be achieved. With advances in laparoscopic surgery, the introduction of a laparoscopic extravesical approach using a bladder neck sling provides a further option with the added advantages of a clear and magnified view of the pelvic cavity. It also allows for other advanced laparoscopic bladder surgery such as laparoscopic bladder augmentation and laparoscopic-assisted Mitrofanoff appendicovesicostomy to be performed as a single-stage operation. It is not uncommon that preoperative urodynamic studies sometimes may not be able to tell whether concurrent bladder neck reconstruction is necessary to achieve continence particularly in those poorly compliant bladders. Therefore some patients may have undergone bladder augmentation and subsequently require a second surgical procedure for bladder neck reconstruction to enhance dryness. This would mean inevitable exploration of areas with dense adhesions and may even carry the risk of injuring the vascular pedicle of the augmented bladder. With the development of a pneumovesical approach to intravesical surgery it is now also possible to perform bladder neck reconstruction without opening up the bladder.

Intravesical Technique: Pneumovesical Bladder Neck Reconstruction

Preoperative Preparation

Before Induction of General Anaesthesia

Patients are prescribed a rectal suppository or enema the night before surgery to reduce faecal loading in the rectum as this may affect the operative field due to the close proximity of the rectum with the posterior wall of the bladder.

After Induction of General Anaesthesia

All patients are placed under general anaesthesia. Prophylactic antibiotic cover with a cephalosporin or aminoglycoside is given on induction. There is no requirement for nasogastric tube placement. Urinary catheters are placed on-table after draping. In older children, preparation of the operative site by shaving of pubic hair is preferable.

Positioning

Patient

For intravesical surgery via pneumovesicum, it is necessary also to perform cystoscopy. Therefore the patient is best placed in the lithotomy position (Fig. 96.1). However, in young children, a supine position with legs spread apart would suffice. The pelvis is tilted with a padding just below the buttocks. As the table may be adjusted to a head-down and slightly right-side position to facilitate the surgeon intraoperatively, the patient is also strapped in on the table over the upper body to prevent slipping during movement of the table. Adequate padding especially of the lower limbs is necessary to make sure all pressure points are covered.

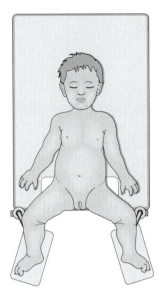

Fig. 96.1. Patient positioning (intravesical technique).

Crew, Monitors and Equipment

The surgeon is usually positioned on the left side of the patient facing the end of the table with a monitor placed next to the patient's right leg (█ Fig. 96.2). The table is therefore tilted head-down and right-side up to turn the patient towards the surgeon. In this position it is also possible for the surgeon to be sitting during the procedure. A robotic arm may be used to hold the camera and would be placed on the right side of the table. This has the advantage of a steady view and allows for fine, precise movements of the camera in a small cavity. If an assistant is used to hold the camera, the assistant would stand/sit to the right of the surgeon so as not to obstruct the surgeon's view. The scrub nurse would sit to the left of the surgeon near the left leg of the patient. Another assistant would sit between the legs of the patient and is responsible for holding the cystoscope at the beginning of the procedure as well as for assisting the operation with the fourth suprapubic port. However, the assistant may alternatively sit out-

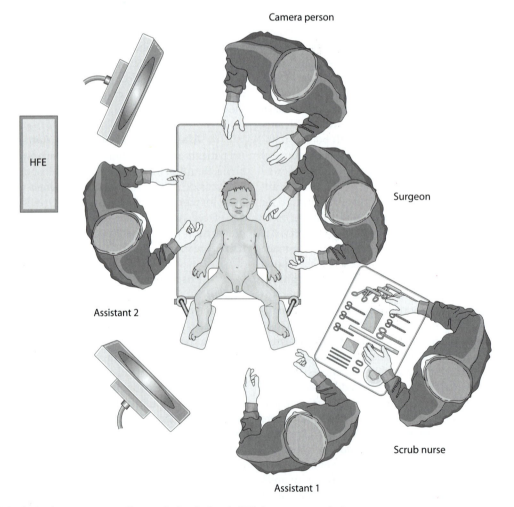

Fig. 96.2. Operating room set-up (intravesical technique). *HFE* electrocautery device

side the legs on the right side of the patient (A2 position) if the surgeon's view is being obstructed. All other equipment is placed on the right side of the patient including the main tower and electrocautery devices.

Technique

Cannulae

Cannula	Method of insertion	Diameter (mm)	Device	Position
1	Closed	5	Camera	Dome of bladder
2	Closed	5	Working port	Left lower bladder
3	Closed	3	Working port	Right lower bladder
4	Closed	3	Retraction	Suprapubic

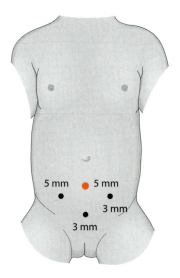

Fig. 96.3. Port placement (intravesical technique)

A 5 mm port is inserted into the dome of the bladder under cystoscopic guidance for placement of a 30° laparoscope (■ Fig. 96.3). Another 5 mm port is inserted into the right lower bladder under laparoscopic guidance as lateral as possible above the level of the ureteric orifice. A 3 mm port is inserted into the left lower bladder in similar fashion. Both these ports are used as the main working ports and therefore should not be placed too close together nor placed too far into the bladder as this would limit its movement. A fourth 3 mm port is placed in the suprapubic region and is used to place a right-angle instrument for retraction of the anterior upper lip of the bladder neck to facilitate dissection and may also be used for intermittent suction and irrigation of the bladder during surgery.

Special Equipment

No special energy requiring systems or other equipment is required. A robotic arm to hold the camera is advantageous.

Procedure

Set-up

Cystoscopy is first performed with a 7.5F cystoscope and fully distending the bladder with normal saline. A small stab incision with a pointed Beaver blade is made just distal to the holding stitch. To permit rapid closure of the bladder wall at port sites at the end of the procedure, a 3/0 polydioxanone (PDS) stitch is placed traversing the stab incision under cystoscopic guidance ensuring that the entry and exit sites of the stitch were below skin level. This stitch is held as a holding stitch and is also used to pull the bladder wall against the anterior abdominal wall during placement of the port. A Veress needle is introduced and a radially expanding 5 mm port is inserted under cystoscopic guidance. Care is taken during port placement as any leakage of gas into the peritoneal cavity may affect the operative field by increasing intra-abdominal pressure and obstructing full distension of the bladder. After placement of the port, the bladder is emptied and the cystoscope removed. An 8F Vygon catheter is inserted in replacement as a urethral stent and connected to a three-way connector to stop leakage of gas from the bladder during insufflation. The bladder is then insufflated via the dome port with carbon dioxide to achieve pneumovesicum up to 12–15 mmHg to facilitate insertion of ports. A 5 mm 30° laparoscope is inserted via the dome port. Another three ports are inserted under laparoscopic guidance in the positions as described above in a similar fashion to the first port. After insertion of all ports, the pneumovesical pressure is reduced to 10–12 mmHg.

Bladder Neck Reconstruction

A mucosal incision is made over the anterior half of the bladder neck incorporating two parallel incisions 1.5 cm apart along the posterior bladder wall and extending cranially up to the level of the interureteric

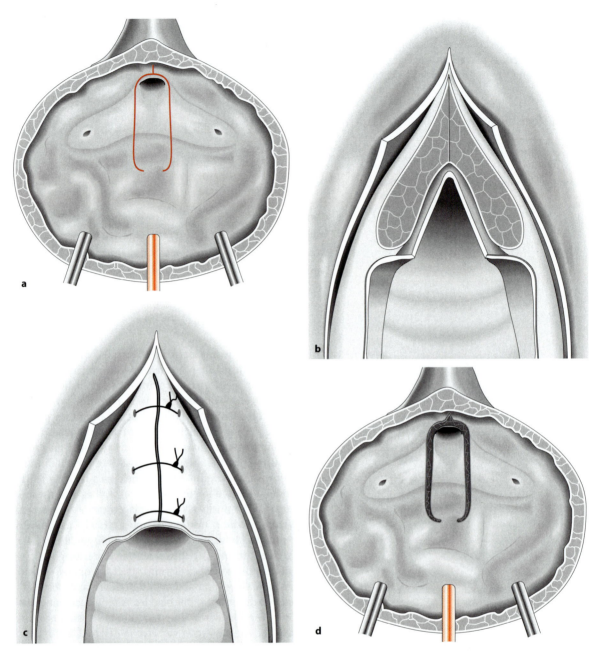

Fig. 96.4 a – d. a Mucosal incision. **b** Incision of proximal urethra. **c** Narrowing of bladder neck. **d** Mucosal strip raised.

bridge using monopolar diathermy (■ Fig. 96.4a). The proximal 1.5 cm of anterior urethra from the bladder neck is incised exposing the detrusor muscle (■ Fig. 96.4b). The urethral stent is advanced through the bladder neck and the bladder neck is narrowed by closing the anterior rim over the stent using interrupted absorbable sutures (■ Fig. 96.4c). The 1.5 cm mucosal strip made at the posterior bladder wall in continuity with the posterior wall of the bladder neck is then lifted off the detrusor muscle on both sides with the aid of endoscopic scissors and electrocautery (■ Fig. 96.4d). The urethral stent is further advanced along the length of the mucosal strip and the mucosal

strip is tubularised around the stent using 5/0 interrupted absorbable sutures (■ Fig. 96.4e). The mucosal edges lateral to the tubularised neourethra are undermined (■ Fig. 96.4f) and the lateral mucosa is closed over the neourethra using 5/0 interrupted absorbable sutures (■ Fig. 96.4g).

Closure

In addition to the urethral stent, a 10F suprapubic catheter is left in situ for postoperative drainage of the bladder. The suprapubic catheter is placed via the supraumbilical port site and the port is removed. The length of suprapubic catheter inside the bladder can be

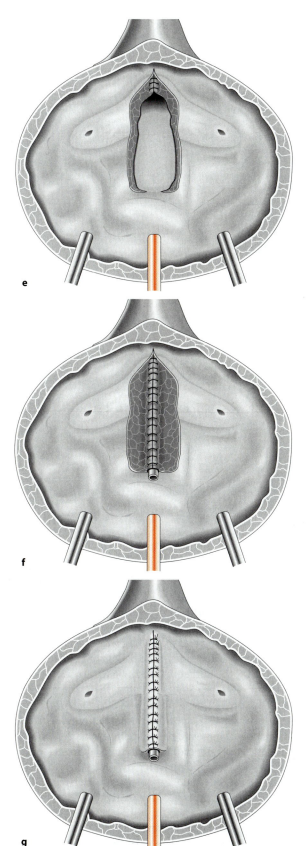

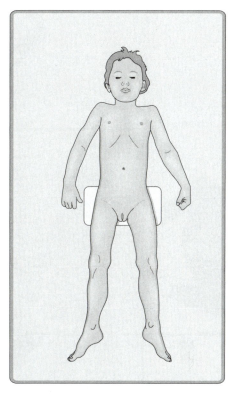

Fig. 96.5. Patient positioning (extravesical technique)

adjusted under laparoscopic guidance. The rest of the ports are removed and the bladder defects closed by tying the preplaced sutures. Local anaesthesia over the port sites is optional. The skin wounds are further closed with a 5/0 subcuticular absorbable monofilament suture.

Postoperative Care

Patients are usually allowed to resume a normal diet once comfortable as the majority of these patients do not develop any ileus postoperatively. Oral analgesia when required is usually sufficient for postoperative wound discomfort. There is usually no need for continuation of antibiotics postoperatively in straightforward procedures. The patient may ambulate once comfortable taking care not to pull out any of the catheters. The two urinary catheters are connected to a bedside bag and left for free drainage for 1 week after surgery. Once the catheters are removed and the patient is able to micturate, the patient may be discharged home. If the patient is on clean intermittent catheterisation (CIC), this may be resumed. The patients are usually followed up in 1 week for wound inspection. Their overall condition and result of surgery is further assessed in 2–3 months time in the outpatient clinic.

Fig. 96.4 e – g. e Tubularisation of mucosal strip. **f** Undermining of mucosal edge. **g** Mucosa closed over neourethra

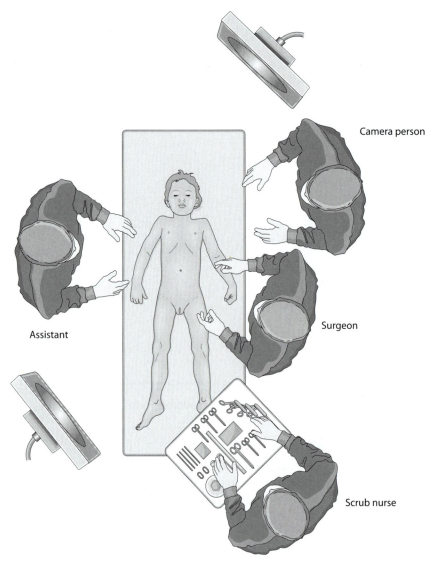

Fig. 96.6. Operating room set-up (extravesical technique)

Camera person

Assistant

Surgeon

Scrub nurse

Extravesical Technique: Laparoscopic Bladder Neck Sling

Preoperative Preparation

As for intravesical technique.

Positioning
Patient
All patients are placed in a supine position (■ Fig. 96.5). This is slightly modified in girls with legs spread to facilitate placing of a urinary catheter on-table. The pelvis is tilted with a padding just below the buttocks. Adequate soft padding to protect pressure points and strapping of the patient to the table to prevent slipping during table movement is ensured.

Crew, Monitors and Equipment
The surgeon is usually positioned on the left side of the patient facing the end of the bed with the main tower placed to the right side of the patient at the end of the bed facing the surgeon (■ Fig. 96.6). An assistant is positioned on the right of the surgeon to hold the camera. The scrub nurse is positioned to the left of the surgeon near the left leg of the patient. Another assistant is positioned opposite the surgeon on the right of the patient. Therefore another monitor may be placed on the left side of the patient for the assistant to see. All other equipment such as the electrocautery device is placed on the right side of the patient.

Special Equipment
No special energy applying systems are required but Hacker staplers and a synthetic SIS sling are available.

Technique

Cannulae

Cannula	Method of insertion	Diameter (mm)	Device	Position
1	Open	5	Camera	Infraumbilical
2	Closed	5	Working port	Right lower quadrant
3	Closed	5	Working port	Left lower quadrant

An infraumbilical incision is made for open insertion of a 5 mm port for placement of a 30° laparoscope (■ Fig. 96.7). Two further 5 mm working ports are inserted into the right and left lower quadrants of the abdomen under laparoscopic guidance.

Procedure

The ports are inserted as described. The Retzius space is entered and pneumo-extraperitoneum is achieved with carbon dioxide insufflation via the infraumbilical port. A pressure of 12 mmHg is usually sufficient. The bladder is first mobilised from the anterior abdominal wall using endoscopic monopolar electrocautery down to the bladder base (■ Fig. 96.8a). In girls it is also necessary to mobilise the posterior wall of the bladder from the vagina to fully expose the entire bladder neck.

To aid dissection a rigid probe, such as a urethral sound, is placed into the bladder transurethrally to act as a retractor for the bladder. During mobilisation of the anterior wall, the probe can be tilted posteriorly for retraction (■ Fig. 96.8b). During mobilisation of the posterior wall in girls, it is also helpful to place another probe into the vagina for further countertraction (■ Fig. 96.8c). The urethral probe is then replaced with a Foley catheter after mobilisation. The size of the Foley catheter is adjusted according to the size and age of the patient.

A synthetic (SIS) sling is prepared and passed into the peritoneal cavity through either port site. It is wrapped around the bladder neck 360° and tightened around the Foley catheter. To prevent loosening, the two ends are stitched together close to the bladder neck using Vicryl sutures (■ Fig. 96.8d). The bladder neck is then hitched anteriorly to either side of the pubic bone using endoscopic Hacker staples (■ Fig. 96.8e).

The ports are removed and port sites closed with 3/0 or 4/0 absorbable interrupted stitches followed by 5/0 subcuticular absorbable monofilament suture. Local anaesthesia at the port site wounds is optional and usually not required. The Foley catheter is left in situ postoperatively for drainage of the bladder.

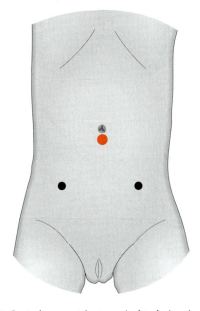

Fig. 96.7. Port placement (extravesical technique)

Postoperative Care

The patient is allowed to resume normal diet once comfortable. Ileus is not usually a problem postoperatively but if abdominal distension is noted then the patient will initially be resumed on fluids building up to a normal diet if tolerated. Oral analgesia as required is usually sufficient. Continuation of antibiotics is not necessary in straightforward procedures. The patient is allowed to ambulate whenever comfortable. A pelvic X-ray is taken postoperatively to document the position of the staples.

As the majority of these patients undergoing laparoscopic bladder neck sling operations have more than one procedure performed at the same setting, removal of the urinary catheter and discharge would depend also on the other procedures performed. For those who have had a bladder augmentation or Mitrofanoff appendicovesicostomy performed at the same setting, for example, their postoperative management and discharge would obviously vary.

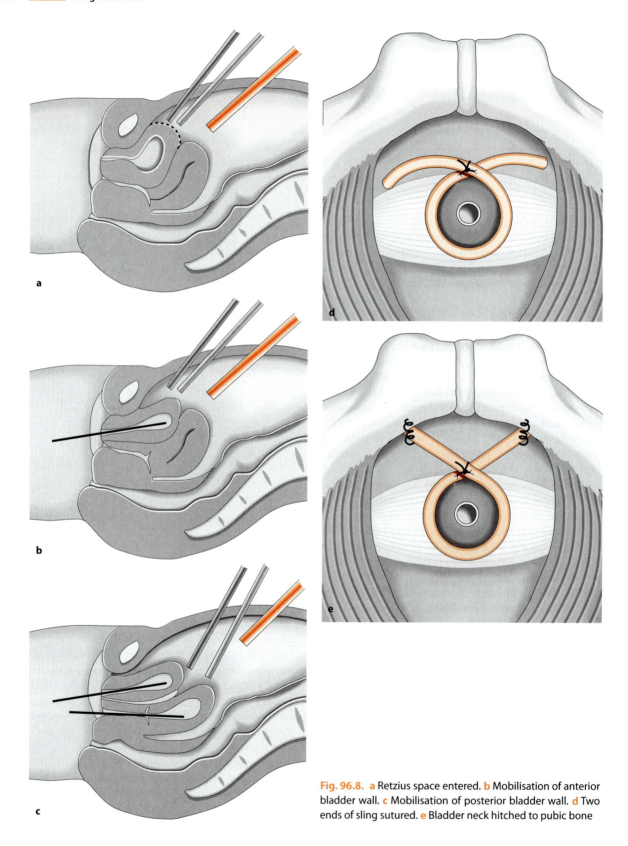

Fig. 96.8. **a** Retzius space entered. **b** Mobilisation of anterior bladder wall. **c** Mobilisation of posterior bladder wall. **d** Two ends of sling sutured. **e** Bladder neck hitched to pubic bone

The patients are usually followed up 1 week after discharge for wound inspection and then in 2 or 3 months for further evaluation of their urinary symptoms.

Results

Bladder neck reconstruction under CO_2 pneumovesicum was performed in five boys aged 4–17 years (mean age 9.8 years) with spina bifida and neuropathic bladder dysfunction who had persistent urinary incontinence despite augmentation enterocystoplasty and Mitrofanoff appendicovesicostomy. Transvesicoscopic bladder neck reconstruction with urethral lengthening was successfully performed in all five patients. The mean operating time was 196 min (range 155–280 min). All patients recovered uneventfully after the procedure. Upon follow-up one boy had persistent occasional urinary leakage. The other four patients had remained completely dry.

Extravesical endoscopic bladder neck sling was successfully performed in three girls aged 5–14 years (mean age 9.5 years) with urinary incontinence and bladder outflow incompetence. The mean operating time was 126 min (range 95–185 min). All patients recovered uneventfully and had remained dry after the procedure.

Discussion

The surgical options to increase bladder outflow resistance include artificial urinary sphincter, urinary diversion, periurethral injection of bulking agents, fascial slings and bladder neck tubularisation. The placement of an artificial sphincter in children has shown good results with achievement of continence. However, with a projected life expectancy of decades in young children, it has been thought to unlikely solve the problem in the long term. Revision of the device may be required resulting in multiple operations in the lifetime of a child (Gonzalez et al. 1995) and the device has been known to cause problems with erosion and infection. The lack of a durable agent for injection and the unpredictable host reaction to the agent has long been the obstacle to the popularity of the use of periurethral injections (Bomalaski et al. 2001). Despite the literature, a consensus on management has yet to be achieved.

Bladder neck sling procedures are relatively simple to carry out with relatively low complication and revision rates. However, there have been previous reports of a lower success rate of sling procedures in boys thus raising concern on its effectiveness in boys (Kurzrock et al. 1996). Therefore this procedure is usually carried out more selectively in girls. Results from the literature have shown achievement of best results of bladder neck sling procedures in combination with bladder augmentations and almost all patients require intermittent catheterisation. Therefore with the introduction of the extravesical laparoscopic bladder neck sling technique, it is possible to perform a relatively simple procedure in a single-stage operation in combination with other laparoscopic surgery.

Bladder neck reconstruction remains to be the most popular surgical treatment for bladder neck incompetence. The principles of bladder neck reconstruction are based on urethral lengthening and the creation of a flap-valve mechanism. The Young-Dees-Leadbetter procedure and its various modifications feature the creation of a neourethra by tubularising the posterior mucosal strip of the bladder and reinforcement by closure of detrusor muscle flaps in a pants-over-vest manner (Ferrer et al. 2001; Jones et al. 1993; Leadbetter 1964). Satisfactory continence rates were reported in patients with bladder exstrophy and epispadias (McMahon et al. 1996). However, lower success rates were reported in patients with bladder neck incompetence secondary to neuropathic bladders (Rink and Mitchell 1987; Tanagho 1981). This has been attributed to the fact that successful bladder neck reconstruction relies on good bladder neck and trigone muscular tone for a resultant sphincteric control. In 1986, Kropp and Angwafo described the creation of an anterior bladder wall tube with a blood supply from the bladder neck, which is passed through a submucosal tunnel between the ureteral orifices on the posterior bladder wall. This method creates a secure flap-valve mechanism that closes off the bladder tube as the intravesical pressure increases. Coupled with intermittent catheterisation through either the urethra or Mitrofanoff stoma over 70% of the patients having undergone this procedure were reported to be dry (Kropp 1999).

The intravesical technique of bladder neck reconstruction via a pneumovesicum described herein is a modified reverse Kropp procedure (Koyle 1998). Intertrigonal posterior mucosal tubularisation is combined with the creation of a flap-valve mechanism by apposing the undermined mucosal edges lateral to the neourethra at the midline. It has been further modified by tightening of the anterior half of the bladder neck and the proximal 1.5 cm of urethra which can further secure a competent bladder neck. Loss of functional bladder capacity by this procedure is minimal. The pneumovesical technique provides an excellent close-up view of the bladder neck and allows for surgery to be performed without opening up of the bladder.

References

Bomalaski MD, Koo HP, Bloom DA (2001) Injectable bulking agents in the treatment of urinary incontinence. In: Gearhart JP, Rink RC, Mouriquand PDE (eds) Pediatric Urology. Saunders, Philadelphia, p 1008

Ferrer FA, Tadros YE, Gearhart J (2001) Modified Young-Dees-Leadbetter bladder neck reconstruction: new concepts about old ideas. Urology 58:791–796

Gonzalez R, Merino FG, Vaughn M (1995) Long-term results of the artificial urinary sphincter in male patients with neurogenic bladder. J Urol 54:769–770

Jones JA, Mitchell ME, Rink RC (1993) Improved results using a modification of the Young-Dees-Leadbetter bladder neck repair. Br J Urol 71:555–561

Koyle MA (1998) Flap valve techniques in bladder neck reconstruction. Dial Pediatr Urol 21:6–7

Kropp KA (1999) Bladder neck reconstruction in children. Urol Clin North Am 26:661–672

Kropp KA, Angwafo FF (1986) Urethral lengthening and reimplantation for neurogenic incontinence in children. J Urol 135:533–536

Kurzrock EA, Lowe P, Hardy BE (1996) Bladder wall pedicle wraparound sling for neurogenic urinary incontinence in children. J Urol 155:305–308

Leadbetter GW Jr (1964) Surgical correction of total urinary incontinence. J Urol 91:261–266

McMahon DR, Cain MP, Husmann DA, et al (1996) Vesical neck reconstruction in patients with exstrophy-epispadias complex. J Urol 155:1411–1413

Rink RC, Mitchell ME (1987) Bladder neck/urethral reconstruction in the neuropathic bladder. Urology 10:5–6

Tanagho EA (1981) Bladder neck reconstruction in total urinary incontinence: 10 years experience. J Urol 125:321–326

Chapter 97

Laparoscopic Ureteric Reimplantation (Extravesical)

Anthony Atala

Introduction

Major advances have been made in the area of laparoscopic surgery since the 1980s. The advantages of this approach include smaller incisions, shorter hospitalizations, a more rapid convalescence, and decreased postoperative discomfort. Laparoscopic antireflux surgery was first described using a modification of the Lich extravesical ureteral approach (Atala et al. 1993; Ehrlich et al. 1994; Lich et al. 1961). Other techniques for laparoscopic ureteral reimplantations, including modifications of the Lich technique (a muscle wrap, an extraperitoneal approach) as well as the use of the Cohen cross-trigonal technique, have also been described (Cohen et al. 1999; Gill et al. 2001; Sakamoto et al. 2003). In this chapter, we describe the Lich extravesical approach, being that it is the most commonly used technique for laparoscopic ureteral reimplantation.

Preoperative Patient Selection and Preparation

Laparoscopic surgical experience is essential for the success of this procedure. As with any laparoscopic technique, the patients should be carefully selected. This procedure should be limited to children with unilateral reflux, in order to minimize postoperative urinary retention.

Before Induction of General Anesthesia

A routine bowel preparation should be performed.

After Induction of General Anesthesia

The same anesthetic protocol is used as for regular reimplantation. Additional epidural anesthesia may be used in certain centers. Nitrous oxide should be avoided as it tends to distend the lower bowel segments adjacent to the bladder.

The bladder should be catheterized, emptied, and the catheter left indwelling for the duration of the surgery. The access to the catheter should be within the sterile field in order to fill and empty the bladder as needed during the procedure.

Broad-spectrum prophylactic perioperative antibiotics (usually cefazolin) are administered intravenously.

Positioning

The patient is placed on the operating room table in the supine and Trendelenburg position.

Technique

A Veress needle is placed in the umbilical region. Pneumoperitoneum is obtained by insufflation of CO_2 (rate 2 L/min) up to a pressure of 15 mmHg. After ad-

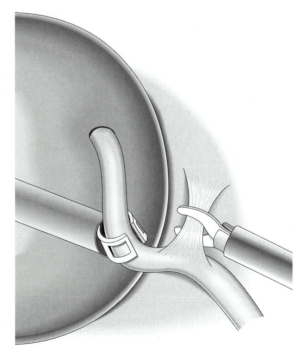

Fig. 97.1. Ureteral mobilization: the obliterated umbilical artery is identified and traced distally until the ureter is seen. The ureter is grasped gently and the periureteral tissue is dissected bluntly toward the ureterovesical junction

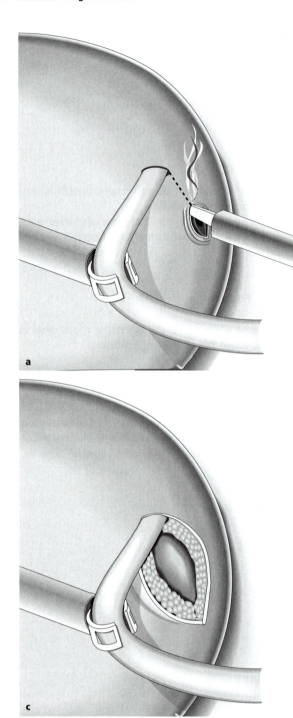

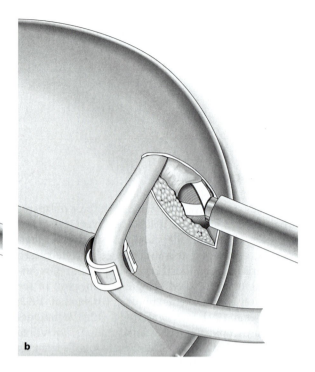

Fig. 97.2. Creation of bladder wall trough: **a** the bladder wall is incised with electrocautery 3 cm proximal to the ureterovesical junction. **b** The muscle fibers are gently cut and spread (*center*). **c** Dissection is complete when mucosal tissue is seen to bulge outward

equate pneumoperitoneum is achieved, two trocars are placed: one in the side opposite the refluxing ureter, at the midclavicular line 1 cm above the umbilicus (for various instruments) and one in the midline subumbilically (camera). Two additional trocars are then positioned in the left and right midclavicular line, 2 cm above the level of the anterior superior iliac spine (dissecting instruments, retractors). A 2/3 mm trocar is used in the periumbilical region for the camera. The rest of the trocars are usually 5 mm. When experience is gained, only three trocars are needed, deleting the placement of the contralateral midclavicular position. The table is laterally rotated with the side of the ureteral repair up, allowing the bladder and viscera to fall away from the area of repair.

Ureteral mobilization is started by identifying the obliterated umbilical artery along the bladder side-wall (■ Fig. 97.1). The bladder is retracted by a grasping

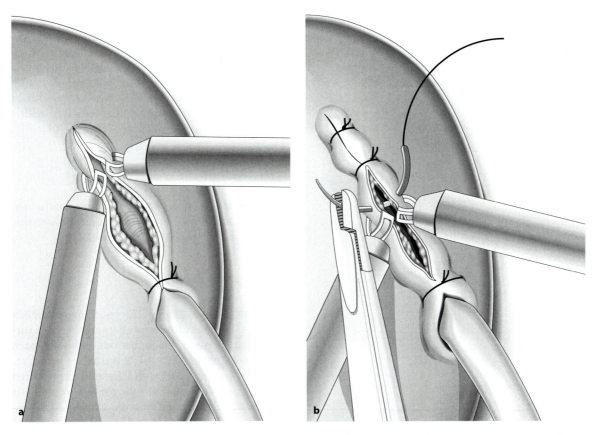

Fig. 97.3. Ureteral tunnel lengthening: the ureter is placed into the trough. **a** Two grasping instruments wrap the superior aspect of the bladder wall around the ureter and a suture is placed proximally, immobilizing the ureter in the trough. **b** Remaining sutures are placed throughout the length of the tunnel

tool at the dome of the bladder, superiorly and away from the operative side. This stretches the obliterated umbilical artery which is traced deep into the pelvis until the ureter is seen passing under it. The obliterated umbilical artery is divided. Periureteral adventitial tissue is used to gently retract the ureter away from the bladder and blunt dissection beneath the ureter begins the mobilization. The aim is to create a window beneath the ureter for a length of 4 cm proximal to the ureterovesical junction (UVJ). This permits placement of the ureter within a bladder wall trough. Mobilization is achieved largely with blunt dissection. Small vessels are bluntly dissected from the ureter and fulgurated with cautery. The UVJ is cleared of any bulky surrounding tissues.

Creation of a bladder wall trough is performed by incising the bladder wall with electrocautery along a line from the UVJ superiorly for approximately 3 cm and inferiorly for 1 cm (■ Fig. 97.2). Gentle spreading of the muscle fibers during dissection opens the trough until mucosal tissue is seen to bulge outward. This level of trough is developed for the entire length of the tunnel. Muscle fibers around the UVJ are spread slight-

ly, but no attempt is made to extensively dissect the UVJ free of bladder wall tissue. This is the most delicate part of the procedure, as the bladder could be inadvertently entered. If the bladder is entered, a suture can be placed to repair the bladder mucosa.

The ureter may be advanced by placing a suture from the lateral bladder muscle tissue at the distal end of the trough to the distal aspect of the ureter, and back through the medial bladder muscle tissue at the distal end of the trough. The ureter is then moved into the trough. The bladder muscle tissue is approximated over the ureter with a continuous long-lasting absorbable suture such as 3-0 polydioxanone (PDS; Ethicon, Cincinnati, Ohio). A Lapra-Ty (Ethicon) is useful for this portion of the procedure. This device applies absorbable anchors laparoscopically onto sutures. The anchor secures the suture in place, acting as a knot. Two grasping instruments are used to wrap the superior aspect of the bladder wall trough around the ureter, and a suture is placed at the most distal point, bringing the edges of the bladder muscle together over the ureter (■ Fig. 97.3). A Lapra-Ty anchor is placed at the end of the suture. This point then serves to main-

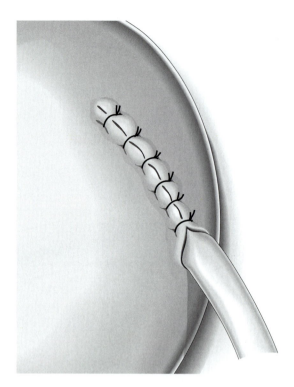

Fig. 97.4. Completed repair

tain traction on the bladder wall trough as the running suture is initiated from the most distal portion of the trough (■ Fig. 97.3). Additional Lapra-Ty anchors are placed throughout the anastomoses in order to keep the suture under appropriate tension during the closure.

After the repair is completed (■ Fig. 97.4), instruments and trocars are removed in the standard fashion to check for trocar site bleeding or visceral injury. The fascial defects in all ports are closed with absorbable sutures. The skin is closed with 4-0 absorbable sutures. A bladder catheter may be kept in place overnight.

Postoperative Care

Pain control is usually managed by the administration of intravenous analgesics for the first 24 h, followed by oral analgesics afterwards. A urinary catheter is left indwelling for 24 h. The patient is allowed to void on their own and is discharged home the following day. The patient's diet is advanced rapidly with the return of bowel sounds. A 3- to 5-day oral broad-spectrum antibiotic regimen is prescribed, to be followed by the patient's regular antibiotic prophylaxis regimen. Regular incision care instructions are provided. Usually the dressings are allowed to fall on their own, or are removed 7 days postoperatively at home, whichever comes first. The patient may start bathing 5 days after surgery. Follow-up care includes a return visit at 4 weeks with an ultrasound, and at 3 months with a cystogram to confirm the absence of reflux.

Results

Results to date at several centers have been satisfactory, with a similar outcome as that expected with open surgery (Ehrlich et al. 1994; Gill et al. 2001).

Discussion

The laparoscopic technique of vesicoureteral reflux correction is a clinically useful alternative to open surgical repair. However, the limitations of this approach must also be recognized. It is a procedure which requires a laparoscopy team with at least two experienced surgeons, and the length of time for the procedure is usually greater than with open techniques. As the instrumentation continues to improve, and greater laparoscopic experience is the norm, operative time has been reduced. As with other laparoscopic procedures, there is a steep learning curve. Extreme caution should be practiced initially, both with patient selection and the procedure itself.

References

Atala A, Kavoussi LR, Goldstein DS, et al (1993) Laparoscopic correction of vesicoureteral reflux. J Urol 150:748–751

Cohen RC, Moores D, Cooke-Yarborough C, et al (1999) Laparoscopic bladder "wrap" technique for repair of vesicoureteral reflux in a porcine model. J Pediatr Surg 34:1668–1671

Ehrlich RM, Gershman A, Fuchs G (1994) Laparoscopic vesicoureteroplasty in children: initial case reports. Urology 43:255–261

Gill IS, Ponsky LE, Desai M, et al (2001) Laparoscopic cross-trigonal Cohen ureteroneocystostomy: novel technique. J Urol 166:1811–1814

Lich R, Howerton LL, Davis LA (1961) Recurrent urosepsis in children. J Urol 86:554–558

Sakamoto W, Nakatani T, Sakakura T, et al (2003) Extraperitoneal laparoscopic Lich-Gregoir antireflux plasty for primary vesicoureteral reflux. Int J Urol 10:94–97

Endoscopic Cross-trigonal Ureteric Reimplantation Under Carbon Dioxide Pneumovesicum

C.K. Yeung

Introduction

Different minimally invasive surgical techniques have been reported for the management of vesicoureteral reflux (VUR). These include cystoscopic subureteric injection of various types of bulking agents, for example, polytetrafluoroethylene (Teflon), collagen, dextranomer/hyaluronic acid copolymer (Deflux), etc., endoscopic ureteral advancement and trigonoplasty, and endoscopic ureteric reimplantation through a transperitoneal extravesical approach (Atala et al. 1993; Lackgren et al. 2001; Lakshmanan and Fung 2000; Okamura et al. 1999; Puri and Granata 1998). Currently, laparoscopic ureteric reimplantation for VUR utilising the Lich-Gregoir technique can be performed in children through a transperitoneal extravesical approach. However, this approach necessitates transgression of the peritoneal cavity and can be technically difficult in the small pelvis of a young child. Furthermore, concerns arose in cases with bilateral reflux as a significant proportion of children developed voiding dysfunction and urinary retention after bilateral laparoscopic extravesical ureteric reimplantation (Lipski et al. 1998).

From a pilot animal model using piglets we have found that under carbon dioxide insufflation of the bladder at around 10 mmHg pressure, a large potential working space could be obtained that would allow various intravesical procedures, including a Cohen's type of cross-trigonal ureteric reimplantation, to be easily conducted endoscopically using standard laparoscopic instruments. In this chapter, we describe our technique of vesicoscopic cross-trigonal ureteric reimplantation under carbon dioxide insufflation of the bladder, or pneumovesicum, in the treatment of VUR in infants and children.

Preoperative Preparation

The surgeon needs to have adequate experience in paediatric laparoscopic surgery and is used to performing intracorporeal suturing in a confined space. The parents are carefully counselled about the pneumovesicum technique and informed consent to the procedure obtained. This is important as the technique is new and long-term data on its potential advantages and disadvantages are not yet available. Unlike the extravesical Lich-Gregoir technique, both unilateral and bilateral reflux can be managed safely using this procedure without the fear of postoperative urinary retention.

Routine bowel preparation with fleet enema is given before surgery to cleanse any pre-existing faecal loading. The patient is prepared for general anaesthesia as usual. Good muscle relaxation is essential to ensure that bladder insufflation is not compromised, and sufficient intravesical operative space can be obtained during the operation. The use of nitrous oxide should be avoided to minimise bowel distension. A nasogastric tube is usually not necessary. A broad-spectrum antibiotic is routinely given intravenously for prophylaxis on induction of anaesthesia.

Positioning of Patient, Crew, Monitors and Equipment

The patient is placed in a supine and slightly Trendelenburg position at the end of the operating table, with the legs separated so that the surgeon can gain access to the urethral orifice for cystoscopy and bladder catheterisation intraoperatively. For small infants the surgeon stands and operates over the patient's head (■ Fig. 98.1), whereas for older children the surgeon usually stands on the patient's left side (■ Fig. 98.2). The video column is placed between the patient's legs at the end of the table, with the cables coming from the patient's right side and fixed to the superior part of the operative field. Similar to open pelvic or bladder surgery, it is preferable for a right-handed surgeon to stand on the patient's left side. After placement of ports, the operating table is laterally rotated with the right side up, so that the patient's body and the bladder will be more aligned with the surgeon's operating angle, thus providing better ergonomics. An AESOP-Hermes system (Computer Motion, USA) is routinely used in the author's institute for optimal positioning of the endoscope, and this is mounted on the right side of the table, opposite to the surgeon.

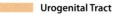

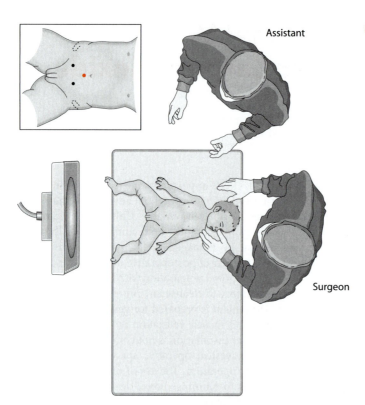

Assistant

Surgeon

Fig. 98.1. Operating room set-up: infants

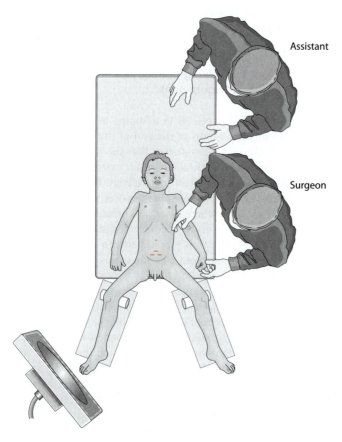

Assistant

Surgeon

Fig. 98.2. Operating room set-up: older children

Special Equipment

In general, ureteric reimplantation under carbon dioxide pneumovesicum can be performed without the need for any special equipment. However, some devices can be helpful:

- Special cannulas with self-retaining devices such as a balloon or umbrella help to prevent any dislodgement, which could be frustrating and even lead to failure of the procedure.
- The AESOP robotic arm gives a remarkable degree of stability and precision in control of the endoscope. This greatly facilitates dissection and reconstruction in the small intravesical space.

Technique

Placement of Ports

The endoscopic procedure is preceded by transurethral cystoscopy to allow placement of the first camera port under cystoscopic guidance. The bladder is first distended with saline and a number 1 monofilament suture is passed percutaneously at the bladder dome under cystoscopic vision, through both the abdominal and bladder walls. This keeps the bladder wall from falling away when the first camera port site incision is made and during insertion of the cannula. A small stab incision carrying right into the bladder wall is then made over the port site. Under cystoscopic guidance, a suture loop is first introduced via a 16-gauge angiocath through the port site and the bladder wall over one side of the stab incision. A 3-0 polydioxanone suture is introduced via a 20-gauge angiocath over the opposite side of the incision, and manipulated to pass through the suture loop. The 3-0 polydioxanone suture is caught by the loop, delivered over the other side of the port site incision and secured at the skin level. This is crucial in keeping the bladder from falling away from the abdominal wall and the cannula intraoperatively, and can be tied at the end of the procedure for port site closure. A 5 mm Step port (Inner Dyne, USA) is inserted under cystoscopic vision through the port site incision, and secured with sutures at the skin level. If a clear cystoscopic view can still be maintained, the procedure is repeated and two more 3- to 5 mm working ports are inserted with cystoscopic guidance while the bladder is still under saline distension. These are inserted on either side along the bikini line on the lateral wall of the bladder, and are also secured as previously described to prevent inadvertent dislodgement of cannula during the procedure. However sometimes blood oozing from the bladder port sites may have clouded the cystoscopic fluid; if this happens the two working ports can be inserted under carbon dioxide bladder

insufflation. A urethral catheter is inserted to drain the bladder and carbon dioxide insufflation to 10–12 mmHg pressure is started. The urethral catheter helps to occlude the internal urethral meatus to secure carbon dioxide pneumovesicum, and can also serve as an additional suction-irrigation device during subsequent dissection and ureteric reimplantation. A 5 mm 30° scope is used to provide intravesical vision.

Ureteric Dissection and Mobilisation

After placement of the ports the pneumovesicum pressure is lowered to 8–10 mmHg. This helps to reduce leakage of carbon dioxide into the extravesical space. A short segment of a 4F suction catheter is inserted into the refluxing ureter and secured by sutures. This serves as a stent to facilitate subsequent ureteric dissection and mobilisation. Intravesical mobilisation of the ureter, repair of the ureteral hiatus, dissection of a submucosal tunnel and a Cohen's type of ureteric reimplantation can then proceed endoscopically in a similar manner to the open procedure. The ureter is mobilised by first circumscribing it around the ureteric orifice using hook electrocautery (■ Fig. 98.3). With traction on the ureteric catheter using a blunt grasper, the fibrovascular tissue surrounding the lower ureter can be seen and divided using fine 3 mm endoscopic scissors and diathermy hook, while preserving the main ureteric blood supply. Mobilisation of the ureter is continued for 2.5–3 cm to the extravesical space. Once adequate ureteric length is obtained, the muscular defect in the ureteric hiatus is repaired using 5-0 absorbable sutures, usually with an extracorporeal knot tying technique (■ Fig. 98.4). This should be done as quickly as possible to avoid excessive leakage of carbon dioxide through the hiatus into the extravesical space, which could in turn result in extrinsic compression of the bladder and compromise of the intravesical space and vision. To ensure that the ureteric hiatus is repaired to appropriate tightness, and to avoid inclusion of ureteric tissue in the knot, the assistant can hold the ureter away with a blunt grasper during the knot tying.

Development of Submucosal Tunnel and Ureteric Reimplantation

A submucosal tunnel is created as in an open Cohen's procedure. Using a diathermy hook, a small incision is made over the future site of the new ureteric orifice, usually chosen to be just lateral and superior to the contralateral ureteric orifice. Dissection of the submucosal tunnel is then started from the medial aspect of the ipsilateral ureteric hiatus towards the new ureteric orifice, using a combination of endoscopic scissors and

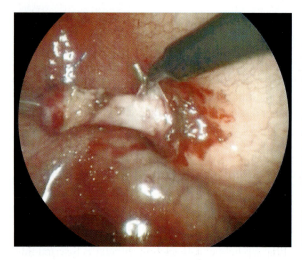

Fig. 98.3. Ureteric mobilisation

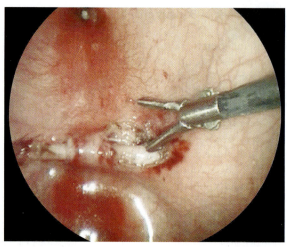

Fig. 98.6. Cross-trigonal ureteric reimplantation

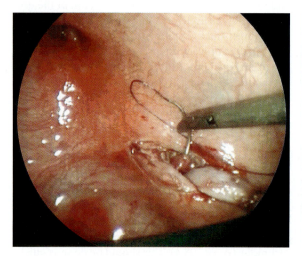

Fig. 98.4. Repair of ureteric hiatus

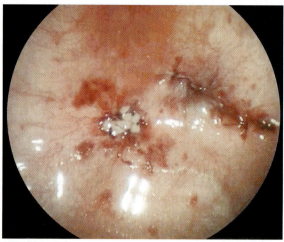

Fig. 98.7. Ureteroneocystostomy completed

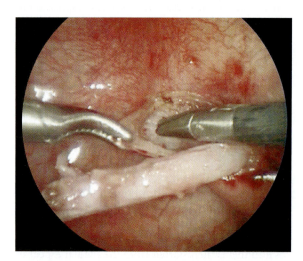

Fig. 98.5. Dissection of submucosal tunnel

diathermy hook for haemostasis (■ Fig. 98.5). Once the submucosal tunnel dissection is completed, a fine grasper is passed and the mobilised ureter is gently drawn through the tunnel. The ureteric catheter is removed. Ureteroneocystostomy is performed under endoscopic guidance with intracorporeal suturing using interrupted 5-0 or 6-0 poliglecaprone or polydioxanone sutures (■ Figs. 98.6, 98.7). A ureteric stent was not used in the early part of the series. This however resulted in a young boy who had gross bilateral reflux and extensive periureteritis developing moderate hydronephrosis postoperatively after bilateral ureteric reimplantation. Hence the policy now is to reserve ureteric stenting with a double pigtail catheter for selected patients undergoing bilateral ureteric reimplantation or those with megaureters requiring tapering ureteroplasty. In unilateral cases a ureteric stent is not required.

The trocar wounds are then closed by simply tying the 3-0 polydioxanone sutures inserted over the port sites at the beginning of the operation. The fascial defects in the trocar wounds are closed with 4-0 absorbable sutures. Local anaesthetics are instilled over the port sites. The skin wounds are closed with 5-0 subcuticular absorbable sutures. A bladder catheter is usually kept in place overnight.

Postoperative Care

Bladder drainage by an indwelling urinary catheter is maintained for 24 h after the operation. Postoperative pain is usually mild and oral analgesics usually suffice. The patient is allowed to void normally and is discharged from hospital usually on the first day after the procedure. A 4- to 5-day course of broad-spectrum oral antibiotic is usually prescribed upon discharge. This is followed by the patient's regular preoperative prophylactic antibiotic regimen. The dressings are either allowed to fall off on their own, or are removed 1 week later upon ward follow-up. A follow-up ultrasound is taken at 1 and 3 months. In view of the very high reflux resolution rate after the operation, a voiding cystogram is now not regarded as a routine, but can be taken at 3 months postoperatively if there is suspicion for persistence of reflux, or if the ultrasound shows abnormal upper urinary tract dilatation.

Results

During a 3.5-year period from August 2000 to March 2004, 58 patients (41 boys, 17 girls) aged 7 months to 14 years with dilating primary VUR (22 bilateral; 80 refluxing ureters), associated with recurrent urinary tract infections and/or multiple pyelonephritic renal scarring, underwent endoscopic Cohen's cross-trigonal ureteric reimplantation with carbon dioxide pneumovesicum. The procedure was successfully completed in all patients. There was no conversion in all except 1 patient who had a working port displaced into the extravesical space shortly after the ureteric reimplantation procedure was completed, and required a small vesicotomy for closure of the mucosal defect. Blood loss was minimal in all cases. The mean operating time was 108 min (range 70–185 min) for unilateral cases, and 162 min for bilateral cases (range 128–265 min). Similar to other novel techniques there was a very steep learning curve, with a much longer operating time at the initial part of the series than in subsequent cases. The mean hospital stay was 1.8 days (range 1–4 days). In the early part of the series when the cannulas were not routinely secured to the bladder wall, displacement of the port outside the bladder wall occurred in 3 pa-

tients. This resulted in gas leakage into the extravesical space, with compromise of the intravesical space and endoscopic vision and thus a prolongation of the operating time, although the procedure could still be completed in each of the 3 cases. Two boys developed mild to moderate scrotal and suprapubic emphysema immediately postoperatively, which subsided spontaneously within 24 h. Persistent mild haematuria for over 72 h was noted in 2 patients. One boy with bilateral ureteric reimplantation developed intermittent right loin pain 1 week postoperatively, but remained otherwise well and afebrile. Urgent ultrasonogram revealed a small submucosal haematoma at the trigone overlying the reimplanted ureters, associated with moderate bilateral hydronephrosis. This was managed by insertion of a double pigtail ureteric catheter on both sides under pneumovesicum, with subsidence of symptoms. There were no other major complications recorded. Of note, bladder spasms were minimal, and were especially so after removal of the urinary catheter. In most cases oral analgesics alone were sufficient and intravenous injections were only very occasionally required. All children returned to normal activities within a week from surgery.

A follow-up cystogram was obtained in 45 patients. Of these, complete resolution of reflux was observed in 43 patients. Two patients with initially grade V reflux were found to have persistent grade I and II reflux, respectively. Two patients developed a febrile urinary infection 5 and 10 months after the ureteric reimplantation. All other patients remained asymptomatic and well at a mean follow-up of 22 months (range 4 months to 3.5 years).

Discussion

The cross-trigonal ureteric reimplantation as first described by Cohen and Politano-Leadbetter has been a time-tested antireflux procedure associated with a high success rate (McCool and Joseph 1995). However, as the technique entails an open vesicotomy, urinary diversion with a bladder catheter is required postoperatively. This is often associated with significant bladder spasms that are severe enough to cause substantial pain and discomfort, thus necessitating prescription of additional analgesics, prolonging hospital stay and delaying return to normal activities (Marotte and Smith 2001). By comparison, the extravesical technique of ureteric reimplantation, initially described by Lich and Gregoir, has been reported to give excellent results that are comparable to the Cohen's intravesical procedure, but is associated with significantly less morbidity (Lapointe et al. 1998; Marotte and Smith 2001). In particular, the often debilitating problem of bladder spasms and intermittent gross haematuria are obviated. Despite these potential advantages, the extravesical technique has not gained universal acceptance because of concerns for the possibility of postoperative voiding dysfunction and urinary retention, especially in patients undergoing bilateral reimplantation (Fung et al. 1995; Lipski et al. 1998).

With the advent of laparoscopic surgery, various minimally invasive surgical techniques have been reported for the management of VUR. Atala et al. have reported their early experience of laparoscopic ureteric reimplantation for VUR in children using the Lich-Gregoir technique through a transperitoneal extravesical approach (Atala et al. 1993). However, this approach necessitates transgression of the peritoneal cavity and can be technically difficult in the small pelvis of a young child. Furthermore, similar to the open procedure, concerns arise in cases with bilateral reflux as a significant proportion of children developed voiding dysfunction and urinary retention after bilateral laparoscopic extravesical ureteric reimplantation (Atala et al. 1993; Fung et al. 1995; Lipski et al. 1998). Other minimal access surgical techniques have also been proposed as possible alternatives to ureteric reimplantation. These include the endoscopic trigonoplasty procedure described by Okamura et al. (1999). However, the results so far reported have been disappointing, with a success rate of only around 70%. In addition, trigonal splitting which resulted in the ureteral orifices receding to their original positions could occur in a substantial proportion of patients (Okamura et al. 1997, 1999). Lakshmanan and Fung (2000) described a total intravesical technique for endoscopic mobilisation of the ureters and trigonoplasty in pigs, but was unable to achieve resolution of reflux (Lakshmanan et al. 1999).

Given the very high success rate in reflux resolution and the minimal morbidity of the conventional open Cohen's technique, the long-term results of any endoscopic antireflux procedure using a minimal access surgical technique must at least be comparable. The intravesical cross-trigonal ureteric reimplantation under carbon dioxide bladder insufflation as described here by the author is in principle identical to, and merely an endoscopic recreation of, the standard open Cohen procedure. Our early experience has shown that it is indeed reproducing the satisfactory results of the open technique. In addition, the pneumovesicum technique with carbon dioxide bladder insufflation has many advantages. Compared with cystoscopy under fluid filling of the bladder, the pneumovesicum technique provides distinctly clearer intravesical vision due to much better light transmission using gas insuffla-

tion. This, together with the optical magnification offered by the laparoscope, allows fine dissection and even meticulous reconstructive procedures to be done inside the bladder without any difficulty. As the urothelial lining is relatively impermeable to carbon dioxide, there are minimal systemic or physiological disturbances due to carbon dioxide absorption. During a Cohen's ureteric reimplantation under pneumovesicum, the small amount of carbon dioxide that will inevitably leak into the extravesical space through the ureteric hiatus will be quickly reabsorbed, causing only a transient increase in carbon dioxide tension. This avoids the problem of fluid extravasation and collection in the extravesical space, which could frequently occur when fluid filling of the bladder was used (Snow 2001). Under normal circumstances, the bladder catheter is kept in place only for 24 h, and no ureteric stent is used. This may contribute to the remarkably few complaints of bladder spasms in our patients.

Introduction of the laparoscope through a suprapubic port provides a familiar forward intravesical view towards the trigone and the ureteric orifices that is similar to that obtained with an open bladder incision. The working instruments are inserted into the bladder with a good working angle in line with the telescope. This greatly enhances operative ergonomics and, in particular, eliminates second-degree paradoxical movements as would be encountered if a cystoscope inserted through the urethra is used to provide intravesical vision (Gill et al. 2001). This significantly reduces the operative technical difficulties and shortens the operative time. With the pneumovesicum technique, no additional laparoscopic instruments are necessary and only standard laparoscopic techniques are required for ureteric mobilisation and intracorporeal suturing.

Conclusions

This preliminary experience illustrates that endoscopic intravesical ureteric mobilisation and a Cohen's type of cross-trigonal ureteric reimplantation can be safely and effectively performed with routine laparoscopic surgical techniques and instruments under carbon dioxide insufflation of the bladder. This pneumovesicum technique also opens the opportunity for other intravesical endoscopic procedures. The long-term outcome and potential physiological effects of carbon dioxide pneumovesicum on the bladder and upper tract function however will need to be further evaluated.

References

Atala A, Kavoussi LR, Goldstein DS, et al (1993) Laparoscopic correction of vesicoureteral reflux. J Urol 50:748–751

Fung LC, McLorie GA, Jain U, et al (1995) Voiding efficiency after ureteral reimplantation: a comparison of extravesical and intravesical techniques. J Urol 153:1972–1975

Gill IS, Ponsky LE, Desai M, et al (2001) Laparoscopic cross-trigonal Cohen ureteroneocystostomy: novel technique. J Urol 166:1811–1814

Lackgren G, Stenberg A, Wahlin N, et al (2001) Long-term follow-up of children treated with dextranomer/hyaluronic acid copolymer for vesicoureteral reflux. J Urol 166:1887–1892

Lakshmanan Y, Fung LC (2000) Laparoscopic extravesicular ureteral reimplantation for vesicoureteral reflux: recent technical advances. J Endourol 14:589–593

Lakshmanan Y, Mathews RI, Cadeddu JA, et al (1999) Feasibility of total intravesical endoscopic surgery using mini-instruments in a porcine model. J Endourol 13:14–15

Lapointe SP, Barrieras D, LeBlanc B, et al (1998) Modified Lich-Gregoir ureteral reimplantation: experience of a Canadian center. J Urol 159:1662–1664

Lipski BA, Mitchell ME, Burns MW (1998) Voiding dysfunction after bilateral extravesical ureteral reimplantation. J Urol 159:1019–1021

Marotte JB, Smith DP (2001) Extravesical ureteral reimplantation for the correction of primary reflux can be done as outpatient procedures. J Urol 165:2223–2228

McCool AC, Joseph DB (1995) Postoperative hospitalization of children undergoing cross-trigonal ureteroneocystostomy. J Urol 154:794–796

Okamura K, Kato N, Takamura S, et al (1997) Trigonal splitting is a major complication of endoscopic trigonoplasty at 1 year follow-up. J Urol 157:1423–1425

Okamura K, Kato N, Tsuji Y, et al (1999) A comparative study of endoscopic trigonoplasty for vesicoureteral reflux in children and adults. J Urol 6:562–566

Puri P, Granata C (1998) Multicenter survey of endoscopic treatment of vesicoureteral reflux using polytetrafluoroethylene. J Urol 160:1007–1011

Snow BW (2001) Percutaneous endoscopic trigonoplasty: experience and modifications. Dialog Pediatr Urol 24:3

Chapter 99

Laparoscopic Treatment of Utricular Cysts

Mario Lima, Antonio Aquino, and Marcello Dòmini

Introduction

In open surgery several ways of approach have been advocated to access the retrourethral space and to remove a utriculus (also called Müllerian duct remnants, MDR): (a) perineal; (b) retropubic or suprapubic extravesical; (c) transvesical transtrigonal; (d) transperitoneal; (e) posterior sagittal transanorectal; (f) anterior sagittal transanorectal (ASTRA); and (g) posterior perirectal or pararectal (Kuhn et al. 1994; Monfort 1982; Rossi 1998; Siegel et al. 1995).

All these procedures are technically challenging and may cause complications such as infection and injury to the pelvic nerve complex resulting in bladder and rectal problems, and in impotence; moreover, they require prolonged hospitalization (Pintér et al. 1996; Ritchey et al. 1988).

Laparoscopic techniques obviate these disadvantages to a large extent because they provide an optimal view, thanks to magnification, and permit a fine dissection of MDR with an excellent exposure of all surrounding structures, with minimal trauma to the peritoneal cavity and low incidence of postoperative adhesions.

McDougal et al. described in 1994 the use of a laparoscopic approach to excise an MDR in a 48-year-old male patient with preservation of continence and potency. In 1998, we first successfully performed a laparoscopic removal of an MDR in a 15-year-old boy (Lima et al. 2000).

In this chapter we present the laparoscopic approach for MDR based on our experience in six boys with MDR.

Preoperative Preparation

Before Induction of General Anesthesia

No bowel preparation is required. Usually these patients take long-term oral antibiotic prophylaxis for urinary tract infections which is stopped the day before the operation.

After Induction of General Anesthesia

The child is intubated endotracheally and mechanically ventilated. We do not use locoregional anesthetic techniques. A nasogastric tube is inserted but will be removed at the end of the operation. Antibiotic prophylaxis is given.

An MDR sometimes hampers bladder catheterization in which case the urinary catheter is placed under urethrocystoscopic guidance.

Positioning

Patient

The child lies supine with the legs stretched out and abducted in order to allow for concomitant cystoscopy. The table is put in Trendelenburg position so that the bowel glides out of the pelvis by gravity.

Crew, Monitors, and Equipment

The monitor for the surgeon is placed at the end of the table, on the left. Another monitor for the assistant and the camera operator is put on the right. All the cables and tubes are fastened to the patient's left leg. The surgeon is positioned to the patient's right, with the scrub nurse to the surgeon's right. The assistant and camera operator stay in front of the surgeon to the patient's left. Another assistant is positioned in between the legs of the patient, to perform the simultaneous cystoscopy (■ Fig. 99.1).

Special Equipment

Bipolar and ultrasonic energy is available as are endolinear staplers and preformed loops of absorbable material.

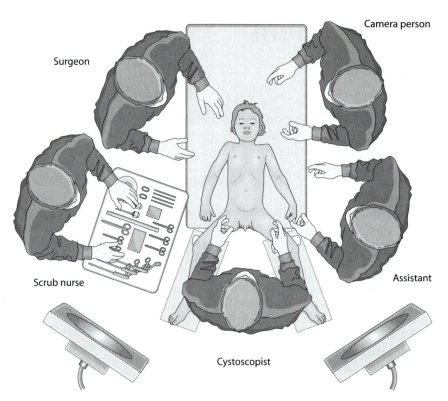

Surgeon

Camera person

Fig. 99.1. Position of the patient and the crew and equipment during the operation. The patient is put in Trendelenburg position

Scrub nurse

Assistant

Cystoscopist

Technique

Cannulae

Cannula	Method of insertion	Diameter (mm)	Device	Position
1	Open	5–10	Optic 0°	Umbilicus
2	Closed	3–5	Forceps and preformed loop	Right iliac fossa
3	Closed	3–5	Forceps and preformed loop	Left iliac fossa
4	Closed	3–5	Forceps	Suprapubic area

Port Positions

Four ports are used: one 5- to 10 mm port for a 0° tele-scope inserted in an open way just below the umbilicus; two secondary 3- to 5 mm ports inserted under endoscopic control in the left and right iliac fossa, respectively; and one more 3- to 5 mm port in the suprapubic area (■ Fig. 99.2).

Procedure

Urethrocystoscopy and visualization of the MDR always precedes the laparoscopic procedure to evaluate its shape, size, and particularly the exact location of the entrance of the MDR in the urethra (■ Fig. 99.3).

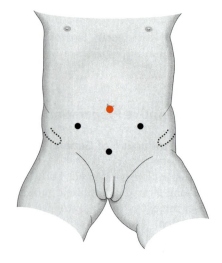

Fig. 99.2. Position of the trocars

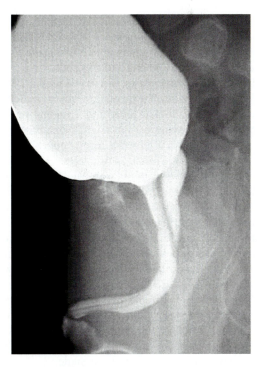

Fig. 99.3. Micturating cystography showing a small Müllerian remnant (MR) in a patient with severe hypospadias

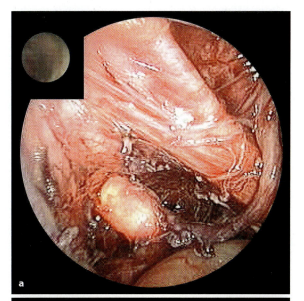

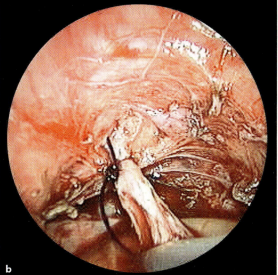

Fig. 99.5 a,b. Laparoscopic view of the same patient. **a** The MR is isolated (see the internal light) and **b** ligated using two endoloops

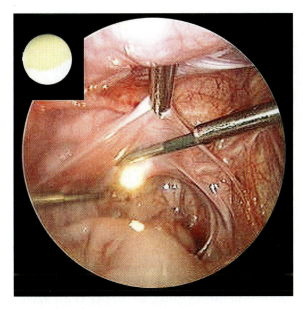

Fig. 99.4. Laparoscopic view of the same patient. Note the light of the cystoscope inserted in the small MR helps to identify it. *Inset* Cystoscopic view

After establishment of the pneumoperitoneum (CO_2 flow 1 L/min and pressure 10 mmHg) the secondary ports are inserted. The boy is then put in Trendelenburg position and the surgeon explores the pelvis looking for the dome of the MDR. At the same time the cystoscope is inserted again into the MDR by the assistant providing transillumination for easy identification, which is particularly useful in those MDR which do not protrude into the peritoneal cavity. The light of the cystoscope is also useful during the dissection of rectourethral space (■ Fig. 99.4).

The peritoneal reflection covering the dome of the MDR or surrounding it is incised and the dome is freed. The dome is then grasped with a forceps introduced through the suprapubic port and carefully freed from the surrounding tissues of the retrovesical space with two instruments, introduced through the iliac fossa ports. Particular attention has to be paid to avoid

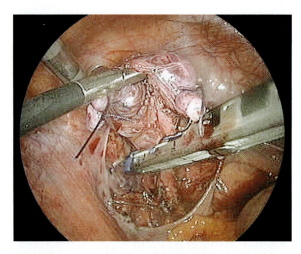

Fig. 99.6. Removal of a huge MR using the Endo-GIA

injury to bladder neck, urethra, rectum, ureters, deferens ducts, prostate, and seminal vesicles. Timely use of a monopolar hook, bipolar grasping forceps, or ultrasonic scissors allows for a complete bloodless dissection of all adhesions without using any clips or ligatures. Once completely dissected, the MDR neck is secured with two preformed loops and resected just above its junction with the urethra (■ Fig. 99.5). In older children an articulating linear endostapler can be used, which is inserted through an 11 mm port that replaces the 5 mm one in the right iliac fossa (■ Fig. 99.6). The specimen is removed through the largest port.

A bladder catheter is left in place at the end of the procedure.

Postoperative Care

The nasogastric tube is removed in the theatre at the end of the procedure. The patient resumes free oral fluid intake on the same day and full oral food intake on the first postoperative day.

Postsurgical discomfort is generally limited to the first and second day and is easily controlled by administration of non-steroidal analgesics.

The bladder catheter is removed on the fourth postoperative day, and discharge follows after a normal micturition.

Results

Six boys with MDR have been treated laparoscopically from February 1998 through February 2003. The mean age was 8.5 years, range 3–18 years. All but one were affected by scrotal hypospadias; two patients also pre-

sented mixed gonadal dysgenesis (MGD) and ambiguous genitalia, one had monolateral cryptorchidism associated with dydimo-epidydimal dissociation and deferential ectopia, and one had anorchia.

In four cases a hypoplastic uterus was present; MDR ended in all cases into the prostatic urethra. In the first case two small fallopian tubes and a vaginal septum were found in the surgical specimen. Deferential ectopia, in which the vasa joined a vaginal pouch and hypoplastic uterus, was found in two cases.

In one of the two patients with MGD bilateral gonadectomy was performed. In order to give the child a chance of later reproduction, the testicular tissue was conserved using cryotechniques.

Mean operating time was about 2 h and no major complications or relevant blood loss were recorded. Histological examination of removed MDRs showed normal features.

All patients are well and free from urogenital tract infections, voiding dysfunction, or urinary incontinence after a follow-up ranging from 6 months to 4 years. As symptoms are completely absent, no further X-ray examinations have been made.

Discussion

In patients with utricular cyst, laparoscopy allows both a diagnostic and a therapeutic purpose. In patients with MGD and ambiguous external genitalia it is possible to explore the abdominal cavity to evaluate and eventually remove the internal gonads. Laparoscopic techniques allow effective dissection of MDR from the retrourethral tissues because they provide clear identification of ureters, seminal vesicle, urethra, and bladder neck. These structures can be gently retracted and preserved.

In small babies the MDR can be excised between two endoloops placed as near to the urethra as possible and cutting in between them. In older patients in whom a large MDR needs to be excised an endolinear stapler can be used to transect the basis. Alternatively the basis can be cut, for example by using ultrasonic energy, and closed with a running suture. By doing this the distal part of the MDR may be left behind. Rather than risking iatrogenic damage to the important structures of the retrourethral space it may be preferable to leave a few millimeters of residual tissue and adopt a policy of precise clinical and ultrasonographic long-term surveillance. Later development of malignant carcinoma in an MDR, however, has been described (Szemes and Rubin 1968). Cystoscopic electrofulguration of the residual MDR mucosa could be a solution to this problem (Husmann and Allen 1997).

The laparoscopic approach does not resolve the problem of the abnormal connection of vas deferens with the MDR. Laparoscopically it is difficult to perform a vasal reimplantation both in bladder or in the urethra.

In conclusion, the laparoscopic approach allows to access the retrovesical space very well. It gives a much better view when compared with open surgery. It allows for very fine dissection, is likely to reduce the incidence of complications, avoids major trauma to the abdominal wall, provides a much faster recovery, and gives a much better cosmetic result.

References

Husmann DA, Allen TD (1997) Endoscopic management of infected enlarged prostatic utricles and remnant of rectourethral fistula tract of high imperforate anus. J Urol 157:1902–1906

Kuhn EJ, Skoog SJ, Nicely ER (1994) The posterior sagittal pararectal approach to posterior urethral anomalies. J Urol 151:1365

Lima M, Morabito A, Libri M et al. (2000) Laparoscopic removal of a persistent Müllerian duct in a male: case report. Eur J Pediatr Surg 10:265–269

McDougall EM, Clayman RV, Bowles W (1994) Laparoscopic excision of Müllerian duct remnant. J Urol 152:482–484

Monfort G (1982) Transvesical approach to utricular cyst. J Pediatr Surg 17:406

Pintér AB, Hock A, Vástyán A et al. (1996) Does the posterior sagittal approach with perirectal dissection impair faecal continence in a normal rectum? J Pediatr Surg 31:1349

Ritchey ML, Benson RC Jr, Kramer SA et al. (1988) Management of Müllerian duct remnants in the male patient. J Urol 140:795–799

Rossi F, De Castro R, Ceccarelli PL et al. (1998) Anterior sagittal transanorectal approach to the posterior urethra in the pediatric age group. J Urol 160:1173–1177

Siegel JF, Brock WA, Peña A (1995) Transanorectal posterior sagittal approach to prostatic utricle (Müllerian duct cysts). J Urol 153:785–787

Szemes GC, Rubin DJ (1968) Squamous cell carcinoma in a Müllerian duct cyst. J Urol 100:40

Chapter 100

Diagnosis of Non-palpable Testis

Fabio Ferro

Introduction

While the laparoscopic female pelvic anatomy has been known for many years, the laparoscopic male pelvic anatomy is a much more recent acquisition. Nowadays not only the normal anatomy but also the anatomy in the non-palpable testis is well known and laparoscopy has become the principal diagnostic tool in impalpable testis, which is the focus of this chapter.

Preoperative Workup

The child with an impalpable testis should be examined in detail preoperatively. A final clinical examination should be performed with the child under general anesthesia. Impalpability of the testes must be confirmed by careful examination, considering the possibility of unusual localizations of the gonad, such as crossed and perineal ectopia, which although they are rare should not be missed by an expert pediatric surgeon. In cases of perineal ectopia a normal spermatic cord can be palpated in the inguinal canal. An interstitial location may be suspected by careful palpation. The interstitial variant may also be seen on ultrasound examination while a preperitoneal gonad may be easily missed by a simple ultrasound examination of the inguinal region. Contralateral testicular hypertrophy is a common finding in patients with a unilateral non-palpable testis and is a strong indicator of monorchia. Only when the atrophy has been precocious, for example antenatally, does hypertrophy of the remaining solitary testis occur. This means that a normal-sized testis does not necessarily mean that the other one is present as well (Perovic and Janic 1994). When a patent processus vaginalis can be palpated one of the following differential diagnoses are possible: a low abdominal, peeping testis, a hypotrophic canalicular testis, or an ectopic testis. Surprisingly, the latter is infrequently referred to in the literature (Baillie et al. 1998). Palpation of a scrotal nubbin stands for a vanishing testis, especially when the nubbin is found on the left side. These data confirm the view of Belman, who considers a vanished testis as a scrotal event, with perinatal torsion occurring after descent but before fixation of tunica vaginalis (Belman and Rushton 2004).

In case of bilateral non-palpable testes, lack of an increase in testosterone level after gonadotrophin stimulation has been considered strongly indicative for anorchia. However, Perovic and Janic (1994) have reported the finding of a normal abdominal testis after such a negative test. Dysgenetic gonads may also not respond to gonadotrophin stimulation, yet they carry a high and rather early risk of malignant degeneration (Bartone et al. 1984). In case of bilateral cryptorchidism in association with severe hypospadias, preoperative workup must include genetic assessment and definition of the pelvic anatomy by diagnostic imaging.

Preoperative Preparation

Informed consent has to include the following topics:
- Possibility of conversion
- Complications directly related to the technique
- Need for orchiectomy (dysgenetic gonad or a testis too high for orchiopexy)
- Need for staged orchiopexy, including section of spermatic vessels and the use of silicon sheet protection (Corkery 1975)
- Insertion of a testicular prosthesis with contralateral fixation of the testis
- Possibility of testicular atrophy after orchiopexy, especially for abdominal testis with short vessels

Previous abdominal surgery is not a contraindication for a laparoscopic approach. The first trocar should be inserted by open technique and the secondary trocars should be inserted under endoscopic control. In case of constipation, which is frequently seen in older boys, an enema is recommended the day before surgery.

Boys should be encouraged to empty their bladder just before induction of anesthesia. We prefer not to catheterize the bladder unless the bladder is palpable, which was only necessary in 2 out of 200 cases. Despite a full bladder in one patient we were able to see the complete anatomy by rotating the child and thus the bladder to the contralateral side. It is unlikely that the bladder will fill during the procedure as the diuresis is hampered by the pneumoperitoneum.

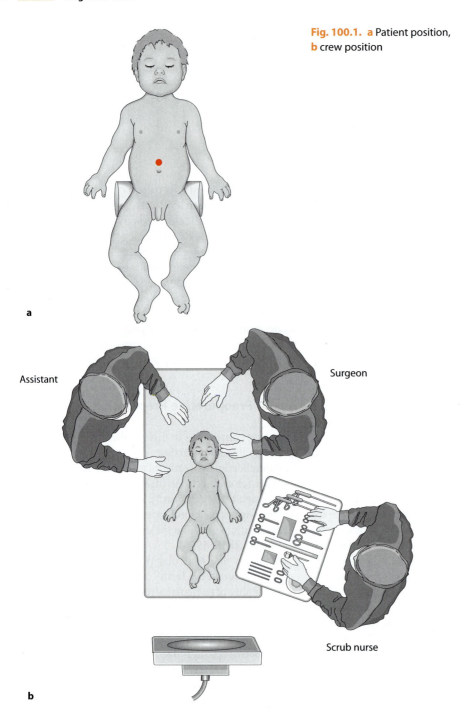

Fig. 100.1. a Patient position,
b crew position

a

Assistant   Surgeon

                                                      Scrub nurse

b

Anesthetic Peculiarities

General anesthesia with endotracheal intubation, mechanical ventilation, and muscle relaxation is given. Postoperative pain may be related to peritoneal irritation due to CO_2 insufflation and of course as a result of the trocar placement. Rectal paracetamol is given after induction and tramadol 3 mg/kg after extubation. Vomiting is counteracted with ondansetron.

The port sites are infiltrated with ropivacain (3 mg/kg), which acts slower (10–20 min) than other local anesthetics but for longer (7–12 h). The infiltration is at the umbilicus administering one third of the total dosage, the remaining to be used for additional ports. In case no extra ports are necessary, the remaining product is injected into the periumbilical region before closure.

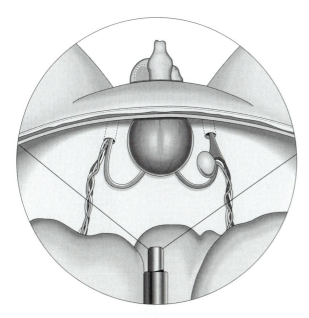

Fig. 100.2. In the patient position outlined and with the telescope in a supraumbilical position both inguinal rings can be seen. The surgeon stands on the left side of the patient

Positioning

The exploration of the abdominal cavity is started with the patient in supine position with the pelvis raised (■ Fig. 100.1a). In the majority of cases both internal rings can be visualized, and the diagnostic laparoscopy is carried out entirely in this position (■ Fig. 100.2). Failure to visualize the spermatic vessels and or vas deferens demands for a 20–30° head-down position and rotation of the table to the side contralateral to the place of interest. Also before inserting a second trocar to lift off obstacles (bowel, bladder) with a grasping forceps, the table is rotated to the contralateral side.

The surgeon should be on the left side of the patient with the scrub nurse at the surgeon's left and the assistant on the opposite side (■ Fig. 100.1b). The column with monitor, light source, CO_2 insufflator, and recorder is positioned at the bottom of the table.

Equipment and Instruments

Standard laparoscopy equipment is used. Recently, ports, optics, and instruments with very small diameters (2–3 mm) have been introduced. However, prefer 5- or 10 mm optic internal much better visualization and image recording.

Equipment for a laparotomy should be available at any time in case conversion to open surgery is necessary.

Technique

Cannula Insertion

Since the umbilicus in infants is contaminated, and sometimes filled with hard incrustations, preparing the umbilical region is important in order to avoid omphalitis.

As the average age of the patients is rather young, we use an open technique for the insertion of the first trocar. We prefer a supraumbilical approach, with a curved incision, which provides good visualization of the linea alba, thereby accessing the abdominal cavity 2–3 cm rostrally when compared to a subumbilical access. A subumbilical approach is adopted in case of concomitant umbilical hernia, which is corrected at the end of exploration. The cannula is secured with a purse-string suture. We presently prefer a slightly different approach. When the linea alba is dissected free, a small vertical incision (1–2 mm) is made and two 2/0 polyglycolic traction sutures are passed at its margins. With the sutures pulled up, the abdomen is palpated to make sure that the deep umbilical region is "free," then the incision is made larger and the peritoneum is opened. After inserting the cannula, the sutures are crossed and tightly twisted, which prevents leaks. At the end of the procedure, the two sutures are pulled while closing.

Insufflation pressure should be approximately 8 mmHg in infants and 10 mmHg in older children with a flow rate of 0.5–1 L/min. Excess CO_2 must be completely eliminated before closing the umbilicus.

Findings

Normal Pelviscopic Anatomy

Differences exist between female laparoscopic pelvic anatomy, as explored by gynecologists for several years, and the male laparoscopic pelvic anatomy which is of more recent acquisition. Several vestigial structures, particularly those related to the umbilical region, are important in the endoscopic examination of the pelvis (Bloom et al. 1994). Umbilical arteries persist in the deep pelvis as the internal iliac and proximal superior vesical artery, whereas the more anterior portions remain as the medial umbilical ligament on each side (■ Fig. 100.3a,b). These are important landmarks, perhaps the best-visualized structures in the pelvis, and enable rapid identification of the internal ring which lies laterally; this is a key point for an accurate diagnosis in a patient with a non-palpable testis. Normal anatomy at the internal ring consists of a substantial leash of that provides spermatic vessels, without attenuation in diameter, proceeding into a closed ring, joining at this level with a vas deferens proceeding from the posterior wall of the bladder and passing over

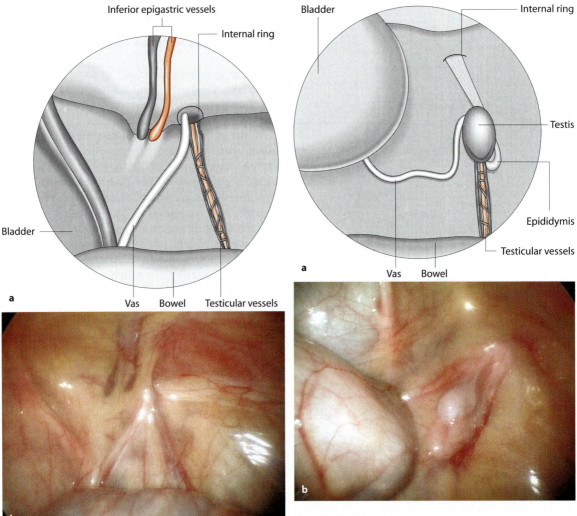

Fig. 100.3. Normal anatomy on the right side. **a** Schematic drawing. **b** Operative view

Fig. 100.4. High abdominal testis without mesorchium on the right. The inguinal ring is closed. **a** Schematic drawing. **b** Operative view

the iliac vessels. Laparoscopically, spermatic vessels and vas are configured like an inverted V. Epigastric artery and vein are visible under the peritoneum of anterior abdominal wall. Another fairly consistent finding in boys is the transverse vesical fold that blends into the anterior margin of the ring and fans out and disappears just above it. The ureter passes from a point medial to the distal spermatic vessels, deviating from them toward the midline across the iliac vessels to pass underneath the vas deferens. Sometimes, the most distal part of the ureter is hidden in fat and it is therefore very important be confident about its position in order to avoid injury. In cases of deficient activity of the müllerian inhibiting factor, uterine or salpingeal structures may be encountered, and, in cases of more complex disorders of sexual differentiation, also ovaries or dysgenetic gonads.

The side of the palpable testis, if so, is explored first: attention is directed to anatomy of the internal inguinal ring (open or closed), to spermatic vessels (normal, hypoplastic, tortuosity) as well to vas deferens. The side of the impalpable testis is explored thereafter.

Pelviscopic Anatomy in Impalpable Testis
Abdominal Testis

High Abdominal Testis with Absent Mesorchium
In most cases the internal ring is closed. Usually the gonad is elongated, and has no mesorchium (▬ Fig. 100.4a,b). The gonad is fixed against the posterior abdominal wall, and may be hidden behind the bowel so that it may not be immediately visualized. Sometimes, the vessels are seen only after mobilization of the colon. The epididymis is frequently abnormally thin, and sometimes rudimentary.

The finding of an irregularly ending vas deferens, resembling an abdominal nubbin, toward which some vascular structures seem to point, requires close evalu-

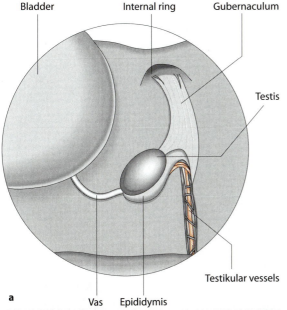

Bladder   Internal ring   Gubernaculum

Testis

Testikular vessels

a

Vas   Epididymis

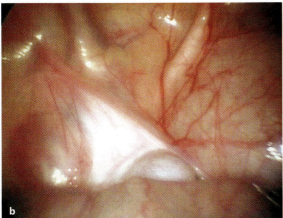

b

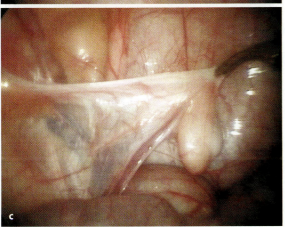

c

Fig. 100.5. Low intra-abdominal testis. **a** Schematic drawing of a right-sided low intra-abdominal testis. The inguinal ring is open. **b** Left-sided low intra-abdominal testis with long mesorchium. **c** Left-sided low intra-abdominal testis with long mesorchium, pulled to the right-sided inguinal ring

ation and insertion of a second trocar and a working instrument. In fact, these structures may be just a folding of the same vas and its vessels, which turn upward to reach a high intra-abdominal testis (Anwar et al. 2002). Such testes always have short vessels that are not long enough to allow a standard orchiopexy. An alternative approach is required to bring them down.

Low Abdominal Testis

The internal inguinal ring is usually open. The mesorchium is elongated and the testis freely mobile, residing behind or laterally to the bladder (Fig. 100.5a). The testis can be moved with the optic but evaluation of the length of the spermatic vessels length may require the introduction of a second trocar with a working instrument. A gonad which can be manipulated up to the contralateral inguinal ring has long been considered amenable to standard orchiopexy (Fig. 100.5b,c). Dissection of spermatic vessels can be carried out laparoscopically, which reduces the surgical trauma. In our experience, bringing such a testis down is easier on the left side than on the right side due to the anatomically shorter vessels on the right side.

Peeping Testis

The testis lies at the internal inguinal ring (Fig. 100.6). External compression of the inguinal region pushes the gonad in the abdominal cavity whereas the traction on the scrotum "milks" the testis into the canal. Standard orchiopexy can be carried out in the vast majority of cases. Occasionally the spermatic cord is too short to allocate the gonad into the scrotum without excessive traction. Under such circumstances a staged orchiopexy with a modified Corkery artifice is our approach of choice (Corkery 1975; Ferro et al. 1990).

No Vas, No Vessels

Such a finding is exceptionally rare (Fig. 100.7). We have found this only once, in a patient with ipsilateral renal dysplasia. The testis was spotted in proximity of the kidney. Cisek et al. (1998) described a similar experience and considers open exploration mandatory. Failure to identify the vas and vessels in intra-abdominal testes laparoscopically has been reported by Elder (1993). Failure of visualization of the intra-abdominal spermatic vessels laparoscopically has also occurred in a patient with Prader-Willi syndrome because of embedding of the vessels in excessive fat (Arnbjornsson et al. 1996).

Vas and Vessels Running Through an Open Internal Ring

A canalicular testis can be visualized by introducing the telescope directly into the processus vaginalis. The processus vaginalis of an infant usually allows only access of a 3- or 5 mm telescope. But even if a testis cannot be

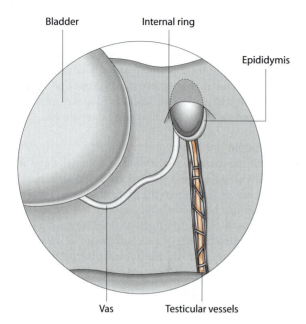

Fig. 100.6. Peeping testis on the right

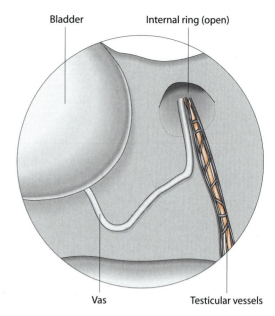

Fig. 100.8. Good caliber vas and vessels enter the open inguinal ring on the right. Inguinal exploration is mandatory if the testis cannot be found

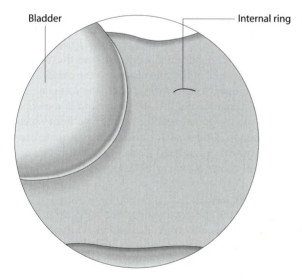

Fig. 100.7. Absent vas and spermatic vessels on the right

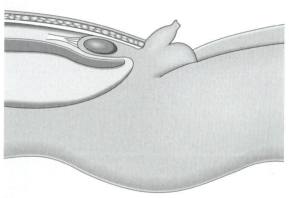

Fig. 100.9. Interstitial testis (between the aponeurosis of the external oblique and the muscle)

seen, surgical exploration should always be carried out in case of an open ring and a cord passing through it (■ Fig. 100.8). We have found cases of interstitial testis (between the aponeurosis of external oblique and muscle) and preperitoneal (between muscle and peritoneum) ectopia (■ Figs. 100.9, 100.10). In the former the testis is usually flat and may therefore be missed on palpation; in the latter the gonad may lie very high, for example at the level of the anterior iliac spine.

The length of spermatic vessels is usually adequate for standard orchiopexy. Testicular atrophy is rare in presence of a patent processus vaginalis. Therefore, palpation of an enlarged spermatic cord is the most important clinical finding to suspect the presence of the gonad.

Vas and Vessels Running Through a Closed Internal Ring

The size of spermatic vessels is here of utmost importance. In case of an atrophic (vanished) testis, the internal ring is generally closed and the spermatic vessels are smaller in caliber (■ Fig. 100.11). Sometimes they

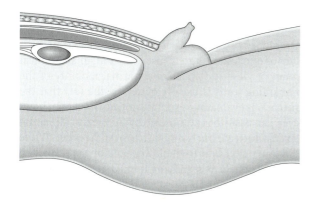

Fig. 100.10. Preperitoneal testis

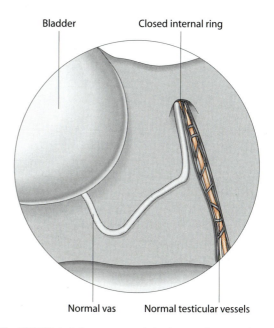

Fig. 100.12. In infants, a normal-sized vas and spermatic vessels may be seen passing through a closed inguinal ring despite complete atrophy of the testis

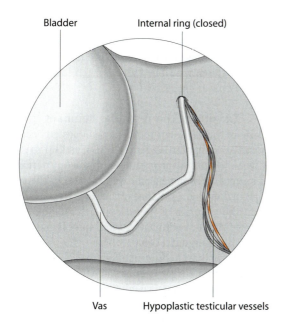

FiFig. 100.11. Small spermatic vessels pass together with the vas through a closed inguinal ring

are hardly visible or end in the proximity of the internal ring, whereas the vas passes through it. This finding should not to be confused with a so-called abdominal vanishing testis, in which both the vas and the vessels end blindly.

In infants the spermatic vessels may appear of normal size even if the testis is completely atrophic (■ Fig. 100.12), which is explained by the short period of time that has elapsed between the testicular atrophy and surgical exploration (Perovic and Janic 1994). In the author's series three impalpable testes, with vas and vessels piercing a closed internal inguinal ring, would have been missed if no surgical exploration had been

carried out. In case of hypotrophic spermatic vessels with hypertrophy of the contralateral testis, a vanished testis has to be suspected. However, even with normal contralateral testis, if the spermatic vessels are small, a vanished testis is the most likely diagnosis. In one patient scheduled for insertion of a testicular prosthesis a testis was found in the inguinal canal and pulled down. Excision of the testicular remnant can be performed later on at the time of implantation of a testicular prosthesis. In one such patient in the author's series, a testis was subsequently palpated by the pediatrician.

Blind-ending Vessels and/or Vas

This finding is the landmark of testicular atrophy (■ Figs. 100.13, 100.14). In contrast to what was previously thought, evidence is now accumulating that any vascular accident leading to atrophy takes place after testicular descent and closure of processus vaginalis. In this context, a testicular nubbin is almost always found in the scrotum during the insertion of a testicular prosthesis. This has been recently substantiated by Belman and Rushton (2004) who recommend a scrotal exploration first, and reserves laparoscopy for those cases in which no nubbin is found or with a patent processus vaginalis (Castilho 1990). However, in view of the short time required for a laparoscopy, we prefer to leave the scrotal wall intact for future implantation of a prosthesis.

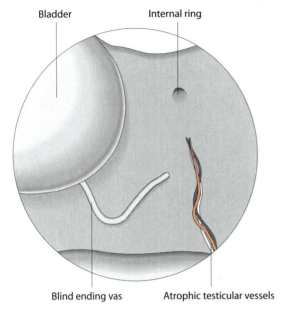

Bladder   Internal ring

Blind ending vas   Atrophic testicular vessels

Fig. 100.13. Blind-ending vas and spermatic vessels

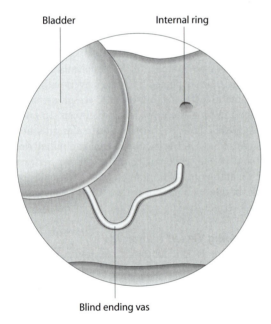

Bladder   Internal ring

Blind ending vas

Fig. 100.14. Blind-ending vas and no spermatic vessels

Contralateral Orchiopexy in Case of a Vanished Testis

Orchiopexy of the contralateral testis in case of atrophy of one testis is rarely justified from an anatomical point of view. Judgment of abnormal mobility of the remaining testis is usually biased by the fact that the surgeon is evaluating a solitary gonad. The testis, however, can easily be exteriorized by incision of all scrotal layers which are freely mobile one over the other. While directing attention to the lower pole of the testis, the tunica vaginalis is seen lying immediately proximal to it which excludes the so-called bell-clapper deformity. Nevertheless when a child has only one testis, that gonad has a value beyond measure and the loss of the solitary remaining testis is a catastrophic event. If removal of the scrotal testicular nubbin is planned, the scrotum can be accessed through the median raphe. Orchiopexy is to be carried out with two sutures between dartoic fascia and incised tunica vaginalis, just proximal to the testis. No sutures should pass through the tunica albuginea since this has been found to impair fertility.

Excision of the Testicular Remnant

Excision of the testicular remnant is suggested because of possible malignant degeneration. Castilho (1990), however, did not find any testicular tissue in spermatic cord structures removed on exploration. On the contrary, Plotzker et al. (1992) advocated surgical exploration on the grounds of microscopic islands of viable tubular epithelium within the small nubbins of tissue residing in the inguinal canal.

We believe that the finding of vanished testis is not an indication for surgery per se since the risk of future malignant degeneration is negligible and no cases have been reported so far. In patients requesting a testicular implant, the nubbin can be removed at the same time as the implantation of the testicular prosthesis.

Postoperative Care

Diagnostic laparoscopy for non-palpable testis is usually done in day care.

Results

The following table gives details of the author's personal experience of the laparoscopic exploration of 202 patients with 219 impalpable testes.

Gonads immediately visualized	95 (43.4%)
Abdomen	76 (34.7%)
Peeping testis	19 (8.7%)
Gonads not immediately visualized	124 (56.6%)
No vas, no vessels (dysplastic kidney) exploration orchiectomy	1 (0.5%)
Vas and vessels through an open internal ring	12 (5.5%)
Testes visualized in the canal; orchiopexy	5 (2.28%)
Testes not visualized; exploration	7 (3.2%)
Orchiopexy (interstitial ectopia)	3
Orchiopexy (preperitoneal ectopia)	3
Remnant excision	1
Vas and vessels through a closed internal ring	84 (38.3%)
Normal vessels	21 (9.6%)
No further surgery (atrophic testis)	18
Orchiopexy (canalicular testes)	1
Orchiopexy (preperitoneal ectopia)	2
Hypotrophic vessels	63 (28,76%)
Contralateral normal testis	30 (13,69%)
No further surgery (atrophic testis)	29
Orchiopexy (canalicular testis)	1
Contralateral hypertrophic testis	33 (15.06%)
Contralateral orchiopexy	33
Exploration when implanting prosthesis	1
Testis subsequently palpated	1
Blind-ending vas and vessels	20 (9.1%)
Blind-ending vas	7 (3.2%)
Exploration, prosthesis	7
Testicular remnant	7

No complications were encountered except for three cases of omphalitis which resolved after a short course of antibiotic therapy. Postoperative ileus with feeding difficulties occurred in three children, requiring intravenous fluid administration for 24 h.

Discussion

Laparoscopy can now be considered to be the principal diagnostic tool in impalpable testis. Moreover laparoscopy may be useful in evaluation of whether an undescended testis should have a standard one-stage orchiopexy or a two-stage approach. The laparoscopic anatomy of the impalpable testis is now well defined and experience has progressed to such an extent that nowadays many authors consider laparoscopic or laparoscopic-assisted orchiopexy superior to conventional approaches (Baillie et al. 1998; Bloom 1991; Diamond and Caldamone 1992; Flett et al. 1999; Poppas et al. 1996; Van Savage 2001; Yu et al. 1995). In the vast majority of children these procedures are carried out in day care (Gill et al. 2000; Soble and Gill 1998).

Laparoscopy is considered advantageous when there is hypertrophy of contralateral testis, since about 50% of patients with a contralateral testicular size greater than 1.8% had blind-ending vessels proximal to the internal ring (Hurwitz and Kaptein 2001). A transscrotal exploration first has been advocated but an abdominal gonad may sometimes be missed since a scrotal nubbin may consist of wolffian structures only (Wolfenbuttel et al. 2000). Moreover, formation of scar tissue in the scrotum may affect subsequent positioning of an implant. Failure to locate vas and vessels laparoscopically has been reported (Arnbjornsson et al. 1996; Elder 1993). Our policy of open surgical exploration (whether immediately or later during implantation of a testicular prosthesis) in all cases in which no clear evidence of a testis during laparoscopy was found, yielded ten gonads. In six the vas and vessels exited an open internal inguinal ring while in four the internal ring was closed. Evaluation of contralateral testicular hypertrophy can be useful in the diagnosis of inguinoscrotal testicular atrophy, especially when hypotrophic vessels and a closed internal ring are seen.

Whether the inguinal region should be explored or not when hypotrophic cord structures and a closed inguinal ring are seen has received much attention in the literature. It has been questioned especially in thin children (Guiney et al. 1989). Some authors did not find any testicular tissue in the cord structures removed at exploration (Castilho 1990), but Plotzker et al. (1992) advocated surgical exploration and removal of all remnants in the inguinal canal based on the finding of microscopic islands of viable tubular epithelium. Of the ten testes in our series with a vas and vessels exiting the internal ring found on open exploration, only two were in an inguinal position while four of the remaining eight were in a preperitoneal position and the other four in an interstitial position. The latter four testes appeared flattened, which explains why they were missed on palpation. An ultrasound scan should diagnose all testes in this anatomical position. According to the literature somewhat less than 5% of the non-palpable testes are found in the inguinal canal during surgical exploration (Gill et al. 2000; Peters 1993).

Laparoscopy can also be used as a tool to evaluate a certain surgical technique. In this respect we have the impression that the maneuver of mobilizing the gonad up to the opposite internal inguinal ring, thereby judging the feasibility of a one-stage orchiopexy, is not entirely reliable. Left-sided intra-abdominal testes, in our opinion, can be more easily brought down than right-sided testes. This may be due to the fact that the vessels on the left side can be dissected free more rostrally and are therefore longer.

Since a one-stage laparoscopic or standard open orchiopexy is a better option for the vast majority of intra-abdominal testes (Flett et al. 1999) and a two-stage orchiopexy offers good results with a modified Corkery artifice (Corkery 1975), there is concern in the literature regarding the high incidence of spermatic vessels division still performed.

References

Anwar A, Kurokava Y, Shintani T, et al (2002) Intraabdominal testis with loop-like epididymis and intracanalicular vas and vessels. Int J Urol 9:528–530

Arnbjornsson F, Mikaelsson C, Lindhagen T, et al (1996) Laparoscopy for nonpalpable testis in childhood: is inguinal exploration necessary when vas and vessels are not seen ? Eur J Pediatr Surg 6:7–9

Baillie CT, Fearns G, Kitteringham I, et al (1998) Management of the impalpable testis: the role of laparoscopy. Arch Dis Child 79:419–422

Bartone FF, Huseman CA, Maizels M, et al (1984) Pitfalls in using chorionic gonadotropin stimulation test to diagnose arnochia. J Urol 132:563–567

Belman AB, Rushton HG (2001) Is the vanishing testis always a scrotal event ? BJU Int 87:480–483

Bloom DA (1991) Two-step orchiopexy with pelviscopic clip ligation of the spermatic vessels. J Urol 145:1030–1033

Bloom DA, Guiney EJ, Ritchey ML (1994) Normal and abnormal pelviscopic anatomy at the internal inguinal ring in boys and the vasal triangle. J Urol 44:905–908

Castilho IN (1990) Laparoscopy for the nonpalpable testis: how to interpret the endoscopic findings. J Urol 144:1215–1218

Cisek LJ, Peters CA, Atala A, Bauer SB, et al (1998) Current findings in diagnostic laparoscopic evaluation of the nonpalpable testis. J Urol 160:1145–1149

Corkery JJ (1975) Staged orchidopexy: a new technique. J Pediatr Surg 10:515–518

Diamond DA, Caldamone AA (1992) The value of laparoscopy for 106 impalpable testes relative to clinical presentation. J Urol 148:632–634

Elder JS (1993) Laparoscopy for the non palpable testis. Semin Pediatr Surg 2:168–173

Ferro F, Inon A, Caterino S, et al (1990) Stage orchidopexy: simplifying the second stage. Pediatr Surg Int 5:10–12

Flett ME, Jones Pf, Youngson GG (1999) Emerging trends in the management of the impalpable testis. Br J Surg 86:1280–1283

Gill IS, Ross JH, Sung GT, et al (2000) Needlescopic surgery for cryptorchidism: the initial series. J Pediatr Surg 35:1426

Guiney EJ, Corbally M, Malone PS (1989) Laparoscopy and the management of the impalpable testis. Br J Urol 63:313–316

Hurwitz RS, Kaptein JS (2001) How well does contralateral hypertrophy predict the absence of the nonpalpable testis. J Urol 165:588–592

Perovic S, Janic N (1994) Laparoscopy in the diagnosis of nonpalpable testes. Br J Urol 73:310–313

Peters CA (1993) Laparoscopy in pediatric urology. Urology 41(1 suppl):33–37

Plotzker ED, Ruschton HG, Belman AB, et al (1992) Laparoscopy for nonpalpable testes in childhood: is inguinal exploration also necessary when vas and vessels exit the internal ring? J Urol 148:635–637

Poppas DP, Lemack GE, Mininberg DT (1996) Laparoscopic orchiopexy. Clinical experience and description of technique. J Urol 155:708–711

Soble JJ, Gill IS (1998) Needlescopic urology incorporating 2mm instrumentation in laparoscopic surgery. Urology 52:187–194

Van Savage JG (2001) Avoidance of inguinal incision in laparoscopically confirmed vanishing testis syndrome. J Urol 166:1421–1424

Wolffenbuttel KP, Kok DJ, Den Hollander JC, et al (2000) Vanished testis: be aware of an abdominal testis. J Urol 163:957–958

Yu TY, Lai MK, Chen WF, et al (1995) Two-stage orchiopexy with laparoscopic clip ligation of the spermatic vessels in prune-belly syndrome. J Pediatr Surg 30:870–872

Chapter 101

Laparoscopic Treatment of Non-palpable Testis

Ciro Esposito

Introduction

There is a variety of therapeutic strategies for the management of non-palpable testes. The surgeon can easily select the most appropriate one based on the laparoscopic findings (Vaysse 1994):

- In case of blind-ending cord structures: no surgical exploration is necessary (Andze et al. 1990).
- In case of cord structures entering the internal inguinal ring: open inguinal exploration may be required to identify and remove, if necessary, an atrophic intracanalicular or ectopic testis. The policy of always performing a surgical exploration, when cord structures enter the internal inguinal ring, based on the fear of malignant degeneration of the remaining testicular tissue is questionable. In fact malignant degeneration of such remaining tissue is very rarely reported in the literature (Esposito et al. 2000).
- In case of an atrophic intra-abdominal testis: a laparoscopic orchiectomy can be performed using clips or simply electrocoagulation (Jordan 1997).

Concerning the optimal surgical treatment of an intra-abdominal testis (IAT), there is no general agreement. Some surgeons prefer to perform an orchidopexy using open surgery, others use microsurgery, but the majority of pediatric surgeons prefer to perform a laparoscopic orchidopexy in case of IAT (Baker et al. 2001).

The main point of discussion in laparoscopic orchidopexy is whether or not the spermatic vessels should be divided or whether they can be spared (Flett et al. 1999). As a matter of fact, there are two main procedures that have been adopted to perform laparoscopic orchidopexy in case of IAT:

1. The Fowler-Stephens (FS) procedure, in which the spermatic vessels are divided. This can be done in one or two steps
2. The laparoscopic-assisted orchidopexy (LAO) where the orchidopexy is performed without sectioning of the spermatic vessels.

Another option, which allows 1 or 2 cm of length to be gained, consists of the creation of a neoinguinal ring medially to the epigastric vessels. This option can be adopted in both the FS procedure and the LAO (Esposito et al. 2002).

Preoperative Preparation

The patient is put under general anesthesia. Postoperative pain is largely abolished if a caudal block is given as well. The patient is asked to empty his bladder immediately before the operation. To make sure that the bladder is empty, the bladder is manually expressed under general anesthesia.

Positioning

Patient

The patient is placed in the supine position, in a 30° Trendelenburg position with the entire abdomen, genitalia, and upper legs included in the operative field.

Team setup

The surgeon stands on the patient's side contralateral to the pathology and the assistant stands on the other side, facing the surgeon. The scrub nurse stands on the same side as the surgeon. The screen is positioned at the patient's feet (Fig. 101.1).

Special Equipment

No special equipment is required.

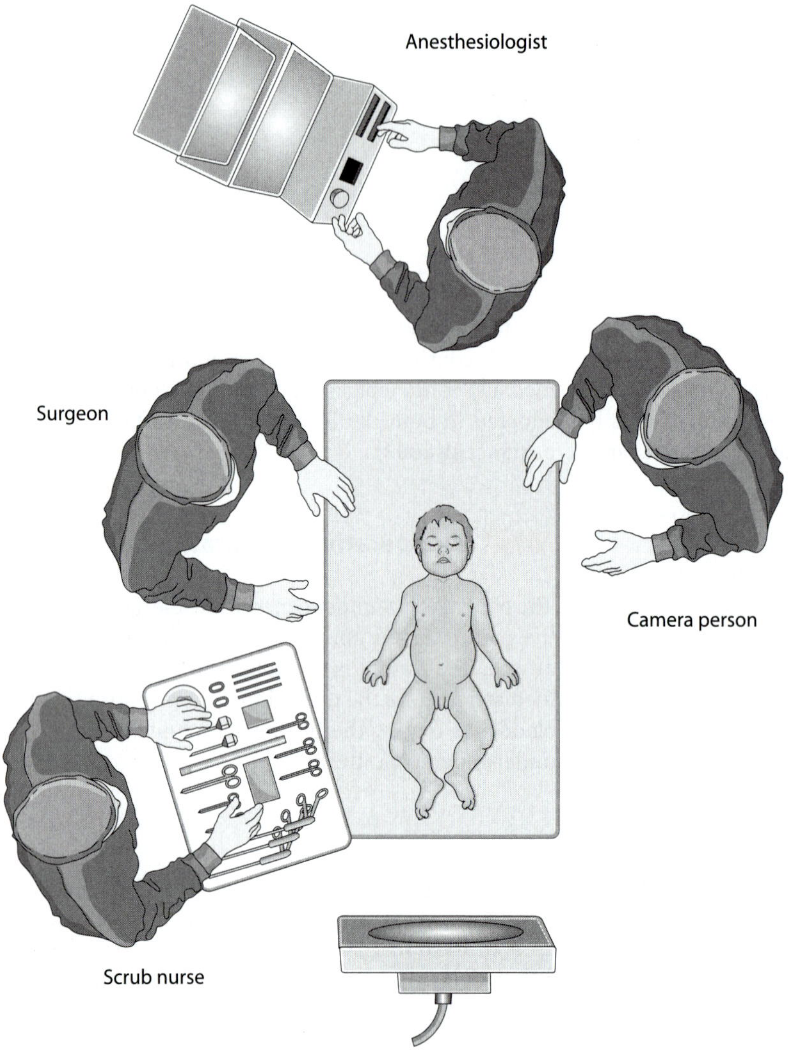

Fig. 101.1. Positioning of the patient, crew and monitor

Anesthesiologist

Surgeon

Camera person

Scrub nurse

Technique

Cannulae

Port	Size (mm)	Instruments	Position
A	5–10	Telescope	Through the umbilicus or infraumbilically
B	3–5	Atraumatic fenestrated grasping forceps	Left iliac fossa
C	3–5	Scissors, needle holder, clips applier	Right iliac fossa
D	–	Grasping forceps	Ipsilateral hemiscrotum

In pediatric patients it is preferable to perform an open procedure to introduce the first umbilical trocar and to achieve the pneumoperitoneum. A 5- or 10 mm blunt-tipped trocar is used. However, several pediatric surgeons use the Veress needle.

A 5- to 10 mm 0° telescope is placed transumbilically or subumbilically and two 3- or 5 mm trocars are placed in the right and left iliac fossa, respectively, about 3–4 cm below the umbilical scar. The exact position of the trocars depends upon the patient's age and size (■ Fig. 101.2). In case of IAT a traditional grasper forceps can be introduced through the scrotum, ipsilateral to the pathology.

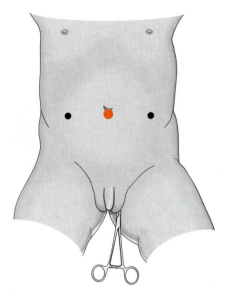

Fig. 101.2. Trocar positions

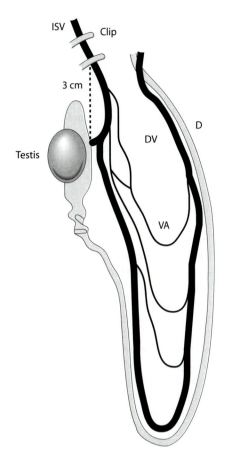

Fig. 101.3. Anatomic principles of the FS procedure. *ISV* Inner spermatic vessels, *D* vas deferens, *DV* deferential vessels, *VA* vascular anastomoses

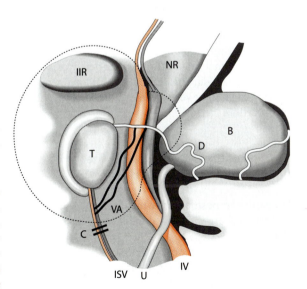

Fig. 101.4. *Dashed lines* indicate peritoneal incision of the two-step FS orchidopexy. *ISV* Inner spermatic vessels, *D* vas deferens, *VA* vascular anastomoses, *U* ureter, *IV* iliac vessels, *C* clips, *IIR* internal inguinal ring, *NR* neoinguinal ring, *B* bladder, *T* testis

Procedure

Laparoscopic Fowler-Stephens Procedure

The principle of the FS procedure is simple; there are several vascular anastomoses between the deferential and inner spermatic vessels close to the testis (■ Fig. 101.3). The inner spermatic vessels are clipped twice 3–4 cm proximally to the testis, according to Fowler-Stephen's description (Elder 1989). The testis will remain viable thanks to the collateral vascularization coming from the deferential vessels which supply now the last 2 cm of the inner spermatic vessels (Thorup et al. 1999) (■ Fig. 101.4).

The FS procedure can be performed in one or two steps (Bloom 1989). In the one-step FS procedure, the vessels are sectioned and the orchidopexy is performed during the same anesthesia. The two-step FS procedure, which is carried out by the majority of authors, consists of two staged surgical procedures (Caldamone and Amaral 1994). During the first step two or three clips are positioned on the inner spermatic vessels 3–4 cm from the testis. The second step of the FS procedure is performed 6–12 months later. This interval is necessary to permit the development of an optimal collateral circulation (Esposito and Garipoli 1997). The technique consists of the creation of a wide peritoneal pedicle using scissors and a blunt dissection laterally to the internal spermatic vessels, near the clips placed during the first operation (■ Fig. 101.4). The dissection is continued distally from the clips and around the internal ring, and is then extended medially to the umbilical ligament as far as 1 cm from the vas deferens. At this point, the inner spermatic vessels are sectioned near the clips and the dissection is extended medially, to as far as 1 cm on the other side of the vas deferens (Lindgren et al. 1999). The testis thus remains pedicled on a peritoneal flap attached to the perideferential peritoneum. A traditional open grasper is inserted through the scrotum, after the creation of a dartos pouch, and is then pushed into the abdominal cavity through the internal inguinal ring. The testis is grasped and brought down into the scrotum, carefully avoiding any torsion of the new vascular pedicle. The internal inguinal ring can be closed using interrupted sutures or a purse-string suture. The sutures are the same as for conventional surgery; they are introduced into the abdomen transparietally.

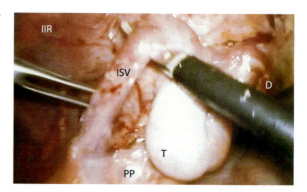

Fig. 101.5. The spermatic vessels are mobilized from the posterior peritoneum. *ISV* Inner spermatic vessels, *T* testis, *D* vas deferens, *PP* posterior peritoneum, *IIR* internal inguinal ring

Laparoscopic-assisted Orchidopexy Leaving the Internal Spermatic Vessels Intact

The gubernaculum, when present, is transected and the posterior peritoneum laterally to the spermatic vessels is opened. The testicular vessels and the vas are then dissected retroperitoneally for about 8–10 cm (■ Fig. 101.5). This dissection is done bluntly using a peanut or grasping forceps, without any type of coagulation. At the end of the dissection, the testis appears free from adhesions to the posterior abdominal wall and is pedunculated onto the inner spermatic vessels and the vas (Youngson and Jones 1991). At this point, if the inner inguinal ring is open, a traditional grasping forceps is introduced through the scrotum into the abdomen (as previously described) (■ Fig. 101.6). If the inner inguinal ring is closed, a neoinguinal ring is created medially to the epigastric vessels, using the same procedure as described above (■ Fig. 101.7). At the end of the procedure the testis is brought down into the scrotum through either through the already open internal inguinal ring or through the newly created inguinal ring (■ Fig. 101.8). The creation of a neoinguinal ring can also be very useful in combination with an FS procedure.

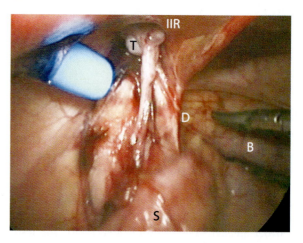

Fig. 101.6. If the inner inguinal ring is open, the testis is pulled down into the scrotum through the internal inguinal ring. *T* Testis, *D* vas deferens, *IIR* internal inguinal ring, *B* bladder, *S* sigmoid colon

Postoperative Management and Complications

No particular postoperative management is necessary, and patients are discharged from hospital on the following day.

The dissection should be done in a very delicate way. Accidental sectioning of the vas deferens or ureter has been reported (Docimo 1995). In case of an LAO with intact spermatic vessels, excessive traction on the inner spermatic vessels may cause iatrogenic rupture of these vessels (Esposito et al. 2000). Other complications include scrotal edema, hydrocele, and inguinal hernia. Atrophy of the testis after a first- or second-step

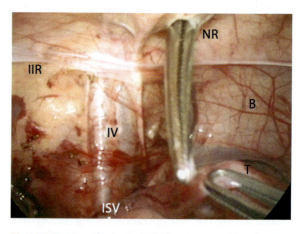

Fig. 101.7. To perform the orchidopexy, a traditional grasping forceps is introduced from the scrotum into the abdomen, in this case through a neoinguinal ring. *IIR* Internal inguinal ring, *NR* neoinguinal ring, *B* bladder, *IV* iliac vessels, *ISV* inner spermatic vessels, *T* testis

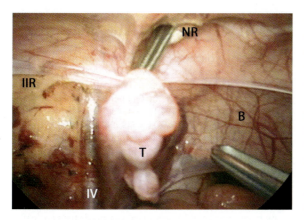

Fig. 101.8. The testis can be brought down into the scrotum also through a newly created inguinal ring. *IIR* Internal inguinal ring, *NR* neoinguinal ring, *B* bladder, *IV* iliac vessels, *T* testis

FS procedure is rarely reported (King 1998). Other late complications are the ascent of the testis or atrophy (Kirsch et al. 1998).

A clinical examination must be performed at 1 week and at 1, 6, and 12 months after surgery. Ultrasonography and an echo-color Doppler study must be performed 6 months after surgery to check the structure of the testis and its vascularization.

Discussion

There are no evidenced-based studies in the literature on the operative management of the non-palpable testis. The choice of one procedure over the other to pull down the testis is based on the surgeon's choice, which depends on knowledge, experience, and laparoscopic skill (Chang et al. 2001).

Concerning the two-staged FS, we reported an 80% success rate (Esposito and Garipoli 1997). Other authors have reported a 70–75% success rate and a 20–25% atrophy rate with the one-stage FS (Canavese et al. 1995). After initial experience with the laparoscopic FS procedure, and based on some reports in the literature, several authors tend nowadays to spare the inner spermatic vessels and to perform an LAO without sectioning the vessels (Esposito et al. 2000). A similar procedure, but using an open preperitoneal approach, has already been described with good results with a mean follow-up period of 11 years by Youngson and Jones (1991).

It is the author's opinion that operative laparoscopy for the non-palpable testis is a logical extension of diagnostic laparoscopy for the non-palpable testis. The main advantage of the laparoscopic orchiopexy without sectioning the spermatic vessels is the mini-inva-

siveness of the procedure in combination with saving of the testicular vascularization (Diamond 1994). The technique of LAO is similar to open orchiopexy but with the advantages that the spermatic vessels can be dissected much higher and over a longer segment. Moreover when the inner inguinal ring is closed, it is possible to create a new inguinal ring laparoscopically medial to the epigastric vessels thus allowing the spermatic vessels and the vas deferens to follow a straight, and thus shorter route.

Long-term follow-up is very important to determine the exact results of these kind of operations (Chang et al. 2001). Clinical examination is not sufficient for this and ultrasonography as well as ultrasound color Doppler examination is essential to evaluate the structure and vascularization of the testis (Esposito et al. 2002).

This author believes that LAO may be used for both the true IAT and the peeping testis, with the same advantages, as reported also by other authors. In any case, when the testis is at more than 3 cm from the internal inguinal ring in younger children, or even closer in children older than 5 years, it may not be possible to bring the testis down with LAO. Under such circumstances a two-steps laparoscopic orchidopexy is advisable.

In conclusion, operative strategy for the non-palpable testis can now be summarized as follows:

- After confirmation of the non-palpability of the testis under general anesthesia, laparoscopic exploration is performed.
- In case of an IAT located near the internal inguinal ring or less than 3 cm from the it, LAO is the procedure of choice.
- In case the IAT is further from the internal ring, a laparoscopic two-step FS procedure is preferable even with the 20% testicular atrophy rate associated with this procedure.
- Long-term follow-up is necessary to control the fate of these testes.

References

Andze GO, Homsy Y, Laberge I, et al (1990) The role of therapeutic laparoscopy in the surgical treatment of intra-abdominal testes in children. Chir Pediatr 31:299–302

Baker LA, Docimo SG, Surer I, et al (2001)A multi-institutional analysis of laparoscopic orchidopexy. Br J Urol 87:484–489

Bloom DA (1989) Two-step orchiopexy with pelviscopic clip ligation of the spermatic vessels. J Urol 145:1030–1033

Caldamone AA, Amaral JF(1994) Laparoscopic stage 2 Fowler-Stephens orchiopexy. J Urol 152:1253–1255

Canavese F, Cortese MG, Gennari F, et al (1995) Non palpable testes: orchiopexy at single stage. Eur J Pediatr Surg 5:104–107

Chang C, Palmer LS, Franco I (2001) Laparoscopic orchidopexy: a review of a large clinical series. Br J Urol 87:490–493

Diamond A (1994) Laparoscopic orchiopexy for the intra-abdominal testis. J Urol 152:1257–1260

Docimo SG (1995) The results of surgical therapy for cryptorchidism: a literature review and analysis. J Urol 154:1148–1152

Elder JS (1989) Laparoscopy and Fowler-Stephens orchiopexy in the management of the impalpable testis. Urol Clin North Am 16:399–411

Esposito C, Garipoli V (1997) The value of 2-step laparoscopic Fowler-Stephens orchiopexy for intrabdominal testes. J Urol 158:1952–1955

Esposito C, Vallone G, Settimi A, et al (2000) Laparoscopic orchiopexy without division of the spermatic vessels: can it be considered the procedure of choice in case of intrabdominal testis? Surg Endosc 7:638–640

Esposito C, Damiano R, Gonzalez Sabin MA, et al (2002) Laparoscopic-assisted orchidopexy: an ideal treatment for children with intra-abdominal testes. J Endourol 16:659–662

Flett ME, Jones PF, Youngson GG (1999) Emerging trends in the management of the impalpable testis. Br J Surg 86:1280–1283

Jordan GH (1997) Will laparoscopic orchiopexy replace open surgery for the non palpable undescended testis? J Urol 158:1956–1958

King LR (1998) Orchiopexy for impalpable testis: high spermatic vessel division is a safe maneuver. J Urol 160:2457–2460

Kirsch AJ, Escala J, Duckett JW, et al (1998) Surgical management of the nonpalpable testis: the Children's Hospital of Philadelphia experience. J Urol 159:1340–1343

Lindgren BW, Franco I, Blick S, et al (1999) Laparoscopic Fowler-Stephens orchiopexy for the high abdominal testis. J Urol 162:990–993

Thorup JM, Cortes D, Visfeldt J (1999) Germ cell may survive clipping and division of the spermatic vessels in surgery for intra-abdominal testes. J Urol 162:872–874

Vaysse P (1994) Laparoscopy and impalpable testis. A prospective multicentric study (232 cases). Geci Groupe d'Etude en Coeliochirurgie Infantile. Eur J Pediatr Surg 4:329–332

Youngson GG, Jones PF (1991) Management of the impalpable testis: long-term results of the preperitoneal approach. J Pediatr Surg 26:618–620

Chapter 102

Transperitoneal Laparoscopic Treatment of Varicocele

Gordon A. MacKinlay

Introduction

The term *varicocele* indicates a dilatation of the testicular veins in the pampiniform plexus caused by a venous reflux. This mainly occurs on the left-hand side (80–90% of cases); bilateral lesions are reported in up to 20% of the cases and right-sided lesions in up to 7% (Saypol 1981) This venous reflux can impair the counter-current heat exchange mechanism within the spermatic vessels, thus causing an increase in testicular and scrotal temperature (Iwata et al. 1992) The abnormally high temperature can subsequently lead to a progressive dysfunction of the testicle and epididymis (Nakamura et al. 1987; Namiki et al. 1987). Testicular atrophy and infertility can be direct consequences of varicocele (Okuyama et al. 1988).

The incidence of varicocele among men in general is 15% and can rise to 20–40% among men presenting to infertility clinics. Varicocele is a rare disorder in prepubertal children with an average incidence of less than 1%. In postpubertal children the incidence is similar to that of adulthood being roughly 15–16%. In the whole of childhood (patients younger than 18 years of age) the incidence of varicocele is 5%, being lower than that of adulthood (Akbay et al. 2000; al-Abbadi and Smadi 2000; Belloli et al. 1993; Camoglio et al. 2001; Liang et al. 1997; Stavropoulos et al. 2002).

Indications for treatment include severe dilatation of testicular vessels (grade II and III varicocele; Lyon et al. 1982), symptoms (discomfort, chronic pain, or dragging sensation), associated testicular atrophy and bilateral varicocele. Although selective embolisation of the enlarged testicular vessels during anterograde or retrograde venography has been proposed (Tauber and Johnsen 1994; Trombetta et al. 2003), varicocele is mainly treated by surgery. Different procedures have been proposed: Ivanissevitch technique (inguinal ligation of enlarged testicular vessels) (Ivanissevich 1960), Palomo technique (retroperitoneal mass ligation of all enlarged vessels above the internal inguinal ring) (Palomo 1949), internal spermatic artery (ISA)-sparing techniques (Lemack et al. 1998), lymphatic-sparing technique (Poddoubnyi et al 2000) and plication of the spermatic fascia over the enlarged vessels (Shafik et al. 1972).

As laparoscopy has gained popularity, many surgeons have used the minimally invasive approach for the treatment of varicocele. Both mass ligation of the spermatic vessels and selective ligation of the enlarged veins with ISA preservation are feasible via a laparoscopic approach (Humphrey and Najmaldin 1997; Martino et al. 2001; Sun et al. 2001; Varlet and Becmeur 2001).

Whatever treatment or approach is chosen, the postoperative complications for varicocele are fairly common and include hydrocele, recurrence, persistence and testicular atrophy (rarely described) (Esposito et al. 2000; Ficarra et al. 2002; Kattan 2001; Pintus et al. 2001; Riccabona et al. 2003).

Preoperative Preparation

Before Induction of General Anaesthesia

Although the risk is small it is advisable that all patients have a preoperative ultrasound scan of the renal tract to exclude a tumour of the kidney. Patients and their parents must be informed of the pros and cons of surgery and the minimal risks of laparoscopic surgery in experienced hands. They must be informed that there is a small risk of testicular atrophy postoperatively although this must be balanced against the risk of infertility.

As this procedure is a day case one, there is very little preoperative preparation required other than the standard for day case surgery. The patient should be asked to void urine prior to induction of anaesthesia.

After Induction of General Anaesthesia

Port sites are infiltrated prior to incision with 0.25% bupivacaine with 1 in 200,000 adrenaline for intraoperative and postoperative pain relief and to minimise bleeding from small vessels.

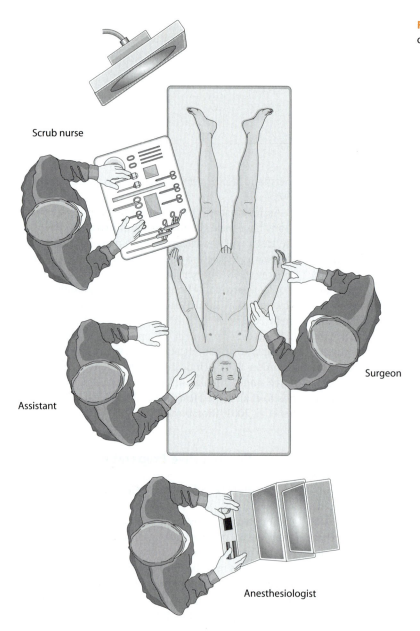

Fig. 102.1. Position of patient, crew and equipment

Scrub nurse

Assistant

Surgeon

Anesthesiologist

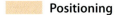

Positioning

Patient

The patient is placed supine on the operating table. Tilting of the table in Trendelenburg and to the right promotes exposure of a left-sided varicocele.

Crew, Monitors and Equipment

The surgeon stands on the patient's right side and the assistant (the camera operator) opposite the surgeon. The scrub nurse stands to the left of the assistant with the instrument trolley towards the foot end of the table. Only one monitor is required for this procedure. It is placed at the foot of the table, facing the head end (■ Fig. 102.1).

Special Equipment and Instruments

No special energy applying systems are needed. A 5 mm clipping device is at hand.

Technique

Cannulae

Cannula	Method of insertion	Diameter (mm)	Device	Position
1	Open	5.5	30° telescope	Subumbilical fold
2	Closed	3.5–5.5	Scissors, clipping device	Suprapubic
3	Closed	3.5–5.5	Grasping forceps	Left iliac fossa

Figure 102.2 shows the port positions.

Procedure

Each port site is first infiltrated with 0.25% Marcaine with adrenaline, partly for postoperative pain relief but also to minimise any bleeding from the port site. The infiltration is from skin to peritoneum. First a 6 mm primary port is placed at the umbilicus, under direct vision. A swab, held firmly against the skin infraumbilically, enables the lower fold of the umbilicus to be everted. Here a 6 mm incision is made using a scalpel with a number 11 blade. A towel clip is used to elevate the umbilicus. Two artery forceps grasp either side of the linea alba and direct vision incision of the peritoneum allows safe introduction of the primary port. If the incision is very small there is no need for a purse-string or other suture to anchor the port. The peritoneal cavity is insufflated with CO_2 at 0.3–1 L/min until the intra-abdominal pressure is 8–10 mmHg. It is maintained at this level with a flow rate of less than 1 L/min. During insufflation a 5 mm laparoscope (preferably 30° viewing) is inserted. Two further ports are then introduced visualising the insertion through the laparoscope. One is placed in the left iliac fossa, above and medial to the anterior superior iliac spine. The other is placed slightly lower and to the right of the midline (■ Fig. 102.2). The left one can be 6 mm or less to accommodate fine grasping forceps. The right one must be 5.5 mm for a 5 mm clip applicator. A smaller one suffices if the vessels are ligated or coagulated.

The internal inguinal ring is identified. A head-down position (Trendelenburg tilt) of the patient facilitates this and occasionally if the sigmoid colon obscures the view, the left side of the table may be slightly elevated. I have never had to mobilise the colon to expose the vessels. The testicular vessels can be seen clearly through the peritoneum above the inguinal ring and the vas with its vessels is seen to join them at the level of the ring.

Using dissecting shears the peritoneum is incised over the testicular vessels a few centimetres above the internal ring. Care must be taken not to damage the underlying veins and an adequate window must be

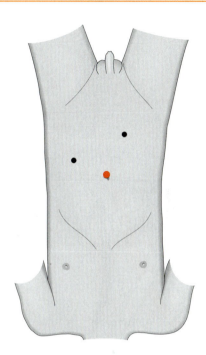

Fig. 102.2. Position of the ports

opened to clearly expose the vessels. Using the scissors the vessels are elevated from the posterior pelvic wall and grasped with the grasping forceps. Once a clear space has been developed behind the vessels the scissors are replaced by a 5 mm clip applicator. Two clips are applied above and two below the grasper prior to changing back to the scissors and dividing the vessels (■ Fig. 102.3). Alternatively the vessels can be electrocoagulated or divided between ligatures. Once they are divided the area behind the vessels is carefully inspected to ensure that no collaterals have been missed. If collaterals are noted then they should be diathermied. Collateral veins are mainly found running parallel to the testicular veins. In the past I endeavoured to preserve the testicular artery but recurrence of the varicocele in one case led to subsequent mass clip ligation of the vessels and 100% success in more than 20 consecutive cases. Fine collateral veins run closely applied to the testicular artery and will open postoperatively if an attempt is made to spare the artery.

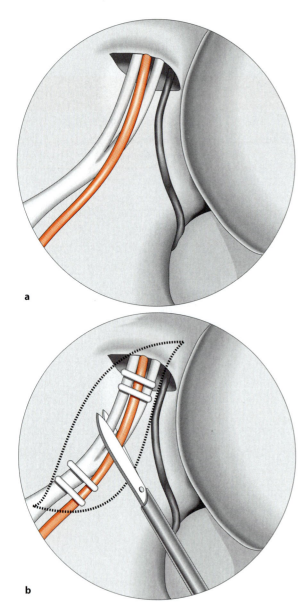

Fig. 102.3. *Top* Identification of internal inguinal ring. *Bottom* Clipping and dividing the testicular vessels

The ports are all removed under direct vision, the abdomen deflated and the wounds closed with subcutaneous 3/0 vicryl and 4/0 subcuticular Dexon to the umbilical wound and subcuticular Dexon alone to the other two. The procedure takes 10–20 min.

Some advocate ligation of additional collateral vessels such as those associated with the vas deferens. Once the main testicular vessels have been ligated the blood has to drain from the testis somehow and to occlude all drainage pathways seems inappropriate. It is inappropriate to perform a procedure laparoscopically that would not be considered in open surgery. To ligate these vessels alongside the vas may lead to venous infarction and testicular loss.

Postoperative Care

The patient may be discharged home within a few hours or remain in overnight. They may eat and drink as soon as they feel able and paracetamol provides sufficient postoperative analgesia. With local anaesthetic wound infiltration often no further analgesia is required. No postoperative complications have been encountered. Outpatient review is carried out at 6 weeks.

Results

Between June 1994 and June 2003, 41 boys with varicocele underwent laparoscopic varicocelectomy. All patients had grade II or III varicocele and 16/41 (40%) patients were noticed to have some degree of testicular atrophy. Ten of 41 (24%) boys were symptomatic.

Mean (±SD) age at operation was 13±1.98 years (range 9–18 years). Thirty-eight of 41 patients (93%) had left-sided varicocele and 3/41 bilateral (7%). Forty of 41 (98%) patients were treated on the left-hand side and 1/41 (2%) was treated only on the right (most severely involved side).

In 6/41 (15%) patients laparoscopy allowed us to identify and also divide enlarged vas vessels along with the testicular vessels. No associated procedures were carried out at the same time of the operation. No conversion to the open approach was required. No perioperative complications occurred.

Mean (±SD) length of hospitalisation was 17±8 h (range 12–48 h) and all the patients were discharged only when completely settled and free of symptoms. Mean (±SD) follow up was 15±13months (range 2–40 months).

The operation proved to be completely successful in 23 patients out of 41 (56%). Ten (62%) out of 16 patients with preoperative testicular atrophy showed catch up growth of the involved testis with an increase in size of more than 50% in the postoperative period. In contrast 6/16 patients (38%) showed no improvement regarding testicular size. Nine out of 10 symptomatic patients improved significantly postoperatively.

Twenty-two complications were identified in 18/41 (44%) patients. One patient of 41 (2%) showed recurrence and therefore underwent inguinal approach with ligation and division of all the enlarged vessels. Seven out of 41 (17%) patients showed some degree of persistently enlarged vessels, which were only observed and settled shortly afterwards (within 12 months of follow up). Fourteen out of 41 (34%) patients developed different degrees of postoperative hydrocele. Six out of 14 were observed and settled on their own while 8/14 patients (8/41 = 19.5%) required some sort of intervention: 3/8 were only aspirated (2 of them finally settled and 1 reaccumulated, on follow up), 1/8 was unsuccessfully aspirated and then underwent Lord's procedure but the hydrocele reaccumulated and he is still followed up, and 4/8 required Lord's procedure and then settled.

Discussion

Many different treatments have been proposed for varicocele but none of them have proved to be completely successful, or free of postoperative complications.

Selective antegrade or retrograde sclerotherapy has a high recurrence rate but a low incidence of postoperative hydrocele. This technique is operator-dependent, requires prolonged radiations exposition and is not feasible for anatomical reasons in up to 15% of the patients. Moreover, testicular atrophy can represent a postoperative complication in around 1% of the patients (Ficarra et al. 2002; Pintus et al. 2001; Tauber et al. 1994). ISA-sparing techniques show low incidence of postoperative hydrocele, but a high recurrence rate (Kattan 2001; Pintus et al. 2001). Ivanissevich and Palomo procedures are, on the one hand, successful as the recurrence rate is low but, on the other hand, they can be commonly complicated by postoperative hydrocele (Esposito et al. 2000; Kass and Marcol 1992; Riccabona et al. 2003). Testicular atrophy is an extremely rare complication for all surgical procedures (Esposito et al. 2000; Kattan 2001; Pintus et al. 2001; Riccabona et al. 2003).

Laparoscopic varicocelectomy is performed with Palomo's concept of mass ligation of all the enlarged testicular vessels above the inguinal ring. Therefore it shares similar results to the open Palomo technique. However, as laparoscopy and its magnification allow careful assessment of the whole pelvic region, this approach makes it possible to identify enlarged vas vessels that can be divided along with the spermatic vessels, thus reducing the risk of recurrence (Humphrey and Najmaldin 1997). Our results confirm this as shown by our very low recurrence rate (1/41, 2%).

Nevertheless, the incidence of postoperative hydrocele in our series is fairly high, accounting for 19.5% of the patients: 8 out of 41 patients required some sort of invasive treatment (aspiration or Lord's procedure). If we consider a hypothetical learning curve for laparoscopic varicocelectomy, it is noted that postoperative hydrocele occurred in around 16% of the cases after 2000, an incidence that is compatible with literature data.

Some authors showed that protein content in hydrocele occurring after varicocelectomy is very high

(Szabo and Kessler 1984). Therefore, postoperative hydrocele seems to be mainly related to some sort of lymphatic obstruction. On the ground of this consideration, microsurgical selective ligation of the enlarged venous vessels with preservation of both lymphatic and arterial supply has been proposed in order to reduce the occurrence of postoperative hydrocele (Lemack et al. 1998; Poddoubnyi et al. 2000). This technique seems to have a fairly low incidence of postoperative hydrocele. However, although available data regarding recurrence rate are not homogeneous, the incidence of postoperative recurrent varicocele seems to be higher in these series of patients (Kattan 2001; Lemack et al. 1998; Poddoubnyi et al. 2000).

In conclusion, thanks to magnification and to the possibility of a careful assessment of the pelvic region, laparoscopic Palomo procedure is the most successful option for the treatment of varicocele. Nevertheless, the high incidence of postoperative hydrocele should lead us to reconsider the sparing procedures, which can be accomplished laparoscopically, although the feasibility and effectiveness of such microsurgical techniques needs to be more carefully evaluated.

References

Akbay E, Cayan S, Doruk E, et al (2000) The prevalence of varicocele and varicocele-related testicular atrophy in Turkish children and adolescents. BJU Int 86:490–493

al-Abbadi K, Smadi SA (2000) Genital abnormalities and groin hernias in elementary-school children in Aqaba: an epidemiological study. East Mediterr Health J 6:293–298

Belloli G, D'Agostino S, Pesce C, et al (1993) Varicocele in childhood and adolescence and other testicular anomalies: an epidemiological study. Pediatr Med Chir 15:159–162

Camoglio FS, Cervellione RM, Dipaola G, et al (2001) Idiopathic varicocele in children. Epidemiological study and surgical approach. Minerva Urol Nefrol 53:189–193

Esposito C, Monguzzi GL, Gonzalez Sabin MA, et al (2000) Laparoscopic treatment of pediatric varicocele: a multicentric study of the Italian society of video surgery in infancy. J Urol 163:1944–1946

Ficarra V, Sarti A, Novara G, Artibani W (2002) Anterograde scrotal sclerotherapy and varicocele. Asian J Androl 4:213–219

Humphrey GM, Najmaldin AS (1997) Laparoscopy in the management of pediatric varicoceles. J Pediatr Surg 32:1470–1472

Ivanissevich O (1960) Left varicocele due to reflux: experience with 4,470 cases in 42 years. J Int Coll Surg 34:742–755

Iwata G, Deguchi E, Nagashima M, et al (1992) Thermography in a child with varicocele. Eur J Pediatr Surg 2:308–310

Kass EJ, Marcol B (1992) Results of varicocele surgery in adolescents: a comparison of techniques. J Urol 148:694–696

Kattan S (2001) The impact of internal spermatic artery ligation during laparoscopic varicocelectomy on recurrence rate and short postoperative outcome. Scand J Urol Nephrol 35:218–221

Lemack GE, Uzzo RG, Schlegel PN, et al (1998) Microsurgical repair of the adolescent varicocele. J Urol 160:179–181

Liang C, Wang K, Chen J (1997) Epidemiological study of external genitalia in 5172 adolescents. Zhonghua Yi Xue Za Zhi 77:15–17

Lyon RP, Marshall S, Scott MP (1982) Varicocele in childhood and adolescence: implication in adulthood infertility? Urology 19:641–644

Martino A, Zamparelli M, Cobellis G, et al (2001) One-trocar surgery: a less invasive videosurgical approach in childhood. J Pediatr Surg 36:811–814

Nakamura M, Namiki M, Okuyama A, et al (1987) Temperature sensitivity of human spermatogonia and spermatocytes in vitro. Arch Androl 19:127–132

Namiki M, Nakamura M, Okuyama A, et al (1987) Influence of temperature on the function of Sertoli and Leydig cells of human testes. Fertil Steril 47:475–480

Okuyama A, Nakamura M, Namiki M, et al (1988) Surgical repair of varicocele at puberty: preventive treatment for fertility improvement. J Urol 139:562–564

Palomo A (1949) Radical cure of varicocele by a new technique: preliminary report. J Urol 61:604–607

Pintus C, Rodriguez Matas MJ, Manzoni C, et al (2001) Varicocele in pediatric patients: comparative assessment of different therapeutic approaches. Urology 57:154–157

Poddoubnyi IV, Dronov AF, Kovarskii SL, et al (2000) Laparoscopic ligation of testicular veins for varicocele in children. A report of 180 cases. Surg Endosc 14:1107–1109

Riccabona M, Oswald J, Koen M, et al (2003) Optimising the operative treatment of boys with varicocele: sequential comparison of 4 techniques. J Urol 169:666–668

Saypol DC (1981) Varicocele. Int J Androl 2:61–71

Shafik A, Khalil AM, Saleh M (1972) The fascio muscular tube of the spermatic cord: a study of its surgical anatomy and relation to varicocele: a new concept for the pathogenesis of varicocele. Br J Urol 44:147

Stavropoulos NE, Mihailidis I, Hastazeris K, et al (2002) Varicocele in schoolboys. Arch Androl 48:187–192

Sun N, Cheung TT, Khong PL, et al (2001) Varicocele. Laparoscopic clipping and color Doppler follow-up. J Pediatr Surg 36:1704–1707

Szabo R, Kessler R (1984) Hydrocele following internal spermatic vein ligation: a retrospective study and review of the literature. J Urol 132:924–925

Tauber R, Johnsen N (1994) Anterograde scrotal sclerotherapy for the treatment of varicocele: technique and late results. J Urol 151:386–390

Trombetta C, Liguori G, Bucci C, et al (2003) Percutaneous treatment of varicocele. Urol Int 70:113–118

Varlet F, Becmeur F (2001) Laparoscopic treatment of varicoceles in children. Multicentric prospective study of 90 cases. Eur J Pediatr Surg 11:399–403

Chapter 103

One-port Retroperitoneoscopic Varicocelectomy in Children and Adolescents

Jean-Stéphane Valla

Introduction

Varicocele is an abnormal dilatation of the veins of the pampiniform plexus. The pathogenesis remains largely unanswered and proper management of the adolescent varicocele is controversial. Since the 1990s, many urologists have adopted the laparoscopic approach for treating varicoceles, and particularly by the transperitoneal approach (Belloli et al. 1996; Hagood et al. 1992; Jarrow et al. 1993; MacKinlay 1999; Matusda et al. 1992), which is never used in classic open surgery. To reproduce the same technique as in open surgery, we have tried to develop a retroperitoneal minimally invasive approach. As we have extensive experience with the use of the operating channel telescope in children (Valla et al. 1999), we have chosen a monotrocar retroperitoneal approach for treating varicoceles (Valla 2003).

Preoperative Preparation

No special preparation is needed, for example no gastric tube and no bladder catheter is inserted and no antibiotics are given.

Positioning

The patient is positioned in a right lateral decubitus position (Fig. 103.1). The surgeon stands behind the patient with the monitor opposite.

Fig. 103.1. Positioning of the patient and equipment. The surgeon stays behind the patient with the monitor opposite

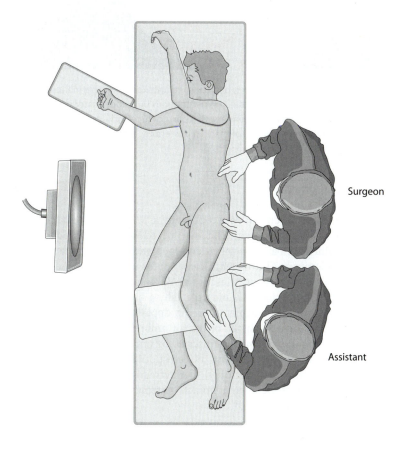

Surgeon

Assistant

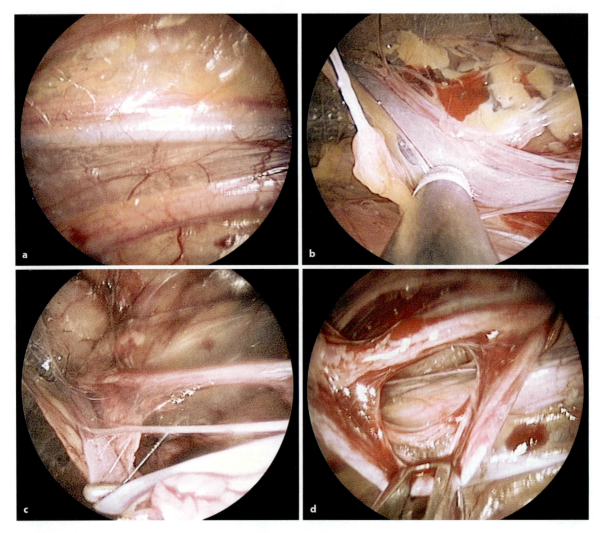

Fig. 103.2. **a** The peritoneum has been pushed anteriorly. The spermatic vessels stick superiorly to the pushed off peritoneum. The ureter also sticks to the pushed off peritoneum but more posteriorly. **b** Dissection of the spermatic vessels with a peanut. **c** The spermatic vessels have been separated: artery superiorly, vein inferiorly, and lymphatics in the middle. **d** Separation of the spermatic artery superiorly and of the vein posteriorly. The ureter is seen in the background

Equipment

We use a short, 27 cm, 0° telescope with a 5.5 mm operating channel (external diameter of telescope 10 mm), which we have specially developed with the Karl Storz Company (Tuttlingen, Germany) for use in pediatric surgery. This short telescope allows to use all the usual 5 mm instruments, and especially a bipolar forceps, or ultrasonic coagulator, or clip applier. The trocar, which is balloon-tipped or has an umbrella in order to prevent dislodgement, is inserted by open approach (see Chapter 86 regarding the retroperitoneoscopic approach for nephrectomy). For retraction of the wound edges of the open approach, narrow deep Farabeuf retractors are useful.

Technique

The same technique of creation of the working space is carried out as described in Chapter 86.

After having created the working space, the spermatic vessels are identified at the place where they cross the ureter (ureterovenous angle) from the anterolateral to the medial side. These vessels stick to the posterior part of the peritoneum. Manual traction on the testicle may help to identify them, and to make sure that they are indeed the spermatic and not the inferior mesenteric vessels. The testicular artery and one or two veins are dissected off from the peritoneum using a 5 mm hook or curved forceps (■ Fig. 103.2a–d). The vessels are then coagulated with monopolar or bipolar electrocautery, or ultrasonic energy, or are clipped, and then divided.

The retroperitoneal space is desufflated. The wound is infiltrated with a local anesthetic and the muscle layers as well as the skin are closed with absorbable sutures. No drain is left behind.

Personal Results

From 1995 to 2003, 60 boys underwent a monotrocar retroperitoneoscopic varicocele treatment. All were on the left side. The mean age of the boys was 14 years (range 11–18 years). All patients were evaluated clinically and by ultrasound-Doppler examination: 36 were grade 2 and 24 were grade 3. Testicular hypotrophy (difference of at least 25%) was recorded in 44 patients (67%).

The testicular artery was identified in all patients at surgery. The artery and veins were divided in 57 cases. In three patients the artery was spared as asked for by the parents. Interruption of the vessels was executed with monopolar coagulation in 20 cases, bipolar coagulation in 17 cases, clips in 19 cases, and ultrasonic coagulation in 4. Peritoneal perforation occurred in two patients early in our experience. In one patient the operation was converted, while in the second one the monotrocar technique was extended to a three-trocar one using two additional 3 mm operating trocars.

The average operation time was 35 min (range 14–70) and the hospital stay 1 day. All but two patients who underwent retroperitoneoscopic varicocelectomy were seen at follow-up, at least 6 months postoperatively. There were no wound complications. There was however one severe postoperative complication: in case 20 the ureter had been electrocoagulated with monopolar electrocautery. The ureter was repaired on the 8th postoperative day with good final result. At an average follow-up of 24 months (range 6–60 months) 54 of the 60 boys were controlled (90%). There were four recurrence (8%): two complete requiring reoperation (one by transperitoneal laparoscopy and one by venous embolization) and two mild recurrences, which are still followed. Six patients developed a hydrocele (10%), of which one required operation. None of the testicles atrophied, and 35 testis out of 44 (79%) had an increased volume.

Discussion

Regarding the Method of Varicocele Repair

Our experience shows that the recurrence rate and complication rate is comparable to that of open surgery or of the intraperitoneal laparoscopic approach. In many series (Esposito et al. 2000; Kass and Marcol

1992), the recurrence rate is lowest when the whole pedicle, artery and veins are interrupted. As a matter of fact, the only recurrences in our series requiring reoperation were seen in patients in which the artery had been spared. Interruption of the whole pedicle also interrupts lymphatic drainage. No wonder that this technique gives the highest incidence of postoperative hydrocele: Glassberg et al. (2000) 28%, Kass and Marcol (1992) 3%, and we 10%. In order to avoid this complication, recent series (Glassberg et al. 2000; Oswald et al. 2000) emphasize lymphatic-sparing surgery. Magnification is essential to do this, which can be provided by the telescope (Kocvara et al. 2001) or operating microscope (Golstein et al. 1992). The future of the retroperitoneoscopic management of varicoceles could be true microdissection using two additional 3 mm-diameter operating devices.

Great care must be taken in the choice of devices for interruption of the spermatic vessels: the monopolar hook is very effective, very cost effective, but also very dangerous for the surrounding structures, which is exemplified by the ureteral burn in one of our patients. In this patient the area of coagulation was 3 cm above the area of the actual coagulation and probably was due to a transmitted electric current. After this accident we have given up the use of monopolar coagulation for this indication and no further accidents have occurred.

Why an Endoscopic Surgical Technique?

The more cranial from the testis, the less plexiform the venous drainage of the testis becomes. Therefore the retroperitoneal dissection of the spermatic vessels is easier a few centimeters above the internal ring than at the internal ring. In my experience there is less hematoma formation, less scrotal edema, and less pain when the vascular pedicle is divided higher up in the retroperitoneum than in its inguinal part. So when comparing a high division of the spermatic vessels by classic open surgery with such a division by an endoscopic approach, it is evident that an endoscopic approach is much less invasive, causing less pain and less scarring.

Why a Retroperitoneal and not a Transperitoneal Endoscopic Surgical Technique?

From the literature the transperitoneal approach is obviously favored: about ten publications regarding more than 500 cases operated on transperitoneally against only three publications (Gaur et al. 1994; Kocvara et al. 2001; Valla 2003) regarding 70 patients operated on retroperitoneally.

The following arguments are helpful in the assessment of the pros and cons. The transperitoneal laparoscopic approach gives access to the spermatic vessels just above the internal inguinal ring and permits dissection of the spermatic vessels and also of the deferential vessels on both sides. The anatomical landmarks are obvious and well known. The working space is large and there is no learning curve with this approach, for example there was no conversion in the 161 cases published by Esposito et al. (2000). Moreover it allows treatment of other intra-abdominal pathological conditions such as an inguinal hernia.

The disadvantages, however, are the following. It is not logical to approach retroperitoneal structures transperitoneally which is also not done in open surgery. There is the risk of injury of intra-abdominal organs, especially in case of previous abdominal surgery. Moreover there is the possibility of postoperative shoulder pain, omental evisceration, and of intra-abdominal adhesions. At least three trocars are needed to open the peritoneum and dissect the vessels. In case of abdominal adhesions between the sigmoid colon and the lateral peritoneum, dissection of the spermatic vessels may be difficult, if not impossible. Belloli had to convert in two patients for this reason (Atassi et al. 1995). Using a transperitoneal approach Jarrow et al. (1993) found that there was a significant learning curve in the ability to spare the testicular artery and they were unable to identify the artery in 11% of cases even when using a Doppler probe. Likewise, Abdulmaaboud et al. (1998) were not able to find the artery in 4.6% of cases, Donovan and Winfield (1992) in 7%, and Ralph et al. (1993) in 20% of cases.

The retroperitoneoscopic approach gives a much higher access to the spermatic vessels than the transperitoneal approach. By going more cranially, an area is encountered in which only one or two major veins running parallel to the testicular artery are encountered. At this level the testicular artery is usually identifiable and easily dissected. The artery was identified and dissected free in 100% of our cases without the help of a Doppler probe (Loughin and Brooks 1992). By using a lateral retroperitoneal approach some other fine retroperitoneal venules, but not the deferential vein can be coagulated. Obviously the contralateral side can not be seen either but a bilateral retroperitoneal approach has been described by Ourpinar et al. (1995). The retroperitoneoscopic approach is logical, anatomical, direct, and fast. Moreover varicocelectomy is possible with one trocar only. Lastly one of the great advantages of retroperitoneoscopic approach, in my mind, is that it provides training in a technique that is very useful in several other indications in pediatric urology.

A first disadvantage of the retroperitoneal approach is the absence of a natural cavity, which means that the working space needs to be created. This poses some difficulties especially at the beginning of the learning curve, which is illustrated by the fact that we, as did Gaur et al. (1994), had two peritoneal perforations in our first ten cases, against none in the rest of the series. The second disadvantage of the retroperitoneal approach is that the working space is smaller than with the transperitoneal approach. When using the operating channel telescope and only one instrument, instead of a three-trocar technique, this reduced working space is not an handicap. Finally, in an obese patient, thick retroperitoneal fat may hinder the dissection, but varicoceles are more common in thin tall boys.

In conclusion, apart from personal preference, for example transperitoneal technique for the general surgeon and retroperitoneal technique for the urologist, a transperitoneal technique is indicated in case of contraindication of the retroperitoneal approach, for example bilateral varicocele, obese patient, and retroperitoneal fibrosis.

Conclusion

There are no evidenced-based studies regarding the best approach toward varicoceles in the adolescent. Only a few comparative studies, mainly in adults, have been published (Abdulmaaboud et al. 1998; Atassi et al. 1995; Kass and Marcol 1992; Lynch et al. 1993; Mandressi et al. 1996; Riccabona et al. 2003). Except for the series of Sayfan et al. (1992) all studies are retrospective comparing only two or three techniques, never including the retroperitoneoscopic approach. Randomized prospective studies are needed to determine the best method, which should fulfill the following criteria: elimination of the varicocele, preservation or even recuperation of testicular function, minimal morbidity, and cost effectiveness (Golstein 1995).

In any case, after a short learning curve and in selected cases, for example a unilateral left varicocele in a non-obese adolescent, which is the usual situation, the retroperitoneoscopic approach allows to reach spermatic vessels quickly, to separate the artery, veins, and lymphatics easily, and to interrupt them as planned.

References

Abdulmaaboud MR, Shokeir A, Farage Y, et al (1998) Treatment of varicocele: a comparative study of conventional open surgery, percutaneous retrograde sclerotherapy and laparoscopy. Urology 52:294–300

Atassi O, Kass EJ, Steneirt BW (1995) Testicular growth after successful varicocele correction in adolescents: comparison of artery sparing technique with Palomo procedure. J Urol 153:482–483

Belloli G, Mussi L, d'Agostino S (1996) Laparoscopic surgery for adolescent varicocele: preliminary report on 80 patients. J Pediatr Surg 31:1488–1490

Donovan JF, Winfield HN (1992) Laparoscopic varix ligation. J Urol 147:77–81

Esposito C, Monguzzi GL, Gonzalez Sabin MA, et al (2000) Laparoscopic treatment of pediatric varicocele: a multicenter study of the Italian society of video surgery in infancy. J Urol 163:1944–1946

Gaur DD, Agarwal DK, Purohit KC (1994) Retroperitoneal laparoscopic varicocelectomy. J Urol 151:895–897

Glassberg KI, Gershbein A, Horowith M (2000) Hydrocele formation after varicocelectomy in adolescents : a long term follow up. Br J Urol 85(suppl 4):36; abstract 63

Golstein M (1995) Editorial: adolescent varicocele. J Urol 153:484–485

Golstein M, Gilvert BR, Dicker AP, et al (1992) Microsurgical inguinal varicocelectomy with delivery of the testis: an artery and lymphatic sparing technique. J Urol 148:1808–1811

Hagood PG, Mehan DJ, Worischeck JH, et al (1992) Laparoscopic varicocelectomy: preliminary reports of a new technique. J Urol 147:73–76

Humphrey GM, Najmaldin AS (1997) Laparoscopy in the management of pediatric varicoceles. J Pediatr Surg 32:1470–1472

Jarrow JP, Assimos DG, Pittaway DE (1993) Effectiveness of laparoscopic varicocelectomy. Urology 42:544–546

Kass EJ, Marcol B (1992) Results of varicocele surgery in adolescents: a comparison of techniques. J Urol 148:694–696

Kocvara R, Koi J, Dite Z, et al (2001) Lymphatic sparing varicocele repair in children and adolescents. A laparoscopic modification. Br J Urol 87(suppl 1):35; abstract E.59

Loughlin KR, Brooks DC (1992) The use of Doppler probe to facilitate varicocele ligation. Surg Gyn Obst 174:326–328

Lynch WJ, Badenoch DF, McAnena OJ (1993) Comparison of laparoscopic and open ligation of the testicular vein. Br J Urol 72:796–798

MacKinlay GA (1999) Laparoscopic varicocele. In: Bax NMA, Georgeson KE, Najmaldin A, Valla JS (eds) Endoscopic Surgery in Children. Springer, Berlin Heidelberg New York, pp 408–414

Mandressi A, Buizza C, Antonelli D, et al (1996) Is laparoscopy a worthy method to treat varicocele? Comparison between 160 cases of two-port laparoscopic and 120 cases of open inguinal spermatic vein ligation. J Endourol 10:435–441

Matusda T, Horii Y, Higashi S, et al (1992) Laparoscopic varicocelectomy: a simple technique for clip ligation of the spermatic vessels. J Urol 147:636–638

Oswald J, Koerner I, Riccabona M (2000) The use of isosulfan blue to identify lymphatic vessels in the high retroperitoneal ligation of adolescent varicocele to avoid post operative hydrocele. Br J Urol 85(suppl 4):34; abstract 64

Ourpinar T, Sariyuce O, Balbay MD, et al (1995) Retroperitoneoscopic bilateral spermatic vein ligation. J Urol 153:127–128

Ralph DJ, Timoney AG, Parker O, et al (1993) Laparoscopic varicocele ligation. Br J Urol 72:230–233

Riccabona M, Oswald J, Koen M, et al (2003) Optimizing the operative treatment of boys with varicocele: sequential comparison of 4 techniques. J Urol 169:666–668

Sayfan J, Soffer Y, Orda R (1992) Varicocele treatment: prospective randomized trial of 3 methods. J Urol 148:1447–1449

Valla JS (2003) Retroperitoneoscopic varicocelectomy in children and adolescents. In: Caione P, Kavonski LR, Micali F (eds) Retroperitoneoscopy and Extraperitoneal Laparoscopy in Pediatric and Adult Patients. Springer, Berlin Heidelberg New York, pp 163–172

Valla JS, Ordorica Flores RM, Steyaert H, et al (1999) Umbilical one puncture laparoscopic assisted appendectomy in children. Surg Endosc 13:83–85

Chapter 104

Laparoscopy in Functional Ovarian Cysts in Neonates

Maria Marcela Bailez

Introduction

There is controversy about the best treatment for fetal ovarian cysts, depending on their ultrasound pattern and diameter. Postnatal therapeutic approaches range from follow-up with ultrasonography alone to open oophorectomy (McKeever and Andrews 1988; Widdowson et al. 1988). We previously presented our experience with the postnatal management of fetal ovarian cysts, using an ovarian conservative approach, that we continue using up till now (Bailez and Martinez Ferro 1997).

All the cysts were diagnosed after 30 weeks gestation by routine prenatal ultrasonography and confirmed postnatally. Diagnostic criteria were: (1) female fetus, (2) absence of urogenital and gastrointestinal anomalies, and (3) presence of a cystic mass in the fetal abdominal cavity. Depending on their ultrasound pattern, the cysts were called simple (completely anechogenic with thin walls) and complex or complicated (presence of septa, fluid/debris, calcification).

The algorithm followed includes ultrasound and/or laparoscopic-guided needle aspiration for non-complicated cysts and laparoscopic oophorectomy for the complicated ones (■ Fig. 104.1).

Preoperative Preparation

There is no need for bowel preparation. After induction of general anesthesia, future port hole sites are infiltrated with bupivacaine 0.2% up to a total dosage of 1.5 mg/kg.

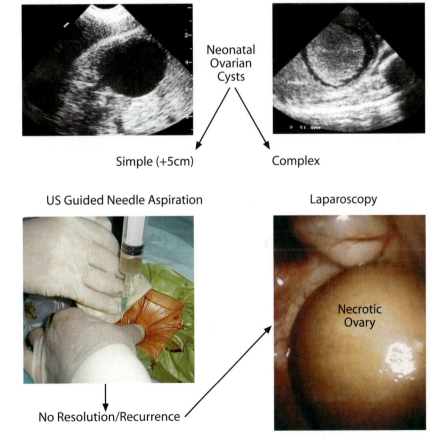

Fig. 104.1. Algorithm that includes ultrasound (*US*) and/or laparoscopic-guided needle aspiration for non-complicated cysts, and laparoscopic oophorectomy for complicated cysts. Note the clear yellow appearance of the fluid coming from a simple cyst

Neonatal Ovarian Cysts

Simple (+5cm)   Complex

US Guided Needle Aspiration   Laparoscopy

Necrotic Ovary

No Resolution/Recurrence

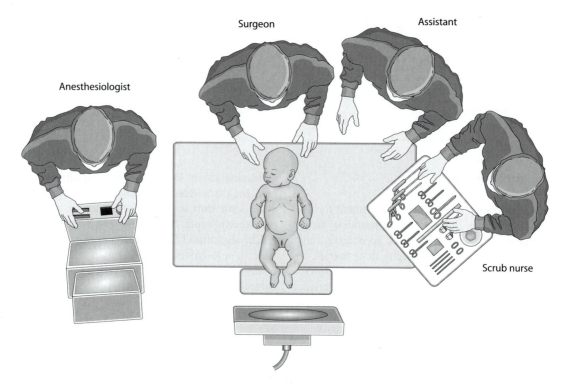

Fig. 104.2. Position of the patient, crew, and monitor. Note the transverse patient position

Positioning

Patient

The patient is placed in a supine position across the operating table, so that surgeon and assistant can work from the head of the patient, on the right side of the table.

Crew, Monitors, and Equipment

Figure 104.2 shows the positions of the crew, monitors, and equipment.

Special Equipment

No special equipment is required except for bipolar electrocoagulation.

Technique

Cannulae

Cannula	Method of insertion	Diameter (mm)	Device	Position
1	Open	4/5	Telescope	Umbilicus
2	Closed	3	Instruments	Right flank
3	Closed	3	Instruments	Left flank

Three ports are used: a 4- or 5-mm umbilical one, and two 3-mm ones in the right and left flank, respectively (Fig. 104.3).

Procedure

Ultrasound-guided needle aspiration is performed in the operating room, under general anesthesia. Estradiol concentrations are measured in the aspirated fluid, to confirm its ovarian origin (Widdowson et al. 1988).

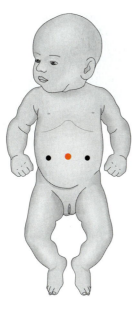

Fig. 104.3. Position of the ports

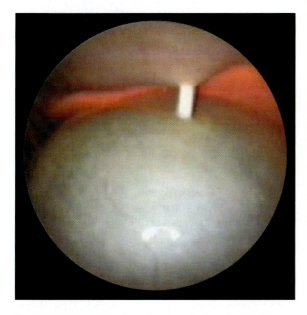

Fig. 104.4. Laparoscopic-assisted aspiration of a simple ovarian cyst

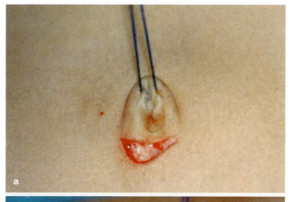

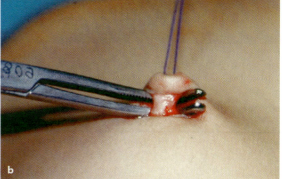

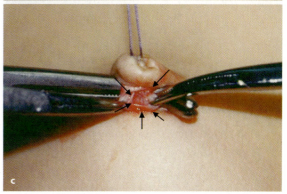

Fig. 104.5. Open technique: "umbilicoplasty smile." **a** A stitch is placed through the umbilicus for umbilical traction. **b** An incision is made around the upper (for lower abdomen procedures) or lower half (for upper abdomen procedures) of the umbilicus. **c** *Arrows* show a patent umbilical process, which is present in most newborns and infants. There is no need to detach the umbilicus for the access

Sometimes laparoscopic assistance is required in which case the smallest available lens (1.5–4 mm) is used (Fig. 104.4). CO_2 is insufflated at a pressure between 5 and 8 mm Hg. The CO_2 status of the child is carefully monitored.

An open technique, which we call "umbilicoplasty smile" (Fig. 104.5) is used for the insertion of the first trocar. Nowadays we use a 4- or 5-mm short device. The second trocar is inserted in one flank. Most of the cystic ovaries in the newborns are out of the pelvis in the middle or upper abdomen and a lower quadrant trocar is usually not ergonomic. Exploratory maneuvers using an atraumatic forceps follow. In the presence of an autoamputated ovary, no additional trocars are inserted (Fig. 104.6). The finding of a missing uterine adnex confirms the diagnosis (Fig. 104.7).

If a formal oophorectomy or lysis of adhesions are required, a third trocar is inserted in the other flank

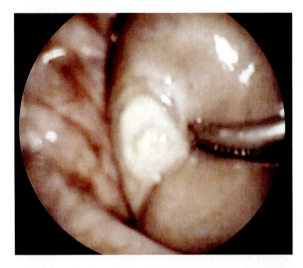

Fig. 104.6. Autoamputated ovary

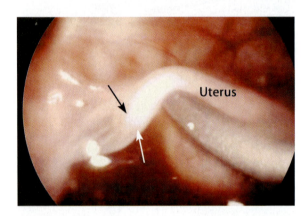

Fig. 104.7. *Arrows* show a missing tube in an autoamputated ovary

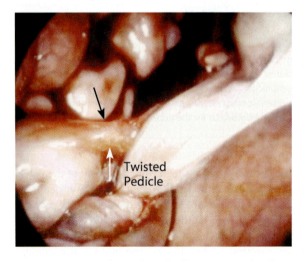

Fig. 104.8. *Arrows* show a bowel adhesion to a twisted pedicle

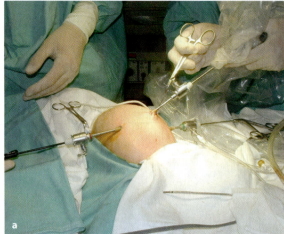

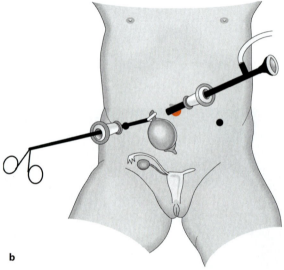

Fig. 104.9 a,b. A grasper is pulling the twisted ovary toward the umbilicus under vision while withdrawing the telescope out of the port. Both ports are aligned to facilitate this maneuver

(■ Fig. 104.8). A bipolar forceps or endoloops are used to complete oophorectomy. As the umbilical incision is very distensible in newborns and shows the best cosmetic results, necrotic ovaries are removed through it. To avoid the use of a second lens, we push the ovary into the umbilical port, aligning one of the operative ports with it while withdrawing the lens and port out guiding its way into the umbilical incision (■ Fig. 104.9). This maneuver is very easy to accomplish in a newborn.

Cysts are punctured under direct vision inside the abdomen. In one patient we punctured the cyst through the umbilical area thus removing the hemorrhagic fluid before removal of the ovary itself (■ Fig. 104.10).

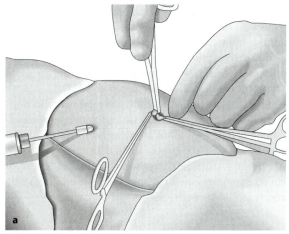

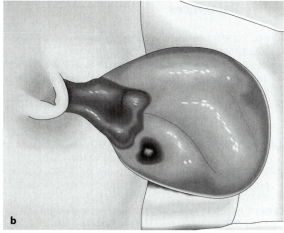

Fig. 104.10 a,b. The necrotic ovary is removed through the umbilicus after previous aspiration of its content

Postoperative Care

Feeding is usually started within the first 6 postoperative hours. The patient is followed clinically and ultrasonographically for 2 years and is seen again close to puberty.

Results

Thirty-two patients have been treated using the proposed algorithm. Ten patients underwent simple cyst needle aspiration, eight under ultrasound guidance and two with laparoscopic assistance. In all these patients a small cystic image persisted for some time during ultrasonographic follow-up. Complete resolution occurred in nine. One patient underwent a laparoscopic-assisted resection of a duplication of the cecum at 2 years of age because of a persistent cystic image on ultrasound. Looking back at the laboratory data, estra-

diol had been undetectable in the aspirated fluid. All ovaries have been preserved.

Of the remaining 22 patients, 20 had ovarian torsion. Nineteen underwent laparoscopic salpingo-oophorectomy (one bilateral) and one ovarian cystectomy. Two cases were misdiagnosed. In one patient, a simple cyst appeared to be complicated, because of associated meconium peritonitis with calcifications. The other patient underwent an initial laparoscopy that unveiled an intestinal duplication, which was excised in an open way.

Three of the nine necrotic ovaries were autoamputated at the time of surgical exploration and presented as a mass with no clear attachment. The finding of a missing uterine adnex confirmed the diagnosis. Bowel adhesions to the affected adnexa were observed and treated in two.

Laparoscopic oophorectomy was completely intraabdominal in all but one patient. In this patient with bilateral involvement excision of one of the twisted ovaries was completed externally through one of the trocar sites.

The mean operative time for laparoscopic approach was 40 min (range 20–60 min). All patients were discharged on the first postoperative day. No complications or recurrences were observed in a follow-up period that ranges from 6 months to 7 years.

Discussion

As a result of placental hormones stimulation of the neonatal ovary is similar to the stimulation which occurs during puberty or adult fertile life. Although small follicular ovarian cysts were found in 34% of necropsies of stillbirths and neonatal deaths (Desa 1975), most of them show spontaneous resolution, without clinical implications.

Occasionally larger ovarian cysts are seen as an abdominal mass in the newborn (Defort et al. 1990; Tjerdman et al. 1988; Valenti et al. 1975). Because of progress in ultrasonography, it is possible to assess the prenatal evolution of these cysts. Differential diagnosis includes mesenteric cysts, mesonephric cysts, hematometra, and duplications (Garner 1957; Jafri et al. 1984). Diagnosis is often made in the third trimester with a range of 27–41 weeks and a median of 34 weeks (Sakala et al. 1991).

Clinical presentation varies from an ultrasound incidental finding to the signs related to complications such as torsion, intestinal obstruction, or respiratory distress. A non-twisted ovarian cyst is usually asymptomatic. A large cyst may result in mechanical complications. The cyst may also rupture or cause intestinal obstruction.

A twisted ovarian cyst may be asymptomatic or be associated with vomiting, fever, abdominal pain, and peritonitis. Infrequently, intestinal obstruction occurs as a result of inflammatory adhesions between the necrotic cyst and the bowel, as in two of our patients. Autoamputation may also occur (Aslam et al. 1995). Because of the small size of the neonatal pelvis and a long cyst pedicle, a completely intra-abdominal location is a common finding as occurred in many of our patients.

There is controversy about the best treatment of these cysts. Timely alertness and a rational approach are required to preserve ovarian tissue and prevent future fertility impairment. The justification for observational management is based on the recognition that fetal ovarian cysts are functional in nature. Once the neonate is moved from the intrauterine environment, spontaneous regression may be expected (Amodio et al. 1987; Meizner et al. 1991; Toma et al. 1988). However, based on the severity of complications (torsion, rupture, intestinal obstruction, hemorrhage, and necrosis) and their unpredictable time of appearance, other authors propose surgical intervention for all of them (Ahmed 1971; Alrabeeah et al. 1988).

Prior to the increased use of prenatal sonography, some of these cysts may have gone undetected as the infants were usually asymptomatic. Even twisted ovaries may not have been resected, ending in an atrophic ovary, resembling a long-term twisted testicle without clinical evidence. However there are cases of deaths related to ovarian torsion in the literature.

We followed the therapeutic regimen proposed by Widdowson et al. (1988), their main objective being the avoidance of unnecessary operations. According to their regimen, the initial approach in simple cysts with a diameter of more than 5 cm is puncture and evacuation under sonographic guidance and follow-up with serial ultrasound scans. This procedure can prevent cystic torsion and avoids surgical accidental removal of normal ovarian tissue. Recurrence of the cyst could be treated by repeated aspiration thus reserving surgical removal for intractable or complicated cases. Estradiol concentrations should be measured in aspirated fluid to confirm its ovarian origin (Widdowson et al. 1988). An initial laparoscopic approach toward simple cysts is indicated when there are diagnostic doubts or when there are technical difficulties in performing the puncture under sonographic guidance, as was the case in three of our patients.

Complicated cysts always require surgery and should be treated with an as conservative operative approach as possible, although in most cases a salpingo-oophorectomy is indicated because of combined ovarian and tubal necrosis. We added the laparoscopy approach to this regimen thus preventing postoperative adhesion formation, a crucial factor in preserving the reproductive future of these girls. This modality is well tolerated by the newborns and infants of this series, as reported by others (van der Zee et al. 1995).

It is possible to preserve the neonatal ovary in noncomplicated cysts. Both ultrasound and laparoscopic-guided needle aspiration are safe and minimum invasive procedures for simple cysts definitive treatment. An initial laparoscopic approach is the procedure of choice in complicated cysts providing both diagnostic and treatment possibilities.

References

Ahmed S (1971) Neonatal and childhood ovarian cysts. J Pediatr Surg 6:702–708

Alrabeeah A, Gallinari C, Giacomantonio M, et al (1988) Neonatal ovarian torsion: report of three cases and review of the literature. Pediatr Pathol 8:143–149

Amodio J, Abramsom S, Berdon W, et al (1987) Postnatal resolution of large ovarian cyst detected in utero. Pediatric Radiol 17:467–469

Aslam A, Wong C, Haworth JM, et al (1995) Autoamputation of ovarian cyst in an infant. J Pediatr Surg 30:1609–1610

Bailez M, Martinez Ferro M (1997) Endosurgical postnatal approach of fetal ovarian cysts. Pediatr Endosurg Innov Tech 2:111–116

Defort P, Thierry M, et al (1990) Ovarian cysts in the fetus and neonate. Z Geburtshilfe Perinatol 194:137–139

Desa DJ (1975) Follicular ovarian cysts in stillbirths and neonates. Arch Dis Child 50:45–50

Garner G (1957) Mesonephric cyst in fetal large ligament. Am J Obstet Gynecol 1957:563

Jafri S, Bree R, Silver J, et al (1984) Fetal ovarian cysts: sonographic detection and association with hypothyroidism. Radiology 150:809–812

McKeever PA, Andrews H (1988) Fetal ovarian cysts: a report of five cases. J Pediatr Surg 23:354–355

Meizner I, Levy A, Katz M, et al (1991) Fetal ovarian cysts: prenatal ultrasonographic detection and postnatal evaluation and treatment. Am J Obstet Gynecol 164:874–878

Sakala EP, Leon ZA, Rouse G (1991) Management of antenatally diagnosed fetal ovarian cysts. Obstet Gynecol Surv 46:407–413

Terdjman P, Taviere V, Pariented, et al (1988) Kystes de l'ovaire neonataux. J Radiol 69:67–70

Toma P, Lituania M, Romano A, et al (1988) Le cisti follicolari dell ovario in eta neonatale. Minerva Pediatr 40:715–718

Valenti C, Kasner G, Yermakov V, et al (1975) Antenatal diagnosis of a fetal ovarian cyst. Am J Obstet Gynecol 15:216

van der Zee DC, Van Seumeren IG, Bax KM, et al (1995) Laparoscopic approach to surgical management of ovarian cysts in the newborn. J Pediatr Surg 30:42–43

Widdowson DJ, Pilling DW, Cook CM (1988) Neonatal ovarian cysts: therapeutic dilemma. Arch Dis Child 63:737–742

Laparoscopy of Functional Ovarian Cysts and Mesosalpinx Cysts in Peripuberal Girls

Maria Marcela Bailez

Introduction

Indications for laparoscopy in functional ovarian cysts (follicular, corpus luteal, and theca lutein cysts) are limited to large cysts (over 5 cm), which persist after 4–8 weeks, or to cysts that are symptomatic (pain, severe dysmenorrhea).

Paraovarian cysts may present as an adnexal mass and are usually detected by pelvic examination and/or sonography as a simple unilocular cystic structure. Indications for laparoscopy are the same as mentioned before.

Preoperative Preparation

No bowel preparation is required. After induction of general anesthesia, future port hole sites are infiltrated with 0.5% bupivacaine to a total dose of 1.5 mg/kg. A urinary catheter is inserted and broad-spectrum prophylactic antibiotics are given.

Positioning

Patient
The patient is placed in a supine Trendelenburg position (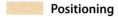 Fig. 105.1).

Crew, Monitors, and Equipment
Figure 105.2 shows positions of crew, monitors, and equipment for a suspected left adnexal mass.

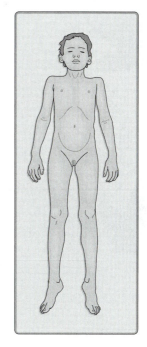

Fig. 105.1. Patient position

Special Equipment

Bipolar electrocautery should be available.

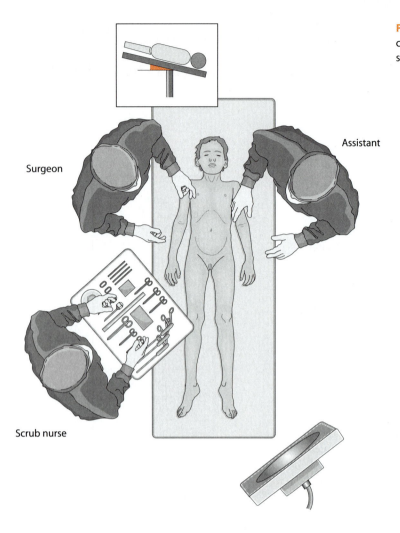

Fig. 105.2. Positioning of the patient, crew, monitor, and equipment for a left sided adnexal mass

Surgeon

Assistant

Scrub nurse

Technique

Cannulae

Cannula	Method of insertion	Diameter (mm)	Device	Position
1	Open/closed	5	Telescope	Umbilicus
2	Closed	5 or 3	Working instruments	Right lower quadrant
3	Closed	5 or 3	Working instruments	Left lower quadrant
4	Closed	5 or 3	Optional: suction/irrigation	Suprapubic area

Port Positions

Three ports are used: a 5 mm umbilical one, and two 5 mm ones (left and right lower quadrant). An alternative position for the working ports is the suprapubic area and the lower quadrant opposite to the ovarian cyst. For example, a right ovarian cyst is operated with a suprapubic port for the surgeon's left hand and a left lower quadrant port for the surgeon's right hand (■ Fig. 105.3). In large cysts a fourth suprapubic port is used for continuous suction and irrigation.

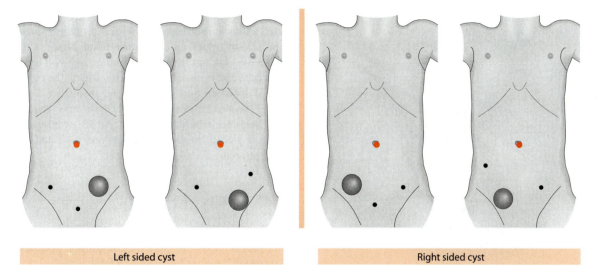

Left sided cyst	Right sided cyst

Fig. 105.3. Position of the operative ports for resection of adnexal peripuberal cyst. The cyst is represented by a *black circle*. Either a suprapubic and a contralateral lower quadrant port or both lower quadrants ports can be used. In large cysts we use three of them, using the suprapubic port for continuous irrigation and suction

Procedure

Laparoscopic removal of an ovarian cyst should be preceded by careful inspection of the pelvic peritoneum, contralateral ovary, and abdominal contents. The ovary is freed from surrounding adhesions and the ureter and pelvic sidewall vessels identified. An incision is made over the cyst with scissors, through the area where the ovarian cortex is maximally thinned. The incision should be parallel to the long axis of the ovary and as far posterior as possible to minimize the possibility of adhesions to the bowel, uterus, or tube. If needed the ovary can be rotated with a blunt probe or with a grasper placed in the utero-ovarian ligament (■ Fig. 105.4). Bluntly, a plane is created between the cyst wall and ovarian cortex by spreading the tip of the scissors. For countertraction, the edge of the cortex can be grasped using a biopsy forceps or grasper. An intact cyst facilitates initial dissection. Once an adequate dissection plane is created circumferentially around the cyst, the cyst is aspirated with an 18- or 16-gauge needle placed transabdominally. We try to avoid spillage by placing a suction cannula near the puncture site. Once open, inspection of the inner aspect of the cyst is performed. The edges of the cyst wall are grasped. Further dissection of the cyst wall is performed using the scissors in blunt fashion (■ Fig. 105.5). After cyst enucleation inspection of the cyst bed should be performed and any remaining fragments removed. Redundant thin ovarian cortex is resected. Hemostasis in the ovary can be obtained with bipolar cautery. Thorough irrigation of the pelvis is performed at the end of the surgery.

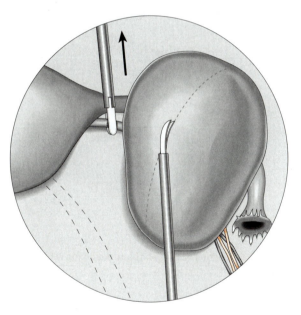

Fig. 105.4. The ovary is rotated with a grasper placed in the utero-ovarian ligament. The ovarian capsule is incised with monopolar cautery

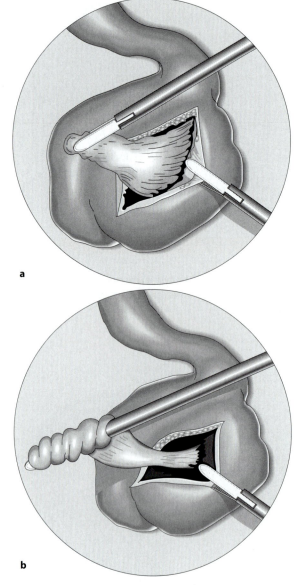

a

b

Fig. 105.5. Countertraction and blunt dissection while grasping the cyst

In the presence of a mesosalpingeal cyst, the peritoneum covering the mesosalpinx is opened and the intact cyst resected, preserving the salpinx and its vessels (■ Fig. 105.6). The incision is performed parallel to the long axis of the tube. Care should be taken not to enter the cystic cavity. The fallopian tube is often stretched and distorted. The surgeon should avoid any manipulation that may endanger this structure, since it returns to normal once the paraovarian cyst is re-

moved. In general, small peritoneal vessels can be transected with minimal bleeding. If there remains a thicker pedicle of coalesced connective tissue between the base of the cyst and the bed, it is cauterized with bipolar forceps and transected. Once enucleated, the cyst is allowed to drain and it is removed through a 5- or 10 mm sleeve. Exceedingly large cysts may require partial aspiration before resection. An 18- or 20-gauge needle is placed through the abdominal wall and the cyst aspirated.

■ Results

Forty-one girls with adnexal cysts have been treated since January 1997: 18 were mesosalpingeal cysts and 23 ovarian (7 corpus luteal and 16 follicular).

Two obese patients developed an umbilical hematoma. Three patients (7%) with follicular cysts required a second procedure because of recurrence. Eight patients (19.5%) had had previous laparotomies that did not interfere with the laparoscopic exploration.

■ Discussion

Functional cysts are the most frequently occurring cysts in the human ovary. They can present as follicular, corpus luteal, and theca lutein cysts. All are benign and are usually self-limiting. The diameter can range up to 8 cm. The majority present as an incidental finding during physical or ultrasonic examination. Large cysts, however, can rupture or twist with loss of the ovary (Horowitz and Sanz de la Cuesta 1992).

Paraovarian cysts are of mesothelial, paramesonephric, or mesonephric origin. They can reach a diameter of 10 cm and present with dysmenorrhea. We prefer to enucleate the cysts without prior drainage as described by Semm (1987). However exceedingly large cysts may require partial aspiration before resection.

A major advantage of laparoscopy, namely the small incisions, necessarily increases the risk of cyst rupture. This has been suggested to increase morbidity in patients with both benign and malignant tumors. The risk of a complication from rupture of benign cysts during laparoscopy is small (Steinkampf and Azziz 1997). Obviously extensive irrigation and aspiration of the pelvis should follow the drainage of cyst contents.

The success of laparoscopy not only depends on the skill of the surgeon but also and even more importantly on the proper preoperative evaluation and patient selection.

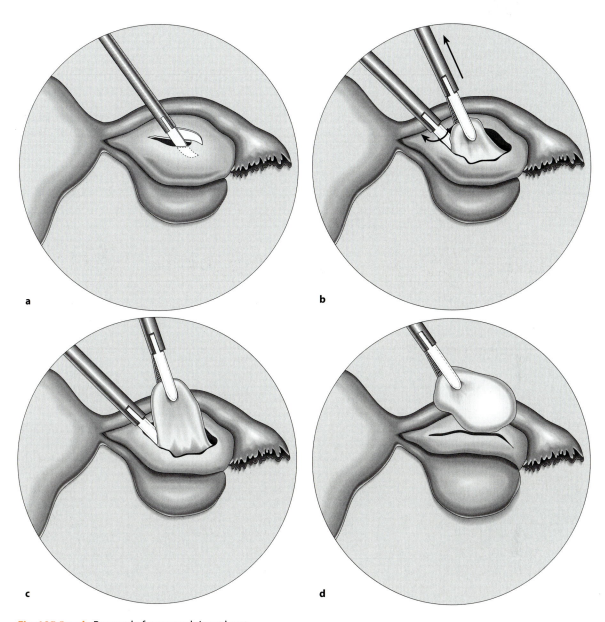

Fig. 105.5 a–d. Removal of a mesosalpingeal cyst

References

Horowitz I, Sanz de la Cuesta R (1992) Benign and malignant tumors of the ovary. In: Carpenter SE, Rock J (eds) Pediatric and Adolescent Gynecology 20. Raven, New York, pp 397–399

Semm K (1987) Operative Manual for Endoscopic Abdominal Surgery. Year Book Medical, Chicago

Steinkampf M, Azziz R (1997) Laparoscopic ovarian and paraovarian surgery. In: Azziz R, Alvarez Murphy A (eds) Practical Manual of Operative Laparoscopy and Hysteroscopy 19. Springer, Berlin Heidelberg New York pp 112–113

Chapter 106

Laparoscopic Ovary-sparing Surgery in Benign Ovarian Neoplasms

Maria Marcela Bailez

Introduction

Mature teratomas are the most common ovarian benign neoplasm in pediatrics (Bailez et al. 1992; Breen and Maxson 1977; Breen et al. 1981). Enucleation of the tumor, preserving the ovary is a current technique in adults. Only a few pediatric cases have been published as case reports in the literature (Garcia et al. 1996; Nehzat et al. 1989). Cystadenomas, although less frequent in the pediatric age group, may occur in adolescents and can be treated by laparoscopically.

Preoperative Preparation

Preoperatively tumor markers such as alpha fetoprotein, CEA 125, and beta HCG are determined but are not elevated. No bowel preparation is needed. After induction of general anesthesia, a urinary catheter is inserted and prophylactic broad-spectrum antibiotics are given. Future port hole sites are infiltrated with 0.5% bupivacaine up to a maximum dose of 1.5 mg/kg.

Positioning

Positioning is as for an ovarian cyst.

Special Equipment

Bipolar electrocautery should be available. All tumors should be removed using a removal bag.

Technique

Cannulae

Cannula	Method of insertion	Diameter (mm)	Device	Position
1	Open/closed	10	Telescope, removal bag	Umbilicus
2	Closed	5 or 3	Working instruments	Right lower quadrant
3	Closed	5 or 3	Working instruments	Left lower quadrant
4	Closed	5 or 3	Optional: suction/irrigation	Midline hypogastrium

Port Positions

Classically three ports are used: a 10 mm umbilical one, and two 3- or 5 mm ones (left and right lower quadrant). An alternative position of the operative ports is one in the suprapubic area and one in the lower quadrant opposite to the ovarian pathology as described above. A fourth 5- or 3 mm midline hypogastric port is used in large tumors for continuous aspiration, irrigation, and retraction.

Procedure

The same technique as described for ovarian cysts is used: the ovarian capsule is opened, and the tumor enucleated. Hemostasis of the ovarian surface is obtained with bipolar electrocoagulation. The pelvis is always thoroughly irrigated (■ Fig. 106.1). Spillage is avoided and all tumors are removed using a bag. The 10 mm umbilical port is used for introduction of the bag and for removal of a tumor that is mostly cystic and not so large. In case of large mainly solid teratomas, we prefer to enlarge one of the low abdomen port sites and to remove the tumor through the enlarged hole.

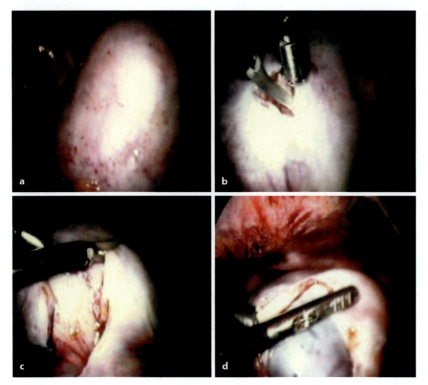

Fig. 106.1. Laparoscopic resection of a mature teratoma. **a** View of an ovary with a mature teratoma. **b,c** Ovarian capsule incision with monopolar scissors. **d** Traction and countertraction maneuver

Results

Twenty-six patients with mature teratomas and a median age of 10 years (range from 4 to 16 years) and six patients with cystadenomas with a median age of 16 years were treated with this approach. Six patients with teratomas (23%) had bilateral tumors. One had bilateral synchronic tumors; two presented with a contralateral ovarian teratoma 2 and 3 years after the first resection, respectively, and three had a previous open oophorectomy.

Preoperative evaluation for patient selection for a laparoscopic approach includes a normal serum value of alpha fetoprotein, beta HCG, and CEA 125. None of them had papillary projections, excrescences, predominantly solid masses, or ascites on pelvic sonography. We found four sonographic patterns in teratomas (■ Fig. 106.2). They usually look like complex adnexal masses with echogenic internal components attributable to the fat and hair, which are often present. Some dermoids may be completely solid, while others may have cystic areas with or without internal septa. All cystadenomas presented as large cystic masses.

Only one patient, who had initial exploratory laparoscopy, required conversion to open because of a suspicious macroscopic appearance. No attempt to open the ovarian capsule was made and the decision was taken with the pathologist in the operative room. She had a dysgerminoma.

The mean maximum tumor diameter on preoperative ultrasound examination was 7.45 cm (range 2.3–17 cm). Mean operative time was 110 min (range 40–180 min). All patients were discharged on the first postoperative day. With a mean follow-up period of 37.5 months (range 4–94 months), two patients required a secondary procedure because of a contralateral ovarian teratoma and one presented with a recurrent teratoma in the single ovary. The latter patient had an open oophorectomy elsewhere for an ovarian teratoma. We performed laparoscopic ovarian-sparing surgery on the single ovary. The recurrent cyst was also dealt with laparoscopically.

Histologic analysis showed a mature teratoma in 26 patients and a serous cystadenoma in six.

Discussion

Mature teratomas are the most common benign ovarian neoplasm in children and adolescents (Bailez et al. 1992; Breen and Maxson 1977; Breen et al. 1981). Among 323 patients with adnexal masses seen in our institution, 79 had neoplasms of which 42 (53.1%) were mature teratomas. Laparoscopic ovarian-sparing surgery is an accepted surgical approach in adults (Nezhat et al. 1989).

Assuming that they are benign tumors and bilateral in 7–10% of the patients, oophorectomy seems an ag-

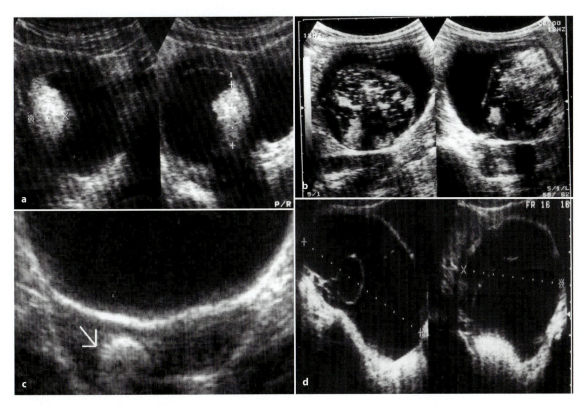

Fig. 106.2. The four most common sonographic patterns in mature teratomas. **a** Hyperechogenic mass in an anechogenic environment. **b** Mixed hyper- and anechogenic mass. **c** Complete hyperechogenic mass. **d** Anechogenic areas

gressive approach (Bailez 1993; Carpenter and Rock 1992; Emans and Goldstein 1990; Garcia et al. 1996). The frequency with which ovarian cancer is encountered during operative laparoscopy of properly selected patients is generally less than 1% (Engel et al. 1965). Furthermore the malignant nature of the tumor is generally recognized at the time of the laparoscopy (Mage et al. 1990).

Although spontaneous or iatrogenic rupture of ovarian teratomas can induce peritoneal granuloma formation and adhesions, such complications have not been reported intraoperatively. Mage and colleagues removed 91 cystic teratomas laparoscopically without complication (Mage et al. 1990). Nezhat et al. (1989) performed second-look laparoscopy on four patients in whom dermoid cysts had been excised laparoscopically and found no evidence of granuloma formation. Our experience suggests that laparoscopic ovarian-sparing surgery in selected pediatric patients is effective and safe.

References

Bailez MM (1993) Conservaciónde la Gonada en la Exéresis de Tumores Benignos del Ovario. Rev Cir Infantil 3:83–85

Bailez MM, Amaral D, González S et al. (1992) Tumores de Ovario en la Infancia y Adolescencia. Experiencia en un sólo centro. Rev Cir Infantil 1:4–9

Breen JL, MaxsonWS (1977) Ovarian tumors in children and adolescents. Clin Obstet Gynecol 20:607–623

Breen JL, Bonano JF, Maxson WS (1981) Genital tract tumors in children. Pediatr Clin North Am 28:355–367

Carpenter SEJ, Rock J (eds) (1992) Pediatric and Adolescent Gynecology. Raven, New York, p 401

Emans JS, Goldstein DP (1990) Pediatric and Adolescent Gynecology, 3rd edn. Little Brown, Boston, p 426

Engel T, Greeley DU, Swenney WJ (1965) Recurrent dermoid cyst of the ovary. Report of 2 cases. Obstet Gynecol 26:757–759

Garcia FA, Lang JF, Childers JM (1996) Laparoscopic ovarian cystectomy for a benign teratoma in a 10-year-old girl. J Am Assoc Gynecol Laparosc 3:321–333

Mage G, Canis M, Manhes H, et al (1990) Laparoscopic management of adnexal cystic masses. J Gynecol Surg 6:71–79

Nezhat C, Winer WK, Nezhat F (1989) Laparoscopic removal of dermoid cysts. Obstet Gynecol 73:278–280

Laparoscopy in (Doubtful) Malignant Adnexal Pathology, Ovarian Torsion Beyond the Neonatal Period, Endometriosis, and Pelvic Inflammatory Disease

Benno M. Ure and Jean-Stéphane Valla

Introduction

In this chapter we address the role of laparoscopy in the management of:

1. Malignant or doubtful malignant ovarian neoplasm
2. Torsion of the adnexa outside the neonatal period
3. Endometriosis
4. Pelvic inflammatory disease

For preoperative preparation, positioning, equipment, and technique, see previous chapter.

Malignant or Doubtful Ovarian Neoplasms

The risk of malignancy for ovarian tumors in girls, including both solid and cystic lesions, is around 10–25%. Malignant or potentially malignant tumors have a good prognosis if the treatment is conducted in close collaboration between surgeons and oncologists. Advances in detection, diagnosis, minimally invasive management, and chemotherapy require a regular review of protocols in order to reduce morbidity without compromising the oncological treatment.

In rare cases the malignant nature of the tumor is obvious, for example in the adolescent patient presenting with a large (>10 cm) solid tumor, which grows rapidly, is poorly delineated (epithelial neoplasm), provokes ascites, gives high levels of tumoral markers, or presents with obvious metastatic disease. A high level of tumoral marker is sufficient for the diagnosis and the level by itself is a prognostic factor. Under such circumstances usually preoperative chemotherapy is needed. If the tumoral marker level is normal, a laparoscopic or percutaneous biopsy is indicated in order to have a precise pathological diagnosis.

Current chemotherapy regimens are effective in treating these tumors. A second surgical evaluation after a complete radiological workup [ultrasound, computed tomography (CT) scan, magnetic resonance imaging (MRI)] may be needed to confirm the complete response to chemotherapy alone. These second-look procedures are performed through laparotomy, but could be preceded by a laparoscopic exploration in order to inspect carefully the superior part of the abdomen including the surface of the diaphragm. By doing so long midline incisions can be avoided and tumor removal can be performed through a Pfannenstiel incision, without jeopardizing oncological treatment principles.

In most situations, the nature of the tumor is confusing. Ultrasound examination is ideal for the identification of ovarian disorders but cannot differentiate well between benign and malignant tumors. Ovarian masses that are solid on ultrasound are more likely to be malignant (30–40%) than either complex masses (10%) or pure cystic masses (3%). Laboratory studies, including tumor markers, may be negative. Moreover the absence of metastatic lesions does not rule out a malignant process. Such an ovarian lesion in the prepubertal or teenage girl has a significant malignant potential and must be managed as such. In the retrospective study of Van Winter et al. (1994) regarding 521 ovarian tumors in infants, children, and adolescents the frequency of malignancy was 8%. Frequency correlated inversely with patient age. During the last decade of their study, ultrasonography and CT did not miss any malignancy.

The use of laparoscopy is controversial but could be very useful as a first explorative step, especially in case of torsion. The surgeon must comply, however, with the guidelines of the Children's Oncologic Group (Bilimire et al. 2004). It is stressed that the staging used for ovarian tumor management in children is a postoperative staging. The guidelines include:

1. Collection of ascites or washing on entering the peritoneal cavity
2. Examination of the peritoneal surfaces including the diaphragm with biopsy or excision of any nodules
3. Inspection and palpation of the omentum with removal of any adherent or abnormal area noted
4. Inspection and palpation of the opposite ovary with biopsy of any abnormal areas

5. Examination and palpation of lymph nodes in the retroperitoneum with sampling of any firm or enlarged nodes
6. Complete resection of the tumor-containing ovary with sparing of the fallopian tube if not involved

Open laparotomy is required for the two last recommendations: palpation of the retroperitoneal lymph nodes and delivery of an intact specimen for the pathologist. Point four is requested as the risk of a contralateral ovarian tumor varies between 5% and 20% according to the histological type. Some have suggested a contralateral bivalving biopsy. But such a procedure may expose the patient to the risk of hemorrhage, infection, and adhesion formation. Furthermore ultrasound is a good predictor of ovarian tumor presence. The study of Bilimire et al. (2004) has demonstrated that in case of a normal-appearing contralateral ovary the biopsy is always negative (21 out of 21 cases), in contrast to the case of a contralateral abnormal-appearing ovary, the biopsy is positive in 50% of cases (11 out of 21 cases). So preoperative ultrasound in combination with careful inspection of the contralateral ovary at the time of surgery offers a safe alternative to systematic contralateral biopsy.

Laparoscopy plays an important role in collecting information regarding the nature of tumors:

- A benign lesion is often cystic, well encapsulated, and less than 8 cm in diameter. The lesion has a smooth regular surface, without adhesions to pelvic organs. Laparoscopy is converted to open surgery in case of large tumor, but even under such circumstances the surgeon would try to enucleate the lesion and to preserve normal ovarian parenchyma.
- A malignant lesion is more often a solid tumor with irregular surface, thick cyst wall, adhesions with adjacent organs, ascites, and or peritoneal implants. It should be kept in mind, however, that 27% of the immature teratomas (Cushing et al. 1999) are associated with diffuse implants of benign glial tissue (gliomatosis peritonei), which do not require complete removal but only biopsy to ensure the proper diagnosis. As there are no clear tumor characteristics that define malignancy and as the risk of malignancy is significant, these doubtful malignant pediatric ovarian lesions should always be managed and completely staged in the assumption that they are malignant. Peroperative frozen section are not reliable, especially not in case of large lesions (Einarsson et al. 2004).

In any case laparoscopy allows the surgeon to judge whether the tumor is removable. If not removable (densely adherent or extensive tumor), a simple laparoscopic biopsy is taken. If it seems removable, a salpingo-oophorectomy is usually performed using classic open surgery. Extensive surgery such as bilateral ovariectomy or hysterectomy should not be performed before definitive histological confirmation. The question of using a laparoscopic technique for the removal of suspicious ovarian lesions that seem resectable is still under debate. With accurate preoperative and intraoperative selection, the rate of unexpected malignancies in the series of Marana et al. (2004), comprising 683 adults, was 1.2% and the laparoscopic management of these adnexal masses did not adversely affect prognosis. In the study of Biran et al. (2002) the risk of unexpected malignancy was 19%. Predictive factors for malignancy in adults (Havrilesky et al. 2003) are not completely transposable to children. The classic adage said that "violating the capsule laparoscopically or rupturing the tumor intra-operatively can result in up-staging of malignant lesions." The capsula can be ruptured preoperatively, incidentally during operative manipulation, or deliberately by puncture or biopsy. As demonstrated by Templeman et al. (2000), the risk of peroperative rupture is higher when using laparoscopy (93% versus 37%) and in cystectomy rather than oophorectomy (92% versus 15%). In the prospective randomized study of Yuen et al. (1997) in adults, the risk of inadvertent rupture was the same by using laparotomy or laparoscopy. Bilimire et al. (2004) reported that assessment of capsula integrity by the surgeon is frequently underappreciated, but that survival was excellent in girls treated with separation to adherent plane or initial biopsy only with delayed resection. The multicentric study of Cushing et al. (1999) showed that the presence of a capsular rupture had no negative impact on survival of patients presenting with an immature teratoma with or without microscopic foci of yolk sac tumor and treated with surgery alone. In recent publications, survival rate is not affected by deviation from classic clinical surgical guidelines (Zanetta et al. 1999) as long as it is adapted to each individual case.

Adnexal Torsion Beyond the Neonatal Period

One third of ovarian masses are discovered because of ovarian torsion, and nearly three quarters of twisted ovaries contain an underlying cystic or solid mass (Steyaert et al. 1998). Preoperative ultrasonography may be unable to distinguish between torsion of a normal adnexa and torsion of an ovary with ovarian mass. Likewise the peroperative aspect can be misleading (Heiss et al. 1994).

Traditionally the management of ovarian torsion has been resection of the twisted adnexa because of: (1) fear for embolic phenomena on detorsion, (2) fear of leaving a malignancy behind, or (3) the belief that leaving an untwisted ovary behind would leave dead tissue behind. Regarding point one, pulmonary embolism has not be reported in the pediatric literature (Beaunoyer et al. 2004). Regarding point two, the concern to leave a malignancy behind is valid but the risk of malignancy in a twisted ovarian mass is small. As said earlier, girls presenting with a non-twisted solid and cystic ovarian mass have a malignancy risk between 10% and 20%. Less than 3% of girls presenting with ovarian torsion have a malignant tumor: 0 cases out of 34 ovarian torsions in the data of Cass et al. (2001); no cases in the data of Steyaert et al. (1998), Beaunoyer et al. (2004), and Aziz et al. (2004). In the study of Sommerville et al. (1991) a benign ovarian neoplasm had a 12.9-fold increased risk of undergoing adnexal torsion when compared with malignant neoplasm. All in all adnexal torsion rarely involves cancer. One explanation is that malignant lesions cause more inflammation and fibrosis leading to adherence to surrounding structures. Regarding point three, the belief that a grossly black hemorrhagic adnex is irreversibly damaged is not true. The time lapse between first symptoms and surgery is not a good criterion. Absence of arterial or venous flow on preoperative Doppler ultrasound is not a good criterion either (Aziz et al. 2004; Templeman et al. 2000). Lastly the degree of ischemia seems difficult to judge by the surgeon. After detorsion of an ischemic ovary, the most common postoperative morbidity is fever. The ovarian viability of an untwisted adnexa can be assessed by postoperative ultrasound (size of ovary, follicles). In the majority of reported cases of detorsion the untwisted ovary appeared viable at follow-up (Aziz et al. 2004; Beaunoyer et al. 2004; Oelsner et al. 1993). So with a low rate of malignancy, difficulty of preoperative and peroperative assessment of potential ovarian survival, and the great efficiency of chemotherapy in treating malignant ovarian tumors, treatment recommendations for adnexal torsion have changed. Nowadays only detorsion of the twisted ovary is recommended. Cystectomy could be performed at the same time in the rare cases where the ovary rapidly shows a good vascular recovery after detorsion. In the majority of cases the ovary is very edematous which makes cystectomy potentially harmful for the ovary. Detorsion alone is therefore preferable followed by elective cystectomy 6–8 weeks later in ovaries with a cystic mass and normal alpha fetoprotein (AFP) levels. Lesions with high AFP levels should be managed with oophorectomy with or without chemotherapy.

What about oophoropexy? There is no definitive answer. There is no clear evidence that oophoropexy is effective in preventing recurrence (Nagel et al. 1997). Theoretically oophoropexy may prevent recurrent (repeat torsion on the same ovary) or sequential (subsequent torsion of the contralateral ovary) ovarian torsion. Different methods of lateral or medial fixation have been proposed (Abes and Sarihan 2004; Davis

and Feins 1990; Righi et al. 1995). A possible disadvantage of oophoropexy is the possibility of an anatomical disturbance between the ovary and the fallopian tube, but there is no medical literature to support this (Aziz et al. 2004; Beaunoyer et al. 2004; Nagel et al. 1997; Shun 1990). However bilateral ovarian loss as a result of contralateral torsion and/or tumor is a real cause of infertility. Hence we could recommend, as in testicular surgery, to fix the ipsilateral gonad in case of sparing surgery and fix the contralateral gonad in case of gonadectomy. Another indication for oophoropexy is protection from radiation (Le Boudec et al. 2000). The position of the fixation depends on the radiation technique, which may be external or vaginal. After fixation, the position of the ovaries may be marked with titanium clips.

Endometriosis

Although endometriosis is mostly diagnosed in women between 20 and 40 years of age, about 10% of all cases of endometriosis occur in girls younger than 20 years of age (about 1% of all women). Most of the women (50–60%) with endometriosis suffer from secondary dysmenorrhea even if the absolute amount of intra-abdominal lesions is low. In contrast, endometriosis may be diagnosed in women who are completely asymptomatic. Endometriosis in adolescent girls is mostly located in the Douglas pouch, but may be found in the uterosacral ligaments, the ovarian fossa, or other peritoneal locations. Laparoscopy is principally indicated to establish the diagnosis. If symptoms are suspicious of involvement of neighboring organs (urinary bladder, colon, etc.) cysto-/ureteroscopy, colonoscopy, or intravenous pyelography/MRI should precede surgical measures. Most importantly, poor response to surgical therapy negates the need for repetitive or radical surgery. The pathological lesion is usually diagnosed as a red superficial lesion. Coagulation, using a monopolar cautery, is preferred to excision. Occasionally, ovarian endometriosis may result in the development of large cysts filled with chocolate-like secretions ("chocolate cysts"). Such cysts should be excised. Extensive tubal endometriosis may result in hematosalpinx, which may require salpingectomy. Care should be taken not to injury the ureter, bowel, and major vessels. Surgical treatment can be followed by hormonal therapy [e.g. gonadotropin-releasing hormone (GnRH) agonist, oral contraceptives].

The role of laparoscopy in the treatment of adolescent endometriosis is still under debate (Attaran and Gidwani 2003; Lauffer et al. 2003). Laparoscopy is well accepted to establish the diagnosis. Repetitive endocoagulation or radical surgery are not indicated. In patients with persisting symptoms after initial laparoscopic coagulation long-term medical therapy is indicated to decrease pain and the progression of the disease.

Pelvic Inflammatory Disease

Pelvic inflammatory disease (PID) has been found to be associated with early sexual activity and number of sexual partners. The major cause is ascending infection. Rarely, adnexal infection and inflammation may be the result of pathological processes in neighboring organs such as ileitis or perityphlitic abscess. The anatomical correlates of PID implicating the adnexa vary from sterile fluid retention within the fallopian tubes (hydrosalpinx) to large tubo-ovarian abscesses. PID should be treated conservatively with antibiotics. Tubo-ovarian abscesses not responding to antibiotic treatment may require salpingotomy depending on the extent as described above.

References

Abes M, Sarihan H (2004) Oophoropexy in children with ovarian torsion. Eur J Pediatr Surg 14:168–171

Attaran M, Gidwani GP (2003) Adolescent endometriosis. Obstet Gynecol Clin North Am 30:379–390

Aziz D, Davis V, Allen L, et al (2004) Ovarian torsion in children: is oophorectomy necessary? J Pediatr Surg 39:750–753

Beaunoyer M, Chapdelaine J, Bouchard S, et al (2004) Asynchronous bilateral ovarian torsion. J Pediatr Surg 39:746–799

Bilimire D, Vinocur C, Rescorla F, et al (2004) Outcome and staging evolution in malignant germ Geil tumors of the ovary in children and adolescents: an intergroup study. J Pediatr Surg 39:424–429

Biran G, Gozan A, Sagi R, et al (2002) Conversion of laparoscopy to laparotomy due to adnexal malignancy. Eur J Gynecol Oncol 23:157–160

Cass DL, Hawkins E, Brandt ML (2001) Surgery for ovarian masses in infants, children and adolescents: 102 consecutives patients treated in a 15 years period. J Pediatr Surg 36:693–699

Cushing B, Giller R, Ablin A, et al (1999) Surgical resection alone is effective treatment for ovarian immature teratoma in children and adolescents: a report of the Pediatric Oncologic Group and the Children's Cancer Group. Am J Obstet Gynecol 181:353–358

Davis AJ, Feins NR (1990) Subsequent asynchronous torsion of normal adnexa in children. J Pediatr Surg 25:687–689

Einarsson JI, Edwards CL, Zurawin RK (2004) Immature ovarian teratoma in adolescent in a case report and review of the literature. J Pediatr Adolesc Gynecol 17:187–189

Havrilesky LJ, Peterson BL, Dryden DK, et al (2003) Predictors of clinical outcomes in the laparoscopic management of adnexal masses. Obstet Gynecol 102:243–251

Heiss KF, Zwiren GT, Winn K (1994) Massive ovarian edema in the pediatric patient: a rare solid tumor. J Pediatr Surg 29:1392–1394

Lauffer MR, Sanfilippino J, Rose G (2003) Adolescent endometriosis: diagnosis and treatment approaches. J Pediatr Adolesc Gynecol 16:83–11

Le Boudec G, Rabischeng B, Canis M, et al (2000) Ovarian transposition by laparoscopy in young women before curietherapy for cervical cancer. J Gynecol Obstet Biol Reprod (Paris) 29:567–570

Marana R, Muzil L, Catalano GF, et al (2004) Laparoscopic excision of adnexal masses. J Am Assoc Gynecol Laparosc 11:162–166

Nagel TC, Sebastian J, Malo JW (1997) Oophoropexy to prevent sequential or recurrent torsion. J Am Assoc Gynecol Laparosc 4:495–498

Oelsner G, Admon D, Bider D, et al (1993) Long term follow-up of the twisted ischemic adnexa managed by detorsion. Fertil Steril 50:976–979

Righi RV, McComb PF, Fluker MR (1995) Laparoscopic oophoropexy for recurrent adnexal torsion. Hum Reprod 10:3136–3138

Shun A (1990) Unilateral childhood ovarian lesions: an indication for contralateral oophoropexy? Aust N Z J Surg 60:791–794

Sommerville M, Grimes DA, Kooning P, et al (1991) Ovarian neoplasm and the risk of adnexal torsion. Am J Obstet Gynecol 164:577–578

Steyaert H, Meynol F, Valla J-S (1998) Torsion of the adnexa in children: the value of laparoscopy. Pediatr Surg Int 13:384–387

Templeman C, Hertweck SP, Fallat ME (2000) The clinical course of unresected ovarian torsion. J Pediatr Surg 35:1385–1387

Templeman C, Hertwaeck SP, Scheetz J, et al (2000) The management of mature cystic teratomas in children and adolescents: a retrospective analysis. Hum Reprod 15:2669–2672

Van Winter JT, Simmons PS, Podratz KC (1994) Surgically treated adnexal masses in infancy, childhood and adolescence. Am J Obstet Gynecol 170:1780–1789

Yuen PM, Yu KM, Lau WC, et al (1997) A randomized prospective study of laparoscopy and laparotomy in the management of benign ovarian masses. Am J Obstect Gynecol 177:109–114

Zanetta G, Ferrari L, Mignini-Renzini M, et al (1999) Laparoscopic excision of ovarian dermoid cyst with controlled intraoperative spillage. Safety and effectiveness. J Reprod Med 44:815–820

Chapter 108

Laparoscopy in Uterovaginal Anomalies

Maria Marcela Bailez

General Introduction

Uterovaginal anomalies are a spectrum of anomalies which are often associated with renal and sometimes with anorectal malformations. In this chapter we will focus on the use of laparoscopy in the diagnosis and treatment of isolated uterovaginal anomalies in the pediatric age group. We use John Rock's modification of the American Fertility Society classification, which is based on embryologic considerations (Tjaden and Rock 1992).

Class I – Dysgenesis of the Müllerian Ducts

Dysgenesis of the müllerian ducts is also known as the Mayer-Rokitansky-Küster-Hauser syndrome. It is characterized by absence of the vagina with or without uterine remnants. Most of the patients in this group are adolescents presenting with primary amenorrhea. We propose a laparoscopic sigmoid vaginal replacement for these patients.

Class II – Disorders of Vertical Fusion of the Müllerian Ducts

These are defects in the fusion between the downgrowing müllerian ducts and the up-growing derivates of the urogenital sinus, and are usually characterized by atresia of a portion of the vagina. The atresia may be a thin membrane (transverse septum) or a thick portion (partial vaginal agenesis while the uterus and cervix are present). Patients with cervical agenesis or dysgenesis are also included in this group.

Most of the patients in this group present in the peripuberal period with acute or subacute abdominal pain and an abdominal tumor. Although most of the vaginal pull-throughs are performed through a perineal approach, we use laparoscopy to define the anomaly, to detect and treat secondary endometriosis, and to perform complete hysterectomy in patients with cervical agenesis.

Class III – Disorders of Lateral Fusion of the Müllerian Ducts

These disorders may be symmetric or asymmetric and may or may not cause obstruction. Most of the patients treated in the pediatric age have obstructed asymmetric anomalies. The most frequent variety is the double uterus with an obstructed hemivagina and ipsilateral renal agenesis (Wunderlich-Heryn-Werner syndrome) (Rock and Jones 1980; Wunderlich 1976) (■ Fig. 108.1). The condition is treated by endovaginal resection of the septum, thus creating one single vagina. Laparoscopy is used to monitor endometriosis.

A higher level of obstruction (uterine cervix) is rare but causes very acute symptoms because of the loss of the reservoir-like action of the duplicated vagina to accommodate the menstrual blood. We propose a combined hysteroscopic and laparoscopic treatment of this anomaly.

Class IV – Unusual Configurations of Vertical/Lateral Fusion Defects

This category includes combined lateral and vertical fusion defects together cloacal as well as urogenital sinus anomalies. These anomalies are addressed in a separate chapter (Chapter 55).

In this chapter we will describe:

1. Laparoscopic sigmoid vaginal replacement
2. Laparoscopic total hysterectomy in cervical aplasia
3. Combined hysteroscopic and laparoscopic treatment of uterine thick obstructive septum

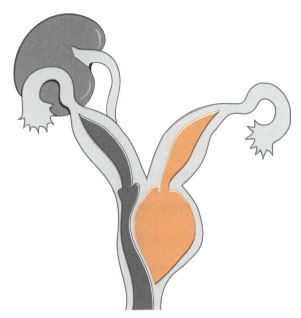

Fig. 108.1. Double uterus with an obstructed hemivagina and ipsilateral renal agenesis

Laparoscopic Sigmoid Vaginal Replacement

Introduction

Sigmoid vaginoplasty is an alternative technique for vaginal replacement. The two major advantages of this procedure are, first, that there is no need for dilatation nor for the use of some kind of a mold in the vagina and, second, that the neovagina has natural lubrication (Novak et al. 1978). One of its major disadvantages is the need for a laparotomy, with associated pain, nasogastric suction, and discomfort. Since the advent of mechanical suturing, we have no longer used routine nasogastric suction. Our next goal has been the avoidance of laparotomy. In the 2000 Annual Meeting of the International Pediatric Endosurgery Group, we reported the first patient who underwent a laparoscopic sigmoid vaginal replacement (Bailez et al. 2000).

Preoperative Preparation

The bowel is well prepared preoperatively. After induction of general anesthesia a nasogastric tube and urinary catheter are inserted. Prophylactic antibiotics are given. Future port holes are infiltrated with bupivacaine.

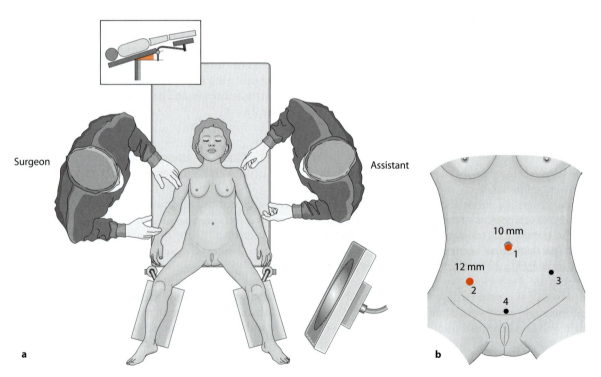

Fig. 108.2. Position of the patient, crew, monitor (**a**), and ports (**b**). *1* Umbilical port. Initial position of the lens and later the port for the surgeon's left-hand instrument after the lens is moved to port 2. *2* Right lower quadrant port. Lens port during isolation of the vascular pedicle (front vision) and endosta- pler port for sigmoid colon (neovagina) isolation. *3* Left lower quadrant port. Assistant port for traction on the sigmoid colon and for vascular transillumination with a second 5 mm lens. *4* Suprapubic port for the surgeon's right-hand instrument

Positioning
Patient
The patient is positioned in a supine lithotomy position. The table is tilted in Trendelenburg.

Crew, Monitors, and Equipment
■ Figure 108.2 shows the positions of the patient, crew, monitors, and ports.

Technique

Cannulae

Cannula	Method of insertion	Diameter (mm)	Device	Position
1	Open	10	Lens	Umbilicus
2	Closed	12/15	Lens, linear stapler, other instruments	Right lower quadrant
3	Closed	5	Instruments	Suprapubic area
4	Closed	5	Instruments	Left lower quadrant

Port Positions
We use four ports: a 10 mm one in the umbilicus, a 12 mm one in the right lower quadrant, and two 5 mm ones, one in the left lower quadrant and one just above the pubic symphysis (■ Fig. 108.2b).

Procedure
The lens is initially introduced through the umbilical port but later on it is moved to the right lower quadrant port in order to achieve better visualization of the vascularization of the sigmoid colon. The sigmoid is transilluminated with a 5 mm lens inserted through the port in the left lower quadrant (■ Fig. 108.3). A segment of the sigmoid colon is isolated using bipolar HFE, ultrasonic energy, or the Ligasure, and two linear endostaplers (■ Fig. 108.4).

Special Equipment
Apart from monopolar and bipolar high-frequency electrocoagulation (HFE), ultrasonic energy or the Ligasure should be available. A linear stapler with 45/60 mm stapling cartridges is at hand as well as an endocircular 28/32 mm stapler.

Next a space is created between the urethra and rectum by perineal dissection but under laparoscopic verification. Colo-colonic continuity is reestablished using a circular mechanical suturing device introduced through the rectum. The proximal end of the colon is exteriorized through the umbilicus, the proximal part of the circular stapling device is inserted, and the colon returned to the abdominal cavity (■ Fig. 108.5). The remaining part of the stapling device is inserted through the rectum. Both parts of the stapling device are assembled intra-abdominally under laparoscopic control, and the stapling device is fired (■ Fig. 108.6).

The peritoneum near the Douglas space is incised in order to allow the passage of a forceps from the perineum, which will enable the descent of the isolated bowel segment (■ Fig. 108.7). The vaginoplasty is completed from the perineal side.

Fig. 108.3. Transillumination of the sigmoid colon. Accessory lens in the left lower quadrant

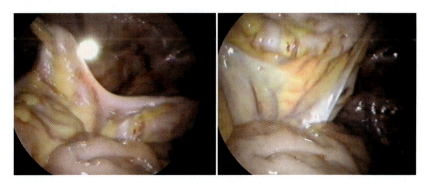

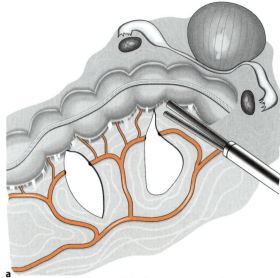

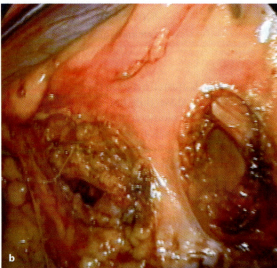

Fig. 108.4. a The sigmoid pedicle has been isolated using a bipolar forceps. With an endostapler both ends of the isolated sigmoid colon will be transected. **b** Intraoperative view

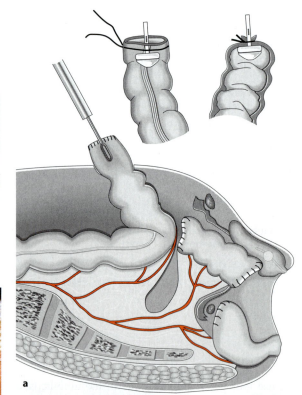

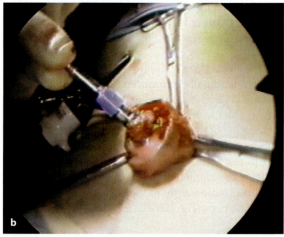

Fig. 108.5. a The sigmoid colon loop has been isolated. The proximal sigmoid colon is exteriorized and the stapler anvil is inserted. **b** Intraoperative view

Postoperative Care

No nasogastric tube is left behind. Feeding is usually started during the first postoperative day. The urinary catheter stays in place for the first 24 h. For pain control, non-steroidal anti-inflammatory drugs are used.

Results

Twenty patients were operated on using this technique. The mean age was 16.3 years (range 15–19 years). Sixteen patients had a Mayer-Rokitansky syndrome and four were male pseudohermaphrodites; two of them had complete androgenic insensitivity and had been previously treated by laparoscopic bilateral orchidec-

tomy. Three patients had a single pelvic kidney. One patient had a previously failed skin vaginoplasty and a laparotomy.

All patients were informed about different treatment modalities and chose to have this procedure. Mean operative time was 3.5 h (range 2–4.5 h). There was one accidental opening of the bladder that was sutured laparoscopically. The urinary catheter was left in for 3 days.

We learned that a complete perineal dissection of the vesicorectal space is required before trying to open

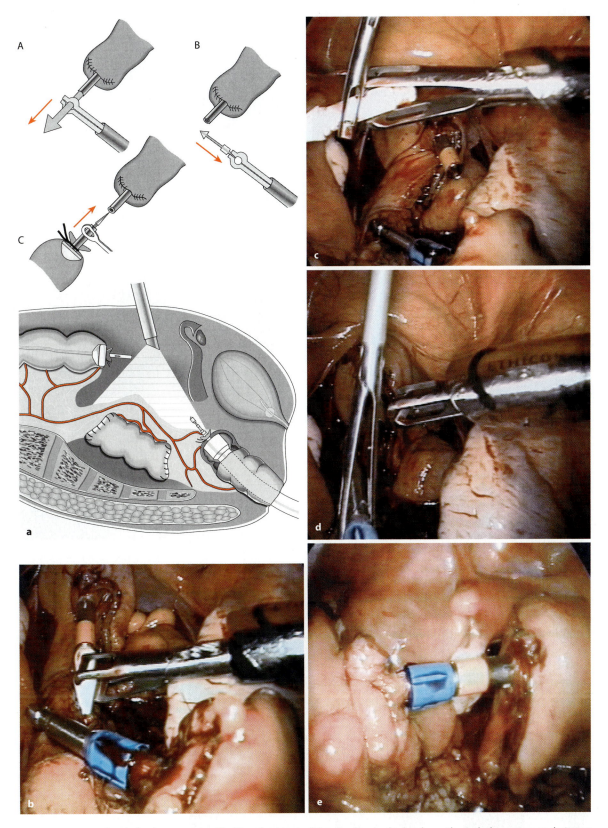

Fig. 108.6 a – e. a Stapled colorectostomy. **b,c** The distal part of the circular stapler has been through the rectum and pierces the rectum. The white piercing end is being removed. **d,e** Both parts of the circular stapler are assembled and the stapler is fired. **f** Completed anastomosis

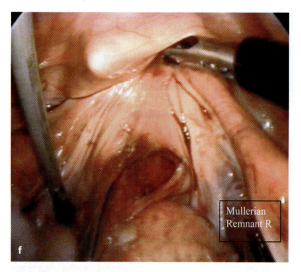

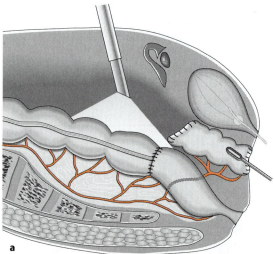

Fig. 108.6. f Completed anastomosis

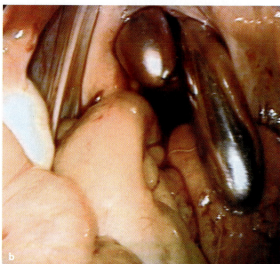

Fig. 108.7. Descent of the sigmoid colon loop. **a** Schematic drawing. **b** The Douglas space has been opened laparoscopically after perineal dissection of the plane between the urethra and rectum became clearly visible. Hegar dilators are used to create an adequate space for sigmoid descent

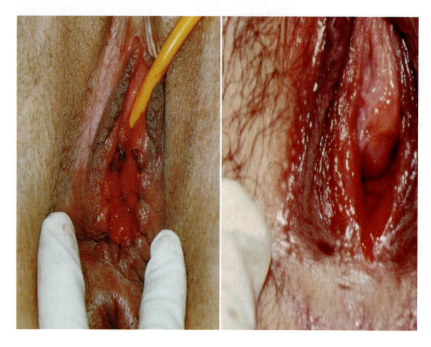

Fig. 108.8. Immediate and long term postoperative aspect of sigmoid vaginoplasty

it from above. Two patients presented transient self-limiting rectal bleeding. A right pelvic kidney made the procedure more difficult and required more "camera work." In contrast, a left pelvic kidney exposed the sigmoidal vessels very well, which made the isolation of a sigmoid colon segment easier.

All patients were able to tolerate food 24 h after the procedure and 17 were discharged within 48 h of the operation. Viability and patency of neovagina are excellent in 17 patients after a mean follow-up of 6 months (range 4–54 months) and 7 patients are sexually active (■ Fig. 108.8). Two patients developed mucosal prolapse.

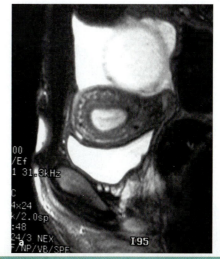

Discussion

There are a variety of conditions with total or partial absence of vagina in which a neovagina has to be created. If a vaginal orifice is present, the treatment of choice is passive or active elongation (Ingram 1981). When this technique fails either because of lack of motivation or in cases of a flat perineum, a surgical correction should be attempted. The surgical approach varies according to the clinical and emotional condition of the affected adolescent and the experience of the surgeon (Tjaden and Rock 1992).

Techniques that have been used more frequently are the McIndoe operation and its modifications and vaginoplasty using an amniotic allograft (McIndoe 1950). Amniotic allografts are used less frequently now because of fear of transmission of human immunodeficiency virus (HIV). Both techniques are successful in 75–85% of the cases (Rock et al. 1983; Strickland et al. 1993). Other techniques described include Williams operation, which uses vulvar skin, Johnson's operation, using skin from the back, Vecchietti's operation (laparoscopic elongation; Vecchietti and Ardillo 1970), or Pratt's operation, which uses sigmoid colon (Ghirardini and Popp 1994; Muran et al. 1992; Pratt 1972; Williams 1964). Even though the use of sigmoid colon is not frequently quoted in the gynecologic literature, the good results obtained with this technique in the repair of complex malformations or those associated with absence of vagina such as a cloaca, or an anorectal malformations with rectovulvar or rectovesicular fistula, which should be repaired in a single operation, encouraged us to optimize this technique for this indication (Bailez et al. 1998; Giovanni et al. 1993; Hendren 1997; Pena 1990). With this technique a tubular vagina with natural lubrication is created, without the need for the use of molds. Excessive mucous drainage was not observed in any of our patients, probably because the bowel descended was not so long. We believe that laparoscopy makes this therapeutic procedure more attractive. With the widespread culturing of vaginal epithelium it is likely that in the future an ideal vaginoplasty material will become available.

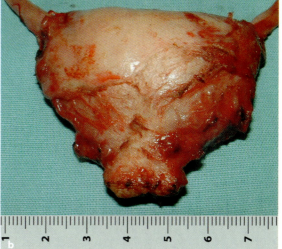

Fig. 108.9. Cervical atresia. **a** MRI. **b** Appearance of a resected uterus with cervical atresia

Laparoscopic Total Hysterectomy

Introduction

Agenesis or atresia of the cervix uteri is an uncommon entity. It is often associated with absence of the vagina (■ Fig. 108.9). The diagnosis is difficult to make prior to surgery. Ultrasonography and magnetic resonance imaging (MRI) show hematometra but sometimes it may be difficult to distinguish between cervical atresia and a high transverse vaginal septum. There is general agreement that if the cervix is absent, without any cervical stroma left, hysterectomy is advisable in order to prevent ovarian endometriosis and pelvic infections (Tjaden and Rock 1992). We treated four patients with combined vaginal and cervical agenesis. We used a combined laparoscopic and perineal approach in the last two patients. Laparoscopy was useful to define the

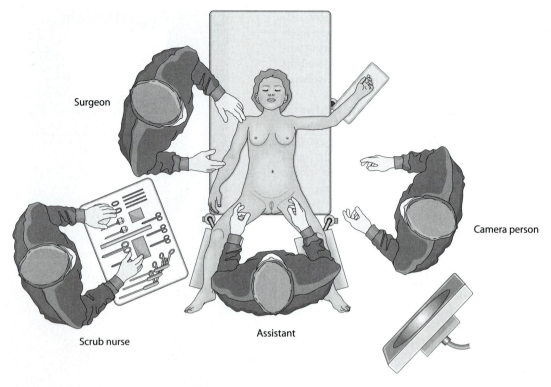

Fig. 108.10. Position of the patient, crew, monitors, and equipment

anomaly and to complete hysterectomy after evidence of total cervical aplasia. In addition, vaginal replacement could be done as described before.

Preoperative preparation

The bowel is well prepared before surgery. After induction of general anesthesia, antibiotics (ampicillin and sulbactam) are given and a urinary catheter is inserted. There is no need for a nasogastric tube. Future port hole sites are infiltrated with 0.5% bupivacaine to a total dose of 1.5 mg/kg.

Positioning
Patient
The patient is placed in a supine lithotomy position and the table is tilted in Trendelenburg.

Crew, Monitors, and Equipment
■ Figure 108.10 shows positions of the patient, crew, monitors, and equipment.

Special Equipment
Apart from monopolar and bipolar HFE, ultrasonic energy or the Ligasure should be available. We particularly like the Ligasure because of the fine beak. Endoloops should be at hand.

Technique

Cannulae

Cannula	Method of insertion	Diameter (mm)	Device	Position
1	Open	5	Lens	Umbilicus
2	Closed	5	Instruments	Right lower quadrant
3	Closed	5	Instruments	Suprapubic area
4	Closed	5	Retractor for the uterus, suction	Left lower quadrant

Port Positions

We used four ports: a 5 mm one at the umbilicus for a 30° lens, a 5 mm one in the right lower quadrant for the instruments in the surgeon's right hand, a 5 mm one in the left lower quadrant for the instruments in the surgeon's left hand, and a last 5 mm one in the hypogastrium for retraction of the uterus and for suction. We prefer a disposable trocar for the right-hand instruments for safer use of monopolar cautery.

Procedure

After insertion of the umbilical port for the lens and of the two working ports, the presence of an obstructed uterus is confirmed. We start to palpate the uterus in order to rule out the presence of a cervix in combination with a distended upper vagina. Next a careful dissection between the bladder and the obstructed uterus is carried out (■ Fig. 108.11). There may be a focus of endometriosis or inflammation depending on the duration of the obstruction.

Under laparoscopic vision a perineal dissection is carried out between the urethra and the rectum to create a space for the neovagina and reach the distal obstructed uterus. The uterus is pushed down with two graspers in order to allow confirmation of aplasia of the cervix by direct palpation and direct visualization thus avoiding a laparotomy.

Only after verification of the diagnosis is laparoscopic hysterectomy conserving the ovaries pursued. The course of the infundibulopelvic ligaments and of the ureters is identified. Coagulation and section of both utero-ovarian ligaments follows, keeping the ovaries out of the way thereby preserving their blood supply (■ Fig. 108.12). We then fulgurate and cut the round ligaments as distally as possible to use them for traction during distal dissection of the uterine pedicle.

We complete anterior and posterior uterine dissection in the midline, which is now easier as perineal dissection has already taken place. The uterine pedicles are dissected very close to the uterus in the area of the fibrotic tissue that replaces the cervix. We use bipolar cautery or the bipolar vessel sealer and place an endoloop depending on the diameter of the vessels. We use both lower quadrant ports for bimanual dissection and the hypogastric port for traction and irrigation. Irrigation is also useful to help in the dissection of the vesicouterine space. The uterus is extracted through the perineum.

Postoperative Care

The patient has no nasogastric tube and most patients start to eat during the first postoperative day. The urinary catheter is left in place for 24 h. Pain is controlled with non-steroidal anti-inflammatory drugs.

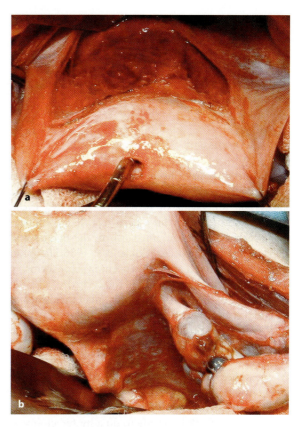

Fig. 108.11. a The bladder has been dissected off the uterus laparoscopically. There is complete absence of the uterine cervix. **b** Secondary endometriosis in the right adnex

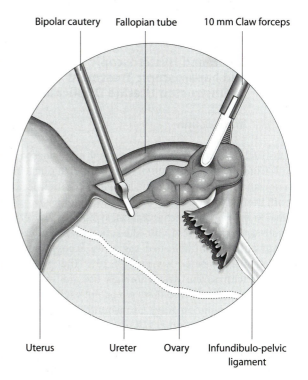

Fig. 108.12. Coagulation and section of the utero-ovarian ligament with bipolar energy

Results

Both patients were able to tolerate food after 24 h and were discharged during the third postoperative day. Histological analysis of the resected uterus confirmed the complete absence of the cervix.

Discussion

Many methods have been tried to create a passage through the dense fibrous tissue between the uterine cavity and the vagina or neovagina. Although cyclic menses and pregnancy have been reported, complications such as severe endometriosis of the ovaries and pelvic infections can occur (Cukier et al. 1986; Hampton et al. 1990). Cervical anomalies occur in three forms:
1. Aplasia (complete absence of the cervix)
2. Absence of the cervix except for small inclusions of endocervical-type tissue in fibrous tissue
3. Presence of an endocervical stroma with complete absence of the cervical canal.

Many authors have recommended early hysterectomy in cervical aplasia to preserve ovarian function.

Even in open surgery with the cervix area in the hands, it is difficult to decide to do a hysterectomy in children or adolescents. We combined the benefits of a very low dissection of the laparoscopic approach with the possibility of direct palpation and direct visualization of the cervix through the perineal dissection made for the creation of a neovagina.

Combined Hysteroscopic and Laparoscopic Treatment of Obstructed Uterine Duplications

Introduction

Obstructed lateral fusion uterovaginal anomalies result from a failure of fusion of both müllerian ducts in association with failure of one lumen to communicate with the outside. When the level of obstruction is proximal to the vagina (uterine cervix), symptoms are very acute as there is no reservoir-like action as seen in case of an obstructed duplicated vagina to accommodate the menstrual blood (Fig. 108.13). The patients present with severe dysmenorrhea but the external genitalia are normal and there is a patent vagina. There is no endovaginal "bulging." Ultrasound shows normal kidneys most of the times but an asymmetric uterine duplication. MRI shows asymmetric hematometria.

In such patients we started to do a laparoscopy to confirm the suspected anomaly and to evaluate endometriosis. Next an operative hysteroscopy is performed through the non-obstructed uterus in order to resect

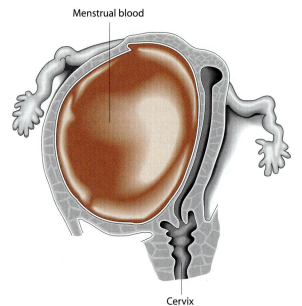

Menstrual blood

Cervix

Fig. 108.13. Obstructed uterine duplication. There is no obstruction in the duplicated vagina. As a result there is no reservoir function of the vagina

the duplicated uterine walls (septum), thus creating one single uterine cavity.

Preoperative preparation

Before Induction of General Anesthesia
The patients should discontinue the use of aspirin or other non-steroidal anti-inflammatory drugs well in advance of surgery. The best timing for the intervention is a time shortly after the patient completes her normal menstrual flow. Endometrial visualization is then optimal. No bowel preparation is needed.

After Induction of General Anesthesia
After induction of general anesthesia, a urinary catheter is inserted and broad-spectrum antibiotics are given. Future port hole sites are infiltrated with 0.5% bupivacaine to a maximal total dose of 1.5 mg/kg.

Positioning
Patient
The patient is placed in a supine lithotomy position with the table tilted in Trendelenburg.

Crew, Monitors, and Equipment
 Figure 108.14 shows positions of the patient, crew, monitors, and equipment.

Special Equipment
Bipolar electrocoagulation should be at hand. The availability of an operating hysteroscope is essential.

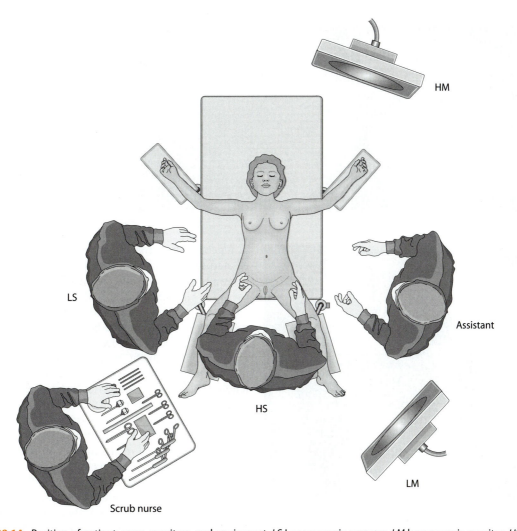

Fig. 108.14. Position of patient, crew, monitors, and equipment. *LS* Laparoscopic surgeon, *LM* laparoscopic monitor, *HS* hysteroscopic surgeon, *HM* hysteroscopic monitor

Technique

Cannulae

Cannula	Method of insertion	Diameter (mm)	Device	Position
1	Open/closed	5	Lens	Umbilicus
2	Closed	5 or 3	Working instruments	Right lower quadrant
3	Closed	5 or 3	Working instruments	Left lower quadrant
Speculum				Vagina
4		7	Sheath of the operative hysteroscope (scope itself 4 mm)	Endocervix

Port Positions

We used three ports: a 5 mm one at the umbilicus, and two 5 mm ones in the right and left lower quadrants, respectively. A speculum is inserted into the vagina and the sheath of the hysteroscope through the uterine cervix.

Procedure

The suspected anomaly is confirmed laparoscopically and the sites and degree of endometriosis are evaluated (■ Fig. 108.15).

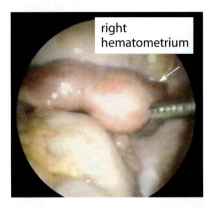
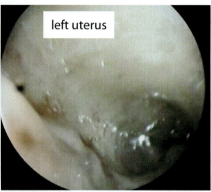

right hematometrium

left uterus

Fig. 108.15. *Left* Laparoscopic vision of a right hematometum. *Right* Hysteroscopic vision of the thick septum from the inside of the patent left uterus. The septum is on the left of the hysteroscopic view

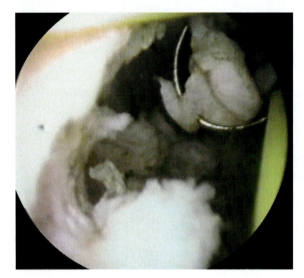

Fig. 108.16. Hysteroscopic resection of the septum using wire loop cautery

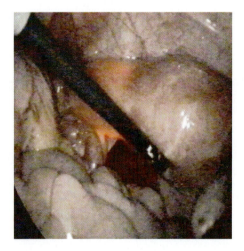

Fig. 108.17. Laparoscopic view of transillumination of the uterine wall by the hysteroscope

Operative hysteroscopy through the non-obstructed uterus follows in order to resect the duplicated uterine walls (septum), thus creating one single uterine cavity (■ Fig. 108.16). A speculum is inserted into the vagina and the cervix exposed and grasped with a tenaculum. The cervix should be dilated only enough to allow the insertion of the hysteroscope into the cavity, maintaining a tight fit around the instrument shaft, which is necessary for good containment of the distending medium. A double-tooth tenaculum or two single-tooth ones, one on each side of the cervix may be used. Alternatively a purse-string suture may be placed around the cervix to serve for traction. It is extremely important to maintain traction on the cervix during the procedure, keeping the long axis of the uterus parallel to the sacrum of the patient. A flexed uterus is more likely to be perforated and reduces visibility when rigid telescopes are used. Two percent glycine is used as distending medium under volume control. Once the hysteroscope is in the uterus, a full inspection of the cavity is performed. The tubal ostium is visualized for proper orientation. The obstructed cavity protrudes into the non-obstructed one.

The hysteroscope should remain relatively fixed just beyond the internal ostium, extending only the instruments. Rigid instruments such as scissors and wire loop cautery are used to incise and resect the large septum that resembles a uterine wall. The laparoscope is left in place to monitor the hysteroscopic operation and to reduce the risk of perforation. The intensity of the laparoscopic illumination is occasionally reduced in order to judge the thickness of the uterine wall as the operation progresses (■ Fig. 108.17). The non-obstructed uterus is thin and displaced by the obstructed one. Caution needs to be taken not to perforate its walls. In contrast the septum is very thick and it may be hard to reach the obstructed cavity, as was the case in our first patient.

Results

Five patients were treated using this approach. The procedure was completed successfully in four. One patient required open surgery as we were not able to dilate the uterine cervix for introduction of the hysteroscope. She underwent a conventional metroplasty and salpingoplasty because of a severe associated hematosalpinx. The mean age of these patients was 13.5 years and the cervix is not always wide enough.

The mean operative time was 90 min, and the mean hospital stay was 1.5 days. All patients are asymptomatic and have regular menses. With a mean follow-up of 40 months (range 37–48 months) there has been no ultrasonic evidence of any further obstruction.

Discussion

These patients represent only 23.8% of all lateral uterovaginal fusion anomalies (class III, n=21 patients) treated at our institution. As we mentioned previously most of the patients in this class have the Wunderlich-Heryn-Werner syndrome. We like to stress the absence of associated renal anomalies in these patients and feel that MRI is a good diagnostic modality. Hysteroscopic treatment of congenital uterine anomalies associated with fetal wastage has been reported in adults (Younger 1992). Although there are no previous reports of this minimally invasive approach in the pediatric age group, we feel that our preliminary data support the further use of this approach.

References

Bailez M, Heinen F, Solana J (1998) Absent vagina in patients with anorectal anomalies. BJU 81:76

Bailez MM, Scherl H, Dibenedetto V, et al (2000) Laparoscopic vaginal replacement with sigmoid colon. Pediatr Endosurg Innov Tech 4:90

Cukier J, Batzofin JH, Conners JS, et al (1986) Genital tract reconstruction in a patient with congenital absence of a vagina and hypoplasia of the cervix. Obstet Gynecol 68(3 suppl):32S–36S

Ghirardini G, Popp LW (1994) New approach to the Mayer-von Rokitansky-Küster-Hauser syndrome. Adolesc Pediatr Gynecol 7:41–43

Giovanni B, Zaffaroni G, Milena D, et al (1993) Proctoperineovaginohysterstomy and sigmoid colon pull-through for vaginal agenesis, hematocervicometra and vestibular anus. Adolesc Pediatr Gynecol 6:95–98

Hampton HL, Meeks RG, Bates GW, et al (1990) Pregnancy after successful vaginoplasty and cervical stenting for partial atresia of the cervix. Obstet Gynecol 76:900–901

Hendren H (1997) Management of cloacal malformations. Semin Pediatr Surg 6:217–227

Ingram JM (1981) The bicycle seat stool in the treatment of vaginal agenesis and stenosis: a preliminary report. Am J Obstet Gynecol 140:867–873

McIndoe A (1950) The treatment of congenital absence and obliterate conditions of the vagina. Br J Plast Surg 2:254–267

Muran D, Frederick R, Shell D (1992) Modified Williams vulvovaginoplasty: the role of tissue expanders. Adolesc Pediatr Gynecol 5:81–83

Novak F, Kos L, Plesko F (1978) The advantages of the artificial vagina derived from sigmoid colon. Acta Obstet Gynecol Scand 57:95–96

Pena A (1990) Atlas of surgical management of anorectal malformations. Springer, Berlin Heidelberg New York, p 19

Pratt JH (1972) Vaginal atresia corrected by use of small and large bowel. Clin Obstet Gynecol 15:639–649

Rock JA, Jones HW Jr (1980) The double uterus associated with an obstructed hemivagina and ipsilateral renal agenesis. Am J Obstet Gynecol 138:339–342

Rock J, Reeves L, Retto H, et al (1983) Success following vaginal creation for müllerian agenesis. Fertil Steril 39:809–813

Strickland JL, Cameron WJ, Krantz KE, et al (1993) Long-term satisfaction of adults undergoing McIndoe vaginoplasty as adolescents. Adolesc Pediatr Gynecol 6:135–137

Tjaden BL, Rock J (1992) Uterovaginal anomalies. In: Carpenter SE, Rock J (eds) Pediatric and Adolescent Gynecology, 20. Raven, New York, pp 313–330

Vecchietti G, Ardillo L (1970) La syndrome di Rokitansky-Küster-Hauser. Fisiopatologia e clinica dell-aplasia vaginale con corni uterini rudimentali. Societá Editrice Universo, Roma

Williams EA (1964) Congenital absence of the vagina: a simple operation for its relief. J Obstet Gynaecol Br Commonw 71:511–512

Wunderlich M (1976) Seltene Variante einer Genitalimissbildung mit Aplasie der rechten Niere. Zentralbl Gynakol 98:559–562

Younger JB (1992) Hysteroscopic treatment of congenital uterine anomalies. In: Azziz R, Alvarez Murphy A (eds) Practical Manual of Operative Laparoscopy and Hysteroscopy, 19. Springer, Berlin Heidelberg New York, pp 183–190

Chapter 109

Laparoscopy in Intersex Patients Raised as Females

Maria Marcela Bailez

Introduction

The newborn with ambiguous genitalia needs a multidisciplinary approach for sex assignment. Gonadal histology is required in some patients with abnormal gonadal development, such as mixed gonadal dysgenesis, true hermaphroditism, and testicular dysgenesis patients. Laparoscopy has been found to be helpful in these conditions where gonads may be inconsistent with the sex of rearing or premalignant (Docimo and Peters 2002). Although sex may be assigned before the biopsy is taken, histology in these patients is necessary for definitive diagnosis. Under such conditions biopsy and eventual gonadal resection may be done at the same time as feminizing genitoplasty. Only in a few patients, mostly true hermaphrodites, is definitive histology required for sex assignment.

Another related indication is complete testicular insensitivity. In such XY females the gonads can be removed laparoscopically (Yu et al. 1995).

The role of laparoscopy in the intersex condition to be raised as males such as excision of müllerian structures, prostatic utricle, and orchidopexy is addressed in other chapters (Chapters 99, 101).

Preoperative Preparation

The patient should be worked up preoperatively according to the intersex protocol. After induction of general anesthesia, future port hole sites are infiltrated with 0.2% bupivacaine up to a maximum dose of 1.5 mg/kg. Prophylactic antibiotics (cephalosporin) are given. A urinary catheter is inserted after disinfection and draping.

Positioning

Patient

Newborns and infants are positioned supine across the operating table. The abdomen and perineum are elevated from the bed with a sterile sheet to permit a more ergonomic use of instruments (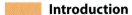 Fig. 109.1a). Adolescents are placed a supine Trendelenburg position (Fig 1b).

Crew, Monitors, and Equipment

In infants, the surgeon and assistant stand at the head of the patient (on the right or left side of the operating table) and the scrub nurse stands to the right of the surgeon. The monitor is at the feet of the patient (■ Fig. 109.1). The positioning of the crew, monitor, and equipment for adolescents is identical to the positioning described for the removal of peripuberal ovarian cysts (Chapter 105).

Special Equipment

We like to use bipolar energy and in the older patient the Ligasure as well. Frozen section analysis should be available.

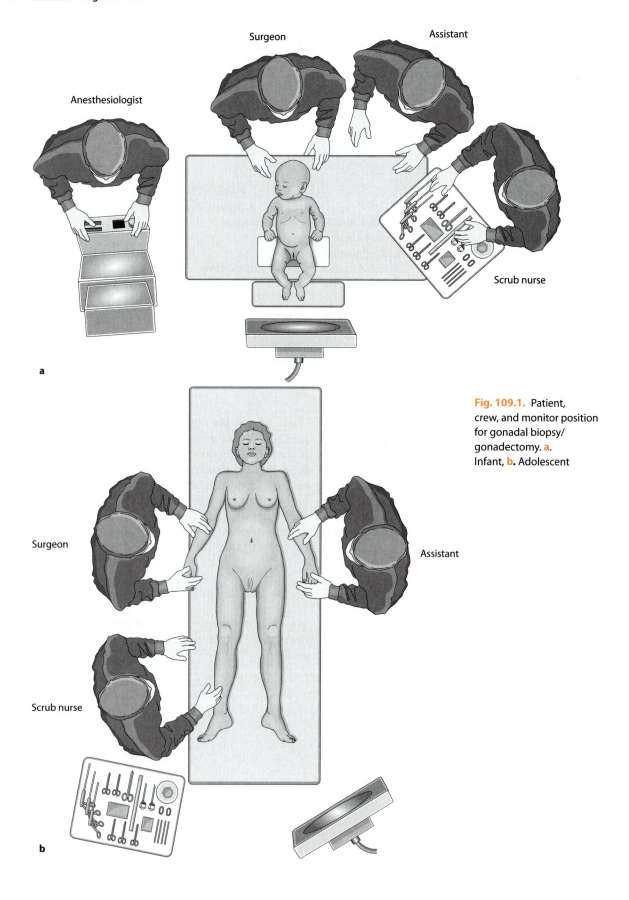

Fig. 109.1. Patient, crew, and monitor position for gonadal biopsy/ gonadectomy. **a.** Infant, **b.** Adolescent

Technique

Cannulae for Newborns and Infants

Cannula	Method of insertion	Diameter (mm)	Device	Position
1	Open	4	Telescope	Umbilicus
2	Closed	3	Instruments	Left flank
3	Closed	5/3	Instruments	Right flank

Cannulae for Adolescents

Cannula	Method of insertion	Diameter (mm)	Device	Position
1	Closed/open	5	Telescope	Umbilicus
2	Closed	5	Instruments	Left lower quadrant
3	Closed	5	Instruments	Right lower quadrant

Fig. 109.2. Port position for gonadal biopsy/gonadectomy. **a**. Infant, **b**. Adolescent

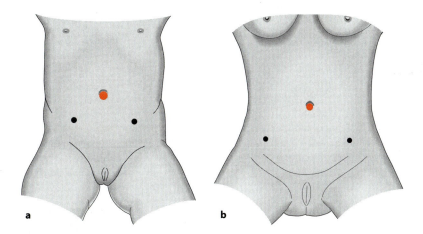

a   b

Port Positions

We use a short 4 mm 30° or 70° lens (arthroscope) in the umbilical port. The working ports are placed in both flanks in the newborn or infant (■ Fig. 109.2a). In adolescents with androgen insensitivity syndrome we use a 5 mm 30° telescope in the umbilicus and two 5 mm working ports in both lower quadrants (■ Fig. 109.2b).

Procedure

The most common laparoscopic procedures are:
1. Gonadal biopsy
2. Resection of intra-abdominal gonads
3. Resection of intrainguinal gonads/hernioplasty
4. Identification of internal ductal system

In newborns and infants we introduce the first port in an open way according to a technique that we call "umbilicoplasty smile" (see Chapter 104). A purse-string suture is put in order to avoid air leakage during the procedure. Moreover this suture facilitates port hole enlargement for gonadal extraction.

Gonadal biopsies are taken along the longitudinal axis of the gonad as both ovarian and testicular tissue may be found at the polar ends of the gonad, for example in case of an ovotestis (■ Fig. 109.3). A 3 mm grasper holds the gonad while 3 mm scissors do the cutting. Hemostasis is achieved with a bipolar forceps. Sometimes the residual gonad is reconstructed. Depending on the patient and the result of the frozen section biopsy, the gonad may be removed. If a streak gonad is recognized it is removed without prior biopsy (■ Fig. 109.4).

A streak gonad is often associated with an intra-abdominal or inguinal dysgenetic testicle, which is also removed at the same time in patients with female sex assignment. Gonadectomy is started by dissecting the peritoneum over the gonadal pedicle. A 3 mm bipolar forceps is used for coagulation and 3 mm scissors for the cutting. Streak gonads are removed en bloc together with the surrounding peritoneum and the ipsilateral gonaduct because of the risk of an in situ gonadoblastoma. An endoloop is tied at the junction of the tube with the uterus before sectioning the tube. The ipsilateral hemiuterus is preserved.

If a dysgenetic testis is found in a hernial sac, it can be pulled into the abdomen and resected en bloc with the peritoneum of the hernial sac. We put one or two sutures (4/0 vicryl on an RV1 needle) at the internal

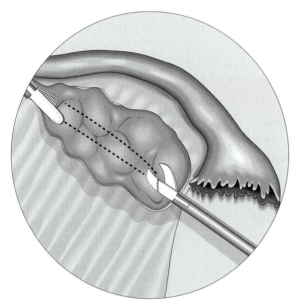

Fig. 109.3. Gonadal biopsies are taken along the longitudinal axis of the gonad. A 3 mm grasper holds the gonad while 3 mm scissors do the cutting

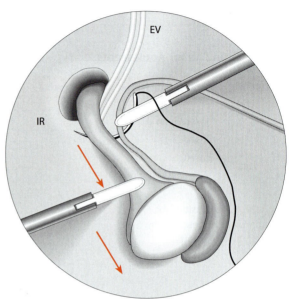

Fig. 109.5. Laparoscopic resection of a left inguinal gonad. The gonad is pulled into the abdomen. A suture is passed at the internal ring closing the defect while resecting the gonad. *IR* Inguinal ring, *EV* epigastric vessels

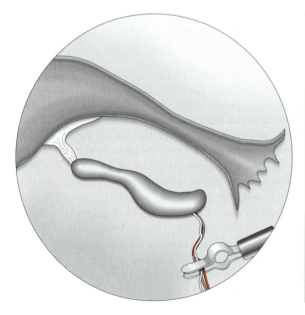

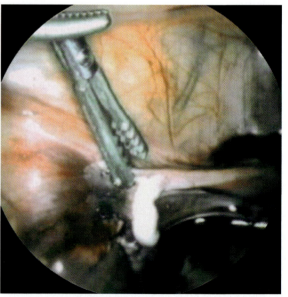

Fig. 109.4. Streak gonad. Bipolar coagulation of the gonadal pedicle. These gonads are resected en bloc together with the surrounding peritoneum

ring while keeping traction on the gonad (■ Fig. 109.5). The suture is either introduced directly through the abdominal wall or through the 5 mm port in the right flank using a 3 mm instrument. The knotting is done intracorporeally.

Gonads are removed through the umbilicus using the same maneuver described for neonatal ovarian complicated cysts (see Chapter 104). In adolescents with androgen insensitivity syndrome we use a closed or open transumbilical approach, but prefer to remove the gonads through one of the operative ports in the lower abdominal quadrants, which is easier and gives better cosmetic results. In these patients we use the 5 mm bipolar sealer to coagulate the three pedicles of the testicle as these testicles are of normal size with a good blood supply. Most of these patients have had a previous hernia repair with surgical introduction of the gonads into the abdominal cavity. As a result there is no need for closure of a hernia during the laparoscopy.

In male pseudohermaphrodites with bilateral inguinal palpable gonads, we start with bilateral inguinotomy for gonadectomy and rule out the presence of müllerian structures by inserting one 3- or 4 mm port in one of the hernial sacs and looking inside.

Postoperative Care

The patients have no nasogastric tube and feeding is resumed within the first 24 postoperative hours. A urinary catheter may be left depending on the associated urogenital reconstruction. Pain is controlled with non-steroidal anti-inflammatory drugs.

Results

Patients treated with a one-stage approach (laparoscopic treatment of gonads and feminizing genitoplasty) are summarized in ■ Table 109.1. Except for one patient, correlation of the karyotype with the macroscopic aspect and frozen section histology was very good. This patient (number 4) had a 45XO/46XY karyotype. The gonads were removed because of their macroscopic appearance. We have not performed separation of the testicular part of an ovotestis yet. This may be the ideal procedure but it is perhaps questionable in a patient with 45XO/46XY because of the risk of development of a neoplasm.

A two-staged approach was used in another patient (■ Table 109.2). Her karyotype was 46XX. She had two palpable gonads with a positive human chorionic gonadotropin (HCG) test. We decided to do gonadal biopsies and to look for müllerian structures before sex assignment. Inguinal exploration including biopsy taking showed bilateral ovotestes and the presence of a uterus. After female sex assignment, unilateral gonadectomy and feminizing genitoplasty were done simultaneously. We still have to do the separation of the testicular from the ovarian tissue.

Ten patients with a mean age of 15 years (6–17 years) with a complete androgen insensitivity underwent bi-

Table 109.1 Patients treated with a one-stage approach. *MGD* Mixed gonadal dysgenesis, *TH* true hermaphroditism

Patient	Diagnosis	Age at surgery (months)	Karyotype	Right gonad Procedure	Left gonad Procedure	Total operative time (with genitoplasty) (min)
1	MGD	3	45XO/46XY	Streak Gonadectomy	Dysgenetic testicle Biopsy/gonadectomy	210
2	MGD	5	45XO/46XY	Streak Gonadectomy	Dysgenetic testicle Biopsy/gonadectomy	240
3	MGD	2	45XO/46XY	Dysgenetic testicle Biopsy/gonadectomy	Streak Gonadectomy	220
4	TH	7	45XO/46XY	Dysgenetic testicle Biopsy/gonadectomy	Ovotestes[a] Gonadectomy	180
5	TH	21	46XX	Testicle Inguinal gonadectomy	Ovary Biopsy	240
6	TH	3	46XX	Ovary Biopsy	Testicle Biopsy gonadectomy	240
7	TH	18	45X/46XX/ 46XY/47XYY	Ovotestes Biopsy gonadectomy	Ovary Biopsy	210

[a] The diagnosis of ovotestes was not expected. The gonad was removed suspecting a streak.

Table 109.2 Patient treated with two-staged approach

Diagnosis	Age (months)	Karyo-type	First procedure	Second procedure	Future procedures
TH	2 and 4	46XX	Inguinal bilateral biopsy Bilateral ovotestes Müller exploration: +	Unilateral gonadectomy Feminizing genitoplasty	Resection of testicular tissue from the ovotestes

lateral gonadectomy. Mean operative time was 40 min. There were no intraoperative or postoperative complications.

Discussion

Sex was assigned prior to laparoscopy in all our patients with 45XO/46XY gonadal dysgenesis. This was based on a functional and psychosocial basis in combination with the results of the karyotyping, HCG testing, and interview of the parents. We scheduled simultaneous laparoscopy and feminizing genitoplasty as early as possible.

Most of the patients with asymmetric gonadal dysgenesis had an intra-abdominal streak gonad. This gonad has to be removed, avoiding previous biopsy, as it has a 25–50% chance to develop a gonadoblastoma and or dysgerminoma and as there is the possibility of an in situ tumor at the time of the procedure. Although there is the same risk of malignancy in the contralateral gonad (dysgenetic testicle) it may biopsied and preserved in the scrotum of patients with male sex assignment because this gonad is functional. We have never found functional ovarian tissue in these patients but we always wait for the result of frozen section biopsy before removing any other gonad than a classic streak.

True hermaphrodite patients do not have such a classic pattern and definitive histology is often necessary for sex assignment. Although the most common karyotype is 46XX and the most common gonadal combination ovary/ovotestes, each case is unique and should be treated on an individual basis. Sometimes the macroscopic aspect of the gonad and gonaduct as well as the result of a frozen section biopsy strongly favors gonadectomy in patients with previous sex assignment. There is an advantage of a laparoscopic approach in these patients requiring secondary pelvic exploration, especially because many of them are potentially fertile.

An inguinal approach may be indicated in patients with palpable gonads. We still prefer a laparoscopic approach in most of them as it enables not only better visualization of potential müllerian structures but also allows for treatment of a patent peritoneal sac, when removing the gonads, with better cosmetic results. In addition, most of these patients have asymmetric gonads with one of them being intra-abdominal. We reserve the inguinal approach for XY patients with symmetric palpable gonads introducing the telescope through the associated hernial sac in order to rule out the presence of müllerian structures.

There is some support in the gynecologic literature for prophylactic gonadectomy late in puberty for the benefit of spontaneous breast development in patients with complete androgen insensitivity. The risk for gonadal malignancy in these patients has been estimated to be 5%. However, we as others recommend gonadectomy at the time of diagnosis. The role of laparoscopy in these patients is resection of intra-abdominal gonads. Most of them were initially palpable in inguinal hernias and introduced into the abdomen during hernioplasty.

References

Docimo SG, Peters C (2002) Endourology and laparoscopy in children. In: Walsh PC, Retik AB, Vaughan CD, Wein AJ (eds) Campbell's Urology, 8th edn. Saunders, Philadelphia

Yu TJ, Shu K, Kung FT, et al (1995) Use of laparoscopy in intersex patients. J Urol 154:1193–1196

Chapter 110

Thoracoscopic Anterior Spinal Procedures in Children

Steven S. Rothenberg

Introduction

Major spinal deformities in children are one of the most difficult and challenging problems faced by the pediatric orthopedic surgeon. Since the early 1980s a combined anterior and posterior approach, performed in concert with a pediatric surgeon, for correction of these severe defects has become the procedure of choice (Burrington et al. 1963; Dwyer and Schafer 1974). However this procedure which requires a large posterolateral thoracotomy incision and in some cases a thoracolumbar incision, followed by an extensive posterior incision can be associated with significant morbidity and pain. Advances in video-assisted thoracic surgery since the 1990s has now allowed the anterior portion of these procedures to be performed thoracoscopically in an attempt to decrease the overall morbidity and recovery period.

Preoperative Preparation

Before Induction of General Anesthesia

Many patients with severe scoliosis also have significant respiratory compromise. A thorough evaluation by a pulmonologist should be carried out to evaluate the patients' ability to tolerate this major surgery. Neurologically impaired children or those with seizures maybe on medications which can cause a coagulopathy. These patients should have a complete coagulation profile done prior to surgery. A type and cross-match should also be done.

After Induction of General Anesthesia

Generally a large-bore central venous line and an arterial line are placed to allow for adequate monitoring and resuscitation. The blood loss associated with the thoracoscopic portion of the spinal fusion is generally minimal but the posterior portion can be quite extensive. It is helpful to have single-lung ventilation. This can be accomplished with a double lumen endotracheal tube, if the patient is large enough, or by a mainstem intubation of the contralateral side. All patients should receive preoperative antibiotics, generally a first- or second-generation cephalosporin. A nasogastric tube and urinary catheter are generally indicated.

Positioning

Patient

The patient is placed in a modified lateral decubitus position tilted 20° to 30° to the prone position (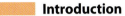 Fig. 110.1). This allows gravity to retract the lung anteriorly giving greater exposure of the spine. The side up should be the convex side of the curve. If the patient is kyphotic without significant scoliosis then the surgeon can pick which side to approach from. In general the right chest gives better access in these cases.

Crews, Monitors, and Equipment

The surgeon and assistant stand in front of the patient facing the spine at chest level (Fig. 110.1). The monitor is placed directly across from them behind the patient. The scrub nurse is also behind the patient below the level of the monitor. A second monitor can be placed above the assistant for the nurse to view, but is not absolutely necessary.

Special Equipment

No special energy applying systems are required. The use of clip, bipolar electrocautery, and or ultrasonic energy is optional. Fluoroscopy may be useful to determine the exact level.

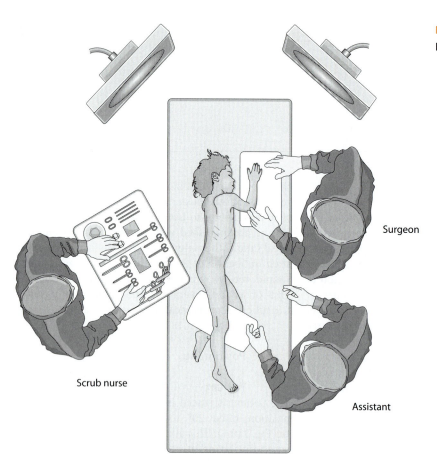

Fig. 110.1. Position of the patient, crew and equipmnent

Surgeon

Scrub nurse

Assistant

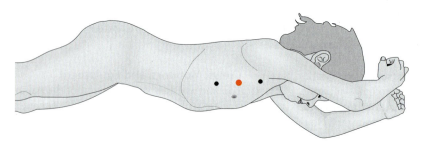

Fig. 110.2. Position of the ports

Technique

Cannulae

Cannula	Method of insertion	Diameter (mm)	Device	Position
1	Closed	5/10	Optic	Midaxillary line, 5th intercostal space
2	Closed	5/10	Harmonic scalpel, curved scissors	Midaxillary line
3–5	Closed	5/10	Diathermia hook, scissors, forceps	Midaxillary line

Procedure

The thoracic cavity is first entered with a Veress needle in the midaxillary line at approximately the 5th or 6th intercostal space. A low flow, low pressure of CO_2 is infused to help collapse the lung. The infusion is continued throughout the case. A 5 mm port is then placed in the midaxillary line at the level of the apex of the curvature.

A 5 mm 30° lens is used for the initial survey and the other ports are placed in a longitudinal plane depending on the levels of the thoracic spine to be manipulated (■ Fig. 110.2). The majority of the ports are 5 mm and provide access for the telescope, suction/irrigator, grasper, scissors, or retractor, as needed. A 10 mm port is necessary for the orthopedic instruments which include 3- and 5 mm straight and angled curettes, straight and angled pituitary rongeurs, and an 8 mm Cobb which has been modified with an extended handle. These instruments have been refined so that the shafts of the instruments resemble standard laparoscopic instruments, thereby maintaining the seal at the trocar valve. Three to seven ports (average 4) are used depending on the number of disc spaces that need to be addressed. Proper positioning of the 10 mm ports allows for manipulation of three to four disc spaces through this one space, thereby limiting the number of larger incisions. However if the angle becomes too great the orthopedic surgeon cannot perform an adequate discectomy.

With the spine visualized the pleura overlying the desired disc spaces is incised and the disc space is cleared. Depending on the surgeon preference the segmental blood vessels are preserved and retracted out of the way, or divided. If the vessels are sacrificed this can be easily accomplished with the hook attachment of the ultrasonic dissector (■ Fig. 110.3). The back of the hook blade is used to compress, seal, and divide the vessels. This avoids the necessity of mobilizing the vessels and attempting ligation and then division. In cases of hemivertebra the overlying segmental vessel is always taken. Dividing the segmental vessels allows the pleura to be cleared widely giving exposure of the anterior longitudinal ligament as well as the majority of the disc circumference anteriorly.

With the interspaces cleared the discectomies are performed by the orthopedic surgeon and the bone graft is applied. If there is significant bleeding Gelfoam is packed in the space to provide hemostasis prior to insertion of the bone graft. With the discectomies complete all instruments and ports are removed and a single chest tube is placed through the most inferior trocar site. The trocar sites are closed with absorbable suture. The lung is re-expanded and the patient is then reposition for the posterior portion of the procedure.

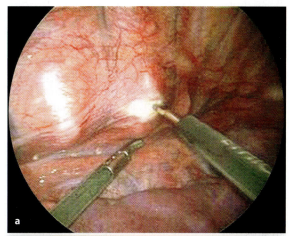

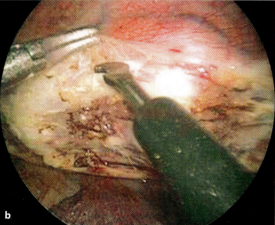

Fig. 110.3. Depending on the surgeon's preference the segmental blood vessels are preserved and retracted out of the way (**a**) or divided with the hook attachment of the ultrasonic dissector (**b**)

Postoperative Care

Most of the postoperative care is dictated by the orthopedic surgeons and by the posterior portion of the fusion as this is the more involved portion of the surgery. The patient often requires ventilation for the first 24–48 h postoperative, especially in patients with cerebral palsy. The patient is given intravenous analgesia and the chest tube is left to suction until the volume drops to 50–60 cc for an 8-h shift. Once the drainage decreases the chest tube is placed to water seal and then removed 6–12 h later if there is no evidence of an effusion or pneumothorax. Patient ambulation and rehabilitation are dictated by the orthopedic surgeon once the chest tube is removed.

Results

Over a 6-year period from February 1997 to February 2003, 77 procedures were performed in children aged 8–17 years. Weight ranged from 25 to 75 kg. Operative times for the thoracoscopic portion ranged from 50 to 165 min (average 105 min). Seventy-six patients had discectomy with anterior release of two to nine levels (average five), 6 patients had hemivertebrectomies, and 4 had epiphysiodesis. Five patients who had a significant lumbar curve contralateral to the thoracic curve also underwent open anterior lumbar release with instrumentation. All 77 patients underwent posterior fusion. Seven patients were extubated at the end of their procedure and 45 on postoperative day 1. Two patients with severe neurologic and pulmonary disability required longer ventilator support, and one required a tracheostomy because of chronic atelectasis. Average chest tube duration was 2.2 days and average intensive care unit (ICU) stay was 1.6 days excluding the aforementioned patients. There were no complications directly related to the thoracoscopic technique used. Hospital stay was primarily dictated by recovery from the posterior portion of their procedure. In follow-up surgical correction was deemed to be acceptable and equivalent to the standard open technique in all cases.

Discussion

One of the most common and most morbid surgeries performed in children requiring a major thoracotomy has been correction of spinal deformities. A combined anterior and posterior approach has been advocated for over 30 years and although the functional results have been excellent the morbidity associated with the procedure has been high. Regan and Mack reported one of the first series of thoracoscopic-assisted procedures for spinal deformity and disc herniation in adults (Mack et al. 1995). Their initial results and improvements in instrumentation and technique encouraged us to try and apply these techniques to children. After our initial learning curve was overcome, the procedures went smoothly and most cases were completed faster than if we had performed a standard thoracotomy (Rothenberg et al. 1998). The pediatric surgeon and pediatric spine surgeon work together throughout the anterior portion of the procedure creating a better flow to the operation. The pediatric surgeon not only creates the initial exposure but helps set up the orientation to each new disc space. The surgeon also protects the segmental vessels, vena cava, aorta, lung, and other structures without the wide exposure and large retractors necessary in standard approach. In cases where an anterior lumbar release was required as well we have chosen to do the thoracic portion video-assisted and the lumbar portion open, thereby avoiding the morbidity of a thoracolumbar incision. Even in these cases operative times have been similar.

The postoperative morbidity has been minimal. Overall the time requiring ventilator support, ICU stay, and length of chest tube drainage are less than those reported in a large series of open spinal fusions (Janik et al. 1997). Hospital stay in most cases is not significantly improved because of the time necessary to recover from the posterior fusion, but in general the patients have been discharged 1–2 days earlier and they seem to recover quicker.

These results confirm our earlier experience and suggest that a thoracoscopic approach for the anterior portion of corrective spine surgery will result in a significant decrease in the morbidity to these patients without sacrificing anatomic and functional results.

References

Burrington JD, Brown C, Odom J (1963) Anterior approach to the thoracolumbar spine. Arch Surg 111:456–463

Dwyer AF, Schafer MF (1974) Anterior approach to scoliosis: results of 51 cases. J Bone Joint Surg 56:218–224

Janik JS, Burrington JD, Janik JE, et al (1997) Anterior exposure of spinal deformities and tumors: a twenty year experience. J Ped Surg 32:852–859

Mack MJ, Regan JJ, McAfee P, et al (1995) Video-assisted thoracic surgery for the anterior approach to the thoracic spine. Ann Thorac Surg 59:1100–1106

Rothenberg SS, Erickson M, Eilert R, et al (1998) Thoracoscopic anterior spinal procedures in children. J Pediatr Surg 33:1168–1171

Fetal Surgery

Chapter 111

Endoscopic Access to the Fetus

Karl G. Sylvester and Craig T. Albanese

Introduction

Endoscopic access to the fetus as a therapeutic option is a technique in evolution. The earliest attempts at fetal access were performed for limited diagnostic procedures via obstetric endoscopes adapted to the unique challenges of the fetal environment. The need for this diagnostic tool was eventually supplanted by ultrasonography. Increasingly accurate ultrasound coupled with a growing knowledge of the natural history of select fetal anomalies led to the establishment of the field of fetal surgical intervention in the early 1980s. This strategy required a hysterotomy which was found to incite vigorous preterm labor (PTL). Open fetal surgery, however, remains constrained by the ever-threatened morbidity of premature rupture of membranes and PTL associated with this approach (Albanese and Harrison 1998). With these limitations, the techniques and technology for endoscopic access to the fetal environ have evolved in an effort to minimize physiologic perturbations to both maternal and fetal patients. As experience has been gained, the application of minimal access fetal surgery (MAFS) techniques has become the preferred approach and may expand the indications for therapeutic fetal interventions.

There are unique challenges inherent to achieving endoscopic access to the fetus, with both maternal- and fetal-specific issues that need to be considered prior to attempted intervention. These are largely conferred by the novel relationship of the "patient within a patient." The protective uterus represents a barrier with obstacles that include variable placental location, a highly vascular and muscular uterine wall that reacts to injury with contraction and hemorrhage, poorly adherent uterine membranes subject to dissection when manipulated, a floating mobile fetus, a relatively opaque operative medium, confined working space, and little ability to monitor the physiologic well-being of the fetal patient (Sydorak and Albanese 2003). Innovations in techniques and instrumentation have allowed many of these seemingly prohibitive obstacles to be overcome. The evolution of these techniques will parallel the ongoing elucidation of fetal pathophysiology.

Preoperative Preparation

Before Induction of General Anesthesia

Preoperative preparations specific to fetal operations include prophylactic measures to prevent uterine hyperactivity in response to operative manipulation. Indomethacin is routinely administered to the mother, given the uterine muscular relaxation achieved with prostaglandin inhibition. Because of the possible effects of prostaglandin on the ductus arteriosus and fetal circulation, a daily echocardiogram is performed after the procedure and for the duration of Indocin therapy which typically is 48 h. Occasionally an intravenous tocolytic infusion of magnesium sulfate is required preoperatively depending on the state of uterine activity as detected by transabdominal uterine monitoring.

With fetoscopic procedures, placental position dictates approach (Fowler et al. 2002; Sydorak and Albanese 2003). Thus, preprocedure mapping of the placenta by ultrasound is an integral part of operative planning. A percutaneous approach is possible with a posterior placenta. With an anterior placenta a maternal laparotomy may be necessary in order to physically elevate the uterus and achieve posterior uterine access free from the highly vascular placenta. The need for a maternal laparotomy will also impact the planning of effective anesthetic management with the possible added benefit of a maternal epidural catheter and a muscle relaxant.

After Induction of General Anesthesia

Most MAFS procedures are performed under general anesthesia. Both mother and fetus are effectively anesthetized with inhaled halogenated agents (Albanese 2002). The advantage to this approach is a desired level of profound uterine relaxation (Albanese 2002). Additional agents utilized for added uterine relaxation include nitroglycerin and sympathomimetics (terbutaline) due to their additive effects on uterine smooth muscle relaxation (Albanese 2002; Fowler et al. 2002; Sydorak and Albanese 2003). These additional agents are most commonly used when a maternal laparotomy is needed for uterine manipulation. Depending on the nature of the case, the fetus can also be given an intraoperative intramuscular injection of a long-acting non-depolarizing muscle relaxant and a short-acting narcotic to further minimize the fetal stress response to operative manipulation (Sydorak and Albanese 2003). A maternal urinary drainage catheter is always placed after induction. Mother, fetus, and their shared environment are administered prophylactic antibiotics prior to any fetal procedure. Skin pathogens are specifically targeted and cefazolin is given for 24 h perioperatively. The incidence of chorioamnionitis with this approach has been kept at a minimum (Albanese 2002; Sydorak and Albanese 2003).

While the approaches above are utilized in the majority of MAFS procedures, there remains a need for case-specific variation in approach given the highly variable indications for fetal interventions. Very specific cases such as selective reduction for anencephalic–acardiac twins require only an epidural catheter, urinary catheter, and local infiltration. Furthermore since a fetoscope is not used and the reduction is performed by ultrasound guidance of a coagulating device with a 16 gauge diameter, placental position is not a strong consideration since the needle can be passed directly through the placenta under ultrasound guidance.

Positioning

Patient

Careful attention to maternal positioning is paramount to successful fetoscopic surgery. The mother is positioned with her right side slightly elevated in order to displace the gravid uterus and relieve anterior compression on the vena cava (■ Fig. 111.1) (Albanese 2002; Sydorak and Albanese 2003). This maneuver effectively prevents unwanted preload reduction and subsequent decreased uterine blood flow which would rapidly lead to fetal distress. The mother is then positioned in a modified lithotomy position with her knees low to allow one of the surgeons to be positioned between the abducted legs (■ Fig. 111.2) (Sydorak and Albanese, 2003; Albanese 2002). This accommodates the increased need for access to the patient at the operating table in consideration of the need for adjunct personnel including a sonologist and perinatologist (■ Fig. 111.2). This relationship of specialists is mandatory in order to provide for maximum expertise in determining placental and fetal position in planning effective interventions. Lower extremity sequential compression devices are placed prior to the induction of anesthesia and remain throughout the operative case and postoperative care.

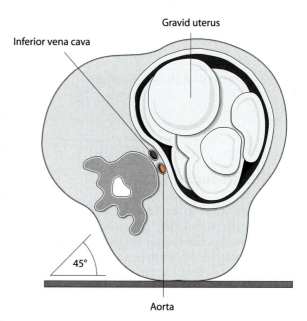

Fig. 111.1. Cross-sectional view of uterine and maternal displacement preventing caval compression

Crew, Monitors, and Equipment

The design of the operating room for fetal interventions is critical to its successful outcome. In order to accommodate the increased need for personnel and equipment, an ergonomic arrangement has to be well planned and is best standardized (■ Fig. 111.2) (Albanese 2002; Sydorak and Albanese 2003). The uniqueness of the technical aspects of fetal manipulation is manifest in the need for guidance from intraoperative ultrasound. Once again two of the factors critical to success are the placental and fetal position (Albanese 2002; Sydorak and Albanese 2003). Furthermore depending on the need for maternal laparotomy, fetal manipulation and version may be necessary and are possible when laparotomy is performed. All of these aspects are accommodated by the operating room configuration depicted in ■ Fig. 111.2.

Special Equipment

As the interest and applicability of fetal endoscopic techniques has increased, the availability and specificity of instruments for these techniques has also expanded. There are a variety of endoscopes available in varying sizes and lens configurations (Albanese 2002; Deprest 2001; Quintero and Morales 2001; Sydorak and Albanese 2003). Most commonly utilized are fixed rod lens systems. The standard telescope is 18 cm in length, 2.7 mm in diameter, and with 30° of angulation (■ Fig. 111.3a). An operative sheath which allows for coaxial deployment of instrumen-

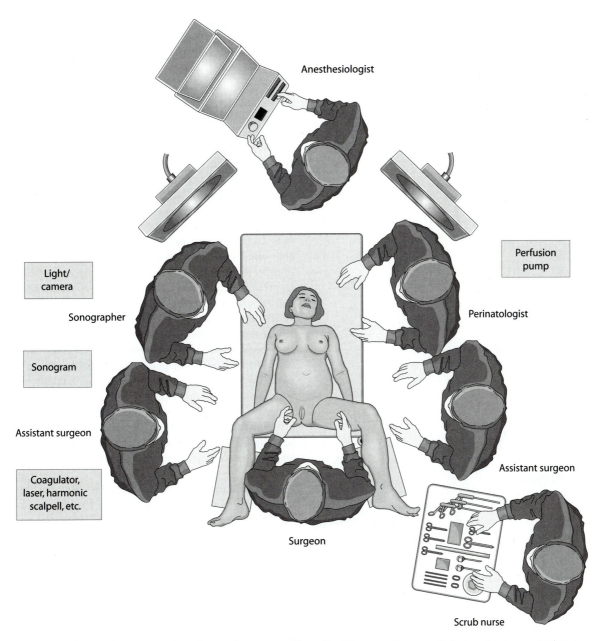

Fig. 111.2. Schematic representation of operating room configuration. The operating room is designed to accommodate numerous personnel and equipment necessitated by the multidisciplinary approach of fetal interventions

tation is also standard (■ Fig. 111.3b). This configuration utilizes the concentric ring design commonly employed in urologic and hysteroscopic procedures. The most commonly utilized operative sheath is 2.7 mm which accommodates a 1.2 mm telescope, coaxial catheter, or small (1 mm) instrument loading and a near constant flow from the uterine fluid exchanger discussed below (■ Fig. 111.3b). Rod lens telescopes larger than 2.0 mm can be angulated providing greater visualization and are preferred. Fiberoptic lens systems have the advantage of greater flexibility, but suffer from greatly inferior optics for visualization

in an already difficult fluid medium with high light scatter.

The uniqueness of the fetal fluid environment necessitates additional special equipment. A mechanized fluid warmer and exchanger is necessary to maintain a relatively constant uterine fluid volume and temperature at or near 37°C (■ Fig. 111.4) (Albanese 2002; Sydorak and Albanese 2003). The exchange of fluid with warmed lactated Ringer's solution also provides for greater operative visibility. This is the secondary effect of replacing the colloid-rich native amniotic fluid with a crystalloid solution. The light scatter in amni-

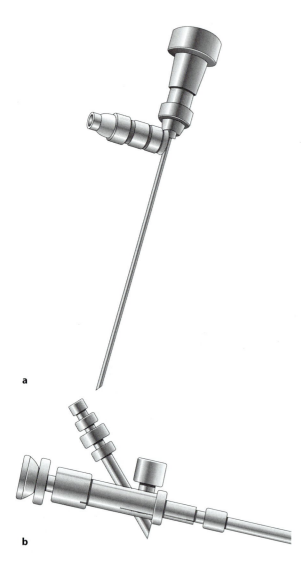

a

b

Fig. 111.3. a Typical operative endoscope measuring between 1.2 and 2.8 mm outside diameter. **b** Operative endoscopic sheath with operative side arm and fluid warmer channel

without amniotic membrane dissection and overt disruption. Toward this end several modified cannulae are available to help control hemorrhage and prevent membrane dissection. Placental positioning is another factor which helps guide the approach to cannulae placement. Depending on the time in gestation and operative objective, the uterus can be approached either percutaneously, through a laparotomy, or a low transverse abdominal incision. In the case of an anterior placenta, uterine manipulation may be necessary to displace the uterus in attempts to identify a safe operative "window" for trocar placement away from both placental and laterally coursing uterine vessels.

For percutaneous access there are a variety of small (1.6- to 5 mm) non-radially expanding trocars available which can be placed with the Seldinger technique in order to avoid membrane dissection (Albanese 2002; Deprest 2001; Quintero and Morales 2001; Sydorak and Albanese 2003). Balloon-tipped trocars exist in a variety of sizes down to 2.5 mm and have the added advantage of controlling both myometrial hemorrhage and amniotic fluid leak. Thus far these cannulae have not been designed to be placed via the Seldinger technique thus complicating their ease of use. Radially expanding trocars which have found common use in pediatric laparoscopic surgery can similarly aid in avoiding uterine bleeding and leak (Sydorak and Albanese 2003). The individual operative case will help determine the choice of trocars and uterine access approach.

There is currently a limited need for extensive dissection in fetal endoscopic cases. Therefore the majority of the other equipment is chosen based on the operative indications. During operative planning it is important to note the ineffectiveness of unipolar cautery in the liquid operating medium. Additionally, bipolar current has been used with variable success depending on the caliber of the target vessel given the tendency of the current to disseminate into the electrolyte-rich amniotic fluid thus limiting its effectiveness. Photocoagulation with Nd-YAG laser for small placental vessels has been successfully utilized for vascular occlusion (De Lia et al. 1990, 1999; Quintero et al. 2001; Sydorak et al. 2002; Ville et al. 1998). Radiofrequency current is being explored as an alternative energy source for vascular obliteration of lesions such as sacrococcygeal teratomas (SCT) and the selective reduction of twins (Paek et al. 2001; Tsao et al. 2002). Finally 5 mm clip appliers may find occasional case-specific utility. Ultimately, other instruments or catheters tailored to the specific needs of the intended intervention will be devised and implemented. A good example of this is the experimental use of coaxially deployed detachable balloon-tipped catheters for tracheal occlusion of fetuses with congenital diaphragmatic hernia (CDH) (Chiba et al. 2000; Harrison et al. 2001).

otic fluid has a dramatic effect on the already constrained visualization in the confined amniotic working environment. The fluid exchange system serves to maintain the fetal fluid environment and warms the fetus while improving visualization. This system can be deployed via a side arm of the operative telescope or trocar (■ Fig. 111.3). The fluid medium also provides an acoustic window for the continued use of intraoperative sonography for operative guidance and fetal monitoring.

A variety of sizes and techniques of introduction for operative trocars have been explored and utilized (Albanese 2002; Fowler et al. 2002; Quintero and Morales 2001; Sydorak and Albanese 2003). The confining factor to be considered in design is ease of introduction

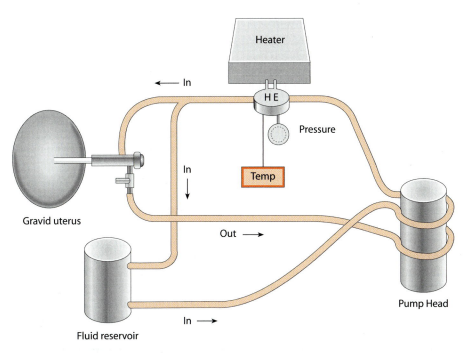

Fig. 111.4. The design of one type of fluid exchange system used during MAFS. This system allows for the amniotic fluid volume to be removed, warmed, returned, or replaced. In addition uterine pressure as a function of fluid volume can be regulated in order to prevent uterine irritability

Energy applying systems are as follows:

Equipment	Requirement
Bipolar high-frequency electro-coagulation (HFE)	Yes
Ultrasonic energy (radiofrequency probe)	Yes
Ligasure	Yes
Argon	No
Laser	Yes
Other	Case specific

Other equipment is as follows:

Equipment	Requirement
Clips	Yes
Staplers	Yes
Bag	No
Hand-assisting port	No
X-ray (ultrasound with Doppler)	Yes
Other	Case specific

Technique

Cannulae

For a discussion of various cannulae and techniques for insertion please see above.

Procedure

Minimal access fetal surgery may have its greatest utility in the treatment of shared placental circulation that can complicate monochorionic twin pregnancies (Allen et al. 2000; Bermudez et al. 2002). In twin-twin transfusion syndrome (TTTS) abnormal vascular connections between twins can result in a hydropic recipient twin with cardiac failure and a donor twin with growth retardation and oligohydramnios. Although the appropriate treatment is controversial, laser photocoagulation of bridging vessels has been successful (De Lia et al. 1990, 1999; Ville et al. 1998). Photocoagulation of abnormal placental vessels with a neodymium: yttrium aluminum garnet (Nd-YAG) laser versus serial amnio-reductions for TTTS is presently being studied in a National Institutes of Health (NIH)-sponsored clinical trial. In the twin reversed arterial perfusion syndrome (TRAP), there is a reversal of blood flow between an advantaged "normal twin" and an acardiac acephalic disadvantaged twin. This physiology threatens the advantaged "normal" twin both with and without demise of the disadvantaged twin. MAFS-guided division of the troublesome umbilical vessels has been performed by either harmonic scalpel ultrasonic cord transection or radiofrequency ablation (RFA) probe (Lopoo et al. 2000; Tsao et al. 2002).

There are several fetal anomalies under study which may have effective interventions performed through specific fetal endoscopic techniques. Fetal obstructive uropathy has been historically treated with ultrasound guided and percutaneously deployed vesicoamniotic shunt placement. These shunts however are beset by frequent dislodgment or obstruction. Fetal cystoscopy with ablation of posterior urethral valves (PUV) and endoscopic suprapubic cystostomy have been described (Quintero et al. 1995, 2000). Since the experimental demonstration of the effectiveness of tracheal occlusion on in utero reduction of diaphragmatic hernia, MAFS approaches have been developed and are now being performed in human fetuses via the detachable occlusive balloon approach deployed during fetal tracheoscopy (Harrison et al. 2001). Also, fetuses with large SCT in mothers who develop the maternal mirror syndrome have had successful feeding vessel ablation using MAFS-guided RFA probe (Tsao et al. 2002). Fetal congenital high airway obstruction syndrome (CHAOS) may be ameliorated by MAFS-directed fetal tracheostomy when lung overdistention results in hydrops (Paek et al. 2002). Fetoscopic procedures have even been successfully adapted to the current in utero approach to myelomeningocele repair (Farmer et al. 2003). Other maladies such as amniotic band syndrome which can cause umbilical cord constriction, have been treated by fetoscopic release (Quintero et al. 1997). Finally, further current investigation may broaden the utility of these techniques toward a previously unheralded approach to fetal cardiac anomalies.

Postoperative Care

In order to monitor postoperative uterine activity an external tocodynamometer is utilized (Albanese 2002; Fowler et al. 2002; Sydorak and Albanese 2003). Well-balanced maternal analgesia is crucial to the success of postoperative management (Albanese 2002; Fowler et al. 2002; Sydorak and Albanese 2003). A combination of intravenous and oral narcotic is utilized. Additionally, if maternal laparotomy was necessary then epidural analgesia is required (Albanese 2002; Fowler et al. 2002; Sydorak and Albanese 2003). Depending on the need for maternal laparotomy or otherwise the postoperative care is case specific. Additional unusual aspects of postoperative care relate to the risk of PTL and its management. Typical approaches implemented to help avoid and treat PTL are bed rest and intravenous

tocolytics including magnesium sulfate (Albanese 2002; Fowler et al. 2002; Sydorak and Albanese 2003). Additional effective agents include intravenous or subcutaneous betamimetics, and oral prostaglandin inhibitors (Albanese 2002; Fowler et al. 2002; Sydorak and Albanese 2003). Several possible side effects of these agents, including maternal tachyphylaxis, pulmonary edema, and constrictive effects on the fetal ductus arteriosus, are all closely monitored postoperatively.

Results

Despite the rational belief that MAFS might prevent PTL altogether, this has not been the case. All fetal operative interventions, both MAFS and open procedures, continue to be beleaguered by postprocedure uterine irritability and PTL. This is likely a much more complicated multifactorial imbalance which results from fetal interventions of any kind. Quite clearly contributing to PTL is the problem of premature rupture of membranes (PROM). Despite meticulous entrance and closure techniques MAFS can experience up to a 40–60% PROM rate (Sydorak and Albanese 2003). The sequelae of PROM are costly and can include PTL, oligohydramnios, chorioamnionitis, and up to 50% fetal demise (Sydorak and Albanese 2003). Investigative efforts continue to address these issues in animal models. Current treatment options remain those which were listed above as PTL continues to hinder a more widespread application of MAFS.

Minimal access fetal surgery has been successful in alleviating much of the bleeding that occurs with open fetal procedures which occurs upon initial uterine entry. The adaptation of Seldinger techniques and radially expanding trocars has dramatically reduced this previously frequently encountered complication. To date there are no large single institutional series of MAFS cases. The indications for the application of these techniques remain limited to a few narrowly defined fetal anomalies with in utero sequelae that threaten fetal viability. For this reason the necessary technical expertise and multidisciplinary infrastructure necessary for accurate diagnosis, treatment, and management will remain confined to a few specialty centers.

Discussion

While fetal surgical interventions including MAFS have historically been performed for otherwise life-threatening maladies, one can anticipate that with improvements in technique and outcome the scope of fetal interventions will continue to evolve. The current NIH-sponsored clinical trial for the treatment of in utero diagnosed myelomeningocele is an example of this technology extended to a highly morbid, but not specifically mortal malformation. A broader understanding of fetal pathophysiology and an ongoing evolution in instrumentation and technique will precede any as yet unforeseen broader applicability. Since MAFS has provided for a diminution in the severity of PROM, PTL, uterine hemorrhage, and overall fetal and maternal morbidity, it seems likely that MAFS will represent the approach of choice to the fetal uterine environment for most fetal therapeutic options of the future. Perhaps the first NIH-sponsored trial of MAFS techniques for TTTS will provide further prospectively gained insight.

References

Albanese CT (2002) Operative fetoscopy. In: Lobe TE (ed) Pediatric Laparoscopy. Lande Bioscience, Georgetown, Texas, pp 239–245

Albanese CT, Harrison MR (1998) Surgical treatment for fetal disease. The state of the art. Ann N Y Acad Sci 847:74–85

Allen MH, Garabelis NS, Bornick PW, et al (2000) Minimally invasive treatment of twin-to-twin transfusion syndrome. AORN J 71:796, 801–810; quiz 811–812, 815–818

Bermudez C, Becerra CH, Bornick PW, et al (2002) Placental types and twin-twin transfusion syndrome. Am J Obstet Gynecol 187:489–494

Chiba T, Albanese CT, Farmer DL, et al (2000) Balloon tracheal occlusion for congenital diaphragmatic hernia: experimental studies. J Pediatr Surg 35:1566–1570

De Lia JE, Cruikshank DP, Keye WR Jr (1990) Fetoscopic neodymium:YAG laser occlusion of placental vessels in severe twin-twin transfusion syndrome. Obstet Gynecol 75:1046–1053

De Lia JE, Kuhlmann RS, Lopez KP (1999) Treating previable twin-twin transfusion syndrome with fetoscopic laser surgery: outcomes following the learning curve. J Perinat Med 27:61–67

Deprest J (2001) Obstetric endoscopy. In: Harrison M, Evans MI, Adzick NS, Holzgreve W (eds) The Unborn Patient. Saunders, Philadelphia, pp 213–231

Farmer DL, von Koch CS, Peacock WJ, et al (2003) In utero repair of myelomeningocele: experimental pathophysiology, natural history, and initial clinical experience. Arch Surg 138:872–878

Fowler SF, Sydorak RM, Albanese CT, et al (2002) Fetal endoscopic surgery: lessons learned and trends reviewed. J Pediatr Surg 37:1700–1702

Harrison MR, Albanese CT, Hawgood SB, et al (2001) Fetoscopic temporary tracheal occlusion by means of detachable balloon for congenital diaphragmatic hernia. Am J Obstet Gynecol 185:730–733

Lopoo JB, Paek BW, Maichin GA, et al (2000) Cord ultrasonic transection procedure for selective termination of a monochorionic twin. Fetal Diagn Ther 15:177–179

Paek BW, Jennings RW, Harrison MR, et al (2001) Radiofrequency ablation of human fetal sacrococcygeal teratoma. Am J Obstet Gynecol 184:503–507

Paek BW, Callen PW, Kitterman J, et al (2002) Successful fetal intervention for congenital high airway obstruction syndrome. Fetal Diagn Ther 17:272–276

Quintero RA, Morales WJ (2001) Percutaneous fetoscopic guided intervention. In: Harrison M, Evans MI, Adzick NS, Holzgreve W (eds) The Unborn Patient. Saunders, Philadelphia, pp 199–207

Quintero RA, Hume R, Smith C, et al (1995) Percutaneous fetal cystoscopy and endoscopic fulguration of posterior urethral valves [comment]. Am J Obstet Gynecol 172:206–209

Quintero RA, Morales WJ, Phillips J, et al (1997) In utero lysis of amniotic bands [comment]. Ultrasound Obstet Gynecol 10:316–320

Quintero RA, Shukla AR, Homsy YL, et al (2000) Successful in utero endoscopic ablation of posterior urethral valves: a new dimension in fetal urology. Urology 55:774

Quintero RA, Bornick PW, Allen MH, et al (2001) Selective laser photocoagulation of communicating vessels in severe twin-twin transfusion syndrome in women with an anterior placenta. Obstet Gynecol 97:477–481

Sydorak RM, Albanese CT (2003) Minimal access techniques for fetal surgery. World J Surg 27:95–102

Sydorak RM, Feldstein V, Machin G, et al (2002) Fetoscopic treatment for discordant twins. J Pediatr Surg 37:1736–1739

Tsao K, Feldstein VA, Albanese CT, et al (2002) Selective reduction of acardiac twin by radiofrequency ablation. Am J Obstet Gynecol 187:635–640

Ville Y, Hecher K, Gagnon A, et al (1998) Endoscopic laser coagulation in the management of severe twin-to-twin transfusion syndrome. Br J Obstet Gynaecol 105:446–453

Subject Index